For Instructors

■ INSTRUCTOR'S ELECTRONIC RESOURCE

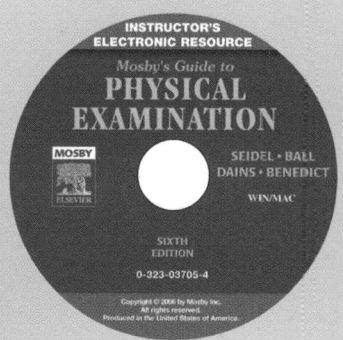

ISBN 0-323-03705-4

Available in CD-ROM and online formats, this helpful instructor's package provides all of the tools needed to develop lectures and student assignments and evaluate student comprehension. The *Instructor's Manual* includes learning objectives, chapter outlines, teaching strategies, critical thinking activities, quizzes, crossword puzzles, and evaluation checklists. The ExamView *Test Bank* contains multiple-choice questions, an answer key with page references to the text, and rationales. Also included are a full-color *Image Collection* and *PowerPoint Lecture Slides* for building presentations and developing lectures.

■ EVOLVE COURSE MANAGEMENT SYSTEM

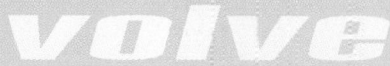

http://evolve.elsevier.com/Seidel

Evolve is an interactive teaching and learning environment coordinated with *Mosby's Guide to Physical Examination* and provides Internet-based course content that reinforces and expands on the concepts delivered in class. In addition to the resources available to students, instructors are able to access all of the components of the *Instructor's Electronic Resource*, including the Test Bank and PowerPoint lecture slides. Instructors can also use Evolve to publish class syllabi, outlines, and lecture notes; set up "virtual office hours" and e-mail communication; share important dates and information through the online class *Calendar*; and encourage student participation through *Chat Rooms* and *Discussion Boards*. Instructors are encouraged to contact their sales representative for more information about integrating Evolve into their curriculum.

■ MOSBY'S GUIDE TO PHYSICAL EXAMINATION VIDEO SERIES

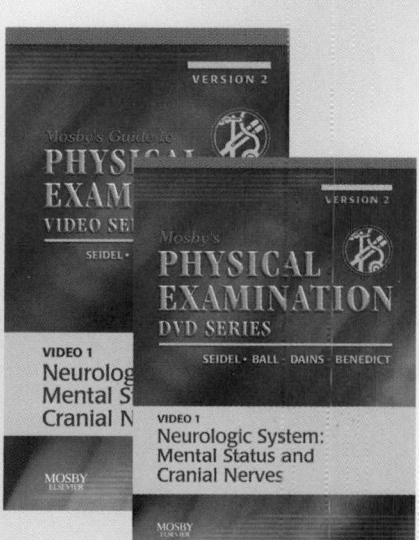

VHS set: ISBN 0-323-03542-6
DVD set: ISBN 0-323-03526-4
Online set: ISBN 0-323-03558-2

Designed to complement *Mosby's Guide to Physical Examination*, this comprehensive video series demonstrates physical examination techniques of the adult for each body system, including life span variations. Tapes are available individually or in sets in VHS, DVD, or online formats. Each 15- to 25-minute video is enhanced by computer animation; introductory remarks and narration; cultural, age, and gender variations where applicable; and a focus on the interaction between examiner and patient. Also available is a separate "Putting It All Together" video that presents a full patient head-to-toe examination, summarizing the key steps in one complete and fluid physical examination. All tapes include closed-captioning.

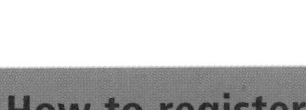
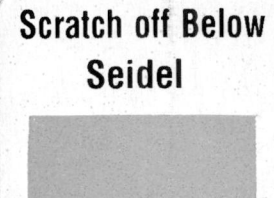

Look for these valuable learning tools hroughout each of the 18 sections on the Companion CD-ROM
- **Sound and Vision Theater:** Vidlips, sound bytes, and images of exam techniques and ings
- **Printouts for Your Practice:** Prble exam guides for you and teaching guides for your pats
- **Interactive Challenge:** Fun exers to enhance your assessment knowledge and skill
- **En Español:** Spanish assessmenms with pronunciation guide
- **Instant Calculators:** Metric corsions and more

Find these unique highlights within individual body systems listed below:

MENTAL STATUS
Sound and Vision Theater: Videclips
- Evaluating Selected Cognitive Abies
- Assessing Memory
- Assessing Emotional Stability

Instant Calculators
- Glasgow Coma Scale
- Pediatric Glasgow Coma Scale
- Six-Item Cognitive Impairment st
- Metric Unit Converter

SKIN, HAIR, AND NAILS
Sound and Vision Theater: Vid Clips
- Assessing a Mole
- Examining the Hair
- Measuring the Angle of the Nabase

Printouts for Your Practice: Pient Teaching Guide
- Cancer: Prevention and Screeng

Interactive Challenge
- Photo Gallery
- Match That Lesion
- Documentation Exercise
- Risk Factor Identification Chalnge

LYMPHATIC SYSTEM
Sound and Vision Theater: Vieo Clips
- Palpating Lymph Nodes in theHead and Neck
- Palpating Lymph Nodes in thArms
- Palpating the Inguinal LymphNodes

Interactive Challenge
- Lymph Nodes: Where Do Th Belong?
- Name That Abnormality
- Ring That Bell
- Risk Factor Identification Chllenge

HEAD AND NECK
Sound and Vision Theater: Video Clips
- Assessing the Temporomandbular Joint
- Inspecting the Thyroid Glard
- Palpating the Thyroid Gland

Interactive Challenge
- Taking a History: Ask the Right Questions
- Examine Katie's Head and Neck: A Beat the Clock Exercise
- The Headache Maze: A Mix and Match Exercise
- Hyperthyroidism vs. Hypothyroidism: Test Your Knowledge

EYES
Sound and Vision Theater: Video Clips
- Assessing the Pupillary Response to Light
- Assessing the Six Cardinal Fields of Gaze
- Examining the Retina

Printouts for Your Practice: Patient Teaching Guide
- Periodic Examinations for Healthy Eyes

Interactive Challenge
- Build the Eye: An Architectural Exercise
- The Six Cardinal Fields of Gaze
- Common Abnormalities and Variations: Photo Gallery

EARS
Sound and Vision Theater: Video Clips
- Assessing the Auricle's Position
- Inspecting the Auditory Canal and Tympanic Membrane
- Performing the Weber and Rinne Tests

Printouts for Your Practice: Patient Teaching Guides
- Foreign Objects in the Ear
- Are Your Ears Protected from Noise?
- Keeping Your Ears Clean

Interactive Challenge
- The Ear Anatomy Challenge
- The Tympanic Membrane Photo Gallery
- Risk Factor Identification Challenge

NOSE AND THROAT
Sound and Vision Theater: Video Clips
- Inspecting the Nasal Cavity
- Inspecting the Buccal Mucosa, Teeth, and Gums
- Assessing the Oropharynx and Gag Reflex

Interactive Challenge
- The Nose and Throat Anatomy Challenge
- Sinus Mapping: An Exercise in Location and Function
- Risk Factor Identification Challenge

CHEST AND LUNGS
Sound and Vision Theater: Video Clips
- Performing Diaphragmatic Excursion
- Palpating for Thoracic Expansion
- Following the Percussion and Auscultation Sequence

Sound Bytes
- Bronchovesicular Sounds (Normal)
- Vesicular Sounds (Normal)
- Bronchial Sounds (Normal)
- High-pitched Crackles (Abnormal)
- Low-pitched Crackles (Abnormal)
- High-pitched Wheezes (Abnormal)
- Low-pitched Wheezes (Abnormal)
- Pleural Friction Rub (Abnormal)

Interactive Challenge
- Breath Sounds: What Is Normal and What Is Not?
- Match That Disorder: A Mix and Match Exercise
- Name That Tone: Percussion Tone Identification
- Risk Factor Identification Challenge

Instant Calculators
- Predicted Peak Flow for Males
- Predicted Peak Flow for Females

HEART
Sound and Vision Theater: Video Clips
- Palpating the Precordium
- Identifying sites for Heart Auscultation
- Auscultating S_1 and S_2

Sound Bytes
- S_1
- S_2
- S_3
- S_4
- Systolic Murmur

Continued

SIXTH EDITION

Mosby's Guide to
PHYSICAL
EXAMINATION

HENRY M. SEIDEL, MD
Professor Emeritus of Pediatrics
The Johns Hopkins University School of Medicine
Baltimore, Maryland

JANE W. BALL, RN, DrPH, CPNP, NAP
Executive Director
National Resource Center
Children's National Medical Center
Washington, DC

JOYCE E. DAINS, DrPH, JD, RN, FNP, BC, NAP
Manager, Professional Education for Prevention and Early Detection
The University of Texas MD Anderson Cancer Center
Houston, Texas

G. WILLIAM BENEDICT, MD, PhD
Assistant Professor, Medicine
The Johns Hopkins University School of Medicine
Baltimore, Maryland

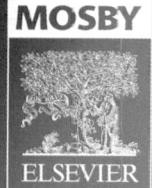

MOSBY

ELSEVIER

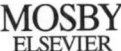

MOSBY
ELSEVIER

11830 Westline Industrial Drive
St. Louis, Missouri 63146

Notice

Neither the Publisher nor the Authors assume any responsibility for any loss or injury and/or damage to persons or property arising out of or related to any use of the material contained in this book. It is the responsibility of the treating practitioner, relying on independent expertise and knowledge of the patient, to determine the best treatment and method of application for the patient.

The Publisher

Executive Publisher: Robin Carter
Associate Developmental Editor: Deanna Davis
Publishing Services Manager: Deborah L. Vogel
Senior Project Manager: Jodi M. Willard
Senior Designer: Jyotika Shroff
Cover Art: Jyotika Shroff

Printed in Canada

Last digit is the print number: 9 8 7 6 5 4 3 2

HENRY M. SEIDEL, MD

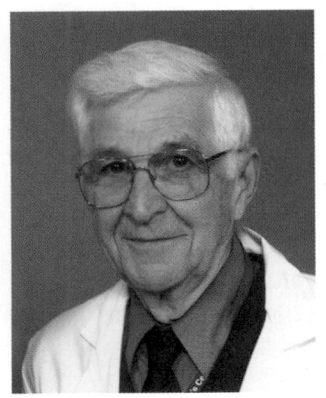

Henry Seidel has spent all of his professional life (except for time served in the U.S. Army)—from college through his appointment as Professor Emeritus of Pediatrics—at The Johns Hopkins University. His effort has included serving patients as a general pediatrician, teaching medical students in their first course concerned with history taking and physical examination, teaching medical students and residents at the bedside on pediatric wards, and conducting investigations concerned with quality essential to the delivery of appropriate medical care. His writings include an Elsevier handbook *Primary Care of the Full-Term Newborn,* a history of the Department of Pediatrics at Johns Hopkins, chapters in several books, and numerous papers published in refereed journals.

It is noteworthy that much of his experience has included service to and the care of adults in Iran during the formation of a new medical school in that country and during work with Project Hope in Nicaragua, Jamaica, and on the Navajo Reservation. Happily, these experiences have preserved and extended his caretaking skills across the full age range.

Numerous awards and a named scholarship at Johns Hopkins have provided abundant recognition of his service at the bedside, in the lecture and seminar rooms and, for 15 years, in the Office of the Dean as Associate Dean for Student Affairs. His experience confirms his absolute conviction that the appropriate care of the sick and the well demands an understanding of the individual patient that can be derived only from a sound and sensitively taken history and a thorough and perceptive physical examination. Our technologic expertise is truly gratifying but is incomplete and will often not succeed without the human skill and art necessary for a healing relationship with the patient.

Henry M. Seidel

JANE W. BALL, RN, DrPH, CPNP, NAP

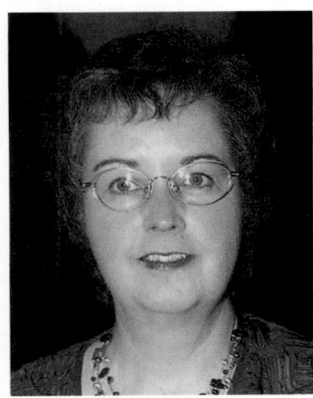

Jane W. Ball graduated from the Johns Hopkins Hospital School of Nursing and subsequently received her Master of Public Health and Doctor of Public Health degrees from the Johns Hopkins University Bloomberg School of Public Health. She began her nursing career as a pediatric nurse and pediatric nurse practitioner in the Johns Hopkins Hospital. Since completing her public health degrees, she has held several positions that enable her to focus on improving the health care of children, such as serving as the Chief of Child Health for the Commonwealth of Pennsylvania Department of Health and as faculty teaching pediatric nursing at the University of Texas at Arlington School of Nursing. Over the past 20 years Jane has focused her efforts on improving the system of emergency medical care for children while employed by Children's National Medical Center in Washington, DC. She currently is the Executive Director of the National Resource Center at Children's National Medical Center, which provides support to two federal programs: Emergency Medical Services for Children and the Trauma-Emergency Medical Services Systems Program. Dr. Ball is also the author of several pediatric nursing textbooks.

Jane W. Ball

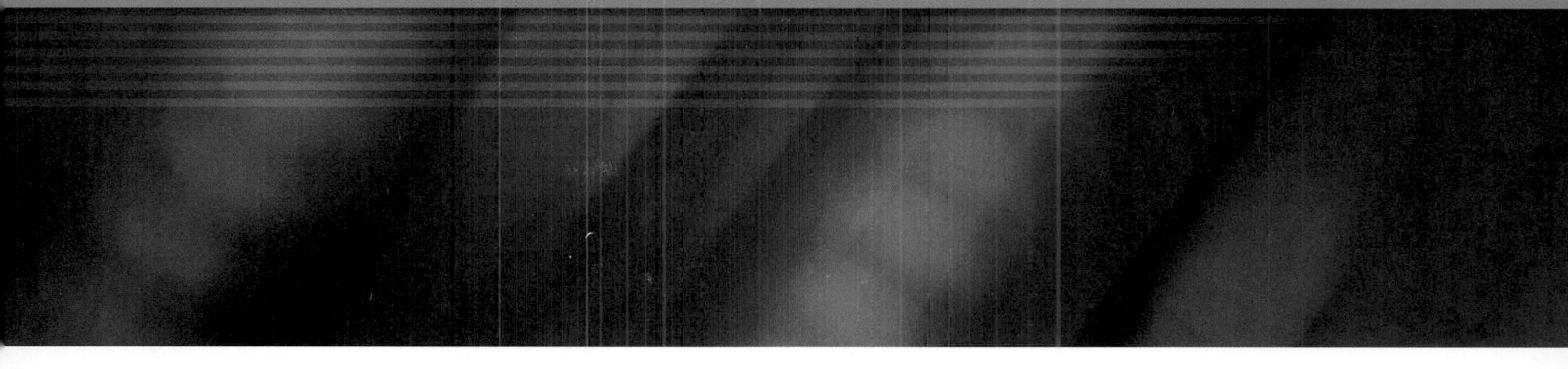

JOYCE E. DAINS, DrPH, JD, RN, FNP, BC, NAP

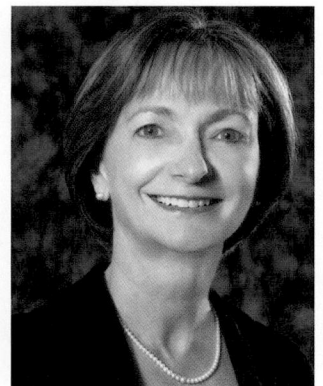

As a board-certified Family Nurse Practitioner with doctorates in both Public Health and Law, Dr. Joyce Dains has had a rich and productive career in education and practice. A graduate of New England Baptist Hospital School of Nursing, she earned a baccalaureate degree in nursing from Boston College, a masters degree in nursing from Case Western Reserve University, and a doctorate in Public Health from the University of Texas—Houston. She earned her law degree at the University of Houston and practiced law for a brief period. Dr. Dains has been in leadership positions at major universities and medical institutions, where she has been instrumental in the education of nursing students, medical students, and other health care professionals. As a family nurse practitioner, she has maintained a clinical practice in a variety of primary care settings. Her numerous presentations, publications, and awards attest to her commitment to professional excellence and productivity. She is currently at The University of Texas M. D. Anderson Cancer Center, where she directs a program for the education of health care professionals in prevention and early detection of cancer and also maintains a clinical practice in the Cancer Prevention Center. Dr. Dains resides in Houston with her husband and teenage children.

Joyce E Dains

G. WILLIAM BENEDICT, MD, PhD

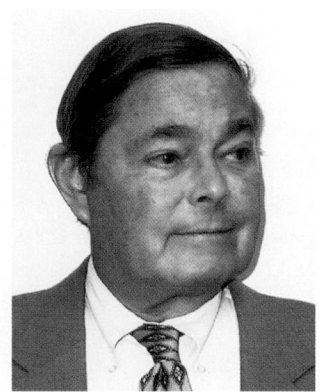

Dr. Benedict graduated from Williams College in Williamstown, Massachusetts. He received his MD from Vanderbilt University School of Medicine in Nashville and his PhD from The Johns Hopkins University in Baltimore. A fellow of the American College of Physicians, he also served as vice president and president of the Central Maryland chapter of the American Heart Association and on the board of directors, as vice president and president, of the Maryland affiliate of the American Diabetes Association. He is the author of numerous chapters in medical textbooks and peer-reviewed journals. Recently retired from practice, Dr. Benedict served as assistant professor of medicine in the division of endocrinology and metabolism at The Johns Hopkins University School of Medicine since the early 1970s.

G William Benedict

CONTRIBUTORS/REVIEWERS

CONTRIBUTORS

Sharon Lechter Smalling, MPH, RD, LD
Clinical Dietitian Specialist IV
Memorial Hermann Hospital
The Texas Medical Center
Houston, Texas

Leah Payne Smith, RNC, MSN, WHNP
Women's Health Nurse Practitioner
Memphis Regional Planned Parenthood;
Adjunct Faculty
University of Tennessee College of Nursing
Memphis, Tennessee

REVIEWERS

Michele F. Bellantoni, MD
Associate Professor of Medicine
Associate Director for Post-Acute and Long-Term Care
Division of Geriatric Medicine & Gerontology
Johns Hopkins University School of Medicine
Baltimore, Maryland

Deborah L. Cross, MPH, CRNP
Lecturer and Course Coordinator
Department of Nursing
University of Pennsylvania
Philadelphia, Pennsylvania

Marye Dorsey Kellermann, RN, MS, CRNP
Adult Nurse Practitioner
Gerontological Nurse Practitioner
Associate Professor
Coppin State College FNP Graduate Program
Baltimore, Maryland

Judy Malkiewicz, RN, PhD
Professor of Nursing
University of Northern Colorado
Greeley, Colorado

Amy Roberts, PhD, RN, FNP-C
Coordinator, Family Nurse Practitioner Program
Assistant Professor
Louise Herrington School of Nursing
Baylor University
Dallas, Texas

Gwen Scarborough, MSN, RN
Assistant Professor of Nursing
The University of Tennessee at Martin
Martin, Tennessee

Leah Payne Smith, RNC, MSN, WHNP
Women's Health Nurse Practitioner
Memphis Regional Planned Parenthood;
Adjunct Faculty
University of Tennessee College of Nursing
Memphis, Tennessee

James M. Wagner, MD
Associate Professor of Internal Medicine
University of Texas Southwestern Medical School
Dallas, Texas

PREFACE

Mosby's Guide to Physical Examination is written primarily for students at the start of their careers in the health professions. The core message of our book is that patients are primary and must be served well. Learning how to take histories and how to perform physical examinations are necessary but not sufficient actions that lead to the full understanding of patients. As in our earlier efforts, the keys to that full understanding are given consistent emphasis throughout this sixth edition. The art and skills involved are common to all of us regardless of our particular health profession.

The relationship with your patients and the development of the trust that doing so requires most often begins with conversation. You need reliable information if you are to serve your patients well. You are, after all, learning the stories of unique individuals, and they involve far more than the sum of body parts and systems.

ORGANIZATION

The achievement of constructive relationships begins with your mastery of sound history taking and physical examination. Chapter 1 offers the vital "getting to know you" guidelines; you need to know the patient, of course, and the patient needs to have a solid sense of you. Chapter 2 stresses that "knowing" is incomplete without the mutual understanding of cultural backgrounds and differences. Chapter 3 then gives an overview of examination processes and the equipment you will need.

The following chapters—4, 5, and 6—introduce important elements of assessment: mental status, growth and development, and nutrition. Chapter 7, new to this edition, highlights your very necessary attention to *pain*. From Chapter 8 and through Chapter 22, specific body systems and body parts are discussed, with each chapter divided into four major sections:

- Anatomy and Physiology
- Review of Related History
- Examination and Findings
- Common Abnormalities

Each of these sections begins with consideration of the adult patient and is completed when appropriate with variations for other age-groups, pregnant women and, also when appropriate, the handicapped.

The Anatomy and Physiology sections begin with the physiologic basis for the interpretation of findings and describe the key anatomic landmarks to guide physical examination. The Review of Related History sections detail a specific method of inquiry when a system or organ-related problem is discovered during the interview or examination. The Examination and Findings sections list needed equipment then describe in detail the procedures for the examination and the expected findings. These sections encourage you to develop an approach and sequence that is comfortable for you and, particularly, for the patient. A summary of the step-by-step examination and a sample write-up of findings conclude these sections. You will note that the terms "normal" and "abnormal" are avoided whenever possible to describe findings because, in our view, these terms suggest a value judgment that may or may not prove valid with experience and additional information. The Common Abnormalities sections provide an overview of diseases and associated problems common to the particular system or body part and conclude these core systems chapters.

A new Chapter 23 details the issues relevant to the sports physical evaluation. In addition, standard approaches are subject to change in emergency and life-threatening situations. Chapter 27 provides guidance for these circumstances. This information is only a beginning and is intended to be useful in your clinical decision making. You will need to add to your base of knowledge with other resources.

The remaining chapters put it all together. Chapter 24 points the way to integrating what you have learned so that it is useful in decision making and problem solving and, with Chapter 25, in thinking critically about clinical challenges. All you have learned, thought, and decided must, of course, be carefully recorded. Chapter 26 shows you how to do this, with particular emphasis on the Problem Oriented Medical Record (POMR) and the use of SOAP (**S**ubjective findings, **O**bjective findings, **A**ssessment and **P**lan) to define a problem completely.

The thoroughly updated appendixes provide the numbers, verbal clues, and charts that can help in fixing the extent of an observation or problem and in preserving a continuous record.

SPECIAL FEATURES

The basic structure of the book—with its consistent chapter organization and the inclusion of special considerations sections for infants, children, adolescents, pregnant women, and older adults, as appropriate to each discussion—facilitates learning. In addition, new "Staying Well" content is a new feature that complements the other features that have proven popular and are retained for this edition:

- Mnemonics boxes in the book's margins provide time-tested memory aids for a new generation of practitioners.
- Physical Variations boxes, also in the book's margins, highlight variations from expected findings.
- Differential Diagnosis content—a hallmark of this text—is highlighted throughout.
- Evidence-Based Practice in Physical Examination boxes are reminders that all we do must—as much as possible—be supported by sound, proven information.
- Risk Factors boxes highlight modifiable and nonmodifiable risk factors for a variety of conditions.
- Sample Documentation and Summary of Examination boxes at the end of each Examination and Findings section model good documentation practice and provide a convenient summary of examination steps.
- Functional Assessment boxes help readers step back from specific physical problems to consider their impact on patient function.

NEW TO THIS EDITION

It is obvious that the entire book has been thoroughly updated for this edition. This includes the replacement of 200 photographs with all new examination photos and the use of new full-color photos and drawings to replace one- and two-color illustrations in the fifth edition. There are a total of approximately 1400 illustrations in addition to the numerous tables and boxes that have traditionally given readers easy access to information. A great deal has also been added to these. Among the many changes:

- Clinical Pearls, Mnemonics, and Physical Variations boxes have been updated and increased in this edition.
- There is an increase in the numbers of Evidence-Based Practice in Physical Examination boxes, which focus on the ongoing need to incorporate research into practice and decision making.
- There are new boxes devoted to "Staying Well," which can be used to encourage health promotion in your patients.
- The newest eye charts for evaluating vision in the young have been added.

- The most recent recommendations for the definition of hypertension in adults and children are included along with a discussion of the types of sphygmomanometers that do not use mercury.
- There is a more comprehensive assessment of the shoulder and of osteoporosis risk in the musculoskeletal chapter.
- The content on upper and lower motor neurons in the neurological chapter has been expanded.
- A video icon has been added to highlight the segments supported by the new interactive CD.
- The content on the use of a SOAP note for documenting has been expanded.
- The chapter on the breast includes a revised approach to examination to reflect practice changes.
- The chapter on nutrition has been reorganized to parallel the format of the body system chapters.

OUR ANCILLARY PACKAGE

Mosby's Physical Examination Handbook is a concise, pocket-sized companion for clinical experiences. It summarizes, reinforces, and serves as a quick reference to the core content of the textbook.

Student Laboratory Manual for Mosby's Guide to Physical Examination is a practical printed workbook that helps readers integrate the content of the textbook and ensure content mastery through a variety of engaging exercises.

Online Faculty Course Resources on the companion EVOLVE site (evolve.elsevier.com/ Seidel) include an Electronic Image Collection and a PowerPoint lecture slide collection that together provide the building blocks for course preparation. Also available on the EVOLVE site is a thoroughly revised Test Bank, in ExamView® format, which faculty can use to create customized exams.

Also for faculty, we have once again provided an *Instructor's Electronic Resource*—now conveniently contained all on one CD-ROM. The "IER" includes an *Instructor's Resource Manual* (which provides learning objectives, chapter highlights, individual student exercises, classroom activities, critical thinking questions, and an open-book quiz for each chapter), the ExamView Computerized Test Bank, PowerPoint collection, and Electronic Image Collection. The *Instructor's Resource Manual* is also being provided in print format for the sixth edition.

Also available, introduced as a groundbreaking new resource with the fifth edition, is the thoroughly revised and expanded online course library entitled *Health Assessment Online*. *Health Assessment Online* is an exhaustive multimedia library of online resources, including animations, video clips, interactive exercises, quizzes, and much more. Available for individual student purchase or as a required course supplement, *Health Assessment Online* unlocks a rich online learning experience with more than 8000 individual assets—second to none.

Two additional electronic offerings new to this edition are inclusion of this book in *Evolve Select* and *Student Consult*, both of which allow for linking and cross-referencing with other online Elsevier textbooks. *Evolve Select* is for nursing students, and *Student Consult* is for medical students. A new video-enhanced Companion CD-ROM packaged with each textbook contains a wide variety of interactive activities, video clips of selected examination procedures, animations depicting content and processes, and illustration overlays showing intricate anatomic details beneath the skin. References throughout the text, signified with this symbol direct the user to the companion CD-ROM for the relevant video clips for a particular exam.

The existing physical examination video series for institutional use has been completely redone and is now being offered in three formats: video (VHS), DVD, and streaming (online). It comprises 14 examination videos, each of which features an examination of a specific body system with animations and illustration overlays to demonstrate examination techniques in greater depth, and a fifteenth "Putting It All Together" video that shows a head-to-toe examination of an adult along with appropriate life span variations.

OUR CORE VALUES

In this sixth edition of *Mosby's Guide to Physical Examination*, we have made every attempt to consider patients in all of their variety and to preserve the fundamental messages explicit in earlier editions. These include the following:

- Respect the patient.
- Achieve the complementary forces of competence and compassion.
- The art and skill essential to history taking and physical examination are the bedrock of care; technologic resources are complements.
- The history and physical examination are inseparable; they are one.
- The computer cannot replace you; it is what you do that builds a trusting, fruitful relationship with the patient.
- That relationship can be indescribably rewarding.

We hope that you will find this a useful text and that it will continue to serve as a resource as your career evolves.

ACKNOWLEDGMENTS

We four, the authors of *Mosby's Guide to Physical Examination*, have worked together for two decades. This sixth edition of our textbook is possible only because of the professionalism and skills of so many others who really know how to fashion a book and its ancillaries so that it is maximally useful to you. First, there are those instructors and students who have so thoughtfully and constructively offered comment over the years. Improvements in content and style stem in large part from their suggestions.

We have, of course, provided the content, but it has to be accessible to the reader. A textbook needs a style that ensures readability, and the folks at Elsevier—easy to work with—have made that happen. Sally Schrefer, our friend and also Executive Vice President, has been with us and guided us from the first day of planning for the first edition. She continues to exercise the wisdom she demonstrated early on without trampling our sometimes tender sensibilities.

Each word, figure, and page needs the artful attention of skilled professionals. The whole is a demanding project requiring effective editing and design. This was assured by Publishing Services Manager Debbie Vogel and Senior Project Manager Jodi Willard. Jodi did a spectacular job of keeping everything moving with her qualitative eye for detail throughout. Jyotika Shroff's design is visually appealing and showcases the content. Glenn Harman's new photographs provide needed insight into what we are about and add significantly to our message.

We also want to recognize the indispensable efforts of the entire marketing team led by Bob Boehringer and Kim Akers, as well as the sales representatives, who make certain that our message is honestly portrayed and that comments and suggestions from the field are candidly reported. Indeed, there are so very many men and women who are essential to the creation and potential success of our sixth edition, and we are indebted to each of them.

The remarkable teaching tools we call the ancillaries need special attention. These are the Laboratory Manual, Handbook, Companion CD-ROM, Instructor's Resource Manual, Test Bank, Health Assessment Online, and Video Series, all demanding an expertise—if they are to be useful—that goes beyond that of the authors. Mary Parker and Denise Vanacore offer theirs for the Laboratory Manual, and Mary worked with Cathy Groeger for the Test Bank. The development of HAO is led by Tab Bates, and Nancy Priff's effort is essential to the success of the Companion CD-ROM and the Video Series.

And then there are Robin Carter, our Executive Publisher, and her Editorial Assistants, Rebecca Williams and, again, Mary Parker. Robin is always quietly there, a firm hand in a velvet glove. A phone call from Robin always ends with the feeling that her suggestion had really originated with us. She made our book better and we thought we were doing it.

Robin worked hand in glove with splendid allies. Kristin Geen, our Developmental Editor, maintained professional skill and calm and taught us that it is possible to do this and keep life at home and office in proper balance. Deanna Davis, our Associate Developmental Editor, is a twin. It is a good world that has two like her in it. And, Jamie Horn ensured that when we used the work of others, it was appropriately acknowledged and recognized.

In addition, we offer many thanks to the following individuals for their contributions of time, talent, expertise, and resources: John S. Andrews; Michelle Bellantoni; Mitchell Blake; Wendy Blake; Abigail E. Bowers; Alan E. Bowers; Anna E. Bowers; Ashley E. Bowers; Carolyn M. Bowers; Chauncey A. Bowers; Moses P. Bowers; Francine Cheese Wethersby; Maureen Clothier; Austin Dains; Carolyn Harvey; David Hunter, MD; Jackson Iliff; Deborah Johnson; Carolyn Kisner; Donna Manello; Wedell Meade; Deborah Nickles; Elba Pacheco; Rachel Rachfal; Dorothy T. Rainwater; John Scruggs; Richard Smalling, MD; Stephanie Smalling; Michelle Thompson; Rebecca Vickers; Elizabeth Vogler; Robert Vogler; and Allen Walker.

Thanks, too, to the following contributors to previous editions: Candis Morrison, Barbara Cousins, Donald P. O'Connor, Kevin Murphy, Samuel Seidel, Adam Seidel, Diane Wind Wardell, George J. Wassilchenko, and Patrick Watson.

And finally—our families! They are patient with our necessary absences, support what we do, and are unstinting in their love. They have our love and our quite special thanks.

HENRY M. SEIDEL, MD

JANE W. BALL, RN, DRPH, CPNP, NAP

JOYCE E. DAINS, DRPH, JD, RN, FNP, BC, NAP

G. WILLIAM BENEDICT, MD, PHD

CONTENTS

THE HISTORY AND INTERVIEWING PROCESS

CLINICAL PEARL

The Special Relationship
You will, in the course of your career, have numerous relationships with patients. Never forget that they are, each time, having with you the one experience that is special for them. Think of actors in a long-running play. They must remember that every performance is new for the persons paying to be in the audience.

CLINICAL PEARL

The Power of the Professional and the Vulnerability of the Patient
"We say to you, 'With so much power, walk carefully and humbly. Do no harm: walk carefully so that the granite weight of that power does not crush. Abide with us.'"

From Berger, 1996.

The purpose of this book is to help you learn about your patients, the well and the sick, when they come to you for care. Patients are patients because of their need. You are available to patients because you have something to give and the ability to give it. You are a presumed authority. Patients, to the extent that they may be willing, recognize your authority, thinking it to be for the potential of good. At the start, you are in a position of strength and your patients in one of vulnerability.

You must, then, understand their need and, often, their suffering. Not easy. To get that special sense of another person, and to realize fully what is sometimes evident and sometimes subtle, demands first that you know yourself and that you cultivate a certain subliminal "feel," a readiness to grasp the clues that patients have to offer. You do not necessarily interpret the world in the same way your patients do, but you do need to get their perspective if you are to discover their concerns, their expectations, and what you can reasonably expect of them. You need, too, to understand the power you have and that that power must be shared with your patients as full partners. Knowing yourself well will defer a possible tendency to use value judgments to excess, to be judgmental, and to preach. Knowing your patients well will go a long way to complementing your competence with compassion.

The history and physical examination are at the heart of the learning process. Ultimately, appropriate assessment based on sound information requires an orderly process and a certain compulsiveness. That does not mean rigidity. All findings, both obvious and subtle, must be recorded precisely. Moreover, because cost containment is essential, the well-done history and physical examination can, in an advantaged society, justify the appropriate and cost-effective use of technologic resources and, in a disadvantaged society, compensate in large part for their absence.

Much has been written about the potential of technology replacing the physical examination and even the history in some part. For example, on August 27, 2003, a headline on CNN read, "Ultrasound May Mean End to Classic Stethoscope." There is no doubting the invaluable benefit of technologic advances, but the care of patients goes far beyond the merely technical. Health professionals, educated and trained to exacting standards, are sanctioned by society to offer advice and the potential of healing to fellow human beings—to offer care to persons not objects. Appropriate care requires a humanism that can be conveyed only by a human touch. That "touch" is essential for the technical aspect to be kept in check, and to be used and interpreted wisely. It must be informed by an experience and judgment that can be derived only from the intimate hearing and seeing of patients, the "laying on of hands." This physical realization of our relationships with our patients, particularly when illness increases their vulnerability, cannot be replaced.

KNOWING YOURSELF

The first step in achieving positive relationships with your patients is to come to a good understanding of yourself. You do not check your beliefs, attitudes, and values at the door when you step into a room with a patient. You do, however, have to discipline them, because it is the patient's needs that must be served and the patient's context of life that must be appreciated if there is to be a favorable outcome.

You will, of course, react differently to different people. Try to understand why and how. What are your deeply felt idiosyncratic needs? Do you too much want to be liked? Do you obsess about how you are doing and does that get in the way of the doing? Do you worry about "catching" something? If a patient makes you angry, why? Is there some underlying frustration in your life? Which of your prejudices may contribute?

The questions are many and the answers may come slowly. Do not hesitate to talk about these issues with a respected colleague or mentor. There is no need to make this a lonely, introspective effort. Your maturity as a care provider will evolve and you will be better able to deal with the many other barriers to successful outcomes that can arise, few of them of your own doing.

You will be better able to serve with candor and relative ease, enhancing your professionalism with its demand for a sound base of knowledge, competence, compassion, honesty, and commitment to quality of care, confidentiality, and trust.

PARTNERSHIP WITH THE PATIENT

The interview with the patient is an extraordinary event. You can, in a relatively brief time, learn so very much, from the facts of the moment to a patient's deepest feelings. Goals of the interview include the following:
- *Discovery:* Glean the information that leads to appropriate assessment and care.
- *Sharing:* Provide the patient with the information that informs your thinking so that the patient can react, ask questions, and offer opinions.
- *Negotiation:* You do not offer an inflexible regime; rather, you arrive at a joint course that respects the patient's feelings, needs, and life situation.
- *Union:* Establish a joint effort regarding all aspects of care during sickness and health.
- *Support:* Define with the patient the basis on which you will be available to bolster the emotional and spiritual needs inherent in the impact of disease and illness.

You and the patient (and, often, others close to the patient) bring much of yourselves to the relationship. The outcome will depend on the honesty, candor, and respect that must prevail if mutual trust is to evolve. The reason the patient came to you, the physical setting, and the economic base on which care is provided are but some of the factors that may help or hinder. From the start, you must listen carefully to what you hear as well as to the silences. There are clues in silence. Unexpressed feelings need evocation and acknowledgment—the patient needs the message that you are trying to understand. The achievement of constructive relationships depends on the honing of your skills and your resistance to the temptation to allow burgeoning technology to take their place uncritically.

AN ETHICAL CONTEXT TO THE PARTNERSHIP WITH THE PATIENT

"Ethics" does not provide answers; rather, it offers a disciplined approach to understanding and determining ultimate behavior. Given a problem—for example, a perceived necessary violation of confidentiality—several concepts must be considered.
- *Autonomy:* The patient's need for self-determination. This definition is clouded when the patient is a child or is incompetent. Parents, guardians, family, and other significant persons in the life of the patient must be included, and the boundaries of their participation must be clearly set, often by an advance directive from the patient. The goals for our efforts are better served if there is a clear understanding of the patient's concept of autonomy. The paternalistic professional, acting as parent or priest, can certainly invade autonomy. Although in recent years there has been considerable constraint placed on pa-

ternalism, it is not always inappropriate; however, the professional must inform and interpret, ensuring a clear understanding of what the information means. The well-informed patient is better able to exercise autonomy.

The concept of autonomy suggests that choices exist and that a patient may choose between alternatives. This, as we have indicated, requires sound information and the competence to use that information. A loss of competence means a loss of autonomy. Determination of competency is not always easy. Both the mental status examination (see Chapter 4) and consultation with other clinicians and with those who know the person well can assist in that determination. Unhappily, the definition of competency may not have consistent agreement among those involved. Wisdom, calm, and a sensitive knowledge of the whole patient are needed.

- *Beneficence:* The clinician needs to do good for the patient. This may be too eagerly pursued and may result in a paternalism that might smother autonomy. "Father" or "mother" may *sometimes* know best, but clearly this is not always the case.
- *Nonmaleficence:* The clinician must do no harm to the patient.
- *Utilitarianism:* The need to consider the appropriate use of resources for the greater good of the larger community.
- *Fairness and justice:* Recognition of the often precarious balance between autonomy and the competing interests of the family and community. Fair treatment has been constrained with the advent of managed care and the increased recognition of our limited resources, issues that are by no means easily resolved.
- *Deontological imperatives:* The duties of care providers established by tradition and in cultural contexts. Such duties appear to have an ordained existence.

Surely, these principles can come into conflict in any given circumstance, for example, the use of limited resources in situations thought to be futile. Consideration of each of them, however, provides a guideline to constructive discussion that can often lead to helpful outcomes. We must accept the patient's major, often decisive contribution and the sometimes competing values that may introduce. Respect and flexibility in attitude are key ingredients in the search for answers, and for the preservation of patient autonomy unconstrained by well-meant but overzealous paternalism.

However, attention to ethical concepts does not always resolve a problem. Although there is no one correct approach to a seemingly intractable issue, we can make sure that we consider the following in each case:

- The problem at hand is truly one of ethics and not a result of poor communication, legal confusion, or personality conflict.
- The facts are as clearly stated as possible.
- The substance of ethical conflict and its sources, possibly cultural, are clearly understood.
- The attitudes of patients or their representatives are clearly communicated.
- There is a reasonable chance for a satisfactory health or medical care outcome.
- External factors such as money, conflict within a family, or conflicting responsibilities outside of the family are properly considered.

In the end, the patient's point of view might well prevail unless there is a compelling argument to do otherwise.

THE VARIETIES OF CARE

| ALLOPATHIC, COMPLEMENTARY, AND ALTERNATIVE CARE | Productive partnerships with patients require an understanding of the many ways in which they may seek care. *Allopathy* is a term incorrectly used to describe the routine health and medical care offered in the United States and most of the Western World. It is more accurately defined as "cure by inducing a pathologic reaction antagonistic to the disease being treated." Alternative care has its roots in the Eastern tradition. Its basic concept is "wholeness" or the unity of the physical, emotional, and spiritual within each of us. These must be balanced and chronic stress eased; if they are not, illness is the result. Maintaining this balance is enabled by deep, personal insight and by taking responsibility for one's own health, concepts compatible |

with allopathy. This compatibility suggests that a term preferable to "alternate care" is "complementary care." This clearly indicates the respect such care is due, recognizes that there is much that can be done to ease human suffering that is not part of the accepted allopathic armamentarium, accepts that approaches to care can be joined and not substituted one for the other, and recognizes the compelling human need to pursue cure.

The modalities of complementary care vary: among others, they include acupuncture, aromatherapy, therapeutic touch, and herbal medications. The potential value of any approach should be appreciated and possible pitfalls understood. For example, the herb Ginkgo biloba, used by many to improve memory, has been associated with thrombocytopenia. Pitfalls, however, cannot obscure the certainty that many of our patients seek a "wholeness" that we do not always appreciate and that they tap into a variety of resources many of us do not fully understand. Grasping this need of the patient and respecting it will go far in validating the partnerships we seek.

COMMUNICATING WITH THE PATIENT

FACTORS THAT ENHANCE COMMUNICATION

Relationships depend on sound communication. You must examine carefully your approaches and habits in this regard and, if necessary, modify them so that your demeanor does not present barriers to effective communication. A stiff, formal approach may inhibit the patient's ability to communicate; a too casual, "laid back" attitude may fail to instill confidence. Because the patient may search for meaning in everything you say, avoid being careless with words. What may seem innocuous to you may seem vitally important to the patient. Begin to understand the intellectual and emotional constraints on the way you ask questions and convey information, how fast you talk, and how often you punctuate speech with "uhs" and "you knows." Similarly, your face need not be a mask, but avoid the extremes of reaction (e.g., startle, surprise, laughter, or grimacing) as the patient provides information. Your nonverbal demeanor matters fully as much as your words.

The maintenance of confidentiality, the basis of a productive relationship, is sometimes difficult. It is the patient who should participate with you if possible. Too often, a parent, spouse, or other person may intervene unless otherwise counseled. However, if you do not speak the patient's language, a family member may be a convenient interpreter but, for reasons unknown to you, this may be a barrier to candid conversation. A stranger might be more appropriate. Interpreters are also helpful when the patient has an incomplete knowledge of the ex-

CLINICAL PEARL

Professional Dress and Grooming
The way you are dressed and groomed will go a long way toward establishing that first good impression with the patient. Some personal habits may intrude on the patient's sensibilities; therefore clean fingernails, modest dress, and neat hair are imperative. Still, you do not have to be stuffy to be neat. Men do not need pinstripes and ties, and women do not need the latest "power" dress to signify respect for the patient. Health professionals can easily avoid extremes in dress and manner so that appearance does not become an obstacle in the patient's response to care.

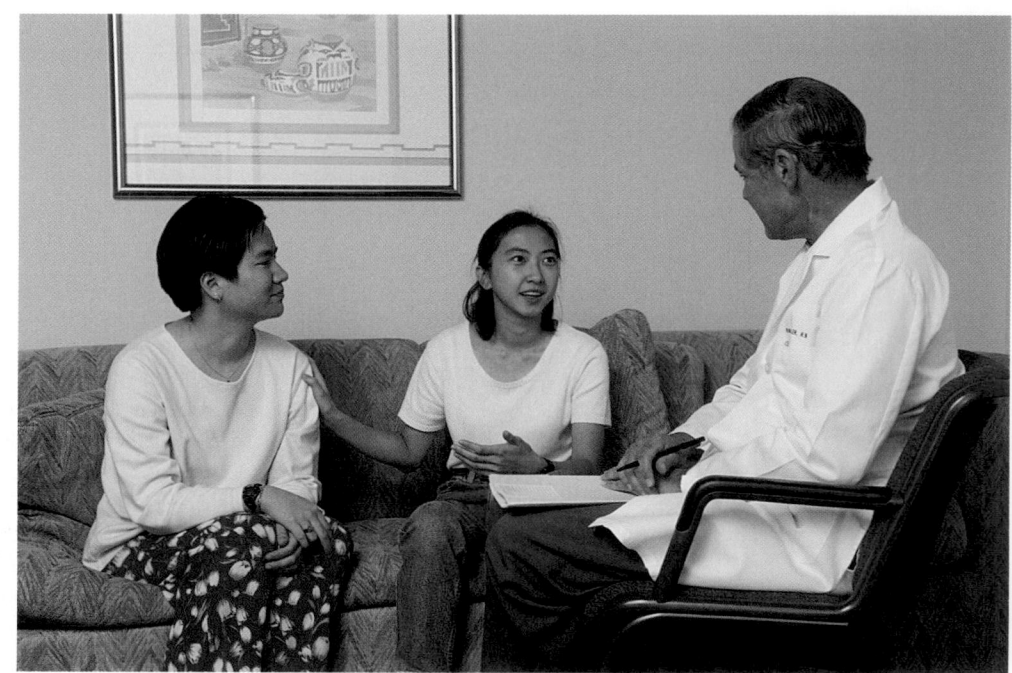

FIGURE 1-1
Interviewing a patient with the help of an interpreter. Someone other than a family member may be preferred when an interpreter is needed to bridge the language difference between examiner and patient.

aminer's language (or vice versa, because idiomatic expression, the "slang" of any language, may need clarification). This is true even in England, where "boot" may not mean "footwear" or a "kick," but rather means part of an automobile (Fig. 1-1).

THE BASIC REQUIREMENTS OF HEALTHY COMMUNICATION

A patient-centered communication has several important elements, informativeness, active encouragement of patient participation and the inclusion of questions and responses addressed to social and emotional issues fully as much as the physical nature of problems. Your nonverbal attitude complements your words. Indeed, communication first means listening—and careful listening leads to successful hearing. Eye contact should be assured and comfortable, and your body language should show that you are really in the room with the patient, comfortably seated, not standing and not reaching for the doorknob. Questions are your essential tools and the patient's responses need your careful interpretation. The way you pose questions can be adapted to persons of any age and circumstance (e.g., older adults, adolescents, or the parents or guardians of an infant or a young child or of an impaired adult). The approach you take to this end requires certain modifiers.

Flexibility. The patient's associations that may often seem like digressions may be important, and you must allow freedom to pursue them. Be flexible! Greet everyone in the room and then begin by asking open-ended questions. ("How have you been feeling since I last saw you?" "What questions do you have for me?" "What do you want to make sure we do today?") Later, as information accumulates, it will be necessary to know precise, measurable details, and you must become more specific. But early in the interview it is entirely appropriate to let it flow, to let the patient tell you what the immediate issues are. You must try to set a tone that will make it more likely that you will uncover hidden concerns. Thus the current visit's agenda may be appropriately set and the collaborative nature of the visit emphasized. You are to be an empathic listener and at the end an accurate recorder (Box 1-1). The written record will help others who become involved to gain a sense of how the patient and the family responded to the experience.

Open-endedness cannot be allowed to go on forever. Telling the patient at the outset the approximate time available for the interview may be helpful. Gentle guidance is sometimes necessary (e.g., "But now let's also talk about . . ." or "I'm sorry to interrupt, but let me make sure I understand . . ."). You cannot assume that a verbose tale is the complete story. (That

---

BOX 1-1

LISTENING: THE ART OF INTELLIGENT REPOSE

To be successful, we must be skilled listeners and observers with a polished sense of timing and a kind of repose that is at once alert and reassuring, and we must have clear goals for each of our interactions. In Robertson Davies' book *World of Wonders* (1977), an experienced actor gives advice to a very young would-be actor. From off stage, the two are watching the "star." It is advice you might take to heart as you enter a space with the patient:

Look at the Guvnor—he hasn't a taut muscle in his body, nor a slack one either. He is in easy control all the time. Have you noticed him standing still when he listens to another actor? Have you noticed how still he is? Look at you now, listening to me; you bob about and twist and turn in a scene, you'd be killing half the value of what I say with all that movement. Just try to sit still. Yes, there you go; you're not still at all, you're frozen. Stillness isn't looking as if you were full of coiled springs. It's repose. Intelligent repose. That's what the Guvnor has. What I have, too, as a matter of fact. What Barnard has. What Milady has. I suppose you think repose means asleep, or dead.

Learn how to listen intently while being still, achieving "intelligent repose." Be open to all the messages in the patient's words and body talk. It will help make your senses—touch, smell, and even taste—more acute. If a patient tells you the food is bad, taste it! Each of your behaviors should contribute to the communication of empathy and the building of the trust that is essential to a therapeutic partnership.

seems to be important but what else is on your mind?") You must be certain that you have asked all the necessary questions.

If the patient makes a reference that is not immediately relevant to your purposes (e.g., introducing a possible problem not previously mentioned), be flexible enough to clarify at least the nature of the irrelevancy. This allows you to make a decision about the need for further exploration. Although too many digressions can lead to the possibility of misspent time, paying attention to a digression of the moment may save a lot of time later.

Specificity. The careless phrasing of questions can lead to inaccurate or misleading patient responses:

- The *open-ended question* gives the patient discretion about the extent of an answer: "And then what happened?" "What are your feelings about this?" "Is that all you wanted to say?" "Is there anything more you need to talk about?"
- The *direct question* seeks specific information: "How long ago did that happen?" "Where does it hurt?" "Please put a finger where it hurts." "How many pills did you take each time, and how many times a day did you take them?"
- The *leading question* is the most risky because it may limit the information provided to what the patient thinks you want to know: "It seems to me that that bothered you a lot. Is that true?" "That wasn't very difficult to do, was it?" "That's a horrible-tasting medicine, isn't it?"

Sometimes the patient does not quite understand what you are asking and says so. Recognize the need at different times and in varying circumstances to perform the following functions:

- *Facilitate:* Encourage your patient to say more, either with your words or with a silence that the patient may break when given the opportunity for reflection.
- *Reflect:* Repeat what you have heard to encourage more detail.
- *Clarify:* Ask "What do you mean?"
- *Empathize:* Show your understanding and acceptance. Do not hesitate to say "I understand," or "I'm sorry" if the moment calls for it.
- *Confront:* Do not hesitate to discuss a patient's disturbing behavior.
- *Interpret:* Repeat what you have heard to confirm the meaning with the patient.

What you ask is complemented by how you ask it. Take the following actions, if necessary, to clarify the patient's point of view:

- Ask often what the patient *thinks and feels* about an issue.
- Make sure you know what the chief *concern* is.
- Make sure that all is well in the patient's life situation, and that nothing major—extraneous to the chief complaint and present illness—has happened recently.
- Suggest at appropriate times that you have the "feeling" that there is more to say or that things may not be as well as they are reported.
- Suggest at appropriate times that it is all right to be angry, sad, or nervous and it is all right to talk about it.
- Make sure that the patient's expectations in the visit are met and that there are no further questions.

Clarity. Take the time to ensure that your questions are clearly understood. Define any words that are not understood. Avoid technical terms if possible. The definitions can be confusing. Be clear and explicit; use the patient's idiom if possible. Meet the level of your patient's ability to understand but do not be patronizing. A patient may not be able to read; giving a handout is clearly not enough. Never assume a patient's every question requires an encyclopedic answer. Be sensitive to the extent of the answer that is being sought. Remember, too, that a patient who is a professional colleague may not be familiar with the jargon of your particular discipline.

Resist the tendency to manipulate. Avoid leading questions. For example, ask how often something happened, allowing the patient to define *often*, rather than asking, "It didn't happen too often, did it?" Pursue the information with short, uncomplicated questions using understandable language. Ask one question at a time, avoiding a barrage that prohibits the patient from being expansive or that limits the patient to simple yes or no answers. It is often better to say, "Tell me about . . ." rather than "Is it . . . ?" Be adaptable to the patient's lan-

CLINICAL PEARL

Mutual Understanding
Do not hesitate to tell patients to interrupt you if they do not understand what you are talking about. Similarly, do the same if you do not grasp a patient's meaning. In one case, a patient said he had "low blood" (anemia), "high blood" (hypertension), "bad blood" (syphilis), and "thin blood" (he was on anticoagulants)! It took a bit of exploring to sort it all out.

guage. If a patient uses a term to describe an event, adopt that term as you attempt to explore further.

Sometimes you will be confused by what the patient tells you. Recognize the confusion as a piece of information and begin to clarify if you can. The confusion may be a clue to a patient's underlying emotional or organic difficulty, or sometimes it may be due to a momentary loss of attention on your part.

Subtlety. Some apparent irrelevancies may provide important background information. A parent, for example, may have died of cancer. The fact itself may not be important at that moment, but the patient's response to the fact and the intensity of feeling associated with it can give important shape to your approaches. Such an insight is vital to your pursuit of understanding. Thus no history is complete without information about the patient's past and present life situation, reaction to earlier events, and coping methods.

Appreciate the subtle as well as the obvious in a question; learn to go far enough but not too far. Your sensitivity must include choosing your words carefully. Most lay people think *tumor* is *synonymous* with cancer. They may interpret your use of the word *nervous* to mean that they have emotional problems. Do not, however, paralyze your spontaneity in a too precise choice of words. If the patient seems to ask a leading question, one you do not feel prepared to answer at the moment, you may respond "Why do you ask?" to seek better understanding. Children need age-appropriate responses to their questions

Empathy. The American Board of Internal Medicine has suggested the following questions that might be asked by an interviewer who seeks an empathic relationship with the patient. We have added one or two. Rarely, if ever, is one patient asked all of these questions; exactly which ones are appropriate must be determined by the particular situation. For example, questions about a living will might alarm a patient seeking a routine checkup, but may relieve a patient hospitalized with a life-threatening disease. In any event, the reactions may appear to be illogical if the patient is cognitively impaired or if emotions such as anxiety, depression, fear, or related feelings dominate the patient's ability to reason. This, as well as racial, gender, ethnic, or other differences, may hinder your effort.

It is easy to be too directive. If advice is asked, be sure you understand the patient's experience and attitudes. Try for an interchange that allows for a decision as free as possible of your value judgment. Avoid this trap and you will remain a health professional and not a preacher. The competent clinician understands that value judgments are not necessarily imbued with wisdom.

- How are you feeling today?
- What can I do for you today?
- What do you think is causing your symptoms?
- What is your understanding of your diagnosis? Its importance? Its need for management?
- How do you feel about your illness? Frightened? Threatened? As a wage earner? As a family member? Angry that you are afflicted? (Be sure, though, to allow a response without putting words in the patient's mouth.)
- Do you believe treatment will help?
- How are you coping with your illness? Crying? Drinking more? Tranquilizers? Talking more? Less? Changing lifestyles?
- Do you want to know all the details about your diagnosis and its effect on your future?
- How important to you is "doing everything possible?"
- How important to you is "quality of life?"
- Have you prepared a living will?
- Do you have people you can talk with about your illness?
- Is there anyone else we should contact about your illness or hospitalization? Family members? Friends? Employer? Religious advisor? Attorney?
- Do you want or expect emotional support from the health care team?
- Are there financial questions about your medical care that trouble you? Insurance coverage? Tests or treatment you may not be able to afford? Timing of payments required from you?

- How would you like to be addressed?
- If you have had previous hospitalizations, does it bother you to be seen by teams of doctors, nurses, and medical students on rounds?
- How private a person are you?
- Are you concerned about the confidentiality of your medical records?
- Would you prefer to talk to an older/younger, male/female clinician?
- Are there medical matters you do not wish disclosed to others?
- Would you prefer to give your history so no one else can hear?

MOMENTS OF TENSION

Curiosity About You. Patients are aware that you are a person with a life of your own. Most of them will at one time or another have some curiosity about aspects of your experience. Sometimes you will be asked about yourself. Often a direct answer, unvarnished by detail, will satisfy the patient's curiosity without significant invasion of your personal life. You may find it comfortable to chat about certain, sometimes relevant, aspects of your own experience ("I have trouble remembering to take medicines, too"). Often, reassurance about personal life events (e.g., illness, pregnancy, and childbirth) can help alleviate fears and—with further exploration—can help in the identification of the patient's concerns. The message that you are a "real" person can lead to a more human and quite possibly trust-enhancing or even therapeutic exchange.

Anxiety. In the context of physical examination, anxiety may be defined as a painful uneasiness of mind resulting from an impending procedure or anticipated diagnosis. The intensity can certainly vary. Some physical disorders are more likely to have intense anxiety as a common accompaniment (e.g., those associated with crushing chest pain or difficulty in breathing). Just seeing a health professional provokes anxiety in some patients. Your approach should be helpful in relieving this anxiety. It pays to answer questions forthrightly, never dissembling. Avoid an overload of information. Pace the conversation. Do not hurry. A calm demeanor—repose—will communicate itself to the patient. This may not be easy to achieve, but pursue it. The patient's vulnerability requires it.

Silence. We are sometimes intimidated by silence, and many of us feel the urge to break it with some kind of chatter. Be patient and do not force the conversation. You may have to edge the patient along with an open-ended question ("What seems to worry you?") or a mild nudge ("And after that?"). Remember, though, that silence may have its uses, such as a moment of reflection or the summoning of courage. Some issues can be so painful and sensitive that the silence becomes necessary and should be allowed. Most people will begin to talk when they are ready. Meanwhile, the quiet listener can be compassionate.

As always, the patient's demeanor, use of hands, and facial expressions contribute to your interpretation of the moment. The eyes may be brimming with tears because of emotions felt so deeply that speech is impossible. Silence may also be cultural: for example, some Native Americans/American Indians take their time, ponder their responses to questions, and answer when they feel ready. Silence is usually a clue for you to go slower, not to push too hard, and to examine your approach. Learn to be comfortable with silence and to give it reasonable bounds.

Depression. Being sick or thinking that you are sick is enough to provoke at least some situational depression. Indeed, serious or chronic, unrelenting illness, or the taking of some prescription drugs (e.g., steroids) is often accompanied by depression. A sense of sluggishness in all of the daily experience; disturbances in sleep, eating, and social contact; and feelings of loss of self-worth can be clues to depression. When any of these happen, it is best to ask specific questions that, when answered, may then allow a more open-ended approach. First ask "When did this problem begin?" Then ask "How do you feel about it?" "Have you stopped enjoying your favorite activities?" "Is your sleep disturbed" "Have you had thoughts about hurting yourself?" A patient in this circumstance cannot be hurried and certainly cannot be relieved by superficial assurance. It is better to say "I understand" than to be falsely reassuring.

Crying. People will cry. Let them. Let the moment pass at the patient's pace. Resume your questioning only when the patient is ready. If you suspect a patient is suppressing the need to cry, give permission. Offer a tissue or simply say "I know you're feeling bad. It's all right to cry."

CLINICAL PEARL

Depression
The lifetime risk of depression ranges from 10% to 25% for women and from 5% to 12% for men.

From Hagman, 2001.

You have respected a need in this way. The responding patient may sense your caring, and the relationship may grow.

Manipulation. Some patients can be excessively flattering. Their illness and insecurity beg for extra-special attention. It is sometimes easy to be taken in by such manipulations. Be aware that it happens, and be aware that it should not encourage you to depart from your professional standard of care. We all like to be liked. The danger is that we may too often try to get patients to like us with our own, perhaps inappropriate, behavior (see Physical and Emotional Intimacy, below).

Physical and Emotional Intimacy. Many of us have grown up in circumstances that tend to increase the difficulty of dealing intimately with the emotions and the bodies of others. The cultural norms, shadings, and behaviors are at once protective of and barriers to good relationships with the patient. We may have powerful feelings, sometimes attracting us, sometimes repelling us.

The patient most likely shares some of the same feelings and may feel an added helplessness induced by the more dependent status. It is all right to acknowledge this and to indicate that you understand. You should then always protect the patient's modesty, using covers appropriately without hampering good examination, and you should always be careful about the ways in which you use words or frame questions. You should not shock the patient.

In particular, you must remember that the patient is generally having an uncommon personal experience and not be "desensitized" to the issues of intimacy as time goes by. Rather, understanding and accepting your own feelings, and keeping them in context will help develop a sensitive, empathic relationship. It is all right to admit that both you and the patient are human (Smith, Kleinman, 1989).

Nevertheless, there are boundaries to professional behavior and they must not be crossed. Patients are variably vulnerable; some are not particularly dependent, and others are deeply dependent. As vulnerability increases and professions of intimacy develop, often urged on by the patient's behavior (see Seduction, below), some professionals slide down the "slippery slope" and cross the boundary that should not be crossed. There is no room for sexual misconduct in the patient relationship, and there can be no tolerance for exploitation of the patient in this regard.

Compassionate Moments. Do not hesitate to say that you feel for the patient, that you are sorry for something that happened, and that you know it may have been painful. Be open and direct about a tender circumstance. At times, the touch of a hand or even a hug is in order. It is all right to bring things out in the open as long as you are gentle and not too aggressive or insistent. Sometimes you must state your concern and confront it (Box 1-2). Sometimes you make an inference and hope that you guessed right in bringing the patient's feelings to the surface. When you are uncertain, ask without imposing your interpretation of what the response might be.

Seduction. There are limits to your expressions of warmth and cordiality. Certainly not all touch is sexually motivated; a heartfelt hug is sometimes just right. Still, you are a professional and you must behave professionally. The insecure, dependent patient is sometimes seductive and often too readily susceptible to manipulation. You must not, either intentionally or unintentionally, fall into the trap of responding to the seductive behavior that so often reflects the patient's insecurity and dependence. Such a situation can be averted by being courteously calm and firm from the start, delivering the clear—and immediate—message that the relationship is and must remain professional. It will take skill to do this, to maintain the patient's dignity, and to seek understanding of the behavior.

Anger. Sometimes those patients who are angriest and most hostile are the ones who may need you the most—and family members and some of our coworkers may also vent strong feelings on us. It is often intimidating. Deal with it by confronting it. It is all right to say "I know you're angry. Please tell me why. I want to hear." Speak calmly and softly and try not to argue the point. After the episode, do not hesitate to talk it over with a trusted colleague and to settle down.

You may sometimes have made the patient angry by being late for an appointment, by taking too long, or by getting in the way of the patient's life or concerns in some way. For all of us, the stress of time, heavy workload, and the tension of caring for the acutely, even fatally, ill

Clinical Pearl

Rules of Thumb: When the Agenda Is the Patient's Emotions

- Thinking does not work well when emotions are in charge.
- Let the patient take the lead: silence on the part of the clinician is a key skill.
- Emotional distress is uncomfortable for the patient: sharing some of it usually leads to a sense of relief.
- When emotions have been disclosed and responded to, the patient usually comes to information-seeking and problem-solving.
- Keep an eye on your own private, emotional response, watching out in particular for defensiveness and judgmental views, even subtle communication of either of these. The patient who may irk you the most may need you the most.

From Barker LR, MD, ScM, Division of General Internal Medicine, Hopkins Bayview Medical Center, Johns Hopkins University School of Medicine.

BOX 1-2

SUICIDE

You may sense that a patient is contemplating suicide. It may not be easy to ask about suicidal ideation directly but you should. There are clues that can support your suspicion:

- Sociodemographic factors

  An older, unmarried male living alone

  An adolescent who has recently "lost face" in an incident that might seem trivial to others

  Successful or attempted suicide of a close relative

- Individual variables

  Possible stressors in family, work, financial factors. Questions to ask include the following: "How are things going in your marriage?" "Your family?" "Your work?"

  Mood disturbance: a lengthy period, 2 weeks or more, of feeling sad, blue, or "empty"; a generally worthless, sinful, guilty feeling, devoid of self-esteem and hope; uninterested in the daily effort and without pleasure in the usual sources of enjoyment; hearing voices

  Changes in habit that may last 2 weeks or more: trouble falling or staying asleep; eating too much or too little; evidence of drinking too much (see the CAGE questionnaire, p. 18) or of present or past substance abuse

  History of affective disorder or psychiatric treatment

- Current concerns

  Patient's understanding of an existing health condition and its implications, concern about becoming a burden to others, fears of nonexisting conditions

Possible change in religious belief

Recent loss of meaningful relationships due to death, divorce, or other separation

Concern about the impact of suicide on survivors and the thought given that problem

Understanding of how to commit suicide: availability of guns, bullets, poisons; history of previous attempts (leaving a note implies a plan and seriousness of intent); history of impulsive behavior and lack of self-control

Deal with the potential of suicide forthrightly. Consultation with others is most often necessary, particularly if the answers to these questions are positive. Just a few questions can begin the discussion (Whooley, Simon, 2000):

- "Have you often been bothered during the past few weeks by feeling down, depressed, or hopeless?"
- "Have you often been bothered during the past few weeks by having little interest or pleasure in doing things?"
- "Have you had any thoughts about not wanting to be alive?"
- And, ultimately, "Have you had any thoughts about suicide or hurting yourself?"

Data from Wagley, 1992; Cooper-Patrick, Crum, & Ford, 1994; Hirschfield, & Russell, 1997; Hagman, 2001.

---

can generate our own impatience and potential for anger. Try to avoid being defensive. After all, it is most often unlikely that you have done anything wrong. Acknowledge the problem and only when appropriate, apologize. The anger generally will not last long. As with crying, the patient or coworker should be given the opportunity to express the feeling and to find that you will not shrink away from it. Often, you can continue on better footing after anger is vented. On occasion, nothing will seem to help. It is all right, if the situation allows, to defer to another time or to suggest a different professional. Successful resolution is not always possible and may be unlikely when illness and uncertainty significantly lower the threshold for anger (Thomas, 2003).

Dissembling. Patients may not always tell the whole story. They may be hiding something, either purposely or unconsciously. Dementia, illness, alcoholism, sexual uncertainties, domestic violence, and child abuse are among the particularly difficult contributing circumstances. Do not push too hard when you think this is happening, but do not neglect it. Allow the interview to go on and then come back to it with gentle questioning. It might become possible to say "I think that you may be more concerned than you are saying." Or you might say "I think you're worried about what we might find out." You must be satisfied that you have learned all that is necessary. But satisfaction may not come in one sitting. You may have to pursue it later that day or the next or perhaps with other members of the family, friends, or associates.

Money. The cost of care and the resulting drain on the resources available to the patient are often sources of stress. These issues are real and they often have an impact on the mindset of the patient. Be prepared to talk about them with candor and accurate knowledge.

EVIDENCE-BASED PRACTICE IN PHYSICAL EXAMINATION

EFFECTIVE COMMUNICATION/EFFECTIVE COUNSELING

Want people to stop smoking? There is abundant evidence that patients in a trusting relationship with nurses, doctors, or other counselors will respond positively to even brief, simple advice about quitting. Twenty-nine pooled studies with nurses, 34 with physicians, and 18 with smoking cessation specialists consistently provide statistical evidence for the same conclusion—it pays to offer even minimal advice if it is given respectfully and earnestly. Of course, not everyone will respond, but the gain is important. The challenge is to incorporate smoking cessation interventions as part of standard practice.

Data from Rice & Stead, 2004; Silagy & Stead, 2004; Lancaster & Stead, 2004.

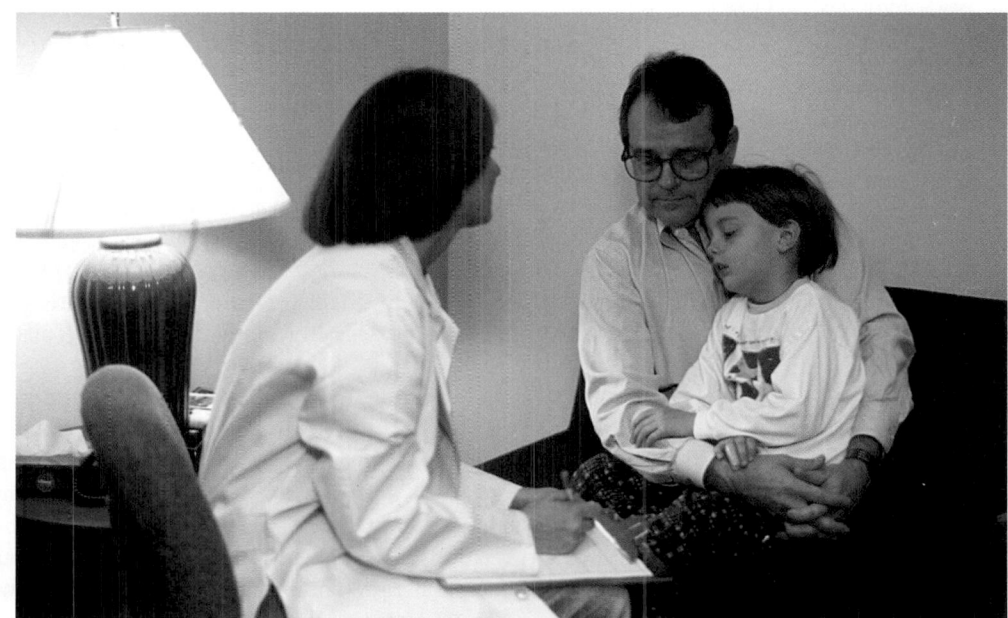

FIGURE 1-2
Interviewing a child with his parent. Note that the interviewer is sitting close to the patient and that the child is secure on his father's lap.

CHILDREN

Children are people. They want to have attention paid to them. They do not want to be patronized, and they love it when you get down on the floor and play with them. They have anxieties and fears that must be anticipated and eased (Fig. 1-2). Talk with them, hold them, reassure them, include them! Use language that is not above them but that does not patronize them. When they are old enough, allow them to be heard fully. The older the child, the more productive it becomes to ask questions directly and to give them information directly. Children and parents may tell a different story: for example, the young understating bad or aggressive behavior and the elder underestimating sadness and the effects of disability. The practical reward is that children who participate are more likely to follow through on your advice. The behavior we suggest holds true for any interaction with a patient accompanied by others. Almost half of adult visits, particularly those with older adults, are "three-party" or triangular visits (Barrone et al, 2003).

The older child and the adolescent require a particular sensitivity. Their hesitancies or passive, sometimes vaguely hostile silences may suggest that they would prefer to be alone with you, free of a parent. Respect the need for separation. This is more common with adolescents, but the need for privacy may also be evident among older preadolescent children. In general, be aware that to get a more complete history it often helps to separate the child from the parent at some point.

The conversation concerning a child (or an infant) can give significant information about the dynamics that prevail within a family and, on occasion, information that may suggest a problem with one of the parents. For example, an excessively tearful mother who does not seem to be having much pleasure in her child and who seems self-absorbed, unresponsive, and uncommunicative, or even hostile may be depressed. Your responsibility goes beyond that for the child. Certainly, in any interaction with any person of any age, clues to possible problems in family, significant others, or friends may become apparent and may demand your action.

ADOLESCENTS

Adolescence, the time between the onset of puberty and maturity, is distinctly different from childhood and adulthood both physically and psychosocially. Ellen (2004) emphasizes that it is a vulnerable time involving a particular tendency to experiment with risky behaviors that lead to a high incidence of morbidity and mortality. Good relationships with adolescents may not come easily. Because adolescents may be reluctant to talk, give clear evidence of your respect for their need for confidentiality and for their impending adulthood. While confidentiality and preventive medicine are at the heart of their care, it may be necessary at times to confirm that there may be state or federal laws that control the degree of confidentiality in certain circumstances, such as pregnancy, abortion, and substance abuse. You should be familiar with these limitations in your area.

If a parent is present at the start of a visit, acknowledge first the patient. It is helpful in the beginning to talk about what is happening in their day-to-day experiences. Do not force conversation, because adolescents do not readily respond to confrontation. On the other hand, you will often sense a need to talk and an inability to get the words out. Silences can be long, sometimes sheepish, occasionally angry, and not always leading to constructive talk. Many of us have found it helpful to have a few cards with subjects common to teenagers noted on them (see the Mnemonics box on p. 31). Simply ask the patient to look at the cards and to indicate silently the ones that note the subjects of present concern. Then you can say the necessary words, phrase the appropriate questions, and make the transition to a verbal discussion reasonably comfortable. Take an open-ended approach, always indicating a sense of alliance and partnership (Ellen, 2004).

CLINICAL PEARL
Adolescent Suicide
Suicide is a major cause of mortality for ages 10 to 18 years, more often in boys. If you think about this when you are with one of them, you can be pretty sure he has too. You can mention it and thereby give permission to talk about it. You will not be suggesting anything new (see Box 1-2).

PREGNANT WOMEN

The first interview provides the foundation for the continuing relationship between the pregnant woman and her health care provider. Care during the prenatal period involves a personal commitment by the woman to her health and that of the fetus, with direction provided by the health care team. Each woman manages her pregnancy according to many factors, including previous experiences with childbearing and childrearing; knowledge, expectations, and perceptions; her relationship with her mother and other significant individuals in her life; her desire for children; and her present life circumstances. It is important to view health care of both the mother and fetus as a complex interactive process. The information obtained during this initial interview includes past history, assessment of health practices, identification of potential risk factors, and assessment of knowledge as it affects pregnancy. It provides a unique opportunity during a receptive time for teaching about health care practices.

OLDER ADULTS

Individual variations in knowledge, experience, cognitive abilities, and personality affect the interview process with older adults, just as with the young. It is certainly important to be knowledgeable about physiologic, sociologic, and psychologic changes associated with aging, and it is appropriate to anticipate what effect these changes may have on the interview. For example, aging increases alcohol risks. The same amount of alcohol does more in the older adult than in the young adult of like weight and height because older tissues hold less water than do younger ones. However, it is equally important to appreciate that not all adults experience the same changes, that such changes do not occur at the same rate, and that some areas do not decline with age. The older patient brings to the interview a lifetime of experience that may be a rich source of wisdom, meaning, and perspective. Do not discount it. Be aware that physiologic age and chronologic age may be disparate.

Some older adults may have sensory losses that make communication more difficult. Some degree of hearing loss is not uncommon. Position yourself so that the patient can see your face. Speak clearly and slowly, taking care not to avert your head while you are talking. Shouting only magnifies the problem by distorting consonants and vowels. In some instances, a written interview may ultimately be less frustrating for both you and the patient. If this becomes necessary, tailor the process to include only the most pertinent questions because this method can be tedious and exhausting for patients.

Conversely, impaired visual perception and light-dark adaptation can adversely affect the interview if written interview forms are used. Provide the patient with a well-illuminated environment and a light source that does not glare or reflect in the eyes.

CLINICAL PEARL
Watch Your Language
Unfortunately, many clinicians often lapse into the use of jargon, the arcane language of their particular profession not understood by the patient. Worse yet are pejorative words that demean patients. Stress, frustration, fatigue, and anger are common underlying causes for these lapses. Still, their very use suggests an attitude that does not speak well for the professional. Know yourself. Understand why you might fall into the habit, and do your best to avoid it.

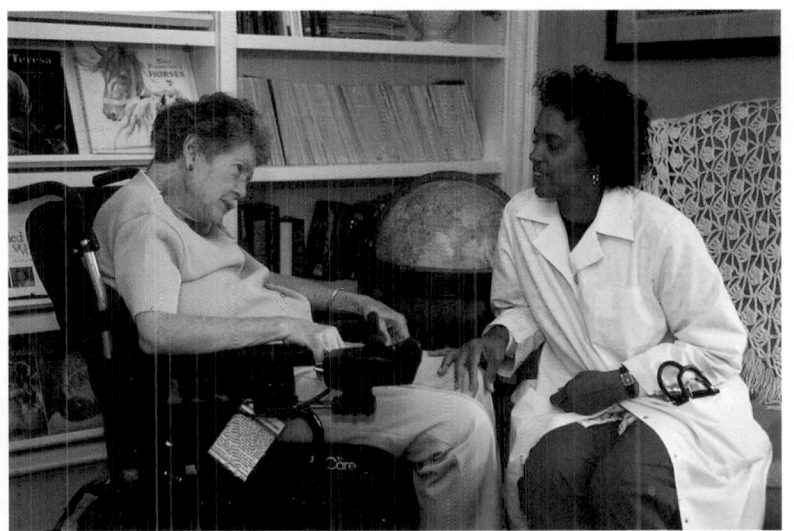

FIGURE 1-3
Interviewing a patient with a physical disability. Note the uncluttered surroundings; be sure the patient in a wheelchair has room to maneuver.

Some older adults may be confused or experience memory loss, particularly for recent events. Take whatever extra time is needed. Ask short (but not leading) questions, and keep your language uncomplicated and free of double negatives. Consult other family members to clarify discrepancies or to fill in the gaps.

PATIENTS WITH DISABILITIES

Patients with serious and disabling physical or emotional disorders (e.g., deafness, blindness, depression, psychosis, developmental delays, or neurologic impairments) require that your approach be adapted to their needs (see Chapter 18). Patients who are thus restricted may not give an effective history, but they must be respected and the history must be obtained from them to the extent possible. Their points of view and their attitudes matter. Every patient must be fully involved to the limit of emotion, mental capacity, or physical ability (Fig. 1-3). Still, when necessary, the family, other health professionals involved in care, and the patient's record must be queried to get a more complete story.

Some of the most common communication barriers can be overcome by keeping the following in mind:

- Families are often available to make the patient more comfortable and to provide you with information.
- Persons with impaired hearing often read, write, and/or read lips, but you must speak slowly and enunciate each word clearly and in full view; a translator who signs may be available.
- Persons with visual impairment usually can hear; talking louder to make a point does not help. Remember, however, that you must always make vocal what you are trying to communicate; gestures may not be seen.

THE HISTORY

Taking the history usually begins your relationship with the patient. A first objective is to identify those matters the patient defines as problems. You must seek out the hidden as well as the obvious concerns, and you need to strive for accuracy. You have to develop a sense of the patient's reliability as an interpreter and reporter of events. Sometimes you will realize that the patient is suppressing some information either intentionally or without realizing it, underreporting other experiences, or giving them a context that is at odds with what you might feel appropriate. You will be in a constant state of subjective evaluation as the history is revealed. Indeed, some circumstances that worry you might not be thought of as unusual by the patient. This is all the more reason to seek an understanding of the patient's perspective. Your attitude of friendliness and obvious respect will go a long way in the pursuit of information and in ensuring your patient's help in obtaining it.

SETTING FOR THE INTERVIEW

The large university teaching hospital, the setting in which most health professionals are educated, is in some ways disadvantageous for a first experience with patient care. You must not allow the profusion of technical competence and the variety of skills to obscure the essential interactions that must take place between you and the patient. There are really few extra aids you need to extend your senses. Even in an empty space, the interview can be a rich and positive interchange, an experience that is rewarding to the patient, to those who accompany the patient, and to you.

Make the setting in which you take the history as comfortable as possible. Often the space provided is small and rather barren. The colors are often not warm, and the chairs are straight-backed and uncomfortable. No matter; you are the focal point of warmth and attention. You can make sure that there are no bulky desks or tables between you and the patient. If possible, have a clock placed where you can see it without obviously looking at your watch (preferably behind the patient's chair). Sit comfortably and at ease, maintaining eye contact and a conversational tone of voice. Your manner can assure the patient that you care and that relieving the patient's worry or pain is your sole concern.

You can do this only with a discipline that allows you to concentrate on the matter at hand, giving it for that moment primacy in your life, and putting aside both personal and professional distractions.

STRUCTURE OF THE HISTORY

Your purposes in taking the history are to establish a relationship and to learn about the patient, so that you might discover *with* the patient the issues and problems that need attention and the assignment of priority. The process has an organization that has been widely accepted for decades. The structure includes the following areas:

- Chief complaint (CC)
- History of present illness or problem (HP1)
- Past medical history (PMH)
- Family history (FH)
- Personal and social history (SH)
- Review of systems (ROS)

Do not forget the identifiers: date, time, age, gender, race, occupation, and referral source.

The *chief complaint* is a brief statement of the reason the patient is seeking health care. Directly quoting the patient is helpful. It is always important, however, to go beyond the given reason and to probe for underlying concerns that cause the patient to seek care rather than do other things (e.g., simply going to work). If the patient has a sore throat, why is he or she seeking help about it? Is it the pain and fever, or is it the concern caused by past experience with a friend or relative who developed rheumatic heart disease? Many interviewers include the *duration of the problem* as part of the chief complaint.

Understanding the *present illness or problem* requires a step-by-step evaluation of the circumstances that surround the primary reason for the patient's visit. The medical history goes beyond this to an exploration of the patient's *overall health before the present problem,* including all of the patient's past medical and surgical experiences. The spiritual, psychosocial, and cultural contexts of the patient's life are essential to a full understanding of these events. Then *the patient's family requires attention:* their health; past medical history; illnesses; deaths; and the genetic, social and environmental circumstances that have influenced the patient's life. The information gained in this context underlies a question that must be implicit in all of your inquiry: *Why is this happening to this particular patient at this particular time?* In other words, if many people are exposed to a potential problem and only some of them succumb to the exposure, what are the factors in the individual circumstance that led to that outcome? A careful inquiry about the *personal and social experience of the patient* should include work habits and the multiplicity of relationships in the family, school, and workplace. Finally, the *systems review* takes a different tack in that it includes a detailed review of possible complaints in each of the body's systems, looking for complementary or seemingly unrelated symptoms that may not have surfaced during the rest of the history.

Be flexible, but also compulsive about achieving as many of your goals as possible while being sensitive to nuance in pursuing each suggestion, however subtle, that information of substance may yet be found.

Provide opportunity for give and take, for the patient to ask questions and to explore feelings. You need not allow the patient to ramble; gentle constraint is most often recognized and successful.

TAKING THE HISTORY

Introduce yourself to the patient, clearly stating your name and your role in the process. If you are a student, do not mask the fact. Be certain that you understand the patient's full name and that you pronounce it correctly.

Address the patient properly (e.g., as Mr., Miss, Mrs., Ms., or using the manner of address preferred by the patient) and repeat the patient's name at appropriate times. Avoid the familiarity of using a first name when you do not expect familiarity in return. Never use a surrogate term for the patient's name; for example, when the patient is a child, do not address the parent as "Mother" or "Father." It is respectful and courteous to take the time to learn a name.

By this time you should *be seated at a comfortable distance from the patient* without furniture barriers between you (Fig. 1-4). Unless you have known the patient in the past and know that there is no matter of great urgency, proceed with reasonable dispatch, asking the patient to state the reason for the visit. *Listen, and do not be too directive* at this point. *Let the patient spill it all out,* and after the first flow of words, begin to shape the direction of the interview. Begin to probe for what has been called the "iatrotropic stimulus," the stimulus to seek health care. If indeed 100 people wake up with a bad headache, and 97 go to work while 3 seek care, what underlying dimension prompted those decisions? Consider, too, the patient's possible use of complementary or alternative care.

This is the point at which you begin *to give structure to the present illness or problem,* giving it a chronologic and sequential framework, fleshing out the bare bones of the chief complaint, probing for the underlying concerns. Unless there is some obvious urgency, go slowly, hear the full story, and refrain from striking out too quickly on what seems the obvious course of questioning. The patient will take cues from you on the amount of leisure you will allow; you must walk a fine line between permitting this leisure and meeting the many time constraints you are apt to have. You do not need a lot of time to let the patient know that you have *enough* time. Lean back, fix your attention on the patient, and *listen;* avoid interrupting unless you really have to, and do not anticipate the next question before you have heard the complete answer.

CLINICAL PEARL

The Humanization of the History

Sadly, the history taking of a patient's health and medical past may follow the routine course we describe so rigidly that little of the patient's substance, little of that which makes the person unique, creeps in. It is all right to speak to and write of the patient beyond the constraints of the outline, to describe what you may hear and see in more than technical language, to lend your own style to the fleshing out of the history, and—as a result, perhaps—to give your patient records a vibrancy that might otherwise be lost. By all means, use the patient's name in the body of the recorded history. It is a particular person's story not meant to be made anonymous with "patient" substituted for the name.

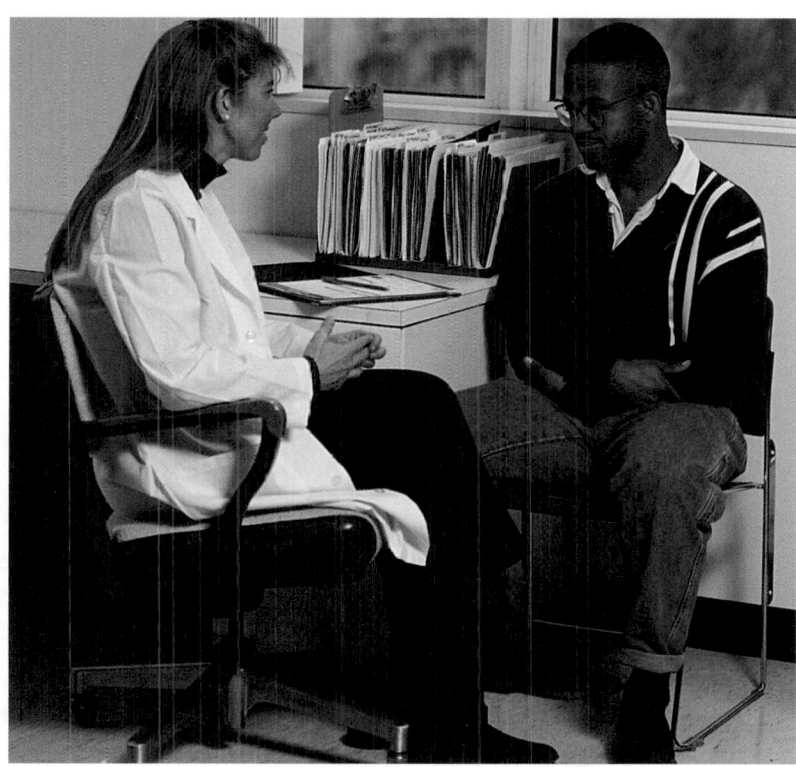

FIGURE 1-4
Interviewing a young adult. Note the absence of an intervening desk or table.

The patient's responses may at times be unclear. Say so and ask questions:

◆ "What of what you've told me concerns you the most?"
◆ "What do you want to make sure we pay attention to today?"
◆ "Do you have any ideas about what we ought to do?"
◆ Or, prompting, "I think _____ worries you the most. Shall we talk about that first?"

Once you have understood the patient's chief complaint and present problem and have obtained a sense of possible underlying concerns, it is time to go on to other segments of the history: the *family and past medical histories; emotional, spiritual, and cultural concerns;* and *social and workplace accompaniments to the present concerns.* Remember that nothing in the patient's experience is isolated. Aspects of the present illness or problem require careful integration with the medical and family history. The life of the patient is not constructed according to your outline, with many factors giving shape to the present illness and with any one chief complaint possibly involving more than one illness.

As the interview proceeds, thoroughly explore each positive response with the following questions:

◆ *Where?* Where are symptoms located, as precisely as possible? If they seem to move, what is the range of their movement? Where is the patient when the complaint occurs—at work or play, active or resting, in the city or country?
◆ *When?* Everything happens in a chronologic sequence. When did it begin? Does it come and go? If so, how often and for how long? What time of day? What day of the week?
◆ *What?* What does it mean to the patient? What is its impact? What does it feel like? What is its quality and intensity? Has it been bad enough to interrupt the flow of the patient's life, or has it been dealt with rather casually? What happened contemporaneously that might be related? What makes it feel better? Worse?
◆ *How?* The background of the symptom becomes important in answering the "how" question. How did it come about? What is the ambiance of the complaint? Are other things going on at the same time, such as work, play, mealtime, or sleep? Is there illness in the family? Have there been similar episodes in the past? Is there concern about similar symptoms in friends or relatives? Are there companion complaints? How is the patient coping? Are there social supports? Again, nothing ever happens in isolation.
◆ *Why?* Of course, the answer to "why" is the solution to the problem. All other questions lead to this one.

When these questions are kept in mind, you will be able to define what you have heard as clearly as possible. You can place it in a context appropriate to the patient's age and gender. You will also be able to determine the size of a complaint—that is, how intense it is, how often it occurs, and how much it affects the patient's life.

As the interview approaches its conclusion, it is possible to return to the more free-flowing, less structured style that might have dominated as the patient first described the present problem. It is a time to review the discussion, to ask the patient to supply any missing details, to ask for questions, and to interpret and summarize what you have heard in a way that communicates your wish to devote whatever time is necessary to achieve comfort with a mutual understanding of the issues.

EVIDENCE-BASED PRACTICE IN PHYSICAL EXAMINATION

ARE THERE GENDER DIFFERENCES?

Digoxin is used for the treatment of heart failure. Women on digoxin therapy have a higher rate and risk of death than do men. There were more than 7000 patients overall in the study at the Yale University School of Medicine. The statistical data revealed an absolute difference of 5.8% between men and women, a significant number. The authors also indicate that sex-based or sex hormone–associated differences have also been demonstrated for myocardial cell function and cardiac cell growth among other influences. The clear message: Gender matters. Never assume as you learn about your patient that what is appropriate for one gender is appropriate for the other. The goose and the gander may require different sauces.

Data from Rathore et al, 2002.

Try to verify that the patient understands what has happened and what you have tried to communicate, and that the patient and family seem to be coping. Repeat instructions, if there are any, and ask to hear them back. Always discuss and explain the next step, whether it is an appointment time, methods of keeping in touch, an exchange of telephone numbers, or planning for the physical examination that will follow the interview.

AN APPROACH TO SENSITIVE ISSUES

It is not always easy to question the patient about sensitive issues (e.g., sex, drug or alcohol use, or concerns about death). Still, these issues must not be avoided. Although there is no specific "right" way to deal with these questions, you must feel comfortable with your approach. The following suggestions are common sense guides that are useful at all times in interviews; they may aid in your discussion of sensitive issues.

- ♦ Privacy is essential. Do not forget that this is as true with the older child and the adolescent as it is with the adult.
- ♦ Do not waffle. Be direct and firm. Avoid asking leading questions.
- ♦ Do not apologize for asking a question. You are doing nothing wrong.
- ♦ Do not preach. Avoid confrontation. You are not there to pass judgment.
- ♦ Use language that is understandable to the patient, yet not patronizing.
- ♦ Do not push too hard. If the patient is defensive, recognize that the patient feels that defense is necessary. Do not demean the behavior; proceed slowly. It is possible to achieve your goals by acknowledging with the patient that you are touching on concerns that are common in society and that therefore need pursuit.
- ♦ Afterward, document carefully, using the patient's words (and those of others with the patient) whenever possible. It is all right to take notes as the conversation progresses, but try to do this sparingly and not at all when particularly sensitive issues are being discussed.

You must always be ready to explain again why you examine sensitive areas. A successful approach will have incorporated four steps:

1. An introduction, the moment when you bring up the issue, alluding to its frequency in society
2. Open-ended questions that first explore the patient's feelings about the issue—whether, for example, it is alcohol, drugs, sex, cigarettes, education, or problems at home—and then the direct exploration of what is actually happening
3. A period in which you thoughtfully attend to what the patient is saying and then repeat the patient's words or offer other forms of feedback, so that the patient agrees that your interpretation is appropriate, thus confirming what you have heard
4. And finally, an opportunity for the patient to ask any questions that might be relevant

Alcohol. The CAGE questionnaire (Box 1-3), advocated by Ewing (1984), is very helpful as a model for approaching a discussion of the use of alcohol. CAGE is an acronym for *C*utting down, *A*nnoyance by criticism, *G*uilty feeling, *E*ye-openers.

The effective use of CAGE does not ensure absolute sensitivity in the detection of a problem. It can be complemented or supplemented by the TACE model (Box 1-4), particularly in the identification of alcoholism in a pregnant woman (because of the potential for damage to the infant), or by CRAFFT, for identification of an alcohol problem in adolescents (Box 1-5).

There is a certain sameness to all of these questionnaires. As you gain experience, you can adapt them to your style and to the particular patient you are serving. You can also adapt them to concerns about drugs other than alcohol.

Domestic Violence. Domestic violence means trouble at home, the kind of trouble that inflicts both physical and emotional pain. It may be assaultive or coercive. It is a problem that affects primarily women and children as victims and, in lesser frequency, men. Intimate partners are most often the perpetrators. Alcohol, even more than other drugs, is a common facilitator. We are sometimes reluctant to screen for such violence for fear of offending patients and families. This misplaced concern is occasionally confounded by an inappropriate response to an abused woman, making too little of her experience or even laying the blame on her. She is, then, twice a victim.

The "she" is used advisably. About 94% of the reported victims of domestic abuse are women and they come from every ethnic and socioeconomic group. Only a relatively few

CLINICAL PEARL

Screening

There is a difference between a screening and an assessment interview. The goal of screening is to find out if a problem exists. This is particularly true of CAGE, CRAFFT, and TACE questionnaires. They are effective, but they are only the start, and assessment goes on from there. Discovering a problem early may lead to a better treatment outcome.

BOX 1-3

CAGE Questionnaire

The following questions are included in the CAGE model:

C-Have you ever been **C**oncerned about your own or someone else's drinking? Have you ever felt the need to **C**ut down on drinking?

Probe: What was it like? Were you successful? Why did you decide to cut down?

A-Have you ever felt **A**nnoyed by criticism of your drinking?

Probe: What caused the worry or concern? Do you ever get irritated by others' worries? Have you ever limited what you drink to please someone?

G-Have you ever felt **G**uilty about your drinking? Have you ever felt **G**uilty about something you said or did while you were drinking?

Probe: Have you ever been bothered by anything you have done or said while you've been drinking? Have you ever regretted anything that has happened to you while you were drinking?

E-Have you ever felt the need for a morning **E**ye-opener?

Probe: Have you ever felt shaky or tremulous after a night of heavy drinking? What did you do to relieve the shakiness? Have you ever had trouble getting back to sleep early in the morning after a night of heavy drinking?

From Ewing, 1984.

BOX 1-4

TACE Questionnaire

The following questions are included in the TACE model:

T-How many drinks does it **T**ake to make you feel high? How many when you first started drinking? "When was that?" "What do you prefer: beer, wine, or liquor? (More than two drinks suggests a tolerance to alcohol that is a red flag.)

A-Have people **A**nnoyed you by criticizing your drinking?

C-Have you felt you ought to **C**ut down on your drinking?

E-Have you ever had an **E**ye-opener drink first thing in the morning to steady your nerves or get rid of a hangover?

A positive answer to T alone or to two of A, C, or E may signal a problem with a high degree of probability. Positive answers to all four signal a problem with great certainty.

From Sokol, Martier, & Ager, 1989.

BOX 1-5

CRAFFT Questionnaire

The following questions are included in the CRAFFT model:

C-Have you ever ridden in a **C**ar with someone who is high on alcohol or other drugs?

R-Do you drink or take drugs to **R**elax, feel better about yourself, or fit in?

A-Do you ever drink or take drugs while you are **A**lone?

F-Do you ever **F**orget things you did while using alcohol or other drugs?

F-Does a **F**amily member or a **F**riend tell you to cut down on drinking or drug use?

T-Have you ever gotten into **T**rouble from drinking or taking drugs?

From Knight et al, 1999.

EVIDENCE-BASED PRACTICE IN PHYSICAL EXAMINATION
PROFESSIONAL RELUCTANCE TO SEEK THE FACTS

Few health professionals who care for children and adolescents make the routine effort to screen for intimate partner violence. Borowsky and Ireland (2002) validated this assumption with a random national survey of 1350 pediatricians and 650 family physicians. The response rate overall was 37%. It would have been preferable to have a greater rate but the problem is clear. Only 5% of pediatricians and 8% of family physicians did this screening routinely. Eighteen percent of family medicine residents did do so. However, with conscientious screening,

Erickson, Hill, and Siegel (2001) found that 40% of mothers will disclose domestic violence by their partner. Their study also involved pediatricians and family physicians. The 310 of 547 questionnaires returned also revealed that routine screening was still at less than 10% despite the recommendation of the American Academy of Pediatrics that all practitioners incorporate domestic violence screening as part of the routine of anticipatory guidance.

Data from Borowsky, Ireland, 2002; Erickson et al, 2001.

MNEMONICS

Domestic Violence: HITS

Verbal abuse is often a proxy for physical violence. HITS is analogous to the CAGE questions for alcohol abuse. HITS stands for **H**urt, **I**nsult, **T**hreaten, or **S**cream. The wording of the question is "In the last year how often did your partner:

- **H**urt you physically?"
- **I**nsult or talk down to you?"
- **T**hreaten you with physical harm?"
- **S**cream or curse at you?"

From Sherin et al, 1998.

choose to discuss it with a clinician and in that event the patient is almost always the initiator of the discussion. If a health professional makes the initial inquiry, it is usually asked in an emergency department of a minority woman or one who is obviously poor. This is a major societal problem that mandates our attention (Mayer, Coulter, 2002).

A female patient should be routinely queried and the questioning should be direct. It is necessary to make time for this. Studies have demonstrated the efficacy of using three questions as a brief screening instrument to detect partner violence. The questions cover two dimensions of partner violence, and a positive response to any one of the following three questions constitutes a positive screen for partner violence:

- Have you been hit, kicked, punched, or otherwise hurt by someone within the past year?
- Do you feel safe in your current relationship?
- Is there a partner from a previous relationship who is making you feel unsafe now?

The first question, which addresses physical violence, has been validated in studies as an accurate measure of 1-year prevalence rates. The latter two questions evaluate the woman's perception of safety, and estimate her short-term risk of further violence and her need for counseling, but reliability and validity evaluations have not yet been established.

Additionally, you may see something suggestive on physical examination and ask the following:

- The bruises I see. How did you get them?

Positive answers require accurate documentation, using words, drawing and, if possible, photographs and the preservation of any tangible evidence. Positive answers require that the patient's safety be ensured. Ask the following:

- Are you afraid to go home?
- Are there guns or knives at home?
- Is alcohol (or other drugs) part of the problem?
- Has it gotten worse lately?
- Are children involved?

A "yes" answer mandates an intervention that needs your knowledge of community resources and your willingness to ask for help. Get the patient's viewpoint and do not be judgmental. Listen. Let her speak; assure her that she is not alone, that there are many who share her experience, and that you will do your best to help her.

A "no" answer may still leave you uncomfortable. Document your concern and your suspicion of injury. Be unafraid to be direct about your suspicion. ("Where did that bruise come from?") Ask her to come back to see you again.

Men may be victims, too, but the facts confirm that perhaps 20 to 30 times more women suffer from abuse than men. Still, if you are worried about a man in this way, the same approach is valid but not necessarily as a routine. His statements or a suspicious injury may trigger your action.

Infants and children have the protection of the legal mandate for you to report your suspicions. Questioning a child about abuse at home or in some other setting can be tricky because you want to avoid suggestion:

- Why did you come to see me today? (Do not mention the concern directly.)
- Tell me everything that happened to you, please. (No leading questions.)

With infants, a bruise of odd shape or location usually suggests a problem. You cannot ignore reporting your concern according to the process in your institution.

Adolescents may endure violence, particularly sexual victimization, at home or in social settings. The clue, particularly with young women but also with young men, may come with obvious behavioral change in the use of dress and makeup, school effort, sleeping, and eating. Alcohol or drugs can become an issue. Friends may be avoided. Most importantly, take your time and listen. Ask the following questions:

- Have you ever had sex?
- When did you start?
- Did you want to, or were you forced or talked into it?
- Do the people you are with ever scare you?
- Did anyone ever touch you in your private places?

Always be available for more conversation and information. The questions are just a start.

Older patients run a greater risk of abuse if they have had a history of mental illness, are physically or cognitively impaired, or are living in a dependent situation with inadequate financial resources. Their abusers may have similar risks and may be alcohol- or drug-addicted. Both groups may well have a past history of some sort of domestic violence. In any event, you must confront your concern using approaches modeled on that for women in difficulty.

Spirituality. The basic condition that life imposes is death. It is exquisitely capable of stirring in us a spiritual or "sacred" feeling, always with us, sometimes sublimated, sometimes not. Illness, even mild illness, stirs that feeling and may carry with it a sense of dread. The faith we and that our patients may or may not have is an intimate contributor to our perspectives on illness and life and death. An understanding of "spirituality" is, then, integral to the care we offer.

Actually, many patients want us to pay attention to this and want us to talk with them about their spiritual needs. Faith is often a key factor in the success of a management plan. Still, there are patients who prefer that you not broach the subject. You should. It is just as appropriate as talking about drugs, cigarettes, sex, and alcohol, and it requires the same great degree of sensitivity and caution.

Some clinicians are inappropriately uncomfortable doing this and back away. That cannot be a deterrent. The questions offered by Puchalski and Romer (2000) with the acronym FICA and adapted by us suggest an approach (Box 1-6).

BOX 1-6

APPROACHING THE SPIRITUAL: FICA

*F*aith, Belief, Meaning
- What is your spiritual or religious heritage? Are the Bible, the Quran, or similar writings important to you?
- Do these beliefs help you cope with stress?

*I*mportance and Influence
- How have these beliefs influenced you in how you handle stress? To what extent?

*C*ommunity
- Do you belong to a formal spiritual or religious community? Does this community support you? In what way? Is there anyone there with whom you would like to talk?

*A*ddress/Action in Care
- How do your religious beliefs affect your health care decisions (e.g., choice of birth control)? How would you like me to support you in this regard when your health is involved?

Modified from Puchalski, Romer, 2000.

The answers to the questions posed by FICA will guide you. They may suggest that you involve the clergy or other spiritual care providers and that you may become more deeply involved. Many clinicians cite empiric evidence, however tenuous, that prayer aids in healing. You may, if you are asked and if you are inclined, pray with a patient although it has been suggested that the professional should not lead the prayer. You may even suggest it if the patient is sorely troubled and you understand the need. The potential relief of stress, if nothing more, may be helpful. There are, however, boundaries. Except for a few of us, we are not theologians and it is inappropriate for us to go beyond the bounds of our professional expertise in counseling patients.

Auster (2004) suggests two circumstances that call for delicacy on our part: (1) patients' queries about our personal beliefs and (2) patients' feelings that they can discuss such matters only with someone of their own faith. As always, the way you respond matters. You may answer the first of these questions by saying "Right now, I'm trying to arrive at the best way to help you so I can't help but wonder why you are asking about my faith." You might answer the second question by saying "I understand that you might prefer to talk with someone of your own faith. Would it help if I found that person for you?" As always, patients' responses and your sense of the situation should guide your next steps (Auster, 2004; Puchalski & Romer, 2000; Fosarelli, 2003).

Sexual History. Questions about the patient's sexual history are often best initiated indirectly, addressing feelings rather than facts. The following is an example of how to address the topic: "Are you satisfied with your sexual life, or do you have worries or concerns? After all, it isn't unusual. Most people do have some." You will recognize in this a trace of a leading question; however, it does not suggest what the patient's feelings should be. Rather, if patients do have concerns about sex, it may comfort them with the realization that they are not alone.

Given the transition into the discussion, it becomes possible very often to gain more direct information, for example, frequency of sexual intercourse, problems in achieving orgasm, variety and numbers of "partners" (a non–gender-linked term), and particular sexual likes and dislikes. Questions about the possibility of exposure to sexually transmitted infections should not be avoided. Age of first intercourse and number of sexual partners can identify risk factors for cervical cancer. Sexual practice (e.g., anal intercourse) can influence your evaluation and management decisions.

Sexual Orientation. The sexual orientation of an adolescent or adult patient must be known if appropriate continuity (or any other kind) of care is to be offered (American Medical Student Association, 1991). About 10% of the persons you serve are likely to be other than heterosexual (i.e., gay men, lesbian women, and bisexual men and women). Armed with this knowledge, you are more likely to serve well during times of stress and illness (by marshaling the patient's support systems), in the provision of gynecologic care (by recognizing the variable need for Pap smears), in the diagnosis and treatment of sexually transmitted infection, and in counseling about a variety of possible issues (such as myths about homosexuality and the development of meaningful relationships). The risk non-heterosexual patients may feel in revealing their sexual preferences should be recognized. It may take courage, given the possibly unacknowledged and sometimes deep-seated feelings of heterosexism and homophobia in some health professionals. Reassuring, nonjudgmental words help: "I'm glad you trust me. Thank you for taking the risk you may have felt in telling me." It is also supportive if the health care setting offers some recognition of the patients involved (e.g., by making relevant informational pamphlets available in waiting areas).

Trust can be better achieved if questions are "gender neutral":

- Tell me about your living situation.
- Are you sexually active?
- In what way?

Rather than:

- Are you married?
- Do you have a boyfriend/girlfriend?

If you use a nonjudgmental approach and have touched an area of need, a variety of questions applicable to any patient and any sexual circumstance becomes possible. The questions should be phrased according to the patient's need and understanding. The vernacular may be necessary. Given a positive response to your first outreach, the following topics for discussion are likely to flow more easily:

- Sexual behavior or feelings that need discussion
- Concerns with sexual identity
- Sexual behavior that increases the risk of disease or of experiences that involve the harassment of or by others
- Worry about masturbating or even touching the body

OUTLINE OF CLINICAL HISTORY

The following outline is a guide for history taking (Griffith, Seidel, 1986). It should not set limits or indicate a rigid pathway; you are the best judge of what will suit your needs as you gain experience. Some ways in which the history may be elaborated are indicated in subsequent chapters. Chapter 26 suggests guidelines for recording the information obtained in the interview.

Chief Complaint (CC) or the Reason for Seeking Care. In brief, this is the answer to the question, "What problem or symptoms brought you here?" The duration of the current illness should next be determined (e.g., "How long has this problem been present?" or "When did these symptoms begin?"). The patient's age, gender, marital status, previous hospital admissions, and occupation should be noted for the record. Other significant complaints often surface while you are taking the history. These seemingly secondary issues may have even greater significance than the original concern, because the driving force for the chief complaint may be found in them (Box 1-7). What really made the patient seek care? Was it a possibly unexpressed fear or concern? Each hint of a care-seeking reason should be thoroughly explored (Box 1-8).

History of Present Illness or Problem (HPI). No outline for the present problem would be applicable to all cases. You will probably find that it is natural and easiest to question the patient on the details of the current problem immediately after obtaining the chief complaint. Others find it of more value to obtain the patient's history and family history before returning to the present. The specific order is not critical; what is important is that you obtain the needed information and organize it before finally recording it. At times it is helpful to let the patient provide an outline of the present problem and then go back to fill in all the pertinent details. This has the advantage of allowing the patient to voice the relative importance of the features surrounding the problem. At other times, experience will dictate that you must obtain the details by specific questions. Nevertheless, leading questions should be avoided. You want the patient's version, although you may ultimately write it in your own words. Box 1-9 suggests many of the variables that can influence the patient's version.

Among the concerns to be explored, you should include the following:

- Ultimately, a chronologic ordering of events
- State of health just before the onset of the present problem
- Complete description of the first symptoms. The question "When did you last feel well?" may help define the time of onset and provide a date on which it was necessary to stop work or school, miss a planned event, or be confined to bed.
- Possible exposure to infection or toxic agents

CLINICAL PEARL

Chief Complaint

Many health professionals prefer to express the "chief complaint" differently, adopting "presenting problem" or "reason for seeking care" as more appropriate terms. Here again, we reject rigidity and suggest that you develop the style that suits you best.

MNEMONICS

How to Characterize Symptoms (e.g., Pain)
PQRST

Precipitating/palliating factors
Quality
Radiation
Severity
Temporal factors

Or, a similar approach:
OLD CARTS

Onset
Location
Duration
Character
Aggravating/associated factors
Relieving factors
Temporal factors
Severity

BOX 1-7

THE BASIS OF UNDERSTANDING

The following are vital questions you must ask yourself that underlie all of your effort to understand a patient:

- Why is this happening in the life of this particular person at this time?
- How is this patient different from all other patients?
- Can I assume that what is generally true for others is necessarily true for this patient?
- How does this bear on my ultimate interpretation of possible problems and solutions?

The unique contribution of the individual must inform your thinking.

BOX 1-8

A REVIEW: GUIDELINES FOR HISTORY TAKING AT THE START, THROUGHOUT, AND AT THE FINISH

- Be courteous. Knock before entering the room. Address the patient formally as Mr., Ms., Miss, or Mrs. Pleasant inquiry about aspects of the patient's life is permissible.
- If the patient is accompanied by a spouse, parent, caretaker, or friend, acknowledge that person, indicating that it is appropriate for the other person to remain in the room and, in time, to participate and to express their views. If there is disagreement among them, encourage them to talk about it with each other but avoid taking sides. They are probable partners in care and your approach should suggest your interest in everyone.
- Ensure everyone's physical comfort including your own. You should be sitting, not standing with one foot in the direction of the door. Try to have as little furniture as possible between you and the patient.
- Look at the patient. Good eye contact facilitates discussion if cultural practices allow.
- Provide good lighting.
- Maintain privacy, using available curtains and shades.
- Provide necessary quiet. Turn off the television set. It is distracting to speak with a patient whose eyes are darting to the television.
- Do not overtire the patient. Come back later to finish the history if possible. During an office or clinic visit, let the circumstance guide the length of the initial interview; it may be appropriate to schedule another appointment to complete the process.
- Always give the patient a chance to say what is the primary concern if several issues are raised.
- Do not dominate the discussion. Listen alertly. Do not let a charged, meaningful word escape your attention.
- Always assure confidentiality and reiterate the assurance whenever appropriate.
- Do not accept a previous diagnosis as the chief complaint. Find out what motivated the patient to seek care if you are not the first person to be involved in his or her treatment. Do not rely on an earlier diagnosis as a firm indicator. Concentrate on what the patient says and not on a diagnosis that may too early lead you down a predetermined and inappropriate path.
- Take the history and do the physical examination before you look at x-ray films, laboratory results, or other studies provided by other professionals. Consider first what the patient has to say.
- Open-ended questions are necessary, particularly at the start of an interview. They often help get conversation moving and guide you in the direction of the more specific and precise. Direct approaches should usually come after the general.
- Avoid being judgmental. You are not a preacher. But an occasional compliment to support a positively expressed feeling will not be amiss.
- Avoid leading questions. They may prompt an answer the patient might think you want to hear.
- Arrive at a conclusion about the patient's ability to be perceptive and articulate.
- Particularly early in an interview, offer thoughtful, respectful silence with gentle encouragement to talk, and listen with obvious interest. Pauses are often productive.
- Be flexible. Be ready to adapt to the unexpected. Rigidity seriously limits the potential of the interview.

- Develop your perception of the patient, never forgetting that you contribute by your responses and demeanor to what you are hearing and seeing as you and the patient continually adjust to each of your contributions.
- If the patient is very talkative or too silent, offer gentle prompts. These verbal behaviors often suggest emotional need. Sharpen the skill it takes to constrain a flood of information that may not be useful at the moment and to define relevance.
- Symptoms can have multiple causes; do not hone in on one possible cause too quickly.
- A chief complaint or a report of a symptom of any kind very often carries with it a hidden concern. Look for underlying and unstated worries. Never trivialize any finding or concern.
- Define any symptom, concern, or finding by as many of the following dimensions as are appropriate: Where is it? What is it like? How bad is it? How long ago was it noted? Does it come and go? In what situation does it happen? Does anything make it better or make it worse? What else happens along with it?
- Watch your language. Avoid jargon, medical terminology, convoluted sentences, and double negatives. Be specific but not patronizingly simplistic. Accurate, understandable information is the goal and your words should not be intimidating or demeaning.
- Avoid asking direct questions that suggest only a "yes" or "no" answer. It helps to maintain eye contact, occasionally nod your head, and simply say "Go on" or "Let me hear more." The patient will often then continue to talk and give a more complete answer.
- Make notes sparingly; jot down key words to help you record the history later, but do not be so intent on note taking that it distracts the patient or interferes with listening and observing.
- Allow the patient the time to be dressed and comfortably settled after the examination. Follow-up discussion with the patient still "on the table" indicates a lack of regard and is often thought to be—and often is—demeaning.
- If you don't know the answer to a question, say so. Then, find out and be sure to get back with the answer.
- If you seem to have made a mistake, admit it and try to repair it.
- The end of an interview can reveal a lot. It should include a summary of what has been discussed, an opportunity for review and elaboration, and an indication of what is to happen next so that the patient clearly understands. The patient, of course, should have the opportunity to express uncertainty and a possible feeling that expectations for the visit have not been met. You allow this by asking a question, "Is there anything else you need to ask about or you want to bring up?" Such an open-ended question voiced with concern can make it easier for the patient to be candid. This takes time, but it may provide clues to previously uncovered resources, and provide better understanding, management, and solutions. Such insights will help your decision making during later meetings, and the patient will be more satisfied.

BOX 1-9

FACTORS THAT AFFECT THE PATIENT'S PERCEPTION OF ILLNESS

An infinite number of variables may convert disease into illness or may cause illness without disease:

- Recent termination of a significant relationship because of death, divorce, or other less obvious intrusions such as moving to a new city
- Physical or emotional illness or disability in family members or other significant individuals
- Inharmonious spousal or family relationships
- School problems and stresses
- Poor self-image
- Drug and alcohol misuse
- Poor understanding of the facts of a physical problem

- Peer pressure (among adults as well as adolescents and children)
- Secondary gains from the complaints of symptoms (e.g., indulgent family response to complaints, providing extra comforts or gifts, solicitous attention from others, distraction from other intimidating problems)

At any age, such circumstances can influence perceptions and contribute to the intensity and persistence of symptoms or, quite the opposite, the denial of an insistent, objective complaint. The patient may then be led to seek help and, at other times, to avoid it.

Modified from Green & Stuy, 1992.

CLINICAL PEARL

Ethnicity

Some conditions are seen more often in certain ethnic groups (e.g., thalassemia in those from the Mediterranean, Tay-Sachs disease in Ashkenazi Jews, and sickle cell disease in blacks). On the other hand, other conditions are not often found in some groups, such as cystic fibrosis in blacks.

Many Jewish people do not know if they are Ashkenazi or Sephardic. They may not even have heard the terms. Ask when their parents, grandparents, or remote ancestors emigrated. If it was in the seventeenth or eighteenth century, the patient is probably Sephardic; if it was in the late nineteenth or twentieth century, the patient is probably Ashkenazi.

- Description of a typical attack. If the present problem involves intermittent attacks separated by an illness-free interval, ask the patient to describe a typical attack (e.g., onset, duration, and associated symptoms, such as pain, chills, fever, jaundice, hematuria, or seizures) and any variations, and to define inciting, exacerbating, or relieving factors such as specific activities, positions, diet, or medications.
- Impact of the illness on the patient's usual lifestyle (e.g., marriage, leisure activity, ability to perform tasks or cope with stress); an assessment of the ability to function in the expected way with an indication of the limitations imposed by illness
- Stability of the problem. Does its intensity vary? Is it getting better, getting worse, or staying the same?
- Immediate reason that prompted the seeking of attention, particularly if the problem has been long-standing
- Compulsive appropriate system review when there is a conspicuous disturbance of a particular organ or system
- Medications: current and recent, including dosage of prescription and home remedies and nonprescription medications
- Use of complementary or alternative therapies and medications
- A review, at the end of the interview, of the chronology of events, seeking the patient's confirmations and corrections. (If there appears to be more than one problem, the process should be repeated for each problem.)
- A summary of problems. In the written history, it is helpful to give a specific number and brief title to each problem and, in a summary, to list the problems in the order of apparent importance (always remember that this can change).

Past Medical History (PMH). The past medical history can be of great value in assessing the present complaint.

- General health and strength
- Childhood illnesses: measles, mumps, whooping cough, chickenpox, smallpox, scarlet fever, acute rheumatic fever, diphtheria, poliomyelitis
- Major adult illnesses: tuberculosis, hepatitis, diabetes, hypertension, myocardial infarction, tropical or parasitic diseases, other infections; any nonsurgical hospital admissions
- Immunizations: polio; diphtheria, pertussis, and tetanus toxoid; influenza; cholera; typhus; typhoid; hepatitis B; pneumococcus; meningococcus; bacille Calmette-Guérin (BCG); last PPD or other skin tests; unusual reactions to immunizations; tetanus or other antitoxin made with horse serum
- Surgery: dates, hospital, diagnosis, complications

CLINICAL PEARL

Family History

The Department of Health and Human Services has designated November 25 as National Family History Day and, in order to emphasize the continuing importance of the family history despite considerable genomic advance, it has set up a Web-based tool (http://www.hhs.gov/familyhistory) to allow individuals to explore for themselves their family histories. This may well be helpful to you. Its potential benefit should be explored.

Data from Guttmacher et al, 2004.

CLINICAL PEARL

Who Am I?

We cannot assume how patients define themselves in terms of their ethnic and cultural background without asking them. Current stereotypes cannot be imposed. Hispanic, "non-Hispanic," "black," "white," and "Latino" among many other designations are subject to a variety of interpretations. The individual patient is the final judge for that person. There is no reason to avoid the subject. Just ask "How do you see yourself?" "How do you define yourself?" "What do you tell others you are?"

- Serious injuries and resulting disability, giving full documentation if the present problem has potential medicolegal relation to an injury
- Limitation of ability to function as desired as a result of past events
- Medications: past, current, and recent medications, including dosage of prescription and home remedies and nonprescription medications (when not mentioned in present problem)
- Allergies, especially to medications, but also to environmental allergens and foods
- Transfusions: reactions, date, and number of units transfused
- Recent screening tests (e.g., cholesterol, Pap smear, prostate specific antigen [PSA], mammogram)
- Emotional status: mood disorders, psychiatric attention

Family History (FH). Ask if there are any blood relatives in the patient's immediate or extended family who have illnesses with features similar to the patient's illness (Box 1-10). Determine the ethnicity, health, and, if applicable, the cause of death of parents and siblings, including their ages at death. Establish whether there is a history of heart disease, high blood pressure, cancer, tuberculosis, stroke, epilepsy, diabetes, gout, kidney disease, thyroid disease, asthma or other allergic state, forms of arthritis, blood diseases, sexually transmitted infections, or any other familial disease. Determine the age and health of the patient's spouse and children.

If there is a hereditary disease—one that "runs in the family," such as sickle cell disease—inquire into the history of the grandparents, aunts, uncles, siblings, and cousins. It pays to review at least two generations on each side of the patient's family and to probe for consanguinity. A pedigree diagram is often helpful in recording this information (Fig. 1-5).

Personal and Social History (SH)
- Personal status: birthplace, where raised, home environment as youth (e.g., parental divorce or separation, socioeconomic class, cultural and ethnic background), education, position in family, marital status, general life satisfaction, hobbies and interests, sources of stress or strain
- Habits: nutrition and diet; regularity and patterns of eating and sleeping; exercise (e.g., quantity and type); quantity of coffee, tea, tobacco, alcohol; use of club or recreational drugs (e.g., frequency, type, and amount); breast or testicular self-examination; use of home, herbal, natural, complementary, or alternative remedies. (The extent of cigarette use can be reported in "pack-years," that is, the number of packs a day times the number of years, e.g., 1.5 packs per day $\times$ 10 years = 15 pack-years.)

BOX I-10

THE FAMILY HISTORY AND GENETIC TESTING

We are reminded by Eugene Rich and his colleagues of the central importance of the family history when genetic testing is thought necessary. There are more than 500 genetic tests currently available and hundreds more on the way. The family history must be exquisitely well taken if our patients are to make proper use of this burgeoning resource. The risks in inappropriate testing include needless anxiety that can at times be overwhelming, the making of perhaps unwarranted decisions that can affect family relationships, lifestyle choice, and reproductive behavior and incur unnecessary cost.

The making of a pedigree diagram, a genogram, is a central need in a family history. The construction of a pedigree diagram involves the use of certain symbols (see Fig. 1-5). It should include three generations if the patient is to get sound advice but it takes an amount of time that current practice styles and reimbursement resources generally do not allow. We must take note of this problem. It will soon escalate. The community will have to decide if inappropriate testing warrants the risks. Health providers must, in the meantime, be aware and strive to do as well as possible, taking great care with the family history and the recommendation of genetic testing.

Rich et al, 2004.

KEY TO THE
PEDIGREE:

☐ Male

○ Female

⬛ } Individual with
⬤ } the particular
    problem

✔ The patient

ADDITIONAL SYMBOLS USED
IN CONSTRUCTION:

◇ Ambiguous or unknown gender

╱ Slash through the symbol: deceased

◇ Pregnancy

⊙ Stillbirth

} Identical twins

} Fraternal twins

☐┅○ Consanguineous union

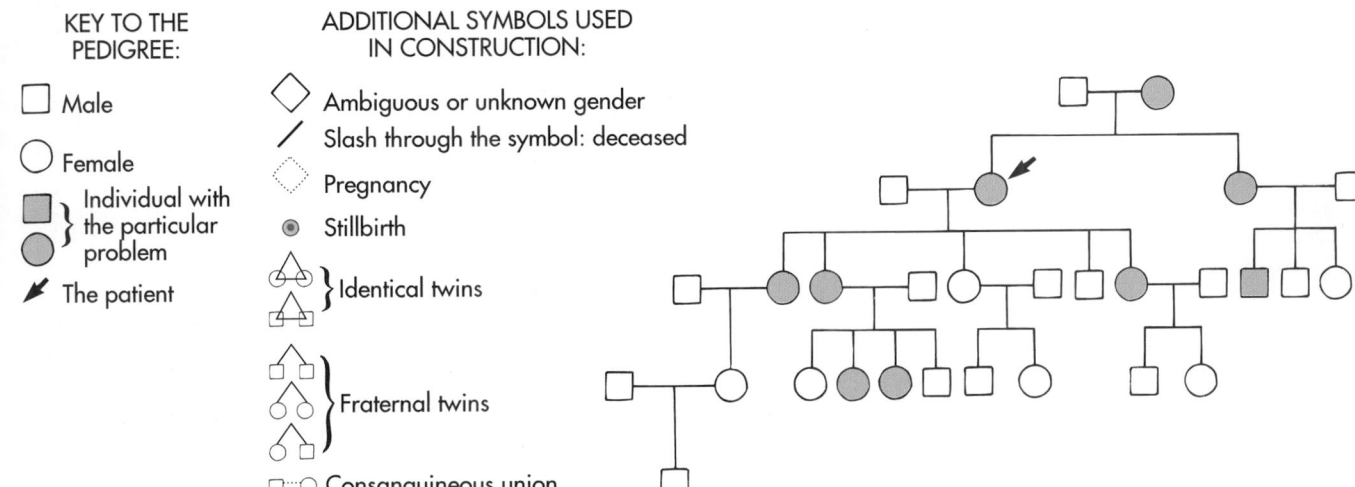

FIGURE 1-5
An example of a pedigree diagram, this one of a patient with Marfan syndrome, an autosomal (non–sex-linked), dominant, single gene disorder characterized by arachnodactyly, subluxation of the lens, and aortic aneurysm. In this pedigree, the mother had Marfan syndrome and passed it on to her daughters. Because it is not sex-linked and is dominant, we find an affected male in a succeeding generation and inheritance based on the gene contributed by only one parent.

- Sexual history: concerns with sexual feelings and performance, frequency of intercourse, ability to achieve orgasm, number and variety of partners. (It is useful to use the term partner, which does not indicate gender, during the early stages of discussion.)
- Home conditions: housing, economic condition, types of furnishings (e.g., carpeting and drapes), pets and their health
- Occupation: description of usual work (and present work if different); list of job changes; work conditions and hours; physical or mental strain; duration of employment; present and past exposure to heat and cold or industrial toxins (especially lead, arsenic, chromium, asbestos, beryllium, poisonous gases, benzene, and polyvinyl chloride or other carcinogens and teratogens); any protective devices required (e.g., goggles or masks)
- Environment: travel and other exposure to contagious diseases, residence in tropics, water and milk supply, other sources of infection if applicable
- Military record: dates and geographic area of assignments
- Religious preference: any religious proscriptions concerning medical care; spiritual needs
- Cultural requirements, possible proscriptions
- Cost of care: resources available to patient, type of health insurance (if any), worries in this regard, candid discussion of issues

Review of Systems (ROS). It is unlikely that all of the questions in each system will be asked each time you take a history. Nevertheless, there are some that generally should be, particularly at the first interview. These are suggested in the outline that follows. More comprehensive questions for particular circumstances in each system are detailed in subsequent chapters.

- General constitutional symptoms: fever, chills, malaise, fatigability, night sweats, sleep patterns, weight (i.e., average, preferred, present, change)
- Skin, hair, and nails: rash or eruption, itching, pigmentation or texture change; excessive sweating, abnormal nail or hair growth
- Head and neck:
  General: frequent or unusual headaches, their location; dizziness, syncope, severe head injuries; periods of loss of consciousness (momentary or prolonged)

Eyes: visual acuity, blurring, diplopia, photophobia, pain, recent change in appearance or vision; glaucoma; use of eye drops or other eye medications; history of trauma or familial eye disease

Ears: hearing loss, pain, discharge, tinnitus, vertigo

Nose: sense of smell, frequency of colds, obstruction, epistaxis, postnasal discharge, sinus pain

Throat and mouth: hoarseness or change in voice; frequent sore throats; bleeding or swelling of gums; recent tooth abscesses or extractions; soreness of tongue or buccal mucosa; ulcers; disturbance of taste

- Lymph nodes: enlargement, tenderness, suppuration
- Chest and lungs: pain related to respiration, dyspnea, cyanosis, wheezing, cough, sputum (character and quantity), hemoptysis, night sweats, exposure to tuberculosis; date and result of last chest x-ray examination
- Breasts: development, pain, tenderness, discharge, lumps, galactorrhea, mammograms (screening or diagnostic), frequency of breast self-examination
- Heart and blood vessels: chest pain or distress, precipitating causes, timing and duration, relieving factors, palpitations, dyspnea, orthopnea (number of pillows needed), edema, hypertension, previous myocardial infarction, estimate of exercise tolerance, past electrocardiogram or other cardiac tests
- Peripheral vasculature: claudication (frequency, severity), tendency to bruise or bleed, thromboses, thrombophlebitis
- Hematologic: anemia, any known abnormality of blood cells, transfusions
- Gastrointestinal: appetite, digestion, intolerance for any class of foods, dysphagia, heartburn, nausea, vomiting, hematemesis; regularity of bowels, constipation, diarrhea, change in stool color or contents (e.g., clay-colored, tarry, fresh blood, mucus, undigested food); flatulence, hemorrhoids; hepatitis, jaundice, dark urine; history of ulcer, gallstones, polyps, tumor; previous x-ray examinations (where, when, findings)
- Diet: appetite, likes and dislikes, restrictions (e.g., because of religion, allergy, or other disease), vitamins and other supplements, use of caffeine-containing beverages (e.g., coffee, tea, and cola); an hour-by-hour detailing of food and liquid intake (sometimes a written diary covering several days of intake may be necessary)
- Endocrine: thyroid enlargement or tenderness, heat or cold intolerance, unexplained weight change, diabetes, polydipsia, polyuria, distribution and changes in facial or body hair, increased hat and glove size, skin striae
- Females

  Menses: onset, regularity, duration and amount of flow, dysmenorrhea, last period (LMP), intermenstrual discharge or bleeding, itching, date of last Pap smear, age at menopause, libido, frequency of intercourse, pain during intercourse, sexual difficulties, infertility

  Pregnancies: number, living children, multiple births, miscarriages, abortions, duration of pregnancy, each type of delivery, any complications during any pregnancy or postpartum period or with neonate; use of oral or other contraceptives; difficulty in getting pregnant
- Males: puberty onset, difficulty with erections, emissions, testicular pain, libido, infertility
- Genitourinary: dysuria, flank or suprapubic pain, urgency, frequency, nocturia, hematuria, polyuria, hesitancy, dribbling, loss in force of stream, passage of stone; edema of face, stress incontinence, hernias, sexually transmitted infection (inquire what type and symptoms, and list results of serologic test for syphilis [STS] if known)
- Musculoskeletal: joint stiffness, pain, restriction of motion, swelling, redness, heat, bony deformity
- Neurologic: syncope, seizures, weakness or paralysis, abnormalities of sensation or coordination, tremors, loss of memory
- Psychiatric: depression, mood changes, difficulty concentrating, nervousness, tension, suicidal thoughts, irritability, sleep disturbances

Concluding Questions. At the conclusion of obtaining the history, ask the patient "Is there anything else that you think would be important for me to know?" If several complaints are mentioned and discussed in the history, it is often useful to ask "What problem concerns you most?" In certain situations, such as vague, complicated, or contradictory histories, it may be helpful to ask "What do you think is the matter with you?" or "What worries you the most about how you are feeling?"

INFANTS AND CHILDREN

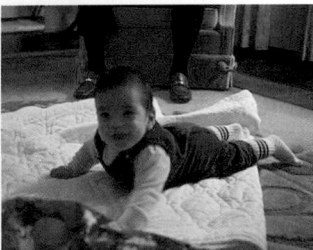

The history for an infant or child is modified according to age. The following is, again, simply a suggested outline.

Chief Complaint. The history may be taken from a parent or other responsible adult (Box 1-11). However, the child should be included as much as is possible and appropriate for his or her age. The latent fears underlying any chief complaint of both parents and children should also be explored. Note the relationship of the person providing the history for the child.

History of Present Illness. The degree and character of the reaction to the problem on the part of parent and child should be noted.

Past Medical History. ◆ General health and strength: Depending on the age of the patient or the nature of the problem, different aspects of the history assume or lose importance. Reserve detailed questioning for those aspects most pertinent to the age of the child.

◆ Mother's health during pregnancy
  ◆ General health as related by the mother if possible, extent of prenatal care
  ◆ Specific diseases or conditions: infectious disease (approximate gestational month), weight gain, edema, hypertension, proteinuria, bleeding (approximate gestational month), preeclampsia

---

BOX 1-11

CONSENT BY PROXY

Infants, children and many adolescents are minors. They may come to you for care accompanied by someone other than their custodial parent or guardian, often a grandparent or other members of their extended family. Sometimes, your informant might be an au pair or nanny or, in the event of divorce and remarriage, a noncustodial parent or stepparent. Does that person have the right to consent to your care for the child? You do need to know. We cannot offer general guidelines for making this judgment because the rules for consent by proxy are not consistent from state to state. A recent good source will help, a clinical report from the American Academy of Pediatrics:

Modified from Berger, The Committee on Medical Liability, 2003.

CLINICAL PEARL

Twins or More
You may have as patients twins, triplets, or more! Each is an individual entitled to separate consideration and a separate record even if they are presumably identical. When they are adolescents—really, always—assure each their own time with you and their confidentiality.

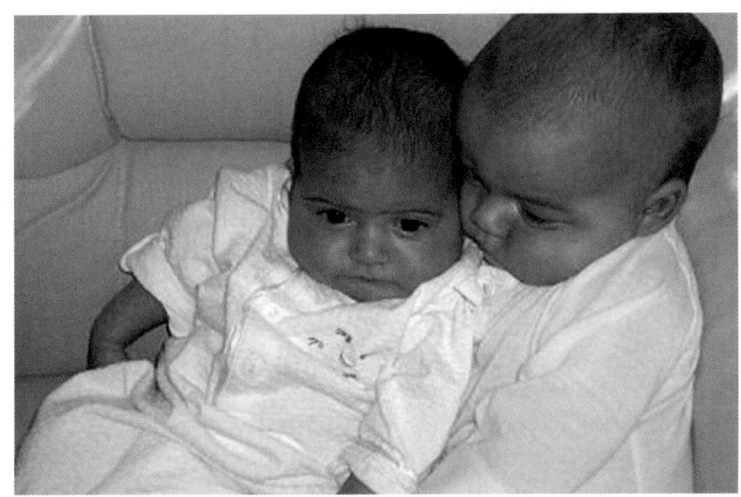

- Medications, hormones, vitamins, special or unusual diet, general nutritional status
  - Quality of fetal movements and time of onset
  - Emotional and behavioral status (e.g., attitudes toward pregnancy and children)
  - Radiation exposure
  - Use of illicit drugs
- Birth
  - Duration of pregnancy
  - Place of delivery
  - Labor: spontaneous or induced, duration, analgesia or anesthesia, complications
  - Delivery: presentation, forceps, vacuum extraction, spontaneous, or cesarean section; complications
  - Condition of infant, time of onset of cry, Apgar scores if available
  - Birth weight of infant
- Neonatal period
  - Congenital anomalies; baby's condition in hospital, oxygen requirements, color, feeding characteristics, vigor, cry; duration of baby's stay in hospital and whether infant was discharged with mother; bilirubin phototherapy, prescriptions (e.g., antibiotics)
  - First month of life: jaundice, color, vigor of crying, bleeding, convulsions, or other evidence of illness
  - Degree of early bonding: opportunities at birth and during the first days of life for the parents to hold, talk to, and caress the infant (i.e., opportunities for both parents to relate to and develop a bond with the baby).
- Feeding
  - Bottle or breast, reason for changes, if any; type of formula used, amounts offered and consumed; frequency of feeding and weight gain
  - Present diet and appetite; age of introduction of solids; age when child achieved three feedings per day; present feeding patterns, with elaboration of any feeding problems; age weaned from bottle or breast; type of milk and daily intake; food preference; ability to feed self; cultural variations
- Development: These are commonly used developmental milestones. The list should be enlarged when indicated. Parents may have baby books, which can stimulate recall, or photographs may be helpful.
  - Age when able to do the following:
    Hold head erect while in sitting position
    Roll over from front to back and back to front
    Sit alone and unsupported
    Stand with support and alone
    Walk with support and alone
    Use words
    Talk in sentences
    Dress self
  - Age when toilet trained: approaches to and attitudes regarding toilet training
  - School: grade, performance, problems
  - Dentition: age of first teeth, loss of deciduous teeth, eruption of first permanent teeth
  - Growth: height and weight in a sequence of ages; changes in rates of growth or weight gain
  - Sexual: present status. In females, development of breasts, nipples, sexual hair, menstruation (description of menses), acne; in males, development of sexual hair, voice changes, acne, nocturnal emissions
- Illnesses: immunizations, communicable diseases, injuries, hospitalizations

Family History. Obtain a maternal gestational history, listing all pregnancies together with the health status of living children. For deceased children, include date, age, cause of death, and dates and duration of pregnancies in the case of miscarriages. Inquire about the mother's health during pregnancies and the ages of parents at the birth of this child. Are the parents cousins or otherwise related? A review of at least two generations on each side of the family is desirable.

CLINICAL PEARL

Putting Prevention into Practice

Advice should often be given along with the questioning. For example, infants should sleep supine to avoid sudden infant death syndrome. And, 90% of the time, child safety seats are used incorrectly when they are used. They should be used and correct use should be discussed.

Personal and Social History

- Personal status: school adjustment, masturbation, nail biting, thumb sucking, breath holding, temper tantrums, pica, tics, rituals; bed wetting, constipation or fecal soiling of pants; playing with fire; reactions to prior illnesses, injuries, or hospitalization. An account of a day in the life of the patient (from parent, child, or both) is often helpful in providing insights. Box 1-12 emphasizes the particular needs of children who are adopted or in foster care.
- Home conditions: father's and mother's occupations, the principal caretakers of child, parents divorced or separated, educational attainment of parents; spiritual orientation; cultural heritage; food preparation and by whom; adequacy of clothing; dependence on relief or social agency; number of rooms in house and number of persons in household; sleep habits, sleeping arrangements available for the child

Review of Systems. In addition to the usual concerns, inquire about any past medical or psychologic testing of the child (Box 1-13). Ask about the following:

- Skin: eczema, seborrhea, "cradle cap"
- Ears: otitis media (frequency, laterality)
- Nose: snoring, mouth breathing, allergic reaction
- Teeth: dental care

BOX 1-12

ADOPTION AND FOSTER CARE

Patients who are adopted or in foster care may not have a sufficient history available for you. Do not hesitate to ask if that information is not immediately forthcoming. The outline of questions we suggest for history taking, however, is still appropriate but should be enhanced by an exploration of the circumstances that have led to adoption or foster care. Do this with care. Some adoptive parents may not yet have shared the knowledge with their children. The trials of the adoptive parents as they sought a child, the process of adoption, the country of origin of the adoptee, and the particular concerns of all involved must be understood.

The needs of foster children vary considerably from those who are adopted. The history may be offered by a social worker, and the issues you encounter may differ in variety and intensity. Foster parents have varying experience, and foster children have often lived in more than one home. Invariably, difficult social circumstances underlie the separation from their parents. The probable lack of stability and security and incomplete knowledge of past illnesses or other conditions make it more difficult to achieve understanding of the full range of the child's needs.

BOX 1-13

A CHILD WHO WITNESSES VIOLENCE OR SERIOUS INJURY TO OTHERS, OR WHO HAS SURVIVED SERIOUS INJURY TO SELF

Witnessing or actually experiencing violence or injury is a fact of life for many children and is a barrier to the smooth evolution of growth and development. Do not avoid talking about it.

Questions should be straightforward, simple, and direct:
- Can you tell me what happened?
- What did you see? What did you hear?
- What scared you the most?
- What were you doing when it happened?
- Do you ever dream about it?
- Do you think about it during the day?
- Do you worry it will happen again?

- Whom do you talk to when you feel worried or scared?
- Why do you think it happened?

For the older child and adolescent:
- How do you think it changed your life?

These questions are not value-laden and are not too constraining. The child is free to talk if you can be comfortable with the silences that may often follow your questions. Parents can also respond to the same questions to fill out the story, and you can then learn how they dealt with the circumstance and what impact they observed on their child's behavior.

Modified from Augustyn et al, 1995.

THE HISTORY AND INTERVIEWING PROCESS

ADOLESCENTS

Adolescence occupies the second decade of life. In *early adolescence,* the body is beginning to change and a degree of independence from parents develops. The peer group and the desire to be like peers becomes important. In a very few years, *middle adolescence,* the peer group takes on a dominant role. Experimentation with risky behaviors begins and frequent arguments with parents are common. This is a time when immature decision making can lead to destructive, life-changing experiences and bad lifelong habits. Later in the decade, *late adolescence,* adult maturity is approached as a more sober consideration of consequences takes hold along with a more secure sense of self, an ability to establish intimate relationships, and to plan a career.

Essentially, the eternal questions—"Who am I?" and "Where am I going?"—are at the heart of the teenage experience. The problem may be illustrated in the example of a youngster who is deciding to smoke. What are the risk factors (Bradford, 1992)?

- Close associations with friends who smoke
- Less attachment to parents
- Poor school performance
- Lack of involvement in school extracurricular activities
- Poor self-esteem
- Need to appear mature, leading to apparent rebelliousness
- Tendency of risk-related, often antisocial behavior to be clustered (e.g., tobacco, alcohol, and sex)
- Peer pressure
- Susceptibility to advertising
- Skewed knowledge, attitudes, and beliefs about smoking

The suggested issues, including self-esteem, acceptance by peers, tensions with parents, and inadequate base of knowledge, can make it very difficult to bridge the barriers created by age differences. Those of you who are not too far removed from that somewhat hazardous time should be aware that you are no longer of that culture. Make generous use of open-ended questions, and do not force an adolescent to talk. Sometimes allowing an opportunity to write a concern or allowing a choice of concerns presented in written, silent fashion may help. For example, a deck of index cards labeled with topics may be offered with the suggestion to select the ones to consider. The following subjects may be included (Green, 1992: adapted from a form used at Stanford Youth Clinic):

- Bed wetting
- Menstrual pain
- Concern with height or weight: too short, too tall, too thin, too fat
- Concern with breast size: too big, too small
- Concern with penis size: too small
- Worry about pregnancy
- Worry about sexual preference
- Sex? Ready or not?
- AIDS
- Parents' attitudes and demands
- Friends and their pressures
- School: not doing well, excessive work
- What am I going to do in life?
- Thoughts about dying

These are highly charged issues requiring sensitivity in discussion, knowledge of the language of the adolescent, and an unforced approach if trust is to be established (Box 1-14). This may not happen at the first meeting. Your consistent availability for talks will be helpful. In time, you may find that the patient, particularly an adolescent woman (but a man, too), would prefer someone of the same gender.

Flexibility, respect, and confidentiality are key. The adolescent must be aware that the respect is there and that confidentiality is appropriately ensured; otherwise, little productive discussion will result.

MNEMONICS

Issues for Adolescents
HEEADSSS

Home environment
Education, employment
Eating
Activities (peer-related), affect, ambitions, anger
Drugs
Sexuality
Suicide/depression
Safety from injury and violence

PACES

Parents, peers
Accidents, alcohol/drugs
Cigarettes
Emotional issues
School, sexuality

NOTE: HEEADSSS and PACES are screening tools and are not substitutes for earnest conversation in a trusting relationship.

From Goldenring & Rosen 2004; DiFrancesco, 1992.

BOX 1-14

THE NEED FOR CONFIDENTIALITY

To The Editor: I am writing to express concern about what I understand to be a standard practice of physicians in dealing with minors. Recently, I was admitted to the hospital for surgery. Before my operation, my anesthesiologist met with me (16 years old) and my parents to review the procedure. At that time, I was asked if I used recreational drugs, smoked, or drank alcohol. Fortunately, my answers put my parents and my doctor at ease.

This apparent formality could prove to be very dangerous if an adolescent who takes drugs, drinks, or smokes is unable to be frank with the doctor while the parents are listening. Kids have the same right of patient confidentiality as adults. I suggest that doctors review their practices so that minors can speak with them privately, to ensure that appropriate safety precautions can be taken during surgery.

From Levin, 1990.

The following sequence suggests the structure of exploratory interviews with adolescents:

- "How are things going at home?" "Tell me about your living situation." Do not assume the traditional family structure. Do not ask directly about who else lives in the house. The open-ended question at the start can lead to greater specifics later on.
- "How is school going?" "Are you working?" "What is it about school that appeals to you?" "What is it about school that doesn't appeal to you?" You may expect to hear somewhat more about jobs outside of school and ideas about the future when the patient approaches the age of 20 years.
- "Tell me about your friends." "Where do you go with them?" "What do you do with them?"

These beginning conversations about home and school and jobs and friends can lead to the many difficult areas that may trouble the adolescent (e.g., sex, drugs, and suicidal ideation). The open-ended question is a prelude to the more complex issues of an age in which talk does not always flow easily as the adolescent moves from dependency to independency, from parents to peer group, and ultimately to self. The process of separation leads to maturity.

PREGNANT WOMEN

An individualized approach is needed in obtaining information appropriate to the age and concerns of the pregnant patient. For example, the very young adolescent may be concerned with the changes that pregnancy will bring to her body and friendships, whereas the older woman may be concerned about the genetic risks of the pregnancy. However, remember that for most women, pregnancy is an expected physiologic event.

Because pregnancy is a "normal" occurrence, the usual format of the clinical history is modified. Many health care providers and institutions use preprinted history forms (e.g., The American College of Obstetricians and Gynecologists Antepartum Record) on which to record information about the current pregnancy and past pregnancies; medical, contraceptive, family, and psychosocial histories; plans for childbirth; and risk factors for the development of complications.

If no standardized history forms are available, the clinical history format can be used.

Chief Complaint. The following information is included:

- Patient's age, ethnicity
- Marital status, partner, or relationship
- Gravidity and parity (Fig. 1-6)
- Last menstrual period (LMP)
- Previous usual/normal menstrual period (PUMP or PNMP)
- Expected date of confinement/delivery (EDC)
- Occupation
- Father of the baby and his occupation

Gravidity and parity	G	T	P	A	L
	# of Pregnancies	# of Term Pregnancies	# of Preterm Pregnancies	# of Abortions/ Miscarriages	# of Living Children

FIGURE 1-6
Gravidity and parity information.

History of Present Illness or Problem. A description of the current pregnancy is obtained, and previous medical care is identified. Attention is given to specific problems (e.g., bleeding or spotting, nausea, vomiting, fatigue, or edema). Include information about illness, injuries, surgeries, or accidents since conception.

Obstetric History. Information on each previous pregnancy includes the date of delivery; length of pregnancy; weight and gender of infant(s); type of delivery (e.g., spontaneous vaginal; cesarean section and type of scar [an evaluation of the competency of the scar is needed for women attempting vaginal birth after cesarean section; the risks and benefits of vaginal birth after cesarean section and repeat cesarean section should be discussed with the patient and documented]; or spontaneous, therapeutic, or elective abortion and the type of procedure); length of labor; and complications in pregnancy or labor, postpartum, or with the infant (Fig. 1-7).

Menstrual History. In addition to previous information, include age at menarche, characteristics of the cycle, unusual bleeding, and associated symptoms. If known, include dates of ovulation and conception, and the use of contraceptives before or during conception.

Gynecologic History. The date of the most recent Pap smear should be ascertained along with any history of abnormalities, treatments, or gynecologic surgery. A sexual history includes age of first intercourse and whether it was consensual, number of sex partners, safe-sex methods, partner orientation and, if a minor, age of partner. Information regarding the types of contraceptives used and reason for discontinuing them with plans for use postpartum is obtained. Any history of infertility and diethylstilbestrol (DES) exposure should be explored. If there has been any occurrence of sexually transmitted infections, then type, dates, treatments, and complications should be discussed. A history of sexual assault should be addressed.

Date of delivery	*Weeks of gestation*	*Weight*	*Gender*	*Type of delivery*	*Length of labor*	*Anesthesia*	Complications	*Condition of infant*
10/05	40	7 6	F	SVD	12 hr	None	None	Good
8/03	36	5	M	LT CS	6 hr	Epidural	Fetal distress, preeclampsia	Infant discharged at 4 wks
6/98	8	—	—	SAB	—	IV	D&C	—

SVD, Spontaneous vaginal delivery; *LT*, low transverse; *CS*, cesarean section; *SAB*, spontaneous abortion; *D&C*, dilation and curettage.

FIGURE 1-7
An example of an obstetric history record.

Past Medical History. The same information identified previously is obtained, with the addition of risk factors for AIDS, hepatitis, tuberculosis, and exposure to environmental and occupational hazards. A mother who herself had intrauterine growth restriction (IUGR) carries this risk factor for her children (Klebanoff et al, 1997).

Family History. In addition to the information obtained previously, a family history of genetic conditions, multiple births, gestational diabetes, preeclampsia/eclampsia or pregnancy-induced hypertension (PIH), and/or congenital anomalies is obtained.

Personal and Social History. Additional information includes feelings toward the pregnancy, whether the pregnancy was planned, possible plans for adoption or abortion, preference for gender of child, social and spiritual supports available, experiences with mothering (of being both mothered and a mother), experience with and plans for labor and breastfeeding, and history of past or present abuse in relationships.

Review of Systems. The effects of pregnancy are seen in all systems; therefore all are reviewed, but special attention is given to the reproductive (including breasts) and cardiovascular systems (documentation of pre-pregnancy blood pressure if possible). The endocrine system is assessed for signs of diabetes and thyroid dysfunction. The urinary tract is assessed for infection, and kidney function is reviewed. Respiratory function is also assessed because it may be compromised later in pregnancy or with tocolytic therapy for preterm labor.

Risk Assessment. Risk assessment encompasses identifying from the history and physical examination those conditions that threaten the well-being of the mother and/or fetus. Various risk assessment categories exist for such conditions as diabetes, preterm labor, and preeclampsia/eclampsia, or PIH.

Postpartum. Postpartum depression occurs in about 1 of every 8 women after delivery. The clues are similar to depression in other circumstances, a sad mood, exceptional anxiety, a feeling of agitation, insomnia, loss of appetite, fatigue, feelings of worthlessness, inappropriate guilt, and suicidal ideation. A cluster of these symptoms should strongly suggest postpartum depression Wisner et al, 2002).

OLDER ADULTS

Older adults may present a challenge in organizing the information obtained from the history. They may have multiple health problems that can be chronic, progressive, and debilitating, and these may overlap with the process of aging. Disease symptoms may be less dramatic in older patients, with vague or nonspecific signs and symptoms. Confusion, for example, may be the only symptom of an infection, hypoxia, or a cerebrovascular accident. Pain is often an unreliable symptom because some older patients seem to lose pain perception and experience pain in a different manner from the classic expectations. The excruciating pain usually associated with pancreatitis, for example, may be perceived by the older patient as a dull ache, and myocardial infarction can occur without the cardinal symptom of pain. Conversely, older patients have a higher risk of developing painful conditions or injuries. Because many conditions may be present simultaneously, the cause of pain may be difficult to isolate.

Some patients may fail to report symptoms either because they expect the complaint to be attributed to old age or because they believe that nothing can be done. They may have lived with a chronic condition, such as urinary incontinence (now much more amenable to treatment than in the past), for so long that they have incorporated the symptoms as part of their expectation of daily living.

The treatment of multiple problems with multiple drugs places the older patient at increased risk for iatrogenic disorders. A complete medication history is essential, with special attention given to interactions of drugs, diseases, and the aging process. This is true for prescription drugs as well as for nonprescription drugs such as laxatives, nonsteroidal antiinflammatory agents, and drugs such as cough suppressants and hypnotics that have anticholinergic side effects. It is particularly helpful to have patients of all ages bring in medication bottles, especially those who have a variety of chronic conditions and a variety of care providers. Older adults and patients with complex medication needs should use a single pharmacy for all prescriptions so that the computer database available to the pharmacist can be queried to determine important, but often unrecognized drug-drug interactions.

Although appropriate at any age when there is apparent disability, the functional assessment outlined in the Functional Assessment box on p. 36 should be routinely included as part of the older patient's history (see Chapter 22 for additional information). These questions, which address functional capacity, should be included in the review of systems.

Other dimensions of functional capacity that should also be explored include social and spiritual resources, economic resources, recreational activity, sleep patterns, environmental control, and use of the health care system. The interrelationship of physical health, mental health, social situation, and the environment is particularly evident in the older population (Box 1-15).

In this regard, catastrophic illness is more likely to be a problem among older adults. For all ages, the prospect of an illness that deprives the patient of the ability to join in the decision-making process emphasizes the need for advance directives. This is a documentation in the medical record of the patient's wishes regarding extraordinary means of life support (e.g., ventilatory supports and feeding tubes). This documentation should be complemented by the appointment of a surrogate (e.g., spouse, child, sibling, or other person with a close relationship) who has a legally executed durable power of attorney for health care. These matters should be considered whenever possible before the onset of catastrophe.

The Frail. There are among the older adults and among the physically or cognitively impaired persons who might be particularly vulnerable and thought of as frail. *Frailty* has its onset with the loss of physical reserve and the increased risk of loss of physical function and independence. Fried and others (2001, 2002, 2004) have characterized it as a state in which muscle weakness, fatigue, a decline in activity, a slow or unsteady gait, and unintentional weight loss may occur and which exists if three or more of these findings are certain. One or two of these findings suggest an intermediate state and suggest the possibility of becoming frail within a few years. Another possible definition suggests that a patient is frail who needs help in two or more of the activities of daily living. Although frailty by either definition increases dramatically with increasing age, age and frailty are not necessarily synonymous. Frailty itself is considered by some to be a disease separate from comorbidity (the compromise imposed on a patient by having more than one chronic condition at a time) and disability (difficulty or dependency in doing what is needed to sustain daily living, the essential roles of self-care and, if necessary, living alone) (Box 1-16). It may well be that these three states may be better distinguished as we learn more. There is, however, quite certainly an interdependency. For our present purposes it is necessary to include the functional assessment as a matter of course in the older adult, the chronically ill, and the physically or emotionally disabled if the obvious problems are to be managed (see the Functional Assessment box on p. 36). (Fried et al, 2001; Fried et al, 2004; Kolata, 2002).

BOX 1-15

COMPETENCY

Adult patients and many youths have the right to decide the extent of care they will accept under your guidance. Many older adults and, given particular health problems, some younger folk, may have lost the ability to make relevant *competent* decisions. To be able to do so and to be able to give consent, they must be well informed about what is proposed, e.g., a procedure or medication, the risks, benefits and alternatives, and they must be able to do so voluntarily. *Competency* is difficult to define and there is not widespread agreement among health professionals. It has been suggested that the ability to handle one's affairs in an adequate manner may suffice for our purposes. The difficulty exacerbates because the capacity to be competent may fluctuate from hour to hour or day to day depending on the age of the patient and the superimposed physical and/or emotional problems. Many of us have found it necessary to seek consultative help in deciding a patient's status. Most often, the law in your state may require this and it may ultimately have to be left to a judge to decide on legal incompetency. *Caution: the patient who disagrees with you is not necessarily incompetent and the patient who agrees with you is not necessarily competent.*

Data from Janofsky et al, 1992.

FUNCTIONAL ASSESSMENT

FUNCTIONAL ASSESSMENT FOR ALL PATIENTS

Quite simply, functional assessment is a disciplined attempt to understand a patient's ability to achieve the basic activities of daily living. This assessment has been best studied and implemented among older adults. However, the same thought should be given to anyone limited not by age but in some way by disease or disability, acute or chronic. It is sometimes difficult to discover just what limits function. A well-taken history and a meticulous physical examination can bring out subtle influences, such as tobacco and alcohol use, sedentary habits, poor food selection, overuse of nonprescription or prescription drugs, and less than obvious emotional distress. Even some physical limitations may not be readily apparent (e.g., limitations of cognitive ability or of the senses).

Whether increasing age or some other factor is the contributor to limitation, your assessment of a patient's response to your questions should be tempered by the knowledge that patients tend to overstate their abilities and, quite often, to obscure reality. You must be cautious in making your judgments.

For the older adult, then, and for those limited by disease or other handicap, consider a variety of disabilities: physical, cognitive, psychologic, social, and sexual. An individual's social and spiritual support system must be as clearly understood as the physical disabilities.

There are a variety of physical disabilities, including the following:

- Mobility
    Difficulty walking standard distances: $\frac{1}{2}$ mile, 2 to 3 blocks, $\frac{1}{3}$ block, across a room
    Difficulty climbing stairs, up and down
    Problems with balance

Modified from Fried, 1992.

- Upper extremity function
    Difficulty grasping small objects, opening jars
    Difficulty reaching out or up overhead, such as to take something off a shelf
- Instrumental activities of daily living (IADLs)
- Housework
    Heavy (vacuuming, scrubbing floors)
    Light (dusting)
    Meal making
    Shopping
    Medication use
    Money management
- Activities of daily living
    Bathing
    Dressing
    Toileting
    Moving from bed to chair, chair to standing
    Eating
    Walking in home

Any limitations, even to a mild degree, in any of these areas will affect a patient's independence and autonomy and, to the extent of the limitation, increase reliance on other people and on assistive devices. These limitations indicate the loss of physical reserve and the potential loss of physical function and independence that indicate the onset of *frailty*. The patient's social support system and material resources are, then, integral to the development of reasonable management plans.

There are a variety of approaches to a finely tuned functional assessment with several available scales and instruments.

BOX 1-16

AT ANY AGE—THE NEED FOR PALLIATIVE CARE

Palliative care means the comprehensive management of the physical, psychologic, social and spiritual needs of patients with life-limiting conditions and their families and other persons significant in their lives. It includes pain control, psychosocial and spiritual support, advance care planning, and bereavement support, and it is intended to achieve the best possible quality of life at a time when life itself is threatened and grieving is perhaps inevitable. There are questions that need to be asked of yourself if you are to judge a patient's need in this regard:

- Does the patient have a life-threatening or life-limiting disease?
- Would you be surprised if the patient died in the next 6 to 12 months?
- Has the frequency of hospitalization increased in the past 6 to 12 months?
- Is the frequency of clinic visits increased because of the

course of the illness?
- Has there been a change or deterioration in the patient's pain intensity, energy, functional status, respiratory function, mental status, or quality of life?
- Has the patient or family voiced concerns about the treatment plan?
- Is there conflict among the family or health care team about the goals of care?

Positive answers to some or all of these questions suggest strongly that you consider the need for palliative care and take advantage of the resources in your setting that may facilitate it. The issues are comprehensive—physical, cultural, ethical, legal, spiritual, psychosocial—and indicate the need for advance planning and the anticipation of a grieving period.

Modified from a lecture and notes by Cynda Rushton and Nancy Hutton, The Johns Hopkins Hospital, March 31, 2004.

THE NEXT STEP

Once the history, in whatever form (Box 1-17), has been taken, it is necessary to move on to the physical examination, the laying on of hands, which is discussed in depth in subsequent chapters. These chapters are necessarily segmented and are not meant to reflect the natural flow that you will develop with experience. We bring it all together in the end and, by then, you will be ready to move on. Do not be intimidated by the realization that your patients expect you to be perfect always. Just be disciplined, alert, and recognize your own humanity.

BOX 1-17

TYPES OF HISTORIES

As your experience with interviewing increases, you will find that a "complete" history is not always necessary. One reason may be that you already know the patient very well or because you may be seeing the patient for the same problem over time. Therefore histories should be adjusted to the need at the moment. The following list explains different forms of histories:

- The complete history is designed to make you as thoroughly familiar with the patient as possible so that you and the patient can begin to seek solutions to problems and initiate the achievement of shared goals in care and prevention. Most often, this history is recorded the first time you see the patient.
- The inventory history is related to but does not replace the complete history. It touches on the major points without going into detail. This history is useful when it is necessary to get a "feel" for the situation, and the entire history taking will be completed in more than one session.
- The problem (or focused) history is taken when the problem is acute, possibly life threatening, requiring immediate attention so that only the need of the moment is given full attention.
- The interim history is designed to chronicle events that have occurred since your last meeting with the patient. The substance of this history is determined by the nature of the problem and the need of the moment. The interim history should always be complemented by the patient's previous record.

ELECTRONIC RESOURCES

For Weblinks and additional resources, go to **evolve**

http://evolve.elsevier.com/Seidel

or to the Companion CD-ROM.

CULTURAL AWARENESS

To be culturally aware is to understand those aspects of the human condition that differentiate individuals and groups and that these differences sometimes have an overpowering effect on their health and medical care. An understanding of a particular culture may often be useful in the solution of problems that may at first seem intractable. They certainly influence patients' decisions to avoid or to seek health care. Box 2-1 suggests ways of developing cultural competence with the caveat that the infinite variety of human experience may sometimes frustrate efforts at understanding. That should not be a barrier to your effort.

Mosby's Cultural Health Assessment, 3rd edition, edited by D'Avanzo and Geissler is a useful source of information about more than 170 cultural entities based on national groups.

CULTURAL COMPETENCE

It may push the envelope to conclude that we can understand persons from another culture with absolute empathy and without bias. We can, however, validate our efforts to do this by bringing to them a respectful curiosity, imagination, and the best possible insight into the self.

BOX 2-1

WAYS OF DEVELOPING CULTURAL COMPETENCE

- Recognize that cultural diversity exists.
- Demonstrate respect for people as unique individuals, with culture as one factor that contributes to their uniqueness.
- Respect the unfamiliar.
- Identify, examine and discipline your own attitudes, biases, and beliefs if you are to work successfully with others; the power we sometimes take for granted in the culture of the caring professions can be matched by that in other groups.
- Recognize that some cultural groups have definitions of health and illness, and practices that attempt to promote health and cure illness, that may differ from your own.
- Be willing to modify health care delivery in keeping with the patient's cultural background; it is better to *mediate* than to be *coercive*.
- Do not expect all members of one cultural group to behave in exactly the same way.
- Appreciate that each person's cultural values are ingrained and therefore very difficult to change.

Modified from Stulc, 1991.

Taken with a conscientious understanding of your patient's culture, these can ensure that we offer better care within differing value systems and act with respect and understanding without imposition of our own attitudes and beliefs. The ability to do this is defined by many as culture competence. This competence does not demean the "other" but allows a clear vision of differences and their value. There is in it esteem for the "other."

A DEFINITION OF CULTURE

Culture, in its broadest sense, reflects the whole of human behavior, including ideas and attitudes; ways of relating to one another; manners of speaking; and the material products of physical effort, ingenuity, and imagination. Language is a part of culture. So, too, are the abstract systems of belief, etiquette, law, morals, entertainment, and education. Within the cultural whole, different populations may exist in groups and subgroups. Each is identified in some way by a particular body of shared traits (e.g., a particular art, ethos, or belief; or a particular behavioral pattern) that is not at all static but rather dynamic in its evolving accommodations with internal and external influences.

Any individual may and probably does belong to more than one group or subgroup. These multiple belongings can be the result of—among others—ethnic origin, religion, gender, occupation, and profession. For example, an Episcopalian, British, white male clinician bears to some degree the cultural imprint of each of these groups; so, too, does a black, Catholic, female clinician. Metaphorically, groups are not impermeable capsules. They are porous and subject to seepage from without and within.

DISTINGUISHING PHYSICAL CHARACTERISTICS

The use of physical characteristics (e.g., gender or skin color) to distinguish a cultural group or subgroup can be a trap. There is a sharp difference between distinguishing cultural characteristics and distinguishing physical characteristics. You should neither confuse the physical with the cultural nor allow the physical to symbolize the cultural. To assume homogeneity in the beliefs, attitudes, and behaviors of all men, or all black individuals, or all health care professionals is to court error and to miss the mark in the effort to understand the individual. The stereotype, a fixed image of any group that rejects the potential of originality or individuality within the group, is itself to be rejected. People can and do respond differently to the same stimuli.

This does not minimize the value of understanding the cultural characteristics of groups; it does deny the use of a physical characteristic, such as gender or race, as a metaphor for the culture of a group. Nor does this deny the interdependence of the physical with the cultural. Genetic imprinting, for example, precedes the development of the intellect, sensitivity, and imagination that allow the creation of a Beethoven sonata or a Miles Davis jazz piece, both of which are genuine cultural achievements. Similarly, skin color precedes most of the experience of life and the subsequent interweaving of color with cultural experience (Box 2-2).

THE IMPACT OF CULTURE

Box 2-2 suggests that social and economic conditions can define many of the subgroups in the United States. Box 2-3 indicates the terms used in addressing these issues. Poverty and inadequate education have a negative cultural impact that is seriously reflected in health and medical care. Although death rates have declined overall in the United States since 1960, the poorly educated and those in poverty still die at higher rates than those who are better educated and economically advantaged. Morbidity, too, is greater among the poor. Recent studies also suggest that racial and gender differences can have an impact on the care of individuals even in the absence of financial differences. White men, for example, are more apt to be subjected to invasive cardiac procedures and tests than are blacks and white women, suggesting that social, cultural, and clinical factors may be weighed differently in different cultural groups

BOX 2-2
THE INFLUENCE OF AGE, RACE, ETHNICITY, AND CULTURE

Age, gender, race, ethnic group and, with these variables, cultural attitudes, regional differences, and socioeconomic status influence the way we serve our patients. Consider, for example, the ethnic, racial and regional disparities in the rates of knee arthroplasty. Non-Hispanic white men and women have a higher annual rate than Hispanic and black men and women. The rate for black men lags far behind. We do not know if some are getting too many arthroplasties and others too few, but cultural attitudes are clearly involved. Also, Elster and colleagues, in the first comprehensive study of racial and ethnic disparities in care for adolescents, demonstrated that differences exist across the age ranges and that black and Hispanic youth have poorer access to needed services than whites. There is a certain need to deal better with the effects of cultural blindness.

Furthermore, the possible beneficial and toxic effects of many culturally important herbal medicines, which are used but not always acknowledged, must be understood and, in trusting relationships, reported to us if we are to guide their appropriate use. Crossing the cultural divide helps, but skepticism is a barrier. For example, many of our colleagues scoff at the notion that osteopathic manipulative treatment might be a helpful adjuvant therapy for recurrent acute otitis media. Mills and colleagues suggest otherwise in the results of a well-done study. The anatomic relationships of the auditory tube appear to make such treatment possible. Skepticism can be put aside, but the need for soundly derived evidence cannot. Cultural competence is entirely consistent with that.

Data from Skinner et al, 2003; Elster et al, 2003; Dasgupta, 2003; Mills et al, 2003.

BOX 2-3
A LEXICON OF CULTURAL CONSIDERATIONS

Acculturation: The process by which an individual accommodates to the traits and behaviors of another culture. The degree of acculturation can vary. The past is rarely, if ever, completely rejected.

Culture: A complex, integrated system reflecting the whole of human behavior and experience; a group's adoption of shared values, the attempt to make sense of their world.

Custom: The habitual activity of a group or subgroup; patterned responses to given occasions, generally passed on from one generation to the next.

Enculturation: The process by which an individual assumes the traits and behaviors of a given culture, adapting to it, adopting its values, and taking on that particular cultural identity.

Ethnocentrism: The belief in the superiority of one's own group and culture, combined with disdain for other groups and cultures. Any degree of ethnocentrism impairs effort to understand patients within the context of their individual cultures.

Ethnos (ethnic group): A group of the same race or nationality, with a common culture and distinctive traits.

Minority: A group that is different from the majority of a population, as with regard to religion, race, or ethnic origin. When the difference is deep-seated in historical relationships or is obvious (e.g., because of skin color), the minority group may be treated unjustly, sometimes obviously, sometimes more subtly.

Norm: A prescribed standard of allowable behavior within a group or subgroup. To the extent that individuals adopt the positive values of their group or groups, and to the extent that they measure up to the norms, they are judged favorably or unfavorably by the other members of the group.

Race: A physical, not a cultural, differentiator based on a common heredity, using as identifier characteristics such as skin color, head shape, and stature.

Rite: A prescribed, formal, customary observance (e.g., ceremonial religious acts, graduation ceremonies).

Ritual: A stereotypic behavior regulating religious, social, and professional behaviors (e.g., the expected use of "please" and "thank you") in a variety of circumstances.

Stereotype: A simplified, generally inflexible conception of the members of a group or subgroup.

Subculture: A group or subgroup having values and behavioral patterns or other distinctive traits that differentiate it from other groups or subgroups within a larger culture. Individuals may share the traits of more than one group or subgroup and may, with adaptation, shed some traits and adopt others.

Values: The ideals, customs, institutions, and behaviors within a group or subgroup for which the members of the group have a respectful regard. Values may be positive or negative and desirable or undesirable (e.g., with regard to charitable donation or criminal behavior, consensual sexual relationships or rape).

(Schulman et al, 1999). These rather stark facts are but the tip of the iceberg; they are, however, sufficient to underscore the need for cultural awareness in health and medical care professionals.

THE BLURRING OF CULTURAL DISTINCTIONS

CLINICAL PEARL
Language Is Not All
A patient who knows the English language, however well, cannot be assumed to know the culture. The absence of a language barrier does not preclude a cultural barrier. You might still have to achieve a "cultural translation."

Cultural differences are malleable in a way that physical characteristics may not be. For example, one nation can be distinguished from another by language. However, change and necessity mandate more and more that we learn one another's languages. We may begin in that way to override political divisions. Modern technology and economics will slowly but inevitably ensure the achievement of universality in language. The changes may be imperceptible, spanning generations, but they are also relentless. However, the resistance to change, driven for better or worse by our culturally derived territorial need to protect individual space, is at the root of social, political, and economic tragedy. This worldwide resistance to develop a true awareness of each other is keenly evident. Still, as health care providers, we must not resist or we will not serve well.

THE PRIMACY OF THE INDIVIDUAL IN HEALTH CARE

CLINICAL PEARL
A Major No-No
It is always dangerous, given the all too human tendency to grasp stereotypes, to attempt a definitive description of any national or ethnic character.

The individual patient may be visualized as being at the center of an indefinite number of concentric circles. The outermost circles represent constraining universal experiences (e.g., death). The circles closest to the center represent the various cultural groups or subgroups to which anyone must, of necessity, belong. The constancy of change forces adaptation and acculturation. The circles are constantly interweaving and overlapping. For example, a common experience in the United States has been the economic gain at the root of the assimilation of many ethnic groups, with greater homogeneity dominating, but not necessarily excluding, earlier ethnic behaviors. However, predicting the individual's character merely on the basis of the common cultural behavior is not appropriate; understanding and taking the common cultural behavior into account are. The stereotype cannot prevail. The individual at the center is unique (Box 2-4).

CLINICAL PEARL
The Impact of Gender
If a female internist or family practitioner serves a woman, then that patient is more apt to be screened with Pap smears and mammograms.

BOX 2-4

QUESTIONS THAT EXPLORE THE PATIENT'S CULTURE

These questions may be addressed directly to the patient or modified for third persons, such as parents and other caretakers who are responsible for and/or involved with the patient. These questions, appropriate in any culture, enable your insights about an individual who is, of course, unique. They help you to avoid the stereotype and lead to a true individualization of care.
- What do you call your problem?
- What do you think caused your problem?
- Why do you think it started when it did?
- What does your sickness do to you?
- How does it work?
- How bad is your sickness?
- How long do you think it will last?
- What should be done to get rid of it?
- Why did you come to me for treatment?
- What benefit will you get from the treatment?
- What are the most important problems your sickness has caused for you?
- What worries you and frightens you the most about your sickness?
- Who else or what else might help you get better?
- Has anyone else helped you with this problem?

Modified from Kleinman, Eisenberg, Good, 1978, and Taylor and Willies-Jacobo, 2003, who remind us that we can substitute "your child" for "your" to adapt these questions for the young.

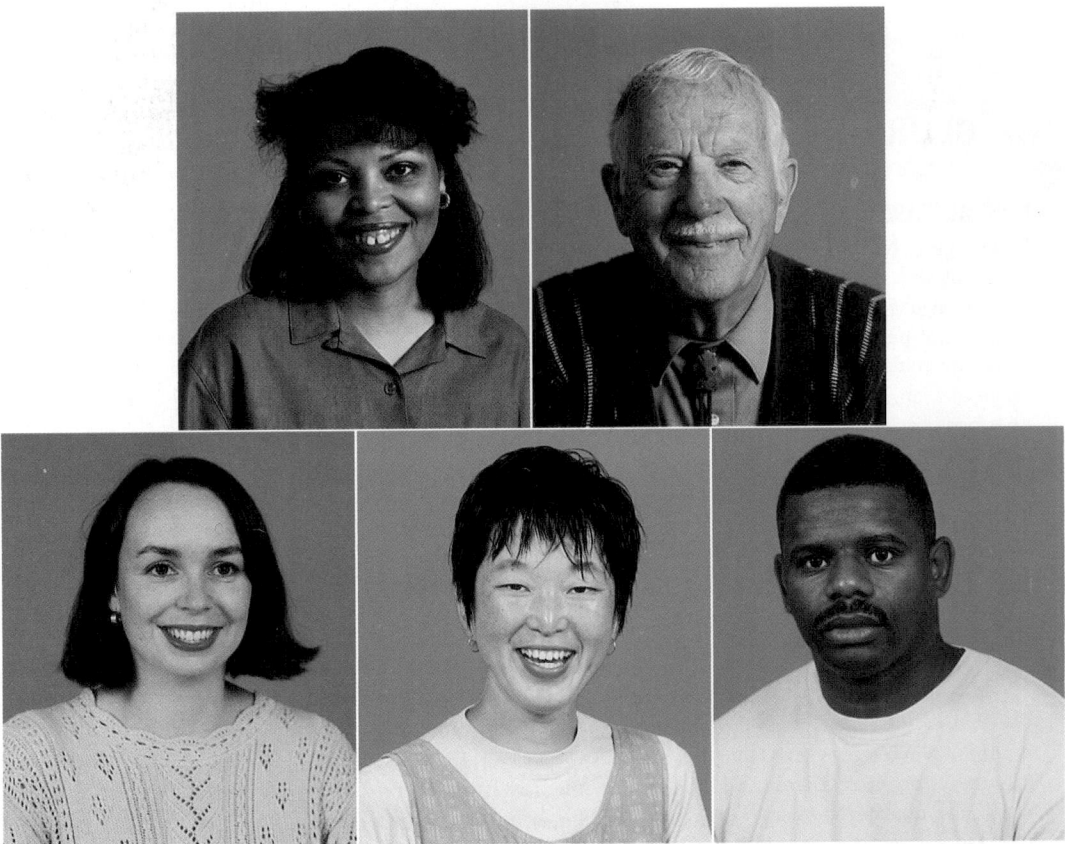

Nevertheless, ethical issues often arise when the care of an individual comes into conflict with the utilitarian needs of the larger community, particularly with the recognition of limited resources and, in the United States, the imposition of managed care. Cultural attitudes, often vague and poorly understood, may constrain our professional behavior and may confuse the context in which we serve the individual. Box 2-5 offers a guide to the understanding of the patient's beliefs and practices and can aid in the relief of confusion.

PROFESSIONAL CULTURES WITHIN THE HEALTH PROFESSIONS

There is a harmony—a unity—in the care of patients that is not constricted by the cultural and administrative boundaries of the individual health professions. Caring and curing, in a practical and a deeply emotional sense, are not the sole provinces of any of them. To the extent that we stake out territories of care, by allowing individual professional cultures and needs to take precedence over patient needs, we impede the achievement of harmony. The blurring of professional cultural borders works to the advantage of the patient, as long as the blurring is motivated by the best interest of the patient. Each of us must understand our professional role and must be adaptable as cultural shifts suggest greater homogeneity in a number of those roles. In addition, Table 2-1 indicates that there are health beliefs and practices that are different from the long-institutionalized Judeo-Christian Western perspective that dominates health education in the United States. Different clinicians in different parts of the world make different decisions. Your ability to understand and to respect differences, and to allow for the blurring of borders, will be a measure of your ability to form reinforcing relationships with other professionals and to care for a wide range of individuals.

BOX 2-5

CULTURAL ASSESSMENT GUIDE: THE MANY ASPECTS OF UNDERSTANDING

Health Beliefs and Practices
- How does the patient define health and illness? How are feelings concerning pain, illness in general, or death expressed?
- Are there particular methods used to help maintain health, such as hygiene and self-care practices?
- Are there particular methods being used by the patient for treatment of illness?
- What is the attitude toward preventive health measures such as immunizations?
- Are there health topics that the patient may be particularly sensitive to or that are considered taboo?
- Are there restrictions imposed by modesty that must be respected; for example, are there constraints related to exposure of parts of the body, discussion of sexual matters in male/female relationships, and attitudes toward various procedures such as termination of pregnancy or vasectomy?
- What are the attitudes toward mental illness, pain, handicapping conditions, chronic disease, death, and dying? Are there constraints in the way these issues are discussed with the patient or with reference to relatives and friends?
- Is there a person in the family responsible for various health-related decisions such as where to go, whom to see, and what advice to follow?
- Does the patient prefer a health professional of the same gender, age, ethnic and racial background, or is this not a significant issue?

Religious Influences and Special Rituals
- Is there a religion to which the patient adheres?
- Is there a significant person to whom the patient looks to for guidance and support?
- Are there any special religious practices or beliefs that may affect health care when the patient is ill or dying?
- What events, rituals, and ceremonies are considered important within the life cycle of birth, baptism, puberty, marriage, and death? What is the culturally appropriate way to respond to these life events? To what extent is an overt expression of emotion and spirituality inherent in that response?

Language and Communication
- What language is spoken in the home?
- How well does the patient understand English, both spoken and written?
- Are there special signs of demonstrating respect or disrespect?
- Is touch involved in communication?

- Are there culturally appropriate ways to enter and leave situations (e.g., greetings and farewells) and convenient times to make a home visit?
- Is an interpreter needed? Should that person be a relative, friend, or a presumably objective stranger? Certainly, whoever it is should be acceptable to the patient.

Parenting Styles and Role of Family
- Who makes the decisions in the family?
- What is the composition of the family? How many generations are considered to be a single family, and which relatives compose the family unit?
- When the marriage custom is practiced, what is the attitude about separation and divorce?
- What is the role of and attitude toward children in the family?
- When do children need to be disciplined or punished, and how is this done (if physical means are used, in what way)?
- Do the parents demonstrate physical affection toward their children and each other?
- What major events are important to the family, and how are they celebrated?
- Are there special beliefs and practices surrounding conception, pregnancy, childbirth, lactation, and childrearing? Is co-sleeping practiced?

Sources of Support Beyond the Family
- Are there ethnic or cultural organizations that may have an influence on the patient's approach to health care?
- Are there individuals in the patient's social network that can influence perception of health and illness?
- Is there a particular cultural group with which the patient identifies? Can this be clarified by where the patient was born and has lived?
- What is the patient's need for relationships with others?
- Is the patient socially gregarious or a loner, and is the preference indicated by behavior before illness?

Dietary Practices
- What does the family like to eat? Does everyone in the family have similar tastes in food?
- Who is responsible for food preparation?
- Are any foods forbidden by the culture, or are some foods a cultural requirement in observance of a rite or ceremony?
- How is food prepared and consumed?
- Are there specific beliefs or preferences concerning food, such as those believed to cause or to cure an illness?
- Are there periods of required fasting? What are they?

Modified from Stulc, 1991.

TABLE 2-1 Comparison of Value Orientations Among Cultural Groups*	
Value Orientation	**Cultural Group**
TIME ORIENTATION	
Present oriented: Accepts each day as it comes; future unpredictable	Black, Hispanic, Native American/American Indian
Past oriented: Maintains traditions that were meaningful in the past; worships ancestors	Eastern Asian
Future oriented: Anticipates bigger and better future; places high value on change	Dominant United States
ACTIVITY ORIENTATION	
"Doing" orientation: Emphasizes accomplishments that are measurable by external standards	Dominant United States
"Being" orientation: Spontaneous expression of self	Black, Hispanic, Native American/American Indian
"Being-in-becoming": Emphasizes self-development of all aspects of self as an integrated whole	Eastern Asian
HUMAN NATURE ORIENTATION	
Human being basically imperfect but with perfectible nature; constant self-control and discipline necessary	Black, dominant United States, Hispanic
Human being as neutral, neither good nor evil	Eastern Asian, Native American/American Indian
HUMAN–NATURE ORIENTATION	
Human being subject to environment with very little control over own destiny	Black, Hispanic
Human being in harmony with nature	Eastern Asian, Native American/American Indian
Human being master over nature	Dominant United States
RELATIONAL ORIENTATION	
Individualistic: Encourages individualism: interpersonal relationships occur more with outsiders and less with family	Dominant United States
Lineal: Group goals dominant over individual goals; ordered positional succession (father to son)	Eastern Asian
Collateral: Group goals dominant over individual goals: more emphasis on relationship with others on one's own level	Black, Hispanic, Native American/American Indian

Modified from Kluckhohn, 1976.

*These are generalizations meant only to be a guide. Do not think of them as stereotypical. Members of any group may and often do hold views and adopt behaviors at variance with their neighbors. The many variables in any one life require that each patient be separately defined.

THE IMPACT OF CULTURE ON ILLNESS

Disease is shaped by illness, and illness—the full expression of the impact of disease on the patient—is shaped by the totality of the patient's experience. Cancers are diseases. The patient dealing with, reacting to, and trying to live with a cancer is having an illness—is "ill" or, in personal terms, is "sick." The definition of "ill" or "sick" is based on the individual's belief system and is determined in large part by his or her enculturation. This is so for a brief, essentially mild episode or for a chronic, debilitating, life-altering condition. If we do not consider the substance of illness—the biologic, emotional, and cultural aspects—we will too often fail to offer complete care. To make the point, imagine that while taking a shower you have done a self-examination and, still young, still looking ahead to your career, you have discovered an unexpected mass in a breast or a testicle. How will you respond? There are components to your response that you can understand and master.

STAYING WELL
CONSIDER THE "NORM" WITH CARE

We often use a variety of screening questionnaires in the effort to help our patients keep well. These screening tools are based on norms that, as Rhodes indicates, "tell us how to place individuals in relation to one another according to some agreed on and standardized measure." Norms, however, may not be consistent across cultures. Problems in one may be the expected in another. This is a trap we can avoid if we

recognize that screening tools are useful and use them with the understanding that they may well not be universally applicable. The human condition is not static. It is in individuals as in cultures dynamic, ever-evolving, and resistant to the inappropriate stereotyping that the careless use of norms may invoke.

From Rhodes, 2003.

THE COMPONENTS OF A CULTURAL RESPONSE

You can understand the culture of another and be emphatic with it. When differences exist, you must be certain that you grasp exactly what the patient means, and know exactly what the patient thinks you mean in words and actions. Asking if you are not sure is far better than making a damaging mistake. Avoid assumptions about cultural beliefs and behaviors made without validation from the patient.

Those that will have an impact on your assessment of the patient include the following:
- Modes of communication: the use of speech, body language, and space
- Health beliefs and practices that may vary from the Judeo-Christian Western model
- Diet and nutritional practices
- The nature of relationships within a family

In particular, there can be a variety of ethnic attitudes toward autonomy. The patient-centered model, still firmly respected in the United States (although subject now to some critical discussion), is at odds with a more family-centered model that is more likely dominant elsewhere. In Japan, for example, the family is generally considered the legitimate decision-making authority for competent and incompetent patients (Fetters, 1998). Many cultures, for example, in the Middle East, believe that a patient should not be told of a diagnosis of a metastatic cancer or a terminal prognosis for any reason, attitudes not likely to be shared by Americans with European or African traditions. The desire to avoid discussing such negative information is particularly strong among the Navajo Native Americans. Traditionally, the Navajo culture holds that thought and language have the power to shape reality. Talking about a possible outcome is thought to ensure the outcome. It is important, then, to avoid thinking or speaking in a negative way. It is important to think and talk "in the Beauty Way" (Carrese, Rhodes, 1995). The situation can be dealt with by talking in terms of a third person or an abstract possibility. You might even refer to an experience you have had in your own family. Obviously, the conflicts that may arise from differing views of autonomy, religion, and information sharing require an effort that is dominated by a clear understanding of the patient's goals and that a patient need not typify the attitudes of the group of origin.

MODES OF COMMUNICATION

Communication and culture are interrelated, particularly in the way feelings are expressed verbally and nonverbally. The same word may have different meanings for different people. For example, in the United States, a "practicing physician" is an experienced, trained person. "Practicing," however, suggests inexperience and the status of a student to an Eskimo or to some Western Europeans. Similarly, touch, facial expressions, eye movement, and body posture all have varying significance.

In the United States, for example, people tend to talk more loudly and to worry less about being overheard than others do. The English, on the other hand, tend to worry more about being overheard and to speak in modulated voices, at a level that might be considered conspiratorial by some. In the United States, people are direct in conversation and are eager to be thought logical, preferring to avoid the subjective and to come to the point quickly. The Japanese tend to do the opposite, using indirection, talking around points, and emphasizing attitudes and feelings. Silence, while sometimes uncomfortable for many of us, affords the Native American/American Indian a time to think; the response should not be forced and the quiet time should be allowed.

Many groups use firm eye contact. The Spanish meet one another's eyes and look for the impact of what is being said. The French, too, have a firm gaze and often stare openly at others. This, however, might be thought rude or immodest in some Asian or Middle Eastern cultures. Americans are more apt to let the eyes wander and to grunt, nod the head, or say, "I see," or "uh huh," to indicate understanding. Americans also tend to avoid touch and are less apt to pat you on the arm in a reassuring way than are, for example, Italians.

These are but a few examples of cultural variation in communication (Hall, 1969). They do, however, suggest a variety of behaviors within groups. As with any example we might use, they are not to be thought of as rigidly characteristic of the indicated groups. Still, the questions suggested in Box 2-6 can at times provide insight to particular situations and can help avoid misunderstanding and miscommunication.

The cultural and physical characteristics of both patient and practitioner may therefore significantly influence communication (Fig. 2-1). Social class, age, and gender are variables

---

BOX 2-6

ASKING QUESTIONS IN THE RIGHT ORDER

Communication when you are exploring differences is made easier if you allow time for thoughtful answers and ask your questions in a comfortable order. A suggested sequence is the following.

When Talking About a Patient's Illness:
• What do you think is wrong with you?
• People have told me that there are sicknesses that doctors and nurses don't know about. Have you heard of them? What are they?
• Have you ever known anyone with one of them?

• Have you ever had one of them?
• Do you think you might have it right now?

When Talking About Treatments:
• People have told me that there are ways of treating sickness that doctors and nurses don't know about. Do you know any of them? What are they?
• Do they work?
• Have you ever tried them?
• Do you use them?
• Are they helpful?

Modified from Pachter, 1997.

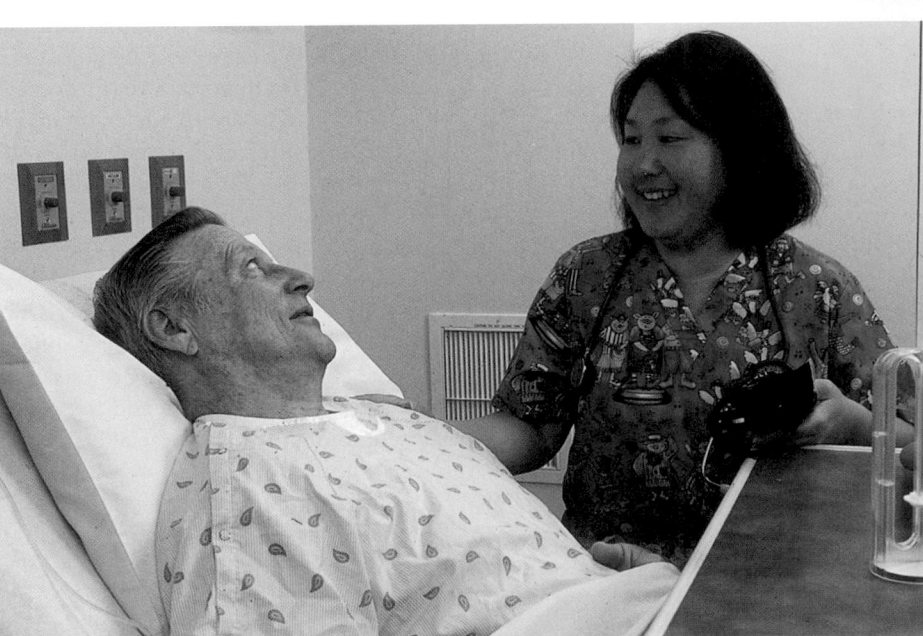

FIGURE 2-1
Being sensitive to cultural differences that may exist between you and the patient can help avoid miscommunication.

that characterize everyone; they can intrude on successful communication if there is no effort for mutual knowledge and understanding. The young student or practitioner and the older adult patient may have an important bridge to cross if they are to work together successfully. If that practitioner is a young woman and that patient is an old man, the crossing may be even more difficult. Recognizing the possible problem and talking about it, evoking feelings sooner rather than later, makes it easier. It is all right to ask if the patient is uncomfortable with any aspect of your person and to talk about it. Also, when any aspect of the patient's person disturbs you, you must try to understand why.

HEALTH BELIEFS AND PRACTICES

The patient may have a view of health and illness and an approach to cure that are shaped by a particular cultural and/or religious belief or paradigm. If that view is "scientific," in the sense that a cause can be determined for every problem in a very precise way, the patient is more apt to be comfortable with Western approaches to health and medical care.

However, the scientific view is reductionist and looks to a very narrow, specific cause and effect. A more naturalistic or "holistic" approach broadens the context. It views our lives as part of a much greater whole (the entire cosmos) that must be in harmony. If the balance is disturbed, illness can result. The goal, then, is to retrieve balance and harmony. Aspects of this concept are evident among the beliefs of many Hispanics, Native Americans/American Indians, Asians, and Arabs, and they are increasingly evident in people of all ethnic groups in the United States today (Box 2-7). There are also those who believe in the supernatural, or forces of good and evil that determine individual fate. In such a context, illness may be thought of as a punishment for wrongdoing.

Clearly, there can be a confusing ambivalence in many of us, patient and provider alike, because our heartfelt and genuine religious or naturalistic beliefs may conflict with the options

CLINICAL PEARL

Chicken Soup

Home-based remedies for common colds are widely used. To some extent, chicken soup complements acetaminophen in European, African-American, Puerto Rican, and West-Indian–Caribbean families.

Pachter et al, 1998.

BOX 2-7

THE BALANCE OF LIFE: THE "HOT" AND THE "COLD"

A naturalistic or holistic approach often assumes that there are external factors—some good, some bad—that must be kept in balance if we are to remain well. The balance of "hot" and "cold" is a part of the belief system in many cultural groups (e.g., Arab, Chinese, Filipino, and Hispanic). To restore a disturbed balance, that is, to treat, requires the use of opposites (e.g., a "hot" remedy for a "cold" problem). Different cultures may define "hot" and "cold" differently, and they may even be defined differently or not at all within what many may wrongly perceive as similar groups. For example, not all Hispanics think the same way. It is not a matter of temperature, and the words used might vary: for example, the Chinese have named the forces yin (cold) and yang (hot). The bottom line: We cannot ignore the naturalistic view if many of our patients are to have appropriate care.

Hot and Cold Conditions and Their Corresponding Treatments

Hot Conditions	Cold Foods	Cold Medicines and Herbs	Cold Conditions	Hot Foods	Hot Medicines and Herbs
Fever	Fresh vegetables	Orange flower water	Cancer	Chocolate	Penicillin
Infection	Tropical fruits	Linden	Pneumonia	Cheese	Tobacco
Diarrhea	Dairy products	Sage	Malaria	Temperate-zone fruit	Ginger root
Kidney problem	Meats such as goat, fish, chicken	Milk of Magnesia	Joint pain	Eggs	Garlic
Rash	Honey	Bicarbonate of soda	Menstrual period	Peas	Cinnamon
Skin ailment	Cod		Teething	Onions	Anise
Sore throat	Raisins		Earache	Aromatic beverages	Vitamins
Liver problem	Bottled milk		Rheumatism	Hard liquor	Iron preparations
Ulcer	Barley water		Tuberculosis	Oils	Cod liver oil
Constipation			Cold	Meats such as beef, water-fowl, mutton	Castor oil
			Headache	Goat's milk	Aspirin
			Paralysis	Cereal grains	
			Stomach cramps	Chili peppers	

Modified from Wilson, Kneisl, 1988.

available for the treatment of illness. Consider, for example, a child with a broken bone, the result of a careless accident that occurred while the child was under the supervision of a babysitter. The first need is to tend the fracture. That done, there is a need to talk with the mother about the guilt she may feel because she was away working, despite her husband's disapproval. She might think this accident must be God's punishment. It is important to be aware of, to respect, and to discuss without belittlement a belief that may vary from yours, in a manner that may still allow you to offer your point of view. This can apply to the guilt of a parent and to the use of herbs, rituals, and religious artifacts. After all, the pharmacopoeia of Western medicine is replete with plants and herbs that we now call drugs. Our inability to understand the belief of another does not invalidate its substance. Nor does a patient's adherence to a particular belief preclude concurrent reliance on allopathic health practitioners.

FAMILY RELATIONSHIPS

Family structure and the social organizations to which a patient belongs (e.g., religious organizations, clubs, and schools) are among the many imprinting and constraining cultural forces. The expectations of children and how they grow and develop are key in this regard and often culturally distinct. This needs emphasis in the United States today, with its shift toward dual-income families, single-parent families, and a significant number of teenage pregnancies. The prevalence of divorce (roughly one for every two marriages) and the increasing involvement of fathers in child care in two-parent families suggest cultural shifts that need to be recognized.

One type of already known behavior may predict another type of behavior. For example, mothers who take advantage of appropriate prenatal care generally take advantage of appropriate infant care, regardless of educational level, marital status, family relationships, or maternal drug use (Butz et al, 1993). Adolescents who are unsupervised after school are more likely to smoke, use alcohol and marijuana, perform poorly in school, be depressed, and take risks than are those who are well supervised (Richardson et al, 1993). Being aware of this sequence of related behaviors is especially important because it often appears unrelated to the integrity of the family structure, gender, or racial or ethnic background. This is particularly true with the American cultural addiction to mass media. Adolescents who spend large amounts of time watching television and listening to "heavy metal" music are more likely to engage in risky behaviors than are those who do not; this, too, is regardless of race, gender, or parents' education (Klein et al, 1993). These examples remind us that one individual may belong to many groups and that the behaviors and attitudes of one of those groups, including pregnant women or adolescents, can override or modify the impact of the cultural values of other groups to which that person belongs.

DIET AND NUTRITIONAL PRACTICES

Beliefs and practices related to food, as well as the social significance of food, play an obvious vital role in everyday life. Some of these beliefs of cultural and/or religious significance may have an impact on your care. An Orthodox Jewish patient will not take some medicines, particularly during a holiday period like Passover, because the preparation of a drug does not meet the religious rules for food during that time. The Muslim woman must respect Halal (prescribed diet) even throughout pregnancy. A Chinese person with hypertension and a salt-restricted diet may need to consider a limited use of monosodium glutamate (MSG) and soy sauce. Attitudes toward vitamins vary greatly, with or without scientific proof, in many of the subgroups in the United States. It is still possible to work out a mutually decided care or management plan if the issues are recognized and freely discussed. This is possible, too, with attitudes toward home, herbal, and natural—complementary or alternative—therapies. Many will have benefit; others may be dangerous. For example, dietary supplements containing ephedra alkaloids may increase the risk of stroke (Haller, Benowitz, 2000; Kernan et al, 2000).

CLINICAL PEARL

Beer

The mother-in-law of one of the authors drank beer while breast-feeding her babies in the belief that beer is a galactagogue, a substance that stimulates the flow of human milk. Whether it does or not, *no one* should use alcohol during pregnancy (and afterward, always in moderation if at all).

BOX 2-8

SUMMING UP

It is not unusual to come across charts that attempt to present succinctly health care–related cultural attitudes along one axis and a variety of the religious and ethnic groups along the other, this to enable quick access to information that might be needed when you are about to meet a patient who appears to belong to a group with which you are not necessarily familiar. You will notice some of this in this chapter. Our experience suggests that there is the danger of a rigid superficiality in this and the parallel danger of a stereotypical picture that too often does not translate to the needs of a particular individual. We are appropriate in cautioning against this repeatedly. Our effort here is to review many of the questions that might be relevant as you prepare to meet the patient, questions that are perhaps not made more explicit in other parts of this chapter. Patient by patient, your insights will develop as you avoid stereotypes, consider the individual, and become increasingly culturally aware.

Communication
- How important are nonverbal clues?
- Are moments of silence valued?
- Is touching to be avoided?
- Are hand-shakes, or even embracing, avoided or desired at meeting and parting?
- What is the attitude toward eye contact?
- Is there a greater than expected need for "personal space?"
- What is the verbal or nonverbal response if your suggestions are not understood?
- Is there candor in admitting lack of understanding?
- What are the attitudes concerning respect for self and for authority figures?
- What are the attitudes toward persons in other groups, such as minorities, majorities?
- What are the language preferences?
- What is the need for "chit-chat" before getting down to the primary concern?
- Is there a relaxed or rigid sense of time?
- What is the degree of trust of health care professionals?
- How easily are personal matters discussed?
- Is there, even with you, a wish to avoid discussing income and other family affairs?

Health Customs/Health Practices
- What is the degree of dependence on the health care system, for illness alone or also for preventive and health maintenance needs?
- What is generally expected of a health professional and what defines a "good one?"
- What defines health?
- Are there particularly common folk practices?
- Is there a greater (or lesser) inclination to invoke self-care and use home remedies?
- Is there a particular suspicion or fear of hospitals?
- What is the tendency to use alternative care approaches and/or herbal remedies exclusively or as a complement?

- What are the tendencies to invoke the magical or meta-physical?
- Who is ultimately responsible for outcomes, you or the patient?
- Who is ultimately responsible for maintaining health, you or the patient?
- Is there a particular fear of painful or intrusive testing?
- Is there a tendency toward stoicism?
- What is the dependence on prayer?
- Is illness thought of as punishment and a means of penance?
- Is there "shame" attached to illness?
- What is the belief about the origins of illness?
- Is illness thought to be preventable and, if so, how?
- What is the attitude toward autopsy?
- Does a belief in reincarnation mandate that the body be left intact?
- Are there particular cultural cooking habits that can influence diagnosis or management?
- Is the degree of modesty in both men and women more than you would generally expect?
- Do women, considering modesty, need a much more cautious and protected approach than usual, for example, during the examination?

Family, Friends, and the Workplace
- How tightly organized (and multigenerational) is the family hierarchy?
- How tight is the family?
- Is social life extended beyond the family and, if so, to what degree?
- Does the family tend to be matriarchal or patriarchal?
- What are the relative roles of women and men?
- Are there particular tasks required of the individual genders, for example, who does the laundry?
- To what extent are older adults and other authority figures given deference and how?
- Who makes decisions for the family?
- To what extent is power shared?
- Who makes decisions for the children and adolescents?
- How strongly are children valued?
- Is there a greater value placed on one of the genders?
- How much are self-reliance and personal discipline valued?
- What is the work ethic?
- What is the sense of obligation to the community?
- How is education sought, from school and reading and/or experience?
- What is the emphasis on tradition and ritual practice?

This is a long list of questions, derived over the years from our experience and a multitude of written and more informal resources, and the human condition is so varied that there are bound to be many more that you will decide are important. There is no need to be intimidated by the apparent mass of "need to know" cultural issues.

SUMMING UP

As clinicians, we face a compelling need to meet each patient on his or her own terms and to resist forming a sense of the patient based on prior knowledge of the culture or cultures from which that patient comes. That knowledge should not be formative in arriving at conclusions; rather, we must draw upon it to help make the questions we ask more constructively probing (Box 2-8). Otherwise, we will see the patient as a stereotype; that is something we must avoid.

You need to understand yourself well. There is no denying that your involvement with any patient gives that interaction a character that is unique, and that the substance you bring to it makes that interaction, to some extent, different from what it might have been with anyone else. If you do not understand this well, your attitudes, which are largely culturally derived, may be so insistent as to overwhelm your better understanding of the patient, and that increases the probability of stereotypic judgment. You must constrain your prejudices and your likes, as well as your tendencies to preach and to be judgmental. Do this and you will be making strides toward cultural competence.

ELECTRONIC RESOURCES

For Weblinks and additional resources, go to

http://evolve.elsevier.com/Seidel

or to the Companion CD-ROM.

EXAMINATION TECHNIQUES AND EQUIPMENT

This chapter provides an overview of the techniques of inspection, palpation, percussion, and auscultation that are used throughout the physical examination. In addition, general use of the equipment for performing these techniques is discussed. Specific details regarding utilization of techniques and equipment as they relate to specific parts of the examination can be found in the appropriate chapters. This chapter also addresses special issues related to the physical examination process.

PRECAUTIONS TO PREVENT INFECTION

Because persons of all ages and backgrounds may be sources of infection for the examiner, it is important to take proper precautions. Universal Precautions (UP), which were introduced in 1985, applied blood and body fluid precautions universally to all persons regardless of their presumed infection status. In addition to emphasizing prevention of needle-stick injuries and the use of traditional barriers such as gloves and gowns, UP expanded the use of masks and eye coverings to prevent mucous membrane exposures during certain procedures, and called for the use of individual ventilation devices for resuscitation. UP applied to blood, to body fluids implicated in or at unknown risk for the transmission of bloodborne infections, and to any other body fluid visibly contaminated with blood. In 1987, Body Substance Isolation (BSI) was proposed. BSI focused on the isolation, primarily through the use of gloves, of all moist and potentially infectious body substances (e.g., blood, feces, urine, sputum, saliva, wound drainage, and other body fluids) from all patients regardless of their presumed infection status.

The guidelines for Standard Precautions, subsequently developed, synthesize the major features of UP and BSI into a single set of precautions to be used for the care of all patients regardless of their presumed infection status. These precautions are designed to reduce the risk of transmission of bloodborne and other infectious pathogens.

Guidelines for Standard Precautions are summarized in Box 3-1. Remember that precautions may be used to protect not only health care workers but also patients with compromised immune systems.

A second tier of precautions, Transmission-Based Precautions, is designed for the care of specified patients who are known or suspected to be infected by epidemiologically important pathogens that are spread by airborne or droplet transmission or by contact with dry skin or contaminated surfaces. Further information regarding the recommendations for Transmission-Based Precautions can be obtained from the Centers for Disease Control and Prevention (CDC, 2005).

BOX 3-1

GUIDELINES FOR STANDARD PRECAUTIONS

Standard Precautions apply to all patients regardless of their diagnosis or presumed infection status. Standard Precautions apply to: (1) blood; (2) all body fluids, secretions, and excretions except sweat, regardless of whether or not they contain visible blood; (3) nonintact skin; and (4) mucous membranes. Standard Precautions are designed to reduce the risk of transmission of microorganisms from both recognized and unrecognized sources of infection.

Standard Precautions

Use Standard Precautions or the equivalent for the care of all patients.

Handwashing

- Wash hands after touching blood, body fluids, secretions, excretions, and contaminated items, whether or not gloves are worn. Wash hands immediately after gloves are removed, between patient contacts, and when otherwise indicated to avoid transfer of microorganisms to other patients or environments. It may be necessary to wash hands between tasks and procedures on the same patient to prevent cross-contamination of different body sites.
- Use a plain (nonantimicrobial) soap for routine handwashing.
- Use an antimicrobial agent or a waterless antiseptic agent for specific circumstances (e.g., control of outbreaks or hyperendemic infections) as defined by the infection control program.

Gloves

Wear gloves (clean, nonsterile gloves are adequate) when touching blood, body fluids, secretions, excretions, and contaminated items. Put on clean gloves just before touching mucous membranes and nonintact skin. Change gloves between tasks and procedures on the same patient after contact with material that may contain a high concentration of microorganisms. Remove gloves promptly after use, before touching noncontaminated items and environmental surfaces, and before going to another patient; and wash hands immediately to avoid transfer of microorganisms to other patients or environments.

Mask, Eye Protection, Face Shield

Wear a mask and eye protection or a face shield to protect mucous membranes of the eyes, nose, and mouth during procedures and patient-care activities that are likely to generate splashes or sprays of blood, body fluids, secretions, and excretions.

Gown

Wear a gown (a clean, nonsterile gown is adequate) to protect skin and to prevent soiling of clothing during procedures and patient-care activities that are likely to generate splashes or sprays of blood, body fluids, secretions, or excretions. Select a gown that is appropriate for the activity and amount of fluid likely to be encountered. Remove a soiled gown as promptly as possible and wash hands to avoid transfer of microorganisms to other patients or environments.

Patient-Care Equipment

Handle used patient-care equipment soiled with blood, body fluids, secretions, and excretions in a manner that prevents skin and mucous membrane exposures, contamination of clothing, and transfer of microorganisms to other patients and environments. Ensure that reusable equipment is not used for the care of another patient until it has been cleaned and reprocessed appropriately. Ensure that single-use items are discarded properly.

Environmental Control

Ensure that the hospital has adequate procedures for the routine care, cleaning, and disinfection of environmental surfaces, beds, bedrails, bedside equipment, and other frequently touched surfaces, and ensure that these procedures are being followed.

Linen

Handle, transport, and process used linen soiled with blood, body fluids, secretions, and excretions in a manner that prevents skin and mucous membrane exposures and contamination of clothing, and that avoids transfer of microorganisms to other patients and environments.

Occupational Health and Bloodborne Pathogens

- Take care to prevent injuries when using needles, scalpels, and other sharp instruments or devices; when handling sharp instruments after procedures; when cleaning used instruments; and when disposing of used needles. Never recap used needles, or otherwise manipulate them using both hands, or use any other technique that involves directing the point of a needle toward any part of the body; rather, use either a one-handed "scoop" technique or a mechanical device designed for holding the needle sheath. Do not remove used needles from disposable syringes by hand, and do not bend, break, or otherwise manipulate used needles by hand. Place used disposable syringes and needles, scalpel blades, and other sharp items in appropriate puncture-resistant containers, which are located as close as practical to the area in which the items were used. Place reusable syringes and needles in a puncture-resistant container for transport to the reprocessing area.
- Use mouthpieces, resuscitation bags, or other ventilation devices as an alternative to mouth-to-mouth resuscitation in areas where the need for resuscitation is predictable.

Patient Placement

Place a patient who contaminates the environment or who does not (or cannot be expected to) assist in maintaining appropriate hygiene or environmental control in a private room. If a private room is not available, consult with infection control professionals regarding patient placement or other alternatives.

From Garner J, 1996a, b.

LATEX ALLERGY

The incidence of serious allergic reaction to latex has increased dramatically in recent years. Latex allergy occurs when the body's immune system reacts to proteins found in natural rubber latex. Latex products also contain added chemicals, such as antioxidants, that can cause irritant or delayed hypersensitivity reactions. Box 3-2 describes the different types of latex reactions.

Health care providers are at risk for developing latex allergy because of their exposure to latex in the form of gloves and other equipment and supplies. Sensitization to the latex proteins occurs by direct skin or mucous membrane contact or through airborne exposure. Examples of workplace and home products that may contain latex, and their suggested nonlatex substitutes, are listed in Table 3-1. The National Institute for Occupational Safety and Health (NIOSH) has issued recommendations for both employers and workers to prevent latex allergy in the workplace. Box 3-3 contains a summary of recommendations to protect yourself from latex exposure in the workplace. Also be aware that some patients who have had multiple procedures or surgeries performed are at higher risk for the development of latex allergy. The patient with latex allergies has the greatest risk of inhaling latex molecules (leading to the more severe reactions) when latex is dispersed in the air after a latex glove is snapped off in the presence of the patient.

STAYING WELL

THE VULNERABILITY OF THE HEALTH PROFESSIONAL

Health professionals do not have better immune systems than other people, although we sometimes behave as if we think we do. Nor are we invincible against the every day work-related injuries. We stand a much better chance of staying well if we are scrupulous in protecting ourselves:

- Follow standard precautions.
- Minimize latex exposure.
- Use good body mechanics in transferring or assisting patients into various positions. NO EXCEPTIONS!

BOX 3-2

TYPES OF LATEX REACTIONS

- *Irritant contact dermatitis*—chemical irritation that does not involve the immune system. Symptoms are usually dry, itching, irritated areas on the skin, usually the hands.
- *Type IV dermatitis (delayed hypersensitivity)*—allergic contact dermatitis that involves the immune system and is caused by the chemicals used in latex products. The skin reaction usually begins 24 to 48 hours after contact and resembles that caused by poison ivy. The reaction may progress to oozing skin blisters.
- *Type I systemic reactions*—true allergic reaction caused by protein antibodies (IgE antibodies) that form as a result of interaction between a foreign protein and the body's immune system. The antigen-antibody reaction causes release of histamine, leukotrienes, prostaglandins, and kinins. These chemicals cause the symptoms of allergic reactions. Type I reactions include the following symptoms: local urticaria (skin wheals), generalized urticaria with angioedema (tissue swelling), asthma, eye/nose itching and gastrointestinal symptoms, anaphylaxis (cardiovascular collapse), chronic asthma, and permanent lung damage.

BOX 3-3

SUMMARY OF RECOMMENDATIONS FOR WORKERS TO PREVENT LATEX ALLERGY

- Use nonlatex gloves for activities not likely to involve infectious materials. Hypoallergenic gloves are not necessarily latex-free, but they may reduce reactions to chemical additives in the latex.
- For barrier protection when handling infectious materials, use powder-free latex gloves with reduced protein content.
- When wearing latex gloves, do not use oil-based hand creams or lotions unless they have been shown to reduce latex-related problems.
- After removing gloves, wash hands with mild soap and dry thoroughly.
- Use good housekeeping practices to remove latex-containing dust from the workplace.
- Take advantage of all latex allergy education and training provided.
- If you develop symptoms of latex allergy, avoid direct contact with latex gloves and products until you can see a health care provider experienced in treating latex allergy.

From NIOSH, 1997a.

TABLE 3-1   **Products Containing Latex and Nonlatex Substitutes***

Products Containing Latex	Nonlatex Substitutes
MEDICAL EQUIPMENT	
Disposable gloves	Vinyl, nitrile, or neoprene gloves
Blood pressure cuffs	Covered cuffs
Stethoscope tubing	Covered tubing
Intravenous injection ports	Needleless system, stopcocks, covered latex ports
Tourniquets	Cloth-covered tourniquets
Syringes	Glass syringes
Adhesive tape	Nonlatex tapes
Oral and nasal airways	Nonlatex tubes
Endotracheal tubes	Hard plastic tubes
Catheters	Silicone catheters
Eye goggles	Silicone eye goggles
Anesthesia masks	Silicone masks
Respirators	Nonlatex respirators
Rubber aprons	Cloth-covered aprons
Wound drains	Silicone drains
Medication vial stoppers	Stoppers removed
HOUSEHOLD ITEMS	
Rubber bands	String
Erasers	Silicone erasers
Automobile tires	(No substitute)
Motorcycle and bicycle handgrips	Handgrips removed or covered
Carpeting	Other types of flooring
Swimming goggles	Silicone construction
Racquet handles	Handles covered
Shoe soles	Leather shoes
Expandable fabric (e.g., waistbands)	Fabric removed or covered
Dishwashing gloves	Vinyl gloves
Hot water bottles	Microwavable, cloth-covered warmers
Condoms	Nonlatex condoms
Diaphragms	Synthetic rubber diaphragms
Balloons	Mylar balloons
Pacifiers and baby bottle nipples	Silicone, plastic, or nonlatex pacifiers and nipples

*This list is intended to provide examples of products. It is not an exhaustive list.

EXAMINATION TECHNIQUE

PATIENT POSITIONS AND DRAPING

Most of the physical examination is conducted with the patient in the seated and supine positions. Other positions are used for specific aspects of the examination. Special positioning requirements are discussed in the relevant chapters.

Seated. When seated, the drape should cover the patient's lap and legs. It can be moved to uncover parts of the body as they are examined.

Supine. In the supine position, the patient lies on his or her back, with arms at the sides and legs extended. The drape should cover the patient from chest to knees or toes. Again, you can move or reposition the drape to give appropriate exposure.

Prone. The patient lies on his or her stomach. This position may be used for special maneuvers as part of the musculoskeletal examination. Drape the patient to cover the torso.

Dorsal Recumbent. The dorsal recumbent position may be used for examination of the genital or rectal areas. The patient lies supine with knees bent and feet flat on the table. Place the drape in a diamond position from chest to toes. Wrap each leg with the corresponding lateral corner of the "diamond". Turn back the distal corner of the drape to perform the examination.

Lateral Recumbent. This is a side-lying position, with legs extended or flexed. The left lateral recumbent position (patient's left side is down) may be used in listening to heart sounds.

Lithotomy. The lithotomy position is generally used for the pelvic examination. Variations of positioning are discussed in Chapter 18. Begin with the patient in the dorsal recumbent position, with feet at the corners of the table. Help the patient to stabilize her feet in the stirrups and slide her buttocks down to the edge of the table. Drape in the diamond position as with the dorsal recumbent position.

Sims. The Sims position can be used for examination of the rectum or obtaining rectal temperature. The patient starts in a lateral recumbent position. The torso is rolled toward a prone position; the top leg is flexed sharply at the hips and knee and the bottom leg is flexed slightly. Drape the patient from shoulders to toes.

INSPECTION

Inspection is the process of observation. Your eyes and nose are sensitive tools for gathering data throughout the examination (Box 3-4). Take time to practice and develop this skill. Challenge yourself to see how much information you can collect through inspection alone. As the patient enters the room, for example, observe the gait and stance and the ease or difficulty with which undressing and getting onto the examining table are accomplished. These observations alone will reveal a great deal about the patient's neurologic and musculoskeletal integrity. Is eye contact made? Is the demeanor appropriate for the situation? Is the clothing appropriate for the weather? The answers to these questions provide clues to the patient's emotional and mental status. Color and moisture of the skin or an unusual odor can alert you to the possibility of underlying disease. These preliminary observations require only a few seconds, yet they provide basic information that can influence the rest of the examination.

Inspection—unlike palpation, percussion, and auscultation—can continue throughout the history-taking process and during the physical examination. With this kind of continuity, what you see about the patient and the patient's demeanor is constantly subject to confirmation or dispute. Be aware of both the patient's verbal statements and body language right up to the end of the appointment. At that point, the stance, stride, strength of a handshake, and eye contact can tell you a great deal about the patient's perception of the encounter. Box 3-5 highlights some cultural aspects to consider when examining patients.

Some general guidelines will be helpful as you proceed through the examination and inspect each area of the body. Adequate lighting is essential. The primary lighting can be either daylight or artificial light, as long as the light is direct enough to reveal color, texture, and mobility without distortion from shadowing. Secondary, tangential lighting from a lamp that casts shadows is also important for observing contour and variations in the body surface. Inspection should be unhurried. Give yourself time to tune in to what you are inspecting. Pay attention to detail and note your findings. An important rule to remember is that you have to

---

BOX 3-4

THE SENSE OF SMELL: THE NOSE AS AN AID TO PHYSICAL EXAMINATION

The first observation when entering an examining room may be an odor, obvious and pervasive. A foreign body that has been present in a child's nose may cause this. Indeed, many problematic conditions can be characterized in this way, but the presentation is rather subtle more often than obvious. Distinctive odors provide clues leading to the diagnosis of certain conditions, some of which need early detection if life-threatening sequelae are to be avoided. Examples of odor clues follow:

	Source of Odor	Type of Odor
Inborn errors of metabolism	Phenylalanine hydroxylase defect	Mousy
	Tyrosinemia	Fishy
Infectious diseases	Tuberculosis	Stale beer
	Diphtheria	Sweetish
Ingestions of poison or intoxication	Cyanide	Bitter almond
	Chloroform and salicylates	Fruity
Physiologic nondisease states	Sweaty feet	Cheesy
Foreign bodies (e.g., in the nose or vagina)	Organic material (e.g., bean in a child's nose)	Foul-smelling discharge

The odors may range from objectionable to bland to rather pleasant. The descriptors include fishy, putrid, fetid, alcoholic, bitter almond, and on and on. The examiner often is the one to determine the characterization of the odor.

In years past, practiced clinicians noted that certain breath and body odors were indicative of a variety of conditions or diseases. Examples follow:

Condition or Disease	Odor
Yellow fever	Butcher shop
Typhoid fever	Fresh-baked bread
Diabetic coma	Fruity
Scurvy	Putrid
Pellagra	Sour, musty bread

These lessons from the past remind us that the nose, fully as much as our other sensors, is portable equipment. We must train ourselves in its use if it is to be of value to us as competent examiners.

Suggested by a Grand Rounds presentation, Rebecca Vickers, MD, May 28, 1997.

BOX 3-5

EXAMINATION TECHNIQUES: CULTURAL CONSIDERATIONS

Nonverbal communication, which includes touch, posture, space, and facial expression, is an integral part of physical examination. Nonverbal communication may have different meanings in different cultures. For example, in North American middle-class culture, direct eye contact is important, whereas in some other cultures (e.g., Asian, Native American/American Indian, Indochinese, Arab, and Appalachian), looking directly at another person may be a sign of disrespect or aggression.

Touch is also subject to varied cultural interpretations. Some groups, such as those of Mediterranean descent, use touch to communicate feelings, whereas other groups view touch as an invasion of privacy. As you become sensitive to cultural variations, remember that individuals are just that—individual—and avoid the pitfall of making decisions based on stereotypes rather than on specifics of the patient and the circumstances.

---

expose what you want to inspect. All too often, necessary exposure is compromised for modesty at the cost of important information. Part of your job is to look and observe critically.

Knowing what to look for is, of course, essential to the process of focused attention. Be willing to validate inspection findings with your patient. The ability to narrow or widen your perceptual field selectively will come with time and experience, but the process must begin right now and will develop only through practice.

PALPATION

Palpation involves the use of the hands and fingers to gather information through the sense of touch. Certain parts of your hands and fingers are better than others for specific types of palpation (Table 3-2). The palmar surface of the fingers and finger pads is more sensitive than the fingertips and is used whenever discriminatory touch is needed for determining position, tex-

CLINICAL PEARL

Right-Sided Examination?
It is the convention, at least in the United States, to teach students to examine patients from the right side and to palpate and percuss with the right hand. We have generally continued with this convention, if only to simplify description of a procedure or technique. We feel no obligation to adhere strictly to the right-sided approach. Our suggestion is that students learn to use both hands for examination and that they be allowed to stand on either side of the patient, depending on both the patient's and examiner's convenience and comfort. The important issue is to develop an approach that is useful and practical and yields the desired results.

TABLE 3-2	Areas of the Hand to Use in Palpation
To Determine	**Use**
Position, texture, size, consistency, fluid, crepitus, form of a mass, or structure	Palmar surface of the fingers and finger pads
Vibration	Ulnar surfaces of hand and fingers
Temperature	Dorsal surface of hand

ture, size, consistency, masses, fluid, and crepitus. The ulnar surface of the hand and fingers is the most sensitive area for distinguishing vibration. The dorsal surface of the hands is best for estimating temperature. Of course, this estimate provides only a crude measure and is best used to detect temperature differences in comparing parts of the body.

Specific techniques of palpation are discussed in more detail as they occur in each part of the examination. Palpation may be either light or deep and is controlled by the amount of pressure applied with the fingers or hand. For light palpation, press in to a depth up to 1 cm; for deep palpation, press in about 4 cm. Light palpation should always precede deep palpation, because the latter may elicit tenderness or disrupt tissue or fluid, thus interfering with your ability to gather information through light palpation. Short fingernails are essential to avoid discomfort or injury to the patient.

Touch is in many ways therapeutic, and palpation is the actuality of the "laying on of hands." It is the moment at which we begin our physical invasion of the patient's body. Our much repeated advice that your approach be gentle and your hands be warm is not only practical but also symbolic of your respect for the patient and for the privilege the patient gives you.

PERCUSSION

Percussion involves striking one object against another to produce vibration and subsequent sound waves. In the physical examination, your finger functions as a hammer, and the vibration is produced by the impact of the finger against underlying tissue. Sound waves are heard as percussion tones (called *resonance*) that arise from vibrations 4 to 6 cm deep in the body tissue. The density of the medium through which the sound waves travel determines the degree of percussion tone. The more dense the medium, the quieter the percussion tone. The percussion tone over air is loud, over fluid less loud, and over solid areas soft. The degree of percussion tone is classified and ordered as listed in Table 3-3 and as follows:

- Tympany
- Hyperresonance
- Resonance
- Dullness
- Flatness

Tympany is the loudest, and flatness is the quietest. Quantification of the percussion tone is difficult, especially for the beginner. For points of reference, as noted in Table 3-3, the gastric bubble is considered to be tympanic; air-filled lungs (as in emphysema) to be hyperresonant;

TABLE 3-3	Percussion Tones				
Tone	**Intensity**	**Pitch**	**Duration**	**Quality**	**Example Where Heard**
Tympanic	Loud	High	Moderate	Drumlike	Gastric bubble
Hyperresonant	Very loud	Low	Long	Boomlike	Emphysematous lungs
Resonant	Loud	Low	Long	Hollow	Healthy lung tissue
Dull	Soft to moderate	Moderate to high	Moderate	Thudlike	Over liver
Flat	Soft	High	Short	Very dull	Over muscle

healthy lungs to be resonant; the liver to be dull; and muscle to be flat. Degree of percussion is more easily distinguished by listening to the sound change as you move from one area to another. Because it is easier to hear the change from resonance to dullness rather than from dullness to resonance, proceed with percussion from areas of resonance to areas of dullness. A partially full milk carton is a good tool for practicing percussion skills. Begin with percussion over the air-filled space of the carton, appreciating its resonant quality. Work your way downward and listen for the change in sound as you encounter the milk. This principle applies in percussion of body tissues and cavities.

The techniques of percussion are the same regardless of the structure you are percussing. Immediate (direct) percussion involves striking the finger or hand directly against the body. Most clinicians use a variant of the technique, mediate or indirect percussion. In this technique the finger of one hand acts as the hammer (plexor) and a finger of the other hand acts as the striking surface. To perform indirect percussion, place your nondominant hand on the surface of the body with the fingers slightly spread. The distal phalanx of the middle finger should be placed firmly on the body surface with the other fingers slightly elevated off the surface. Snap the wrist of your other hand downward, and with the tip of the middle finger sharply tap the interphalangeal joint of the finger that is on the body surface (Fig. 3-1). You may tap just distal to the interphalangeal joint if you choose, but decide on one and be consistent because the sound varies from one to the other. If you are not able to hear the percussion tone try pressing harder against the patient's skin with your finger that lies on the body surface. Failing to press firmly enough is a common error. On the other hand, pressing too hard on an infant or very young chest can be obscuring.

Several points are essential in developing the technique of percussion. The downward snap of the striking finger originates from the wrist and not the forearm or shoulder. The tap should be sharp and rapid; once the finger has struck, snap the wrist back, quickly lifting the finger to prevent dampening the sound. Use the tip and not the pad of the plexor finger (hence short fingernails are again a necessity). Percuss one location several times to facilitate interpretation of the tone. Like other techniques, percussion requires practice to obtain the skill needed to produce the desired result. Box 3-6 describes common percussion errors. In learning to distinguish between the tones, it may be helpful to close your eyes to block out other sensory stimuli, concentrating exclusively on the tone you are hearing.

The fist may also be used in percussion. Fist percussion is most commonly used to elicit tenderness arising from the liver, gallbladder, or kidneys. In this technique, use the ulnar aspect of the fist to deliver a firm blow to the area. Too gentle a blow will not produce enough force to stimulate the tenderness, but too hearty a blow can create unnecessary discomfort even in a well patient. The force of a direct blow can be mediated by use of a second hand placed over the area. Practice on yourself or a colleague until you achieve the desired middle ground.

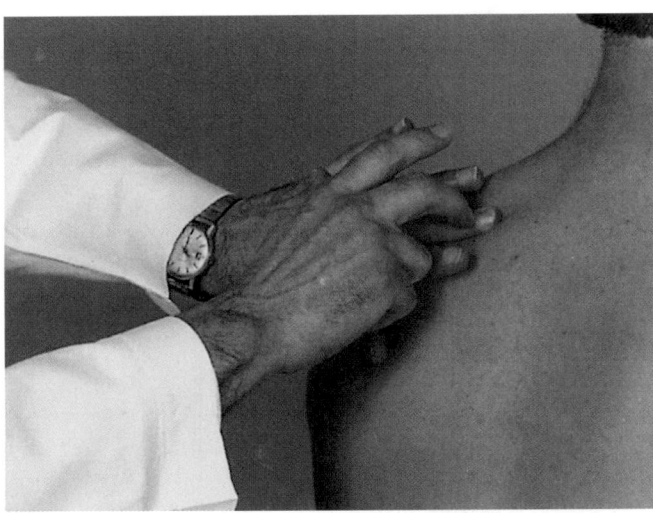

FIGURE 3-1
Percussion technique: tapping the interphalangeal joint. Only the middle finger of the examiner's nondominant hand should be in contact with the patient's skin surface.

BOX 3-6

COMMON PERCUSSION ERRORS

Percussion requires practice, but practice of incorrect techniques will not assist in obtaining the desired results. In learning percussion, beginning practitioners often make the following errors:
- Failing to exert firm pressure with the finger placed on the skin surface
- Failing to separate the hammer finger from other fingers
- Snapping downward from the elbow or shoulder rather than from the wrist
- Tapping by moving just the hammer finger rather than the whole hand
- Striking with the finger pad rather than the fingertip of the hammer finger

---

AUSCULTATION

Auscultation involves listening for sounds produced by the body. Some sounds, such as speech, are audible to the unassisted ear. Most others require a stethoscope to augment the sound. Specific types of stethoscopes, their use, and desired characteristics are discussed later in the section on stethoscopes.

Although what you are listening for will depend on the specific part of the examination, there are some general principles that apply to all auscultatory procedures. The environment should be quiet and free from distracting noises. Place the stethoscope on the naked skin, because clothing obscures the sound. Listen not only for the presence of sound but also its characteristics: intensity, pitch, duration, and quality. The sounds are often subtle or transitory, and you must listen intently to hear the nuances. Closing your eyes may prevent distraction by visual stimuli and narrow your perceptual field to help you focus on the sound. Try to target and isolate each sound, concentrating on one sound at a time. Take enough time to identify all the characteristics of each sound. Auscultation should be carried out last, except with the abdominal examination, after other techniques have provided information that will assist in interpreting what you hear. Too often the temptation is to rush right in with the stethoscope, thus missing the opportunity to gather other data that would be useful.

One of the most difficult achievements in auscultation is learning to isolate sounds. You cannot hear everything all at once. Whether it is a breath sound, or a heartbeat, or the sequence of respirations and heartbeats, each segment of the cycle must be isolated and listened to specifically. After the individual sounds are identified, they are put together. Do not anticipate the next sound; concentrate on the one at hand. Auscultation of the lungs is discussed in Chapter 13, the heart in Chapter 14, and the abdomen in Chapter 17.

CLINICAL PEARL

Unexpected Findings

The key (one among several) to a successful physical examination is to respect your judgment and your instinct whenever you find that which you had not expected to find—that is, when your sense of the expected or of what you might call the "normal" has been violated. Pay attention when that happens even if it does not seem to make sense or you cannot explain it easily.

MEASUREMENT OF VITAL SIGNS

The pulse, respiration, blood pressure, and temperature are considered the baseline indicators of a patient's health status: this is why they are called *vital signs*. They may be measured early in the physical examination or integrated into separate aspects of the examination.

PULSE

The pulse may be palpated in several different areas; however, the radial pulse is most often used as the screening measure for heart rate, which is the number of cardiac cycles per minute. With the pads of your second and third fingers, palpate the radial pulse on the flexor surface of the wrist laterally. Count the pulsations, also noting their rhythm, amplitude, and contour. A detailed discussion of evaluation of arterial pulses is found in Chapter 15.

RESPIRATIONS

Respirations are counted and evaluated by inspection. Observe the rise and fall of the patient's chest and the ease with which breathing is accomplished. Count the number of respiratory cycles (i.e., inspiration and expiration) that occur in 1 minute to determine the respiratory rate. In infants the rise and fall of the abdomen with respiration facilitates the count. Also observe the regularity and rhythm of the breathing pattern. Note the depth of respirations and whether the patient uses accessory muscles. A more thorough evaluation of respiration is described in Chapter 13.

BLOOD PRESSURE

Blood pressure is a peripheral measurement of cardiovascular function. Indirect measures of blood pressure are made with a stethoscope and either an aneroid or mercury sphygmomanometer. Electronic sphygmomanometers, which do not require the use of a stethoscope, are also available. Each sphygmomanometer is composed of a cuff with an inflatable bladder, a pressure manometer, and a rubber hand bulb with a pressure control valve to inflate and deflate the bladder. The electronic sphygmomanometer senses vibrations and converts them into electric impulses. The impulses are transmitted to a device that translates them into a digital readout. The instrument is relatively sensitive and is also capable of simultaneously measuring the pulse rate. It does not, however, indicate the quality, rhythm, and other characteristics of a pulse and should not be used in place of your touch in assessing pulse.

Cuffs are available in a number of sizes; the appropriate size is determined by the size of the patient's limb (Fig. 3-2). For adults, choose a width that is one-third to one-half the circumference of the limb. The length of the bladder should be twice the width (about 80% of the limb circumference), not quite enough to completely encircle the limb. For children, the cuff width should cover approximately two thirds of the upper arm or thigh. For both adults and children, cuffs that are too wide will underestimate blood pressure, and those that are too narrow will give an artificially high measurement. The correct cuff size ensures that equal pressure will be exerted around the artery, thus resulting in an accurate measurement.

Other pointers for using blood pressure equipment are as follows:

- If you are using a mercury sphygmomanometer, keep the manometer vertical and make all readings at eye level, no more than 3 feet away.
- If you are using an aneroid instrument, position the dial so it faces you directly, no more than 3 feet away. An aneroid manometer becomes inaccurate with repeated use and needs periodic calibration.
- If the patient has an obese arm, substitute a larger cuff, using the cuff size principles to choose the appropriate size. If a sufficiently large cuff is unavailable, a standard cuff can be wrapped around the forearm and a stethoscope placed over the radial artery. The size of the cuff and the site of auscultation should be recorded.
- If the adult patient is very thin, a pediatric cuff may be necessary.

CLINICAL PEARL

Choosing the Right Blood Pressure Cuff for a Child

Because children (even those of the same age) vary markedly in build, choosing the correct blood pressure cuff is more than a matter of size-for-age recommendations. The following guidelines will assist you in choosing an appropriately sized cuff to obtain the most accurate blood pressure reading:

- The bladder width should not exceed two-thirds the length of the upper or lower arm.
- The bladder length should not completely wrap around or overlap the extremity used to take the measurement, but ideally should cover three-fourths the circumference of the extremity.

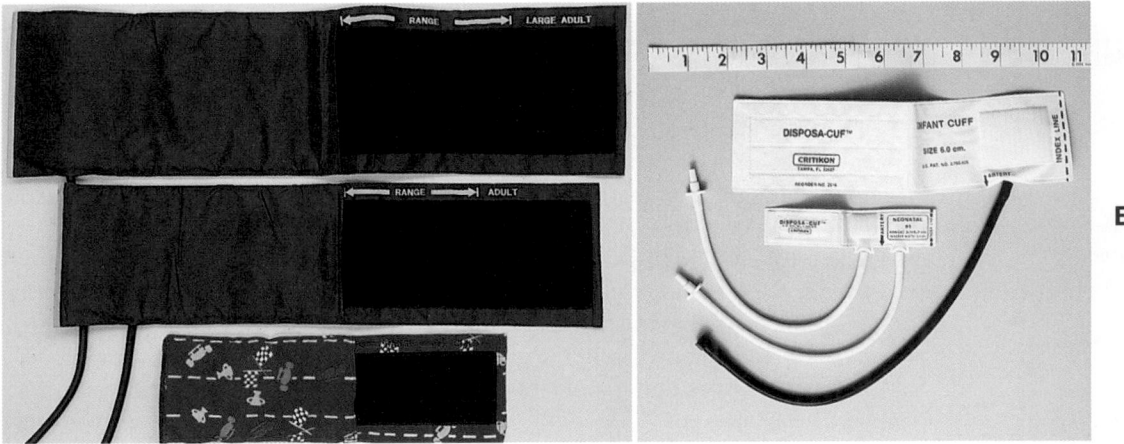

FIGURE 3-2
Select the appropriately sized blood pressure cuff. **A,** *(From top)* large adult, adult, and child cuffs.
B, Infant cuff *(top)* and neonatal cuff for use with Dinamap vital signs monitor *(bottom).*
A *from Thompson, Wilson, 1996.*

◆ Avoid slow or repeated inflations of the cuff, which can cause venous congestion and result in inaccurate readings. If repeated measurements are needed, wait at least 15 seconds between readings, with the cuff fully deflated. You can also remove the cuff and elevate the arm for 1 or 2 minutes.

◆ Auscultatory systolic readings tend to be somewhat lower than those of oscillometric devices. They are not interchangeable.

The specific technique for measuring blood pressure is described in Chapter 15.

TEMPERATURE

The assessment of body temperature may often provide an important clue to the severity of a patient's illness. In cases of bacterial infection it may well be the most critical diagnostic indicator, especially with infants, toddlers, and older adults. Temperature measurement can be accomplished through several different routes, most commonly oral, rectal, axillary, and tympanic.

Electronic temperature measurement has decreased the time required for accurate temperature readings (Fig. 3-3, *A*). One piece of equipment that contains an electronic sensing probe can be used for measurement of rectal, oral, and axillary temperatures. The probe, covered by a disposable sheath, is placed either under the tongue with the mouth tightly closed; in the rectum; or in the axillary space with the arm held close to the torso. A temperature reading (in either Fahrenheit or Celsius) is revealed on a liquid crystal display (LCD) screen within 15 to 60 seconds, depending on the model used.

The measurements obtained from tympanic thermometers vary somewhat from those obtained by oral or rectal routes (Fig. 3-3, *B* and *C*). In some situations, as with very young infants, traditional routes of measurement may be more accurate; in other situations, such as with children in an outpatient setting, the tympanic route is preferred. Although tympanic thermometers are simple to use, accurate measurement depends on correct technique, so be sure to follow the manufacturer's instructions.

For tympanic membrane temperature measurement, a specially designed probe similar in shape to an otoscope is required. Gently place the covered probe tip at the external opening of

A	B	C
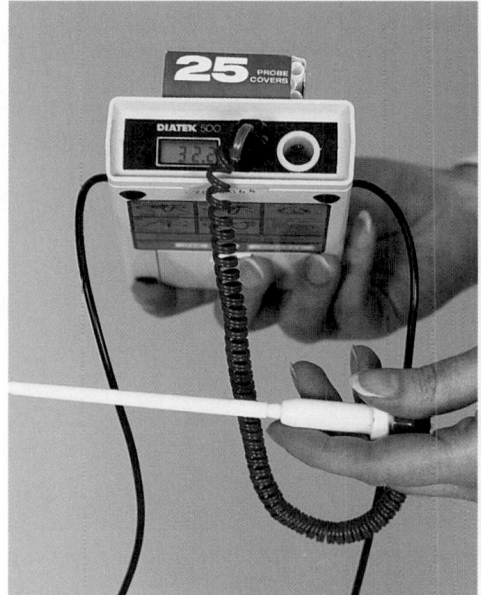	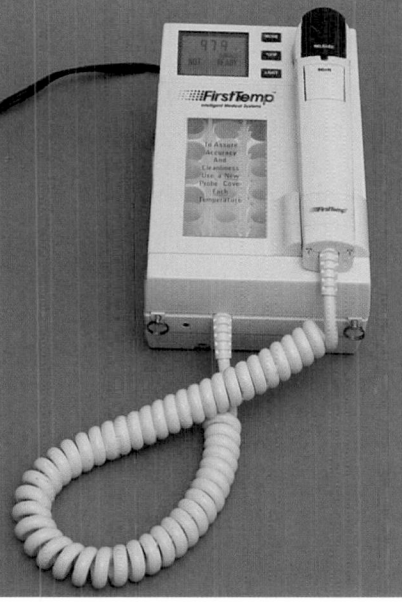	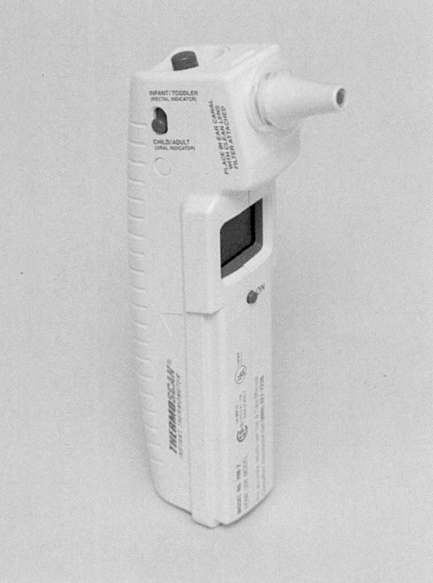

FIGURE 3-3
Devices for electronic temperature measurement. **A,** Rectal, oral, or axillary thermometer.
B and **C,** Tympanic membrane thermometers.

the ear canal. Do not try to force the probe into the canal or to occlude it. Infrared technology provides a temperature reading on the LCD screen in approximately 2 seconds. Ear temperature reflects the body's temperature because the tympanic membrane shares its blood supply with the hypothalamus in the brain.

Infrared axillary thermometers for neonates are available. Axillary measurements correlate well with core temperatures of newborns because of the infant's small body mass and uniform skin blood flow. A recessed reflective cup on the probe protects the measurement from the effects of external heat sources, making these thermometers suitable for use in incubators and under radiant warmers or phototherapy lights.

PAIN

Pain, because of its ubiquitous nature, its universality as a distress signal, and its frequency as a chief complaint, is more and more often being recognized as the fifth vital sign. Throughout the text we have included assessment of pain as it pertains to the specific body systems. Chapter 7 describes specific history questions, cues to watch for in the physical examination, and pain assessment scales.

MEASUREMENT OF HEIGHT AND WEIGHT

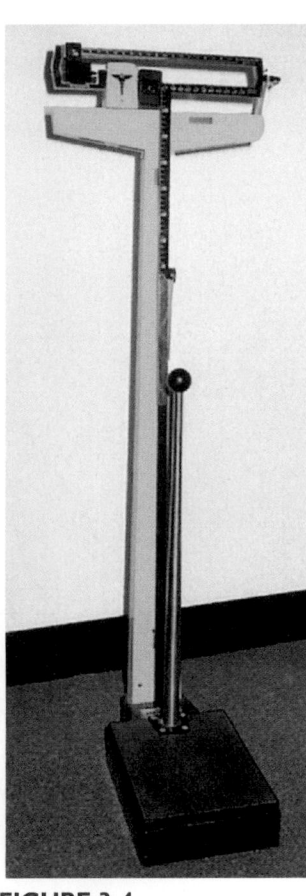

FIGURE 3-4
Platform scale with height attachment.

Height and weight of adults are measured on a standing platform scale with a height attachment. The scale uses a system of adding and subtracting weight in increments as small as ¼ lb or 0.1 kg to counterbalance the weight placed on the scale platform. The scale needs to be manually calibrated each time it is used.

Calibrate the scale to zero before the patient mounts the platform by moving both the large and small weights to zero. The balance beam should be made level and steady by adjusting the calibrating knob. Pull up the height attachment, and position the headpiece at the patient's crown (Fig. 3-4). The height attachment should be pulled up before the patient steps on the scale to avoid a jab with the horizontal piece. Place a paper towel on the platform before the patient steps on it to avoid the potential transmission of organisms from bare feet.

With electronic scales, weight is calculated electronically and provided as a digital readout. These scales are automatically calibrated each time they are used.

The infant platform scale is used for measuring weights of infants and small children (Fig. 3-5). It works the same as the adult scale but can measure in ounces or grams. The scale has a platform with curved sides in which the child may sit or lie. Place paper under the child, and use caution to never leave the child unattended on the scale.

Infant lengths can be measured by using an infant measuring device that comes with a rigid headboard and movable footboard (Fig. 3-6, A). An alternative to the rigid measuring device is a commercially available measure mat, consisting of a soft rubber graduated mat attached to a plastic headboard and footboard (Fig. 3-6, B). The measuring board is placed on the table so that the headboard and footboard are perpendicular to the table. The infant lies supine on the measuring board with the head against the headboard. The footboard is moved until it touches the bottom of the infant's feet. The baby's length can be read in either inches or centimeters. Be sure to clean the mat between uses.

An infant can also be measured by placing the baby on a pad, putting one pin into the pad at the top of the head and another at the heel of the extended leg. The length is then measured from pin to pin. The same technique can be used with a marking pen if the infant is lying on a disposable paper sheet.

Once a child is able to stand erect without support, a stature-measuring device is used to measure height. The device consists of a movable headpiece attached to a rigid measurement bar and platform. A tape measure attached to the wall and a movable headpiece can also be used (Fig. 3-7).

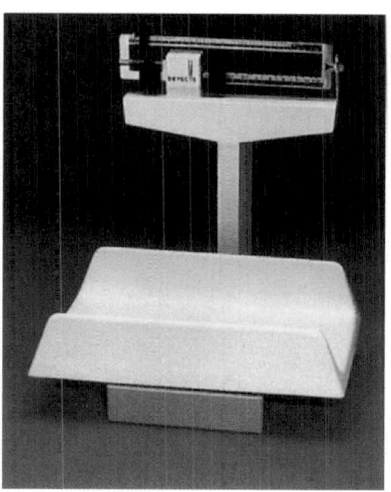

FIGURE 3-5
Infant platform scale.

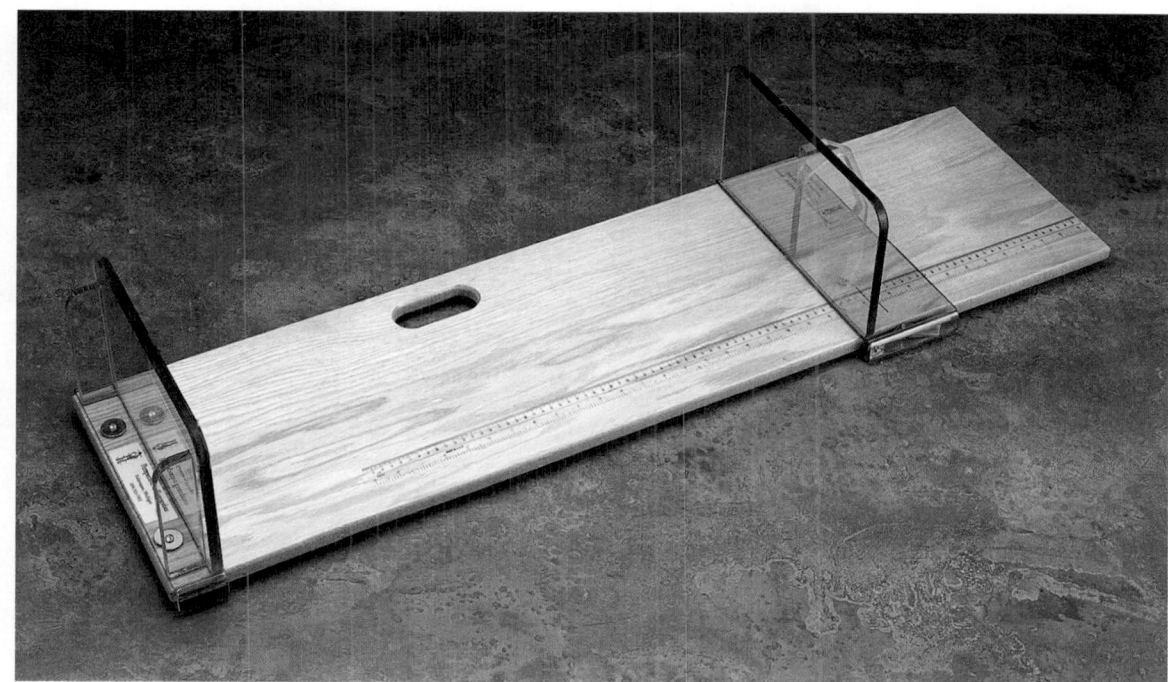

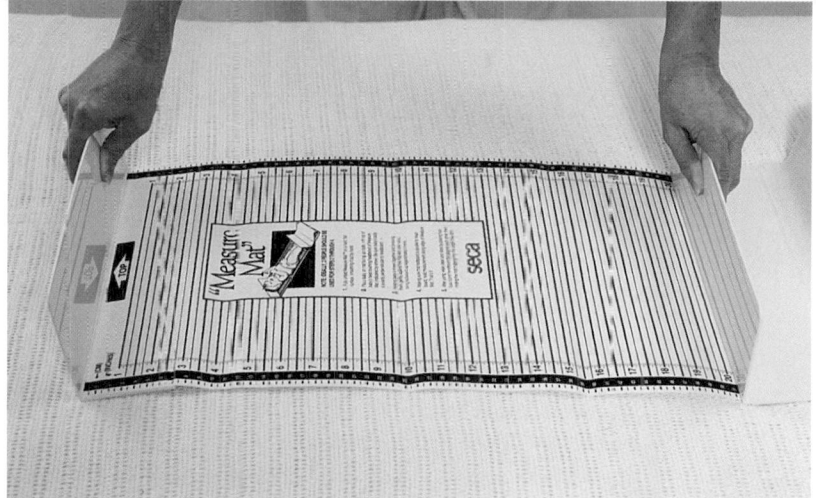

A

B

FIGURE 3-6
Devices used to measure length of an infant. **A,** Infant length board. **B,** Measure mat.
B *Courtesy of Perspective Enterprises, Inc., Portage, MI.*

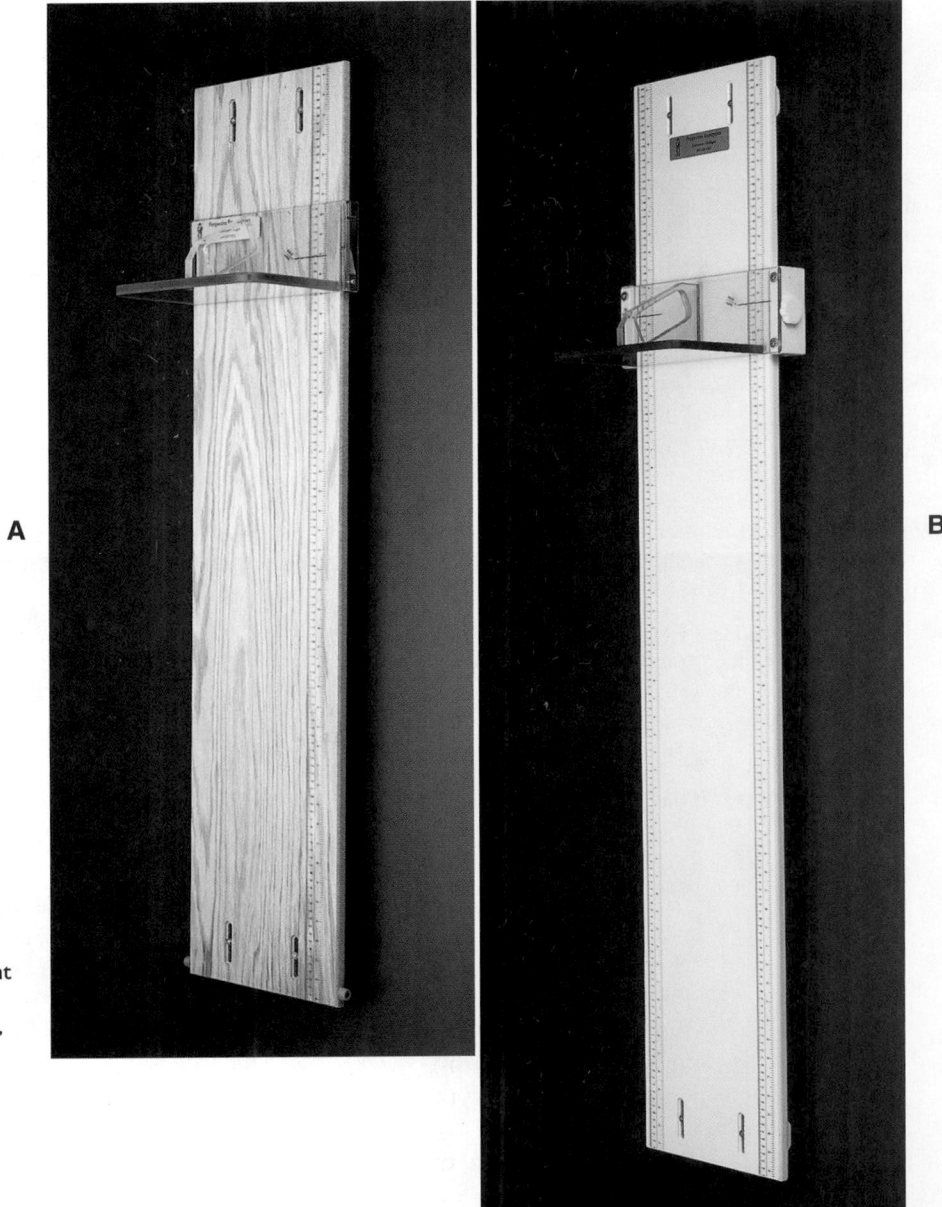

A

B

FIGURE 3-7
Devices used to measure height
of a child.
Courtesy of Perspective Enterprises,
Inc., Portage, MI.

MODIFICATIONS FOR PATIENTS WITH DISABILITIES

Each disability affects each person differently; therefore it is important for clinicians to educate themselves about relevant aspects of a patient's disability. A clinician's sensitivity in asking only pertinent questions about the disability will increase the patient's comfort and cooperation.

Keep some considerations in mind about the environment and the encounter. Speak directly to the patient. Often people will address a disabled person's friend, attendant, or an interpreter instead of speaking directly to the person. Removing or rearranging the furnishings in the examination room will provide the space needed for a wheelchair or for an interpreter to be seen. The paper covering can be taken off the examination table if it is a bother during transfers and positioning. Equipment such as a high-low examination table or a particularly wide examination table or a slide board can be obtained to facilitate safer, easier transfers and positioning. Obstetric or foot stirrups can be padded or equipped with a strap to increase the

---

BOX 3-7

TRANSFER GUIDELINES

Guidelines for the Lifter

- The patient should direct the transfer and positioning process.
- Assistants should not overestimate their ability to lift.
- Keep in mind that not all nonambulatory patients need assistance.
- Assistants should keep their backs straight, bend their knees, and lift with their legs.
- It may be helpful to perform a test lift or to practice the transfer by lifting the patient just over the wheelchair before attempting a complete transfer.
- Assistants who feel that they may drop a patient during a transfer should not panic. It is important, whenever possible, to explain what is happening to reassure the patient throughout the situation. Assistants will usually have time to lower the patient safely to the floor until they can get additional help.

Guidelines for the Disabled Patient

- Explain clearly the preferred transfer method and direct the clinician and assistants during the process.
- Assistants can help by preparing equipment. Because many people are not familiar with wheelchairs or supportive de-

vices, the patient may need to explain to the clinicians and assistants how they can handle belongings. Patients who use wheelchairs should explain how to apply the brakes, detach the footrests and armrests, or turn off the motor of an electric wheelchair. Have the patient who wears adaptive devices (e.g., leg braces or supportive undergarments) explain how to remove them, if necessary, and where to put them if the patient cannot do so.

- Patients who use urinary equipment should direct assistants in the moving or straightening of catheter tubing. The patient may wish to unstrap the leg bag and place it on the table beside or across the abdomen for proper drainage while supine. Assistants should be reminded not to pull on the tubing or allow kinks to develop.
- Have the patient inform the clinician and assistants when he or she is comfortable and balanced, after the transfer is completed.
- All parties should be aware of jewelry, clothing, tubing, or equipment that might catch or otherwise interfere with the transfer.

---

patient's comfort and safety during a pelvic examination. If a urine sample is required, a patient with mobility impairment (e.g., spinal cord injury, polio, or cerebral palsy) should be given the option of bringing a urine sample to the appointment. Because it is not necessary for patients to remove all their clothes for all examinations, partial undressing can conserve time and energy. For the pelvic examination, a woman can wear an easily removable skirt or pair of pants. A button-up or zippered shirt will facilitate the breast examination. It is appropriate to suggest to your patient or the caregiver that such clothing be worn.

PATIENTS WITH MOBILITY IMPAIRMENTS

The patient is the expert in transferring from the wheelchair or in using assistants to climb onto the examination table. Transfers are relatively simple if the patient, assistant, and clinician all understand the method that will best suit the patient's disability, the room space, and the examination table (Box 3-7).

Pivot Transfer. Standing in front of the patient, the assistant takes the patient's knees between his or her own knees, grasps the patient around the back and under the arms, raises the patient to a vertical position, and then pivots from wheelchair to the table. The examination table must be low enough for the patient to sit on; therefore a hydraulic high-low table may be needed when using this transfer method.

Cradle Transfer. While bending or squatting beside the patient, the assistant puts one arm under both of the patient's knees and the other arm around the back and under the armpits. The assistant stands and carries the patient to the table. If one assistant cannot do it alone, two assistants can grasp each other's arms behind the patient's back and under the knees. It is important that both assistants work together.

Two-Person Transfer. In all two-person transfers, the assistants must be careful to work together to lift the patient over the arms of the wheelchair from a sitting position onto the examination table. A stronger, taller person should always lift the upper half of the patient's body. There are two ways to perform a two-person transfer.

- *Method 1* requires the patient to fold the arms across the chest. The assistant standing behind the patient kneels down, putting his or her elbows under the patient's armpits, and grasps the patient's opposite wrists. The second assistant lifts and supports the patient under the knees.

- *Method 2* can be used if the patient cannot fold the arms. The assistant standing behind the patient puts his or her own hands together around the patient if possible so there is less likelihood of losing hold of the patient. The second assistant lifts and supports the patient under the knees.

Equipment. Some disabled persons use a slide board, which forms a bridge to slide across from the wheelchair to the examination table. For this method to work, the table and chair must be approximately the same height. Most examination tables, however, are quite a bit higher than wheelchairs. Some examining rooms have high-low examination tables that can be adjusted to a height that will facilitate the safest and easiest transfer. A wider table, even if it is not adjustable in height, can also make transfers and positioning easier.

PATIENTS WITH SENSORY IMPAIRMENT

At the beginning of the visit by a hearing-impaired or speech-impaired patient, discuss the communication system that will be used (e.g., a sign language interpreter, word board, or talk box). Specialized educational materials (e.g., braille or audiotaped information, or three-dimensional anatomic models) can be acquired to make information accessible to sensory-impaired patients.

Impaired Vision. Clinicians or assistants should remember to identify themselves upon entering the examination room and inform the patient when they are leaving the room. A red-tipped white cane and guide animal are mobility aids used by many visually impaired people. If a patient is accompanied by a guide animal, do not pet or distract the animal, which is trained to respond only to its owner. A patient may prefer to keep the guide animal or white cane nearby in the examination room. Do not move either of these without the patient's permission. Before the examination, ask whether the patient would like to examine any equipment or instruments that will be used during the examination. If three-dimensional models are available, they can be used to acquaint the patient with the examination process (e.g., with the genital examination). During the examination, the patient may feel more at ease if you maintain continuous tactile or verbal contact; for example, by keeping a hand on the arm or by narrating what is taking place during the examination.

Some visually impaired patients will want to be oriented to their surroundings, whereas others may not. Each should be encouraged to specify the kind of orientation and mobility assistance needed. Verbally describe and assist the patient in locating where to put the clothes, where the various furnishings are positioned, how to approach the examination table, and how to get positioned on the table.

Impaired Hearing or Speech. The patient should choose which form of communication to use during the examination (e.g., a sign language interpreter, lip reading, or writing). Although a patient may use an interpreter throughout most of the visit, she or he may decide not to use the interpreter during parts of the actual examination. If an interpreter is used, the patient and the clinician should decide where the interpreter should stand. When working with an interpreter, speak at a regular speed and directly to the patient instead of to the interpreter. If a patient wishes to lip-read, be careful not to move your face out of sight of the patient without first explaining what you are doing. Look directly at the patient and enunciate words clearly. Some patients may wish to view a pelvic examination with a mirror while it is happening.

SPECIAL CONCERNS FOR PATIENTS WITH DISABILITIES

Bowel and bladder concerns such as hyperreflexia, hypersensitivity, and spasticity are conditions common to many disabled people and should be given special attention during the examination process.

Bowel and Bladder Concerns. Some disabled patients (e.g., those with spinal cord injuries or spina bifida) do not have voluntary bladder or bowel movements. A bladder or bowel routine could affect the pelvic or rectal examination. The physical stimulation of a speculum, bimanual, or rectal examination can mimic the stimulation for the bowel routine and cause a bowel movement during the examination. An indwelling catheter need not be removed during the examination unless it is not working; if it is removed, another catheter should be available for insertion. If a woman is catheterized, it is not necessary to remove the catheter during the pelvic examination because it will not interfere in any way.

If a patient uses intermittent catheterization to manually open the bladder sphincter at regular intervals during the day, tactile stimulation in the pelvic area during the examination could cause the bladder sphincter to open and produce incontinence.

Autonomic Hyperreflexia. Autonomic hyperreflexia, also called hyperflexia or dysreflexia, describes a set of symptoms common to people with spinal cord injury. It is often due to stimulation of the bowel, bladder, or skin below the spinal lesion. Some causes of hyperreflexia that may occur during the physical examination include reactions to a cold, hard examination table or cold stirrups; insertion and manipulation of a speculum; pressure during the bimanual or rectal examination; or tactile contact with hypersensitive areas. Common symptoms may include high blood pressure, sweating, blotchy skin, nausea, or goose bumps. If the patient experiences hyperreflexic high blood pressure, identify and remove the source of the stimulation. Once the hyperreflexia ceases, the patient and clinician should mutually decide whether to continue the examination. If the examination is continued and hyperreflexia recurs, another examination should be scheduled. If the blood pressure does not decrease with removal of stimulus, or if the hyperreflexic symptoms persist and lead to a throbbing headache or nasal obstruction, treat the situation as a medical emergency. A patient experiencing any degree of hyperreflexia should not be left unaccompanied.

Hypersensitivity. To help prevent possible discomfort or spasms, ask the patient about hypersensitive areas of the body before the examination. Some patients may experience variable responses (e.g., spasms or pain) to ordinary tactile stimulation. Often, sensitive areas can be avoided or an extra amount of lubricant jelly can be used to decrease friction or pressure.

Spasticity. Spasms may be a common aspect of a disability, ranging from slight tremors to quick, violent contractions. Spasms may occur during a transfer, while assuming an awkward or uncomfortable position, or from stimulation of the skin with an instrument. If spasm occurs during the examination, gently support the area (usually a leg, arm, or the abdominal region) to avoid any injury to the patient. Spasms should be allowed to resolve before the examination is continued.

A feeling of physical security can decrease spasm intensity or frequency. A disabled patient who experiences spasms should never be left alone on the examination table. An assistant should stand near the examination table and maintain physical contact with the patient to provide a feeling of safety.

INSTRUMENTATION

STETHOSCOPE

Auscultation of most sounds requires a stethoscope. Three basic types are available: acoustic, magnetic, and electronic.

The acoustic stethoscope is a closed cylinder that transmits sound waves from their source and along its column to the ear (Fig. 3-8). Its rigid diaphragm has a natural frequency of around 300 Hz. It screens out low-pitched sounds and best transmits high-pitched sounds such as the second heart sound. The bell endpiece, with which the skin acts as the diaphragm, has a natural frequency varying with the amount of pressure exerted. It transmits low-pitched sounds when very light pressure is used. With firm pressure, it converts to a diaphragm endpiece. The chestpiece contains a closure valve so that only one endpiece, either the diaphragm or bell, is operational at any one time (thus preventing inadvertent dissipation of sound waves).

The magnetic stethoscope has a single endpiece that is a diaphragm. It contains an iron disk on the interior surface; behind this is a permanent magnet. A strong spring keeps the diaphragm bowed outward when it is not compressed against a body surface. Compression of the diaphragm activates the air column as magnetic attraction is established between the iron disk and the magnet. Rotation of a dial adjusts for high, low, and full frequency sounds.

The electronic stethoscope picks up vibrations transmitted to the surface of the body and converts them into electrical impulses. The impulses are amplified and transmitted to a speaker where they are reconverted to sound. Newer versions of the electronic stethoscope can also provide additional features such as extended listening ranges, digital readout, sound recording and storage, playback, and computer linkage.

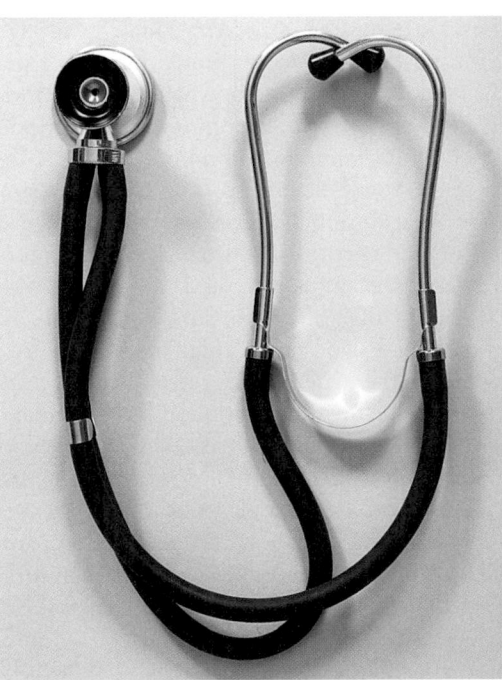

FIGURE 3-8
Acoustic stethoscope.

Of these, the most commonly used is the acoustic stethoscope, which comes in several models. The ability to auscultate accurately depends in part on the quality of the instrument, so it is important that the stethoscope have the following characteristics:

- The diaphragm and bell are heavy enough to lie firmly on the body surface.
- The diaphragm cover is rigid.
- The bell is large enough in diameter to span an intercostal space in an adult and deep enough so that it will not fill with tissue.
- A rubber or plastic ring is around the bell edges to ensure secure contact with the body surface.
- The tubing is thick, stiff, and heavy; this conducts better than thin, elastic, or very flexible tubing.
- The length of the tubing is between 30.5 and 40 cm (12 and 18 inches) to minimize distortion.
- The earpieces fit snugly and comfortably. Some instruments have several sizes of earpieces and some have hard and soft earpieces. The determining factors are how they fit and feel. The earpieces should be large enough to occlude the meatus, thus blocking outside sound. If they are too small, they will slip into the ear canal and be painful.
- Angled binaurals point the earpieces toward the nose so that sound is projected toward the tympanic membrane.

To stabilize the stethoscope when it is in place, hold the endpiece between the fingers, pressing the diaphragm firmly against the skin (Fig. 3-9). The diaphragm "piece" should never be used without the diaphragm. Because the bell functions by picking up vibrations, it must be positioned so that the vibrations are not dampened. Place the bell evenly and lightly on the skin, making sure there is skin contact around the entire edge. To prevent extraneous noise, avoid touching the tubing with your hands or allowing the tubing to rub against any surfaces.

A fourth type of stethoscope, the stereophonic stethoscope, is becoming more widely available (Fig. 3-10). With a single tube, diaphragm, and bell, it looks and functions like an acoustic stethoscope. However, a two-channel design allows the stethoscope to differentiate between the right and left auscultatory sounds. The right and left ear tubes are independently connected to right and left semicircular microphones in the chestpiece.

Many pediatric specialists have found that a tiny, virtually weightless doll clinging to the structure of a stethoscope provides a diversion for the young child without interfering with the examination. Decoration and color will not interfere with what you hear.

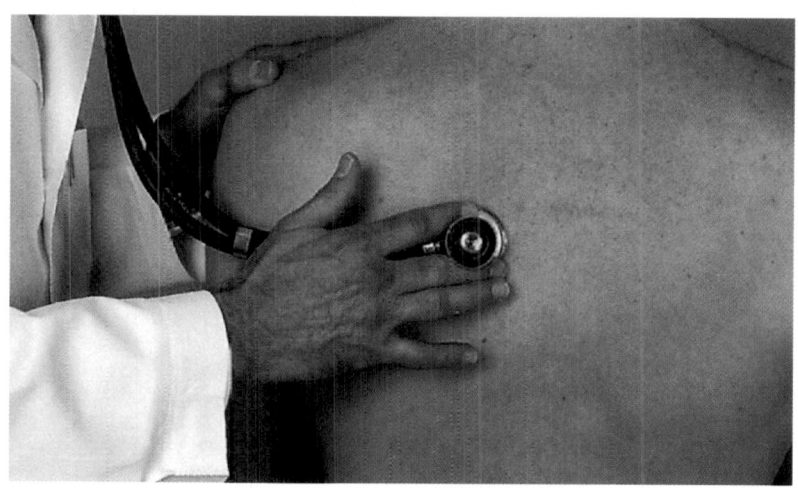

FIGURE 3-9
Position the stethoscope between the index and middle fingers.

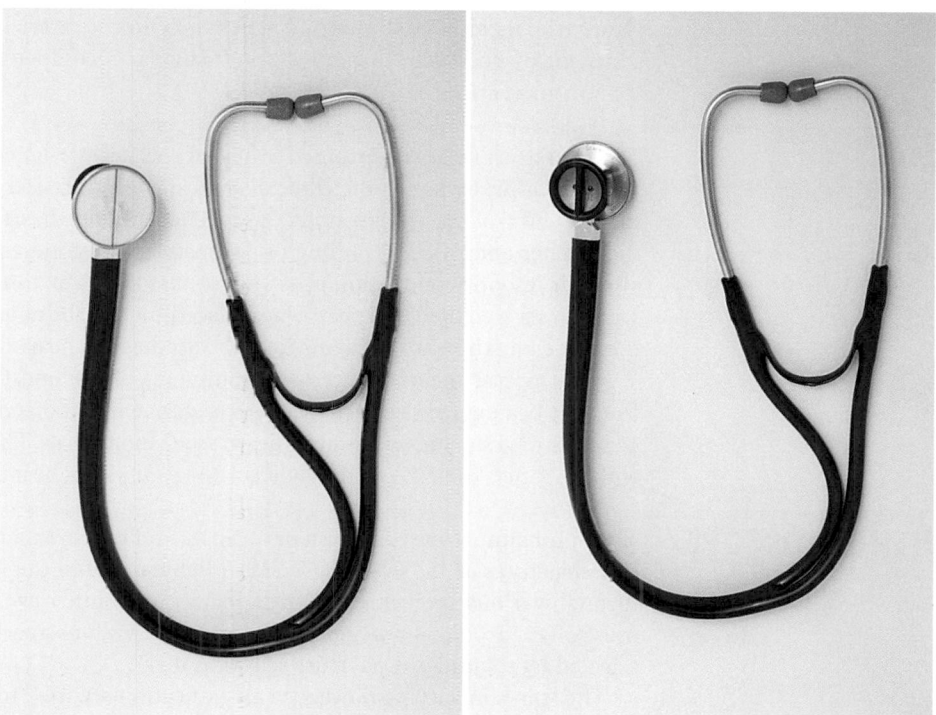

FIGURE 3-10
Stereophonic stethoscope. Note divided bell and diaphragm.

DOPPLER

Some sounds are so difficult to auscultate that a regular stethoscope will not suffice. Dopplers are useful at these times (Fig. 3-11). Dopplers are ultrasonic stethoscopes that detect blood flow rather than amplify sounds, and they vary in frequency from 2 to 10 MHz. The use of a Doppler requires that you first place transmission gel over the skin area where you will be listening. Then place the tip of the instrument directly over the area being examined. Tilt the tip at an angle along the axis of blood flow to obtain the best signal. Arterial flow is heard as a pulsatile pumping sound, and venous flow resembles the sound of rushing wind. When using a Doppler, do not press so hard as to impede blood flow.

The mechanism of action for a Doppler is known as the "Doppler shift" principle: a low-power sound wave of very high ultrasonic frequency is directed into the body; reflections occur at the various tissue interfaces. If an object is moving relative to the instrument, these reflections will have their frequency shifted slightly, resulting in audible sounds.

The Doppler has many uses. It can be used to detect systolic blood pressures in patients with weak or difficult-to-hear sounds (e.g., patients in shock, infants, or obese persons). It is

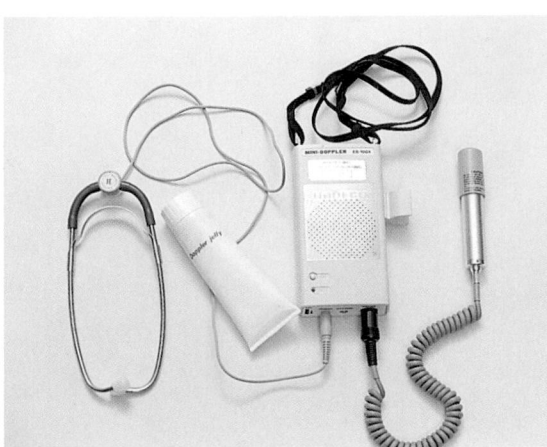

FIGURE 3-11
Doppler.

used to auscultate fetal heart activity, locate vessels, take weak pulses, and assess vessel patency. Other uses include localization of acute and chronic arterial occlusions in the extremities, assessment of deep vein thrombosis and valvular incompetency, and assessment of testicular torsion and varicocele.

FETAL MONITORING EQUIPMENT

The fetal heart rate is determined by use of specially designed instruments called the *fetoscope* and *Leff scope*; by use of the clinical stethoscope, addressed previously; or with an electronic instrument that uses the Doppler effect. The fetoscope has a band that fits against the head of the listener and makes handling of the instrument unnecessary (Fig. 3-12). The metal band also aids in bone conduction of sound, so that the heart tones are heard more easily. The Leff scope has a weighted end that, when placed on the abdomen, does not need stabilization by the clinician. These instruments can pick up the fetal heart rate at 17 to 19 weeks of gestation.

The Doppler method employs a continuous ultrasound that picks up differing frequencies from the beating fetal heart. It is a more sensitive method and can detect the fetal heart at 10 to 12 weeks of gestation, and even earlier in some individuals. These instruments are often supplied with amplifiers so that both the clinician and parents can hear the fetal heartbeat at the same time.

OPHTHALMOSCOPE

The ophthalmoscope has a system of lenses and mirrors that enables visualization of the interior structures of the eye (Fig. 3-13). A light source in the instrument provides illumination through various apertures while you focus on the inner eye. The large aperture, the one used most often, produces a large round beam. The various apertures (described in Table 3-4) are selected by rotating the aperture selection dial.

The lenses in varying powers of magnification are used to bring the structure under examination into focus by converging or diverging light. On the front of the ophthalmoscope is an illuminating lens indicator that displays the number of the lens positioned in the viewing aperture. The number, ranging from about ±20 to ±140, corresponds to the magnification power (diopter) of the lens. The positive numbers (plus lenses) are shown in black, and the negative numbers (minus lenses) are shown in red. A way to remember this is that when you are using a minus lens, you are in the red. Clockwise rotation of the lens selector brings the plus sphere lenses into place. Counterclockwise rotation brings the minus sphere lenses into place. Fig. 3-14 shows the expected lens diopters to focus on eye structures. The system of plus and minus lenses can compensate for myopia or hyperopia in both the examiner and the patient. There is no compensation for astigmatism.

The ophthalmoscope head is seated in the handle by fitting the adapter of the handle into the head receptacle and pushing downward while turning the head in a clockwise direction. The two pieces lock into place.

Turn on the ophthalmoscope by depressing the on/off switch and turning the rheostat control clockwise to the desired intensity of light. Turn the instrument off when you have finished using it to preserve the life of the bulb.

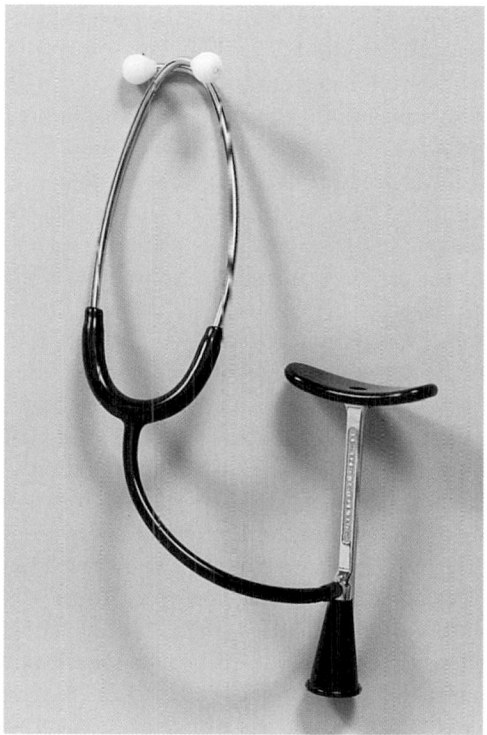

FIGURE 3-12
Fetoscope.

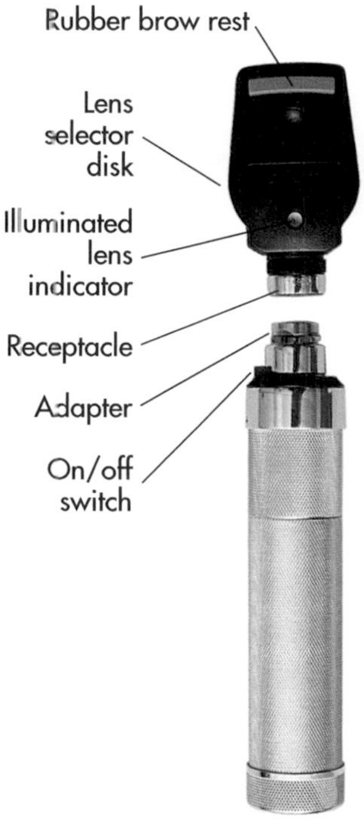

Rubber brow rest

Lens selector disk

Illuminated lens indicator

Receptacle

Adapter

On/off switch

FIGURE 3-13
Ophthalmoscope.

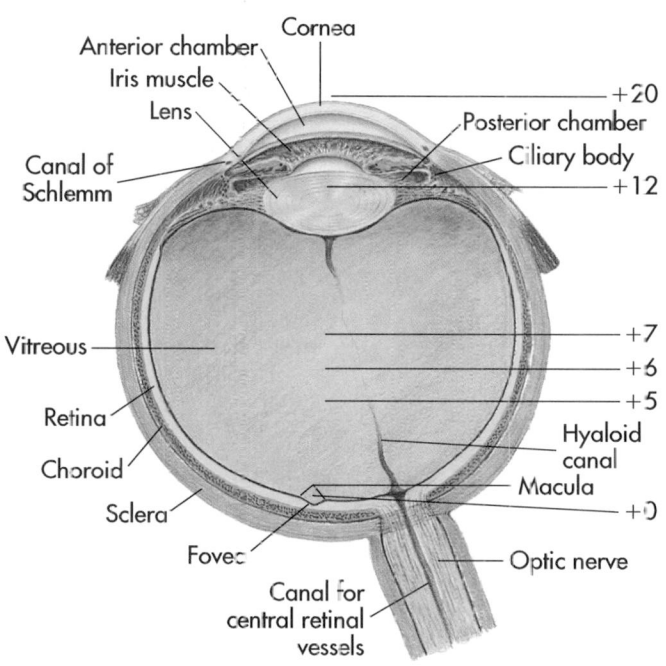

Cornea
Anterior chamber
Iris muscle
Lens
Canal of Schlemm
+20
Posterior chamber
Ciliary body
+12

Vitreous
+7
+6
+5

Retina
Choroid
Sclera
Fovea
Hyaloid canal
Macula
+0
Optic nerve
Canal for central retinal vessels

FIGURE 3-14
Longitudinal cross section of eye showing lens diopters to focus eye structures.

TABLE 3-4	Apertures of the Ophthalmoscope
Aperture	**Examination Use**
Small aperture	Small pupils
Red-free filter	Produces a green beam for examination of the optic disc for pallor and minute vessel changes; also permits recognition of retinal hemorrhages, with blood appearing black
Slit	Examination of the anterior eye and determination of the elevation of lesions
Grid	Estimation of the size of fundal lesions

An optional "panoramic" head allows a larger field of view and increases magnification. As a result, the view of the fundus is five times larger than the view achieved with the standard ophthalmoscope in an undilated eye.

The ophthalmoscopic examination is discussed in more detail in Chapter 11.

STRABISMOSCOPE

The strabismoscope is used for detecting strabismus and can be used as part of routine eye testing in children (Fig. 3-15). Instruct the child to focus on an accommodative target. Turn on the strabismoscope and place it over the patient's eye. Because of a one-way mirror, you are able to see in but the patient is not able to see out. As a result, subtle eye movements associated with strabismus are more easily detected. With the strabismoscope in place, watch for movement in both the covered and uncovered eye. Repeat with the other eye. The instrument comes with a wall poster with test instructions and a guide to interpretation of test results.

VISUAL ACUITY CHARTS

Snellen Alphabet. The Snellen alphabet chart is used for a screening examination of far vision (Fig. 3-16, *A*) for literate, verbal, and English speaking adults and school-age children. The chart contains letters of graduated sizes with standardized numbers at the end of each line of letters. These numbers indicate the degree of visual acuity when read from a distance of 20 feet.

Test visual acuity for each eye using the standardized numbers on the chart. Visual acuity is recorded as a fraction, with the numerator of 20 (the distance in feet between the patient and the chart) and the denominator as the distance from which a person with normal vision could read the lettering. The larger the denominator, the poorer the vision. The standard used for normal vision is 20/20. Measurement other than 20/20 indicates either a refractive error or an optic disorder. Record the smallest complete line that the patient can read accurately without missing any letters. If the patient is able to read some but not all letters of the next smaller line, indicate this by adding the number of letters read correctly on that next line, for example, 20/25 +2. This would indicate that the patient read all of the letters in the 20/25 line correctly and also two of the letters of the 20/20 line correctly.

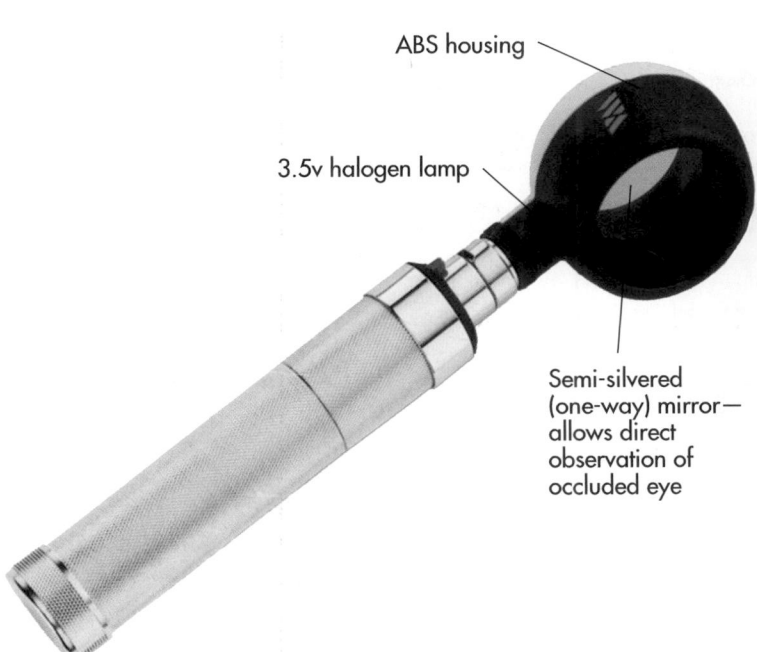

ABS housing

3.5v halogen lamp

Semi-silvered (one-way) mirror— allows direct observation of occluded eye

FIGURE 3-15
Strabismoscope.
Courtesy Welch Allyn, Skaneateles Falls, NY.

For young children or adults not able to use the Snellen chart, several options are available. The highest difficulty of test that the child is capable of performing should be used. In general, the tumbling E or the HOTV test should be used for children 3 to 5 years of age and Snellen letters or numbers for children 6 years and older. For children, cover the nontested eye by an occluder held by the examiner or by an adhesive occluder patch applied to eye. Ensure that it is not possible to peek with the nontested eye. Children usually stand 10 feet (3 m) away from the visual chart to minimize distraction. Young children require training before testing.

Tumbling E. A non-alphabet version of the Snellen chart, the Tumbling E chart has the capital letter "E" facing in different directions. (Fig. 3-16, *B*). The person being tested must determine which direction the "E" is pointing—up, down, left, or right—by holding out three or four fingers to mimic the letter.

A

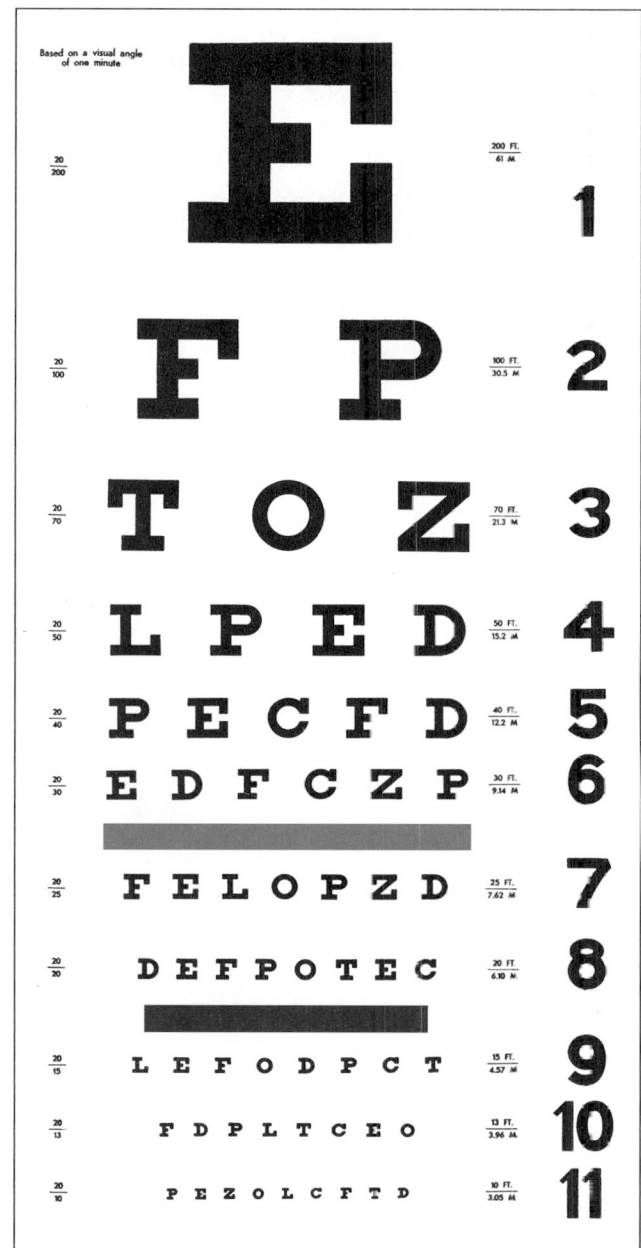

B

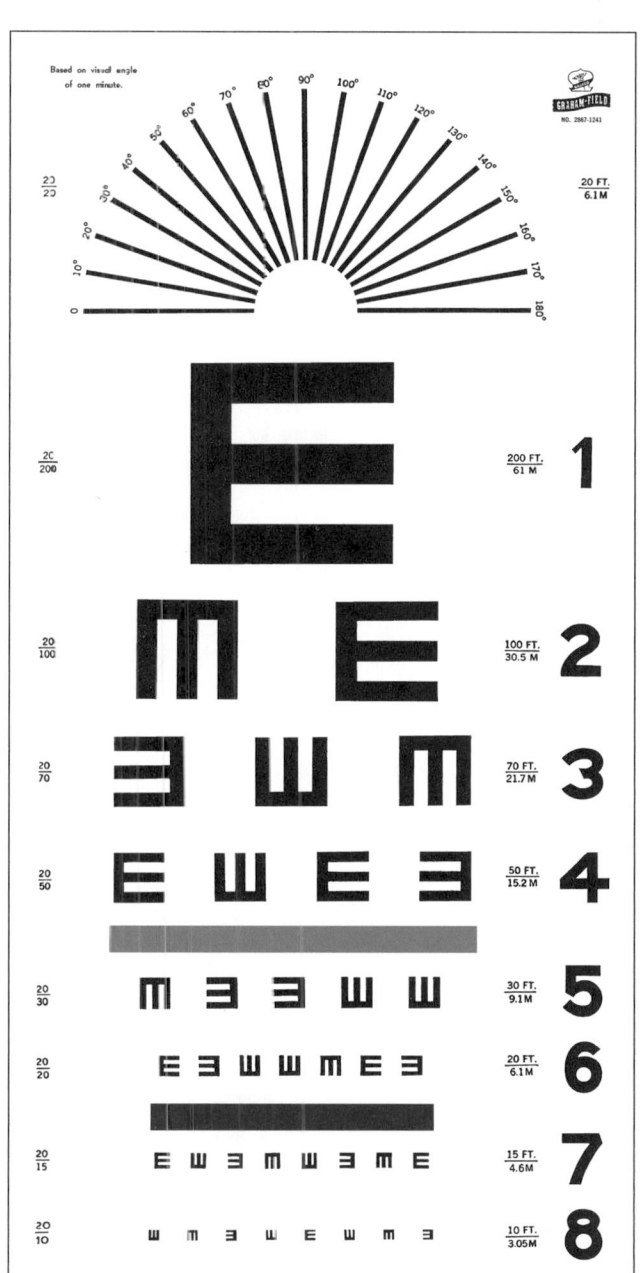

FIGURE 3-16
Charts for testing distant vision. **A,** Snellen chart. **B,** Tumbling E chart.

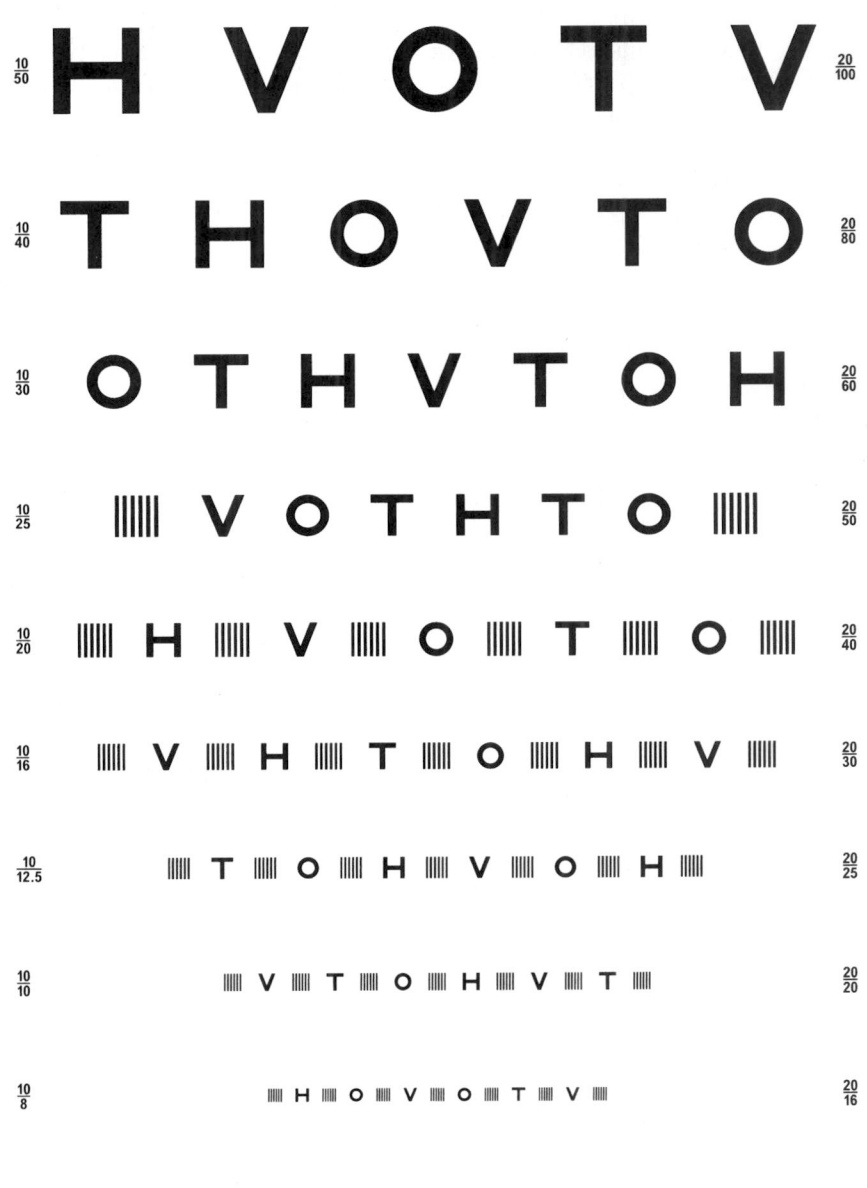

FIGURE 3-17
The HOTV set includes a translucent chart (shown above), a four-object response panel, and a set of training flash cards.

HOTV. This test consists of a wall chart composed only of Hs, Os, Ts, and Vs (Fig. 3-17). The child is given a testing board containing a large H, O, T, and V. The examiner points to a letter on the wall chart, and the child points to (matches) the correct letter on the testing board.

LH Symbols (LEA Symbols). The Lea Symbols chart consists of four optotypes (circle, square, apple, house) that blur equally. The child has to find a matching block or point to the shape that matches the target presented. The visual acuity is determined by the smallest symbols that the child is able to identify accurately at 10 feet. For example, if the child is able

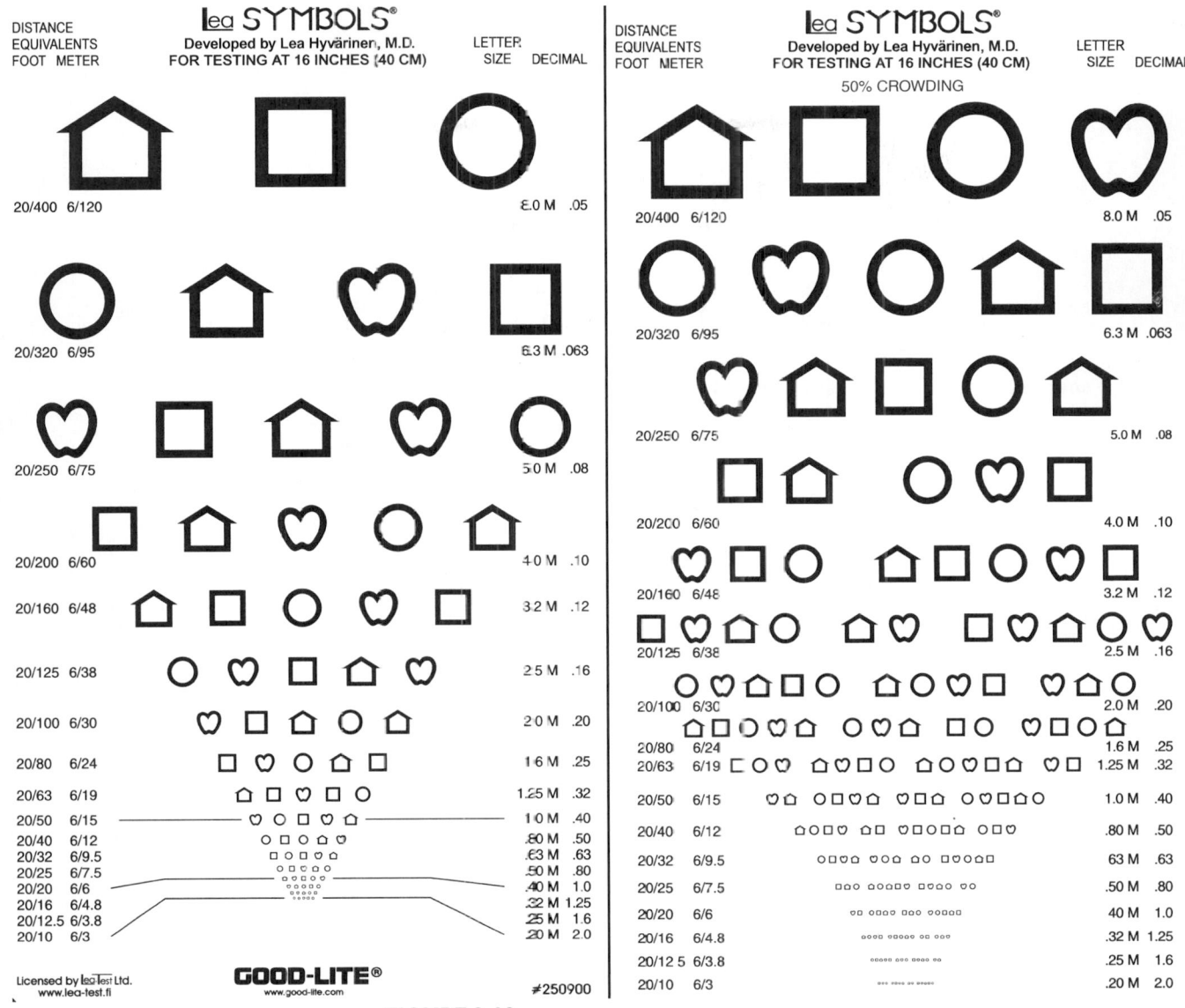

FIGURE 3-18
Lea (LH) cards (front and back are shown above).

to identify the 10/15 symbols at 10 feet, then the child's visual acuity is 10/15 or 20/30. If it is not possible to perform testing at 10 feet, move closer to the child until he or she correctly identifies the largest symbol. Proceed down in size to the smallest symbols the child is consistently able to correctly identify. Record the acuity as the smallest symbol identified (bottom number) at the testing distance (top number). For example, correctly identifying the 10/15 symbols at 5 feet is recorded as 5/15 or 20/60 (Fig. 3-18).

Broken Wheel Cards. The Broken wheel test consists of six pairs of cards with the following acuities: 20/100, 20/80, 20/60, 20/40, 20/30, and 20/20. In each pair, one card has solid wheels while the other has Landolt C or "broken" wheels. The child identifies the card that has the broken wheels on the pictured car. Record the acuity of the card with the smallest car for which the child can distinguish the broken wheels (Fig. 3-19).

EXAMINATION TECHNIQUES AND EQUIPMENT

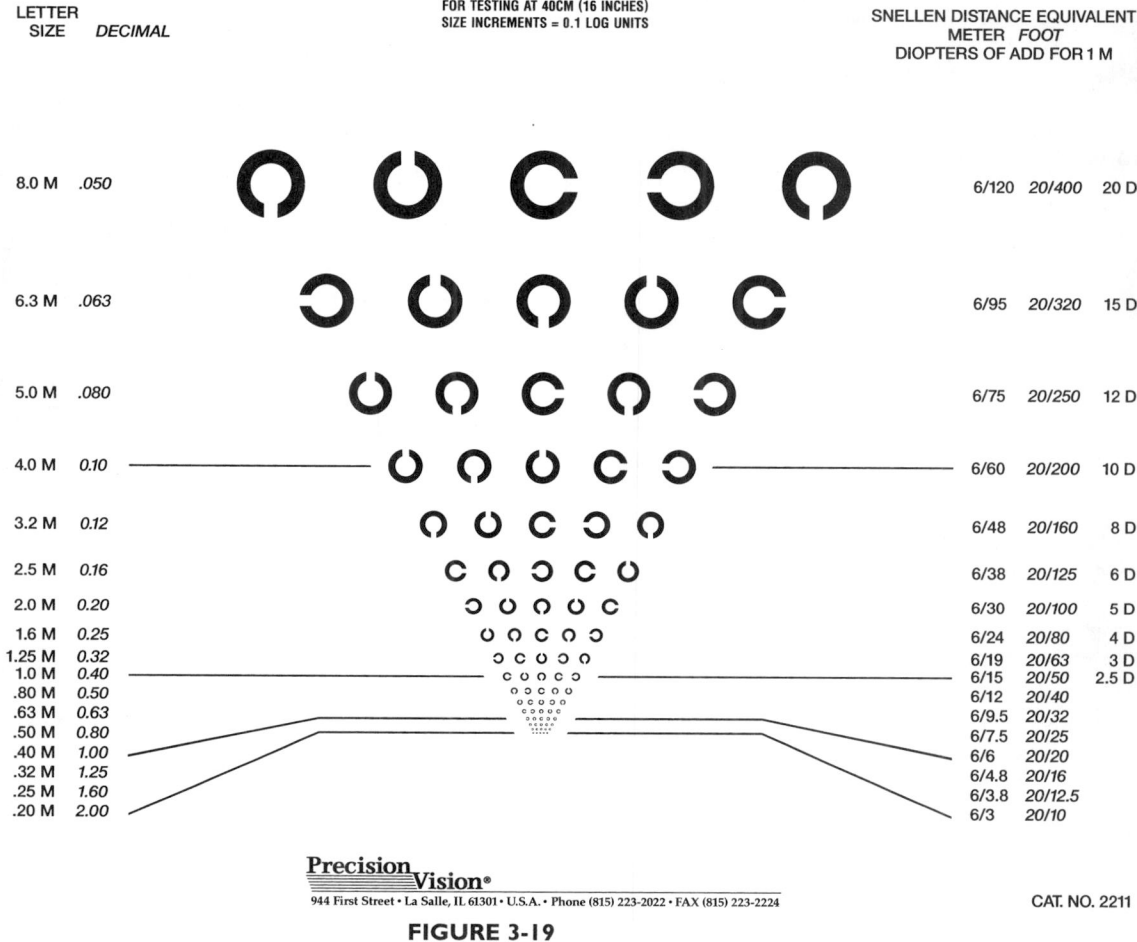

FIGURE 3-19
Landolt C (Broken Wheel) cards.

NEAR VISION CHARTS

To assess near vision, a specially designed chart such as the Rosenbaum or Jaeger chart can be used, or simply use newsprint. The Rosenbaum chart contains a series of numbers, Es, Xs, and Os in graduated sizes (Fig. 3-20). Test and record vision for each eye separately. Acuity is recorded as either distance equivalents such as 20/20 or Jaeger equivalents such as J-2. Both these measures are indicated on the chart. If newsprint is used, the patient should be able to read it without difficulty.

AMSLER GRID

A screening test for use with individuals at risk of macular degeneration is provided with the Amsler grid (Fig. 3-21). The grid monitors about 10 degrees of central vision and is used when retinal drusen bodies are seen during an ophthalmologic examination or when there is a strong family history of macular degeneration. The grid consists of straight lines that resemble graph paper. At the center of the grid is a black dot that acts as a fixation point. The patient views the grid with one eye at a time and notes the occurrence of line distortion or actual scotoma (see Chapter 11).

OTOSCOPE

The otoscope provides illumination for examining the external auditory canal and the tympanic membrane (Fig. 3-22). The otoscope head is seated in the handle in the same manner as the ophthalmoscope and is turned on the same way. An attached speculum narrows and directs the beam of light. Select the largest size speculum that will fit comfortably into the patient's ear canal. A glass plate magnifies and acts as a viewing window. In many models, the glass plate slides aside, allowing insertion of a cerumen spoon or forceps while the otoscope remains in place. Chapter 12 discusses the specific techniques of examination.

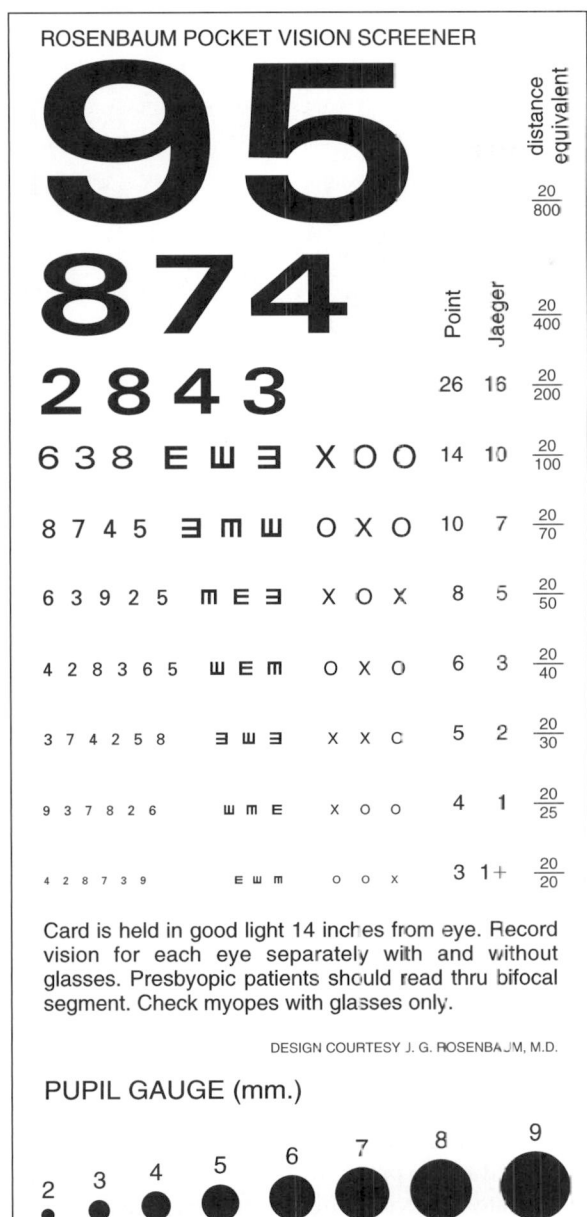

FIGURE 3-20
Rosenbaum chart for testing near vision.

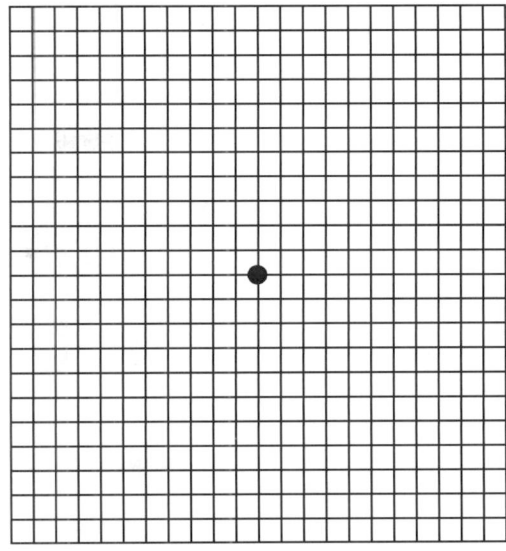

FIGURE 3-21
Amsler grid.
From Palay, Krachmer, 1997.

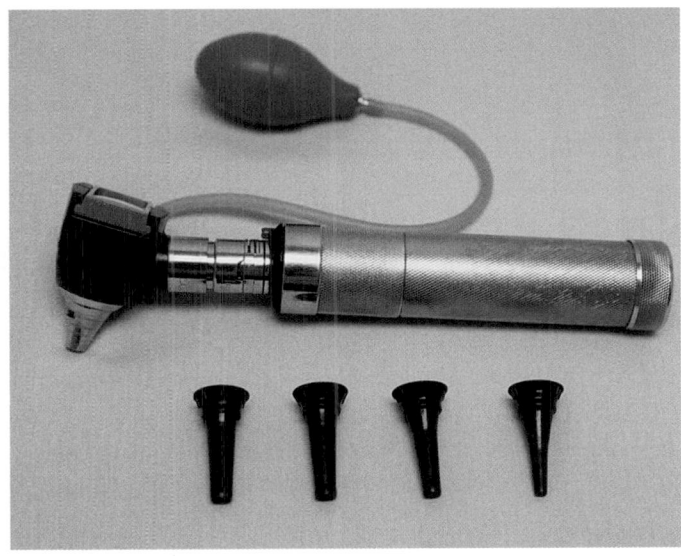

FIGURE 3-22
Otoscope with various sizes of specula and a pneumatic attachment.

The otoscope can also be used for the nasal examination if a nasal speculum is not available. Use the shortest, widest speculum and insert it gently into the patient's naris.

The pneumatic attachment for the otoscope is used to evaluate the fluctuating capacity of the tympanic membrane. A short piece of rubber tubing is attached to the head of the otoscope. A handbulb attached to the other end of the tubing, when squeezed, produces puffs of air that cause the tympanic membrane to move.

TYMPANOMETER

Various instruments are used to perform screening tympanometry. Tympanometry is a simple, reliable, and objective means of assessing the functions of the ossicular chain, eustachian tube, and tympanic membrane, as well as the interrelation of these parts.

Position the probe at the opening of the ear canal (Fig. 3-23). When a tight seal is obtained, a known quantity of sound energy is introduced into the ear. The amount of the sound energy transmitted is the amount of sound energy introduced minus the amount of sound energy that

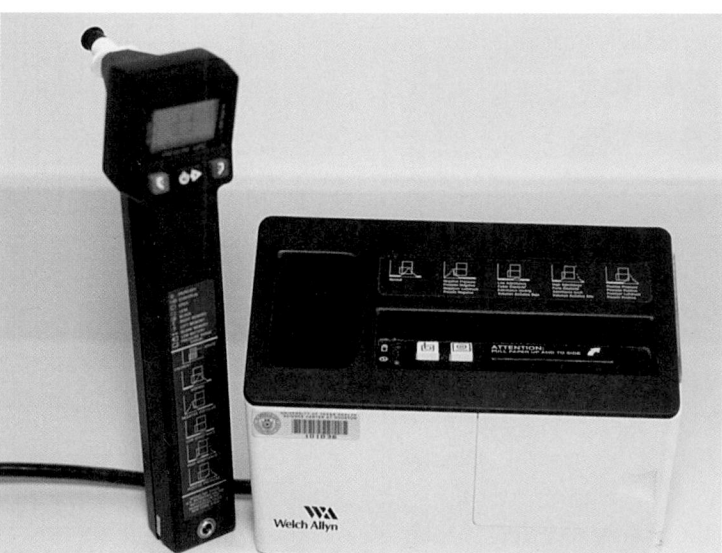

FIGURE 3-23
Tympanometer.

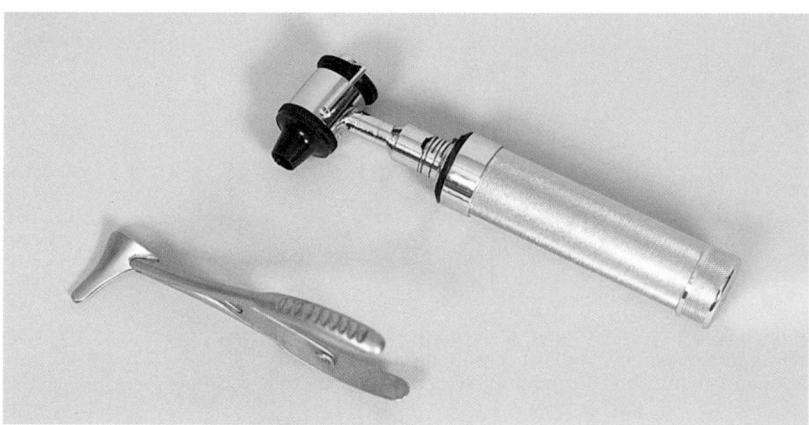

FIGURE 3-24
Nasal specula.

returns to the probe microphone. The amount of energy transmitted is directly related to the compliance of the system. Compliance (measured in milliliters or cubic centimeters of equivalent volume) indicates the amount of mobility in the middle ear. A low compliance measurement indicates that more energy has returned to the probe, with less energy admitted to the middle ear. A high compliance reading indicates a flaccid or highly mobile system.

At this point, the probe introduces a pressure of 200 daPa (decaPascals; a measurement of air pressure) to the middle ear canal. This positive pressure forces the tympanic membrane inward, and the approximate ear canal volume is recorded. This volume gives a baseline from which the compliance curve is drawn. The pressure is then varied in the negative direction, constantly monitoring the compliance of the system. The pressure continues toward the negative direction until a pressure peak has been detected or until a pressure of 2400 daPa is present in the ear canal, whichever comes first. The point of peak compliance occurs once the pressure is equalized on both sides of the tympanic membrane.

A tympanogram is a graphic representation of the change in compliance of the middle ear system as air pressure is varied. The tympanogram results are displayed on the probe monitor or can be printed out for a hard copy.

NASAL SPECULUM

The nasal speculum is used with a penlight to visualize the lower and middle turbinates of the nose (Fig. 3-24). Be sure that the patient is in a comfortable position. The head may need to be supported, or you can have the patient lie down. You will need to tilt the patient's head at various angles for a complete nasal examination. Stabilize the speculum with your index finger to avoid contact of the blades with the nasal septum, which can cause discomfort. Squeezing the handles of the instrument opens the blades.

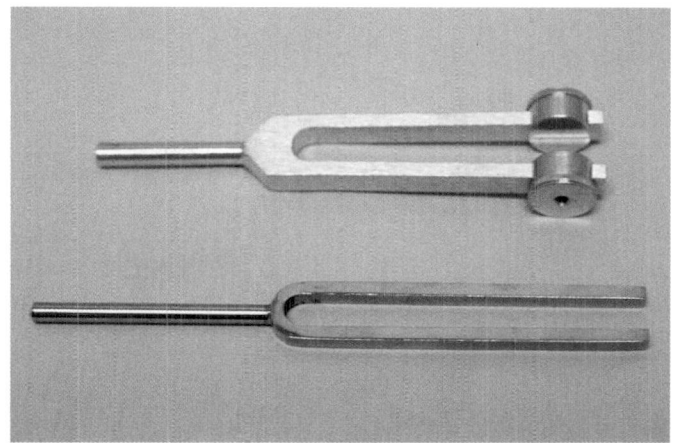

FIGURE 3-25
Tuning forks for testing vibratory sensation *(top)* and auditory screening *(bottom)*.

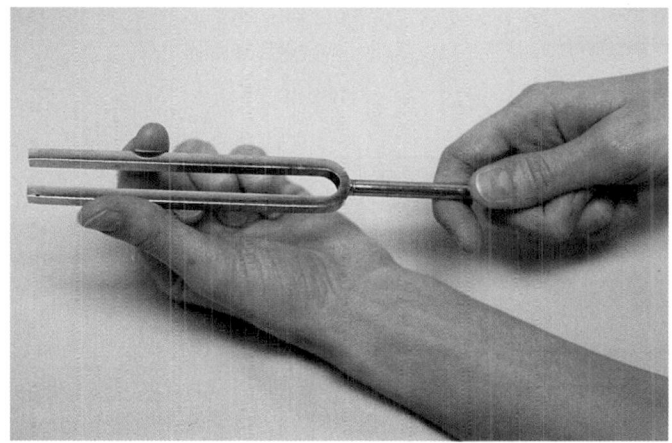

FIGURE 3-26
Squeezing and stroking the tuning fork to activate it.

TUNING FORK

Tuning forks are used in screening tests for auditory function and for vibratory sensation as part of the neurologic examination (Fig. 3-25). As tuning forks are activated, vibrations are created that produce a particular frequency of sound wave, expressed as cycles per second (cps) or Hertz (Hz). Thus a fork of 512 Hz vibrates 512 cycles per second.

For auditory evaluation use a fork with a frequency of 500 to 1000 Hz, because it can estimate hearing loss in the range of normal speech, approximately 300 to 3000 Hz. Forks of lower frequency can cause you to overestimate bone conduction and can be felt as vibration as well as heard. Activate the fork by gently squeezing and stroking the prongs or by tapping them against the knuckles of your hand so that they ring softly (Fig. 3-26). Because touching the tines will dampen the sound, the fork must be held at the base. Hearing is tested at near-threshold level; this is the lowest intensity of sound at which an auditory stimulus can be heard. Striking the prongs too vigorously results in a loud tone that is above the threshold level and requires time to quiet to a tone appropriate for auditory testing. The specific tuning fork tests for hearing are described in Chapter 12.

For vibratory sensation, use a fork of lower frequency. The greatest sensitivity to vibration occurs when the fork is vibrating between 100 and 400 Hz. Activate the tuning fork by tapping it against the heel of your hand, then apply the base of the fork to a bony prominence. The patient feels the vibration as a buzzing or tingling sensation. The specific areas of testing are described in Chapter 22.

PERCUSSION (REFLEX) HAMMER

The percussion hammer is used to test deep tendon reflexes. Hold the hammer loosely between the thumb and index finger so that the hammer moves in a swift arc and in a controlled direction. As you tap the tendon, use a rapid downward snap of the wrist; tap quickly and

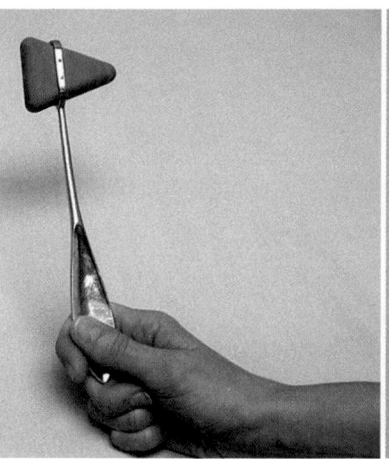
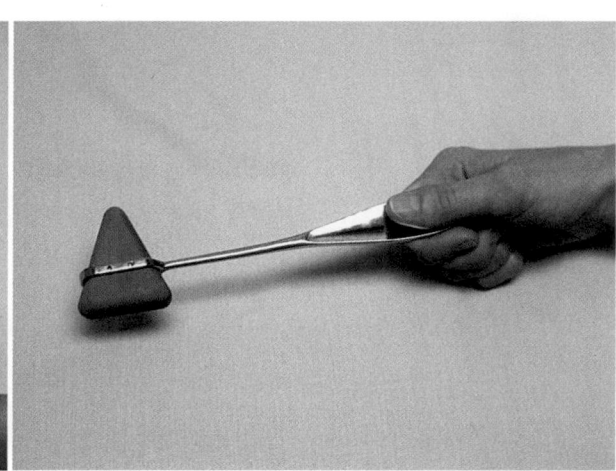

FIGURE 3-27
A, Reflex hammer. **B,** Use a rapid downward snap of the wrist.

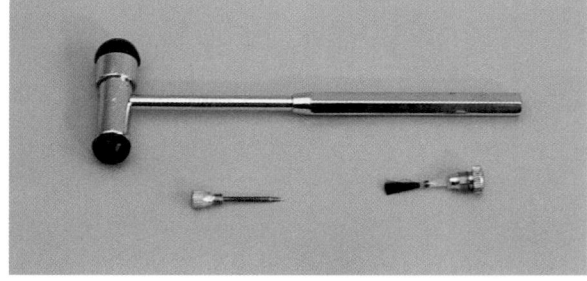

FIGURE 3-28
Neurologic hammer. Note the brush and needle. The needle should not be used.

firmly; then snap your wrist back so that the hammer does not linger on the tendon (Fig. 3-27). The tap should be brisk and direct. Practice this action to achieve smooth, rapid, and controlled motion. You can use either the pointed or flat end of the hammer. The flat end is more comfortable when striking the patient directly; the pointed end is useful in small areas, such as on your finger placed over the patient's biceps tendon. Chapter 22 contains a detailed discussion of evaluation of deep tendon reflexes.

Your finger can also act as a reflex hammer; this can be particularly useful when you are examining very young patients. Certainly it is less threatening to a child than a hammer. Many pediatric specialists let the child hold the hammer while they use their fingers.

NEUROLOGIC HAMMER

A variant of the percussion hammer is the neurologic hammer, which is also used for testing deep tendon reflexes (Fig. 3-28). The hammer has two additional features that make it a multipurpose neurologic instrument. The base of the handle unscrews, revealing a soft brush. A tiny knob on the head also unscrews, to which is attached a sharp needle. These additional implements were designed to determine sensory perception as part of the neurologic examination. The brush can still be used for that purpose; however, because of the possibility of cross infection, the needle should not be used at all. Instead, use a disposable needle, pin, or the sharp end of a broken tongue blade. The procedure for testing sensory perception is described in detail in Chapter 22.

TAPE MEASURE

A tape measure 7 to 12 mm wide is used for determining circumference, length, and diameter. It may be helpful to have one that measures in both inches and metric units. Tape measures are available in a variety of materials, including paper (disposable) and cloth. The tape measure should be nonstretchable for accuracy and pliable for circumference measurement. Because it is placed against the skin, beware of edges that are sharp and can cut.

When measuring, make sure that the tape is not caught or wrinkled beneath the patient. Pull the tape closely but not tightly enough to cause depression of the skin when measuring circumference.

CLINICAL PEARL

The Transience of Memory

I saw a patient today who had a swollen elbow. Was it less swollen than it was 2 days ago? Hard to tell. It would have been much better if the person who first saw that patient had measured the circumference of the elbow and also of the other one. Use a tape measure! It should always be with you. (A small ruler, too!) Don't rely on memory for judging such observations.

CLINICAL PEARL

Transillumination

Compared to radiologic imaging technology, transillumination may seem archaic and imprecise. Radiologic imaging is to be used when necessary, of course, but transillumination maintains its value as a clinical tool and is far less expensive.

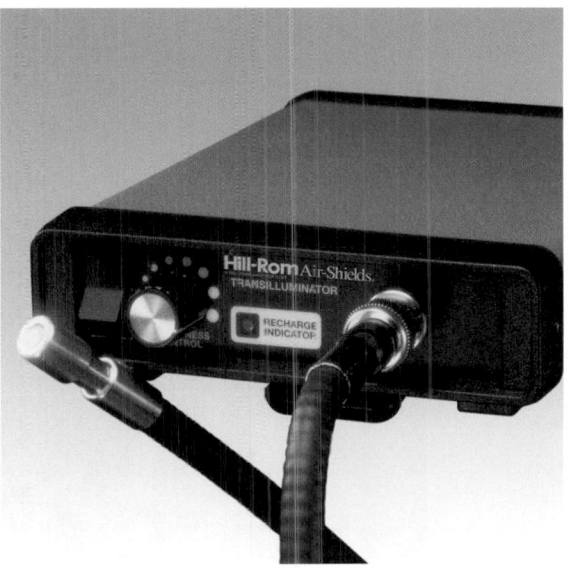

FIGURE 3-29
Transilluminator.
Courtesy of Hill-Rom Air-Shields, Hatboro, PA.

When monitoring serial measures, such as head circumferences or abdominal girth, it is important to place the tape measure in the same position each time. If serial measures are made over a period of days, an easy way to ensure accurate placement is to use a pen to mark the borders of the tape at several intervals on the skin. Subsequently, the tape can be placed within the markings. Accurate placement of the tape for specific measurements is described in Chapter 5 and related chapters.

TRANSILLUMINATOR

A transilluminator consists of a strong light source with a narrow beam. The beam is directed to a particular body cavity and is used to differentiate between various media present in that cavity. Air, fluid, and tissue differentially transmit light; this allows you to detect the presence of fluid in sinuses, the presence of blood or masses in the scrotum, and abnormalities in the cranium of infants.

Specific transilluminating instruments are available (Fig. 3-29). Or a flashlight with a rubber adapter can be used. It is fine, when situations demand, to use a plain flashlight or penlight. Do not use a light source with a halogen bulb because this can burn the patient's skin. In any case, transillumination should be performed in a darkened room. Place the beam of light directly against the area to be observed, shielding the beam with your hand if necessary. Watch for the red glow of light through the body cavity. Note the presence or absence of illumination and any irregularities.

VAGINAL SPECULUM

A vaginal speculum is composed of two blades and a handle. There are three basic types of vaginal specula, which are used to view the vaginal canal and cervix. The Graves speculum is available in a variety of sizes with blades ranging from 3½ to 5 inches in length and ¾ to 1¼ inches in width. The blades are curved with a space between the closed blades. The bottom blade is about ¼ inch longer than the top blade to conform to the longer posterior vaginal wall and to aid in visualization. The Pederson speculum has blades that are as long as those of the Graves speculum but are both narrower and flatter. It is used for women with small vaginal openings. Pediatric or virginal specula are smaller in all dimensions with short, narrow, flat blades (Fig. 3-30).

Specula are available in either disposable plastic or reusable metal. The metal speculum has two positioning devices. The top blade is hinged and has a positioning thumbpiece lever attached. By pressing down on the thumbpiece, the distal end of the blade rises, thus opening

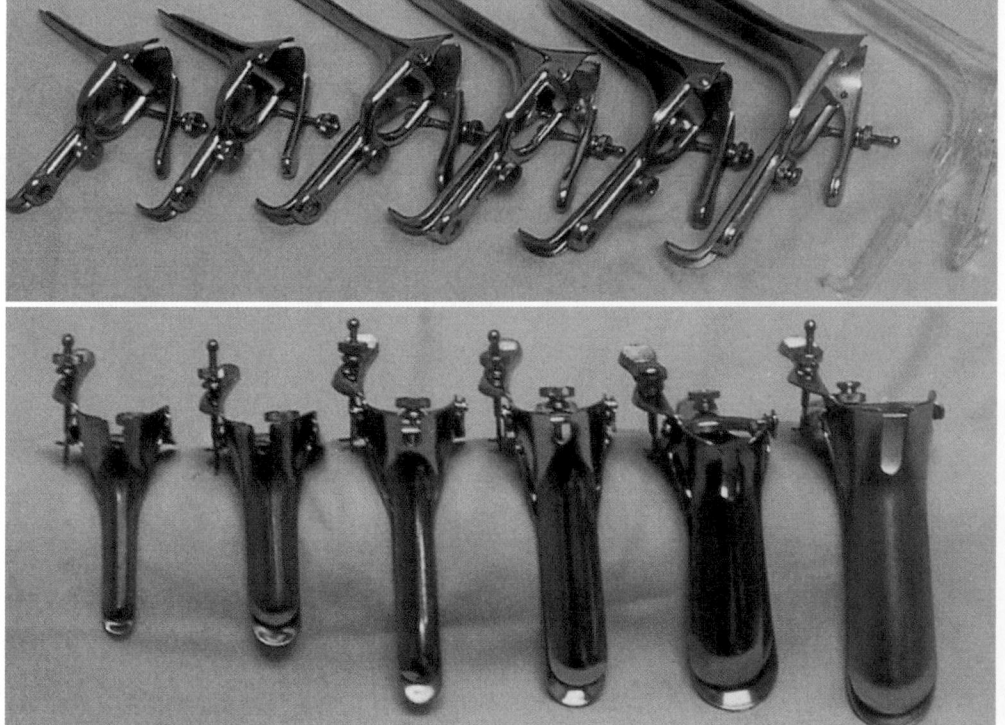

A

B

FIGURE 3-30
Vaginal specula. **A,** *from left:* Short-billed pediatric, pediatric, small Pederson, Pederson, small Graves, large Graves, plastic Graves. **B,** *from left:* Short-billed pediatric, pediatric, small Pederson, Pederson, small Graves, large Graves.

the speculum. The blade can be locked in an open position by tightening the thumbscrew on the thumbpiece. Moving the top blade up or down controls the degree of opening of the proximal end of the blades; it is locked in place by another thumbscrew, which is on the handle.

The plastic speculum operates in a different way. The bottom blade is fixed to a posterior handle, and an anterior lever handle controls the top blade. As you press on the lever, the distal end of the top blade elevates. At the same time, the base of the speculum also widens. The speculum is locked into position with a catch on the lever handle that snaps into place in a positioning groove.

You will need to become familiar with and practice with both types of specula to feel comfortable with them. Do not wait until you are in the process of doing your first examination, or you are likely to be embarrassed and cause discomfort to the woman because of your initial clumsiness in handling (or mishandling) the instrument.

The procedure for performing the speculum examination is described in detail in Chapter 18.

GONIOMETER

The goniometer is used to determine the degree of joint flexion and extension. The instrument consists of two straight arms that intersect and that can be angled and rotated around a protractor marked with degrees (Fig. 3-31). Place the center of the protractor over the joint and align the straight arms with the long axes of the extremities. The degree of angle flexion or extension is indicated on the protractor. The specific joint examinations are discussed in Chapter 21.

WOOD'S LAMP

The Wood's lamp contains a light source with a wavelength of 360 nm (Fig. 3-32). This is the "black light" that causes certain substances to fluoresce. It is used primarily to determine the presence of fungi on skin lesions. Darken the room, turn on the Wood's lamp, and shine it on the area or lesion you are evaluating. A yellow-green fluorescence indicates the presence of fungi.

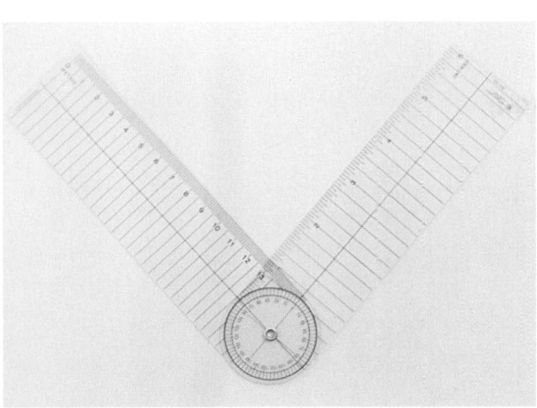

FIGURE 3-31
Goniometer.

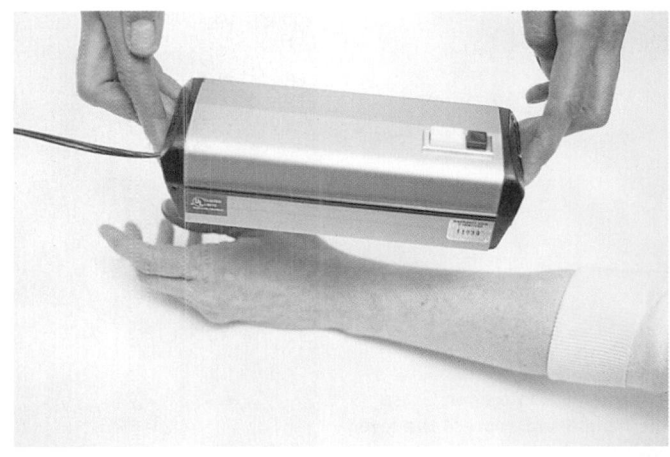

FIGURE 3-32
Wood's lamp. The purple color on the skin indicates no fungal infection is present.
From Thompson, Wilson, 1996.

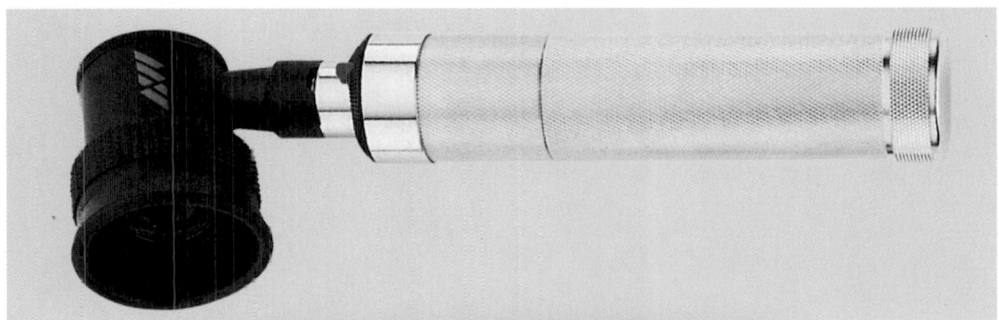

A

B

FIGURE 3-33
Dermatoscopes. **A,** Epiluminescence microscope. **B,** Digital epiluminesence microscope.
A *courtesy Welch Allyn, Skaneateles Falls, NY.* **B** *courtesy of 3Gen LLC, Dana Point, CA.*

Darkening the room can sometimes be intimidating, particularly to children. Children and their parents react positively when they know what to expect. You can accomplish this by shining the lamp on something fluorescent (such as a nondigital watch) to give them the sense of what you are looking for.

DERMATOSCOPE

A dermatoscope is a skin surface microscope that uses epiluminescence microscopy (ELM) with or without the application of oil on a skin lesion to illuminate and magnify a lesion to allow for a more detailed inspection of the surface of pigmented skin lesions (Fig. 3-33, *A*). Digital epiluminescence microscopy (DELM) uses technology to not only examine the skin's surface but also to view, image, record, and document subsurface layers and structures of the skin (Fig. 3-33, *B*). *Dermoscopy* is used to confirm a diagnosis or determine which skin lesions require biopsy or removal and requires special training and expertise.

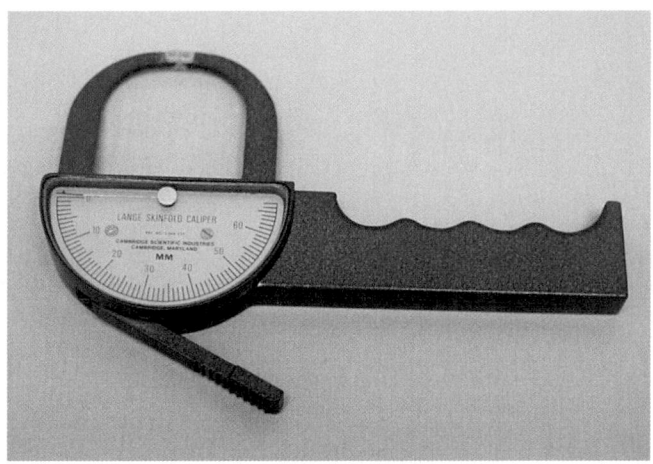

FIGURE 3-34
Triceps skinfold caliper. Grasp the handle and depress the lever with thumb.

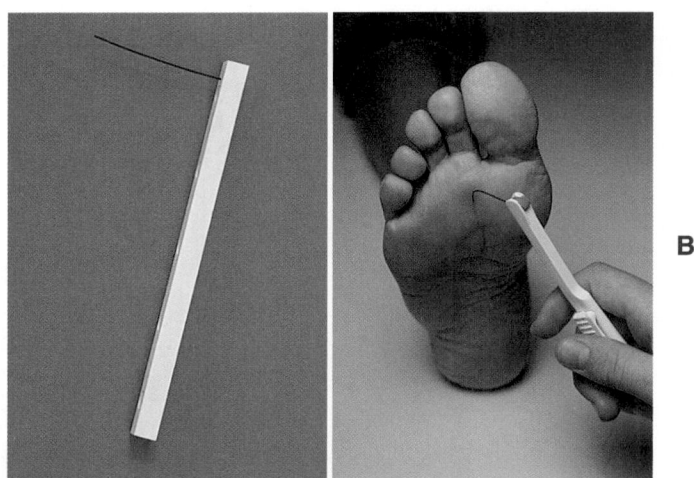

A

B

FIGURE 3-35
A, Monofilament. **B,** Press the monofilament against the skin hard enough to allow it to bend.

CALIPERS FOR SKINFOLD THICKNESS

Skinfold thickness calipers are designed to measure the thickness of subcutaneous tissue at certain points of the body (Fig. 3-34). Specifically calibrated and tested calipers, such as the Lange and Harpenden models, are used. The skinfold is pinched up so the sides of the skin are parallel. Place the caliper edges at the base of the fold, being careful not to capture bone or muscle. Tighten the calipers so that they are grasping the skinfold but not compressing it. The specific technique for triceps skinfold thickness measurement is described in Chapter 5.

MONOFILAMENT

The monofilament is a device designed to test for loss of protective sensation, particularly on the plantar surface of the foot (Fig. 3-35, A). It bends at 10 g of linear pressure. Patients who cannot feel the application of the monofilament at the point that it bends have lost their protective sense and are at increased risk for injury.

Test intact skin on the plantar surface of the foot at various areas, including the great toe, heel, and ball of the foot (Fig. 3-35, B). Lock the monofilament in its handle at a 90-degree angle. With the patient's eyes closed, apply the monofilament perpendicular to the surface of the skin. Press hard enough to allow the monofilament to bend. Application at test sites should be in random order and last approximately 1.5 seconds. Have the patient indicate whether the monofilament is felt. Vary the interval between applications. Note the response at each location in the patient record. Clean the monofilament with alcohol. For a further discussion of skin testing with the monofilament, see Chapter 22.

BOX 3-8

WHAT EQUIPMENT DO YOU NEED TO PURCHASE?

Students are confronted by a large number and variety of pieces of equipment for physical examination. A commonly asked question is "What do I really need to buy?" The answer depends somewhat on where you will be practicing. If you are in a clinic setting, for example, wall-mounted ophthalmoscopes and otoscopes are provided. This is not necessarily true in a hospital setting.

The following list is intended only as a guideline to the equipment that you will use most often and should personally own. The price of stethoscopes, otoscopes, ophthalmoscopes, and blood pressure equipment can vary markedly. Different models, many with optional features, can affect the price. Because these pieces of equipment represent a significant monetary investment, evaluate the quality of the instrument con-sider the manufacturer's warranty and support, and decide on the features that you will need.

- Stethoscope
- Ophthalmoscope
- Otoscope
- Blood pressure cuff and manometer
- Centimeter ruler
- Tape measure
- Reflex hammer
- Tuning forks: 500 to 1000 Hz for auditory screening; 100 to 400 Hz for vibratory sensation
- Penlight
- Near vision screening chart

ELECTRONIC RESOURCES

For Weblinks and additional resources, go to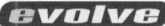

http://evolve.elsevier.com/Seidel

or to the Companion CD-ROM.

MENTAL STATUS

Mental status is the total expression of a person's emotional responses, mood, cognitive functioning, and personality. It is closely linked to the individual's executive functioning that involves motivation and initiative, goal formation, planning and performing of work or activities, self-monitoring, and integration of feedback from multiple sources to refine or redirect energy. The mental status portion of the neurologic examination is performed continuously throughout the entire interaction with a patient. A major focus of the examination is identification of the individual's strengths and capabilities for interaction with the environment.

ANATOMY AND PHYSIOLOGY

The cerebrum of the brain is primarily responsible for a person's mental status. Many areas in the cerebrum contribute to the total functioning of a person's mental processes. Two cerebral hemispheres, each divided into lobes, comprise the cerebrum. The gray outer layer, the cerebral cortex, houses the higher mental functions and is responsible for perception and behavior (Fig. 4-1).

The frontal lobe, containing the motor cortex, is associated with speech formation (in the Broca area). Associated areas related to emotions, affect, drive, and awareness of self, and the autonomic responses related to emotional states also originate in the frontal lobe. Goal-oriented behavior (e.g., ability to concentrate) and short-term memory are also associated with this section of the brain.

The parietal lobe is primarily responsible for processing sensory data as they are received.

The temporal lobe is responsible for perception and interpretation of sounds and determination of their source. It contains the Wernicke speech area, which permits comprehension of spoken and written language. It is also involved in the integration of behavior, emotion, and personality. Long-term memory is associated with this area.

The limbic system mediates certain patterns of behavior that determine survival (e.g., mating, aggression, fear, and affection). Reactions to emotions such as anger, love, hostility, and envy originate here. Expression of affect is mediated by connections between the limbic system and the frontal lobe.

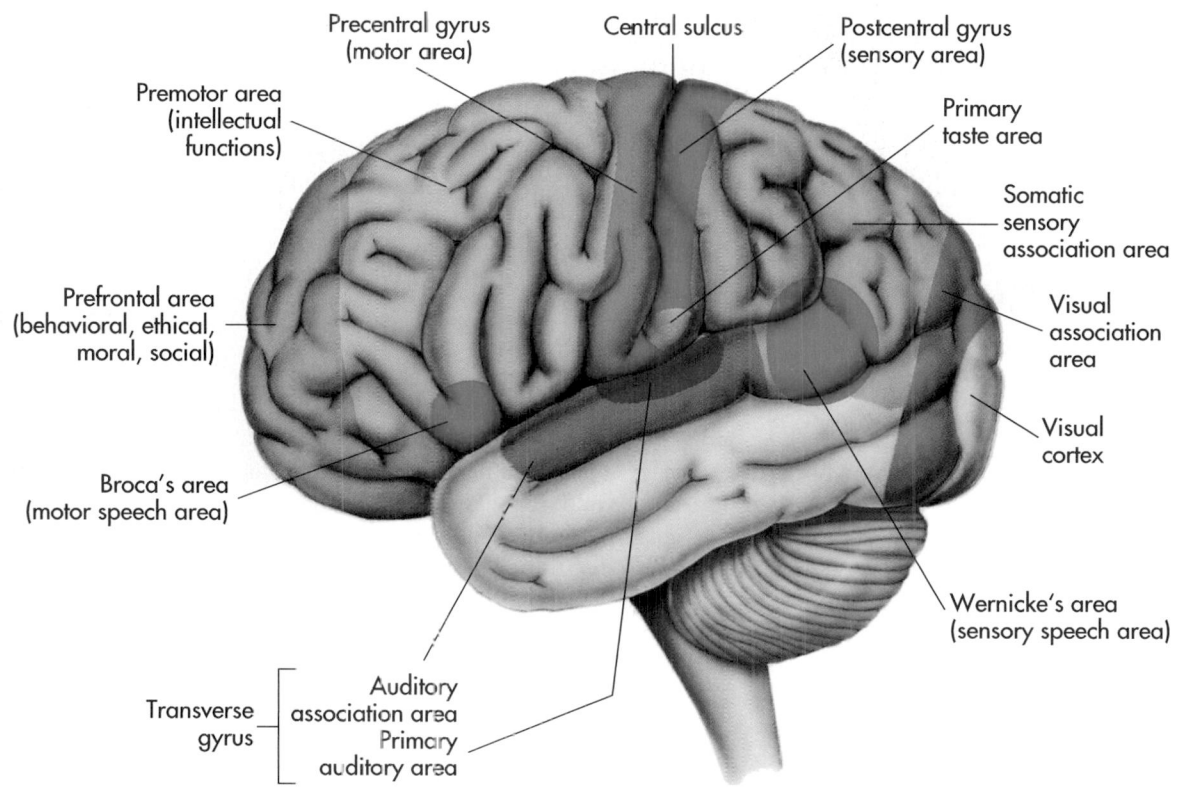

FIGURE 4-1
Functional subdivisions of the cerebral cortex.
Modified from Thibodeau, Patton, 2003.

INFANTS AND CHILDREN All brain cells are present at birth, but it takes the first years of life for the brain cells to fully develop and myelinize. Factors such as infection, trauma, or chemical imbalance—insults to the brain—can damage brain cells, leading to potentially serious dysfunction in mental status. Environmental influences may promote or impair intellectual development.

ADOLESCENTS Intellectual maturation continues with greater capacity for information and vocabulary development. Abstract thinking (i.e., the ability to develop theories, use logical reasoning, make future plans, use generalizations, and consider risks and possibilities) develops during this period. Judgment begins to develop with education, intelligence, and experience. A set of values is eventually reflected in thinking and action.

OLDER ADULTS No decline in general intelligence is evident in older adults unless a systemic or neurologic disorder develops. Problem-solving skills may decline, probably from disuse, but vocabulary skills and inventories of available information do not significantly change. Aging is associated with an expected slower recall of new data and more problems with nonverbal memory, such as misplacing items, but these changes are not severe enough to interfere with daily functioning (Cullum & Rosenberg, 1996). Remote memory may be more efficient than recent memory, but that may be a function of the individual's overall health.

With aging, there is a decline in synthesis and metabolism of neurotransmitters. In times of stress, the metabolism is inadequate to respond to heightened pressures. This often results in an increased risk of delirium with acute illness or metabolic derangement.

REVIEW OF RELATED HISTORY

For each of the conditions discussed in this section, targeted topics to include in the history of the present illness are listed. Responses to questions about these topics help fully assess the patient's condition and provide clues for focusing the physical examination.

HISTORY OF PRESENT ILLNESS

- Disorientation and confusion
  - Onset: abrupt or insidious, associated with physical condition, time of day
  - Duration: hours, days, or persistent
  - Associated problems: loss of vision or hearing, neurologic disorder, brain injury, systemic infection, withdrawal from alcohol, metabolic or electrolyte disorder, vascular occlusion, or overwhelming emotional crisis
  - Associated symptoms: delusions, hallucinations, mood swings, anxiety, sadness, lethargy or agitation, insomnia, change in appetite, drug toxicity
  - Medications: anticholinergics, benzodiazepines, opioid analgesics, tricyclic antidepressants, levodopa or amantadine, diuretics, digoxin, antiarrhythmics, sedatives, hypnotics, or alternative and complementary therapies such as gingko biloba and St. John's wort
- Depression
  - Troubling thoughts or feelings, constant worry; change in outlook on life; change in feelings or always feel troubled; feelings of hopelessness; inability to control feelings
  - Energy level; agitation; feels best in the morning or at night; awakens feeling fatigued
  - Recent cause of grief; changes in lifestyle or living situation; death or relocation of friends or family members; change in physical health
  - Feels like hurting self; any plans for harming self; any thoughts about dying; no plans for the future
  - Medications: antidepressants, prescription or nonprescription; alternative or complementary therapies
- Anxiety
  - Sudden, unexplained attacks of intense fear, anxiety or panic for no apparent reason; afraid of not being able to get help or of not being able to escape in certain situations; difficulty controlling worrying; more time spent than necessary doing or checking things over and over again
  - Avoids or feels uncomfortable in situations or events that involve being with people
  - Experienced an extremely frightening, traumatic, or horrible event
  - Associated symptoms: panic attacks, obsessive thoughts, or compulsive behaviors
  - Medications: antidepressants, benzodiazepines, prescription or nonprescription; alternative or complementary therapies

PAST MEDICAL HISTORY

- Neurologic disorder, brain surgery, brain injury, residual effects, chronic disease, or debilitating condition
- Psychiatric therapy or hospitalization

FAMILY HISTORY

- Psychiatric disorders, mental illness, alcoholism
- Mental retardation, autism
- Alzheimer disease
- Learning disorders

PERSONAL AND SOCIAL HISTORY

- Emotional status: feelings about self; ability to cope with current stressors in life; level of stress; anxiety or irritability; restlessness; decreased sexual activity; problems with money, job, marriage, or children
- Discouragement, life goals, frustrations, attitudes, relationship with family members
- Intellectual level: educational history, any cognitive changes, communication pattern (e.g., able to understand questions, speech is coherent and appropriate), change in memory or thought processes, access to information
- Sleeping or eating patterns; appetite, weight loss or gain; anxiety
- Use of alcohol
- Use of street drugs, especially "club" drugs or mood-altering drugs

CHILDREN

- Speech and language: first words, intelligibility, quality of sounds, progression to phrases and sentences
- Behavior: temper tantrums, breath-holding, hyperactivity, limited attention span, ability to separate from family and adjust to new situations
- Performance of self-care activities: dressing, toileting, feeding
- Personality and behavior patterns: changes related to any specific event, fever of unknown origin, trauma
- Learning or school difficulties: associated with attention, interest, activity level, or ability to concentrate

ADOLESCENTS

- Risk-taking behaviors
- School performance
- Family interactions, reluctance to communicate and to speak of attitudes and experience

OLDER ADULTS

- Changes in mental functions: cognitive functioning, thought process, memory, sudden or gradual confusion
- Depression: somatic complaints, hopelessness, helplessness, thoughts of dying, lack of interest in personal care

EXAMINATION AND FINDINGS

Mental status (cerebral function) is assessed throughout the physical examination by evaluating the patient's awareness, orientation, cognitive abilities, and affect (Box 4-1). Observe the patient's physical appearance, behavior, and responses to questions asked during the history

---

BOX 4-1

PROCEDURES OF THE MENTAL STATUS SCREENING EXAMINATION

The shorter screening examination is commonly used for health visits when no known neurologic problem is apparent. Information is generally obtained during the history in the following areas (pp. 90-97):

Appearance and Behavior
- Grooming
- Emotional status
- Body language

Emotional Stability
- Mood and feelings
- Thought processes

Cognitive Abilities
- State of consciousness
- Memory
- Attention span
- Judgment

Speech and Language
- Voice quality
- Articulation
- Comprehension
- Coherence
- Aphasia

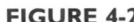

CLINICAL PEARL

The Importance of Validation

If you have concerns about any of the patient's responses or behaviors, it is important to interview a family member or other independent observer, especially if this is your first visit with the patient.

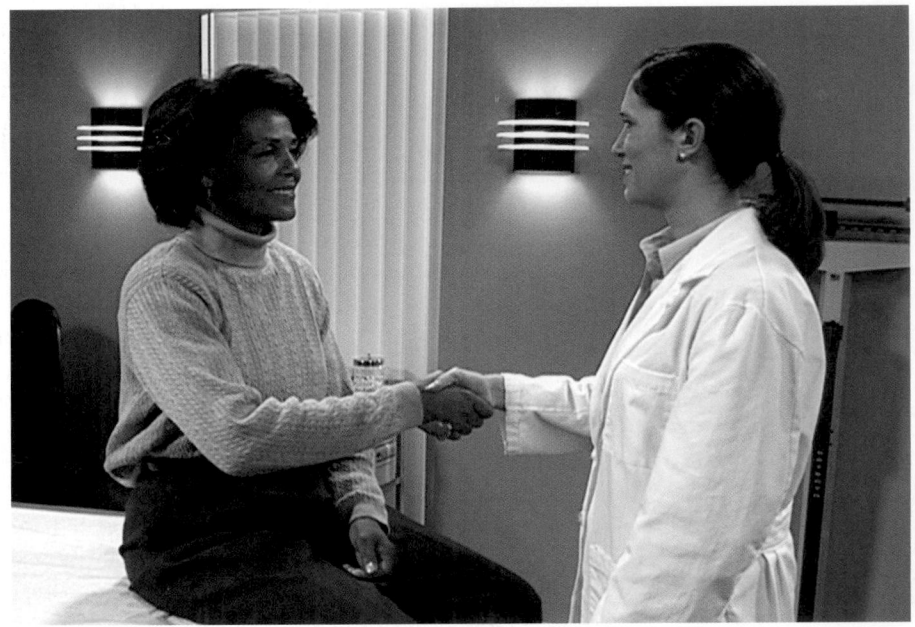

FIGURE 4-2

During the initial greeting, observe the patient for behavior, emotional status, grooming, and body language.

(Fig. 4-2). Note any variations in response to questions of differing complexity. Speech should be clearly articulated. Questions should be answered appropriately, with ideas expressed logically, relating current and past events.

PHYSICAL APPEARANCE AND BEHAVIOR

| GROOMING | Poor hygiene; lack of concern with appearance; or inappropriate dress for season, gender, or occasion in a previously well-groomed individual may indicate depression, psychiatric disturbance, or dementia. |

| EMOTIONAL STATUS | The patient should behave in a manner expressing concern appropriate for the emotional content of topics discussed in the visit. Consider cultural variations when assessing emotional responses. Note behavior that conveys carelessness, apathy, inability to sense emotions in others, loss of sympathetic reactions, unusual docility, rage reactions, or excessive irritability. |

| BODY LANGUAGE | Posture should be erect, and the patient should make eye contact with you (Fig. 4-3). Slumped posture and a lack of facial expression may indicate depression or a neurologic condition such as Parkinson disease. Excessively energetic movements or constantly watchful eyes suggest tension, anxiety, or a metabolic disorder. |

COGNITIVE ABILITIES

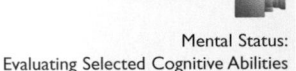

Mental Status:
Evaluating Selected Cognitive Abilities

Cognitive functions are evaluated while the patient responds to your questions during the history-taking process. Specific questions and specific tasks can provide detailed assessment of cognition. The six-item Cognitive Impairment Test is a simple tool to assess cognition (Fig. 4-4; see the Evidence-Based Practice in Physical Examination box on p. 91).

The Mini-Mental State Examination (MMSE) is a standardized tool that may be used to quantitatively estimate cognitive function or to serially document cognitive changes (Fig. 4-5). It is a good tool for detecting the progression of organic disease. The 11 questions take approximately 5 to 10 minutes to administer. Scores on the MMSE vary in the population by age and education, with lower scores seen with advancing age and low levels of education (Crum et al., 1993; Folstein et al., 1985). Fig. 4-6 shows testing the copying skill under the language portion of the MMSE.

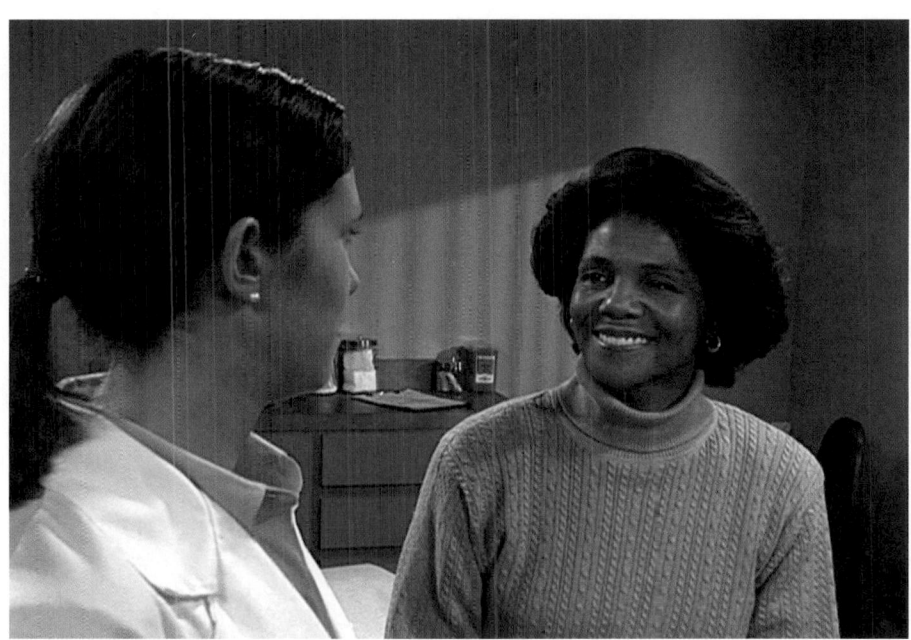

FIGURE 4-3
Note the patient's body posture and ability to make eye contact.

EVIDENCE-BASED PRACTICE IN PHYSICAL EXAMINATION

THE COGNITIVE IMPAIRMENT TEST

The Cognitive Impairment Test is a simple six-item screening test to assess cognition (Fig. 4-4). This test correlates well with the Mini-Mental State Examination (MMSE) but performs better than the MMSE in detecting milder forms of dementia. It has a sensitivity of 78.57% and a specificity of 100% for individuals with dementia (Brooke, Bullock, 1999).

Six-Item Cognitive Impairment Test

Item	Maximum Error	Score	Weight	Final Item Score
1. What *year* is it now?	1		4	
2. What *month* is it now?	1		3	
Memory phrase: Repeat this phrase after me: *"John Brown, 42 Market Street, Chicago"*				
3. About what time is it now? (within an hour)	1		3	
4. Count backwards 20 to 1	2		2	
5. Say the months in reverse order	2		2	
6. Repeat the memory phrase	5		2	

FIGURE 4-4
The six-item Cognitive Impairment Test. Assign 0 for a correct score, and assign 1 for each incorrect score up to the maximum number of errors permitted. Multiply the item score by the item weight to obtain the final item score. The maximum total score possible is 28. A score of 10 or higher is significant, indicating the need for referral.
From Brooke, Bullock, 1999.

Signs of possible cognitive impairment include the following: significant memory loss, confusion (e.g., getting lost in familiar territory or at night), impaired communication, inappropriate affect, personal care difficulties, hazardous behavior, agitation, and suspiciousness.

STATE OF CONSCIOUSNESS

The patient should be oriented to time, place, and person and be able to respond appropriately to questions and environmental stimuli (Box 4-2). Time disorientation is associated with anxiety, depression, and organic brain syndrome. Place disorientation occurs with psychiatric disorders and organic brain syndromes. Person disorientation results from cerebral trauma, seizures, or amnesia.

FIGURE 4-5
Sample items from the MMSE. For a full copy of the MMSE, administration instructions, and scoring guidelines, contact Psychological Assessment Resources.
© 1975, 1998, 2001 by MiniMental, LLC. All rights reserved. Published 2001 by Psychological Assessment Resources, Inc. May not be reproduced in whole or in part in any form or by any means without written permission of Psychological Assessment Resources, Inc., 16204 N. Florida Ave., Lutz, FL 33549; phone 1-800-331-8378 or (813) 968-3003; http://www.minimental.com. From Folstein et al., 1985.

Mini-Mental State Examination Sample Items

Orientation to Time
"What is the date?"

Registration
"Listen carefully, I am going to say three words. You say them back after I stop. Ready? Here they are . . .
HOUSE (pause), CAR (pause), LAKE (pause). Now repeat those words back to me."
[Repeat up to five times, but score only the first trial.]

Naming
"What is this?" [Point to a pencil or pen.]

Reading
"Please read this and do what it says." [Show examinee the words on the stimulus form.]
CLOSE YOUR EYES

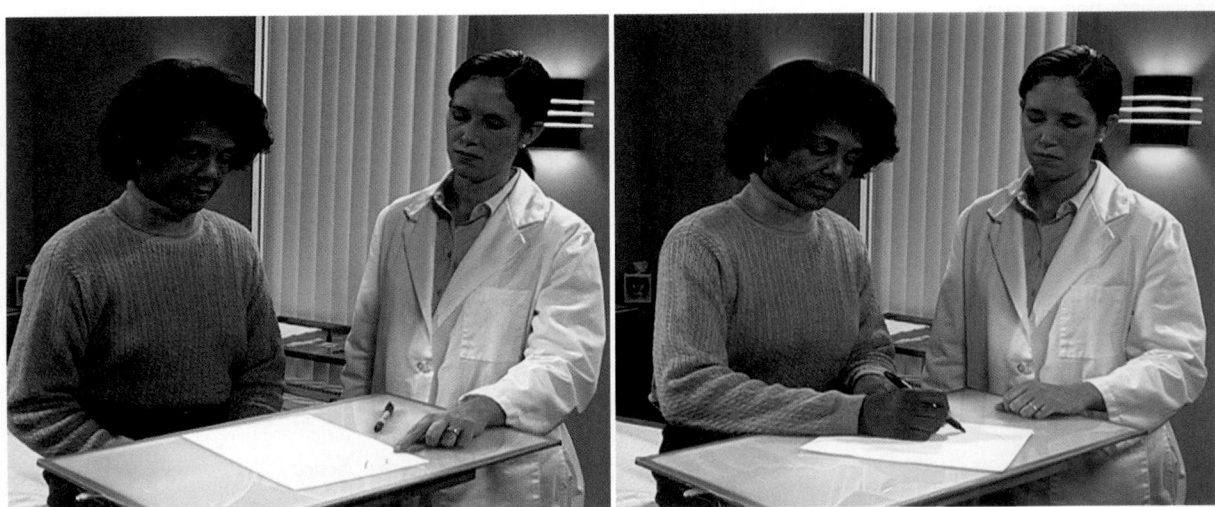

A   B

FIGURE 4-6
Copying is one of the tasks on the MMSE. **A,** Draw intersecting pentagons. **B,** Have the patient copy them.

BOX 4-2

UNEXPECTED LEVELS OF CONSCIOUSNESS

Confusion	Inappropriate response to question Decreased attention span and memory
Lethargy	Drowsy, falls asleep quickly Once aroused, responds appropriately
Delirium	Confusion with disordered perceptions and decreased attention span Marked anxiety with motor and sensory excitement Inappropriate reactions to stimuli
Stupor	Arousable for short periods to visual, verbal, or painful stimuli Simple motor or moaning responses to stimuli Slow responses
Coma	Neither awake nor aware Decerebrate posturing to painful stimuli

ANALOGIES

Ask the patient to describe simple analogies first and then more complex analogies:
- What is similar about these objects: peaches and lemons; ocean and lake; trumpet and flute?
- Complete this comparison: An engine is to an airplane as an oar is to a _____.
- What is different about these two objects: a magazine and a telephone book; a bush and a tree?

Correct responses should be given when the patient has average intelligence. An inability to describe similarities or differences may indicate a lesion of the left or dominant cerebral hemisphere.

ABSTRACT REASONING

Ask the patient to tell you the meaning of a fable, proverb, or metaphor, such as the following:
- A stitch in time saves nine.
- A bird in a hand is worth two in a bush.
- A rolling stone gathers no moss.

An adequate interpretation of these phrases should be given when the patient has average intelligence. An inability to give adequate explanation may indicate dementia, brain damage, schizophrenia, or a lack of intelligence or sophistication.

ARITHMETIC CALCULATIONS

Ask the patient to do simple arithmetic without paper and pencil, such as the following:
- Subtract 7 from 50; subtract 7 from that answer; and so on until the answer is 8.
- Add 8 to 50; add 8 to that total; and so on until the answer is 98.

The calculations should be completed with few errors and within a minute when the patient has average intelligence. Impairment of arithmetic skills is associated with depression and diffuse brain disease.

WRITING ABILITY

The patient should be asked to write his or her name and address, or a dictated phrase. Omission or addition of letters, syllables, words, or mirror writing may indicate aphasia. If the patient is illiterate, ask him or her to draw simple geometric figures (e.g., a triangle, circle, or square) and then more complex figures such as a clock face, a house, or a flower (Fig. 4-7). Uncoordinated writing or drawing may indicate dementia, parietal lobe damage, a cerebellar lesion, or peripheral neuropathy.

EXECUTION OF MOTOR SKILLS

Ask the female patient to put on her lipstick or the patient to comb his or her hair (Fig. 4-8). Apraxia, or the inability to complete a task that is unrelated to paralysis or lack of comprehension, may indicate a cerebral disorder.

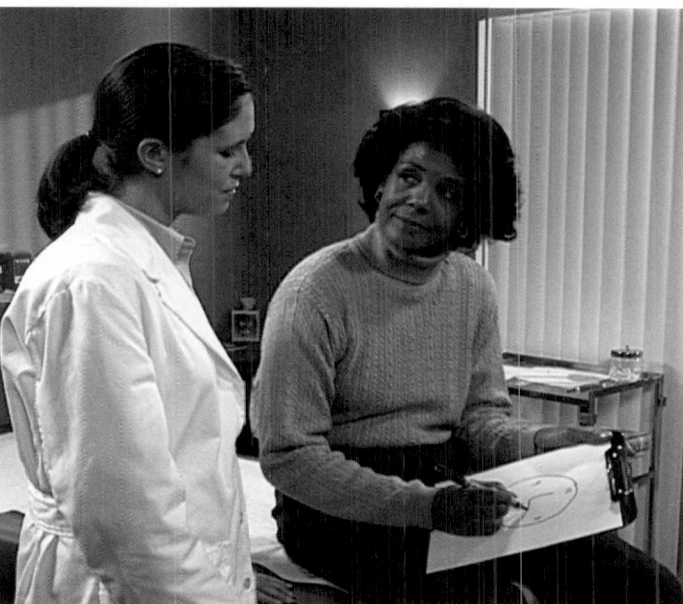

FIGURE 4-7
Ask the patient to draw a clock face.

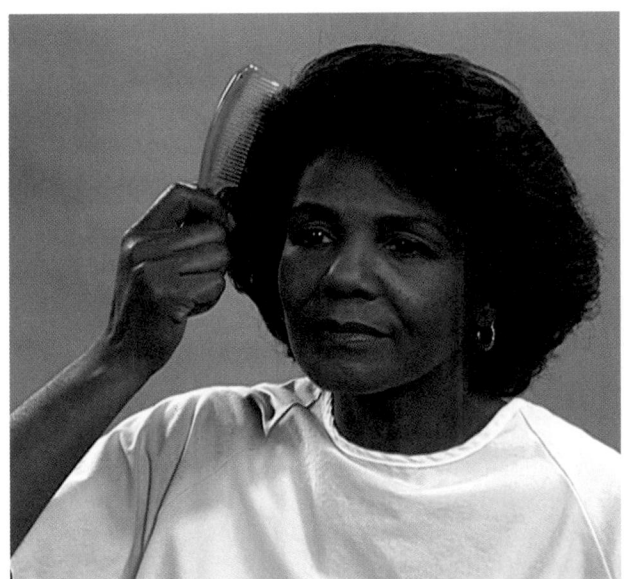

FIGURE 4-8
Ask the patient to complete a simple task such as combing the hair.

MEMORY

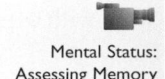

Mental Status:
Assessing Memory

Immediate recall or new learning is tested by asking the patient to listen and then repeat a sentence or a series of numbers. Five to eight numbers forward or four to six numbers backward can usually be repeated. Test recent memory by showing the patient four or five test objects, saying you will ask about them in a few minutes (Fig. 4-9). Ten minutes later, ask the patient to list the objects. All objects should be remembered. To test remote memory, ask the patient about verifiable past events such as his or her mother's maiden name, high school attended, or a subject of common knowledge.

Memory loss may result from disease, infection, or temporal lobe trauma. Impaired memory occurs with various neurologic or psychiatric disorders, such as anxiety and depression. Loss of immediate and recent memory with retention of remote memory suggests dementia.

ATTENTION SPAN

Ask the patient to follow a series of short commands or to repeat a short story you relate. The patient should respond to directions appropriately. Ability to perform arithmetic calculations is another test of attention span. Easy distraction, confusion, negativism, and impairment of

CLINICAL PEARL

Testing Memory in the Visually Impaired
When a patient is visually impaired, test recent memory by using unrelated words rather than test objects. Pick four unrelated words that have distinct sound differences, such as green, daffodil, hero, and sofa; or bird, carpet, treasure, and orange. Tell the patient to remember these words. After 5 minutes, ask the patient to list the four words.

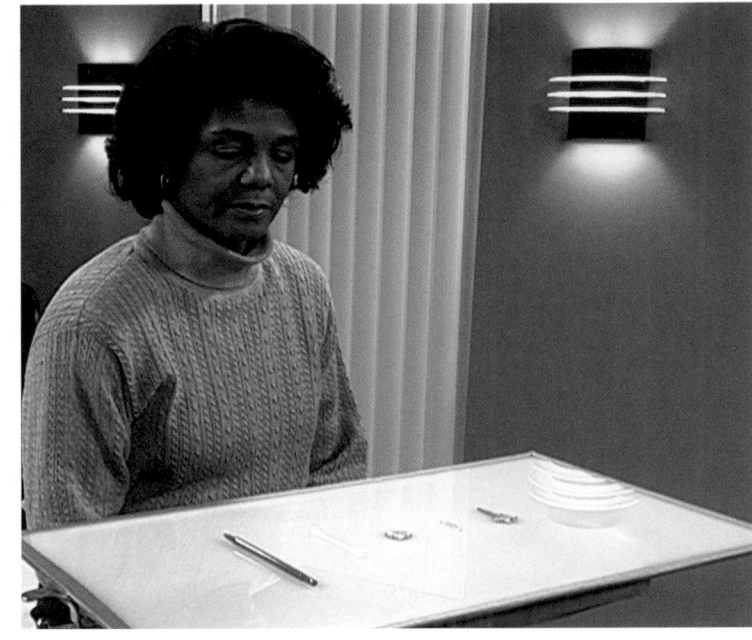

FIGURE 4-9
To test memory, show the patient four or five objects for later recall.

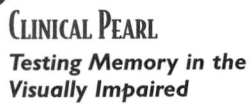

STAYING WELL
PROMOTING MEMORY AND COGNITIVE FUNCTIONING

A variety of mental exercises help keep the brain active. Encourage patients to keep their brain active with card games, crossword puzzles, classes, working on the computer, doing volunteer work, and reading. Many older adults self-assess their cognitive function through regular efforts to complete crossword puzzles.

recent and remote memory may all indicate a decreased attention span. This may be related to fatigue, anxiety, or medication in an otherwise healthy patient.

JUDGMENT

Determine the patient's reasoning skills by exploring the following areas:
- How is the patient meeting social and family obligations?
- What are the patient's plans for the future? Do they seem appropriate?
- Ask the patient to provide solutions to hypothetical situations, such as: "What would you do if you found a stamped envelope?" "What would you do if a policeman stopped you after you drove through a red light?"
- Have the patient explain fables (e.g., the Tortoise and the Hare) or metaphors.

The patient should be able to evaluate the situations presented and provide appropriate responses. If the patient is meeting social and family obligations and adequately dealing with business affairs, judgment is considered intact. Impaired judgment may indicate mental retardation, emotional disturbance, frontal lobe injury, dementia, or psychosis.

EMOTIONAL STABILITY

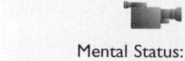

Mental Status:
Assessing Emotional Stability

Emotional stability is evaluated when the patient does not seem to be coping well or does not have resources to meet his or her personal needs.

MOOD AND FEELINGS

During the physical examination, observe the mood and emotional expression evident from the patient's verbal and nonverbal behaviors. Note any mood swings or behaviors indicating anxiety, depression, anger, hostility, or hyperalertness.

Ask the patient how he or she feels right now; whether feelings are a problem in daily life; and whether there are times or experiences that are particularly difficult for the patient.

The patient should express appropriate feelings that correspond to the situation. Unresponsiveness, hopelessness, agitation, aggression, anger, euphoria, irritability, or wide mood swings indicate disturbances in mood, affect, and feelings. Determine whether there are risk factors for suicide. (See Box 1-2.)

THOUGHT PROCESS AND CONTENT

During the examination, observe the patient's patterns of thinking, especially the appropriateness of sequence, logic, coherence, and relevance to the topics discussed. You should be able to follow the patient's thought processes, and the ideas expressed should be logical and goal directed.

Illogical or unrealistic thought processes, blocking (i.e., an inappropriate pause in the middle of a thought, phrase, or sentence), or disturbance in the stream of thinking (e.g., repeti-

CLINICAL PEARL

Distorted Thinking
A patient who evidences an unrealistic sense of persecution, jealousy, grandiose ideas, or ideas of reference (e.g., neutral things in the environment have a special meaning to the person) may be experiencing distorted thinking.

tion of a word, phrase, or behavior) indicates an emotional disturbance or a psychiatric disorder. Disturbance in thought content is evaluated by asking the patient about obsessive thoughts related to making decisions, fears, or guilt. Does the patient ever feel like he or she is being watched or followed, is controlled or manipulated, or loses touch with reality? Does the patient compulsively repeat actions, or check and recheck something to make sure it is done? Obsessive thoughts, compulsive behaviors, phobias, or anxieties that interfere with daily life or that are disabling indicate mental dysfunction or a psychiatric disorder. Does the patient have delusions (false personal beliefs not shared by others in the same culture), such as delusions of grandeur or of being controlled by an outside force, or does the patient feel unrealistic persecution or jealousy? Delusions are often associated with psychiatric disorders, delirium, and dementia.

PERCEPTUAL DISTORTIONS AND HALLUCINATIONS

Determine whether the patient perceives any sensations that are not caused by external stimuli (e.g., hears voices, sees vivid images or shadowy figures, smells offensive odors, tastes offensive flavors, feels worms crawling on skin). Find out when these experiences occur.

Auditory and visual hallucinations are associated with psychiatric disorders, organic conditions, and psychedelic drug ingestion. Tactile hallucinations are most commonly associated with alcohol withdrawal.

SPEECH AND LANGUAGE SKILLS

Detailed evaluation of the patient's communication skills, both receptive and expressive, should be performed if the patient has difficulty communicating during the history. The patient's voice should have inflections, be clear and strong, and be able to increase in volume. Speech should be fluent and articulate, with clear expression of thoughts.

VOICE QUALITY

Determine whether there is any difficulty or discomfort in making laryngeal speech sounds. Dysphonia, a disorder of voice volume, quality (e.g., nasal, slurred, or indistinct), or pitch (e.g., monotone), suggests a problem with laryngeal innervation or disease of the larynx.

ARTICULATION

Evaluate spontaneous speech for pronunciation, fluency, rhythm, and ease of expression. Abnormal articulation includes imperfect pronunciation of words; difficulty articulating a single speech sound; rapid-fire delivery; or speech with hesitancy, stuttering, repetitions, or slow utterances. Dysarthria, a defect in articulation, is associated with a motor deficit of the lips, tongue, palate, or pharynx. Cerebellar dysarthria, which is poorly coordinated, irregular speech with unnatural separation of syllables (scanning), is associated with multiple sclerosis.

COMPREHENSION

Ask the patient to follow simple one- and two-step directions during the examination. The patient should be able to follow simple instructions.

COHERENCE

The patient's intentions or perceptions should be clearly conveyed to you. Circumlocutions and perseveration (i.e., repetition of a word, phrase, or gesture) should not be present. Words or sentences that proceed in disorderly fashion (e.g., a flight of ideas or loosening of associations), word salad (e.g., meaningless, disconnected word choices), neologisms, clang association (i.e., word choice based on sound so that words rhyme in a nonsensical way), echolalia (i.e., repetition of another person's words), and utterances of unusual sounds are associated with psychiatric disorders.

APHASIA

Listen for an omission or addition of letters, syllables, and words; or the misuse or transposition of words. Indications of aphasia include hesitations, omissions, inappropriate word substitutions, circumlocutions, creation of new words, and disturbance of rhythm of words in sequence. Aphasia can result from facial muscle or tongue weakness, or from neurologic damage to brain regions controlling speech and language. Table 4-1 lists the characteristics of different types of aphasia.

TABLE 4-1	Differentiating Types of Aphasia		
Characteristics	**Broca Aphasia**	**Wernicke Aphasia**	**Global Aphasia**
Word comprehension	Fair to good	Can hear words but cannot relate them to previous experiences	Absent or reduced to person's own name, few select words
Spontaneous speech	Cannot express self using language few words; laborious effort; primarily uses nouns and verbs (e.g., eat pie, get mail)	Fluent, effortless speech; words are malformed, may be totally incomprehensible	Absent or reduced to only a few words or sounds
Reading comprehension	Intact	Impaired	Severely impaired
Writing	Impaired	Impaired	Severely impaired

BOX 4-3

GLASGOW COMA SCALE

Assessed Behavior	Adult Criteria	Infant and Young Child Criteria	Score
Eye opening	Spontaneous opening	Spontaneous opening	4
	To verbal stimuli	To loud noise	3
	To pain	To pain	2
	No response	No response	1
Verbal response	Oriented to appropriate stimulation	Smiles, coos, cries	5
	Confused	Irritable, cries	4
	Inappropriate words	Inappropriate crying	3
	Incoherent	Grunts, moans	2
	None	No response	1
Motor response	Obeys commands	Spontaneous movement	6
	Localizes pain	Withdraws to touch	5
	Withdraws from pain	Withdraws to pain	4
	Flexion to pain (decorticate)	Abnormal flexion (decorticate)	3
	Extension to pain (decerebrate)	Abnormal extension (decerebrate)	2
	None	No response	1

Add the numbers from each category. Maximum score = 15, minimum score = 3.

Modified from Teasdale, Jennett, 1974; and James, 1986.

ADDITIONAL PROCEDURES

GLASGOW COMA SCALE

When a patient has an altered level of consciousness because of brain trauma or another hypoxic event, the Glasgow Coma Scale is often used to quantify consciousness. Versions for both the adult and for the infant and young child are available. This instrument assesses the function of the cerebral cortex and brainstem through the patient's verbal, motor, and eye opening responses to specific stimuli (Box 4-3). This assessment can be repeated at intervals to detect improvement or deterioration in the patient's level of consciousness. The instrument was initially developed to predict mortality associated with brain injuries, but it is now widely used in coma assessment.

The patient's best response in each category is matched to the criteria for scoring. Appropriate verbal stimuli are questions eliciting the patient's level of orientation to person, place, and time. Painful stimuli are used when necessary to obtain eye opening and motor responses. Begin with less painful stimuli (e.g., pinching the skin) and progress to squeezing muscle mass or tendons if there is no response. Table 4-2 describes the postures found in unresponsive patients.

TABLE 4-2	Postures Often Found in Unresponsive Patients
Posture and Site of Lesion	**Characteristics**
DECORTICATE Corticospinal tracts above the brainstem	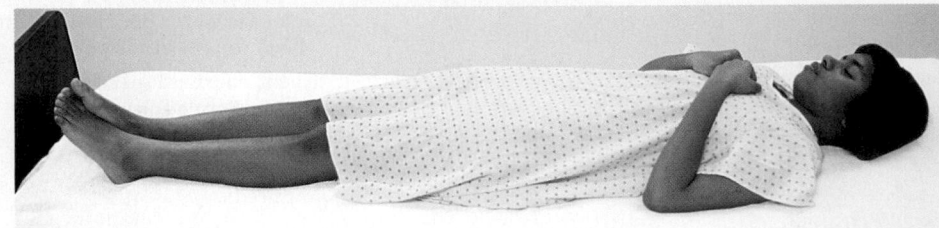 Rigid flexion; upper arms held tightly to the sides of body; elbows, wrists, and fingers flexed; feet plantar flexed, legs extended and internally rotated; may have fine tremors or intense stiffness
DECEREBRATE Brainstem	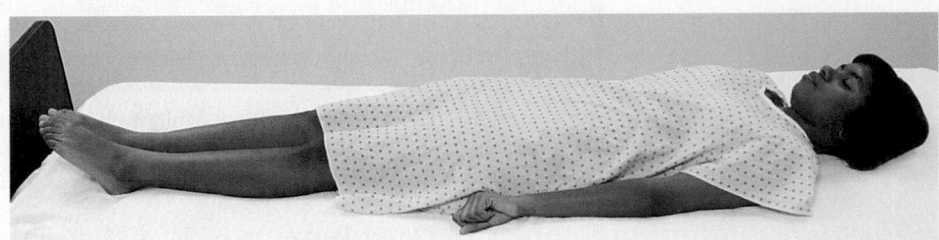 Rigid extension; arms fully extended; forearms pronated; wrists and finger flexed; jaws clenched, neck extended, back may be arched; feet plantar flexed; posturing may occur spontaneously, intermittently, or in response to a stimulus
HEMIPLEGIA Corticospinal tract	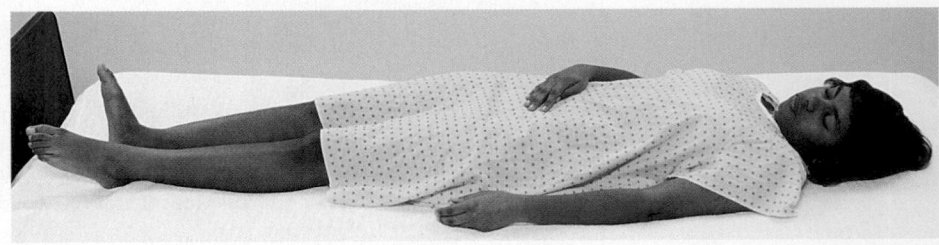 Unilateral flaccidity or spasticity; voluntary movement on unaffected side

Three scores are added to produce the Glasgow Coma Score. The maximum score of 15 indicates the optimal level of consciousness. The lower the score, the more severe the impairment in consciousness. The lowest score possible is 3, indicating deepest coma. Box 4-4 lists the common causes of unresponsiveness.

INFANTS AND CHILDREN   The infant's general behavior and level of consciousness are evaluated by observing the level of activity and responsiveness to environmental stimuli. Note whether the baby is lethargic, drowsy, stuporous, alert, active, or irritable (Fig. 4-10). By 2 months of age, the infant should appear alert, quiet, and content and should recognize the face of a significant other (Fig. 4-11).

By the time an infant is 2 to 3 months old, it is reasonable to expect that a careful examiner who devotes time to developing a relationship with the baby could coax a smile. If it is difficult or impossible to elicit a social smile, there should be concern about the child's immediate health and neurologic competence.

In the first year of life, drooling is often attributed to teething. After the age of 1 year, drooling becomes much less common; by age 2 it generally disappears. If drooling persists, the examiner should be concerned about some neurologic handicap (perhaps mental retardation) or anomalies of the teeth or the upper gastrointestinal tract.

Because language has not yet developed, crying and other vocal sounds are evaluated. The infant's cry should be loud and angry, not high pitched or hoarse. A shrill or whiny high-pitched cry or catlike screeching cry suggests a central nervous system deficit. Cooing and bab-

BOX 4-4

COMMON CAUSES OF UNRESPONSIVENESS

Type of Disorder	Cause
Focal structural lesions of the brain	Hemorrhage, hematoma, infarction, tumor, abscess, trauma
Diffuse brain disease	Drug intoxications
	Metabolic disorders such as hypoglycemia, ketoacidosis, hypernatremia or hyponatremia, renal failure, myxedema, hypercalcemia or hypocalcemia, pulmonary insufficiency
	Hypothermia, hyperthermia
	Hypoxemia—strangulation, drowning, cardiopulmonary arrest, pulmonary embolism
	Encephalitis, meningitis
	Seizures
Psychogenic unresponsiveness	Dementia

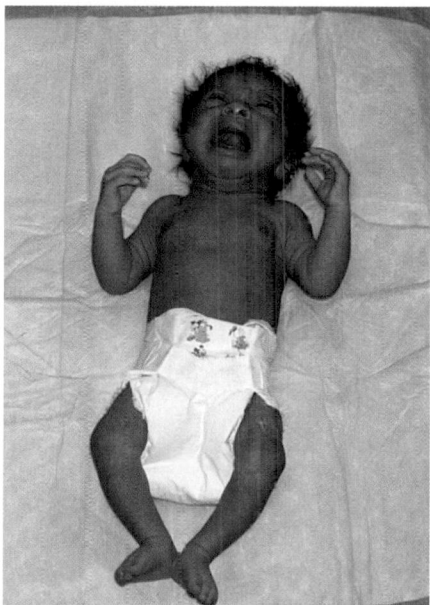

FIGURE 4-10
Note the level of irritability and posturing expressed by this newborn with cocaine withdrawal.

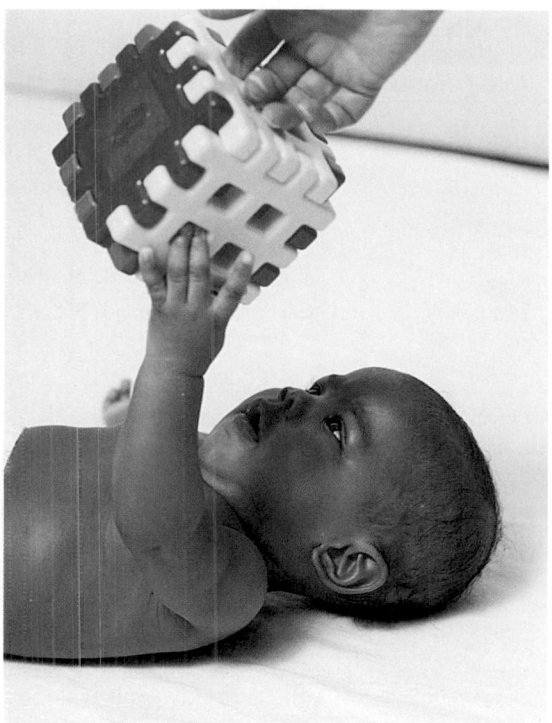

FIGURE 4-11
Note the level of alertness and interest in various objects and people.

bling are expected after 3 and 4 months of age, respectively. One or two words (e.g., "mama," "dada," or "bye-bye") should be distinct by 9 to 10 months of age.

The Denver II tool is useful for determining whether the child is developing fine and gross motor skills, language, and personal-social skills as expected (see Appendix D). Older children can be asked to draw a picture of a person to assess cognitive development with the Goodenough-Harris Drawing Test (Fig. 4-12). In addition, parents can be asked to respond to specific tools that identify their concerns or judgments about the child's developmental and behavioral development.

Observe the child's mood, activity level, communication pattern, preferences, and responsiveness to and ability to separate from the parent. Observe behaviors during the interview to identify self-comforting measures, and whether the child can play and have fun. (See Box 24-9.)

Evaluate the types of words and speech patterns used. The child's language and speech should be appropriate for age. Table 4-3 describes expressive language milestones for toddlers. Articula-

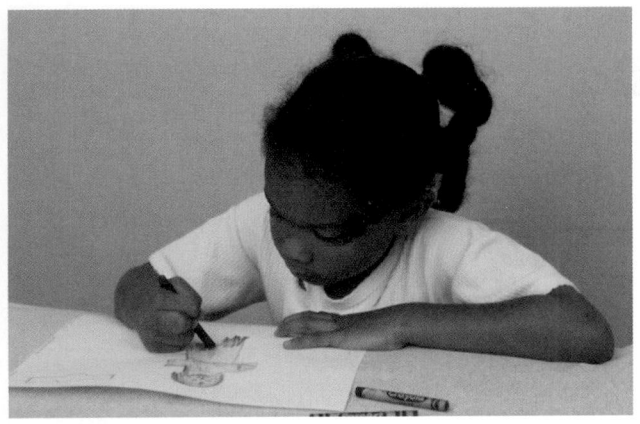

FIGURE 4-12
Ask the child to draw a picture of a man or woman. The presence and form of body parts provide a clue about the child's development when following the scoring criteria of the Goodenough-Harris Drawing Test.

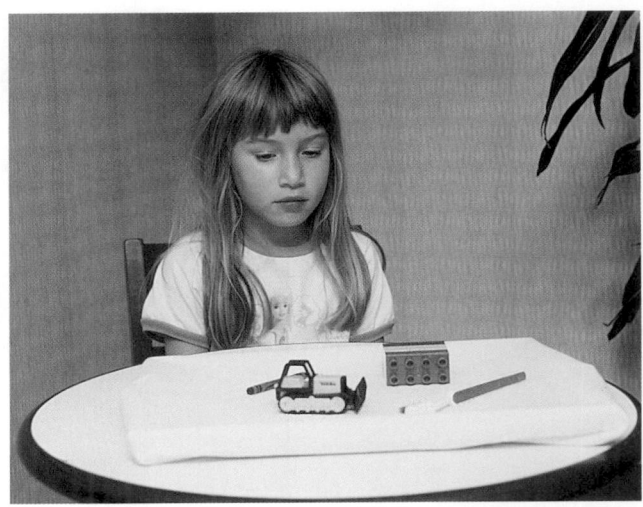

FIGURE 4-13
Test memory recall using familiar objects.

TABLE 4-3	Expressive Language Milestones for Toddlers
Age (months)	**Expressive Language Milestones**
12 to 15	Says three or four words appropriately, including names; uses flow of connected sounds that have inflection and seem like a sentence
15 to 18	Uses 10 words including names; makes requests by naming objects; begins to repeat words heard in adult conversations
18 to 24	Uses short sentences (three or four words); uses pronouns but some syntax errors; tells full name; echoes last two or three words of a rhyme
24 to 36	Caregiver understands 90% of speech; uses noun-verb combinations with correct verb tense; repeats three numbers

Modified from Krajicek, Tomlinson, 1983.

tion is a fine motor skill, and speech should be more clearly understandable with advancing age. Articulation milestones may be evaluated with the Denver Articulate Screening Exam (DASE).

Memory testing may be attempted at about 4 years of age, if the child pays attention and is not too anxious. Expected memory skills vary with the age of the child. Test immediate recall by asking the child to repeat either numbers or words. A 4-year-old can repeat three digits or words, a 5-year-old can repeat four digits or words, and a 6-year-old can repeat five digits or words. Recent memory is not usually tested in children but may be done with modification. Show the child only familiar objects, and wait no longer than 5 minutes to ask the child to recall what objects were shown (Fig. 4-13). Older preschoolers will be more skilled with this test. Test remote memory by asking the child what he or she had for dinner the previous night, what his or her address is, or to recite a nursery rhyme.

OLDER ADULTS

There is little evidence that personality changes with age, in the absence of other health problems. Older adults are expected to maintain the same level of interpersonal skills. Existing personality traits may become exaggerated, however. Paranoid thought is the most striking alteration in personality. Attempt to determine whether the thought process is accurate or a paranoid ideation, keeping in mind that the incidence of abuse of the older adult is increasing.

Deterioration of intellectual function should not be found until 70 years of age unless the patient has a central nervous system disease or a disease that affects the central nervous system. Ask the patient to draw a clock as one method to help identify early stages of cognitive impairment. Two or more errors in drawing a clock (such as numbers are not in correct sequence around clock face or numbers are significantly out of position on the clock face) is a sign of cognitive impairment (Esteban-Santillan et al, 1998). Determine whether any changes in cere-

FUNCTIONAL ASSESSMENT

ABILITY TO PERFORM ADLs RELATED TO MENTAL STATUS

The ability to perform instrumental activities of daily living (ADLs) depends on the patient's mental status. When talking with patients, attempt to determine the patient's ability to perform the following ADLs:

- Manage personal finances and business affairs
- Shop, cook, and prepare balanced meals
- Use problem-solving skills

- Manage medications
- Understand spoken and written language
- Speak and write
- Remember appointments, family occasions, holidays, household tasks

Ask the patient to choose the best answer for how he or she felt over the preceding week.

1. Are you basically satisfied with your life?	Yes/No
2. Have you dropped many of your activities and interests?	Yes/No
3. Do you feel that your life is empty?	Yes/No
4. Do you often get bored?	Yes/No
5. Are you in good spirits most of the time?	Yes/No
6. Are you afraid that something bad is going to happen to you?	Yes/No
7. Do you feel happy most of the time?	Yes/No
8. Do you feel helpless?	Yes/No
9. Do you prefer to stay at home rather than going out and doing new things?	Yes/No
10. Do you feel you have more problems with memory than most people?	Yes/No
11. Do you think it is wonderful to be alive now?	Yes/No
12. Do you feel pretty worthless the way you are now?	Yes/No
13. Do you feel full of energy?	Yes/No
14. Do your feel that your situation is hopeless?	Yes/No
15. Do you think most people are better off than you are?	Yes/No

FIGURE 4-14
Geriatric Depression Scale (short form).
From Sheikh, Yesavage, 1986.

Correct responses are the following:
Yes for questions 2, 3, 4, 6, 8, 9, 10, 12, 14, and 15.
No for questions 1, 5, 7, 11, and 13.
Give one point for each correct answer. A score greater than 5 suggests depression.

bral function could be the consequence of cardiovascular, hepatic, renal, or metabolic disease. Depression, one of the most common conditions in older adults, may contribute to cognitive impairment. Depression can be identified with the Geriatric Depression Scale (Fig. 4-14).

Medications can also impair central nervous system function, causing slowed reaction time, disorientation, confusion, loss of memory, tremors, and anxiety. Problems may develop because of the dosage, number, or interaction of medications prescribed or purchased over the counter. Review the patient's ability to perform activities of daily living associated with mental status functioning.

Some problem-solving skills deteriorate with age, but this may be related to disuse. Skills involving vocabulary and inventories of available information are expected to remain at younger adult levels of performance. Recent memory for important events and conversations is usually not impaired. The older adult may complain about memory loss, but be able to provide substantial detail about episodes of forgetfulness (Rabins, 2004). Recent memory is believed to deteriorate before remote memory. Most older adults comment that their remembrance of distant events actually improves. When close family members are more concerned about memory loss than the patient, be concerned about cognitive impairment and dementia (Rabins, 2004). Because the ability to perceive spatial relationships and to reason abstractly declines with age, some patients may have a problem understanding new concepts by 80 years of age.

Mental function as a whole may be evaluated in about 5 minutes with the Set Test. Ask the patient to name 10 items in each of four groups: *Fruits, Animals, Colors,* and *Towns/cities* (FACT). Do not prompt or rush the patient. The patient's ability to respond demonstrates motivation, alertness, concentration, short-term memory, and problem-solving. In addition, the patient has had to categorize, count, name, and remember the items listed. Each of these skills is important to enable older people to adapt to a new environment and learn new self-care skills. To score, give each item 1 point. A maximum of 40 points is possible. Scores less than 15 are associated with dementia. Scores greater than 25 are not associated with dementia. Scores between 15 and 25 need further investigation to distinguish between mental changes and cultural, educational, or social factors.

Facial expressions that are masklike or overly dramatic, or a stance that is stooped and fearful, may indicate a progressive disease in the older adult.

SAMPLE DOCUMENTATION

HISTORY AND PHYSICAL EXAMINATION

Subjective
A 16-year-old male fell playing basketball and struck the back of his head on a wooden floor. No loss of consciousness, got up and walked immediately, dazed and confused for a few moments, has a headache.

Objective
Oriented to time, place, and person. Reasoning and arithmetic calculation abilities intact. Immediate, recent, and remote memory intact. Appropriate mood and feelings expressed. Speech clearly and smoothly enunciated. Comprehends direction.

For additional sample documentation, see Chapter 26.

SUMMARY OF EXAMINATION

MENTAL STATUS

1. Observe physical appearance and behavior (p. 90).
2. Investigate cognitive abilities by assessing the following (pp. 90-95):
   • State of consciousness
   • Response to questions
   • Reasoning
   • Arithmetic ability
   • Memory
   • Attention span
3. Evaluate emotional stability from the following (pp. 95-96):
   • Signs of depression or anxiety
   • Disturbance in thought content
   • Hallucinations
4. Observe speech and language by the following (pp. 96-97):
   • Voice quality
   • Articulation
   • Coherence
   • Comprehension

COMMON ABNORMALITIES

DISORDERS OF ALTERED MENTAL STATUS

DELIRIUM

Delirium is an acute confusional state accompanied by a disorder of perception. Symptoms include acute alterations in mental status, attention span, sleep patterns, and affect. The person is unable to orient to time, place, or circumstance, but maintains orientation to person. Behavior may vary from intense agitation, frenzied excitement, and trembling; to decreased motor activity and sluggishness. Hallucinations, vivid dreams, absurd fantasies, and delusions

MNEMONICS

Causes of Dementia: DEMENTIA

D Drugs, medications
E Emotional illness, depression
M Metabolic, endocrine disorders
E Eye/ear involvement, environmental
N Nutritional, neurologic
T Tumor, trauma
I Infection
A Alcoholism, anemia, atherosclerosis

From Dains, et al, 1998.

TABLE 4-4	Distinguishing Characteristics of Delirium and Dementia	
Characteristic	**Delirium**	**Dementia**
Onset	Sudden	Insidious, relentless, or sporadic
Duration	Hours, days	Persistent
Time of day	Worse at night and when drug levels peak, sleep-wake cycle disturbed	Stable, no change
Cognition	Impairment of memory, attentiveness, consciousness, calculations	Impairment of abstract thinking, judgment, memory, thought patterns, calculations, agnosia, permanent and progressive
Activity	Increased or decreased, may fluctuate; tremors, spastic movements	Unchanged from usual behavior
Speech/language	Rambling and irrelevant conversation, illogical flow of ideas, incoherent	Disordered, rambling, incoherent; struggles to find words
Mood and affect	Rapid mood swings; fearful, suspicious	Depressed, apathetic, uninterested
Delusions/hallucinations	Visual, auditory, tactile hallucinations, delusions	Delusions, no hallucinations
Associated factors or triggers	Physical condition, drug toxicity, brain injury, change in environment, vision or hearing problems	Chronic alcoholism, vitamin B_{12} deficiency, Huntington chorea, vascular infarcts, HIV encephalopathy, Alzheimer disease
Reversibility	Potential	No, progressive

may also be experienced. Delirium may be associated with a withdrawal from an excessive intake of alcohol or other drugs, age-related impairment of drug metabolism, neurologic or neoplastic disorders, infections, trauma, toxins, or diminished reserves in responding to physiologic stress. Other characteristics are described in Table 4-4.

DELIRIUM TREMENS

Delirium tremens is the brain's response to withdrawal of alcohol that was consumed in large quantities over time. Once the central nervous system depressant effects of the alcohol dissipate, the brain experiences a rebound excitation. Signs of alcohol withdrawal include elevated vital signs, irritability, anxiety, restlessness, and anorexia. Signs of delirium tremens include agitation, confusion, combativeness, panic, seizures, hallucinations, and illusions.

DEMENTIA

Dementia is a clinical syndrome of failing memory and cognitive impairment, behavioral abnormalities, and personality changes resulting from a chronic progressive deterioration of the brain. It is usually related to obvious structural diseases of the brain tissue. Classic signs include memory impairment, disturbance in executive functioning, and one or more of the following: aphasia, apraxia, or agnosia. Impairment in social and occupational functioning is present (Lyketsos, 2004). Other characteristics are described in Table 4-4.

CONCUSSION

A concussion is a temporary alteration in mental status resulting from brain injury (e.g., head trauma). Common causes include sports injuries, motor vehicle crashes, and falls. Immediate signs and symptoms may include any or all of the following: headache, dizziness, a dazed look, slurred speech, slow motor and verbal responses, emotional lability, restlessness, irritability, nausea and vomiting, blurred vision, tinnitus, hypersensitivity to stimuli, amnesia, and deficits in coordination, cognition, memory, and attention. Loss of consciousness, even for a few seconds, indicates a more severe injury. Symptoms may disappear within 15 minutes or persist for several weeks.

DISORDERS OF MOOD

DEPRESSION	Depression is a common psychiatric disorder resulting from a lack of important neurotransmitters that function at the synapses between neurons in the brain. Symptoms range from mild to a major depressive disorder that is characterized by feelings of helplessness and hopelessness and recurrent suicidal thoughts. Mood and affect are altered, with extreme sadness or anxiety and agitation expressed. Somatic complaints may include altered appetite, problems sleeping, constipation, headache, and fatigue. The patient may complain of memory loss, poor concentration, lack of motivation, and indecisiveness. Speech may be slow and sluggish. Delusions of worthlessness or paranoid ideation may be present. The disorder may result from grief, reaction to medical or neurologic diseases, or a change in lifestyle. See risk factors for suicide in Box 1-2.
MANIA	Mania is a persistently elevated, expansive, or irritable mood lasting longer than a week; it is caused by a biochemical imbalance in the brain. Symptoms include periods of hyperactivity, overconfidence, an exaggerated view of one's own abilities, grandiose or persecutory delusions, a decreased need for sleep, and poor social judgment. The person has racing thoughts, flights of ideas, and rapid-fire speech that is loud and may involve excessive rhyming or punning. Impairments in social, occupational, and interpersonal functioning are seen. The person appears involved in pleasurable activities, but no pleasure appears to be associated with them.

ANXIETY DISORDERS

Anxiety disorders are a group of disorders with marked anxiety or fear at such a high level that significant interference is noted with personal, social, and occupational functioning. Specific disorders include panic attacks, panic disorders, agoraphobia, specific phobias, obsessive-compulsive disorder, and acute and post-traumatic stress disorder. Signs and symptoms of panic attacks include palpitations, tachycardia, sweating, shaking, trembling, choking, chest pain or discomfort, nausea, abdominal distress, dizziness, faintness, feeling unreal or detached from self, "going crazy," and paresthesias. Many people suffering from these disorders recognize that their fear or anxiety is unreasonable, such as chronic social avoidance because they fear being embarrassed or humiliated. These are the most common psychiatric disorders, and people who suffer from them may have problems throughout their lifetime.

SCHIZOPHRENIA

Schizophrenia is a severe, persistent, psychotic disorder that is a neuroanatomic and neurochemical abnormality; it may be either genetically or environmentally induced. It typically has an adolescent or early adult onset. Schizophrenia affects a person's perceptions, thinking, language, emotions, and social behavior. Major symptoms include hallucinations, delusions, and disordered thinking, speech, and behavior. The disorder is characterized by relapses and persists throughout life. The several subtypes include paranoid, disorganized, catatonia, mixed type, and residual (no active symptoms).

INFANTS AND CHILDREN

MENTAL RETARDATION	Mental retardation is manifested during the child's development by significant subaverage general intellectual functioning, existing concurrently with deficits in adaptive behavior. Signs and symptoms include delayed developmental milestones, inability to discriminate between two or more stimuli, impaired short-term memory, and lack of motivation.
ATTENTION DEFICIT HYPERACTIVITY DISORDER	In attention deficit hyperactivity disorder (ADHD), a combination of behavior problems interfere with the child's ability to learn; these include developmentally inappropriate inattention, impulsivity, and hyperactivity. Other symptoms may include temper outbursts, labile moods, and poor self-esteem. Onset is before 7 years of age and is more common in boys than girls. It is not related to mental retardation or a psychiatric disorder.

AUTISTIC DISORDER

Autistic disorder is a pervasive developmental disorder that may result from left brain dysfunction; it includes a combination of behavioral traits and communication deficits that begins before age 3 years. The child has a deficit in at least one of three areas: social interaction, language for social purposes, or symbolic and imaginative play. Language is delayed or does not develop. Echolalia (parrot speech) is common. Behavioral traits associated with this condition may include a lack of awareness of others, an aversion to touch or being held, odd or repetitive behaviors, or preoccupation with parts of objects. Motor development often progresses normally. The majority of autistic children are mentally retarded. This condition is more common in boys than girls with a ratio of 4:1, and may occur in a familial pattern. Only 1% to 2% of affected children progress to function independently as adults.

OLDER ADULTS

DEMENTIA OF ALZHEIMER TYPE

Dementia of Alzheimer type accounts for approximately 60% to 70% of dementia cases. There is severe progressive deterioration in mental functions with a subtle, insidious onset. The duration and rate of progression varies. Impaired ability to learn new information or to recall previously learned information is present. At least one of the following signs is also present: aphasia, apraxia, agnosia, or a disturbance in executive functioning. The disorder leads to profound disintegration of personality and to eventual complete disorientation. Cognitive deficits are not caused by other central nervous system or systemic conditions. It is present in approximately 3% to 11% of people older than 65 years of age and in 25% to 47% of people older than 85 years (Boustani et al., 2003). Women, especially those with a positive family history, are at greatest risk.

VASCULAR DEMENTIA (MULTI-INFARCT DEMENTIA)

Vascular dementia has a rapid onset with deterioration in cognitive ability, often related to a series of infarcts in the cerebral blood vessels. The patient has impaired memory, leading to an inability to learn new information or to recall previously learned information. In addition, the patient has aphasia, apraxia, agnosia, or a disturbance in executive functioning. Other focal neurologic signs are usually present. Risks include long-standing hypertension and small strokes often without significant loss of muscle strength. Symptom onset may be sudden or subtle depending upon the location, size, and frequency of the infarct. A stepwise deterioration of cognitive function occurs with plateaus and occasional episodes of improvement.

ELECTRONIC RESOURCES

For Weblinks and additional resources, go to   **evolve**

http://evolve.elsevier.com/Seidel

or to the Companion CD-ROM.

Additional information related to the content in Chapter 4 can be found on the companion website at evolve.elsevier.com/Seidel/ or on the interactive companion CD-ROM. Resources and activities for Chapter 4 include:
- Sound and Vision theater
- Printouts for Your Practice
- Spanish Assessment Terms with Pronunciation Guide
- Instant Calculators

GROWTH AND MEASUREMENT

Weight and body composition offer much information about an individual's health status and often provide a clue to the presence of disease when they are out of balance. The care of children is exciting because of the constancy of change that is explicit in growth and development. Children just do not stay the same. Measuring their weights and heights and giving careful attention to the sequence of their achievements is gratifying as you get to know a child over time. When all goes well and the child grows and develops as expected, there is great pleasure; but when all is not well, your careful attention and early detection can often correct or at least ameliorate a problem.

The focus of this chapter is the evaluation of an individual's anthropometric parameters and the examination for growth, gestational age, and pubertal development. Nutritional assessment is discussed in Chapter 6. Neurologic and motor development of children is discussed in Chapters 21 and 22. For specific age-related milestones, see Tables 21-4 and 22-13.

ANATOMY AND PHYSIOLOGY

Growth, the increase in size of an individual or of a single organ, is dependent on a sequence of endocrine, genetic, constitutional, environmental, and nutritional influences. Through the biologic process of development and maturation, individual organ systems acquire function.

The growth process requires the interaction and balance of many hormones for normal growth and development to proceed (Fig. 5-1).

Growth hormone is secreted by the pituitary gland under the neuroendocrine control of two hormones of the hypothalamus. Growth hormone–releasing hormone (GHRH) stimulates the pituitary to release the growth hormone; somatostatin inhibits the secretion of both GHRH and thyroid-stimulating hormone.

Growth hormone needs the insulin-like growth factor I (IGF I), produced by the liver, to stimulate muscle and skeletal growth. The production of IGF I is regulated by growth hormone, the thyroid hormones, and possibly insulin. IGF I acts by stimulating target cells that control connective tissue growth and ossification. Growth hormone also has a direct effect on the growth of other tissues. Insulin-like growth factors act primarily as local regulators of cell growth and differentiation.

The trigger for puberty is potentially linked to the concentration of leptin, a hormone produced by adipose tissue, which informs the central nervous system that adequate nutritional

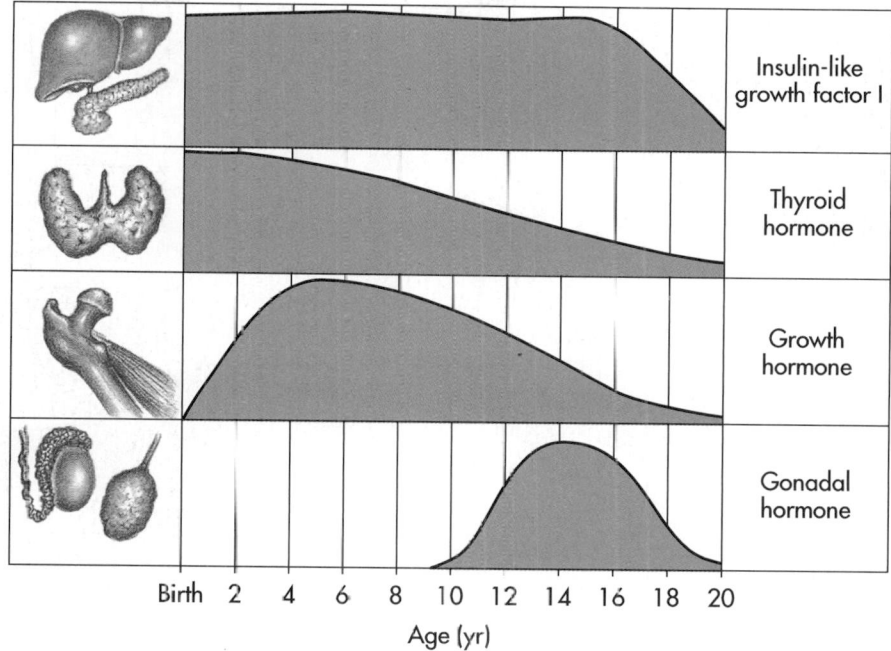

FIGURE 5-1
Hormones affecting growth during childhood and the ages at which they are most influential. *Redrawn from Hughes, 1984.*

status and body fat mass are present to support pubertal changes and growth (Mann & Plant, 2002). G protein–coupled receptor gene is another required factor for puberty to begin (Crowley et al, 2003). The gonads begin to secrete testosterone and estrogen during puberty. Rising levels of these hormones trigger the release of gonadotropins (luteinizing hormone and follicle-stimulating hormone) that stimulate the gonads to release more sex hormones. The genitalia begin growing to adult proportions. Testosterone enhances muscular development and sexual maturation, and promotes bone maturation and epiphyseal closure. Estrogen stimulates the development of female secondary sexual characteristics and linear growth by the acceleration of skeletal maturation and epiphyseal fusion. Androgens, secreted by the adrenal glands, promote masculinization of the secondary sex characteristics and skeletal maturation.

Growth at puberty is dependent on the interaction of growth hormone, IGF I, and the sex steroids (androgens). The sex steroids stimulate an increased secretion of the growth hormone, which in turn mediates the dramatic increase in IGF I. This leads to the adolescent growth spurt. Thyroid hormones play a central role in skeletal maturation by stimulating growth hormone secretion and by controlling the effect of growth hormone on IGF I production. Thyroid hormones also affect the growth and maturation of other body tissues.

DIFFERENCES IN GROWTH BY ORGAN SYSTEM

Each organ or organ system has its particular period of rapid growth, marked by rapid cell differentiation and changes in form that is influenced by the physical and environmental factors to which it is exposed. Each individual has a unique growth timetable and final growth outcome; however, the sequential patterns are consistent for all, unless some external environmental or inherent pathophysiologic process intervenes (Figs. 5-2 and 5-3).

General growth encompasses most body measurements and organ growth, specifically the musculoskeletal system, liver, and kidneys. Their growth approximates the growth curves described for stature.

Skeletal growth is considered complete when the epiphyses of long bones have completely fused. The mean age for this event in males is 17.5 years (±2 years) and in females is 14.5 years (±2 years) or 2 years after menarche. However, skeletal growth continues until 30 years of age with the apposition of bone to the upper and lower surfaces of the vertebral bodies. The increase in stature is only 3 to 5 mm during this time. Stature is stationary between the ages of 30 and 50 years and then begins to decline (Tanner, 1990).

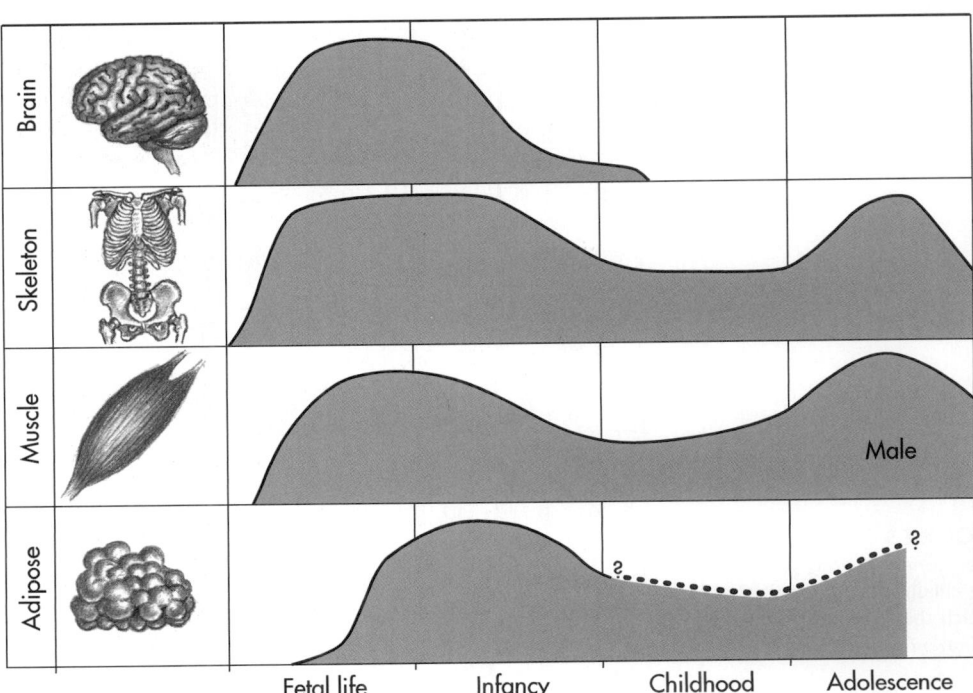

FIGURE 5-2
Rates of growth in various tissues between fetal development and adolescence.
Redrawn from Smith, 1977.

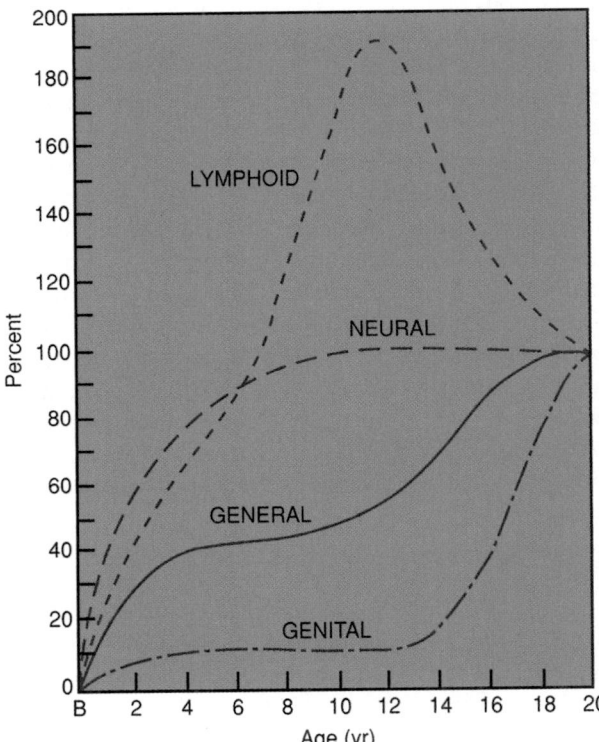

FIGURE 5-3
Growth rates for the body as a whole and three types of tissues. Lymphoid type: thymus, lymph nodes, and intestinal lymph masses. Neural type: brain, dura, spinal cord, optic apparatus, and head dimensions. General type: body as a whole; external dimensions; and respiratory, digestive, renal, circulatory, and musculoskeletal systems. Genital type: includes the reproductive organ system.
From Wong, 1999. Modified from Harris et al, 1930.

Weight is closely related to growth in stature and organ development. Growth and development are influenced by nutritional adequacy, which contributes to the number and size of adipose cells. The number of adipose cells increases throughout childhood. Gender-related differences in fat deposition appear in infancy and continue through adolescence.

Lymphatic tissues (i.e., lymph nodes, spleen, tonsils, adenoids, and blood lymphocytes) are small in relation to total body size but are well developed at birth. These tissues grow rapidly to reach adult dimensions by 6 years of age. By age 10 to 12 years, the lymphatic tissues are at their peak, about double adult size. During adolescence, they decrease in size until stable adult dimensions are reached.

The reproductive organs, both internal and external, have a slow prepubertal growth. With the interaction of the hypothalamus, pituitary, and gonadal hormones, the reproductive organs double in size during adolescence, achieving maturation and function.

The brain is a marvelous organ, so fully developed at an early age that it provides infants and young children opportunities to sense and appreciate the world and to learn an enormous amount. We often fail to appreciate the sophistication of the brain in the body of a baby or a toddler and thus tend to underestimate the ability of the very young to sense their environment and to process a myriad of constant inputs.

The brain, along with the skull, eyes, and ears, completes physical development more quickly than any other body part. The most rapid and critical period of brain growth occurs between conception and 2 years of age. Most of the neurons are present by 18 to 20 weeks of gestation, and two thirds of brain cells are present at birth. Glial cells, dendrites, and myelin continue to develop after birth, and by 10 months of age, new cell development is complete. Cell size continues to increase, and at 2 years of age, 80% of the brain growth is completed (Trauner, 1979). Brain growth continues until about 12 to 15 years of age. During adolescence, the size of the head further increases because of development of air sinuses and thickening of the scalp and skull.

INFANTS AND CHILDREN

As the child grows from infancy to adulthood, the change in body proportion is related to the pattern of skeletal growth (Fig. 5-4).

Growth of the head predominates during the fetal period. Fetal weight gain naturally follows growth in length, but weight reaches its peak during the third trimester with the increase in organ size. The birth weight of the infant is in large part determined by the mother's prepregnancy weight and the weight gained by the mother during pregnancy, by the placental function, and by the gestational age (Fig. 5-5).

During infancy, the growth of the trunk predominates, and weight gain velocity proceeds at a rapid but decelerating rate. The fat content of the body increases slowly during early fetal development and then rapidly accelerates during infancy until approximately 9 months of age.

The legs are the fastest growing body part during childhood, and weight is gained at a steady rate. Fat tissue increases slowly until 7 years of age, at which time a prepubertal fat spurt occurs before the true growth spurt.

The trunk and the legs elongate during adolescence. During this period about 50% of the individual's ideal weight is gained, and the skeletal mass and organ systems double in size. Of adults who become obese, 30% are obese during childhood and 70% are obese during adolescence (Subcommittee on Military Weight Management, Committee on Military Nutrition Research, and Food and Nutrition Board of the Institute of Medicine, 2003).

It is during adolescence that males develop broader shoulders and greater musculature; females develop a wider pelvic outlet. Males have a slight increase in body fat during early adolescence and then have a proportionate gain in lean body tissue. Females have a persistent increase in fat tissue throughout adolescence, occurring after the peak growth spurt (Peck, Ullrich, 1985).

PREGNANT WOMEN

Progressive weight gain is expected during pregnancy, but the amount varies among women. The growing fetus accounts for only 5 to 10 pounds of the total weight gained. The remainder results from an increase in maternal tissues (i.e., placenta, amniotic fluid, uterus, blood and fluid volume, breasts, and fat reserves) (Fig. 5-6).

Desirable weight gain follows a curve through the trimesters of pregnancy. The rate of weight gain is slow during the first trimester, rapid during the second trimester, and less rapid during the third trimester. Maternal tissue growth accounts for most of the weight gained in the first and second trimesters, whereas fetal growth accounts for weight gained during the third trimester. Pregnant adolescents younger than 16 years, or less than 2 years after menarche, may still be in their growth spurt. They may require higher weight gains during pregnancy to achieve an optimal infant birth weight (Stang, 2000).

Maternal nutrition before and during pregnancy and during lactation may have subtle effects on the developing brain of the infant and on the outcome of the pregnancy. Women who have inadequate weight gain are at risk for delivering a low-birth-weight or intrauterine

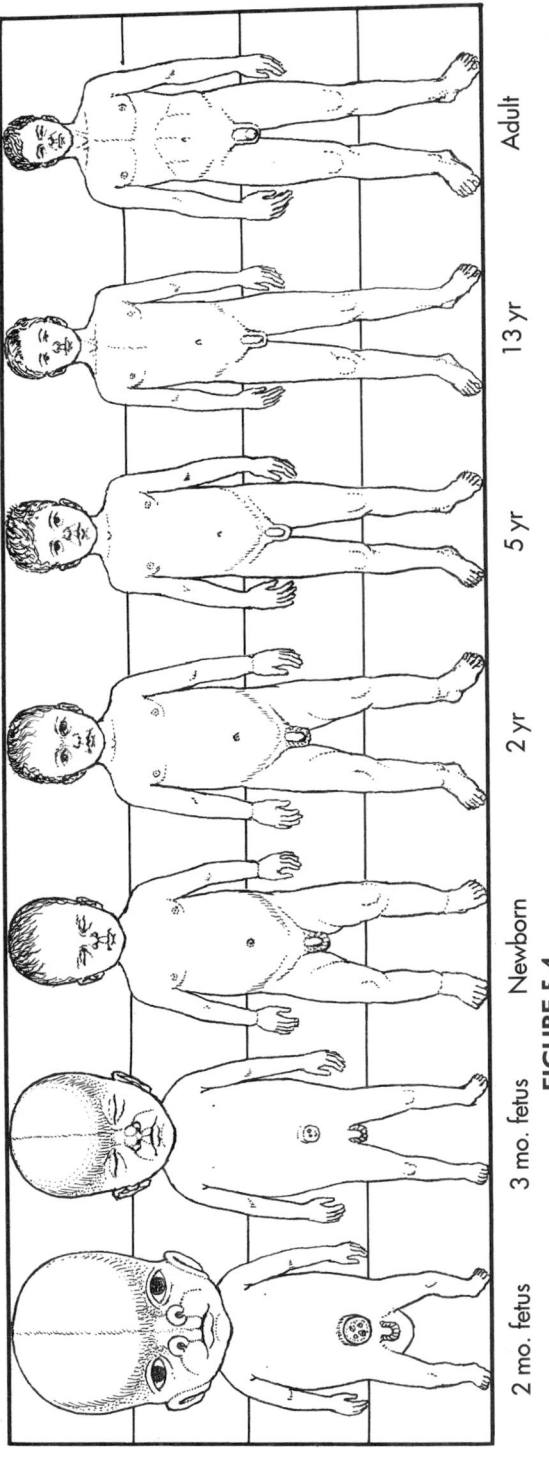

FIGURE 5-4
Changes in body proportions from 8 weeks of gestation through adulthood.
Redrawn from Crouch, McClintic, 1976.

GROWTH AND MEASUREMENT
Anatomy and Physiology

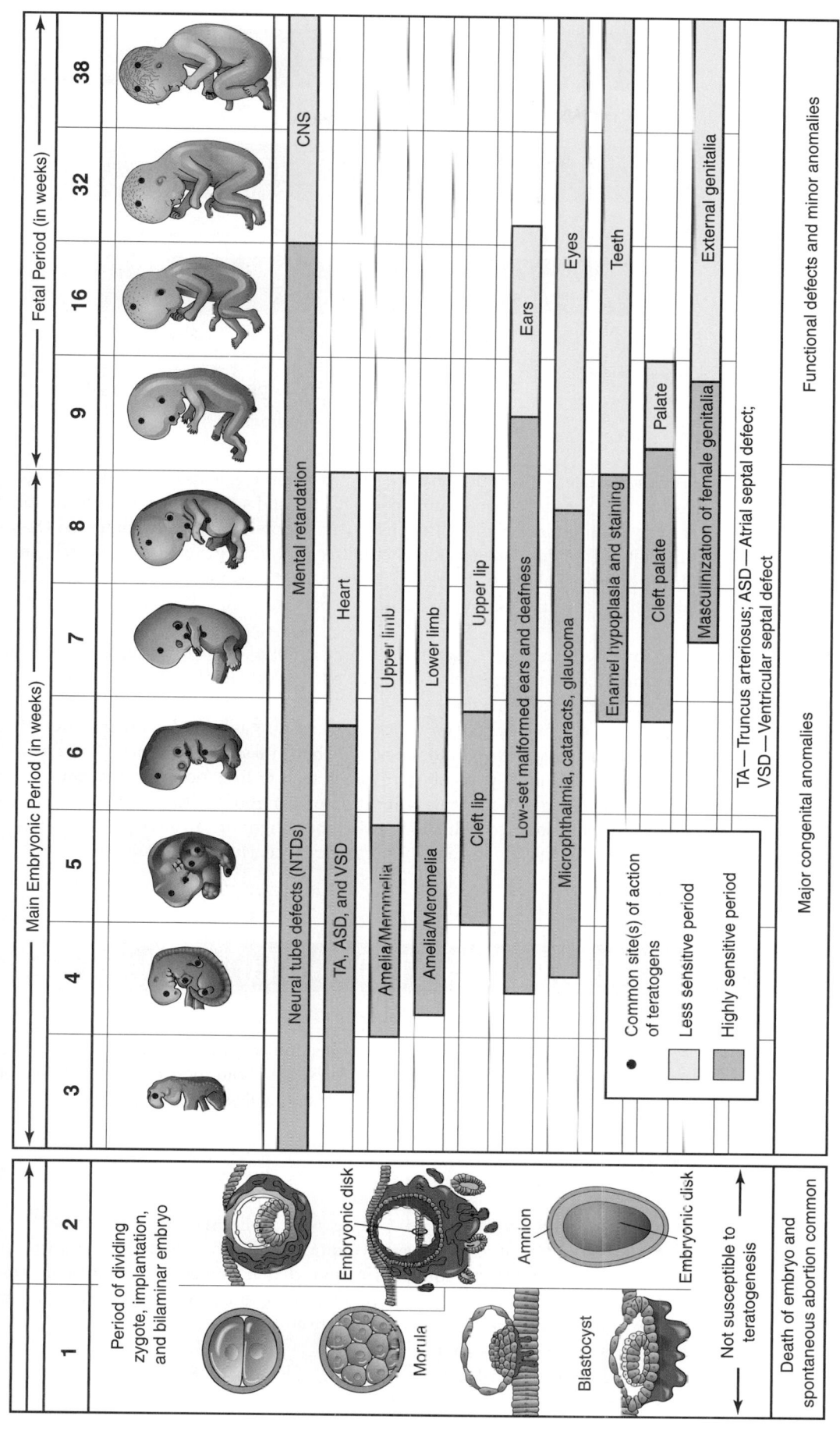

FIGURE 5-5
Sensitive or critical periods in human development.
From Moore, 1977.

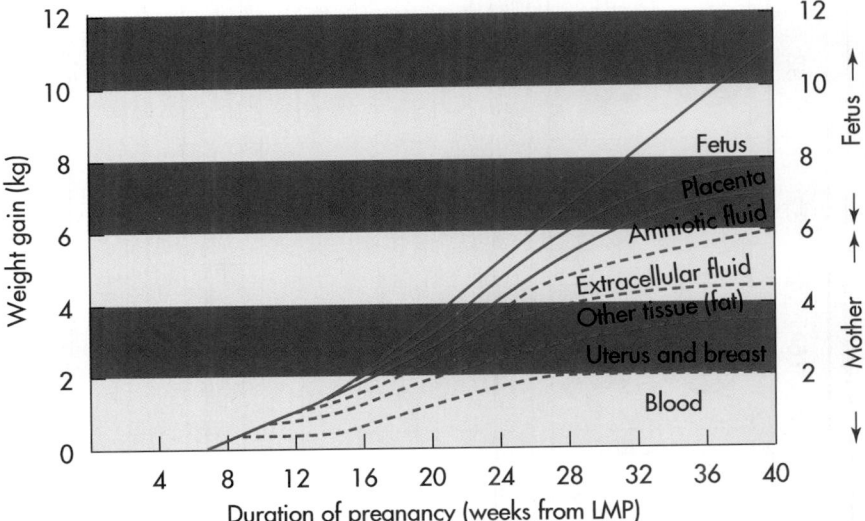

FIGURE 5-6
Weight gain during pregnancy and tissue growth contribute to the total weight gained.
From Schneide et al, 1977.

growth–restricted infant and lack of plasma volume expansion (Johnson & Niebyl, 2002). Postpartum weight retention ranges between 0.5 and 4.8 kg for most women; however, black women retain more weight in the postpartum period than white women do (Subcommittee on Military Weight Management, Committee on Military Nutrition Research, and Food and Nutrition Board of the Institute of Medicine, 2003). Women who gain excess weight may be susceptible to future obesity and its health consequences.

OLDER ADULTS

Stature declines in older adults beginning at approximately 50 years of age. This is caused by a thinning of the intervertebral disks and by the development of kyphosis with osteoporotic vertebral compression.

An increase in overweight and obese older adults has been documented over the past 15 to 20 years. A decrease in weight for height and body mass index has been found with increasing age between 70 and 89 years of age. Women tend to lose more subcutaneous fat rather than muscle mass. Men lose a greater proportion of arm muscle (Kuczmarski, Kuczmarski, Najjar, 2000). An age-associated reduction in size and weight of various organs has been identified, especially of the liver, lungs, and kidneys (McCance, Huether, 2006).

REVIEW OF RELATED HISTORY

For each of the conditions discussed in this section, targeted topics to include in the history of the present illness are listed. Responses to questions about these topics help fully assess the patient's condition and provide clues for focusing the physical examination.

HISTORY OF PRESENT ILLNESS

- Weight loss and weight gain (see Chapter 6 for additional suggested targeted topics)
    - Undesired weight loss: anorexia; vomiting or diarrhea, frequency, consistency, time period; excessive thirst, frequent urination; change in lifestyle; activity and stress levels
    - Medications: chemotherapy, diuretics, insulin, fluoxetine (Prozac); nonprescription diet pills, laxatives, steroids, oral contraceptives
- Changes in body proportions
    - Coarsening of facial features, enlarging of hands and feet, moon facies
    - Change in fat distribution: trunk-girdle versus generalized
    - Medication: steroids

PAST MEDICAL HISTORY

- Chronic illness: gastrointestinal, renal, pulmonary, cardiac, cancer, infections, allergies
- Previous weight loss or gain efforts: weight at 21 years, maximum body weight

FAMILY HISTORY

- Obesity
- Constitutionally short or tall stature, precocious or delayed puberty
- Genetic or metabolic disorder: cystic fibrosis, dwarfism

PERSONAL AND SOCIAL HISTORY

- Usual weight and height
- Activity or exercise pattern
- Use of alcohol
- Use of club (street) drugs

INFANTS

- Estimated gestational age, birth weight
- Following an established percentile growth curve
  - Unexplained changes in length, weight, or head circumference
  - Poor growth: falling one or more standard deviations off growth curve pattern; below fifth percentile for weight and height; infant small for gestational age; quality of mother-infant interaction
- Development: achieving milestones at appropriate ages
- Congenital anomaly or chronic illness: heart defect, hydrocephalus, microcephalus, malabsorption syndrome, urinary tract infection, others

CHILDREN AND ADOLESCENTS

- Sexual maturation of girls: early (before 7 years) or delayed (beyond 13 years); signs of breast development and pubic hair, age at menarche
- Sexual maturation of boys: early (before 9 years) or delayed (beyond 14 years); signs of genital development and pubic hair
- Short stature: not growing as fast as peers, change in shoe and clothing size in past year, extremities short or long for size of trunk, height of parents, size of head disproportionate to body
- Tall stature: growing faster than peers, height of parents, signs of sexual maturation
- Medications: steroids, growth hormones

PREGNANT WOMEN

- Prepregnancy weight, dietary intake
- Age at menarche
- Date of last menstrual period, weight gain pattern, following established weight gain curve for gestational course
- Eating disorders
- History of pica (eating laundry starch, ice, clay, raw icing)
- Nausea and vomiting

OLDER ADULTS

- Chronic debilitating illness: problems with meal preparation; problems eating; poorly fitting dentures; ability to follow prescribed diet; difficulty with chewing, swallowing, or digestion
- See Chapter 6 for nutrition topics to discuss.

EXAMINATION AND FINDINGS

EQUIPMENT

- ◆ Standing platform scale with height attachment
- ◆ Skinfold thickness calipers
- ◆ Measuring tape, nonstretching
- ◆ Infant scale
- ◆ Recumbent measuring device (for infants)
- ◆ Stature measuring device (for children)

WEIGHT AND STANDING HEIGHT

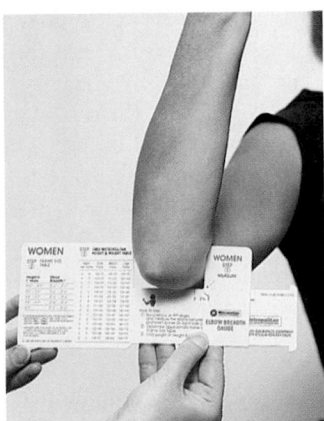

FIGURE 5-7
Measurement of elbow breadth using sliding calipers.

To measure weight, have the patient stand in the middle of the scale platform while you balance the scale. Move the largest weight to the last 50-pound or 10-kg increment under the patient's weight. Adjust the smaller weight to balance the scale. Read the weight to the nearest 0.1 kg or ¼ pound. Weight variations occur during the day and from day to day with changes in fluid and intestinal contents of the body. When monitoring a patient's weight daily or weekly, weigh the patient at the same time each day.

To measure height, have the patient stand erect with his or her back to the scale. Pull up the height attachment and position the headpiece at the patient's crown. Make the reading at the nearest centimeter or ½ inch.

Measurement of the elbow breadth provides an estimate of frame size. Have the patient extend the right arm and flex the elbow to 90 degrees. The patient's thumb should be pointing up with the palm turned laterally. Facing the patient, place the elbow-breadth measuring device or skinfold calipers, held on the same plane as the upper arm, on the two most prominent bones of the elbow to measure the elbow breadth (Fig. 5-7). (Sliding calipers may be needed if the skinfold calipers do not extend to the breadth of the elbow.) Read the patient's measurement in centimeters and compare it with the table of elbow breadth measurements for age and gender (Table 5-1).

When calipers are not available, another method for determining frame size is to measure the patient's wrist circumference. This measurement is used with the patient's height to create a ratio. Place the measuring tape around the smallest part of the wrist distal to the styloid process of the radius and ulna. Obtain the measurement in centimeters to the nearest millimeter. The wrist circumference ratio is the patient's height in centimeters divided by the

TABLE 5-1	**Elbow Breadth Measurements for Age and Gender (Medium Frame)**[*][†]		
Men		**Women**	
Age (yr)	**Elbow Breadth (cm)**	**Age (yr)**	**Elbow Breadth (cm)**
18-24	6.6-7.6	18-24	5.6-6.4
25-34	6.7-7.8	25-34	5.7-6.7
35-44	6.7-7.9	35-44	5.7-7.0
45-54	6.7-8.0	45-54	5.7-7.1
55-74	6.7-8.0	55-74	5.8-7.1

Modified from Frisancho, 1984.
*Data from National Center for Health Statistics, 1981.
†Measurements lower than ranges given indicate a small frame, whereas higher measurements indicate a large frame.

wrist circumference in centimeters. Table 5-2 describes how to determine the body frame size based on the wrist circumference ratio.

Once the frame size has been determined, the appropriateness of the patient's weight for gender, height, and frame size can be evaluated (see Appendix C, Tables C-1 and C-2). It is necessary to convert the patient's weight to kilograms to use the tables.

The prevalence of obesity among adults is increasing, with approximately 65% of adults in the United States being overweight, 30% being obese, and 5% being extremely obese (Hedley, et al, 2004). Severe weight loss and wasting are usually associated with a debilitating disease or self-starvation.

WAIST-TO-HIP CIRCUMFERENCE RATIO

The waist-to-hip circumference ratio is a measure of fat distribution by body type. It is not as helpful as the body mass index in assessing total body fat (see Chapter 6). An excess proportion of trunk and abdominal fat (e.g., an ovoid or apple-shaped body) has a higher risk association with diabetes mellitus, hyperlipidemia, stroke, and ischemic heart disease than does a larger proportion of gluteal fat (e.g., a pear-shaped body). Using a tape measure with millimeter marks, measure the waist at a midpoint between the costal margin and the iliac crest. Then measure the hip at the widest part of the gluteal region (Fig. 5-8). Divide the waist circumference by the hip circumference to obtain the ratio. Ratios greater than 1.0 in men and more than 0.85 in women indicate increased risk of diseases identified above (McGee, 2001). This measurement is an indicator of central fat distribution and seems predictive of certain disease risk for both whites and blacks.

TRICEPS SKINFOLD THICKNESS

The measurement of skinfold or fatfold thickness provides another parameter to evaluate the nutritional status of the patient. The jaws of skinfold thickness calipers must be correctly placed to get an accurate reading.

TABLE 5-2	Determining Body Frame Size from the Wrist Circumference Ratio*	
Frame Size	**Ratio for Men**	**Ratio for Women**
Small	>10.4	>10.9
Medium	10.4-9.6	10.9-9.9
Large	<9.6	<9.9

*Height (cm) ÷ wrist circumference (cm).

STAYING WELL

CONTROLLING WEIGHT

Exercise is a key factor in maintaining body weight or in reducing body weight. Regular exercise such as 30 minutes of walking or other aerobic exercise several times a week is recommended. Look for ways to increase activity such as walking up stairs instead of taking elevators, or parking a distance from the doors to businesses and work places. Children should have video, television, and computer hours limited and be encouraged to walk, ride a bicycle, and participate in sports and recreational activities.

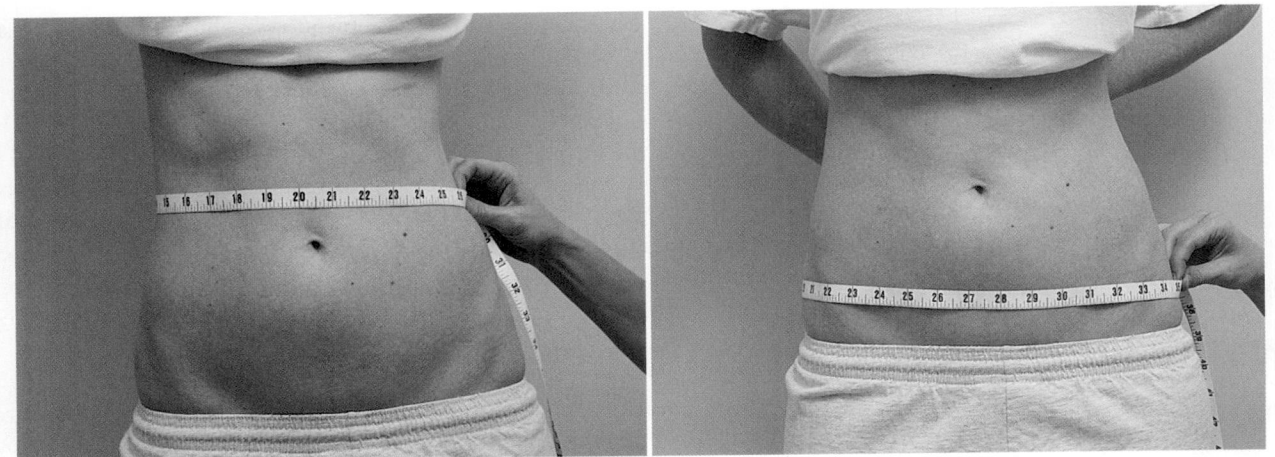

A   B

FIGURE 5-8
Measurement of waist circumference **(A)** and hip circumference **(B)** to calculate the waist-to-hip circumference ratio. Waist circumference (cm) ÷ Hip circumference (cm) = Waist-to-hip ratio.

To determine the site of the triceps skinfold thickness measurement, have the patient flex the right arm at a right angle. Position yourself behind the patient and using a measuring tape, make a horizontal mark halfway between the tips of the olecranon and acromial processes on the posterior aspect of the arm. Then draw a line along the vertical plane of the arm to cross the midpoint. Allowing the patient's arm to hang relaxed, use your thumb and forefinger to grasp and lift the triceps skinfold about ½ inch (1.27 cm) proximal to the marked cross. Make sure you feel the main bulk of the triceps muscle, identifying the muscle's subcutaneous interface between your fingers deep to the skinfold. (If you do not feel the muscle bulk, you may be too medial or lateral to the muscle mass and need to reposition your fingers.) Place the caliper jaws on each side of the raised skinfold at the marked cross, but not so tightly as to cause an indentation (Fig. 5-9). With the gauge at eye level, make two readings to the nearest millimeter at the same site and derive an average.

Because approximately 50% of the body fat is present in the subcutaneous tissue layers, a correlation exists between the triceps skinfold thickness and the body's fat content. Therefore the triceps skinfold measurement may be used in the diagnosis of obesity. Compare the patient's measurement with the percentiles of triceps skinfold thickness by age and gender (see Appendix C, Tables C-1 and C-2).

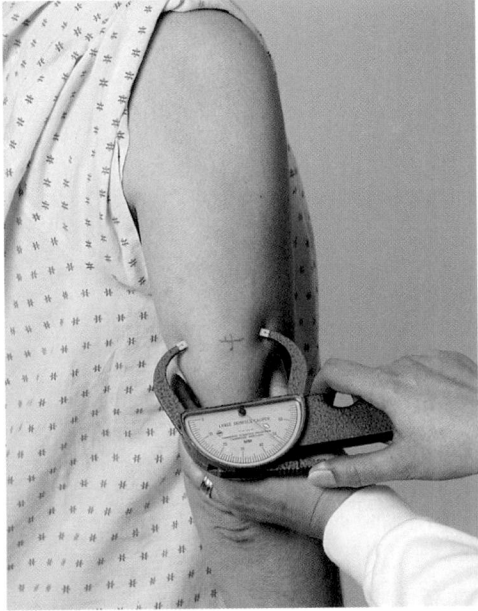

FIGURE 5-9
Placement of calipers for triceps skinfold thickness measurement.

Measuring skinfold thickness in the very obese is difficult because calipers are not large enough for some skinfolds. The thickness of adipose tissue in the obese also makes it more difficult to raise the skinfold with parallel sides for the measurement.

INFANTS

PHYSICAL VARIATIONS
Birth Weight
Black infants generally weigh 181 to 240 g less than white infants at birth. Asian, Filipino, Hawaiian, and Puerto Rican babies generally also weigh less than white infants. However, the birth weights of Native American/American Indian infants vary a great deal: as much as 362 g separates the mean birth weights of various tribes.

Data from Hulsey, Levkoff, Alexander, 1991; National Center for Health Statistics, 1981; Yip, Li, Chong, 1991; Crowell et al, 1992; Adams, Niswander, 1973; Thomson, 1990.

A baby born at term who is the size and proportion expected (i.e., not too big and not too small) and is free of a history of prenatal or perinatal difficulty has the best chance to be a healthy neonate and infant. Unexpected deviations during the first few days of life must always be given serious attention because they may be clues to potential problems. This is true whether the deviation is one of measurement or is suspected because of a subjective impression on physical examination of the baby's vibrancy and interest in life, particularly in feeding.

Most babies born at full term to the same parents weigh within 6 ounces of each other at birth. If the baby has a lower birth weight than older siblings, suspect an undisclosed congenital abnormality or intrauterine growth retardation. Babies with a larger birth weight than older siblings, at 10 pounds or greater, are at risk for acute lymphatic leukemia.

There is real excitement in watching an infant's growth and development. It is not just a measurement of weight and height and other growth parameters that provides such feelings, but also careful attention to the sequence of these measurements and to the child's progressive achievements that is exciting about the care of children.

RECUMBENT LENGTH

CLINICAL PEARL
Reliability of Length Measurements
The reliability of length measurements in newborns is difficult because of the natural flexion of the infant and the molding of the head. Use a consistent technique to increase reliability between examiners, and verify the length with a second measurement.

Johnson et al, 1999.

Recumbent length is the measurement of choice for infants between birth and 24 to 36 months of age (Fig. 5-10). Place the infant supine on the measuring device and have the parent hold the infant's head against the headboard. Hold the infant's legs straight at the knees and place the footboard against the bottom of the infant's feet. Read the length measurement to the nearest 0.5 cm or ¼ inch. Compare the infant's length to the population standard, using the appropriate growth curve for age and gender, and identify the infant's percentile placement (see Appendix C, Figs. C-1 and C-2; for very-low-birthweight (VLBW) infants from birth to 12 months, see Appendix C, Fig. C-3).

At birth, healthy term newborns have length variations between 45 and 55 cm (18 and 22 inches). Length increases by 50% in the first year of life.

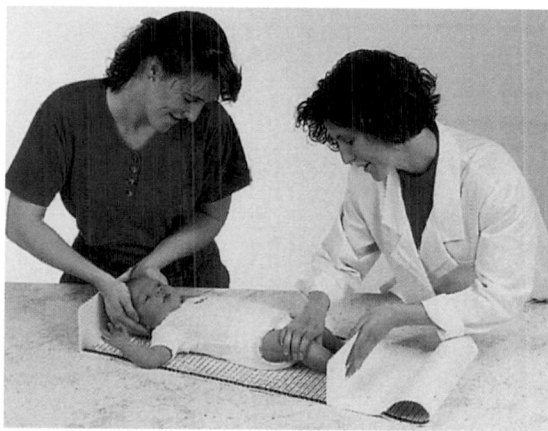

FIGURE 5-10
Measurement of infant length.
Courtesy Seca Corporation., Hanover, MD.

WEIGHT

CLINICAL PEARL

Uses of Growth Charts
Growth charts are designed to plot and track anthropometric data to screen for unusual size and growth patterns, as well as to make an overall clinical assessment. For example, growth charts for children between birth and 36 months of age make it possible to identify excessive weight gain for length. A separate growth curve for VLBW infants compares the growth of these infants with growth of other low birth weight infants, although the Centers for Disease Control and Prevention growth charts may also be used to evaluate the growth of these infants.

Sherry, Mei, Grummer-Strawn, Dietz, 2003.

Use an infant scale, measuring weight in ounces or grams for infants and small children. Distract the infant and balance the scale as you would for a standing scale. Read the weight to the nearest 10 g or ½ ounce when the infant is most still. Plot the infant's weight on the appropriate growth curve for age and gender, comparing the infant's weight to the population standard. Identify the infant's percentile placement (see Appendix C, Figs. C-1 and C-2).

Healthy term newborns vary in weight between 2500 and 4000 g (5 pounds and 8 ounces to 8 pounds and 13 ounces). In general, they double their birth weight by 4 to 5 months of age and triple their birth weight by 12 months of age. Formula-fed infants are heavier after the first 6 months of life than breast-fed infants; they grow faster in the first 6 months of life, with slower growth in the second 6 months of the first year (Binns et al., 1996). VLBW infants tend to be heavier for length than non-VLBW infants until they reach 65 cm in length when they are thinner than non-VLBW infants according to the growth chart percentile lines (Guo et al, 1996).

HEAD CIRCUMFERENCE

CLINICAL PEARL

Paper Tape
Use of paper tape improves intraexaminer and interexaminer reliability.

Sutter et al, 1997.

Measure the infant's head circumference at every health visit until 2 years of age, and then measure the young child's head circumference yearly until 6 years of age. Wrap the measuring tape snugly around the child's head at the occipital protuberance and the supraorbital prominence to find the point of largest circumference, taking care not to cut the skin (Fig. 5-11). Make the reading to the nearest 0.5 cm or ¼ inch. (Remeasure the head circumference at least one time to check the accuracy of your measurement.)

Plot the infant's head circumference on the appropriate growth curve, comparing the infant's measurement with expected measurements for the population (see Appendix C, Figs. C-1 and C-2).

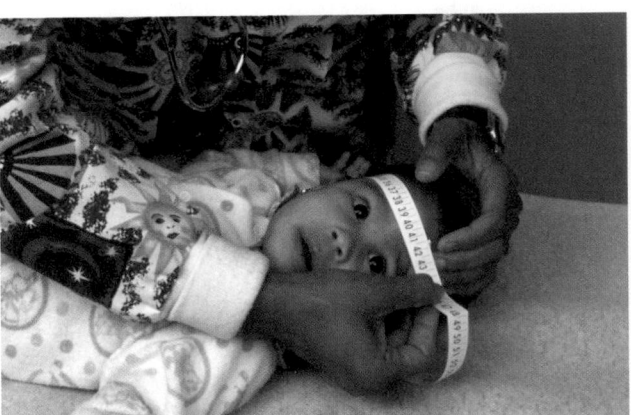

FIGURE 5-11
Place the measuring tape around the largest circumference of the infant's head, across the occiput and the forehead.

Expected head circumferences for term newborns range between 32.5 and 37.5 cm (12½ to 14½ inches) with a mean of 33 to 35 cm (13 to 14 inches). At 2 years of age, the child's head circumference is two-thirds its adult size. A head circumference increasing rapidly and rising above percentile curves suggests increased intracranial pressure. A head circumference growing slowly enough to fall off percentile curves suggests microcephaly.

CHEST CIRCUMFERENCE

Although the chest circumference is not used universally, it is a useful measurement for comparison with the head circumference when you suspect a problem in either head size or chest size. Wrap the measuring tape around the infant's chest at the nipple line, firmly but not tight enough to cause an indentation of the skin (Fig. 5-12). The chest circumference measurement is ideally taken midway between inspiration and expiration and read to the nearest 0.5 cm or ¼ inch.

The newborn's head circumference may equal or exceed the chest circumference by 2 cm (¾ inch) for the first 5 months of age. Between the ages of 5 months and 2 years, the infant's chest circumference should closely approximate the head circumference. When an infant's head circumference is smaller than the chest circumference, consider microcephaly as a potential cause. After 2 years of age, the chest circumference should exceed the head circumference because the chest grows faster than the head (Table 5-3).

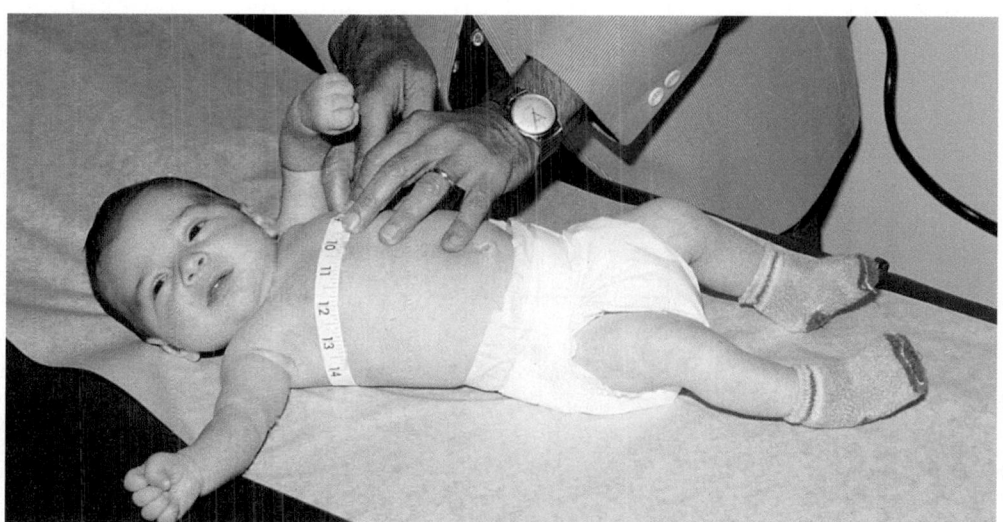

FIGURE 5-12
Measurement of infant chest circumference with the measuring tape at the level of the nipple line.

TABLE 5-3	Average Chest and Head Circumference for Children in the United States		

| Age | Chest Circumference (cm) | Head Circumference (cm) | |
		Males	Females
Birth	35	35.3	34.7
3 months	40	40.9	40.0
6 months	44	43.9	42.8
12 months	47	47.3	45.8
18 months	48	48.7	47.1
2 years	50	49.7	48.1
3 years	52	50.4	49.3

Data from Lowrey, 1986; Waring, Jeansonne, 1982.

NEUROMUSCULAR MATURITY

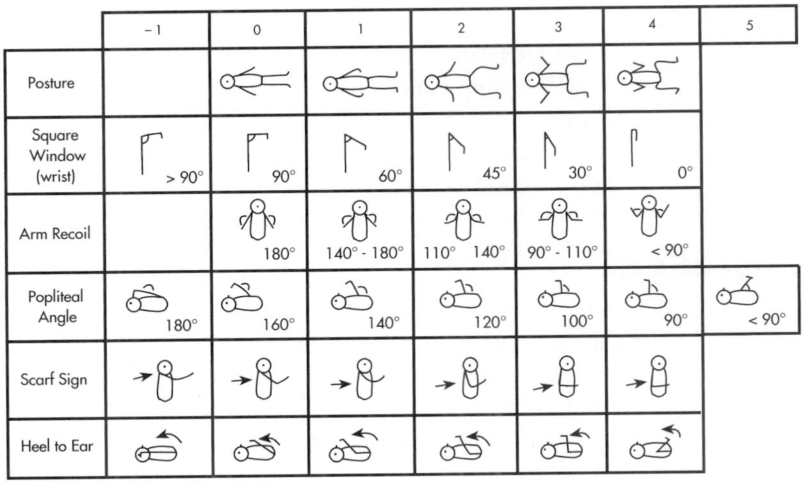

	−1	0	1	2	3	4	5
Posture							
Square Window (wrist)	> 90°	90°	60°	45°	30°	0°	
Arm Recoil		180°	140° - 180°	110° 140°	90° - 110°	< 90°	
Popliteal Angle	180°	160°	140°	120°	100°	90°	< 90°
Scarf Sign							
Heel to Ear							

A

PHYSICAL MATURITY

Skin	sticky friable transparent	gelatinous red, translucent	smooth pink, visible veins	superficial peeling &/or rash, few veins	cracking pale areas rare veins	parchment deep cracking no vessels	leathery cracked wrinkled
Lanugo	none	sparse	abundant	thinning	bald areas	mostly bald	
Plantar Surface	heel-toe 40-50 mm: -1 <40 mm: -2	>50 mm no crease	faint red marks	anterior transverse crease only	creases ant. 2/3	creases over entire sole	
Breast	imperceptible	barely perceptible	flat areola no bud	stippled areola 1-2 mm bud	raised areola 3-4 mm bud	full areola 5-10 mm bud	
Eye/Ear	lids fused loosely: -1 tightly: -2	lids open pinna flat stays folded	sl. curved pinna; soft; slow recoil	well-curved pinna; soft but ready recoil	formed & firm instant recoil	thick cartilage ear stiff	
Genitals (male)	scrotum flat, smooth	scrotum empty faint rugae	testes in upper canal rare rugae	testes descending few rugae	testes down good rugae	testes pendulous deep rugae	
Genitals (female)	clitoris prominent labia flat	prominent clitoris small labia minora	prominent clitoris enlarging minora	majora & minora equally prominent	majora large minora small	majora cover clitoris & minora	

B

MATURITY RATING

score	weeks
-10	20
-5	22
0	24
5	26
10	28
15	30
20	32
25	34
30	36
35	38
40	40
45	42
50	44

C

FIGURE 5-13
Assessment of gestational age by maturity rating. Following the directions for assessment, assign a score for each of the 12 physical signs based on the descriptions for each. If a characteristic falls halfway between scoring options, a half score is assigned. **A,** Scoring system of physical signs. **B,** Scoring system of neuromuscular signs. **C,** Add the scores from the 12 signs and compare the total with this table to determine the neonate's gestational age in weeks.
From Ballard et al, 1991.

Examination for Gestational Maturity
Procedures for assessing the 12 characteristics that indicate gestational age are explained below. Scoring of maturity is presented in **C.**

Neuromuscular Maturity
Posture is the position the baby naturally assumes when lying quietly on his back. A very premature infant will lie with arms and legs extended or in whatever posture he is placed. As intrauterine development progresses, the fetus is capable of more and more flexion. When born at term, an infant lies with his arms flexed to his chest, his hands fisted, and his legs flexed toward his abdomen. To assign a posture score, the scorer compares infant's position with those pictured above.

Square window (wrist) is the angle achieved when the infant's palm is flexed toward his forearm. A premature infant's wrist exhibits poor flexion and makes a 90 degree angle with the arm. An extremely immature infant has no flexor tone and cannot achieve even 90-degree flexion. A term infant's wrist will flex completely against the forearm.

Arm recoil is elicited by first flexing the arms at the elbows to the chest, then fully extending them and releasing. Term infants will resist extension and briskly return their arms to the flexed position. Very preterm infants will not resist extension and respond with weak and delayed flexion in a small arc. The flexion angle of the elbow is estimated.

Popliteal angle is assessed with the infant lying supine. Keeping his pelvis flat, flex his thigh to his abdomen and hold it there while extending his leg at the knee. The angle at the knee is estimated. The preterm infant will achieve greater extension.

Scarf sign is elicited by moving the baby's arm across his chest as far toward the opposite shoulder as possible while he is lying supine. The term infant's elbow will not cross midline, but it will be possible to bring the preterm infant's elbow much farther toward the opposite shoulder. The score is based on comparison to the drawings above.

Heel to ear is similar to popliteal angle, but the knee and thigh are not held in place. The baby's foot is drawn as near to the head or ear as possible. Scoring is based on the distance from heel to head. The premature baby will be able to get his foot closer to his head.

Physical Maturity
Skin is assessed for thickness, transparency, and texture. Premature skin is thin, with visible vessels, and smooth. Extremely preterm infants have sticky, transparent skin. A term infant's skin is thick, veins are difficult to see, and the texture may be flaky.

Lanugo is the fine hair seen over the back of premature babies by 24 weeks. It begins to thin over lower back first and disappears last over the shoulders.

Plantar creases are the deep folds and creases seen over the bottom of the foot. One or two appear over the pad of the foot at approximately 32 weeks. At 36 weeks, the creases cover the anterior two-thirds of the foot. At term, they cover the whole foot. At very early gestation, the length of the sole is measured. For extremely immature infants, this item was expanded to include foot length measured from the tip of the great toe to the back of the heel.

Breast tissue is examined for visibility of nipple and areola and size of bud when grasped between thumb and forefinger. The very premature infant will not have visible nipples or areola. These become more defined and then raised by 34 weeks, with a small bud appearing at 36 weeks and growing to 5–10 mm by term.

Ear formation includes the development of cartilage and the curving of the pinnae. Lack of cartilage in earlier gestation results in the ear folding easily and retaining this fold. As gestation progresses, soft cartilage can be felt with increasing resistance to folding and increasing recoil. The pinnae are flat in very preterm infants. Incurving proceeds from the top down toward the lobes as gestation advances.

Eyes in the extremely immature infant are examined, and the degree of eyelid fusion is assessed with gentle traction.

Genitalia are virtually indistinguishable at 20 weeks. In males, the testes are in the inguinal canal around 28 weeks, and rugae are beginning to be visible. By 36 weeks, the testes are in the upper scrotum, and rugae cover the anterior portion of the scrotum. At term, rugae cover the scrotum, and at postterm, the testes are pendulous. In females, the clitoris is initially prominent and the labia minora are flat. By 36 weeks, the labia majora are larger and the clitoris is nearly covered.

GESTATIONAL AGE

Gestational age is an indicator of a newborn's maturity. One method of determining gestational age is to calculate the number of completed weeks between the first day of the mother's last menstrual period and the date of birth. An estimate of gestational age is used for evaluating an infant's developmental progress and for differentiating between preterm newborns of appropriate size and term newborns that are small for gestational age.

The Ballard Gestational Age Assessment Tool is used to evaluate six physical and six neuromuscular newborn characteristics within 36 hours of birth, establishing or confirming the newborn's gestational age. Fig. 5-13 provides directions and criteria for scoring each characteristic. The assessment is accurate within 2 weeks of the assigned gestational age. Scores are more accurate for extremely preterm newborns when the assessment occurs within 12 hours of birth, but accuracy is not associated with time of assessment in other newborns.

The gestational ages of 37 through 41 weeks, which are considered term, are associated with the best health outcomes. Infants born before 37 weeks of gestation are preterm, whereas infants born after 41 completed weeks of gestation are postterm.

SIZE FOR GESTATIONAL AGE

A newborn's fetal growth pattern and size for gestational age can be determined once gestational age is assigned. Standardized intrauterine growth curves are used to plot the newborn's birth weight, length, and head circumference (Fig. 5-14). The infant is then classified as small, appropriate, or large for gestational age by percentile curve placement for weeks of gestation (Fig. 5-15). The classification system is as follows:

Classification	Weight Percentiles
Appropriate for gestational age (AGA)	10th to 90th
Small for gestational age (SGA)	Less than 10th
Large for gestational age (LGA)	Greater than 90th

There is an associated risk of morbidity and mortality with infants that are either small or large for gestational age. Risks increase if the infant is preterm and small for gestational age for such conditions as respiratory distress syndrome, bronchopulmonary dysplasia, and intraventricular hemorrhage.

CHILDREN

STATURE AND WEIGHT

Standing height is obtained beginning at 24 to 36 months when the child is walking well. To get the most accurate measurement, use a stature-measuring device (stadiometer) mounted on the wall rather than the height-measurement device on a scale. Have the child stand erect with heels, buttocks, and shoulders against the wall or freestanding stadiometer, looking straight ahead (Fig. 5-16). The outer canthus of the eye should be on the same horizontal plane as the external auditory canal while you position the headpiece at the crown. The stature reading is made to the nearest 0.5 cm or ¼ inch. Table 5-4 lists the expected yearly stature growth, or height velocity, for age and gender.

CLASSIFICATION OF NEWBORNS –
BASED ON MATURITY AND INTRAUTERINE GROWTH
Symbols: X-1st Exam O-2nd Exam

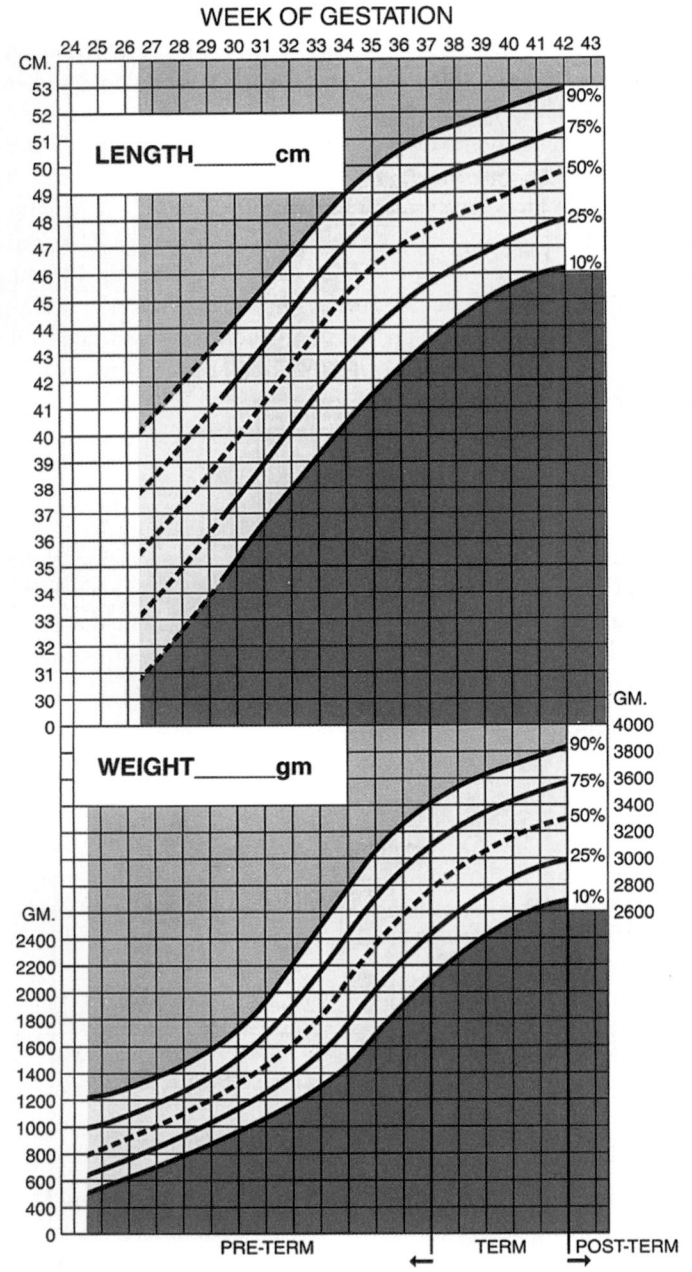

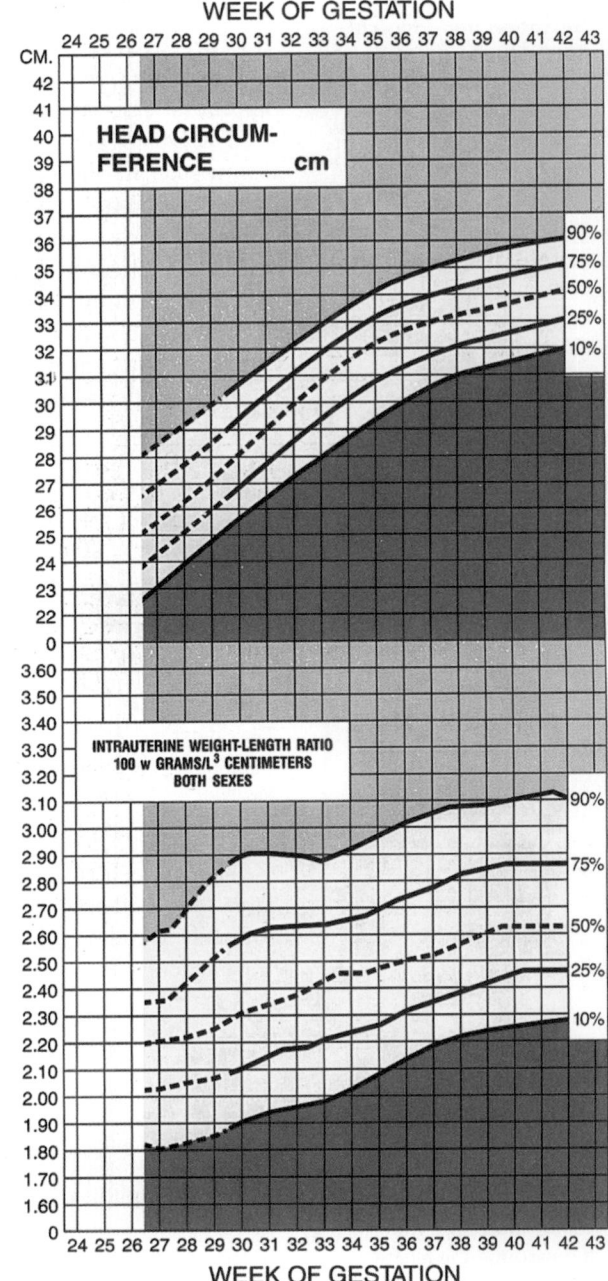

	1st Exam (X)	2nd Exam (O)
LARGE FOR GESTATIONAL AGE **(LGA)**		
APPROPRIATE FOR GESTATIONAL AGE **(AGA)**		
SMALL FOR GESTATIONAL AGE **(SGA)**		
Age at Exam	hrs	hrs
Signature of Examiner	M.D.	M.D.

FIGURE 5-14
Intrauterine growth curves for length, weight, and head circumference by weeks of gestation.
Redrawn from Lubchenco et al, 1966; and Battaglia & Lubchenco, 1967.

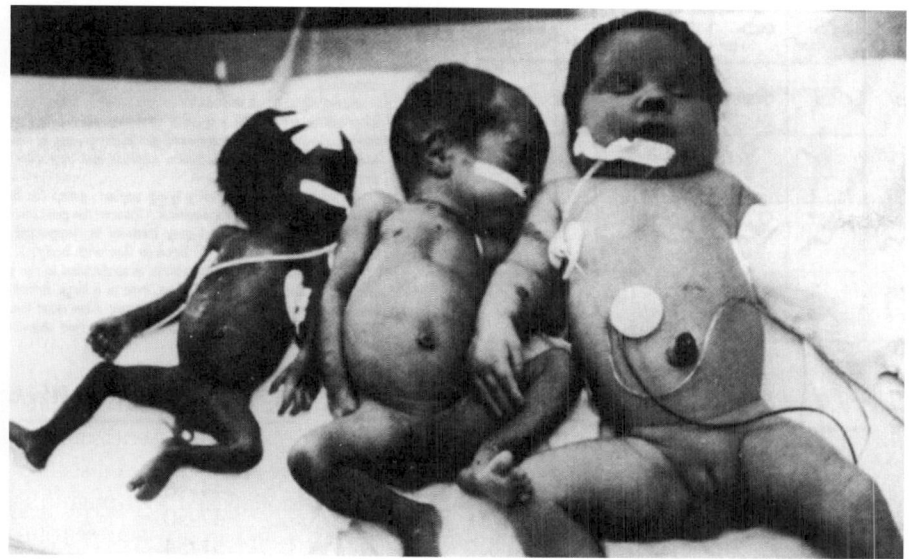

FIGURE 5-15
Three infants, each at 32 weeks of gestational age, demonstrating the difference in size between SGA, AGA, and LGA newborns. Birth weights are 600, 1400, and 2750 g, respectively, from left.
From Korones, 1986.

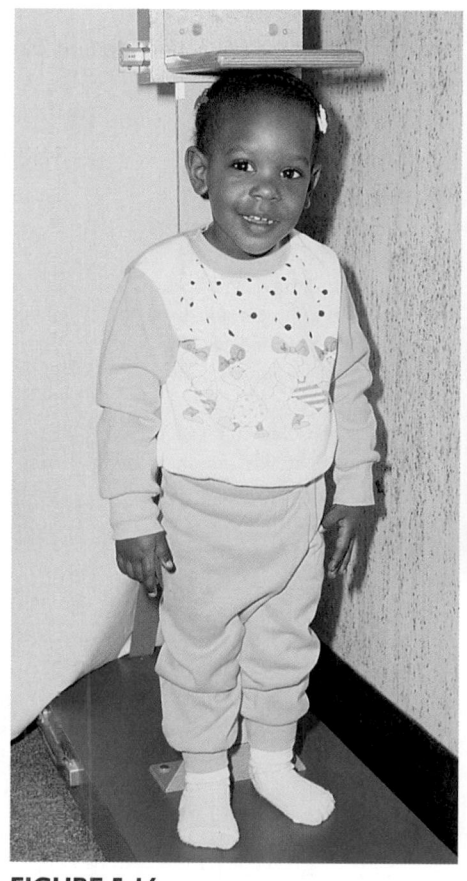

FIGURE 5-16
Measuring the stature of a child.

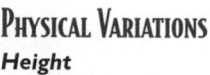

PHYSICAL VARIATIONS

Height

Children of different races vary in height. Tallest are black and white children, followed by Native American/American Indian children, who are similar or a little shorter. Next in height are Mexican-American children, followed by the shortest group— Asian children. Black children achieve their growth earlier than white children—white boys catch up with black boys around 9 or 10 years; white girls catch up to black girls around 14 to 15 years. Within the same racial group, children from families with higher socioeconomic status are taller than those from families of lower socioeconomic status. Obese children are taller than lean children, and the difference in height can be as much as one standard deviation above their leaner cohorts.

Data from Foster et al, 1977; Strauss, 1993; Dewey et al, 1986; Roche et al, 1990; Lin, 1992; Malina, Hamill, Lemeshow, 1974; Hamill, Johnston, Lemeshow, 1973; Schutte, 1980; Chrzastek-Spruch, Wolanski, Wrebiakowski, 1984; Garn, Clark, Guire, 1974.

TABLE 5-4 Expected Height Velocity for Specified Time Intervals During Childhood*

| | Height Velocity (cm) | |
Age (yr)	Males	Females
2-3	8.3	8.6
3-4	7.4	7.6
4-5	6.8	6.8
5-6	6.4	6.4
6-7	6.0	6.1
7-8	5.8	5.9
8-9	5.4	5.7
9-10	5.2	5.8
10-11	5.1	6.7
11-12	5.3	8.3
12-13	6.8	5.9
13-14	9.5	3.0
14-15	6.5	0.9
15-16	3.3	0.1
16-17	1.5	
17-18	0.5	

Modified from Tanner, Davies, 1985.
*Peak height velocity during adolescence is given for average times (13.5 years in males and 11.5 years in females).

PHYSICAL VARIATIONS

Weight

Weight-for-height measures are affected by bone density, musculature, and body fat. Children in the extreme percentiles should be assessed to see which components predominate. Heavily muscled children or those with sturdy bones should not be considered obese. With the above cautions, children of various races can be grouped from lightest to heaviest. Asian and black children are generally the lightest, followed by white children, who are a little heavier; Native American/American Indian children come next, followed by Mexican-American children as the heaviest.

Data from Strauss, 1993; Ryan et al, 1990.

CLINICAL PEARL

Special Growth Charts

Special growth charts do exist for children with specific conditions such as achondroplasia, Down syndrome, cerebral palsy, and Marfan syndrome, but they should be used in association with Centers for Disease Control and Prevention standardized charts.

Weigh young children older than age 2 years of age on a standing scale, in standard light garments. Read the weight to the nearest 0.1 kg or ¼ pound. Remember to measure the child's head circumference once a year.

Plot the child's height, weight, and head circumference measurements on the appropriate growth curves for gender and age, comparing the child's growth with the population standards. (See Appendix C, Figs. C-4 and C-5, for physical growth curves for height and weight of children 2 through 20 years of age.) Population standards reflecting various times of the growth spurt for adolescents can be found in the physical growth curves for height and sexual development of children and adolescents 2 through 19 years of age in Appendix C, Fig. C-6. Obesity is present in approximately 16% of children and adolescents 5 to 20 years of age, and an additional 31% are at risk for being overweight (Hedley et al, 2004). See Chapter 6 for a discussion of body mass index use and interpretation in children older than 2 years of age.

To calculate height velocity, determine the change in height over a time interval (e.g., 1 year). Shorter time intervals may reflect seasonal variations in growth. Make height measurements as close to 12 months apart as possible, no fewer than 10 months and no more than 14 months. (See Appendix C, Fig. C-7, for the gender-specific height velocity curves.)

Over time, interval measurements should demonstrate that the child has established a growth pattern, indicated by consistently following a percentile curve on the growth chart. Children of first generation immigrants may not fit the U.S. population standard, but should follow a growth pattern consistent with other children, even if it is near or below the fifth percentile. Infants and children who suddenly fall below or rise above their established percentile growth curve should be examined more closely to determine the cause.

SKINFOLD THICKNESS

Triceps skinfold thickness measurement is not routinely recommended for children, being reserved for those children who have weight for stature greater than the 90th percentile. It is often difficult to differentiate fatfolds from lean muscle tissue in children. This measurement is more commonly used with adolescents. Using the technique described for adults, take the triceps skinfold measurement and compare the reading to that on the gender-appropriate triceps skinfold thickness table for children and adolescents (Fig. 5-17).

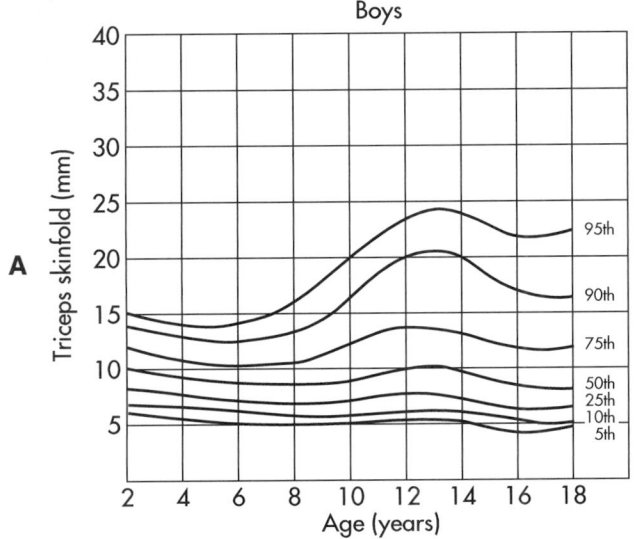
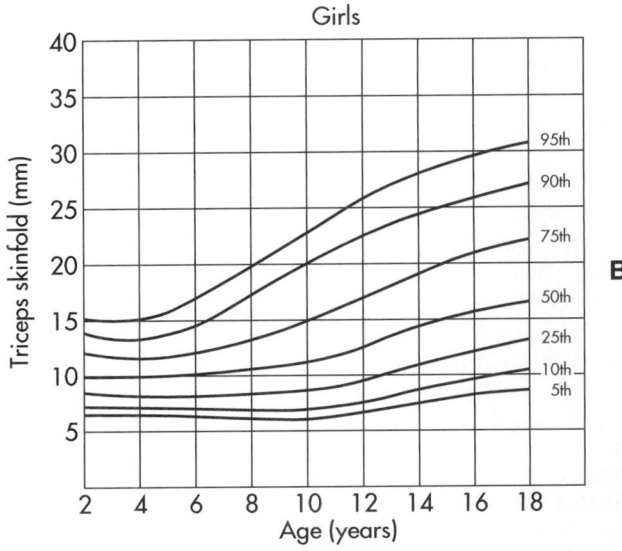

FIGURE 5-17
Skinfold thickness curves for children, ages 2 to 18 years. **A,** Boys. **B,** Girls.
Redrawn from Owen, 1982.

UPPER-TO-LOWER SEGMENT RATIO

Measure the distance from the symphysis pubis to the floor when a child is suspected of having a growth problem or unusual body proportions. Calculate the ratio with the following formula:

[Total height − Lower segment measurement] ÷ Lower segment measurement

Compare the ratio with the findings for age and gender to determine whether the child is within the expected range (Fig. 5-18).

ARM SPAN

The arm-span measurement, although not routinely obtained, may be useful when evaluating a child with tall stature. Have the child hold his or her arms fully extended from the sides of the body. Measure the distance from the middle fingertip of one hand to that of the other hand. The arm span should equal the child's height or stature. Arm span that exceeds height is associated with Marfan syndrome.

ADOLESCENTS

The changes of puberty do not occur at exactly the same age in each boy and girl; this can cause great concern when adolescents feel they are growing too fast or too slow. This is a good time to share your knowledge about the various rates of speed in human development, reassuring adolescents that almost all of them get there in good time. The Tanner charts are valuable for explaining to older children, particularly adolescents, where they are in reference to others and where they are going. Show them the pictures and talk about them. Adolescents are curious and will gain from your respectful candor.

Assessing growth and development of the older child and adolescent includes evaluating the patient's sexual maturation. In girls, breast and pubic hair development are evaluated; in boys, genital and pubic hair development are evaluated. The expected stages of pubertal changes for each secondary sexual characteristic are described in Figs. 5-19 through 5-22. The duration and tempo of each sequence are quite variable between individuals.

A sexual maturity rating (SMR) may be assigned, or each secondary sexual characteristic may be rated separately to determine the child's pubertal development. The SMR is calculated by averaging the girl's stages of pubic hair and breast development or the boy's stages of pubic hair and genital development. The stage of each secondary sexual characteristic is then related to the timing of other physiologic events occurring during puberty.

The stage of breast and pubic hair development in the female is related to chronologic age, age at menarche, and evidence of the height spurt. In two thirds of girls, breasts begin developing before pubic hair appears. The breasts do not always develop at the same rate, so some asymmetry is common. Menarche generally occurs in SMR 4 or breast stage 3 to 4. These

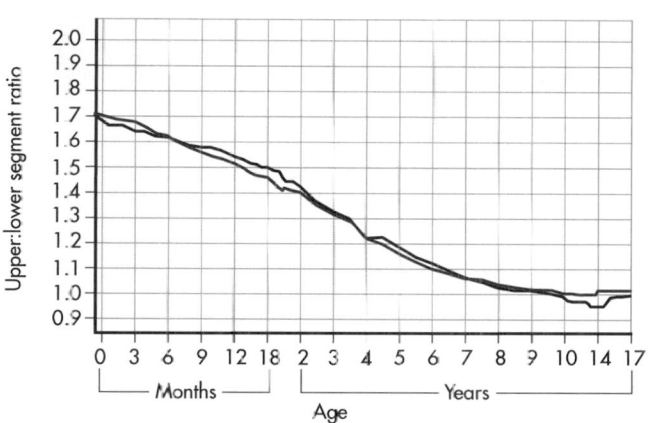

FIGURE 5-18
Normal upper-to-lower segment ratio by age and gender.
From The Johns Hopkins Hospital, 2000.

P₁—Tanner 1 (preadolescent). No growth of pubic hair; that is, hair in pubic area no different from that on the rest of the abdomen.

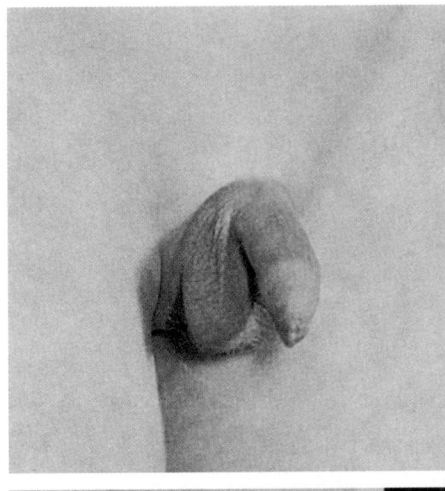

P₂—Tanner 2. Slightly pigmented, longer, straight hair, often still downy; usually at base of penis, sometimes on scrotum. Stage is difficult to photograph.

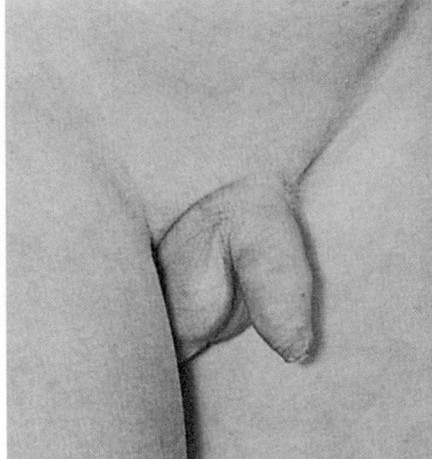

P₃—Tanner 3. Dark, definitely pigmented, curly pubic hair around base of penis. Stage 3 can be photographed.

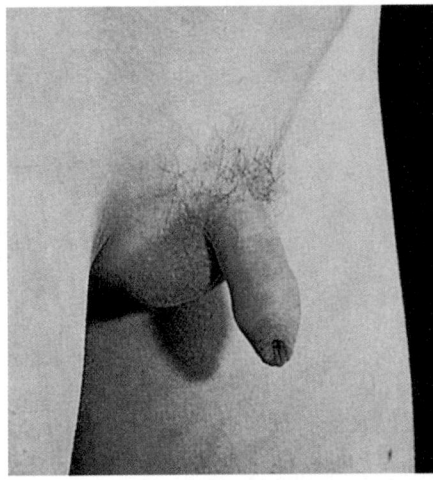

P₄—Tanner 4. Pubic hair definitely adult in type but not in extent (no further than inguinal fold).

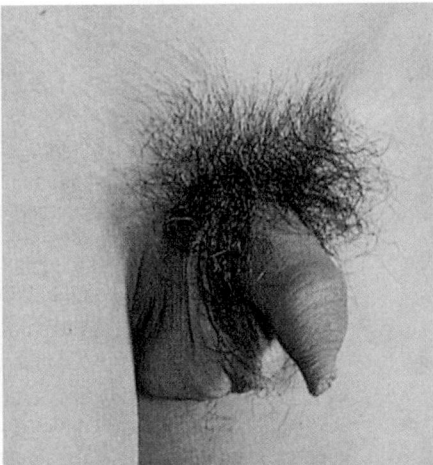

P₅—Tanner 5 (adult distribution). Hair spread to medial surface of thighs, but not upward.

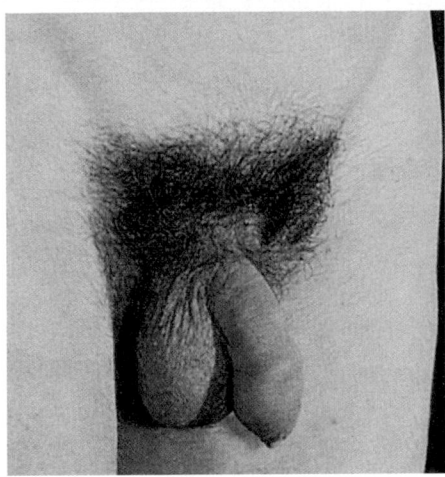

P₆—Hair spread along linea alba (occurs in 80% of men).

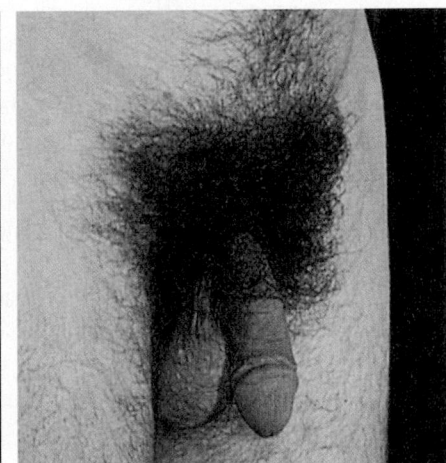

FIGURE 5-19
Six stages of pubic hair development in males.
Photographs from Van Wieringen JC: Growth diagrams 1965 Netherlands, Second national survey on 0-24-year-olds, Groningen, Netherlands, 1971, Wolters-Noordhoff. *Reprinted by permission of Kluwer Academic Publishers.*

G₁—Tanner 1. Testes, scrotum, and penis are the same size and shape as in the young child.

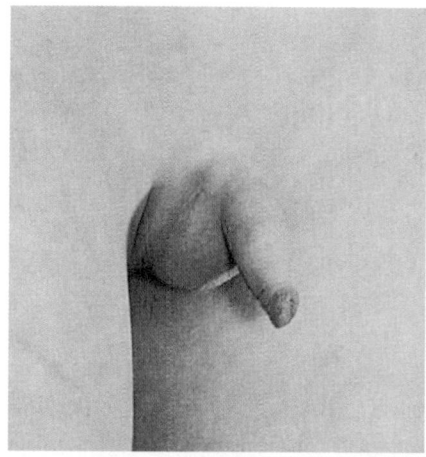

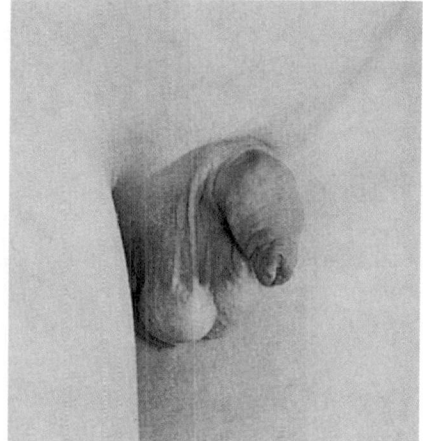

G₂—Tanner 2. Enlargement of scrotum and testes. The skin of the scrotum becomes redder, thinner, and wrinkled. Penis no larger or scarcely so.

G₃—Tanner 3. Enlargement of the penis, especially in length; further enlargement of testes; descent of scrotum.

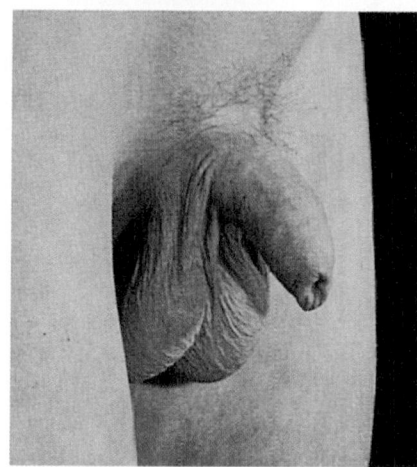

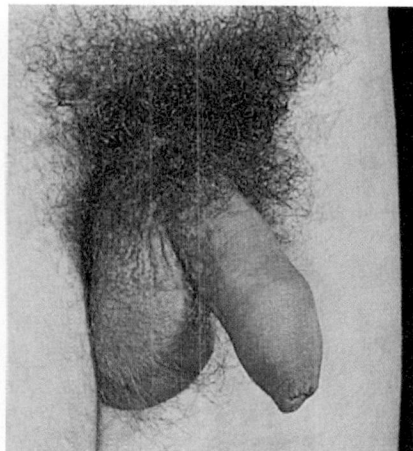

G₄—Tanner 4. Continued enlargement of the penis and sculpturing of the glans; increased pigmentation of scrotum. This stage is sometimes best described as "not quite adult."

G₅—Tanner 5 (adult stage). Scrotum ample, penis reaching nearly to bottom of scrotum.

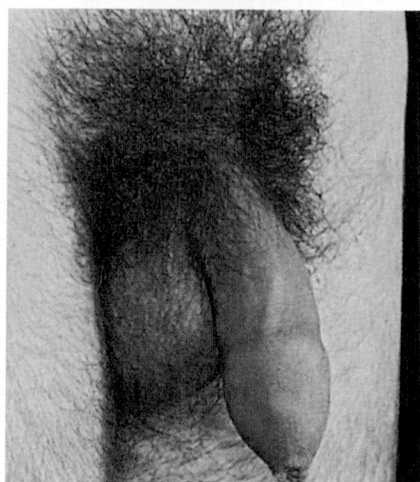

FIGURE 5-20
Five stages of penis and testes/scrotum development in males.
Photographs from Van Wieringen JC: Growth diagrams 1965 Netherlands, Second national survey on 0-24-year-olds, Groningen, Netherlands, 1971, Wolters-Noordhoff. Reprinted by permission of Kluwer Academic Publishers.

P₁—Tanner 1 (preadolescent). No growth of pubic hair.

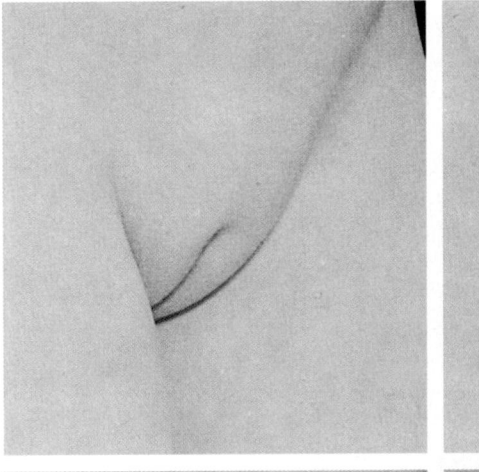

P₂—Tanner 2. Initial, scarcely pigmented straight hair, especially along medial border of the labia.

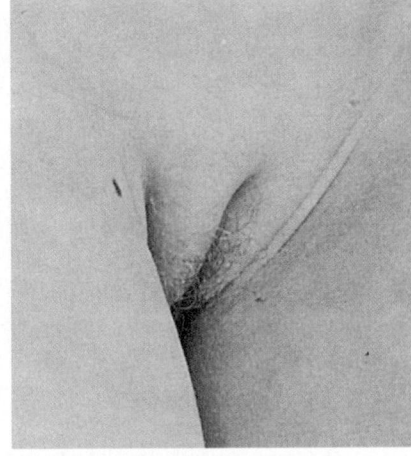

P₃—Tanner 3. Sparse, dark, visibly pigmented, curly pubic hair on labia.

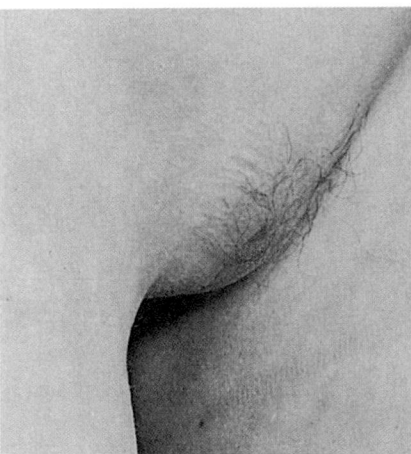

P₄—Tanner 4. Hair coarse and curly, abundant but less than adult.

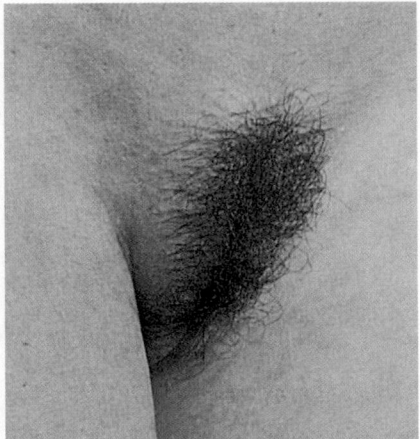

P₅—Tanner 5. Lateral spreading; type and triangle spread of adult hair to medial surface of thighs.

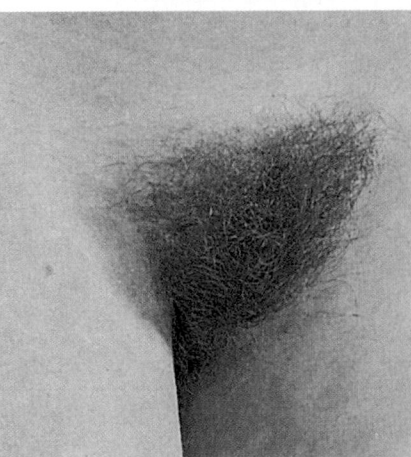

P₆—Tanner 6. Further extension laterally, upward, or dispersed (occurs in only 10% of women).

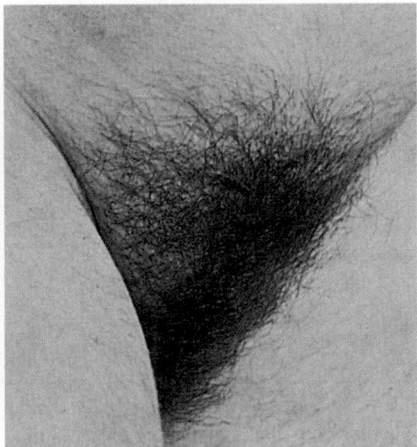

FIGURE 5-21
Six stages of pubic hair development in females.
Photographs from Van Wieringen JC: Growth diagrams 1965 Netherlands, Second national survey on 0-24-year-olds, *Groningen, Netherlands, 1971, Wolters-Noordhoff. Reprinted by permission of Kluwer Academic Publishers.*

M₁—Tanner 1 (preadolescent). Only the nipple is raised above the level of the breast, as in the child.

M₂—Tanner 2. Budding stage; bud-shaped elevation of the areola; areola increased in diameter and surrounding area slightly elevated.

M₃—Tanner 3. Breast and areola enlarged. No contour separation.

M₄—Tanner 4. Increasing fat deposits. The areola forms a secondary elevation above that of the breast. This secondary mound occurs in approximately half of all girls and in some cases persists in adulthood.

M₅—Tanner 5 (adult stage). The areola is (usually) part of general breast contour and is strongly pigmented. Nipple projects.

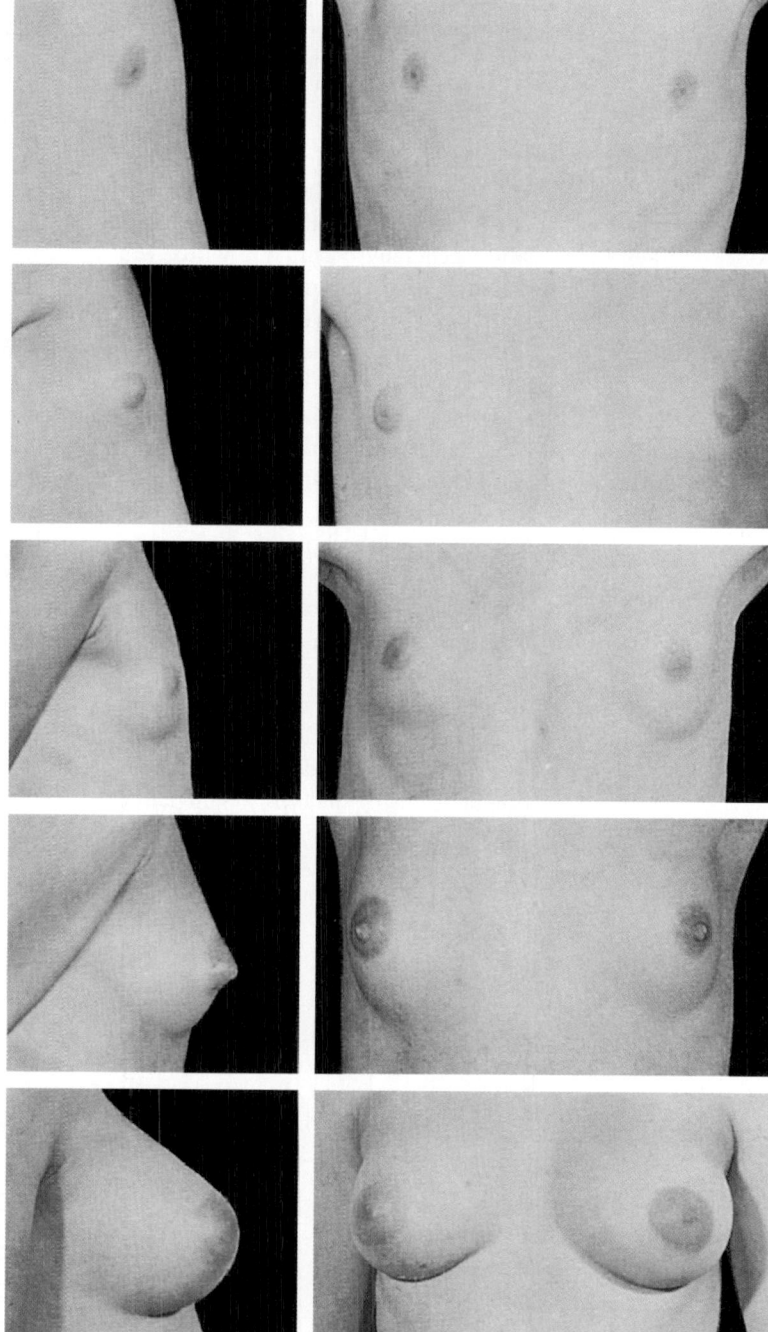

FIGURE 5-22
Five stages of breast development in females.
Photographs from Van Wieringen JC: Growth diagrams 1965 Netherlands, Second national survey on 0-24-year-olds, *Groningen, Netherlands, 1971, Wolters-Noordhoff. Reprinted by permission of Kluwer Academic Publishers.*

physiologic events may be plotted on the growth curve (see Appendix C, Fig. C-6). The peak height velocity occurs about a year before menarche at a mean age of 11.5 years (Chang, Tzeng, Cheng, & Chie, 2000). Development of breast tissue or pubic hair in prepubertal girls younger than 6 (for black females) or 7 years of age (for white females) should be further investigated for cause (Kaplowitz, Oberfield, Lawson Wilkins Pediatric Endocrine Society, 1999).

The stage of genital and pubic hair development in the male is related to age and evidence of the height spurt. External genital changes usually precede pubic hair development. Ejaculation generally occurs at SMR 3, with semen appearing between SMR 3 and 4. The peak height velocity occurs at a mean age of 13.5 years, usually in SMR 4 or genital development stage 4 to 5. These events may be plotted on the standardized height velocity growth chart for adolescents (see Appendix C, Fig. C-6). Development of genitals or pubic hair in prepubertal boys younger than 9 years should be further investigated for cause.

Delayed onset of adolescence, in which the secondary sexual characteristics begin development at an age later than the average, is often a normal variant in both boys and girls. It is accompanied by a lag of stature growth. Parents often had a similar adolescent pattern. Once pubertal changes begin, the sequence of development is the same as for other adolescents, but it may occur over a shorter time span. Ultimate height may still be the same.

Early development of sexual hair without signs of sexual maturation may be an indication of premature pubarche. In these children, pubescence usually occurs at the expected time as with healthy children.

PREGNANT WOMEN

Weight gain during pregnancy should be calculated from the woman's prepregnant weight (Fig. 5-23). To provide guidance in weight gain during pregnancy, first determine the prepregnancy body mass index (BMI) (see Box 6-4). Then monitor the woman's weight throughout pregnancy using the BMI weight gain curve guidelines on the prenatal weight gain chart. Note any variation from the expected weight gain. Consider the woman's age, weight, dietary habits, source of calories, and health status.

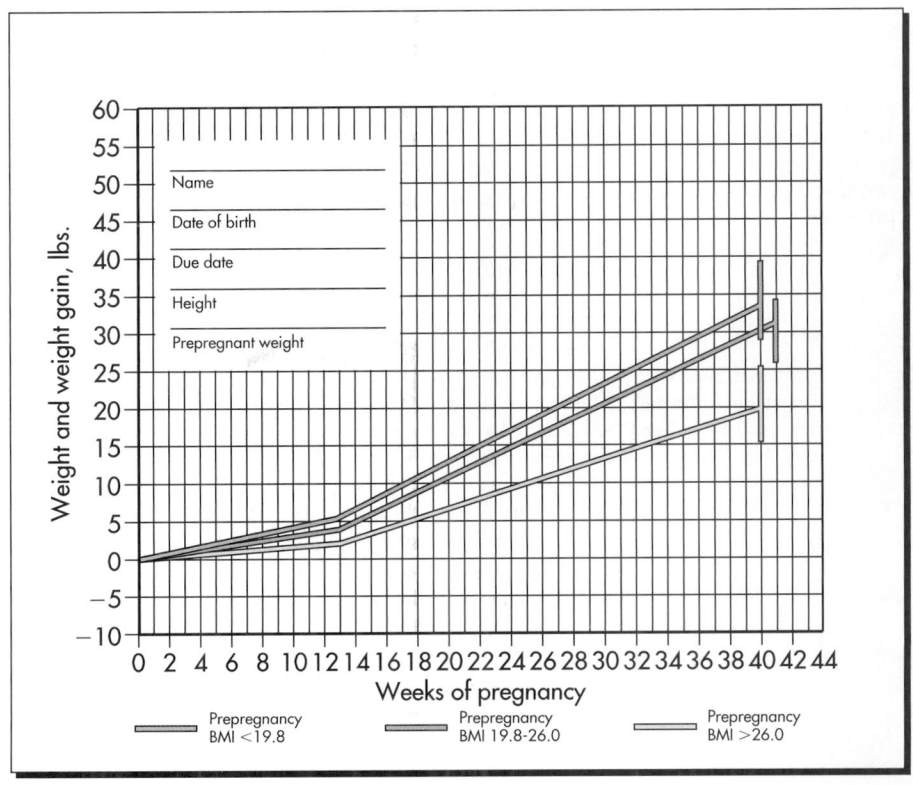

FIGURE 5-23
Prenatal weight gain curve by weeks of gestation.
From Food and Nutrition Board, 1992.

Women with a wide variation in weight gain during pregnancy have good reproductive outcomes. Women with an appropriate weight for height or prepregnancy BMI of 19.8 to 26.0 should gain 11.5 to 16 kg (25 to 35 pounds) over the entire pregnancy. Overweight women (i.e., BMI 26.1 to 29) should gain 7 to 11.5 kg (15 to 25 pounds). Those who are obese (i.e., BMI >29) should gain no more than 7 kg (15 pounds). Obese women who lose or do not gain weight are at an increased risk for a small for gestational age infant. If they gain more than 16 kg (35 pounds), they have an increased risk for a large for gestational age infant (Reifsnider, Gill, 2000; Edwards et al, 1996). Obese women are more at risk for maternal complications such as hypertension, diabetes, complications of labor and delivery, fetal complications, and fetal death (Abrams & Pickett, 1999).

First trimester gain is variable, from 1 to 2 kg (2 to 4 pounds). In the second and third trimester, weekly weight gain should be approximately 0.45 kg (1 pound) per week. Underweight women should gain 2 to 3 kg (5 pounds) during the first trimester, and slightly more than 0.45 kg (1 pound) per week through the remainder of the pregnancy. Overweight women should gain 1.0 kg (2 pounds) during the first trimester and slightly less than 0.45 kg (1 pound) per week through the remainder of the pregnancy. Women with a twin pregnancy are recommended to gain 16 to 20.4 kg (35 to 45 pounds), with approximately 0.68 kg (1½ pounds) per week gained during the second and third trimesters. Women with a triplet pregnancy are recommended to gain 22.7 kg (50 pounds), with a steady 0.68 kg (1½ pounds) weight gain throughout the pregnancy (Brown, Carlson, 2000).

OLDER ADULTS

Measurement procedures for the older adult are the same as those used for the general population. Compare the individual's weight for height and triceps skinfold thickness by gender and age category on the tables found in Appendix C, Tables C-3 to C-6.

SAMPLE DOCUMENTATION
HISTORY AND PHYSICAL EXAMINATION

Subjective
A 4-month-old female infant in for routine health examination and immunizations. Breast-fed, no other foods introduced. Good appetite. No illnesses.

Objective
Weight 6.2 kg (13½ pounds) 50th percentile; length 62 cm (24.5 inches) 50th percentile; head circumference 41 cm (16 inches) 50th percentile; maintaining growth curve at 50th percentile since visit 2 months ago.

For additional sample documentation, see Chapter 26.

SUMMARY OF EXAMINATION
GROWTH AND MEASUREMENT

1. From the history, assess the patient's size (pp. 112-113), including the following:
   - Recent growth, weight gain, or weight loss
   - Chronic illnesses affecting weight gain or loss
2. Obtain the following anthropometric measurements (pp. 114-117), and compare them to those in standardized tables:
   - Standing height
   - Weight
   - Frame size
   - Skinfold thickness

COMMON ABNORMALITIES

METABOLIC DISORDERS

ACROMEGALY

Gradual marked enlargement and elongation of the bones of the face, jaw, and extremities are indicative of acromegaly. This disorder is associated with a pituitary tumor that causes excessive production of growth hormone in middle-aged adults. It is characterized by facial feature exaggeration and massive hands and feet, but no change in height (Fig. 5-24; see also Fig. 10-23).

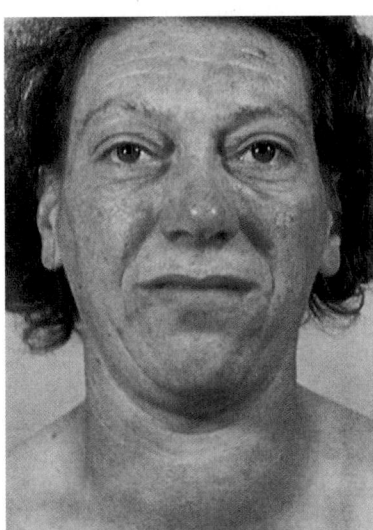

FIGURE 5-24
Acromegaly. Note the large head, forward projection of jaw, and protrusion of frontal bone.
From 400 More Self-Assessment Picture Tests in Clinical Medicine, 1988.

CUSHING SYNDROME

This disorder results from chronic excessive cortisol production by the adrenal cortex or from the long-term administration of large doses of glucocorticoids. Cushing syndrome is seen most commonly with steroid therapy; however, on rare occasions it is the result of pituitary adenoma in adults or an adrenal malignancy in children. It is characterized by weight gain, muscle weakness, hyperpigmentation, oligomenorrhea or decreased testosterone levels, and abnormally pigmented, fragile skin. There is a redistribution of fat tissue to include a pendulous pad of fat on the chest and abdomen covered with striae, as well as supraclavicular fat pads, moon facies, and thin extremities (see Fig. 10-17).

OTHER DISORDERS

CHILDREN

HYDROCEPHALUS

Hydrocephalus originates when an imbalance occurs between the production and absorption of cerebrospinal fluid that circulates between the brain and the dura mater and within the ventricular system. The condition is often associated with central nervous system anomalies. The excess cerebrospinal fluid causes increased intracranial pressure, head enlargement, widening sutures and fontanels, lethargy, irritability, weakness, and "setting sun" eyes. Without intervention, irreversible neurologic damage results (Fig. 5-25).

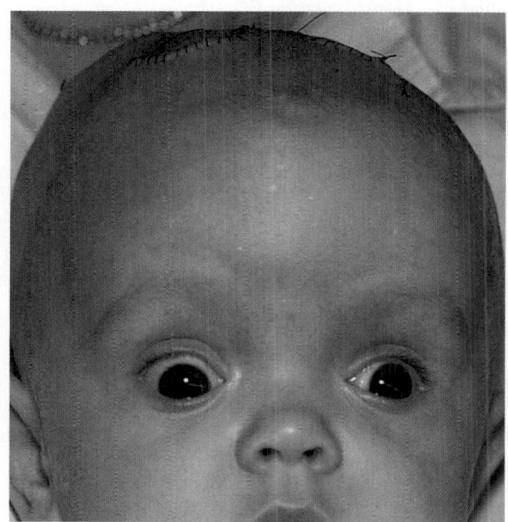

FIGURE 5-25
Infantile hydrocephalus. Paresis of the upward gaze is seen in an infant with hydrocephalus resulting from aqueductal stenosis. It appears more apparent on the right. This phenomenon is often termed the *sunsetting sign.*
From Zitelli, Davis, 1997. Courtesy Dr. Albert Biglan, Children's Hospital of Pittsburgh.

FAILURE TO THRIVE

The failure of an infant to grow at rates considered appropriate for the population occurs for several reasons. It may be related to chronic disease that increases metabolic requirements; inadequate calories and protein in the diet; inability to feed properly due to neurologic dysfunction, gastroesophageal reflux, or cleft palate; or malabsorption that interferes with utilization of adequate nutrients. It is also possible that there are social and emotional causes. An emotionally deprived infant—one who is hungry for affection—will not grow. Growth hormone is not released (Fig. 5-26). Failure to thrive may result in behavioral, cognitive, language, and motor development delays. It is also associated with increased susceptibility to infections (Agency for Healthcare Research and Quality, 2003).

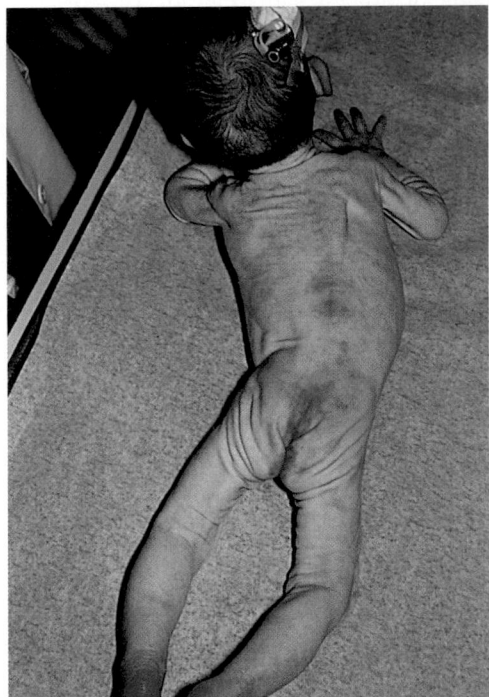

FIGURE 5-26
Psychosocial failure to thrive as the result of neglect. This 4-month-old infant was brought to the emergency department because of congestion. She was found to be below weight and suffering from severe developmental delay. Note the marked loss of subcutaneous tissue manifested by the wrinkled skinfolds over the buttocks, shoulders, and upper arms.
From Zitelli, Davis, 1997.

ACHONDROPLASIA

This genetic disorder causes abnormalities in endochondral ossification. It is characterized by dwarfism with short, curved arms and legs; a long narrow trunk, midfacial hypoplasia, and a prominent forehead. Spinal canal stenosis may be present and compress the spinal cord, resulting in hypotonia, paresis, and central and obstructive apnea (Fig. 5-27).

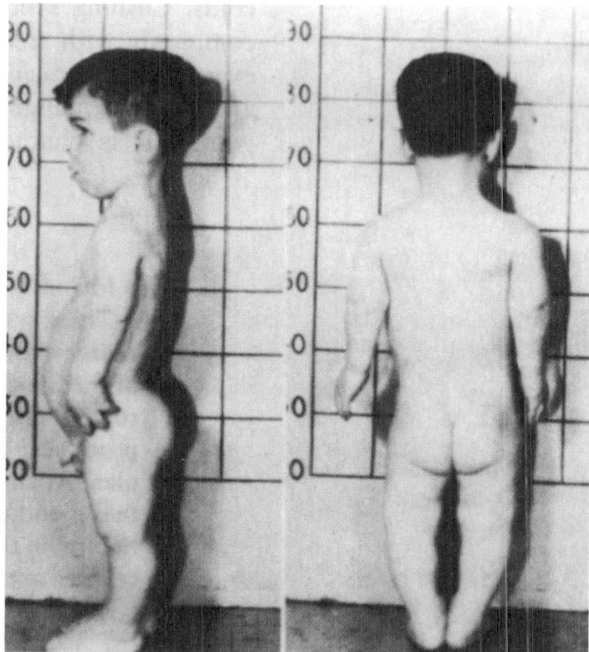

FIGURE 5-27
Achondroplasia.
From McKusick, 1972.

HYPOPITUITARY DWARFISM

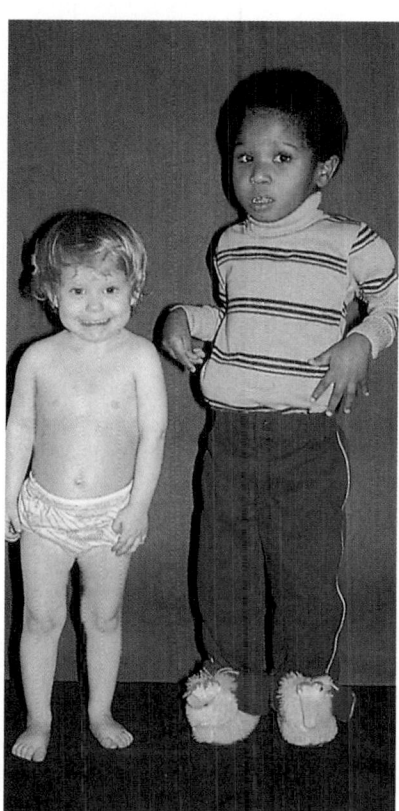

This growth hormone deficiency results in a child with short stature who appears younger than his or her chronologic age. The affected child is usually of normal size and weight at birth. Length or height growth then is slower than expected, with children and infants with severe growth hormone deficiencies being several standard deviations below the mean by 1 year of age. Dwarfism results unless treated (Fig. 5-28).

FIGURE 5-28
The normal 3-year-old boy is in the 50th percentile for height. The short 3-year-old girl exhibits the characteristic "Kewpie doll" appearance, suggesting a diagnosis of growth hormone deficiency.
From Zitelli, Davis, 1997.

PRECOCIOUS PUBERTY

This disorder is characterized by development with all secondary sexual characteristics and advancement in skeletal maturation before age 8 years in females and age 9 years in males (Kakarla & Bradshaw, 2003). Precocious puberty is usually idiopathic, but it may be related to central nervous system or gonadal neoplasm, or to McCune-Albright syndrome (Fig. 5-29).

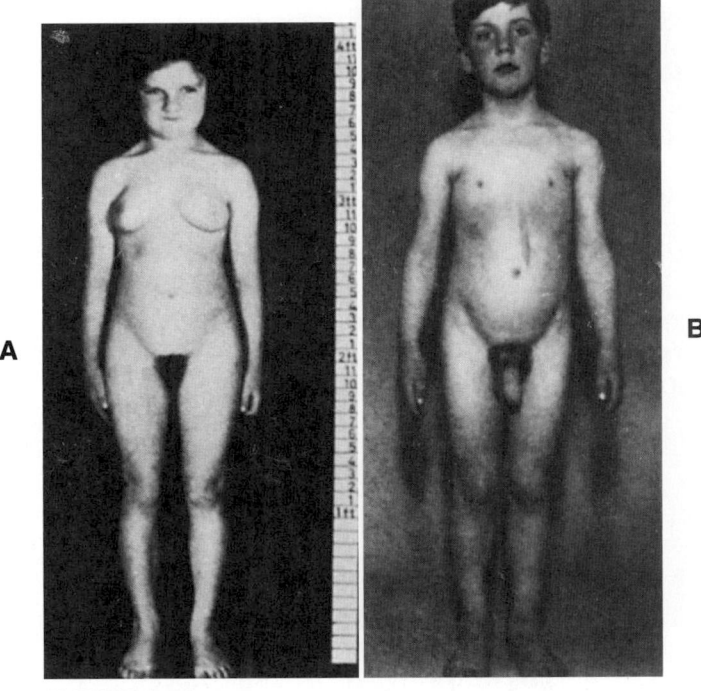

FIGURE 5-29
A, Constitutional sexual precocity in a 5-year-old girl. **B,** Constitutional sexual precocity in a 5-year-old boy.
From Jolly, 1981.

TURNER SYNDROME

This syndrome results from complete or partial absence of the second X chromosome and results in a phenotypic female. The affected child is often identified during adolescence because of the absence of sexual development. Common clinical manifestations in an affected child include: webbed neck, low posterior hairline, small mandible, epicanthal folds, high arched palate, increased carrying angle of the elbow, shield-shaped chest deformity with hypoplastic nipples, short stature, and congenital anomalies of heart or urinary tract (Fig. 5-30).

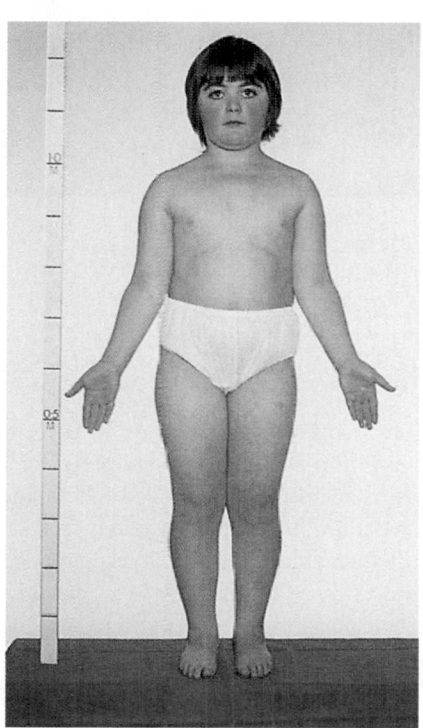

FIGURE 5-30
Turner syndrome.
From Thibodeau, Patton, 2003.

ELECTRONIC RESOURCES

For Weblinks and additional resources, go to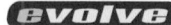
http://evolve.elsevier.com/Seidel

or to the Companion CD-ROM.

NUTRITION

Nutrition may be defined as the science of food as it relates to optimal health and performance. Nutritional intake and status may therefore offer insight into an individual's total health status. In some instances, abnormalities such as anemia and hyperlipidemia may at least in part be a direct result of food intake. A nutritional assessment encompasses analysis of an individual's approximate nutrient intake and relates it to the review of related history, physical examination and findings, and anthropometric and biochemical measures. This chapter reviews the use of nutrients for growth, development, and maintenance of health and provides guidelines for assessing an individual's intake. Use of related history, anthropometric (see Chapter 5) and biochemical measures, and physical findings to complete a nutrition assessment are discussed in detail for the pediatric and adult populations.

ANATOMY AND PHYSIOLOGY

Food nourishes the body by supplying necessary nutrients and calories to function in one or all of three ways:
1. To provide energy for necessary activities
2. To provide for the building and maintenance of body tissues
3. To regulate body processes

The nutrients necessary to the body are classified as macronutrients, micronutrients, and water. Energy requirements are based on the balance of energy expenditure associated with an individual's body size and composition and the level of physical activity. An appropriate balance contributes to long-term health and allows for the maintenance of desirable physical activity.

MACRONUTRIENTS

Carbohydrate, protein, and fat are referred to as macronutrients because they are required in large amounts. These three macronutrients provide the calories needed to produce energy in the human body. Even though alcohol also provides calories (7 per gram), it is not required for any physiologic processes by the body and therefore is not discussed in detail in this chapter.

CARBOHYDRATE

Carbohydrate, a nutrient found mostly in plants and in milk, is considered the body's main source of energy. About 365 g are stored as glycogen in the liver and muscle tissues and is present in circulating blood, but this amount provides energy for only about 13 hours of moderate activity. Moderate amounts of carbohydrate must be ingested at frequent intervals to meet the energy demands of the body. Carbohydrate also serves major functions in vital organs:

- The liver—sparing the use of protein for energy and participating in specific detoxifying metabolic pathways
- The heart—as glycogen stored in cardiac muscle
- The central nervous system—as the only energy source to the brain.

If more carbohydrate is eaten than is needed for energy, the excess is stored in fatty tissues throughout the body. It is recommended that carbohydrate content of the diet be at least 50% of total calories, with no less than 100 g being consumed per day. Refer to Appendix E for the 2002 Dietary Reference Intakes for carbohydrate needs from birth to adult as established by the Food and Nutrition Board, Institute of Medicine. One gram of carbohydrate supplies 4 calories.

PROTEIN

Protein, present in all animal and plant products, is essential to life. It is a part of more than half the organic matter in the body, including hair, skin, nails, muscle, glandular organs, connective tissue, blood plasma, and hemoglobin. In all, 20 different amino acids combine in different ways to form proteins. Eight amino acids are considered essential because they cannot be manufactured by the body and are essential for normal growth and development. During the digestion process, protein is broken down into amino acids, the building blocks of the protein molecule, and absorbed into the bloodstream where they are carried to the tissues. Each tissue uses a specific amino acid to build its individual protein. The major functions of protein include the following:

- Building and maintaining tissues
- Regulating internal water and acid-base balances
- Acting as a precursor for enzymes, antibodies, and several hormones

If more protein is eaten than is needed for these major functions, the surplus is either used to supply energy or is stored as body fat if total calorie intake is in excess of needs. It is recommended that protein content of the diet be 14% to 20% of total calories, or a daily minimum of 13 g in infants, 25 g in children, and 45 g in adults. Refer to Appendix E for the 2002 Dietary Reference Intakes for protein needs, from birth to adult, as established by the Food and Nutrition Board, Institute of Medicine. One gram of protein supplies 4 calories.

FAT

Fat, which is present in animal and some plant products (particularly the seeds of plants), is necessary as the main source of linoleic acid, a fatty acid essential for normal growth and development. Other major functions of fat include the following:

- Synthesis and regulation of certain hormones
- Maintenance of tissue structure
- Nerve impulse transmission
- Memory storage
- Energy metabolism

Again, if more fat is eaten than is needed for these functions, the extra is stored in fatty tissues in the body. Some of these fatty tissues, especially those under the skin and around the abdominal organs, serve a purpose (e.g., as a reserve store of fuel to be used when calorie intake does not meet needs, to support and protect organs from injury, and to prevent undue loss of heat from the body surface). It is recommended that fat content of the diet be 25% to 35% of total calories, or at least 20 to 35 g per day. Refer to Appendix E for the 2002 Dietary Reference Intakes for fat from birth to adult as established by the Food and Nutrition Board, Institute of Medicine. One gram of fat supplies 9 calories.

MICRONUTRIENTS

Vitamins, minerals (elements), and electrolytes are known as *micronutrients* because they are required and stored in very small quantities by the body. Even though they are not used as a source of energy, they are essential for growth, development, and hundreds of metabolic processes that occur daily. Vitamins and minerals must be taken in either through food or by supplement. With the exception of vitamin K and biotin (produced by certain intestinal microorganisms), vitamin D (synthesized from cholesterol), and niacin (synthesized from tryptophan), micronutrients cannot be metabolized by the body. Refer to Appendix E for the 2002 Dietary Reference Intakes (DRIs) as established by the Food and Nutrition Board, Institute of Medicine, for selected vitamins and minerals (elements).

WATER

Water, although listed last in this section, is the most vital nutrient. An individual can exist without food for several weeks, but without water, an individual would last only a few days. The body of an adult is about 55% to 65% water. The major functions of water include the following:

- ✦ Providing turgor to body tissues
- ✦ Altering dissolved substances to make them available for metabolic processes
- ✦ Transporting dissolved nutrients and wastes throughout the body
- ✦ Maintaining a stable body temperature

There is a continual loss of water from the body by the kidneys as urine, by the lungs as water vapor in expired air, and by the skin as perspiration. Approximately 2 to 2½ liters of water are lost daily. This loss of water is replaced by fluids taken in, water contained in solid foods eaten, and water produced in the body as a result of oxidative processes. The body is able to maintain a fluid balance except during some acute or chronic illnesses. Although no recommended dietary allowance has been established, refer to Appendix E for the 2004 Adequate Intake Values for recommended water intake goals for healthy individuals as established by the Food and Nutrition Board, Institute of Medicine.

ENERGY REQUIREMENTS

A day's total energy expenditures include the energy used at rest; energy used in physical activity; and energy used as a result of thermogenesis, the metabolic response to food intake. Affecting these components are age, gender, body size and composition, genetics, physiologic state (e.g., rapid growth, pregnancy, or lactation), presence of disease, and body temperature. At all ages, a change in body energy stored as fat occurs if energy in the form of calories taken in through food either exceeds or is deficient to meet an individual's needs.

RESTING ENERGY EXPENDITURE

Resting energy expenditure (REE) contributes the largest proportion of total energy expenditure by the body. REE represents the energy expended by a person at rest under conditions of stable temperature. Although basal metabolic rate (BMR) is defined as the REE measured soon after awakening in the morning (12 hours after the last meal), these two values are often interchangeable (their variability is less than 10%). Table 6-1 presents equations developed by the World Health Organization (WHO, 1985). These equations are meant to serve as a guide; they are not completely accurate for all individuals but can assist in determining approximate energy needs. The table accounts for age, weight, and gender, but not height. Height does not appear to affect the accuracy of the calculation.

PHYSICAL ACTIVITY

Physical activity constitutes the second largest proportion of total energy expenditure by the body. The energy expended by numerous activities has been studied thoroughly by researchers. The energy expended by a given activity can vary greatly among individuals and is most affected by body weight and muscle mass. A heavier person will expend more energy for a given task than a lighter individual. This often makes calculating exact energy expenditure difficult and time consuming. Table 6-2 provides estimates of energy needs for infants

TABLE 6-1	Equations for Predicting Resting Energy Expenditure (REE) from Body Weight*
Gender and Age (yr)	**Equation to Derive REE in kcal/day**
MALES	
0-3	$(60.9 \times wt^\dagger) - 54$
3-10	$(22.7 \times wt) + 495$
10-18	$(17.5 \times wt) + 651$
18-30	$(15.3 \times wt) + 679$
30-60	$(11.6 \times wt) + 879$
>60	$(13.5 \times wt) + 487$
FEMALES	
0-3	$(61.0 \times wt) - 51$
3-10	$(22.4 \times wt) + 499$
10-18	$(12.2 \times wt) + 746$
18-30	$(14.7 \times wt) + 496$
30-60	$(8.7 \times wt) + 829$
>60	$(10.5 \times wt) + 596$

Modified from Subcommittee on the Tenth Edition of the RDAs, 1989.
*From WHO, 1985. These equations were derived from BMR data.
†Weight of person in kilograms.

TABLE 6-2	Median Heights and Weights and Recommended Energy Intake

Category	Age (yr) or Condition	Weight (kg)	Weight (lb)	Height (cm)	Height (inches)	REE (kcal/day)	Multiples of REE	Per kg Body Weight	Per Day*
Infants	0.0-0.5	6	13	60	24	320		108	650
	0.5-1.0	9	20	71	28	500		98	850
Children	1-3	13	29	90	35	740		102	1300
	4-6	20	44	112	44	950		90	1800
	7-10	28	62	132	52	1130		70	2000
Males	11-14	45	99	157	62	1440	1.70	55	2500
	15-18	66	145	176	69	1760	1.67	45	3000
	19-24	72	160	177	70	1780	1.67	40	2900
	25-50	79	174	176	70	1800	1.60	37	2900
	51+	77	170	173	68	1530	1.50	30	2300
Females	11-14	46	101	157	62	1310	1.67	47	2200
	15-18	55	120	163	64	1370	1.60	40	2200
	19-24	58	128	164	65	1350	1.60	38	2200
	25-50	63	138	163	64	1380	1.55	36	2200
	51+	65	143	160	63	1280	1.50	30	1900
Pregnant	1st trimester								+0
	2nd trimester								+300
	3rd trimester								+300
Lactating	1st 6 months								+500
	2nd 6 months								+500

From Wardlaw, Insel, Seyler, 1994.
REE, Resting energy expenditure: calculation based on equations from the FAO (Food and Agriculture Organization of the United Nations), then rounded. This is the same as resting metabolic rate (RMR).
*Figure is rounded.

through adults and is based on a light to moderate activity level. These estimates should be adjusted for individuals with higher activity levels and for greater or smaller body size. The WHO derived these energy requirements for infants and children from estimates of intake associated with normal growth. The estimated energy requirements for pregnancy and lactation also come from the WHO and are based on the increase in energy expenditure during both physiologic states.

THERMOGENESIS

After eating, the metabolic rate increases, depending on the size and composition of the meal. This accounts for about 7% of the total energy expended during a day. The increased rate peaks after about 1 hour and disappears after 4 hours. It has little long-term effect on energy requirements, being lost in the day-to-day variations in energy metabolism.

REVIEW OF RELATED HISTORY

For each of the conditions discussed in this section, targeted topics to include in the history of the present illness are listed. Responses to questions about these topics help fully assess the patient's condition and provide clues for focusing the physical examination.

HISTORY OF PRESENT ILLNESS

- Weight loss
  - Total weight lost, compared with usual weight; time period (sudden, gradual); desired or undesired
  - Desired weight loss: eating habits; diet plan used; medical nutrition therapy guidelines followed; food preparation; food group avoidance; calorie intake; appetite; exercise pattern; support group participation; weight goal
  - Undesired weight loss: anorexia; vomiting or diarrhea, other illness symptoms, time period; frequent urination, excessive thirst; change in lifestyle, activity, and stress levels
  - Preoccupation with body weight or body shape: never feeling thin enough, fasting, unusually strict caloric intake; unusual food restrictions or cravings; laxative abuse, induced vomiting; amenorrhea; excessive exercise; alcohol intake
  - Medications: chemotherapy, diuretics, insulin, fluoxetine; prescription and nonprescription appetite suppressants; laxatives; oral hypoglycemics; herbal supplements
- Weight gain
  - Total weight gained: time period, sudden or gradual, desired or undesired, possibility of pregnancy
  - Change in lifestyle: change in social aspects of eating; more meals eaten out of the home; meals eaten quickly and "on the go"; change in meal preparation patterns; change in exercise patterns, stress level, or alcohol intake
  - Medications: steroids, oral contraceptives, antidepressants, insulin
- Increased metabolic requirements
  - Fever, infection, burns, trauma, pregnancy, infancy, hyperthyroidism, cancer
  - External losses (e.g., fistulas, wounds, abscesses, chronic blood loss, chronic dialysis)

PAST MEDICAL HISTORY

- Chronic illness: cystic fibrosis, phenylketonuria (PKU), maple syrup urine disease, inborn errors of carbohydrate metabolism, tyrosinemia, Prader-Willi syndrome, Wilson's disease, homocystinuria, diabetes, congestive heart failure, hypothyroidism, hyperthyroidism, pancreatic insufficiency, celiac disease, Crohn's disease, surgical resection of gastrointestinal tract

- Previous weight loss or gain efforts: weight at 25 years, maximum body weight, minimum weight as an adult
- Previously diagnosed eating disorder, hypoglycemia

FAMILY HISTORY

- Obesity
- Constitutionally short or tall stature
- Genetic or metabolic disorder: diabetes; see Chronic Illness under Past Medical History
- Eating disorder: anorexia, bulimia
- Alcoholism

PERSONAL AND SOCIAL HISTORY

- Nutrition: appetite; usual calorie intake; vegetarianism; medical nutrition therapy guidelines followed; religious/cultural food practices; proportion of fat, protein, carbohydrate in the diet; intake of major vitamins and minerals (e.g., A, C, iron, calcium, folate).
- Use of vitamin, mineral, and herbal supplements
- Usual weight and height; current weight and height; ability to maintain weight, goal weight
- Use of alcohol
- Use of recreational/club drugs
- Adequate income for food purchases; limited/fixed income; need to choose between medications or food
- Ability to shop/prepare foods; food storage/preparation equipment (refrigerator, stove, oven)
- Typical mealtime situations; companions; living environment
- Use of oral supplements, tube feedings, parenteral nutrition
- Dentition: dentures, missing teeth, gum disease

(Refer to Determine Your Nutritional Health and Level I Screen in Appendix F.)

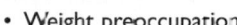 **INFANTS AND CHILDREN**

- Nutrition: breast-feeding frequency; type and amount of infant formula; time it takes to drink one feeding; intake of protein, calories, vitamins, and minerals adequate for growth; vegetarianism; food allergies; vitamin and mineral supplements
- Chronic illness: PKU, maple syrup urine disease, inborn errors of carbohydrate metabolism, tyrosinemia, homocystinuria, Wilson's disease, cystic fibrosis
- Congenital anomalies: prematurity, cleft palate, malformed palate, tongue thrust, swallowing disorders, neurologic disorders, gastrointestinal reflux, severe congenital heart defect

RISK FACTORS

EATING DISORDERS

- Weight preoccupation
- Poor self-esteem, perfectionist personality
- Self-image perceptual disturbances
- Chronic medical illness (insulin-dependent diabetes)
- Family history of eating disorders, obesity, alcoholism, or affective disorders
- Cultural pressure for thinness or outstanding performance
- Athlete driven to excel in sports (particularly females)
- Food cravings, restrictions
- Compulsive/binge eating
- Difficulties with communication and conflict resolution; separation from families
- Use of appetite suppressants and/or laxatives

ADOLESCENTS

- Nutrition: intake of protein, calories, vitamins, and minerals adequate for growth; vegetarianism; fast food intake; fad diets; food allergies; vitamin and mineral supplements; herbal supplements; appetite suppressants; laxative use; alcohol use
- Preoccupation with weight (not limited to girls)
- Overconcern with developing muscle mass, losing body fat
- Excessive exercise
- Weighs self daily, boasts about weight loss
- Omits perceived fattening foods and food groups from diet

CLINICAL PEARL

Eating Disorders
A major risk factor for developing an eating disorder (e.g., anorexia or bulimia) is having a first-degree relative with an eating disorder.

PREGNANT WOMEN

- Prepregnancy weight, age, eating patterns/disorders, folic acid
- Weight gain during pregnancy; nutrient intake during pregnancy (particularly protein, calories, iron, folate, calcium); supplementation with vitamins, iron, folic acid
- Potential risks: pica, alcohol, inadequate weight gain, and known teratogens (e.g., certain drugs such as some acne medications, some antihypertensive agents, anticonvulsants, some antibiotics)
- Lactation: nutrient intake during lactation (particularly protein, calories, calcium, vitamins A and C); fluid intake (water, juice, milk, caffeine)
- Influence of disorders: diabetes, renal disease, others

OLDER ADULTS

- Nutrition: weight gain or loss, adequate income for food purchases, interest in meal preparation, medical nutrition therapy needs, participant in older adult feeding programs, social interaction at mealtime, number of daily meals and snacks, transportation to grocery stores (Refer to the Level II Nutrition Screen in Appendix F.)
- Energy level, regular exercise/activities
- Chronic illnesses: diabetes, renal disease, cancer, heart disease, others
- Food/nutrient/medication interactions (Box 6-1)

BOX 6-1

FOOD/NUTRIENT/MEDICATION INTERACTIONS

Medication can affect nutritional intake and status just as some foods, and the nutrients contained in them, can affect absorption, metabolism, and excretion of medications. For example, a consistently high intake of grapefruit juice while taking simvastatin increases the bioavailability of the medication, often resulting in an increased risk of myopathy. It is important to assess the medications that a patient is taking to determine appropriateness and whether there are any possible interactions. The term *medications* should be interpreted to include those by prescription as well as those purchased over-the-counter. Often patients are taking vitamin, mineral, herbal, and protein supplements that they do not consider to be medication; thus they do not remember to relate these during the examination unless specifically asked about them.

RISK FACTORS

POSSIBLE MEDICATION EFFECTS ON NUTRITIONAL INTAKE AND STATUS

- Altered food intake resulting from altered taste/smell, "drug mouth," gastric irritation, bezoars (foodball often found in the stomach and/or intestines), appetite increase/decrease, nausea/vomiting
- Modified nutrient absorption resulting from altered gastrointestinal pH, increased/decreased bile acid activity, altered gastrointestinal motility, inhibited enzymes, damaged mucosal cell walls, insoluble nutrient-drug complexes
- Modified nutrient metabolism resulting from vitamin antagonism, vitamin inactivation
- Modified nutrient excretion resulting from urinary loss, fecal loss

EXAMINATION AND FINDINGS

EQUIPMENT

- Tape measure with millimeter markings
- Calculator
- Standing platform scale with height attachment

ANTHROPOMETRICS

Procedures for accurately measuring height, weight, and triceps skinfold, and the tables of the norms for the relevant age and gender groups are addressed in Chapter 5. These measures are useful in assessing a patient's nutritional status and possible disease risk. Refer to Box 6-2 to perform measures and calculations. See Box 6-3 for adjusting desirable weights for amputations and paraplegia/quadriplegia.

BODY MASS INDEX

The body mass index (BMI) is a formula used to assess nutritional status and total body fat (Box 6-4). It is a measure of kilograms per meter squared. For adult men and women, a BMI between 18.5 and 24.9 is expected. Track the change of a patient's BMI over time to identify nutritional problems or illness. Refer to Table 6-3 for the classification of overweight and obesity by BMI and waist circumference. See Box 6-4 or Appendix G for calculating BMI using pounds and inches. A nomogram for calculating BMI is available on the Level II Nutrition Screen form in Appendix F.

BOX 6-2

ASSESSING HEIGHT AND WEIGHT

Current Weight	_____	Current Height _____
Usual Weight	_____	
Desirable		(Women: 100 pounds for first 5 feet; plus 5
Body Weight	_____	pounds for each inch thereafter)
		(Men: 106 pounds for first 5 feet; plus 6 pounds
		for each inch thereafter)
		This is a quick method for determining desirable
		weight.
		(See Chapter 5 for height/weight tables and Box
		6-4 for body mass index measurements.)
		Add 10% for a large frame; subtract 10% for a
		small frame. Refer to Chapter 5 for methods
		used to determine body frame size.
% Desirable Weight	_____	*current weight* × 100 divided by desirable body
		weight
% Usual Weight	_____	*current weight* × 100 divided by usual weight
% Weight Change	_____	(*usual weight* minus *current weight*) × 100 divided
		by usual weight

A significant weight loss equals or exceeds:

    1% to 2% in 1 week

    5% in 1 month

    7.5% in 3 months

    10% in 6 months

For pediatric patients (birth to age 18), refer to the growth charts in Appendix C.

BOX 6-3

DESIRABLE BODY WEIGHT (DBW) ADJUSTMENTS

Adjustment for Amputation

To make adjustments for amputation, subtract the percent weight contributed by the amputated body part(s).

Trunk without limbs	42.7%
Entire upper extremity	6.6%
Hand	0.8%
Forearm	2.3%
Upper arm	3.5%
Entire lower extremity	18.7%
Foot	1.8%
Lower leg	5.3%
Thigh	11.6%

Adjustment for Paraplegia/Quadriplegia

To make adjustment for paraplegia: subtract 5% to 10% from calculated DBW.
To make adjustment for quadriplegia: subtract 10% to 15% from calculated DBW.

BOX 6-4

CALCULATING BODY MASS INDEX

Quick calculation for BMI:

$$BMI = \left(\frac{\text{Weight in pounds}}{[\text{Height in inches}] \times [\text{Height in inches}]} \right) \times 703$$

The following is a simpler way of writing this formula:
[(Weight in pounds $\times$ 703) $\div$ Height in inches] $\div$ Height in inches

Example: A man 6 feet tall weighing 185 pounds has a BMI of 25.1
185 $\times$ 703 = 130,055
130,055 $\div$ 72 = 1806.3194
1806.3194 $\div$ 72 = 25.1

See the Companion CD-ROM accompanying this text to test some of your own calculations on the BMI Calculator.

TABLE 6-3   **Classification of Overweight and Obesity by BMI, Waist Circumference, and Associated Disease Risks**

	BMI	Obesity Class	Disease Risk Relative to Normal Weight and Waist Circumference	
			Men <102 cm (<40 inches) Women <88 cm (<35 inches)	>102 cm (>40 inches) >88 cm (>35 inches)
Underweight	<18.5		—	—
Normal	18.5-24.9		—	—
Overweight	25-29.9		Increased	High
Obesity	30-34.9	I	High	Very high
	35-39.9	II	Very high	Very high
Extreme obesity	≥40	III	Extremely high	Extremely high

TABLE 6-4	Interpretation of Body Mass Index for Age in Children and Adolescents
BMI Category	**BMI Percentile**
Underweight	BMI-for-age <5th percentile
At risk of overweight	BMI-for-age >85th percentile
Overweight	BMI-for-age >95th percentile

The BMI is now standardized for use in children and adolescents. As children grow, their body fatness changes over the years; therefore interpretation of BMI depends on the child's age. Additionally, boys and girls differ in their body fatness as they mature, so the BMI-for-age is plotted according to gender-specific charts. Use the BMI gender-specific growth charts in Appendix C to assess appropriate height and weight relevant to age and gender. Established cutoff points are used to identify underweight and overweight children and adolescents (Table 6-4).

WAIST CIRCUMFERENCE

Persons of normal weight who have increased waist circumferences often fall into a higher disease risk classification. A large waist circumference (>35 inches in women; >40 inches in men) is often associated with increased risk for type 2 diabetes, dyslipidemia, hypertension, and cardiovascular disease (National Institutes of Health, *Practical Guide to the Identification, Evaluation, and Treatment of Overweight and Obesity in Adults, 2000*). Monitoring changes in a person's waist circumference over time, with or without changes in BMI, may aid in predicting relative disease risk in terms of cardiovascular risk factors and obesity-related diseases. Refer to Chapter 5 for guidelines for measuring waist circumference and waist-hip ratio.

DETERMINATION OF DIET ADEQUACY

The history of an individual's food intake allows estimation of the adequacy of the diet. Histories may be obtained through 24-hour diet recalls or with a 3- or 4-day food diary that includes 1 weekend day. Various methods for measuring nutrient intake are available.

24-HOUR RECALL DIET

The 24-hour recall is the quickest and most simple method for obtaining a food intake history. Ask the patient to complete a 24-hour food recall using the form in Appendix F, listing all foods, beverages, and snacks eaten during the last 24 hours. Alternatively, ask the patient to tell you what he or she ate and drank during the last 24 hours. Remember to ask specific questions about the method of food preparation, portion sizes, types of added fat, and use of salt. This method, however, provides a very limited view of an individual's actual intake over time and may be misleading. Most individuals also are unable to accurately remember everything they ate the day before, causing further inaccuracies in interpreting the information.

FOOD DIARY

The food diary is both the most accurate and the most time-consuming method for the patient and health professional. It provides a retrospective view of an individual's eating habits and dietary intake, recorded as it happened. It can also collect relevant data that may aid in identifying problem areas. The patient is provided the food diary form found in Appendix F and requested to record specific food and beverage intake for at least 3 days, including 1 weekend day.

MEASURES OF NUTRIENT ANALYSIS

Complete a nutrient analysis by using a method of diet history or recall. Appendix F contains three nutrition screening forms that can be used to obtain specific information about current nutrition status and intake and to determine whether problem areas exist. Select the screening form that corresponds to the preferred depth of assessment and the availability of anthropometric and laboratory values. The questions can be modified for infants, children, older adults, or particular circumstances.

Computerized nutrient analysis programs offer the quickest and most efficient method of analyzing an individual's nutrient intake. Analysis may be performed for 1 or more days to obtain averages for all or selected nutrients. A nutrition textbook containing food composition tables may also be used; however, it is time consuming, and the tables found in these books are often not as complete as those in computerized programs. The quickest method of estimating adequacy with reliable accuracy is simply to compare the individual's intake with the recommended servings and portions listed in the MyPyramid Food Guide (Fig. 6-1).

MYPYRAMID FOOD GUIDE

A method to estimate dietary adequacy is to use the MyPyramid Food Guide (see Fig. 6-1), which indicates the number of servings to eat from each food group. The MyPyramid Food Guidance System provides food-based guidance to help implement the recommendations of the 2005 *Dietary Guidelines for Americans*. Based on the latest scientific evidence, the Guidelines, published by the U.S. Department of Health and Human Services (HHS) and the U.S. Department of Agriculture (USDA) provide information and advice for choosing a nutritious diet, maintaining a healthy weight, achieving adequate exercise, and keeping foods safe to avoid foodborne illness. The full guidelines are available at http://www.health.gov/dietaryguidelines/dga2005/document/

MyPyramid (http://www.mypyramid.gov) provides web-based interactive and print materials for consumers and professionals. The system can be used to track and analyze individual eating and physical activity habits and can generate an individualized dietary plan based on age, gender, and physical activity level.

When using the MyPyramid guide, remember the following:
- The guide does not deal with infant feeding.
- No one food is absolutely essential to good nutrition. Each food is low in at least one essential nutrient.
- No one food group provides all essential nutrients in adequate amounts. Each food group makes an important and distinct contribution to nutritional intake.
- Variety is the key. Variety is guaranteed by using all the groups. Furthermore, one should consume a variety of foods within each group.

VEGETARIAN DIETS

Vegetarian diets can meet all the recommendations for nutrients. The key is to consume a variety of foods and the right amount of foods to meet calorie needs. Five nutrients may be deficient in a vegetarian diet if it is not carefully planned: protein, calcium (lacto-ovo and vegan), iron, vitamin B_{12} (vegan), and vitamin D.

ETHNIC FOOD GUIDE PYRAMIDS

Ethnic Food Guide Pyramids are culturally sensitive (e.g., Mediterranean, Indian, Mexican, and Asian). To see examples of ethnic food guide pyramids, go to http://www.nal.usda.gov/fnic, then select Topics A-Z, Food Guide Pyramid, Other Food Guide Pyramids, Ethnic/Cultural Food Guide Pyramids. In addition, contact Oldways Preservation & Exchange Trust at http://www.oldwayspt.org or phone 617-421-5500.

MEASURES OF NUTRIENT ADEQUACY

Nutrition can be assessed through many body systems. Summaries of the functions/metabolism/utilization, deficiencies/excesses, and food sources of fat- and water-soluble vitamins and minerals are provided in Tables 6-5 through 6-7. The clinical findings often associated with nutrient deficiencies are indicated in Table 6-8. The section that follows discusses methods of measuring nutrient intake and adequacy along with specific anthropometric and biochemical measures of nutritional status.

An individual's diet can be measured for nutritional adequacy based on energy needs and/or a variety of macronutrients or micronutrients.
- Energy: A variety of methods can be used for calculating an individual's energy needs. The "rule of thumb" calculations also offer a quick estimate for energy needs for those

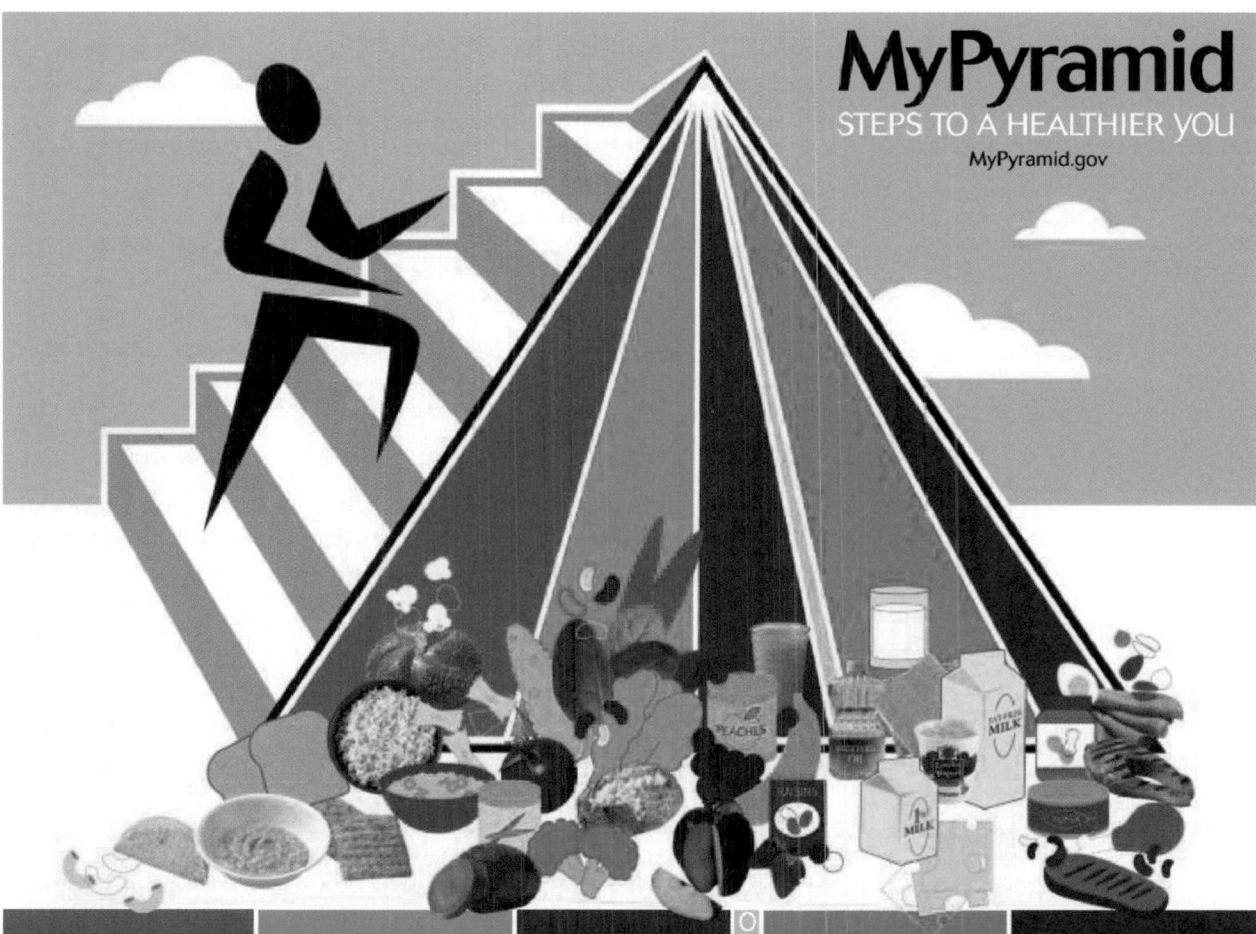

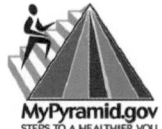

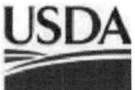

FIGURE 6-1
MyPyramid Food Guide.
From the U.S. Department of Agriculture, Center for Nutrition Policy and Promotion, http://www.Mypyramid.gov, April 2005.

TABLE 6-5	Fat-Soluble Vitamin Summary		
Vitamins	**Metabolism**	**Deficiency or Excess**	**Food Sources**
VITAMIN A Retinol Retinal Retinoic acid	Bile needed for absorption Mineral oil prevents absorption Stored in liver	Night blindness Keratomalacia Lowered resistance to infection Severe drying and scaling of skin; eye infections; blindness	Liver, kidney
PROVITAMIN A Carotenes	Bone and tooth structure Healthy skin and mucous membranes Vision in dim light	Overdoses are toxic: skin, hair, and bone changes; petechiae	Egg yolk, butter, fortified margarine Milk, cream, cheese Dark-green leafy and deep-yellow vegetables Deep-yellow fruits
VITAMIN D Precursors: Ergosterol in plants 7-dehydrocholesterol; in skin	Some storage in liver Liver synthesizes calcidiol Kidney converts calcidiol to calcitriol Functions as hormone in absorption of calcium and phosphorus Mobilization and mineralization of bone	*Rickets* • Soft bones • Enlarged joints • Enlarged skull • Deformed chest • Spinal curvature • Bowed leg *Osteomalacia* *Renal osteodystrophy* Even small excess is toxic	*Fortified milk* Concentrates: calciferol; viosterol Fish-liver oils Exposure to ultraviolet rays of sun
VITAMIN E Tocopherols	Prevents oxidation of vitamin A in intestine Protects cell membranes against oxidation Protects red blood cells Limited stores in body Polyunsaturated fats increase need	Deficiency not common Red cell homolysis in malnourished infants Low toxicity	Salad oils, shortenings, margarines Whole grains, legumes, nuts, dark leafy vegetables
VITAMIN K	Forms prothrombin for normal blood clotting Synthesized in intestines	Prolonged clotting time Hemorrhage, especially in newborn infants Biliary tract disease Large amounts are toxic	Synthesized by intestinal bacteria Dark-green leafy vegetables

Modified from Robinson, Weigley, Mueller, 1993.

TABLE 6-6	Water-Soluble Vitamin Summary		
Vitamins	**Metabolism/Function**	**Deficiency**	**Food Sources**

ASCORBIC ACID
Vitamin C
	Forms collagen
	Keeps teeth firm in gums
	Hormone synthesis
	Resistance to infection
	Improves iron absorption
		Poor wound healing
		Poor bone, tooth development
		Scurvy
		  Bruising and hemorrhage
		  Bleeding gums
		  Loose teeth
			Citrus fruits
			Strawberries, cantaloupe
			Tomatoes, broccoli
			Raw green vegetables

THIAMIN
Vitamin B$_1$
	Coenzyme for breakdown of glucose for energy
	Healthy nerves
	Good digestion
	Normal appetite
	Good mental outlook
	Angular stomatitis
		Beriberi
		  Fatigue
		  Poor appetite
		  Constipation
		  Depression
		  Neuropathy
		  Polyneuritis
		  Edema
		  Heart failure
			Pork, liver, other meats, poultry
			Dry beans and peas, peanut butter
			Enriched and whole-grain bread
			Milk, eggs

RIBOFLAVIN
Vitamin B$_2$
	Coenzymes for protein and glucose metabolism
	Fatty acid synthesis
	Healthy skin
	Normal vision in bright light
		Cheilosis
		  Scaling skin
		  Burning, itching, sensitive eyes
			Dairy products
			Meat, poultry, fish
			Dark-green leafy vegetables
			Enriched and whole-grain breads, cereals

NIACIN
Nicotinic acid
Niacinamide
	Coenzymes for energy metabolism
	Normal digestion
	Healthy nervous system
	Healthy skin
	Tryptophan a precursor:
	60 mg = 1 mg niacin
		Pellagra
		  Dermatitis
		  Angular stomatitis
		  Diarrhea
		  Depression
		  Disorientation
		  Delirium
			Meat, poultry, fish
			Dark-green leafy vegetables
			Whole-grain or enriched breads, cereals

VITAMIN B$_6$ Pyridoxine Pyridoxal Pyridoxamine	Coenzymes for protein metabolism Conversion of tryptophan to niacin Formation of heme	Cheilosis Gastrointestinal upsets Weak gait Irritability Neuropathy Convulsions	Meat Whole-grain cereals Dark-green leafy vegetables Potatoes
VITAMIN B$_{12}$	Formation of mature red blood cells Synthesis of DNA, RNA Requires intrinsic factor from stomach for absorption	Pernicious anemia: lack of intrinsic factor, or after gastrectomy Macrocytic anemia: neurologic degeneration, pallor	Animal foods only: milk, eggs, meat, poultry, fish
FOLATE Folacin Folic acid	Maturation of red blood cells Synthesis of DNA, RNA	Macrocytic anemia in pregnancy, sprue, pallor	Dark-green leafy vegetables Meat, fish, poultry, eggs Whole-grain cereals
BIOTIN	Components of coenzymes in energy metabolism Some synthesis in intestine Avidin, a protein in raw egg white, interferes with absorption	Deficiency occurs only when large amounts of raw egg whites are eaten Dermatitis, loss of hair	Organ meats Egg yolk Legumes, nuts
PANTOTHENIC ACID	Component of coenzyme A Synthesis of sterols, fatty acids, heme	Deficiency occurs rarely Neuritis of arms, legs; burning sensation of feet	Meat, poultry, fish, legumes, whole-grain cereals Lesser amounts in milk, fruits, and vegetables

Modified from Robinson, Weigley, Mueller, 1993.

TABLE 6-7	Mineral Summary		
Element	**Function**	**Utilization/Deficiency**	**Food Sources**
CALCIUM	99% in bones, teeth Nervous stimulation Muscle contraction Blood clotting Activates enzymes	10%-40% absorbed Aided by vitamin D and lactose; hindered by oxalic acid Parathyroid hormone regulates blood levels *Deficiency:* fragile bones, osteoporosis	Dairy products Mustard and turnip greens Cabbage, broccoli Clams, oysters, salmon
PHOSPHORUS	80%-90% in bones, teeth Acid-balance Transport of fats Enzymes for energy metabolism; protein synthesis	Vitamin D favors absorption and use by bones Dietary deficiency unlikely	Dairy products Meat, poultry, fish Whole-grain cereals, nuts, legumes
MAGNESIUM	60% in bones, teeth Transmits nerve impulses Muscle contraction Enzymes for energy metabolism	Salts relatively insoluble Acid favors absorption Dietary deficiency unlikely; occurs in alcoholism, renal failure	Milk, meat, green-leafy vegetables, legumes, whole-grain cereals
SODIUM	Extracellular fluid Water balance Acid-base balance Nervous stimulation Muscle contraction	Almost completely absorbed Body levels regulated by adrenal; excess excreted in urine and by skin *Deficiency:* rare, occurs with excessive perspiration	Table salt Baking powder, baking soda Milk, meat, poultry, fish, eggs
POTASSIUM	Intracellular fluid Protein and glycogen synthesis Water balance Transmits nerve impulse Muscle contraction	Almost completely absorbed Body levels regulated by adrenal; excess excreted in urine *Deficiency:* occurs with starvation, diuretic therapy	Ample amounts in meat, cereals, fruits, fruit juices, vegetables
IRON	Mostly in hemoglobin Muscle myoglobin Oxidizing enzymes for release of energy	5%-20% absorption Acid and vitamin C aid absorption Daily losses in urine and feces Menstrual loss *Deficiency:* anemia, cheilosis, pallor	Organ meats, meat, fish, poultry Whole-grain and enriched cereal Green vegetables, dried fruits
IODINE	Forms thyroxine for energy metabolism	Chiefly in thyroid gland *Deficiency:* endemic goiter	Iodized salt Shellfish, saltwater fish
FLUORIDE	Prevents tooth decay	Storage in bones and teeth Excess leads to tooth mottling	Fluoridated water
COPPER	Utilization of iron for hemoglobin formation Pigment formation	In form of ceruloplasmin in blood Abnormal storage in Wilson's disease *Deficiency:* rare	Liver, shellfish, meats, nuts, legumes, whole-grain cereals
ZINC	Enzymes for transfer of carbon dioxide Taste, protein synthesis	*Deficiency:* growth retardation; altered taste	Plant and animal proteins

From Robinson, Weigley, Mueller, 1993.

TABLE 6-8	Clinical Signs and Symptoms of Various Nutrient Deficiencies	
Examination	**Sign/Symptom**	**Deficiency**
Hair	Alopecia	Zinc, essential fatty acids
	Easy pluckability	Protein, essential fatty acids
	Lackluster	Protein, zinc
	"Corkscrew" hair	Vitamin C, vitamin A
	Decreased pigmentation	Protein, copper
Eyes	Xerosis of conjunctiva	Vitamin A
	Corneal vascularization	Riboflavin
	Keratomalacia	Vitamin A
	Bitot spots	Vitamin A
Gastrointestinal tract	Nausea, vomiting	Pyridoxine
	Diarrhea	Zinc, niacin
	Stomatitis	Pyridoxine, riboflavin, iron
	Cheilosis	Pyridoxine, iron
	Glossitis	Pyridoxine, zinc, niacin, folate, vitamin B_{12}
		Riboflavin
		Vitamin C
		Niacin
		Protein
Skin	Dry and scaling	Vitamin A, essential fatty acids, zinc
	Petechiae/ecchymoses	Vitamin C, vitamin K
	Follicular hyperkeratosis	Vitamin A, essential fatty acids
	Nasolabial seborrhea	Niacin, pyridoxine, riboflavin
	Bilateral dermatitis	Niacin, zinc
Extremities	Subcutaneous fat loss	Calories
	Muscle wastage	Calories, protein
	Edema	Protein
	Osteomalacia, bone pain, rickets	Vitamin D
	Arthralgia	Vitamin C
Neurologic	Disorientation	Niacin, thiamin
	Confabulation	Thiamin
	Neuropathy	Thiamin, pyridoxine, chromium
	Paresthesia	Thiamin, pyridoxine, vitamin B_{12}
Cardiovascular	Congestive heart failure, cardiomegaly, tachycardia	Thiamin
	Cardiomyopathy	Selenium

Data from Ross Products Division, Abbott Laboratories, Inc.

CLINICAL PEARL

"Rule of Thumb" Estimates for Calculating Daily Energy Needs

Healthy Adults	**kcal/kg body weight**
To promote weight loss	25
To promote weight maintenance	30
To promote weight gain	35
To promote weight maintenance and/or weight gain in hypermetabolic and malnourished patients	35-50

Use adjusted weight for patients who are greater than 125% of their DBW.

Adjustment for obese patients (for energy if 125% of DBW):

Adjusted weight = [(ABW − DBW) × 325%] + DBW

Pediatric Patients:
1000 Kcal + 100 Kcal/year of age up to age 12

ABW, Actual body weight; DBW, desirable body weight.

---

needing to gain, maintain, or lose weight. Adjustments to the calculations may be made to meet the needs of certain individuals (e.g., those who appear to have a higher metabolic rate and continue to lose weight even when the higher calculation is used). It is important to note that overweight individuals underreport their energy intake by 30% to 55% and lean individuals by only 0% to 20%.

♦ Fat: For those older than 2 years of age, a diet should have 25% to 35% of the daily calories consumed coming from fat, with a distribution of less than 7% saturated fat, less than 10% polyunsaturated fat, and the rest in monounsaturated fat. Before 2 years of age, fat intake may reach 35% to 40% of calories. To obtain essential fatty acids, an intake of at least 20 g per day is recommended. Refer to Appendix E for the Dietary Reference Intakes (DRI) for fat for all individuals, including infants, children, and adolescents.

♦ Protein: For adults, an average of 0.8 g per kilogram body weight is sufficient to meet needs. Refer to Appendix E for the Dietary Reference Intakes for protein needs for all individuals, including infants, children, and adolescents.

◆ Vitamins, minerals and electrolytes: An individual who eats a variety of foods from the food groups will meet his or her needs for most vitamins and minerals. Several that may be of concern if food intake is restricted include vitamins C, E, and A; calcium; iron; and folate. Refer to Appendix E for the suggested Dietary Reference Intakes for all individuals, including infants, children and adolescents.

◆ Fiber: Although fiber is not classified as a nutrient, it is recommended that an adult obtain 25 to 30 g of fiber per day. In children 3 to 18 years of age the formula "age + 5 g" should be used to determine fiber needs. Refer to Appendix E for the suggested Dietary Reference Intakes for total fiber for all individuals, including infants, children, and adolescents.

SPECIAL PROCEDURES

MID–UPPER ARM CIRCUMFERENCE

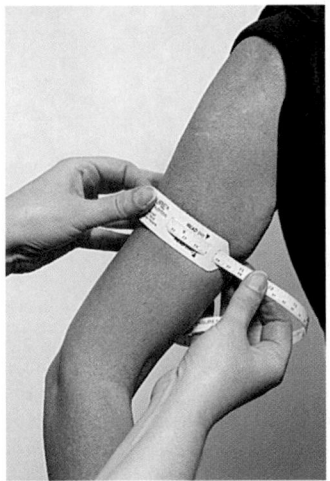

FIGURE 6-2
Measurement of mid–upper arm circumference.

The mid–upper arm circumference (MAC), not routinely obtained, provides a rough estimate of muscle mass and available fat and protein stores. A depressed value, however, is usually found only in the most severe forms of protein-calorie malnutrition. The measurement is of more value in the calculation of arm muscle circumference and arm muscle mass, both of which are sensitive to changes in muscle and/or protein stores. Select the patient's bare right arm for measurement. (**NOTE:** Use the same side of the body for all anthropometric measures.) Place the millimeter measuring tape around the patient's upper arm, midway between the tips of the olecranon and acromial processes (Fig. 6-2), the same location where the triceps skinfold (TSF) thickness measurement is made (see Chapter 5). Hold the measuring tape snugly, but not tight enough to cause an indentation, and make the reading to the nearest 5 mm (0.5 cm). Use the value obtained along with the triceps skinfold measure (see Chapter 5) to calculate midarm muscle circumference (MAMC).

MIDARM MUSCLE CIRCUMFERENCE/ MIDARM MUSCLE AREA

Midarm muscle circumference and arm muscle area are estimated from measures of MAC and TSF. The midarm muscle circumference is well accepted as a sensitive index of body protein reserves. The cross-sectional midarm muscle area (MAMA) can also be estimated. Both measures are commonly decreased in the presence of protein malnutrition. Arm muscle area is useful in children because the muscle area changes more with age than does arm muscle circumference. This measure of arm muscle is only an estimate because the thickness of the humerus is not taken into account and upper arms are not perfectly round as the formula assumes. Tables G-2 through G-5 (Appendix G) show the percentiles for both of these measures for men, women, and children ages 1 to 55 years. In order to accurately assess the nutritional status of older adults 60 years of age and older, age- and gender-specific data derived from the National Health and Nutrition Examination Survey (NHANES III) database was used to prepare new tables for BMI, MAC, TSF, and MAMC for this subgroup of the population (see Chapter 5 and Appendix G). The Level II Nutrition Screen (Appendix F) provides a summary for the percentiles for these measurements (MAC, MAMC, and TSF) for men and women 55 to 75 years of age based on older data.

Calculations:
MAMC: MAC (in mm) − [3.14 × TSF (in mm)]
MAMA: MAC (in mm) − [3.14 × TSF (in mm)]^2 ÷12.56

BIOCHEMICAL MEASUREMENT

This list is intended as a guideline. Not all indicators may be necessary or appropriate for a given patient. Likewise, other laboratory measures not listed here may be useful or necessary in a particular situation. Compare laboratory data to the norms for the relevant age and gender group (Table 6-9). A laboratory may have established different reference ranges based on testing equipment and procedure.

Biochemical measurement:

- Hemoglobin (g/100 mL)
- Hematocrit (%)
- Transferrin saturation (%)
- Serum albumin (g/100 mL)
- Serum cholesterol (CHOL) (mg/100 mL)
- Serum triglycerides (TRI) (mg/100 mL)
- High-density lipoproteins (HDL) (mg/100 mL)
- Low-density lipoproteins (LDL) (mg/100 mL)
- CHOL/HDL ratio
- Serum glucose (mg/100 mL)
- Hemoglobin A1C (%)
- Serum folate (ng/mL)

TABLE 6-9	Biochemical Indicators of Good Nutrition Status			
Nutrient or Measurement	**Test**	**Age Group**	**Male**	**Female**
Iron	Hemoglobin (g/100 mL)	Adults	≥14.0	≥12.0
		Infants (<2 yr)	≥10.0	≥10.0
		Children (2-5 yr)	≥11.0	≥11.0
		Adolescents (13-16 yr)	≥13.5	≥11.5
		Pregnancy		
		(2nd trimester)		≥11.0
		(3rd trimester)		≥10.5
	Hematocrit (%)	Adults	≥40.0	≥37.0
		Infants (<2 yr)	≥31.0	≥31.0
		Children (2-5 yr)	≥34.0	≥34.0
		Adolescents (13-16 yr)	≥40.0	≥36.0
	Transferrin saturation (%)	Adults	≥20.0	≥20.0
		Infants (<2 yr)	≥15.0	≥15.0
		Children (2-12 yr)	≥20.0	≥15.0
		Adolescents (12+ yr)	≥20.0	≥15.0
Protein	Serum albumin (g/100 mL)	Adults	3.4-5.4	3.4-5.4
		Children	3.0-5.0	3.0-5.0
Normal lipid metabolism	Serum cholesterol (mg/100 mL)	Adults	<200	<200
		Children and adolescents	<170	<170
	Serum triglyceride (mg/100 mL)		<150	<150
	High-density lipoprotein (mg/100 mL)		>40	>40
	Low-density lipoprotein (mg/100 mL)	Adults	<130	<130
		Children and adolescents	<110	<110
	Cholesterol/high density lipoprotein ratio		<4.5	<4.5
Normal carbohydrate metabolism	Serum glucose (mg/100 mL)		75-110	75-110
	Hemoglobin A1C (%)		6 or less	6 or less
Folate (ng/mL)	Serum folate		3.6-20	3.6-20

SAMPLE DOCUMENTATION

HISTORY AND PHYSICAL EXAMINATION

Subjective

A 45-year-old businessman with steady weight gain over the past 5 years. Seeks nutrition counseling for weight loss plan. Eats three full meals per day with snacking in-between, eats breakfast and dinner at home, wife prepares meals. Often eats lunch (fast foods) on the run. Alcohol intake: 1 or 2 glasses of wine daily with dinner. No regular exercise. Has never kept a meal log. No change in lifestyle, moderate stress.

For additional sample documentation, see Chapter 26.

Objective

Height: 173 cm (68 inches); weight: 90.9 kg (200 pounds); 123% of desirable body weight; BMI 30.5; triceps skinfold thickness 20 mm, 90th percentile, midarm circumference 327.8 mm; midarm muscle circumference 265 mm, 25th percentile, waist circumference 42 inches; hip circumference 41 inches; waist-hip ratio 1.02; 2200 calories daily, estimated for appropriate weight loss

SUMMARY OF EXAMINATION

NUTRITION ASSESSMENT

1. From the history and physical examination, assess the patient's nutritional status, including the following:
   - Nutrition screen (p. 147)
   - Assessment of nutrient intake (pp. 147-154)
   - Recent growth, weight loss, or weight gain (p. 142)
   - Chronic illnesses affecting nutritional status or intake (p. 142)
   - Laboratory values (p. 155)
   - Clinical signs or symptoms of nutrient or energy deficiency (p. 153)
   - Medication and supplement use (p. 144)

2. Obtain the following anthropometric measurements and compare them to standardized tables:
   - Standing height (p. 145, see Chapter 5)
   - Weight (p. 145, see Chapter 5)
   - Calculate body mass index (p. 146, see Chapter 5)
   - Waist circumference (p. 147, see Chapter 5)
   - Hip circumference (p. 147, see Chapter 5)
   - Calculate waist-hip ratio (p. 147, see Chapter 5)
   - Triceps skin fold thickness and mid–upper arm circumference measurements; calculate MAMC and MAMA (p. 154)

COMMON ABNORMALITIES

OBESITY

Two types of obesity are defined based on the characteristics of the adipose tissue and the area of fat distribution. In exogenous obesity there is an increase in the number of fat cells (i.e., hyperplasia), as much as three to five times normal. The cells may or may not be enlarged. This is the type of obesity most often found in children and women. Excess fat tissue is generally located in the breasts, buttocks, and thighs and is associated with excessive caloric intake, thick skin, pale striae, preservation of muscle strength, and no evidence of osteoporosis. Exogenous obesity is associated with a higher risk of breast cancer (Fig. 6-3, *A*).

In endogenous obesity, the fat cells are greatly enlarged (i.e., hypertrophied). The actual number of cells may be normal or increased. Excess fat tissue is distributed to certain regions of the body, such as the trunk or abdominal area. Men are more likely to have this type of obesity, although it is seen in women as well. This type of obesity is associated with a higher risk of diabetes, heart disease, high blood pressure, and stroke (Fig. 6-3, *B*). Table 6-3 summarizes the classification of obesity and overweight by BMI, waist circumference, and associated disease risk.

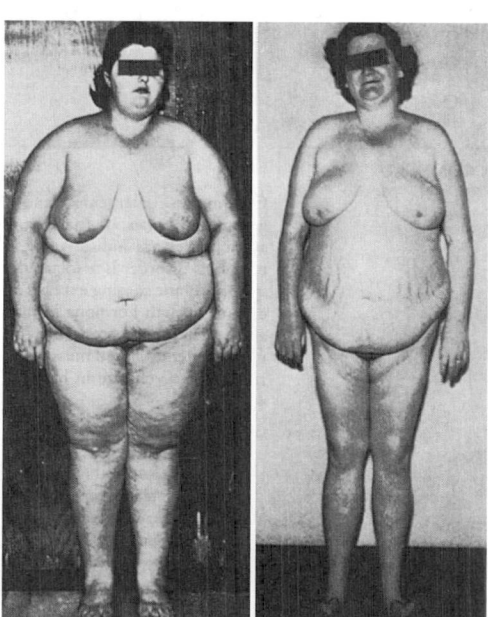

FIGURE 6-3
A, Fat distribution associated with exogenous obesity (female pattern). **B,** Fat distribution associated with endogenous obesity (Cushing syndrome).
From Prior et al, 1981.

ANOREXIA NERVOSA

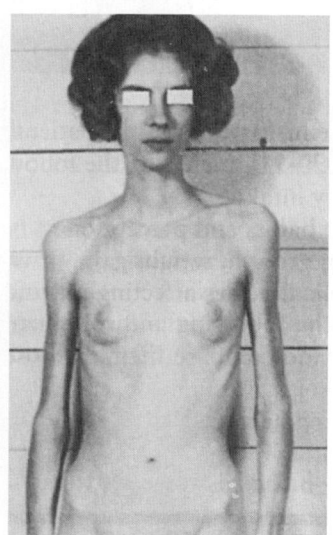

FIGURE 6-4
Wasting associated with anorexia nervosa.
From Ezrein, Godden, Volpe, 1979.

Anorexia nervosa is a psychologic disorder in which the patient has a perceptual distortion of body shape, with a relentless drive for thinness through self-imposed starvation, bizarre food habits, obsessive exercise, and self-induced vomiting or laxative abuse. Adolescent and young adult women, usually from middle and upper class families, are most commonly involved. Males at risk for an eating disorder include those who participate in certain sports (e.g., wrestling, gymnastics, or track), are homosexual, or have problems with addiction and personality disorders. In young adults, the individual usually has a history of being overweight as a child. Anorexia nervosa is characterized by weight loss to 85% or less of expected weight, or failure to attain expected weight. Common signs and symptoms include those of starvation: dry skin, lanugo hair, brittle nails, bloating, constipation, slow heart rate, orthostatic hypotension, stunted growth, amenorrhea, intolerance to cold, carotene (orange) pigmentation, food preoccupation, depression or irritability, decreased libido, and interrupted sleep. Visceral protein levels are adequate. Anemia is not common because serum iron and folate levels are usually at expected levels (Fig. 6-4).

BULIMIA

Bulimia is characterized by binge eating (i.e., the rapid intake of a large amount of food), usually consisting of high-calorie sweets or high-carbohydrate foods. Laxative or diuretic abuse often follows the bingeing episode. If binge eating is followed by self-induced vomiting, it is termed *bulimarexia*. Bulimic individuals, both male and female, are usually in their late teens or early 20s and may have a history of substance (i.e., alcohol or drug) abuse. Generally the bingeing occurs during a time when the individual is trying to lose weight, but the repeated episodes become habitual. Bulimic individuals do not usually become malnourished unless their body weight continues to drop to less than 85% of their expected weight.

NUTRITION
Common Abnormalities

ANEMIAS

Several types of anemias exist; each is dependent on which nutrient is deficient, but all are associated with a lowering of serum hemoglobin and hematocrit levels and a change in the size, appearance, and production of red blood cells. Symptoms of severe anemias include skin pallor, weakness, easy fatigability, headaches, dizziness, sensitivity to cold, paresthesia, cheilosis, glossitis, loss of appetite, and concave fingernails with longitudinal ridging. With increasing severity, tachycardia, palpitations, and shortness of breath may occur. Refer to Table 6-10 to determine type of anemia based on laboratory testing.

TABLE 6-10	**Comparison of Laboratory Test Results for Anemias**			
Test	**Normal Value**	**Iron Deficiency Anemia**	**Folic Acid Deficiency Anemia**	**Vitamin B$_{12}$ Deficiency Anemia**
Hemoglobin, g/100 mL	Men: 14-16 Women: 12-14	Decreased	Decreased	Decreased
Hematocrit, %	Men: 40-54 Women: 37-47	Decreased	Decreased	Decreased
MCV, femtoliters or cubic micrograms/cell	82-92	↓ (<80)	↑ (>92)	↑ (>92)
MCH, picograms/cell	27-31	↓ (<27)	↑ (>35)	↑ (>35)
MCHC, %	32-36	↓ (<32)	Normal	Normal
Serum iron, mcg/100 mL	60-180	Decreased	Increased	Increased
TIBC, mcg/100 mL	250-450	↑ (>350)	Normal	Normal
Transferrin saturation, %	20-55	↓ (<20)	Normal	Normal

MCH, Mean corpuscular hemoglobin; *MCV*, mean corpuscular volume; *MCHC*, mean corpuscular hemoglobin concentration; *TIBC*, total iron binding capacity.

HYPERLIPIDEMIA

High blood cholesterol (240 g/100 mL) is defined as values above which the risk for coronary heart disease (CHD) rises more steeply; this corresponds approximately to the 80th percentile of the adult U.S. population (NHANES III). For patients with blood cholesterol values between 200 and 239 g/100 mL, the appropriate therapy is determined by the presence or absence of other risk factors for CHD and the blood levels of HDL and LDL cholesterol. The Differential Diagnosis box on p. 159 lists the categories of risk and risk factors that modify LDL cholesterol goals.

In children and adolescents, the aim is to identify and treat individuals at the greatest risk of having high blood cholesterol and an increased risk of CHD as adults. This would include selective screening of those with a family history of premature cardiovascular disease or at least one parent with high blood cholesterol. Universal screening of all children is not currently recommended. See the Differential Diagnosis box on p. 159 for the diagnosis of hyperlipidemia in children and adolescents.

DIFFERENTIAL DIAGNOSIS

RISK CATEGORIES AND ASSOCIATED LDL-C GOALS FROM THE ATP (ADULT TREATMENT PANEL) III UPDATE 2004*

Risk Category	Risk Quantification	Factors	LDL-C Goal
High risk	Coronary heart disease (CHD) (10-year risk >20%)† or CHD risk equivalents‡ (10-year risk >20%)	History of myocardial infarction, unstable angina, stable angina, coronary artery procedures (angioplasty or bypass surgery), or Evidence of clinically significant myocardial ischemia. Clinical manifestations of noncoronary forms of atherosclerotic disease (peripheral arterial disease, abdominal aortic aneurysm, and carotid artery disease [transient ischemic attacks or stroke of carotid origin or >50% obstruction of a carotid artery]), diabetes 2+ risk factors with 10-year risk for hard CHD§ >20%.	<100 mg/dL (optional goals: <70 mg/dL) <100 mg/dL (optional goals: <70 mg/dL)
Moderately high risk	2+ risk factors (10-year risk 10%-20%)	Cigarette smoking Hypertension (BP >140/90 mm Hg or on antihypertensive medication)	<130 mg/dL (optional goal < 100 mg/dL)
Moderate risk	2+ risk factors (10-year risk <10%)	Low HDL cholesterol (<40 mg/dL)	<130 mg/dL
Low risk	0 to 1 risk factors	Family history of premature CHD (CHD in male first-degree relative <55 years of age; CHD in female first-degree relative <65 years of age) Age (men >45 years; women >55 years)	<160 mg/dL

Modified from Grundy et al, 2004

*HDL cholesterol > 60 mg/dL counts as a negative risk factor; its presence removes one risk factor from the total count.

†Electronic 10-year risk calculators are available at http://www.nhlbi.nih.gov/guidelines/cholesterol.

‡In ATP III diabetes is regarded as a CHD risk equivalent.

§Hard CHD = Myocardial infarction + CHD deaths.

DIFFERENTIAL DIAGNOSIS

CLASSIFICATION OF TOTAL AND LDL CHOLESTEROL LEVELS IN CHILDREN AND ADOLESCENTS FROM FAMILIES WITH HYPERCHOLESTEROLEMIA OR PREMATURE CARDIOVASCULAR DISEASE

Category	Total Cholesterol	LDL Cholesterol
Acceptable	<170 mg/100 mL	<110 mg/100 mL
Borderline	170-199 mg/100 mL	110-129 mg/100 mL
High	≥200 mg/100 mL	≥130 mg/100 mL

From National Cholesterol Education Program Coordinating Committee, 1991.

STAYING WELL

THERAPEUTIC LIFESTYLE CHANGES

ATP III recommends a multifaceted lifestyle approach to reduce risk for CHD. This approach is designated *therapeutic lifestyle changes (TLC)*. Its essential features are the following:

- Reduced intake of saturated fats (<7% of total calories) and cholesterol (<200 mg per day) (see nutrient composition of the TLC Diet, below)
- Therapeutic options for enhancing LDL lowering such as plant stanols/sterols (2 g/day) and increased viscous (soluble) fiber (10 to 25 g/day)
- Weight reduction
- Increased physical activity

Nutrient Composition of the TLC Diet

Nutrient	Recommended Intake
Saturated fat*	Less than 7% of total calories
Polyunsaturated fat	Up to 10% of total calories
Monounsaturated fat	Up to 20% of total calories
Total fat	25%-35% of total calories
Carbohydrate†	50%-60% of total calories
Fiber	20-30 g/day
Protein	Approximately 15% of total calories
Cholesterol	Less than 200 mg/day
Total calories (energy)‡	Balance energy intake and expenditure to maintain desirable body weight/prevent weight gain

From *ATP III, JAMA 2001*.

*Trans fatty acids are another LDL-raising fat that should be kept at a low intake.

†Carbohydrate should be derived predominantly from foods rich in complex carbohydrates including grains, especially whole grains, fruits, and vegetables.

‡Daily energy expenditure should include at least moderate physical activity (contributing approximately 200 Kcal per day).

STAYING WELL

DIETARY GUIDELINES FOR AMERICANS 2005

Dietary Guidelines for Americans is published jointly every 5 years by the Department of Health and Human Services (HHS) and the Department of Agriculture (USDA). The guidelines provide evidence-based advice to promote health and to reduce risk for major chronic diseases through diet and physical activity. The recommendations are targeted to the general public older than 2 years of age who are living in the United States, and they are intended as a guide for health care providers, nutritionists, and nutrition educators as well as policy makers. The *Dietary Guidelines for Americans 2005* contains additional recommendations for specific populations. The full document is available at http://www.healthierus.gov/dietaryguidelines.

ELECTRONIC RESOURCES

For Weblinks and additional resources, go to   evolve

http://evolve.elsevier.com/Seidel

or to the Companion CD-ROM.

ASSESSMENT OF PAIN

CLINICAL PEARL

An "Ouch" Trial

Pain can do odd things. Try this: Put a very small pebble in your shoe when you dress in the morning. Walk around with it all day. By night, if you can last that long, you will have an assortment of aches and pains from head to toe. There is nothing that goes on in one part of the body that does not have some impact on the whole body and mind. "The head bone is connected to the neck bone" and so on.

Pain is a common, uncomfortable sensation and emotional experience associated with actual or potential tissue damage. Acute pain is sudden and of short duration, and it is usually associated with surgery, injury, or an acute illness episode. Chronic pain is persistent, lasting many weeks and even many months or longer, and is usually associated with a prolonged disease process.

Persons have individualized responses to pain because it is a physiologic, behavioral, and emotional phenomenon. The threshold at which pain is perceived, and the tolerance level for pain, vary widely among individuals. Because of the subjective nature of pain, assessment is based mostly on history and patient responses to various scales that evaluate pain intensity and quality. The ubiquitous nature of pain and its universality and frequency as a distress signal suggest that it be referred to as the fifth vital sign. That is an appropriate reminder. Pain, however, should have status beyond temperature, pulse, respiration, and blood pressure. It should always be a compelling concern and it is the patient who should decide whether the pain is at an unacceptable level. There is no universal standard.

When the chief complaint is pain, the location and related symptoms may assist in the diagnosis of a patient's condition. If the pain is related to a diagnosed condition (e.g., trauma, surgery, or cancer), assessment of its character and intensity is necessary for pain control.

Unfortunately, control of pain is often poor because there is inadequate determination of the intensity; uncertainty about the etiologic factors; and, at times, misplaced concern about the potential for addiction, tolerance, or other side effects relative to medications for pain. Patients, as well as health professionals, share many of these concerns, and if they are worried about this, they may not fully express or at times even admit the intensity of discomfort they are experiencing. This often strong possibility requires direct inquiry about the possible presence of pain and its intensity and character. Remember that there may be more than one cause of pain.

AN IMPORTANT REMINDER

The Joint Commission on Accreditation of Healthcare Organizations (JCAHO) requires that pain be assessed in all patients and that the assessment be conscientiously recorded. They must be asked on admission to a hospital or other health care facility if they have pain or a persistent pain problem. There must then be, for each patient, consistent attention and repeated assessment whether or not there has been an initial complaint. Prompt treatment of reported pain must be assured and the intensity repeatedly recorded to follow its course and to validate relief.

ANATOMY AND PHYSIOLOGY

Peripheral pain receptors transmit sensation to the spinal cord through sensory nerve fibers. Sensory fibers are specialized for rapidly transmitted, sharp, well-localized pain. For more slowly transmitted, dull, burning, diffusely localized pain, the sensory nerve cell bodies are located in the dorsal root ganglia.

If the pain sensation is not blocked by physiologically produced interceptors, opioids, or stimulation, it is relayed from the spinal cord to the brain through the spinothalamic and spinoreticular nerve pathways. Emotions, cultural background, sleep deprivation, previous pain experience, and age are among those factors that have an impact on the perception and interpretation of pain.

Neonates feel pain. The nervous system is adequately developed for pain perception by at least 26 weeks of gestation and probably sooner. Needle-sticks and other greater or lesser injuries evoke responses indicating pain with demonstrable specific behaviors and with autonomic, hormonal, and metabolic signs of stress and distress. Berde and Sethna (2002) and Taddio and colleagues (1997) also remind us that infant boys circumcised without analgesia show greater distress later during their subsequent routine immunizations than do those who had the procedure with a topical local anesthetic. We cannot make too much of such findings until further studies are done, but it is clear that newborns, along with everyone else, do feel pain and deserve attention to their pain and relief from it.

REVIEW OF RELATED HISTORY

PRESENT PROBLEM

+ Onset: date of onset, sudden or slow, time of day, duration, variation, rhythm (constant or intermittent)
+ Quality: throbbing, shooting, stabbing, sharp, cramping, gnawing, hot or burning, aching, heavy, tender, splitting, tiring or exhausting, sickening, fear producing, punishing or cruel
+ Intensity: Ranges from slight to severe using one of the pain scales we suggest, if possible
+ Precipitating factors: causes of increases or decreases in pain
+ Location: Where is the pain? Can the patient point a finger to it? Does it travel or radiate?
+ Effect of pain on daily activities: limitation of activity, interruption of sleep, increased need for rest periods, change in appetite
+ Effect of pain on psyche: change in mood or social interactions, poor concentration, can think only about pain; irritability
+ Pain control measures: distraction, relaxation, heat, electrical stimulation
+ Medications: opioids, anxiolytics, nonsteroidal antiinflammatories; nonprescription medication

PERSONAL AND SOCIAL HISTORY

+ Previous experiences with pain and its effect; typical coping strategies for pain control
+ Family's concerns and cultural beliefs about pain: expect or tolerate pain in certain situations
+ Attitude toward the use of opioids, anxiolytics, and other pain medications for pain control; fear of addiction
+ Current or past use of illicit substances

CHILDREN

- Word(s) the child uses for pain, such as "ouch" or "hurt"
- The child's response when suddenly hurt (e.g., falling down)
- The child's response with longer lasting pain (e.g., an earache)
- How the child or parent rates pain

OLDER ADULTS

- Older adults often use "aching," "cramping," or "sore" to describe pain.
- Older adults may minimize pain, saying "it's just pain" even if it is severe.
- Older adults, who are often beset with multiple complaints, may accept pain as "natural" and not report it. They should be asked about their pain routinely.
- Dementia occurs in as many as 5 in 10 patients older than 85 years of age and delirium occurs in 14% to 18% of older adult patients hospitalized for illness. That makes it difficult to assess pain in many. Nevertheless, the cognitively impaired at any age may well be able to respond to simple questioning and may differentiate the usual pain from the worst. They, too, should be asked, best in the present tense, because recollection of past pain is often not readily achieved (Herr, 2002).

PREGNANT WOMEN

Investigators Melzack, Taenzer, Feldman and Kinch used the McGill Pain Questionnaire to evaluate pain in labor of 87 nulliparous and 54 parous patients. The pain rating index scores compared labor pain with different kinds of pain. Fifty-nine percent of nulliparous and 43% of parous women in labor described their pain as more severe that those patients suffering back and cancer pain. Greater that 50% of all laboring women described their pain as sharp, cramping, and intense and more than 33% said it was aching, throbbing, stabbing, shooting, heavy, and exhaustive. Twenty-five percent of nulliparous and 9% of parous women described the pain as horrible or excruciating. Childbirth training classes seemed to make little difference in pain perception. Better predictors were socioeconomic status and prior menstrual history (Melzack et al, 1981; Gabbe et al, 2002).

During pregnancy:

- Camping or pressure may be signs of Braxton Hicks contractions or preterm labor contractions.
- Epigastric pain may occur from the pressure of the gravid uterus.
- Round ligament pain may occur from the stretching of the ligaments by the enlarging uterus.
- Pressure on the bladder may occur from the weight of the enlarging uterus.

During labor:

- Pain may be related to dilatation of the cervix, uterine contractions, and stretching of the pelvic floor, vagina, and perineum.

EXAMINATION AND FINDINGS

Throughout your examination of the patient, be alert to signs of pain, which may include any combination on the following list. When communication is a problem, as with the cognitively impaired, young children, and older adults, have a family member describe known cues to the patient's expression of pain. It is often likely that an individual patient will repeat a behavior pattern from one episode of pain to the next.

- Guarding, protective behavior, hands over painful area, distorted posture, irritability
- Facial mask of pain: lackluster eyes, "beaten look," wrinkled forehead, tightly closed or opened eyes, fixed or scattered movement, grimace or other distorted expression, a sad or frightened look
- Vocalizations: grunting, groaning, crying, talkative patient becomes quiet
- Body movements such as head rocking, pacing, or rubbing; an inability to keep the hands still

- Changes in vital signs: blood pressure, pulse, respiratory rate and depth, with acute exacerbations of pain; fewer changes in vital signs found in cases of chronic pain
- Pallor and diaphoresis
- Pupil dilation
- Dry mouth
- Decreased attention span, greater confusion

There are a number of classic pain patterns that provide valuable clues to underlying conditions:

- Bone and soft tissue pain may be tender, deep, and aching.
- Heavy, throbbing, and aching pain may be associated with a tumor pressing on a cavity.
- Burning, shocklike pain may indicate nerve tissue damage.
- A clenched fist over the chest with diaphoresis and grimacing is the classic picture of myocardial infarction. Even a mild pain can require immediate attention in this regard.
- Cramping spasms may define visceral or colic pain

PAIN ASSESSMENT SCALES

A variety of scales and instruments have been developed to obtain and measure a patient's perception of pain intensity and quality; only a sample is presented here (Figs. 7-1 through 7-5). Very few of the instruments widely used include the patient's emotional response to pain. Remember that the patient's perception may not compare with expected pain intensity identified by other individuals. It is the patient's perception, however, that should be the "gold standard," or the controlling variable. The use of scales also permits the very important day-to-day documentation of the response to therapy.

FIGURE 7-1
Descriptive Pain Intensity Scale.

None   Slight   Mild   Moderate   Severe   Worst Pain

0   1   2   3   4   5   6   7   8   9   10

FIGURE 7-2
Numeric Pain Intensity Scale.

No Pain   Moderate Pain   Worst Pain

FIGURE 7-3
Visual Analogic Scale.

No Pain   Worst Pain

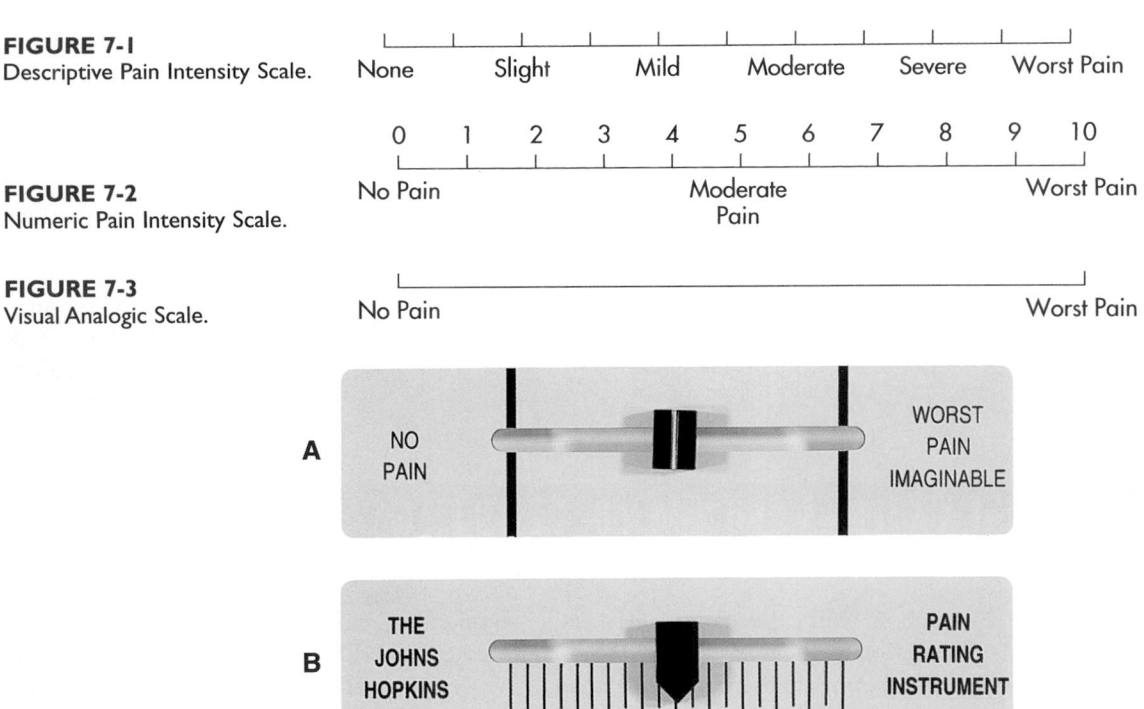

A NO PAIN   WORST PAIN IMAGINABLE

B THE JOHNS HOPKINS   10 9 8 7 6 5 4 3 2 1 0   PAIN RATING INSTRUMENT

FIGURE 7-4
Self-contained, portable, pain-rating instrument that can provide an immediate assessment of pain. It is a 5 cm × 20 cm plastic visual analogue scale with a sliding marker that moves within a 10-cm groove. The side facing the patient (**A**) resembles a traditional visual analogue scale, whereas the opposite side (**B**) is marked in centimeters to quantify pain intensity. The scale has been shown to be a valid tool to measure pain intensity. It facilitates the documentation of pain and the monitoring of pain relief interventions.
From Grossman et al, 1992.

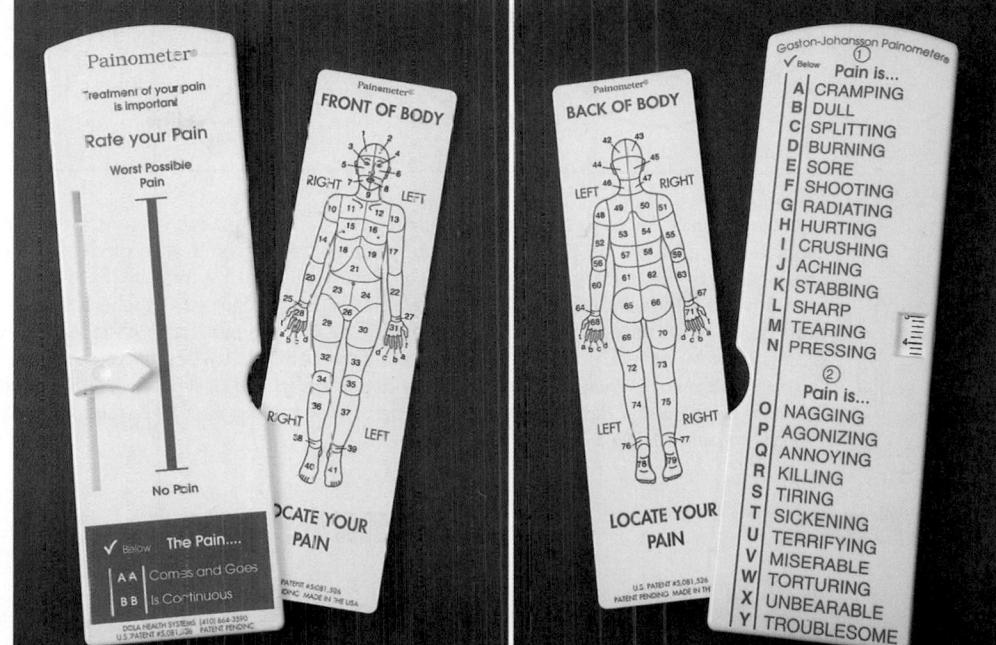

FIGURE 7-5
The "pain-o-meter." A multidimensional measure of pain, allowing a measure of intensity and quality and an opportunity for localization. It is the first handheld instrument that meets the standards of the Joint Commission for Accreditation of Healthcare Organizations (JCAHO).
Courtesy of Dr. Fannie Gaston-Johansson, School of Nursing, The Johns Hopkins University, Baltimore.

Introducing the patient to the appropriate use of any scale requires a patient and clear explanation of the purposes of the scale and the meanings of the numbers or figures on the scale. It helps, too, to learn the patient's customary terminology for different kinds of pain (e.g., "aching," "burning," "stabbing," "sharp," or "dull"). A dry run considering a past experience with pain (e.g., a headache or a particular trauma) might precede the scaling of the present hurt. The young, the older adult, and the cognitively impaired will benefit from a scale in which the figures are large and easily discerned.

It is helpful to pick from among the several available scales a few that are most comfortable for you and your colleagues. Their consistent use will result in consistent interpretation. If you have more than one scale available, ask the patient to pick the scale he or she prefers to use. Document the selection and use it in all of that patient's subsequent assessments.

When assessing pain, remember that intensity may vary in different sites. Intensity may also vary with routine activity such as moving, coughing, or deep breathing. Be sure to link pain intensity reported with location and activity. Use body drawings to have the patient identify the sites. Be sure to reassess regularly the degree of pain until and even after the problem is solved.

CHILDREN

The history and physical examination provides much information about a child's pain. Some children as young as 3 years of age have adequate communication skills to respond to pediatric pain assessment scales. Those who do not yet have such skills can be evaluated the same way as an infant would (see the next section). Be sure a child understands concepts of higher/lower and more/less in order to use the scales. Children do best when given an opportunity to practice the chosen scale using selected examples of past painful experiences (e.g., a finger prick, earache, or skinned knee). You and your colleagues may differ in the way you approach children. The effort should be made to be as consistent as possible so that there might be a degree of reliability from one assessment to another when more than one caregiver is involved.

The Wong/Baker Faces Rating Scale (Fig. 7-6) and the Oucher Scale (Figs. 7-7, 7-8, and 7-9) are examples of pain scales that are reliable and valid for children. Pain rating scales that use facial expressions are not designed for comparison of the child's facial expression with those on the scale. The face should be selected that the child feels best represents the amount of pain being felt at that particular time.

Using Figs. 7-7, 7-8, and 7-9, ask the child to select the face that fits his or her level of pain. Use the version that best fits the child's cultural identity (e.g., white, black, or Hispanic).

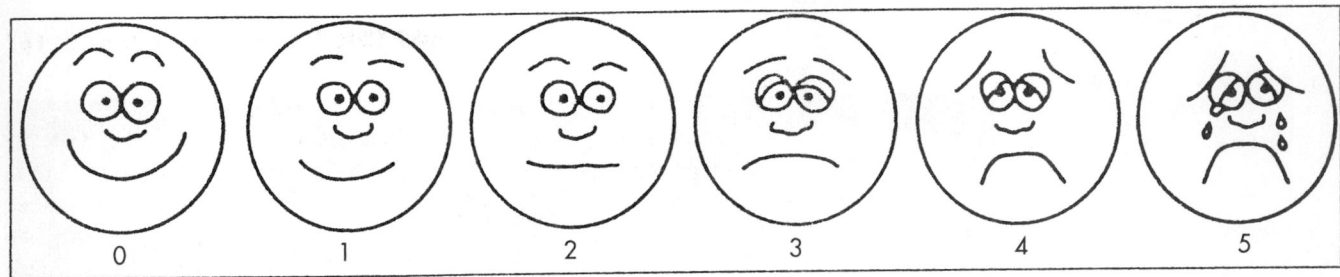

FIGURE 7-6

The Wong/Baker Faces Rating Scale. Explain to the patient that each face is for a person who feels happy because he has no pain (hurt) or sad because he has some or a lot of pain. Face 0 is very happy because the person doesn't hurt at all. Face 1 hurts just a little bit. Face 2 hurts a little more. Face 3 hurts a little more. Face 4 hurts a whole lot. Face 5 hurts as much as you can imagine, although you don't have to be crying to feel this bad. Ask the patient to choose the face that best describes how he or she is feeling. Recommended for persons 3 years and older.

Originally published in Whaley L, Wong D: Nursing care of infants and children, ed 3, St Louis, 1987, Mosby. Reprinted by permission. Research reported in Wong D, Backer C: Pain in children: comparison of assessment scales, Pediatric Nursing 14(1):9-17, 1988.

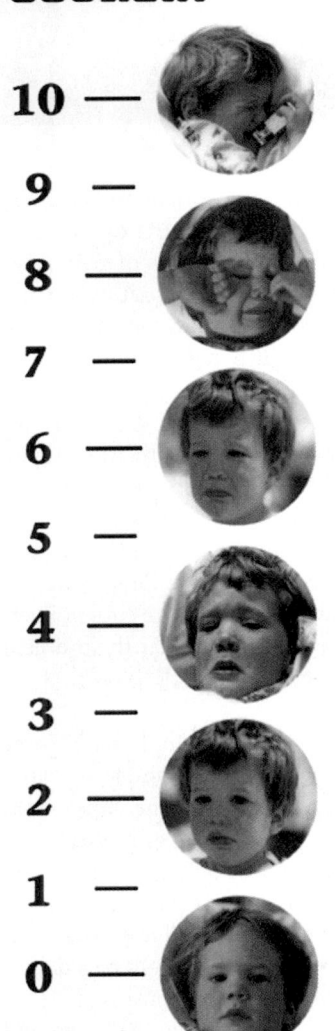

http://www.oucher.org

FIGURE 7-7

Caucasian version of the Oucher.

Developed and copyrighted in 1983 by Judith E. Beyer, PhD, RN (University of Missouri-Kansas City School of Nursing).

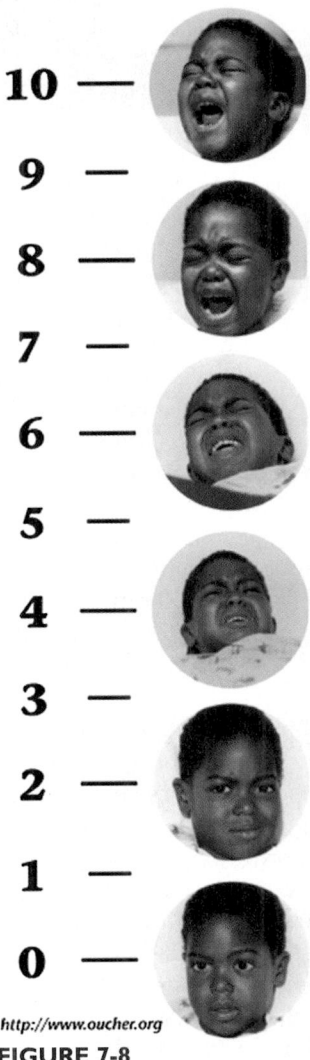

http://www.oucher.org

FIGURE 7-8

African-American version of the Oucher.

Developed and copyrighted in 1990 by Mary J. Denyes, PhD, RN (Wayne State University), and Antonia M. Villarruel, PhD, RN (University of Michigan). Cornelia P. Porter, PhD, RN, and Charlotta Marshall, RN, MSN, contributed to the development of this scale.

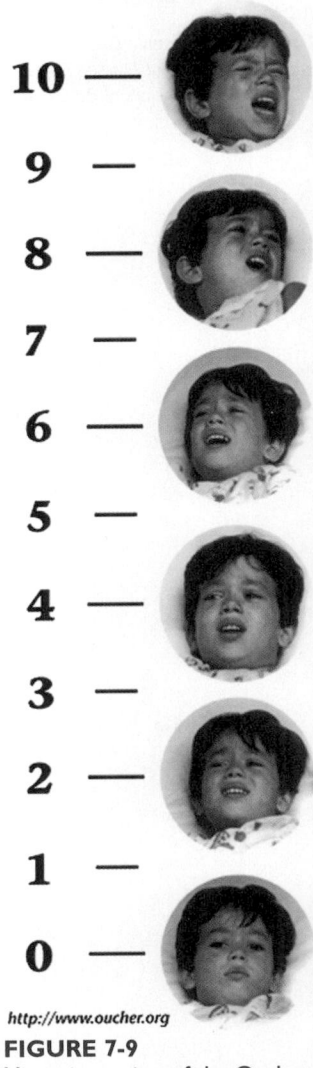

http://www.oucher.org

FIGURE 7-9

Hispanic version of the Oucher.

Developed and copyrighted in 1990 by Antonia M. Villarruel, PhD, RN (University of Michigan) and Mary J. Denyes, PhD, RN (Wayne State University).

INFANTS

Pain scales can also be used for neonates and infants. Stevens and colleagues developed the Premature Infant Pain Profile (PIPP) in 1996. It is best validated for premature infants, but the observations are also appropriate for judging pain in full-term neonates and young infants. Similarly, the Neonatal Infant Pain Scale (NIPS) developed by Lawrence and others requires careful observation of the infant. You can readily assess the cry (often high-pitched and shrill), sleep patterns (disturbed, fussy, even thrashing), facial expressions (tightly closed eyes, wide open mouth, and wrinkled brow), feeding and sucking, overall tone, and consolability. A crying, hypertonic, sleepless baby who is unable to suck and unable to be consoled is hurting. Changes can be observed and documented. The Individualized Numeric Rating Scale (INRS) initiated by Solodiuk and Curley for use with nonverbal children appeals to us the most. It recognizes the necessary observations and presents them in a manner that makes recording and follow-up easy (Fig. 7-10). In our view, the INRS is a good guide to assessing pain in the nonverbal or otherwise compromised patient at any age and in a variety of circumstances, whether it is a neurologic or cognitive handicap, an intubation, or a serious injury. Parents and those familiar with the patient can be enlisted to complement your observations, using the scale suggested in Fig. 7-10 (Stevens et al, 1996; Lawrence et al, 1993).

CLINICAL PEARL

Assess the Patient, Not the Age

The severely cognitively impaired at any age, unable to respond in the expected manner, may be assessed for pain as with the newborn, infant, or young child.

OLDER ADULTS

Pain scales are certainly appropriate for use with older adults. Battista suggests using a Geriatric Pain Assessment Tool developed by Herr and colleagues (Fig. 7-11). It combines aspects of the scales we have already demonstrated and provides a suggested chart for recording your findings.

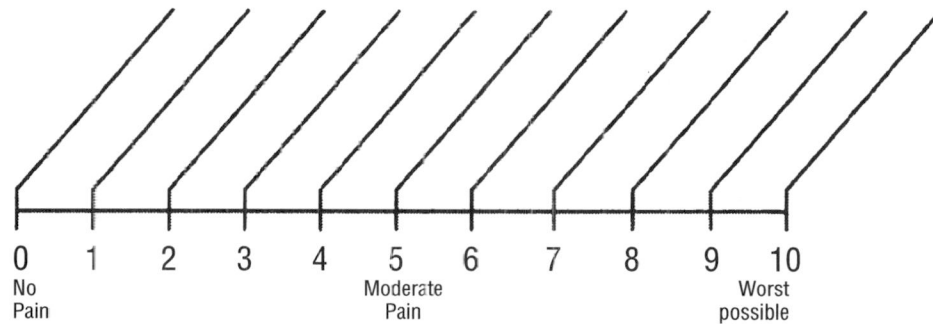

FIGURE 7-10
The Individualized Numeric Rating Scale (INRS).
From Solodiuk and Curley, 2003.

0 1 2 3 4 5 6 7 8 9 10
No Pain   Moderate Pain   Worst possible

STAYING WELL

THINK SUGAR WATER!!

One way to keep well is to be freed of the prospect of pain. This is true for people of any age and it is certainly true of newborns. Venipuncture hurts and babies let us know by crying. Some people believe that a local anesthetic cream rubbed on the area of the procedure might relieve the pain. Others think that orally administered sweet-tasting solutions reduce signs of pain during painful procedures. Gradin and colleagues compared the two approaches in a randomized, controlled, double-blind study in which 30% glucose water was preferred over the anesthetic cream. Carbajal and colleagues matched 30% glucose water against a pacifier to ease the pain of subcutaneous injections in very preterm neonates, and the glucose water was preferred again. Sugar water—cheap, tasty, inexpensive, and noninvasive—prevents pain and contributes to wellness!

Gradin et al, 2002; Carbajal et al, 2002.

ASSESSMENT OF PAIN
Examination and Findings

Geriatric Pain Assessment Tool

Date:_____

Medical Record Number:_____

Patient's Name:_____

Problem List:_____

Medications:_____

_____

_____

_____

_____

PAIN DESCRIPTION:

Pattern: Constant   Intermittent

Duration:_____

Location:_____

Character:

Piercing/Stabbing   Burning   Stinging

Radiating   Shooting   Tingling

Pain Intensity:

0   1   2   3   4   5   6   7   8   9   10

None   Moderate   Severe

Worst Pain in Last 24 Hours:

0   1   2   3   4   5   6   7   8   9   10

None   Moderate   Severe

Other Descriptors:_____

_____

_____

Exacerbating Factors:_____

_____

Relieving Factors:_____

_____

Other Assessments or Comments:_____

_____

Most Likely Cause of Pain:_____

Plans:_____

_____

Mood:_____

Depression Screening Score:_____

Gait and Balance Score:_____

Impaired Activities:_____

_____

Sleep Quality:_____

Bowel Habits:_____

Adapted from Stein W, Ferrell BA. Pain in the nursing home. *Clinics in Geriatric Med.* 1996;12:29-38.

FIGURE 7-11
Geriatric Pain Assessment Tool.
From Battista, 2002.

ELECTRONIC RESOURCES

For Weblinks and additional resources, go to   **evolve**

http://evolve.elsevier.com/Seidel

or to the Companion CD-ROM.

SKIN, HAIR, AND NAILS

ANATOMY AND PHYSIOLOGY

Skin provides an elastic, rugged, self-regenerating, protective covering for the body. However, it has another important function: the skin and its appendages are our primary physical presentation to the world.

The skin is a stratified structure composed of several functionally related layers. Fig. 8-1 shows the main structural components and their approximate spatial relationships. The anatomy of the skin varies somewhat from one part of the body to another.

Skin structure and physiologic processes perform the following integral functions:

- Protect against microbial and foreign substance invasion and minor physical trauma
- Retard body fluid loss by providing a mechanical barrier
- Regulate body temperature through radiation, conduction, convection, and evaporation
- Provide sensory perception via free nerve endings and specialized receptors
- Produce vitamin D from precursors in the skin
- Contribute to blood pressure regulation through constriction of skin blood vessels
- Repair surface wounds by exaggerating the normal process of cell replacement
- Excrete sweat, urea, and lactic acid
- Express emotions

EPIDERMIS

The epidermis, the outermost portion of the skin, consists of two major layers: the stratum corneum, which protects the body against harmful environmental substances and restricts water loss, and the cellular stratum, in which the keratin cells are synthesized. The basement membrane lies beneath the cellular stratum and connects the epidermis to the dermis. The epidermis is avascular and depends on the underlying dermis for its nutrition.

The stratum corneum consists of closely packed, dead squamous cells that contain the waterproofing protein keratin; these form the protective barrier of the skin. These keratin cells are formed in the deepest sublayer of the cellular stratum, the stratum germinativum. The keratinocytes mature as they make their way to the surface through the stratum spinosum and stratum granulosum to replace the cells in the stratum corneum. The stratum germinativum also contains melanocytes, the cells that synthesize melanin, which gives the skin its color. An

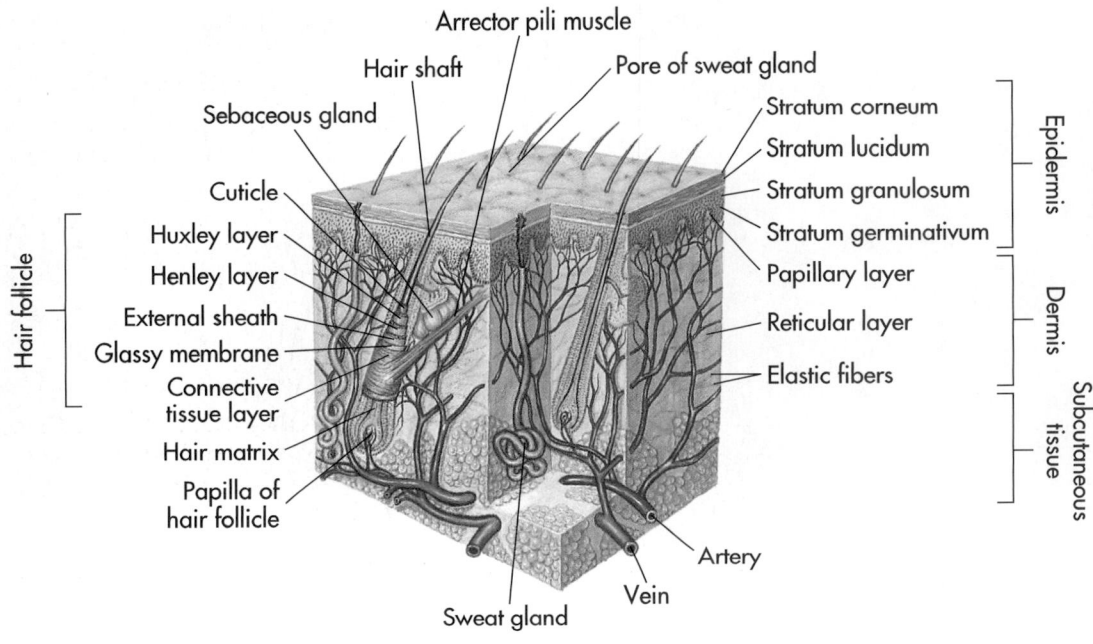

FIGURE 8-1
Anatomic structures of the skin.

additional sublayer of the cellular stratum, the stratum lucidum, is present only in the thicker skin of the palms and soles and lies just below the stratum corneum.

DERMIS

The dermis is the richly vascular connective tissue layer of the skin that supports and separates the epidermis from the cutaneous adipose tissue. Upward projecting papillae penetrate the epidermis and provide nourishment for the living epidermal cells. Elastin, collagen, and reticulum fibers provide resilience, strength, and stability. Sensory nerve fibers located in the dermis form a complex network to provide sensations of pain, touch, and temperature. The dermis also contains autonomic motor nerves that innervate blood vessels, glands, and the arrectores pilorum muscles.

HYPODERMIS

The dermis is connected to underlying organs by the hypodermis, a subcutaneous layer that consists of loose connective tissue filled with fatty cells. This adipose layer generates heat and provides insulation, shock absorption, and a reserve of calories.

APPENDAGES

The epidermis invaginates into the dermis at myriad points and forms the following appendages: eccrine sweat glands, apocrine sweat glands, sebaceous glands, hair, and nails.

The eccrine sweat glands open directly onto the surface of the skin and regulate body temperature through water secretion. The glands are distributed throughout the body except at the lip margins, eardrums, nail beds, inner surface of the prepuce, and the glans penis.

The apocrine glands are specialized structures found only in the axillae, nipples, areolae, anogenital area, eyelids, and external ears. These glands are larger and located more deeply than the eccrine glands. In response to emotional stimuli, the glands secrete a white fluid containing protein, carbohydrate, and other substances. Secretions from these glands are odorless. Bacterial decomposition of apocrine sweat produces a characteristic adult body odor in blacks and whites.

The sebaceous glands secrete sebum, a lipid-rich substance that keeps the skin and hair from drying out. Secretory activity, which is stimulated by sex hormones (primarily testosterone), varies according to hormonal levels throughout the life span.

Hair is formed by epidermal cells that invaginate into the dermal layers. Hair consists of a root, a shaft, and a follicle (i.e., the root and its covering). The papilla, a loop of capillaries at the base of the follicle, supplies nourishment for growth. Melanocytes in the shaft provide its color. Adults have two kinds of hair: vellus and terminal. Vellus hair is short, fine, soft, and nonpigmented. Terminal hair is coarser, longer, thicker, and usually pigmented. Each hair goes through cyclic changes: anagen (growth), catagen (atrophy), and telogen (rest), after which the hair is shed. Males and females have about the same number of hair follicles that are stimulated to differential growth by hormones.

The nails are epidermal cells converted to hard plates of keratin. The highly vascular nail bed lies beneath the plate, giving the nail its pink color. The white crescent-shaped area extending beyond the proximal nail fold marks the end of the nail matrix, the site of nail growth. The stratum corneum layer of skin covering the nail root is the cuticle, or eponychium, which pushes up and over the lower part of the nail body. The paronychium is the soft tissue surrounding the nail border. Fig. 8-2 shows the structures of the nail.

INFANTS AND CHILDREN

The skin of infants and children appears smoother than that of adults, partly because of the relative absence of coarse terminal hair and partly because the skin has not been subjected to years of exposure to the elements. Desquamation of the stratum corneum may be present at birth or very shortly after. The degree of desquamation varies from mild flakiness to shedding of large sheets of cornified epidermis. Vernix caseosa, a mixture of sebum and cornified epidermis, covers the infant's body at birth. The subcutaneous fat layer is poorly developed in newborns, predisposing them to hypothermia. The newborn's body, particularly the shoulders and back, is also covered with fine, silky hair called lanugo. This hair is shed within 10 to 14 days. Some newborns are bald, whereas others have a large amount of head hair. Either way, most of the hair is shed by about 2 to 3 months of age, to be replaced by more permanent hair with a new texture and often a different color.

The eccrine sweat glands begin to function after the first month of life. Apocrine function has not yet begun, giving the skin a less oily texture and resulting in characteristic inoffensive perspiration.

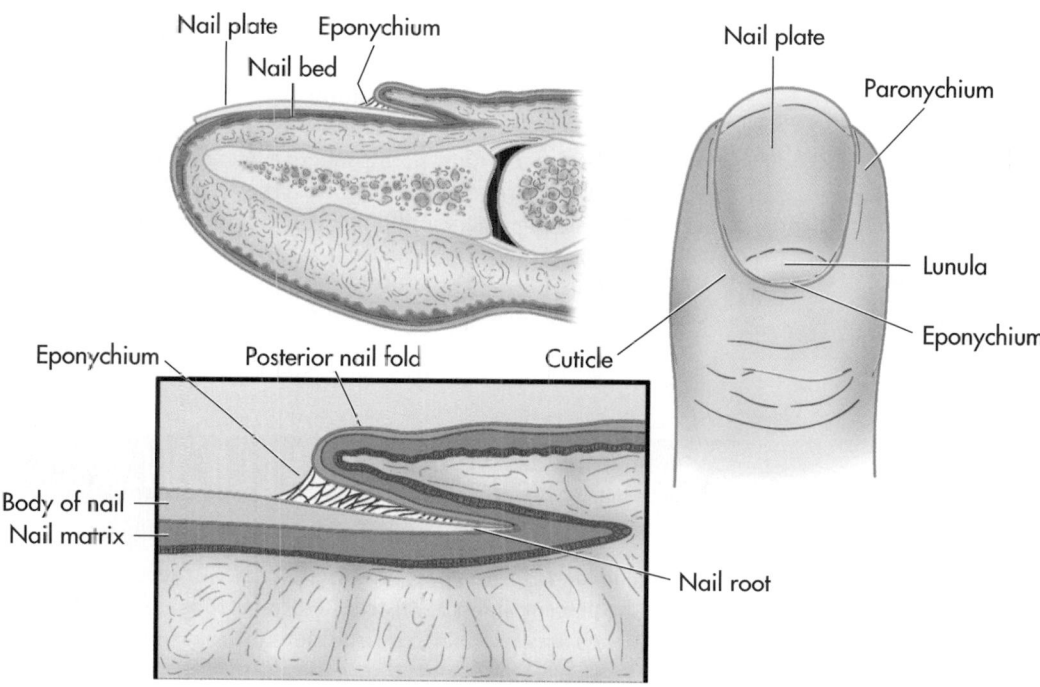

FIGURE 8-2
Anatomic structures of the nail.
Modified from Thompson et al, 1997.

ADOLESCENTS

During adolescence the apocrine glands enlarge and become active, causing increased axillary sweating and sometimes body odor. Sebaceous glands increase sebum production in response to increased hormone levels, primarily androgen, giving the skin an oily appearance and predisposing the individual to acne.

Coarse terminal hair appears in the axillae and pubic areas of both female and male adolescents and on the face of males. Hair production is one response to changing androgen levels. Refer to Chapter 5 for a more thorough discussion of maturational changes during adolescence.

PREGNANT WOMEN

Increased blood flow to the skin, especially that of the hands and feet, results from peripheral vasodilation and increased numbers of capillaries. Acceleration of sweat and sebaceous gland activity occurs. Both processes assist in dissipating the excess heat caused by the increased metabolism during pregnancy. Vascular spiders and hemangiomas that are present may increase in size.

The skin thickens, and fat is deposited in the subdermal layers. Because of increased fragility of connective tissues, separation may occur with stretching. Most (about 90%) pregnant women have some degree of skin darkening beginning in early pregnancy. This increased pigmentation is seen on the face, nipples, areolae, axillae, vulva, perianal skin and umbilicus. During pregnancy, some nevi may grow and new nevi may appear.

OLDER ADULTS

Sebaceous and sweat gland activity decreases in older adults, and as a result the skin becomes drier with less perspiration produced. The epidermis begins to thin and flatten, taking on the look of parchment as the vascularity of the dermis decreases. Epidermal permeability is increased, reducing the efficiency of the barrier function of the stratum corneum.

The dermis becomes less elastic, loses collagen and elastic fibers, and shrinks, causing the epidermis to fold and assume a wrinkled appearance. A lifetime of exposure to the sun also predisposes the skin to wrinkling. Wrinkling is less marked in individuals with black and yellow skins and in those who are obese.

Subcutaneous tissue also decreases, particularly in the extremities, giving joints and bony prominences a sharp, angular appearance. The hollows in the thoracic, axillary, and supraclavicular regions deepen.

Gray hair results from a decrease in the number of functioning melanocytes. The hair of whites turns gray before the hair of blacks and Asians does. Axillary and pubic hair production declines because of reduced hormonal functioning. The density and rate of scalp hair growth (anagen phrase) declines with age. The size of hair follicles also changes, and terminal scalp hair progressively transitions into vellus hair, causing age-associated baldness in both men and women. The opposite transition, from vellus to terminal, occurs in the hair of the nares and on the tragus of men's ears. Women produce increased coarse facial hair because of higher androgen/estrogen ratios. Both genders experience overall loss of hair from the trunk and extremities. Peripheral extremity hair loss may also occur when peripheral vascular disease is present. The loss of axillary and pubic hair results from diminished androgen production.

Nail growth slows because of decreased peripheral circulation. The nails, particularly the toenails, become thicker, brittle, hard, and yellowish. They develop longitudinal ridges and are prone to splitting into layers.

REVIEW OF RELATED HISTORY

For each of the conditions discussed in this section, targeted topics to include in the history of the present illness are listed. Responses to questions about these topics help fully assess the patient's condition and provide clues for focusing the physical examination.

HISTORY OF PRESENT ILLNESS

- Skin
  - Changes in skin: dryness, pruritus, sores, rashes, lumps, color, texture, odor, amount of perspiration; changes in wart or mole; lesion that does not heal or is chronically irritated
  - Temporal sequence: date of initial onset; time sequence of occurrence and development; sudden or gradual onset; date of recurrence, if any
  - Symptoms: itching, pain, exudate, bleeding, color changes, seasonal or climate variations
  - Location: skinfolds, extensor or flexor surfaces, localized or generalized
  - Associated symptoms: presence of systemic disease or high fever, relationship to stress or leisure activities
  - Recent exposure to drugs, environmental or occupational toxins or chemicals, to persons with similar skin condition
  - Apparent cause, patient's perception of cause
  - Travel history: where, when, length of stay, exposure to diseases, contact with travelers
  - What the patient has been doing for the problem, response to treatment, what makes the condition worse or better
  - How the patient is adjusting to the problem
  - Medications: topical or systemic, nonprescription or prescription
- Hair
  - Changes in hair: loss or growth, distribution, texture, color
  - Occurrence: sudden or gradual onset, symmetric or asymmetric pattern, recurrence
  - Associated symptoms: pain, itching, lesions, presence of systemic disease or high fever, recent psychologic or physical stress
  - Exposure to drugs, environmental or occupational toxins or chemicals, commercial hair care chemicals
  - Nutrition: dietary changes, dieting
  - What the patient has been doing for the problem, response to treatment, what makes the problem worse or better
  - How the patient is adjusting to the problem
  - Medications: nonprescription or prescription; drugs or preparations for hair loss (minoxidil, Propecia, dihydrotestosterone [DHT] inhibitors)
- Nails
  - Changes in nails: splitting, breaking, discoloration, ridging, thickening, markings, separation from nail bed
  - Recent history: systemic illness, high fever, trauma, psychologic or physical stress
  - Associated symptoms: pain, swelling, exudate
  - Temporal sequence: sudden or gradual onset, relationship to injury of nail or finger
  - Recent exposure to drugs, environmental or occupational toxins or chemicals; frequent immersion in water
  - What the patient has been doing for the problem, response to treatment, what makes the problem worse or better
  - Medications: nonprescription or prescription

PAST MEDICAL HISTORY

- Skin
  - Previous skin problems: sensitivities, allergic skin reactions, allergic skin disorders (e.g., infantile eczema), lesions, treatment
  - Tolerance to sunlight
  - Diminished or heightened sensitivity to sensory stimuli
  - Cardiac, respiratory, liver, endocrine, or other systemic diseases

◆ Hair
  ◆ Previous hair problems: loss, thinning, unusual growth or distribution, brittleness, breakage, treatment
  ◆ Systemic problems: thyroid or liver disorder, any severe illness, malnutrition, associated skin disorder
◆ Nails
  ◆ Previous nail problems: injury; bacterial, fungal, or viral infection
  ◆ Systemic problems: associated skin disorder; congenital anomalies; respiratory, cardiac, endocrine, hematologic, or other systemic disease

FAMILY HISTORY

◆ Current or past dermatologic diseases or disorders in family members; melanoma; psoriasis; allergic skin disorders; infestations; bacterial, fungal, or viral infections
◆ Allergic hereditary diseases such as asthma or hay fever
◆ Familial hair loss or coloration patterns

PERSONAL AND SOCIAL HISTORY

CLINICAL PEARL

Sunscreen

Surprise! Do you ask if your patients use sunscreens? Keep this in mind when they respond: Those who use sunscreens with a protection factor of 15 or even more will more often get a more significant sunburn than those who do not use or hardly ever use a sunscreen. Why? Those who are users do not use enough; they think they are protected, and stay out in the noonday sun too long. It is necessary to use a lot of sunscreen and to reapply it after being in the water.

◆ Skin care habits: cleansing routine; soaps, oils, lotions, or local applications used; cosmetics; home remedies or preparations used; sun exposure patterns and history; sunburn history; use of sunscreen agents; recent changes in skin care habits
◆ Skin self-examination (Box 8-1)
◆ Hair care habits: cleansing routine, shampoos and rinses used, coloring preparations used, permanents, recent changes in hair care habits
◆ Nail care habits: any difficulty in clipping or trimming nails, instruments used; biting nails
◆ Exposure to environmental or occupational hazards: dyes, chemicals, plants, toxic substances, frequent immersion of hands in water, frequent sun exposure
◆ Recent psychologic or physiologic stress
◆ Use of alcohol
◆ Use of club/recreational drugs

BOX 8-1

PATIENT INSTRUCTIONS FOR SKIN SELF-EXAMINATION

- Always use a good light, positioned to minimize distracting glare. Look for a new growth or any skin change.
- Be aware of the locations and appearance of moles and birthmarks.
- Examine your back and other hard-to-see areas of the body using full-length and handheld mirrors. Ask a friend or relative to help inspect those areas that are difficult to see, such as the scalp and back.
- Begin with your face and scalp using one or more mirrors. Proceed downward, focusing on neck, chest, and torso. Women, check under breasts. With back to the mirror, use hand mirror to inspect back of neck, shoulders, upper arms, back, buttocks, legs. Concentrate especially on areas where dysplastic nevi (those with unexpected changes) are most common—the shoulders and back; and areas where ordinary moles are rarely found—the scalp, breast, and buttocks. Check hands, including nails. In a full-length mirror, examine elbows, arms, underarms. Sitting down, check legs and feet, including soles, heels, nails, and between the toes. Use a hand mirror to examine genitals. See rather than feel any early signs of a mole change. Compare photographs of your moles (if you have them) with the appearance of those same moles on self-examination. Monitor change in size by measuring. It can be simply done with a small ruler or even by comparing them to the size of your thumb or fingernail.
- Consult your health care provider promptly if any pigmented skin spots look like melanoma, if new moles have appeared, or if any existing moles have changed.

INFANTS

- Feeding history: breast or formula, type of formula, what foods introduced and when
- Diaper history: type of diapers used, skin cleansing routines, use of rubber pants, use of washable diapers, and methods of cleaning
- Types of clothing and washing practices: soaps and detergents used, new blanket or clothing
- Bath practices: types of soap, oils, or lotions used
- Dress habits: amount and type of clothing in relation to environmental temperature
- Temperature and humidity of the home environment: air conditioning, heating system (drying or humidified)
- Rubbing head against mattress, rug, furniture, wall

CHILDREN

- Eating habits and types of food including chocolate, candy, soft drinks, bubble gum
- Exposure to communicable diseases
- Allergic disorders: eczema, urticaria, pruritus, hay fever, asthma, other chronic respiratory disorders
- Pets or animal exposure
- Outdoor exposures such as play areas, hiking, camping, picnics
- Skin injury history: frequency of falls, cuts, abrasions; repeated history of unexplained injuries
- Chronic manipulation of hair
- Nail biting

PREGNANT WOMEN

- Weeks of gestation or postpartum
- Hygiene practices
- Exposure to irritants
- Presence of skin problems before pregnancy (e.g., acne may worsen)
- Effects of pregnancy on preexisting conditions (e.g., psoriasis may remit; condylomata acuminata commonly become larger and more numerous)

OLDER ADULTS

- Increased or decreased sensation to touch or the environment
- Generalized chronic itching; exposure to skin irritants, detergents, lotions with high alcohol content, woolen clothing, humidity of environment
- Susceptibility to skin infections
- Healing response: delayed or interrupted
- Frequent falls resulting in multiple cuts or bruises
- History of diabetes mellitus or peripheral vascular disease
- Hair loss history: gradual versus sudden onset, loss pattern (symmetric or asymmetric)

EXAMINATION AND FINDINGS

EQUIPMENT

- Centimeter ruler (flexible, clear)
- Wood's lamp (to view fluorescing lesions)
- Flashlight with transilluminator
- Handheld magnifying lens (optional)

SKIN

Examination of the skin is performed by inspection and palpation. The most important tools are your own eyes and powers of observation. Sometimes, when gross inspection leaves you uncertain, a handheld magnifying glass or episcope may help.

INSPECTION

PHYSICAL VARIATIONS

Pigmentary Demarcation Lines

Individuals with dark skin often show pigmentary demarcation lines. These lines, a normal variation, mark the border between the darker skin of outward facing surfaces and the lighter skin of inward facing surfaces. They are seen on the arms, legs, chest, and back. About 70% of black adults have such lines compared with 11% of whites. Statistics for Asian and Native Americans/American Indians fall between these two figures.

Data from Rampen, 1988; James, Carter, Rodman, 1987.

Skin, Hair, and Nails: Assessing a Mole

Adequate lighting is essential. Daylight provides the best illumination for determining color variations, particularly jaundice. If daylight is unavailable or insufficient, supplement it with overhead fluorescent lighting. Tangential lighting is helpful in assessing contour, but inadequate lighting can result in inadequate assessment.

Although the skin is commonly observed as each part of the body is examined, it is important to make a brief but careful overall visual sweep of the entire body. This "bird's-eye view" gives a good idea of the distribution and extent of any lesions. It also allows you to observe skin symmetry, to detect differences between body areas, and to compare sun-exposed to non–sun-exposed areas. You can also be alert for special conditions that require attention as the examination progresses (Box 8-2).

Adequate exposure of the skin is necessary. It is essential to remove encumbering clothing and to fully remove drapes or coverings as each section of the body is examined. Make sure that the room temperature is comfortable. Look carefully at areas not usually exposed such as the axillae, buttocks, perineum, backs of thighs, and inner upper thighs. Remove shoes and socks to look at the feet. Pay careful attention to intertriginous surfaces, especially in older and bedridden patients. As the examination is completed for each area, the patient should be re-draped or covered. Begin by inspecting the skin and mucous membranes (especially oral) for color and uniform appearance, thickness, symmetry, hygiene, and the presence of any lesions.

Skin thickness varies over the body, with the thinnest skin on the eyelids and the thickest at areas of pressure or rubbing, most notably the soles, palms, and elbows. Note callusing on the hands or feet.

The range of expected skin color varies from dark brown to light tan with pink or yellow overtones. Although color should assume an overall uniformity, there may be sun-darkened areas and darker skin around knees and elbows. Knuckles may be darker in dark-skinned patients. Callused areas may appear yellow. Vascular flush areas (e.g., cheeks, neck, upper chest, and genital area) may appear pink or red, especially with anxiety or excitement. Be aware that skin color may be masked by cosmetics and tanning agents. Look for localized areas of discoloration.

Nevi (moles) occur in forms that vary in size and degree of pigmentation. Nevi are present on most persons regardless of skin color, and may occur anywhere on the body. They may be flat, slightly raised, dome-shaped, smooth, rough, or hairy. Their color ranges from tan, gray, and shades of brown to black. Table 8-1 describes the features and occurrence of various types of pigmented nevi.

BOX 8-2

CUTANEOUS MANIFESTATIONS OF TRADITIONAL HEALTH PRACTICES

The use of certain traditional health practices by various cultural groups can produce cutaneous manifestations that could be wrongly confused with disease or physical abuse. Two such practices are that of "coining" and "cupping" as used by some Asian subcultures. In coining, a coin dipped in mentholated oil is vigorously rubbed across the skin in a prescribed manner, causing a mild dermabrasion. This practice is believed to release excess force from the body and hence restore balance. In cupping, a series of small, heated glasses are placed on the skin, forming a suction that leaves a red circular mark, drawing out the bad force. The skin markings may alarm the clinician who is unaware of such practices. The lesson: In the history, ask about home remedies or practices. Be aware of and open to traditional modalities that may conflict with your own experience.

While most nevi are harmless, some may be dysplastic, precancerous, or cancerous. Table 8-2 describes differences in the features of normal and dysplastic moles. Dysplastic nevi tend to occur on the upper back in men and on the legs in women (see pp. 213 to 216 for malignant abnormalities).

Several variations in skin color occur in almost all healthy adults and children, including nonpigmented striae (i.e., silver or pink "stretch marks" that occur during pregnancy or weight gain), freckles in sun-exposed areas, some birthmarks, and some nevi (Fig. 8-3). Adult women will commonly have chloasma (also called melasma), areas of hyperpigmentation on

TABLE 8-1	Features and Occurrence of Various Types of Pigmented Nevi		
Type	**Features**	**Occurrence**	**Comments**
Halo nevus	Sharp, oval, or circular; de-pigmented halo around mole; may undergo many morphologic changes; usually disappears and halo repigments (may take years)	Usually on back in young adult	Usually benign; biopsy indicated because same process can occur around melanoma
Intradermal nevus	Dome shaped; raised; flesh to black color; may be pedunculated or hair bearing	Cells limited to dermis	No indication for removal other than cosmetic
Junction nevus	Flat or slightly elevated; dark brown	Nevus cells lining dermoepidermal junction	Should be removed if exposed to repeated trauma
Compound nevus	Slightly elevated brownish papule; indistinct border	Nevus cells in dermis and lining dermoepidermal junction	Should be removed if exposed to repeated trauma
Hairy nevus	May be present at birth; may cover large area; hair growth may occur after several years		Should be removed if changes occur

From Wilson, Giddens, 2005.

TABLE 8-2	Features of Normal and Dysplastic Moles	
Feature	**Normal Mole**	**Dysplastic Mole**
Color	Uniformly tan or brown; all moles on one person tend to look alike	Mixture of tan, brown, black, and red/pink; moles on one person often do not look alike
Shape	Round or oval with a clearly defined border that separates the mole from surrounding skin	Irregular borders may include notches; may fade into surrounding skin and include a flat portion level with skin
Surface	Begins as flat, smooth spot on skin; becomes raised; forms a smooth bump	May be smooth, slightly scaly, or have a rough, irregular, "pebbly" appearance
Size	Usually less than 6 mm (size of a pencil eraser)	Often larger than 6 mm and sometimes larger than 10 mm
Number	Typical adult has 10 to 40 moles scattered over the body	Many persons do not have increased number; however, persons severely affected may have more than 100 moles
Location	Usually above the waist on sun-exposed surfaces of the body; scalp, breast, and buttocks rarely have normal moles	May occur anywhere on the body, but most commonly on back; may also appear below the waist and on scalp, breast, and buttocks

TABLE 8-3	Cutaneous Color Changes		
Color	**Cause**	**Distribution**	**Select Conditions**
Brown	Darkening of melanin pigment	Generalized Localized	Pituitary, adrenal, liver disease Nevi, neurofibromatosis
White	Absence of melanin	Generalized Localized	Albinism Vitiligo
Red (erythema)	Increased cutaneous blood flow	Localized Generalized	Inflammation Fever, viral exanthem, urticaria
Yellow	Increased intravascular red blood cells Increased bile pigmentation (jaundice) Increased carotene pigmentation Decreased visibility of oxyhemoglobin	Generalized Generalized Generalized (except sclera) Generalized	Polycythemia Liver disease Hypothyroidism, increased intake of vegetables containing carotene Anemia, chronic renal disease
Blue	Increased unsaturated hemoglobin secondary to hypoxia	Lips, mouth, nail beds	Cardiovascular and pulmonary diseases

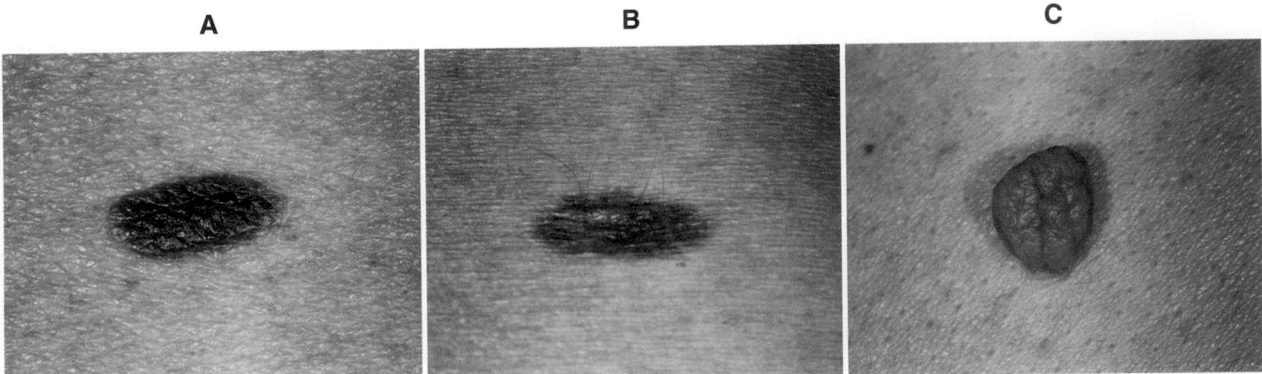

A **B** **C**

FIGURE 8-3
Commonly occurring nevi. **A,** Junction nevus. Color and shape of this black lesion are uniform.
B, Compound nevus. Center is elevated and surrounding area is flat, retaining features of a junction nevus. **C,** Dermal nevus. Papillomatous with soft, flabby, wrinkled surface.
From Habif, 2004.

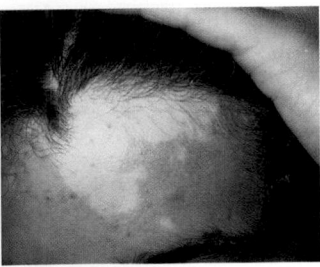

FIGURE 8-4
Vitiligo.
Courtesy Jaime A. Tschen, BD, Baylor College of Medicine, Department of Dermatology, Houston; from Thompson et al, 1993.

the face and neck that are associated with pregnancy or the use of hormones. This condition is more noticeable in darker-skinned women. The absence of melanin produces patches of unpigmented skin or hair (Fig. 8-4).

Color hues in dark-skinned persons are best seen in the sclera, conjunctiva, buccal mucosa, tongue, lips, nail beds, and palms. Be aware, however, that heavily callused palms in dark-skinned persons have an opaque yellow cast. Particular variations in skin color may be the result of physiologic pigment distribution. The palms and soles are lighter in color than the rest of the body. Hyperpigmented macules on the soles of the feet are common. Freckling of the buccal cavity, gums, and tongue is common. The sclera may appear yellowish brown (often described as "muddy") or may contain brownish pigment that looks like petechiae. A bluish hue of the lips and gums can be a normal finding in persons with dark skin. Some dark-skinned persons have very blue lips, giving a false impression of cyanosis.

Systemic disorders can produce generalized or localized color changes; these are described in Table 8-3. Localized redness often results from an inflammatory process. Pale, shiny skin of the lower extremities may reflect peripheral changes that occur with systemic diseases such as diabetes mellitus and cardiovascular disease. Injury, steroids, vasculitis, and several systemic disorders can cause localized hemorrhage into cutaneous tissues, producing red-purple discolorations. The discolorations produced by injury are called ecchymoses; when produced by other causes they are called petechiae if smaller than 0.5 cm in diameter (Fig. 8-5) or purpura if larger than 0.5 cm in diameter (Fig. 8-6). Vascular skin lesions are characterized in Fig. 8-7. Box 8-3 describes some characteristic odors that you may note as you examine the skin.

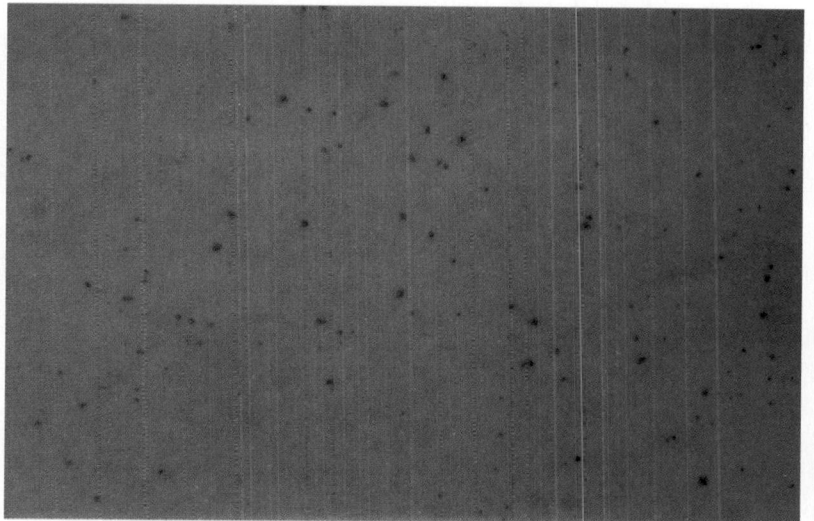

FIGURE 8-5
Petechiae on abdomen.
From Lemmi, Lemmi, 2000.

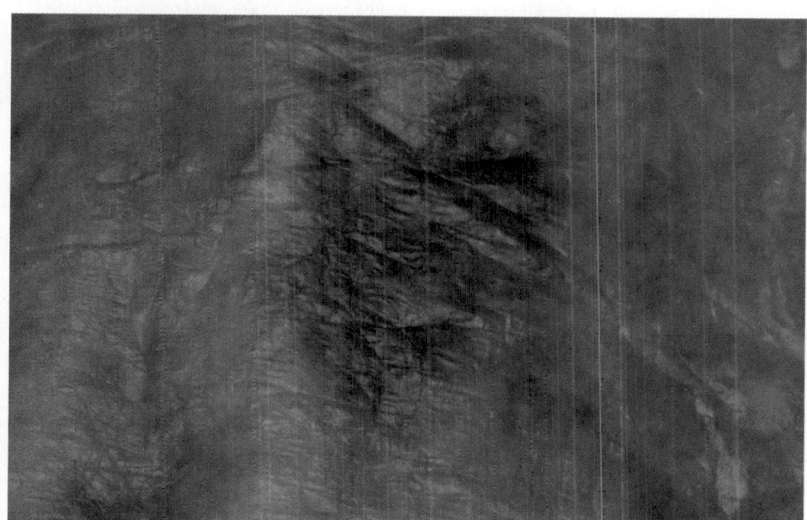

FIGURE 8-6
Senile purpura.
From Lemmi, Lemmi, 2000.

Purpura—red-purple nonblanchable discoloration greater than 0.5 cm diameter.
Cause: Intravascular defects, infection

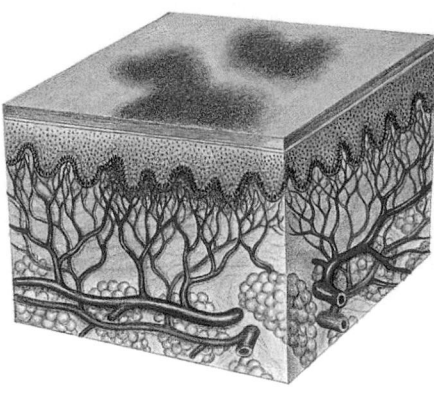

Petechiae—red-purple nonblanchable discoloration less than 0.5 cm diameter
Cause: Intravascular defects, infection

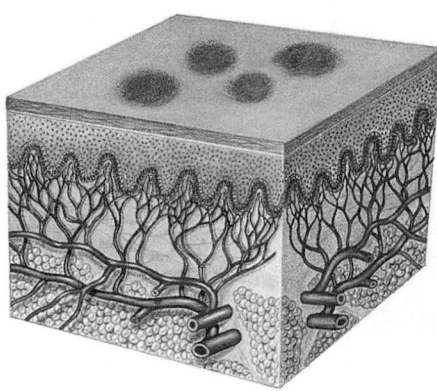

Ecchymoses—red-purple nonblanchable discoloration of variable size
Cause: Vascular wall destruction, trauma, vasculitis

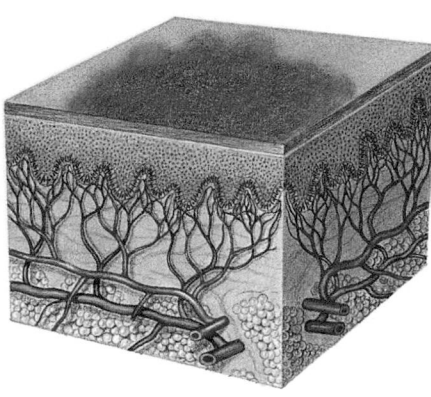

Spider angioma—red central body with radiating spiderlike legs that blanch with pressure to the central body
Cause: Liver disease, vitamin B deficiency, idiopathic

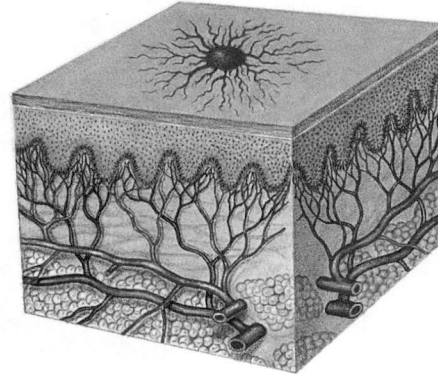

Venous star—bluish spider, linear or irregularly shaped; does not blanch with pressure
Cause: Increased pressure in superficial veins

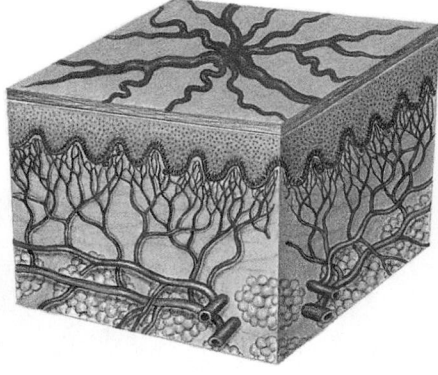

Telangiectasia—fine, irregular red line
Cause: Dilation of capillaries

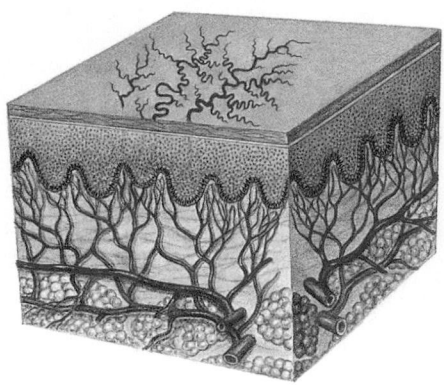

Capillary hemangioma (nevus flammeus)—red irregular macular patches
Cause: Dilation of dermal capillaries

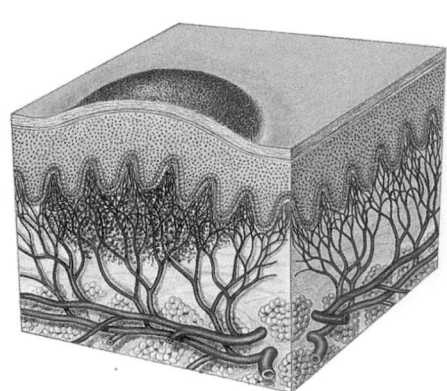

FIGURE 8-7
Characteristics and causes of vascular skin lesions.

CLINICAL PEARL

Mercury Poisoning

A patient presents with a generalized red flush or a widespread miliarial rash, really does not feel well, and is sweating profusely. Consider mercury poisoning.

BOX 8-3

SMELL THE SKIN

Even the skin may have odors suggesting a variety of problems: infectious, metabolic, or neurologic. Sweatiness intensifies the smell.

Cause of Odor	Type of Odor
Clostridium gas gangrene	Rotten apples
Proteus infection	Mousy
Pseudomonas infection (especially burns)	Grapelike
Schizophrenia	Pungent
Tuberculous lymphadenitis (scrofula)	Stale beer
Anaerobic infection; scurvy	Putrid
Intestinal obstruction, peritonitis	Feculent
Phenylketonuria	Mousy, musty

Modified from Wilson, 1997.

PALPATION

As you inspect, palpate the skin for moisture, temperature, texture, turgor, and mobility. Palpation may yield additional data for describing lesions, particularly in relation to elevation or depression.

Minimal perspiration or oiliness should be present. Increased perspiration may be associated with activity, warm environment, obesity, anxiety, or excitement; it may be especially noticeable on the palms, scalp, forehead, and in the axillae (usually the dampest areas). The intertriginous areas should evidence minimal dampness. Pay particular attention to areas that get little or no exposure to circulating air such as in the folds of large breasts or obese abdomens or in the inguinal area (Fig. 8-8).

The skin should range from cool to warm to the touch. Use the dorsal surface of your hands or fingers because these areas are most sensitive to temperature perception. At best, this assessment is a rough estimate of skin temperature; what you are really looking for is bilateral symmetry. Environmental conditions, including the temperature of the examining room, may affect surface temperature.

The texture should feel smooth, soft, and even. Roughness on exposed areas or areas of pressure (particularly the elbows, soles, and palms) may be caused by heavy or woolen clothing, cold weather, or soap. Extensive or widespread roughness may be the result of a keratinization disorder or healing lesions. Hyperkeratoses, especially of the palms and soles, may be the sign of a systemic disorder such as arsenic or other toxic exposure.

To assess turgor and mobility, gently pinch a small section of skin on the forearm or sternal area between the thumb and forefinger and then release the skin (Fig. 8-9). Turgor should not be tested on the back of a patient's hand because of the looseness and thinness of the skin in that area. The skin should feel resilient, move easily when pinched, and return to place immediately when released. Turgor will be altered if the patient is substantially dehydrated or if edema is present. For example, turgor is decreased in a dehydrated patient as evidenced by the pinched skin's failing to spring back to place after release. Some connective tissue diseases, notably the forms of scleroderma, affect skin mobility.

CLINICAL PEARL

Telangiectases/Vascular Spiders

How do you tell the difference between telangiectases and vascular spiders? Telangiectases are little masses of venules. When you blanch them, they will refill in an erratic, not-at-all-organized way. Vascular spiders are arterial. Blanch the center and they will refill in a very organized way, from the center out and evenly in all directions.

SKIN LESIONS

As you assess the skin, pay particular attention to any lesions that may be present. "Skin lesion" is a catchall term that collectively describes any pathologic skin change or occurrence. Lesions may be primary (i.e., those that occur as initial spontaneous manifestations of a pathologic process) or secondary (i.e., those that result from later evolution of or external trauma to a primary lesion).

Tables 8-4 and 8-5 show the characteristics of primary and secondary lesions. The nomenclature is often used inaccurately; if you are uncertain about a lesion, use the descriptors rather than the name. Be aware that several types of lesions may occur concurrently and that secondary changes may obscure primary characteristics.

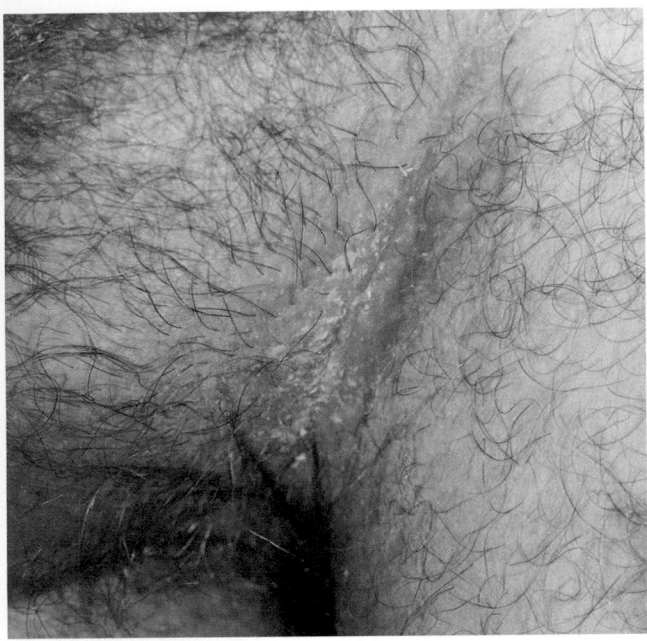

FIGURE 8-8
Examining an intertriginous area. Note fissure and maceration in the crural fold.
From Habif, 2004.

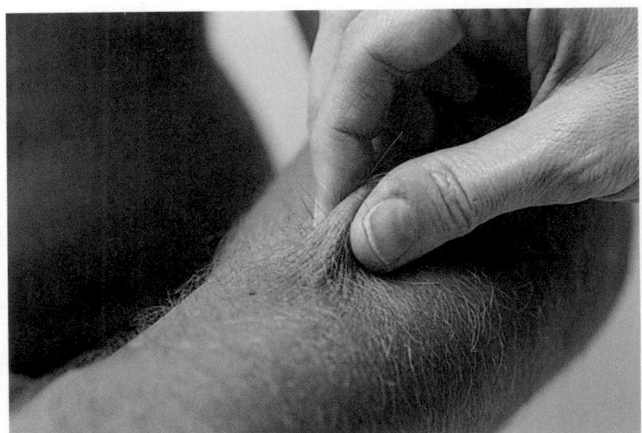

FIGURE 8-9
Testing skin turgor.

Describe lesions according to characteristics (Table 8-6), exudates, configuration, and location and distribution:

Characteristics

- Size (measure all dimensions)
- Shape
- Color
- Texture
- Elevation or depression
- Pedunculation
- Exudates
  - Color
  - Odor
  - Amount
  - Consistency
- Configuration
  - Annular (rings)
  - Grouped
  - Linear
  - Arciform (bow-shaped)
  - Diffuse
- Location and distribution
  - Generalized or localized
  - Region of the body (Box 8-4)
  - Patterns (Figs. 8-10 to 8-12)
  - Discrete or confluent

A small, clear, flexible ruler is necessary for measuring the size of lesions. Examiners often rely on household measures such as fruit, vegetables, and coins to estimate the size of lesions, nodules, or eruptions, but the resulting descriptions can be as inaccurate as they are interesting. Subjective estimates should not be used as measures of size; instead, use the ruler and report sizes in centimeters (inches may also be used, but centimeters is the preferred unit of measure). Try to measure size in all dimensions (i.e., height, width, and depth) when possible.

TABLE 8-4	Primary Skin Lesions	
Description	**Examples**	

MACULE

A flat, circumscribed area that is a change in the color of the skin; less than 1 cm in diameter

Freckles, flat moles (nevi), petechiae, measles, scarlet fever

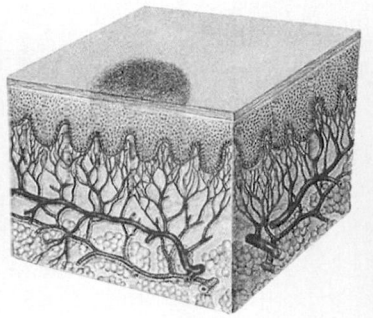

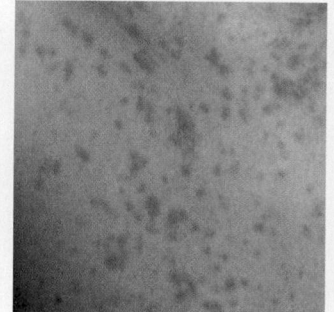

Measles. (From Habif, 2004.)

PAPULE

An elevated, firm, circumscribed area; less than 1 cm in diameter

Wart (verruca), elevated moles, lichen planus

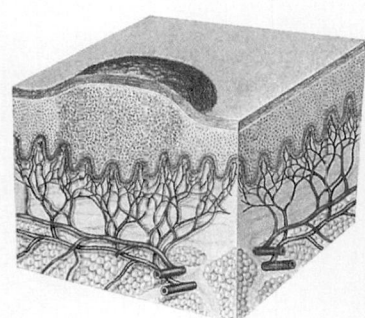

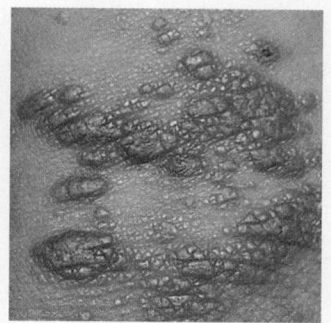

Lichen planus. (From Weston, Lane, Morelli, 1996.)

PATCH

A flat, nonpalpable, irregular-shaped macule greater than 1 cm in diameter

Vitiligo, port-wine stains, Mongolian spots, café au lait patch

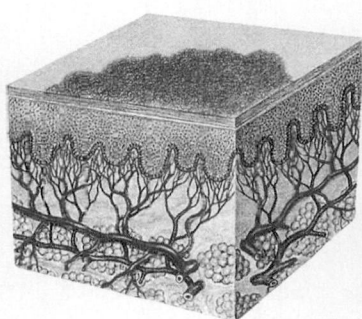

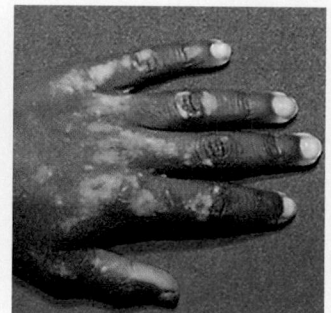

Vitiligo. (From Weston, Lane, 1991.)

PLAQUE

Elevated, firm, and rough lesion with flat top surface greater than 1 cm in diameter

Psoriasis, seborrheic and actinic keratoses

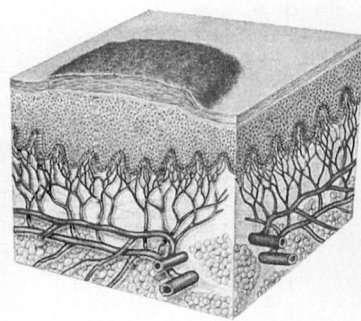

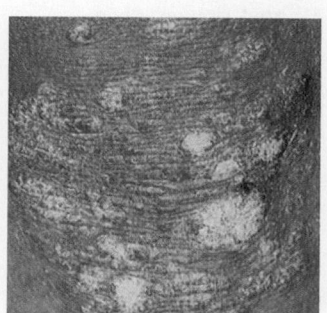

Plaque. (From Habif, 2004.)

Modified from Thompson, Wilson, 1996.

Continued

TABLE 8-4	Primary Skin Lesions—cont'd

Description	Examples		
WHEAL Elevated, irregular-shaped area of cutaneous edema; solid, transient, variable diameter	Insect bites, urticaria, allergic reaction	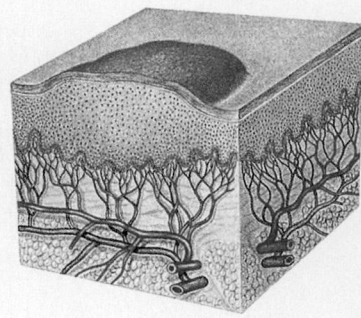	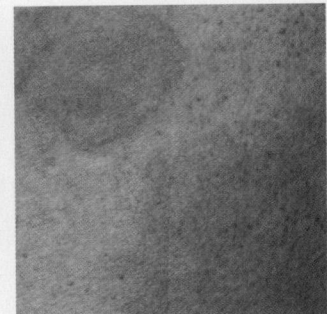 Wheal. (From Farrar et al, 1992.)
NODULE Elevated, firm, circumscribed lesion; deeper in dermis than a papule; 1 to 2 cm in diameter	Erythema nodosum, lipomas	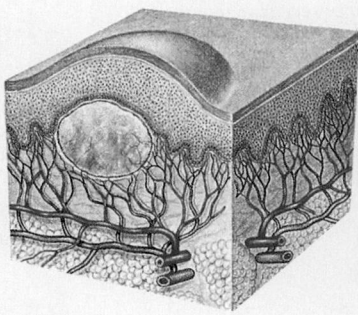	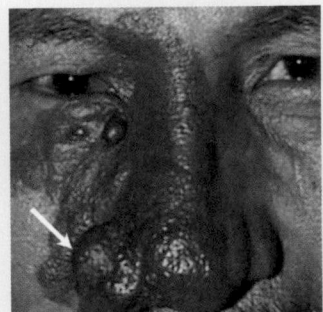 Hypertrophic nodule. (From Goldman, Fitzpatrick, 1994.)
TUMOR Elevated and solid lesion; may or may not be clearly demarcated; deeper in dermis; greater than 2 cm in diameter	Neoplasms, benign tumor, lipoma,	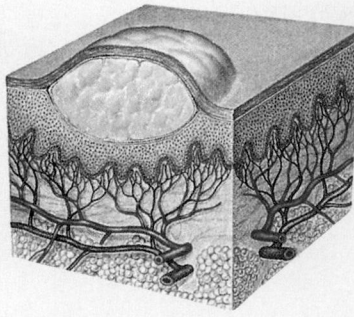	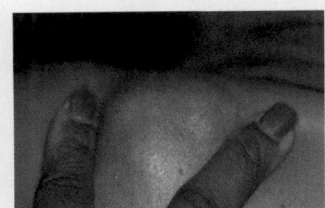 Lipoma. (From Lemmi, Lemmi, 2000.)
VESICLE Elevated, circumscribed, superficial, not into dermis; filled with serous fluid; less than 1 cm in diameter	Varicella (chickenpox), herpes zoster (shingles)	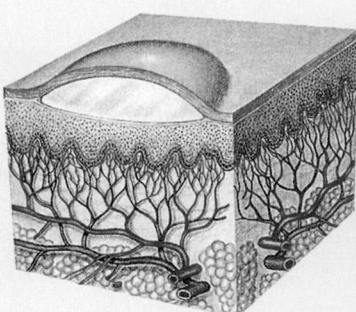	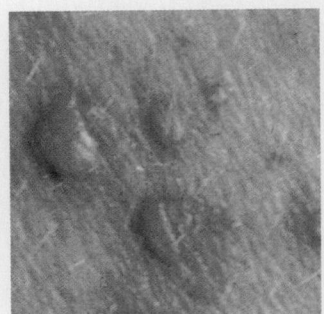 Vesicles caused by varicella. (From Farrar et al, 1992.)

Modified from Thompson, Wilson, 1996.

TABLE 8-4	Primary Skin Lesions—cont'd

Description	Examples		
BULLA Vesicle greater than 1 cm in diameter	Blister, pemphigus vulgaris	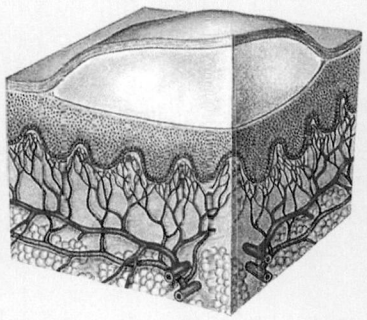	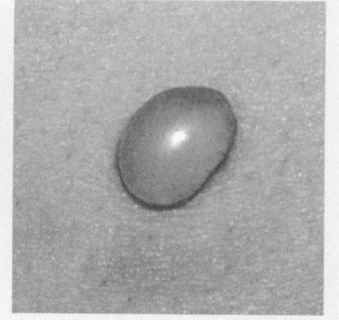 Blister. (From White, 1994.)
PUSTULE Elevated, superficial lesion; similar to a vesicle but filled with purulent fluid	Impetigo, acne	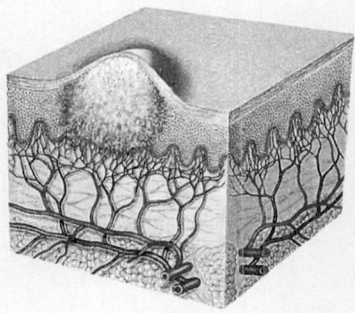	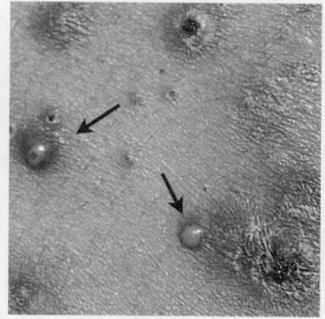 Acne. (From Weston, Lane, Morelli, 1996.)
CYST Elevated, circumscribed, encapsulated lesion; in dermis or subcutaneous layer; filled with liquid or semi-solid material	Sebaceous cyst, cystic acne	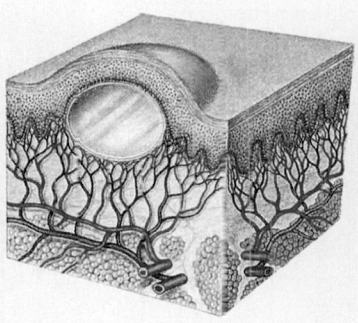	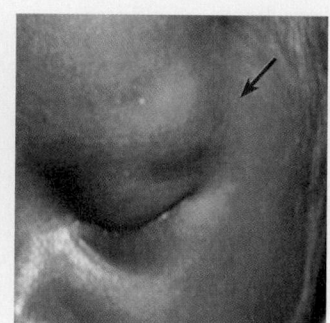 Sebaceous cyst. (From Weston, Lane, Morelli, 1996.)
TELANGIECTASIA Fine, irregular, red lines produced by capillary dilation	Telangiectasia in rosacea	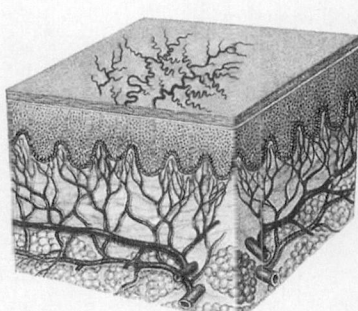	 Telangiectasia. (From Lemmi, Lemmi, 2000.)

TABLE 8-5	**Secondary Skin Lesions**

Description	Examples

SCALE

Heaped-up, keratinized cells; flaky skin; irregular; thick or thin; dry or oily; variation in size

Flaking of skin with seborrheic dermatitis following scarlet fever, or flaking of skin following a drug reaction; dry skin

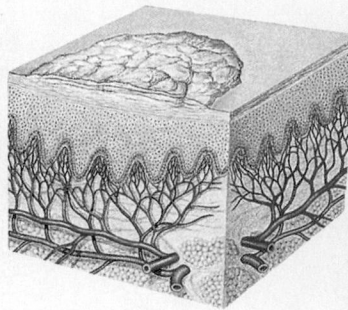

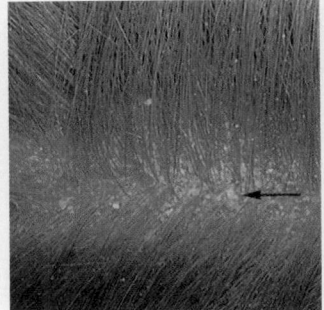

Fine scaling. (From Baran, Dawher, Levene, 1991.)

LICHENIFICATION

Rough, thickened epidermis secondary to persistent rubbing, itching, or skin irritation; often involves flexor surface of extremity

Chronic dermatitis

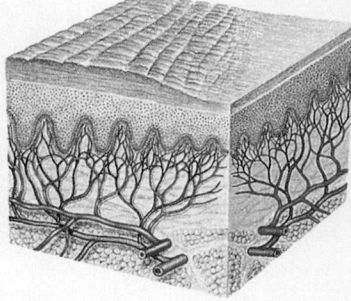

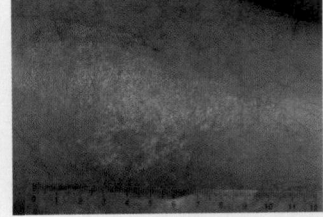

Lichenification. (From Lemmi, Lemmi, 2000.)

KELOID

Irregular-shaped, elevated, progressively enlarging scar; grows beyond the boundaries of the wound; caused by excessive collagen formation during healing

Keloid formation following surgery

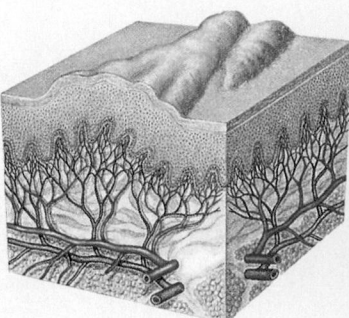

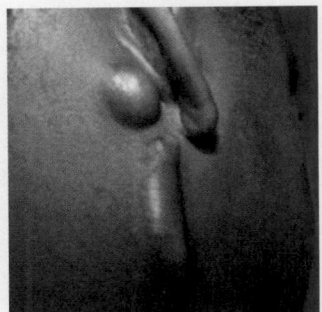

Keloid. (From Weston, Lane, Morelli, 1996.)

SCAR

Thin to thick fibrous tissue that replaces normal skin following injury or laceration to the dermis

Healed wound or surgical incision

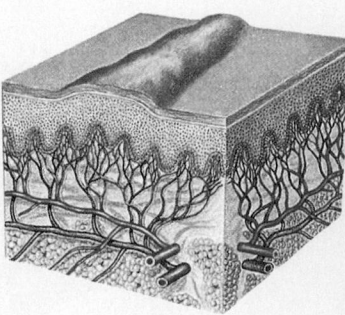

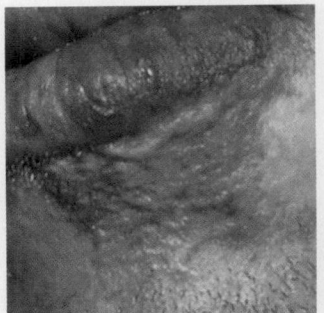

Hypertrophic scar. (From Goldman, Fitzpatrick, 1994.)

Modified from Wilson, Giddens, 2005.

TABLE 8-5	Secondary Skin Lesions—cont'd

Description	Examples		

EXCORIATION

Loss of the epidermis; linear hollowed-out, crusted area

Abrasion or scratch, scabies

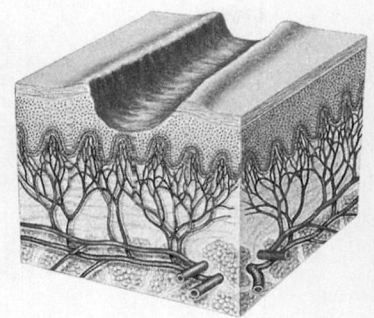 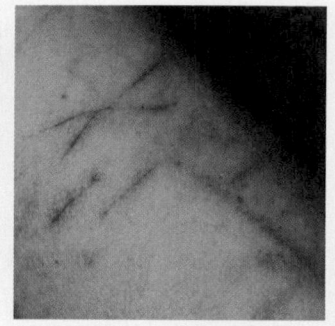

Excoriation from a tree branch. (From Lemmi, Lemmi, 2000.)

FISSURE

Linear crack or break from the epidermis to the dermis; may be moist or dry

Athlete's foot, cracks at the corner of the mouth

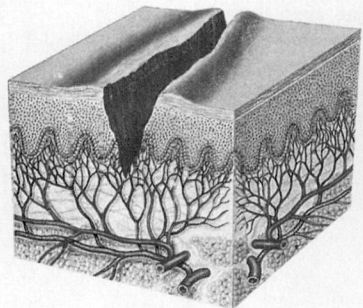 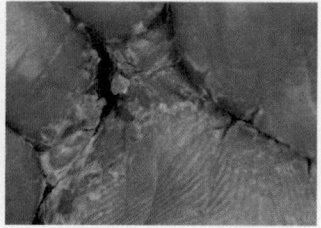

Scaling and fissures of tinea pedis. (From Lemmi, Lemmi, 2000.)

EROSION

Loss of part of the epidermis; depressed, moist, glistening; follows rupture of a vesicle or bulla

Varicella, variola after rupture

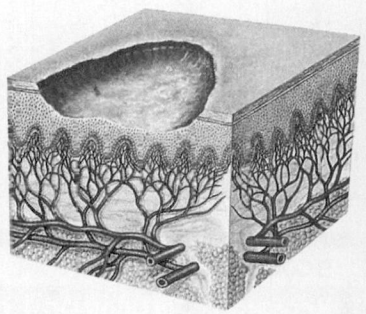 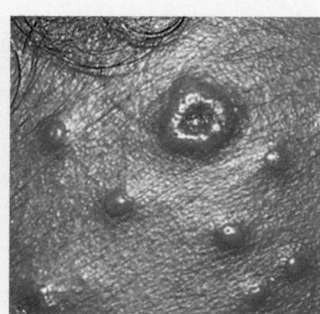

Erosion. (From Cohen, 1993.)

ULCER

Loss of epidermis and dermis; concave; varies in size

Decubiti, stasis ulcers

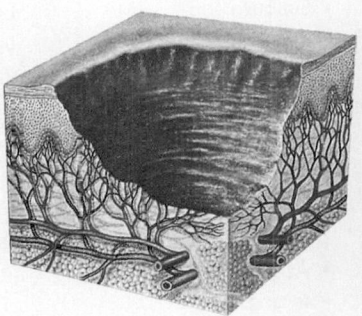 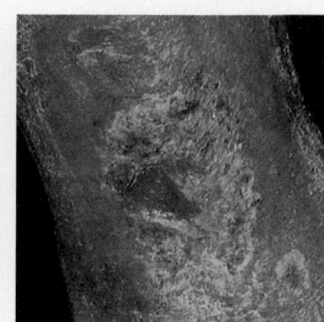

Stasis ulcer. (From Habif, 2004.)

Continued

TABLE 8-5	Secondary Skin Lesions—cont'd	
Description	**Examples**	
CRUST Dried serum, blood, or purulent exudates; slightly elevated; size varies; brown, red, black, tan, or straw-colored	Scab on abrasion, eczema	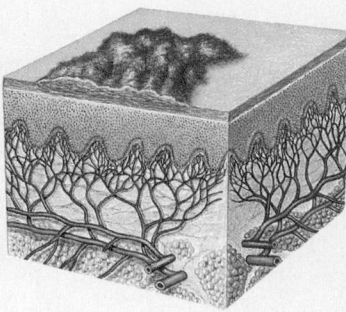 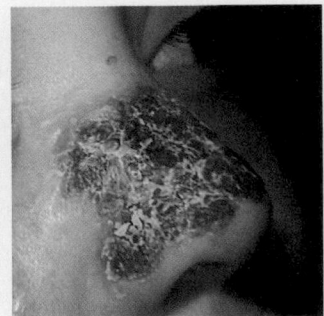 Scab.
ATROPHY Thinning of skin surface and loss of skin markings; skin translucent and paper-like	Striae; aged skin	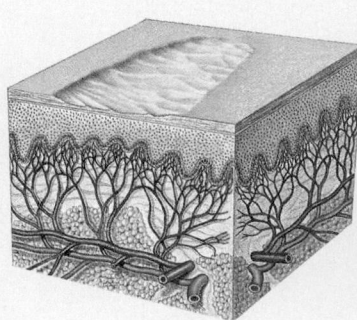 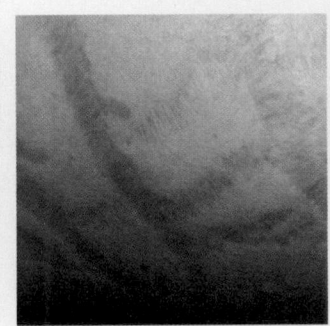 Striae. (Courtesy Antoinette Hood, MD, Department of Dermatology, University of Indiana, Department of Medicine, Indianapolis).

Modified from Wilson, Giddens, 2001.

TABLE 8-6	Morphologic Characteristics of Skin Lesions	
Characteristic	**Description**	**Examples**
DISTRIBUTION		
Localized	Lesion appears in one small area	Impetigo, herpes simplex (e.g., labialis), tinea corporis ("ringworm")
Regional	Lesions involve a specific region of the body	Acne vulgaris (pilosebaceous gland distribution), herpes zoster (nerve dermatomal distribution), psoriasis (flexural surfaces and skin folds)
Generalized	Lesions appear widely distributed or in numerous areas simultaneously	Urticaria, disseminated drug eruptions
SHAPE/ARRANGEMENT		
Round/discoid	Coin- or fine-shaped (no central clearing)	Nummular eczema
Oval	Ovoid shape	Pityriasis rosea
Annular	Round, active margins with central clearing	Tinea corporis, sarcoidosis
Zosteriform (dermatomal)	Following a nerve or segment of the body	Herpes zoster
Polycyclic	Interlocking or coalesced circles (formed by enlargement of annular lesions)	Psoriases, urticaria
Linear	In a line	Contact dermatitis
Iris/target lesion	Pink macules with purple central papules	Erythema multiforme
Stellate	Star-shaped	Meningococcal septicemia
Serpiginous	Snakelike or wavy line track	Cutanea larva migrans
Reticulate	Netlike or lacy	Polyarteritis nodosa, lichen planus lesions of erythema infectiosum
Morbilliform	Measles-like: maculopapular lesions that become confluent on the face and body	Measles, roseola
BORDER/MARGIN		
Discrete	Well demarcated or defined, able to draw a line around it with confidence	Psoriasis
Indistinct	Poorly defined, have borders that merge into normal skin or outlying ill-defined papules	Nummular eczema
Active	Margin of lesion shows greater activity than center	Tinea eruptions
Irregular	Nonsmooth or notched margin	Malignant melanoma
Border raised above center	Center of lesion is depressed compared to the edge	Basal cell carcinoma
Advancing	Expanding at margins	Cellulitis
ASSOCIATED CHANGES WITHIN LESIONS		
Central clearing	An erythematous border surrounds lighter skin	Tinea eruptions
Desquamation	Peeling or sloughing of skin	Rash of toxic shock syndrome
Keratotic	Hypertrophic stratum corneum	Calluses, warts
Punctation	Central umbilication or dimpling	Basal cell carcinoma
Telangiectasias	Dilated blood vessels within lesion blanch completely, may be markers of systemic disease	Basal cell carcinoma, actinic keratosis
PIGMENTATION		
Flesh	Same tone as the surrounding skin	Neurofibroma, some nevi
Pink	Light red undertones	Eczema, pityriasis rosea
Erythematous	Dark pink to red	Tinea eruptions, psoriasis
Salmon	Orange-pink	Psoriasis
Tan-brown	Light to dark brown	Most nevi, pityriasis versicolor
Black	Black or blue-black	Malignant melanoma
Pearly	Shiny white, almost iridescent	Basal cell carcinoma
Purple	Dark red-blue-violet	Purpura, Kaposi sarcoma
Violaceous	Light violet	Erysipelas
Yellow	Waxy	Lipoma
White	Absent of color	Lichen planus

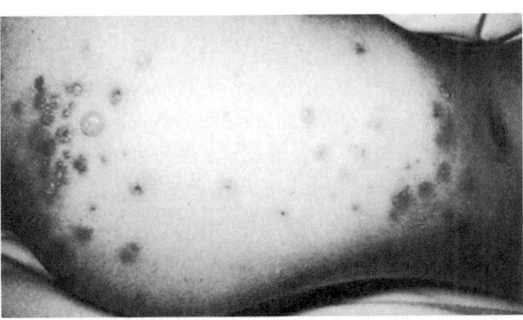

FIGURE 8-10
Clustering of lesions.
Reproduced by permission of the Wellcome Foundation, Ltd.

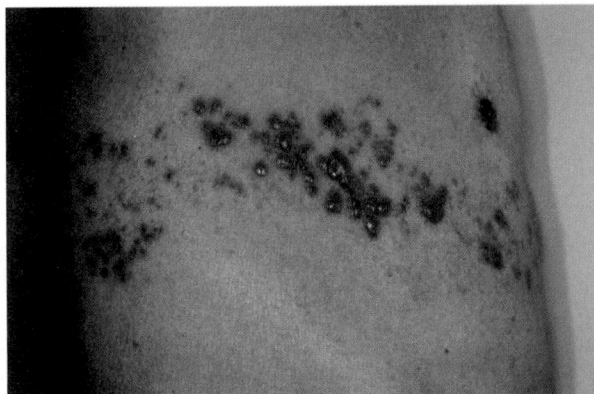

FIGURE 8-11
Linear formation of lesions (herpes zoster).
From Lemmi, Lemmi, 2000.

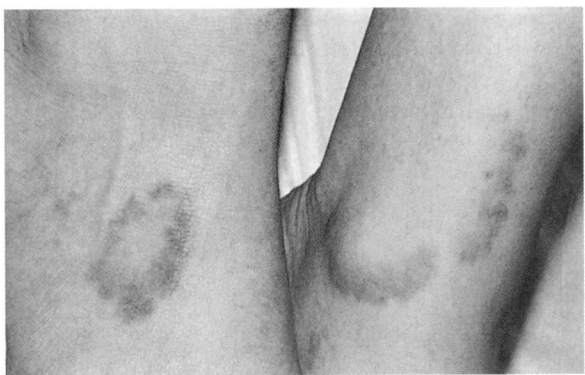

FIGURE 8-12
Annular formation of lesions (granuloma annulare). An annular plaque or plaques may occur on the dorsa of the feet or hands as a manifestation of granuloma annulare.
From White, 1994.

STAYING WELL

PRACTICE SUN SAFETY

- Do not sunbathe.
- Avoid unnecessary sun exposure, especially between 10:00 AM and 4:00 PM, the peak hours for harmful ultraviolet (UV) radiation.
- When outdoors, use a sunscreen rated SPF 15 or higher that blocks both UVB and UVA. Apply it liberally, uniformly, and frequently. Reapply after swimming, sweating, or toweling dry.
- When exposed to sunlight, wear protective clothing such as long pants, long-sleeved shirts, broad-brimmed hats, and UV-protective sunglasses.

- Avoid tanning booths.
- Teach children good sun protection habits at an early age: The damage that leads to adult skin cancers starts in childhood.

The American Cancer Society advocates "Slip! Slop! Slap! . . . and Wrap" as a catch phrase for kids that works well for adults, too. It reminds people to use four key methods to protect themselves: Slip on a shirt, slop on sunscreen, slap on a hat, and wrap on sunglasses to protect the eyes and sensitive skin around them from ultraviolet light.

Use a light for closer inspection of a particular lesion to detect its nuances of color, elevation, and borders. A 5-10 power handheld magnifying lens is useful in evaluating the subtle details of a lesion. Transillumination may be used to determine the presence of fluid in cysts and masses. Darken the room and place the tip of the transilluminator against the side of the cyst or mass. Fluid-filled lesions will transilluminate with a red glow, whereas solid lesions will not.

The Wood's lamp can be used to distinguish fluorescing lesions. Darken the room and shine the light on the area to be examined. Look for the characteristic yellow-green fluorescence that indicates the presence of some types of fungal infection.

HAIR

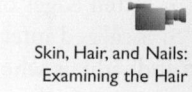

Skin, Hair, and Nails:
Examining the Hair

Palpate the hair for texture, while at the same time inspecting it for color, distribution, and quantity. The scalp hair may be coarse or fine, curly or straight, and should be shiny, smooth, and resilient. Palpate the scalp hair for dryness and brittleness that could indicate a systemic disorder. Color will vary from very light blond to black to gray and may show alterations with rinses, dyes, or permanents.

The quantity and distribution of hair vary according to individual genetic makeup. Hair is commonly present on the scalp, lower face, neck, nares, ears, chest, axillae, back and shoulders, arms, legs, toes, pubic area, and around the nipples. Note hair loss, which can be either generalized or localized. Inspect the feet and toes for hair loss that may indicate poor circulation or nutritional deficit. Look for any inflammation or scarring that accompanies hair loss, particularly when it is localized. Diffuse hair loss usually occurs without inflammation and scarring. The presence of scarring is helpful in diagnosis. Note whether the hair shafts are broken off or are completely absent.

Genetically predisposed men often display a gradual symmetric hair loss on the scalp during adulthood as a response to elevated androgen levels. Asymmetric hair loss may indicate a pathologic condition. Women in their 20s and 30s may also develop adrenal androgenic female-pattern alopecia (hair loss), with a gradual loss of hair from the central scalp.

Fine vellus hair covers the body, whereas coarse terminal hair occurs on the scalp, pubic, and axillary areas, on the arms and legs (to some extent), and in the beard of men. The male pubic hair configuration is an upright triangle with the hair extending midline to the umbilicus. The female pubic configuration is an inverted triangle; the hair may extend midline to the umbilicus. Look for hirsutism in women—growth of terminal hair in a male distribution pattern on the face, body, and pubic area. Hirsutism, by itself or associated with other signs of virilization, may be a sign of an endocrine disorder.

NAILS

INSPECTION

Inspect the nails for color, length, configuration, symmetry, and cleanliness. The condition of the fingernails can provide important insight to the patient's sense of self. Are they bitten down to the quick? Are they clean? Are they kept smooth and neat, or do they look unkempt? There are, of course, physical clues to pathophysiologic problems in the nails, just as in the hair. The condition of the hair and nails gives a clue about the patient's level of self-care and some sense of emotional order and social integration.

The shape and opacity of nails vary considerably among individuals. Nail bed color should be variations of pink. Pigment deposits or bands may be present in the nail beds of persons with dark skin (Fig. 8-13). The sudden appearance of such a band in whites may indicate melanoma. Yellow discoloration occurs with several nail diseases, including psoriasis and fungal infections, and may also occur with chronic respiratory disease. Proximal subungual fungal infection is associated with human immunodeficiency virus (HIV) infection. Diffuse darkening of the nails may arise from antimalarial drug therapy, candidal infection, hyperbilirubinemia, and chronic trauma, such as occurs from tight-fitting shoes. Green-black discoloration, which is associated with *Pseudomonas* infection, may be confused with similar discoloration caused by injury to the nail bed (subungual hematoma). Nail beds that are blue

PHYSICAL VARIATIONS

Pigment in the Nail Beds
Pigmented deposits or bands may be present in the nail beds of persons with dark skin. The sudden appearance of such a band in whites may indicate melanoma.

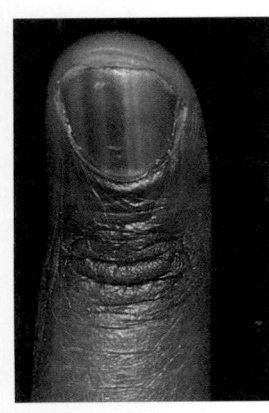

FIGURE 8-13
Pigmented bands in nails are expected in persons with dark skin.
From Habif, 2004.

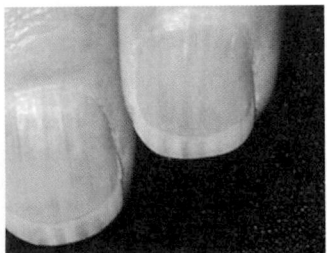

FIGURE 8-14
Aging nails. Longitudinal ridging of the nail is a common expected variation.
From White, 1994.

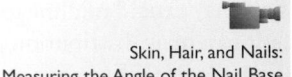

Skin, Hair, and Nails:
Measuring the Angle of the Nail Base

may be a transient response to a cold examining room. A single blue or black nail may indicate melanoma or bruising/bleeding from trauma. Generalized blue nails may be caused by conditions that produce cyanosis such as asthma, cardiac disorders, or severe anemia. Other causes of blue nails include silver poisoning, medication side effects, and Wilson disease, an inherited disorder. Pain accompanies a subungual hematoma, whereas *Pseudomonas* infection is painless. Splinter hemorrhages, longitudinal red or brown streaks, may occur with severe psoriasis of the nail matrix or as the result of minor injury to the proximal nail fold (habit-tic deformity). White spots in the nail plate, a common finding, result from cuticle manipulation or other forms of mild trauma. These spots need to be differentiated from longitudinal white streaks or transverse white bands that are indicative of a systemic disorder. Separation of the nail plate from the bed produces a white, yellow, or green tinge on the nonadherent portion of the nail.

Nail edges should be smooth and rounded. Jagged, broken, or bitten edges or cuticles are indicators of poor care habits and may predispose the patient to localized infection. Peeling nails (from the plate splitting into layers) are usually found in individuals whose hands are subject to repeated water immersion.

The nail plate should appear smooth and flat or slightly convex. Complete absence of the nail (anonychia) may occur as a congenital condition. Look for nail ridging, grooves, depressions, and pitting. Longitudinal ridging and beading are common expected variants (Fig. 8-14). Longitudinal ridges and grooves may also occur with lichen planus of the nail. Transverse grooves result from repeated injury to the nail, usually the thumb, as with chronic manipulation to the proximal nail fold. The most common cause is picking at the thumb with the index finger (habit-tic deformity). Chronic inflammation, such as occurs with chronic paronychia or chronic eczema, produces transverse rippling of the nail plate. Transverse depressions that appear at the base of the lunula occur after stress that temporarily interrupts nail formation. Involvement of a single nail usually points to an injury to the nail matrix. Assure the patient that the nail will grow out and assume normal appearance in about 6 months. Depressions that occur in all the nails are usually a response to systemic disease, including syphilis, disorders producing high fevers, peripheral vascular disease, and uncontrolled diabetes mellitus. Pitting is seen most commonly with psoriasis. Broadening and flattening of the nail plate may be seen in secondary syphilis. Fig. 8-15 illustrates unexpected nail findings.

The nail base angle should measure 160 degrees. One way to observe this is to place a ruler or a sheet of paper across the nail and dorsal surface of the finger and examine the angle formed by the proximal nail fold and nail plate. In clubbing, the angle increases and approaches or exceeds 180 degrees. Another method of assessment is the Schamroth technique (Fig. 8-16). Have the patient place together the nail (dorsal) surfaces of the fingertips of corresponding fingers from the right and left hands. When the nails are clubbed, the diamond-shaped window at the base of the nails disappears, and the angle between the distal tips increases. Clubbing is associated with a variety of respiratory and cardiovascular diseases, cirrhosis, colitis, and thyroid disease (Fig. 8-17).

Examine the proximal and lateral nail folds for redness, swelling, pus, warts, cysts, and tumors. Pain usually accompanies ingrown nails and infections.

PALPATION

The nail plates should feel hard and smooth with a uniform thickness. Thickening of the nail may occur from tight-fitting shoes, chronic trauma, and some fungal infections. Thinning of the nail plate may also accompany some nail diseases. Pain in the area of a nail groove may be secondary to ischemia.

Gently squeeze the nail between your thumb and the pad of your finger to test for adherence of the nail to the nail bed. Separation of the nail plate from the bed is common with psoriasis, trauma, candidal or *Pseudomonas* infections, and some medications. The nail base should feel firm (Fig. 8-18). A boggy nail base accompanies clubbing.

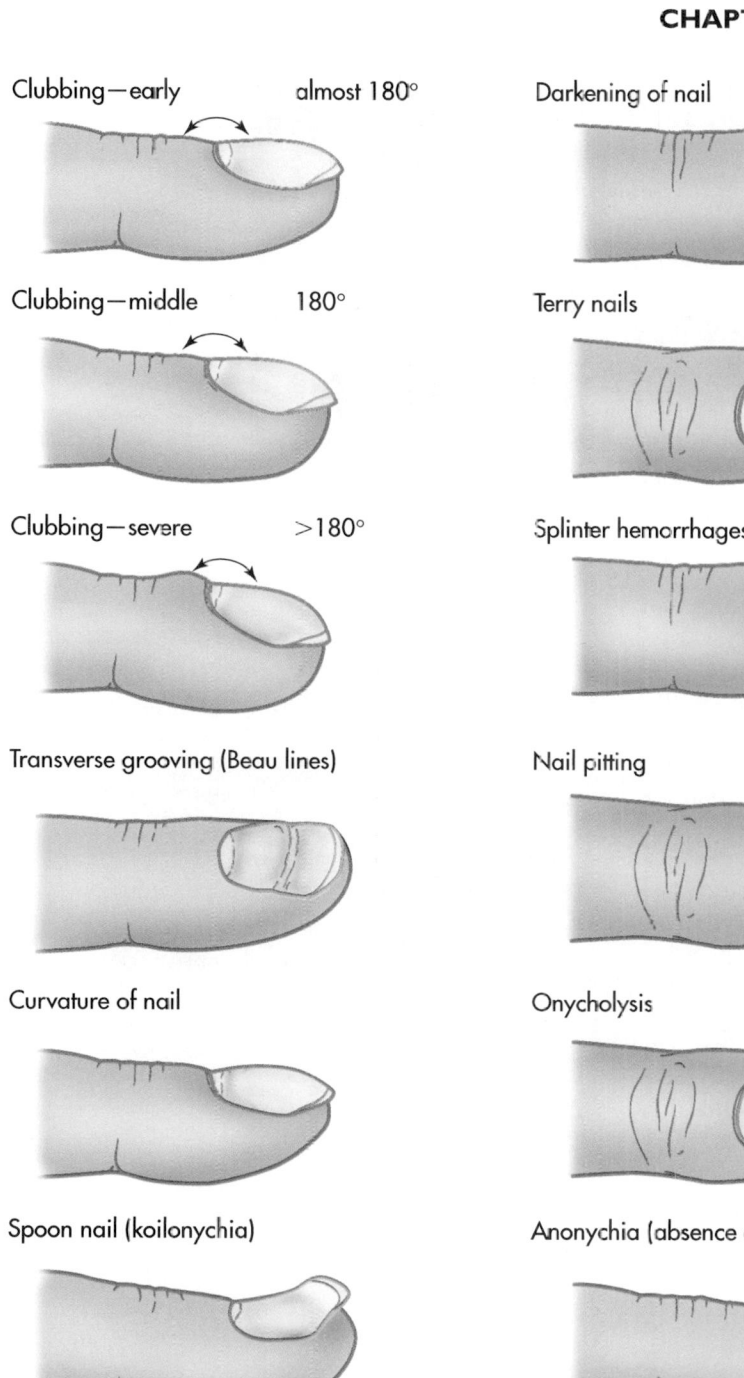

Clubbing—early   almost 180°

Clubbing—middle   180°

Clubbing—severe   >180°

Transverse grooving (Beau lines)

Curvature of nail

Spoon nail (koilonychia)

Broadening of nail

Darkening of nail

Terry nails

Splinter hemorrhages

Nail pitting

Onycholysis

Anonychia (absence of nail)

Paronychia

FIGURE 8-15
Nails: unexpected findings and appearance.

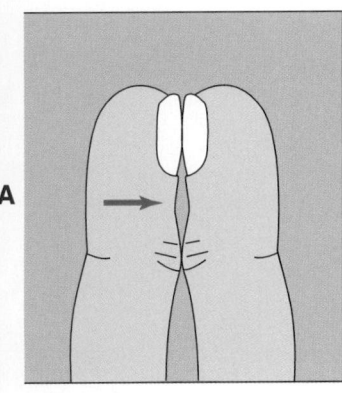

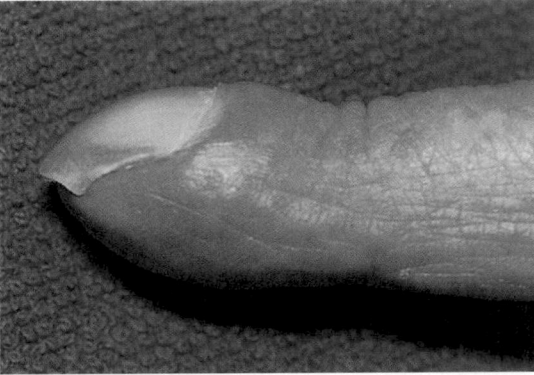

FIGURE 8-17
Finger clubbing. Nail is enlarged and curved.
From Lawrence, Cox, 1993.

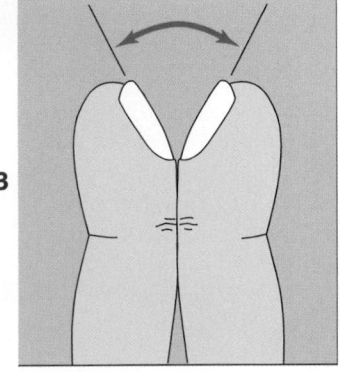

FIGURE 8-16
Schamroth technique. **A,** Patient with healthy nails, illustrating window. **B,** Patient with nail clubbing, illustrating loss of the window and prominent distal angle *(arrows).*

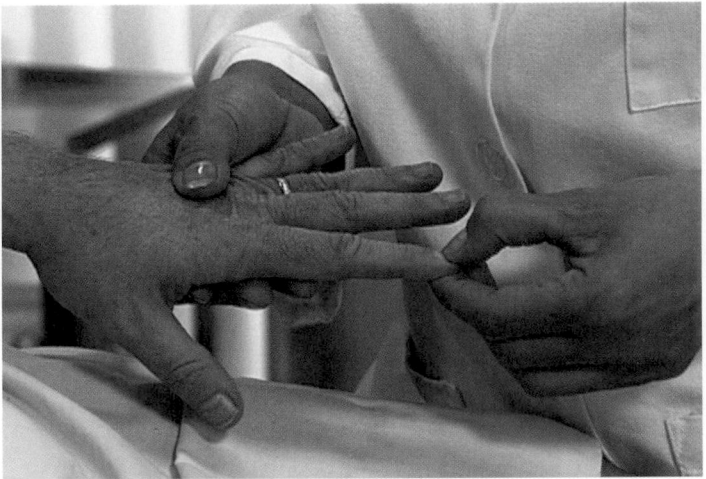

FIGURE 8-18
Testing nail bed adherence.

INFANTS AND CHILDREN

INSPECTION AND PALPATION

In the first few hours of life, the infant's skin may look very red (Fig. 8-19). The more gentle pink coloring that predominates in infancy usually surfaces in the first day after birth. Skin color is partly determined by chubbiness; the less subcutaneous fat, the redder and more transparent the skin. Dark-skinned newborns do not always manifest the intensity of melanosis that will be readily evident in 2 to 3 months. The exceptions in this regard are the nail beds and skin of the scrotum. The expected color changes in newborns are described in Box 8-5.

Physiologic jaundice may be present to a mild degree in as many as 50% or more of newborn infants. It usually starts after the first day of life and disappears by the eighth to tenth day, but may persist for as long as 3 to 4 weeks. Intense and persistent jaundice should suggest liver disease or severe, overwhelming infection. Risk factors for hyperbilirubinemia in the newborn are listed in the Risk Factors box on p. 195.

In examining the newborn for hyperbilirubinemia, look at the whole body. Jaundice begins on the face and descends. The bilirubin level is not high if only the face is involved; however, the bilirubin may well be at a worrisome level if the jaundice descends below the nipples. Be

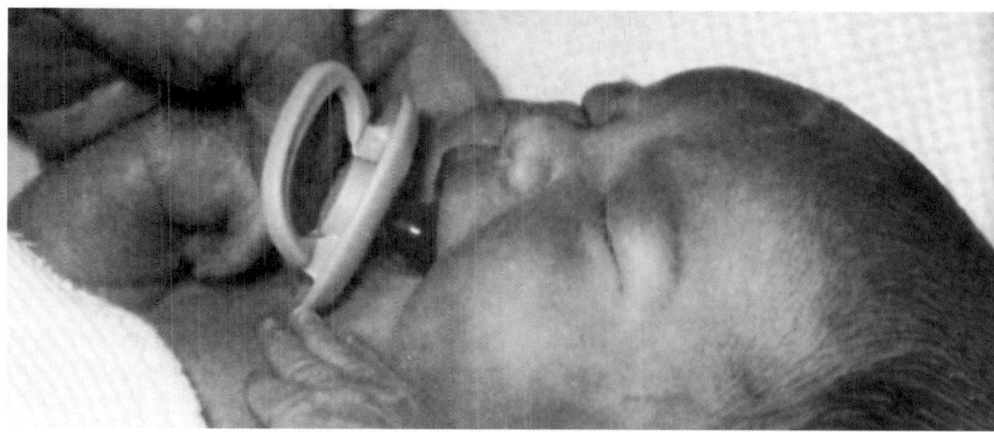

FIGURE 8-19
Ruddy color of newborn.

BOX 8-5

EXPECTED COLOR CHANGES IN THE NEWBORN

Acrocyanosis: Cyanosis of hands and feet

Cutis marmorata: Transient mottling when infant is exposed to decreased temperature

Erythema toxicum: Pink papular rash with vesicles superimposed on thorax, back, buttocks, and abdomen; may appear in 24 to 48 hours and resolves after several days

Harlequin color change: Clearly outlined color change as infant lies on side; dependent lower half of body becomes pink and upper half is pale

Mongolian spots: Irregular areas of deep blue pigmentation, usually in the sacral and gluteal regions; seen predominantly in newborns of African, Native American/American Indian, Asian, or Latin descent

Telangiectatic nevi ("stork bites"): Flat, deep pink localized areas usually seen on back of neck

From Wong et al, 1999.

RISK FACTORS

HYPERBILIRUBINEMIA IN THE NEWBORN

- Breast-feeding (possibly because of β-glucuronidase in breast milk)
- Cephalhematoma or other cutaneous or subcutaneous bleeds
- Infrequent feedings
- Hemolytic disease
- Infection

---

sure to examine the oral mucosa and sclera of the eyes, because jaundice can be detected more easily there than in the skin. Examine the baby in natural daylight if possible. Both artificial light and environmental colors (e.g., orange drapes) can produce a false color.

The skin of the newborn should be checked carefully for small defects, especially over the entire length of the spine; the midline of the head, from the nape of the neck to the bridge of the nose; and the neck extending to the ear. This may offer a clue to sinus tracts, brachial clefts, or cysts. The skin should feel soft and smooth. Also look for skin findings that may signal underlying systemic conditions (Box 8-6).

Inspect the skin for distortions in contour suggestive of hygromas, fluid-containing masses, subcutaneous angiomas, lymphangiomas, hemangiomas, nodules, and tumors. Transillumination may help if there is a question about the density of the mass or the amount of fluid. With more density and less fluid, there is less tendency to glow on transillumination.

BOX 8-6

SKIN LESIONS: EXTERNAL CLUES TO INTERNAL PROBLEMS

Many systemic conditions or disorders may present congenital external clues that are apparent on physical examination. The following are a few examples of cutaneous markers that may signal underlying disease. A thorough evaluation is necessary, although some clues may be isolated findings and may require no intervention, follow-up, or treatment.

Faun tail nevus: Tuft of hair overlying the spinal column at birth, usually in the lumbosacral area; may be associated with spina bifida occulta

Epidermal verrucous nevi: Warty lesions in a linear or whorled pattern that may be pigmented or skin colored; present at birth or in early childhood; associated most commonly with skeletal, central nervous system, and ocular abnormalities

Café au lait patches: Flat, evenly pigmented spots varying in color from light brown to dark brown or black in dark skin; larger than 5 mm in diameter; present at birth or shortly thereafter; may be associated with neurofibromatosis or miscellaneous other conditions including pulmonary stenosis, temporal lobe dysrhythmia, and tuberous sclerosis

Freckling in the axillary or inguinal area: Multiple flat pigmented macules associated with neurofibromatosis; may occur in conjunction with café au lait spots

Facial port-wine stain: When it involves the ophthalmic division of trigeminal nerve, may be associated with ocular defects, most notably glaucoma; or may be accompanied by angiomatous malformation of the meninges (Sturge-Kalischer-Weber syndrome), resulting in atrophy and calcification of the adjacent cerebral cortex

Port-wine stain of limb and/or trunk: When accompanied by venous varicosities and hypertrophy of underlying soft tissues and bones, may be associated with visceral involvement, resulting in bleeding, and/or with limb hypertrophy, resulting in orthopedic problems (Klippel-Trenaunay-Weber syndrome)

Congenital lymphedema with or without transient hemangiomas: May be associated with gonadal dysgenesis caused by absence of an X chromosome, producing an XO karyotype (Turner syndrome)

Supernumerary nipples: Congenital accessory nipples with or without glandular tissue, located along the mammary ridge (see Chapter 16); may be associated with renal abnormalities, especially in the presence of other minor anomalies, particularly in whites

"Hair collar" sign: A ring of long, dark, coarse hair surrounding a midline scalp nodule in infants may indicate neural tube closure defects of the scalp

Persistent pruritus: Persistent pruritus in the absence of skin disease may indicate chronic renal failure, cholestatic liver disease, Hodgkin disease, or diabetes mellitus

---

Examine the hands and feet of newborns for skin creases. Flexion results in creases that are readily discernible on the fingers, palms, and soles (Fig. 8-20). One indicator of maturity is the number of creases; the older the baby, the more creases. Examine the crease patterns of the fingers and palms because certain abnormalities are associated with specific derangements of the patterns (the study of which is known as *dermatoglyphics*). The most commonly recognized crease is the simian line, a single transverse crease in the palm that may be seen in individuals who are otherwise well; however, it is also commonly seen in children with Down syndrome (Fig. 8-21).

All newborn infants are covered to some degree by vernix caseosa, a whitish, moist, cheeselike substance. Transient puffiness of the hands, feet, eyelids, legs, pubis, or sacrum occurs in some newborns. It has no discernible cause and should not create concern if it disappears within 2 to 3 days.

Newborn infants are particularly susceptible to hypothermia, partly because of their poorly developed subcutaneous fat. In addition, infants have a relatively large body surface area, providing greater area for heat loss. Combined with an inability to shiver, these factors cause term newborns to lose heat at a rate four times that of an adult, per unit of body weight.

Cutis marmorata, a mottled appearance of the body and extremities, is part of the newborn's response to changes in ambient temperature, whether cooling or heating. It is more

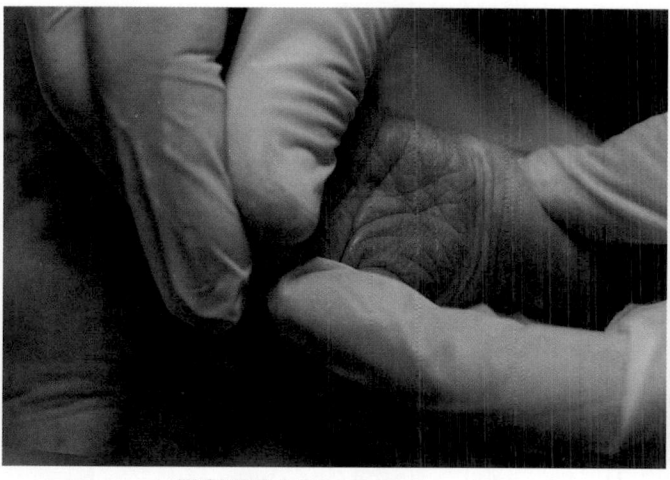
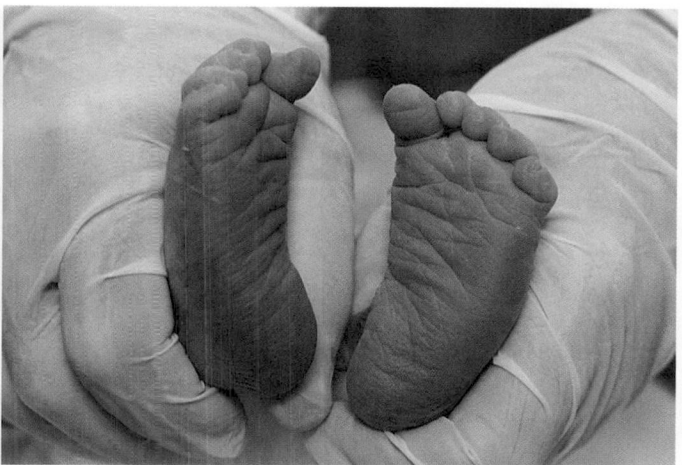

A   B

FIGURE 8-20
Expected creases of newborn's hands (**A**) and feet (**B**).

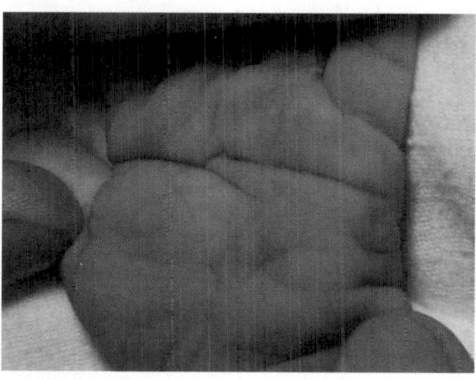

FIGURE 8-21
Unexpected palmar crease.
Simian crease in child with
Down syndrome. Compare to
Fig. 8-20, A.
From Zitelli, Davis, 1997.

common in premature infants and children with Down syndrome and hypothyroidism (Fig. 8-22). Cyanosis of the hands and feet (acrocyanosis) may be present at birth and may persist for several days or longer if the newborn is kept in cool ambient temperatures. It often recurs when the baby is chilled. Generally, when the cyanosis persists, it is more intense in the feet than in the hands, and an underlying cardiac defect should be suspected (Fig. 8-23).

Harlequin color change (dyschromia) often occurs in the normal newborn. One half of the body is more red than the other, with a rather sharp demarcation down the midline. The condition is self-resolving and does not last long.

Bluish-black to slate-gray spots are sometimes seen on the back, buttocks, shoulders, and legs of well babies. These patches, called mongolian spots, occur most often in babies with dark skin and usually disappear in the preschool years. Mongolian spots are easily mistaken for bruises by the inexperienced examiner (Fig. 8-24).

Milia are small whitish, discrete papules on the face; they are commonly found during the first 2 to 3 months of life. The sebaceous glands function in an immature fashion at this age and are easily plugged by sebum (Fig. 8-25).

Sebaceous hyperplasia produces numerous tiny yellow macules and papules in the newborn, probably the result of androgen stimulation from the mother. It commonly occurs on the forehead, cheeks, nose, and chin of the full-term infant. Sebaceous hyperplasia disappears quickly within 1 to 2 months of life.

Mothers and fathers sometimes define the excellence of their parenting by the condition of their baby's skin. Diaper rashes are distressing; a false message to the world that parents may not be clean or knowledgeable about baby care. When you notice a skin problem such as diaper rash or impetigo, try to avoid comments or questions that imply that the parent has done something wrong.

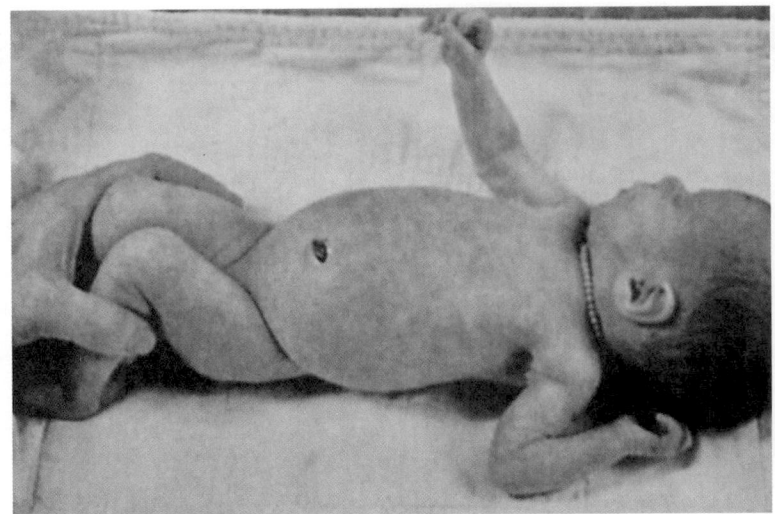

FIGURE 8-22
Mottling (cutis marmorata).
*Courtesy Mead Johnson & Co.,
Evansville, IN.*

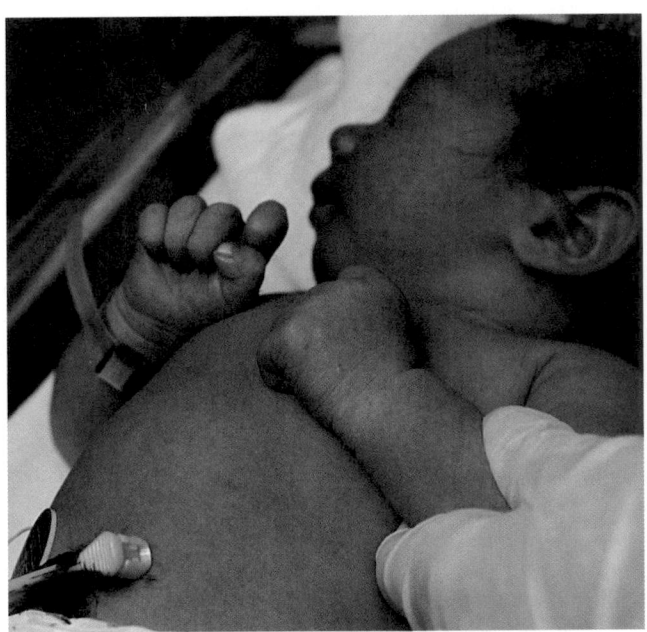

FIGURE 8-23
Acrocyanosis of hands in newborn.

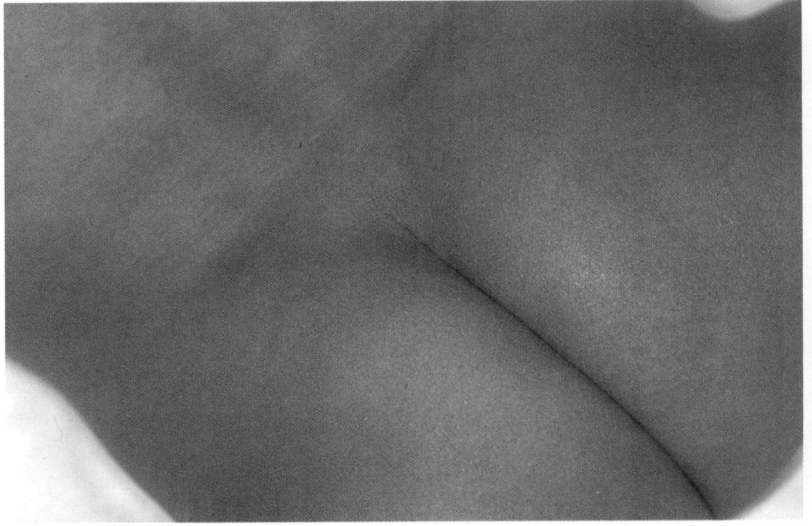

FIGURE 8-24
Mongolian spots are common in
babies with dark skin.
From Lemmi, Lemmi, 2000.

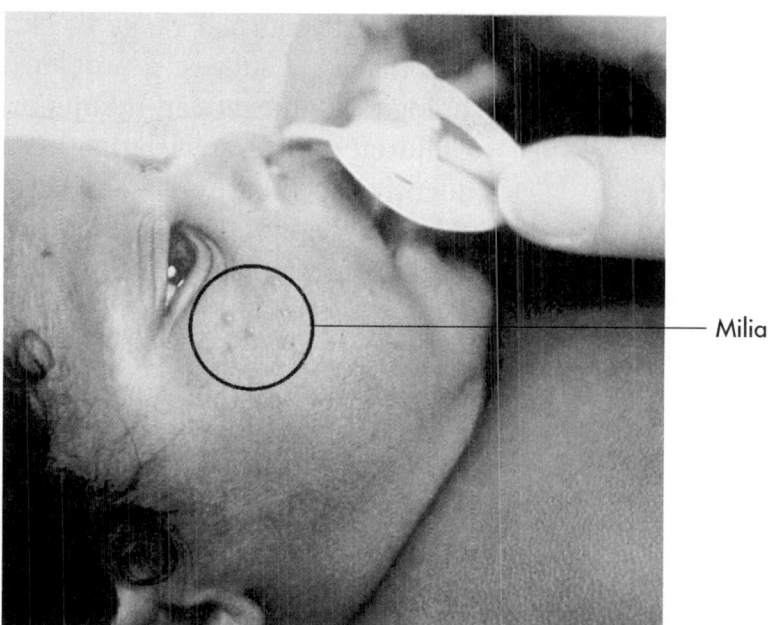

—— Milia

FIGURE 8-25
Milia in infant.

TURGOR

The skin and subcutaneous tissues of an infant and young child, more readily than in the older child and adolescent, can give an important indication of the state of hydration and nutrition (Table 8-7). The tissue turgor is best evaluated by gently pinching a fold of the abdominal skin between the index finger and thumb. As with the adult, resiliency allows it to return to its undisturbed state when released. A child who is seriously dehydrated (i.e., more than 3% to 5% of body weight) or very poorly nourished will have skin that retains "tenting" after it is pinched. How quickly the tent disappears provides a clue to the degree of dehydration or malnutrition (Fig. 8-26).

TABLE 8-7	Estimating Dehydration
Return to Normal After the Pinch	**Degree of Dehydration**
<2 seconds	<5% loss of body weight
2 to 3 seconds	5% to 8% loss of body weight
3 to 4 seconds	9% to 10% loss of body weight
>4 seconds	>10% loss of body weight

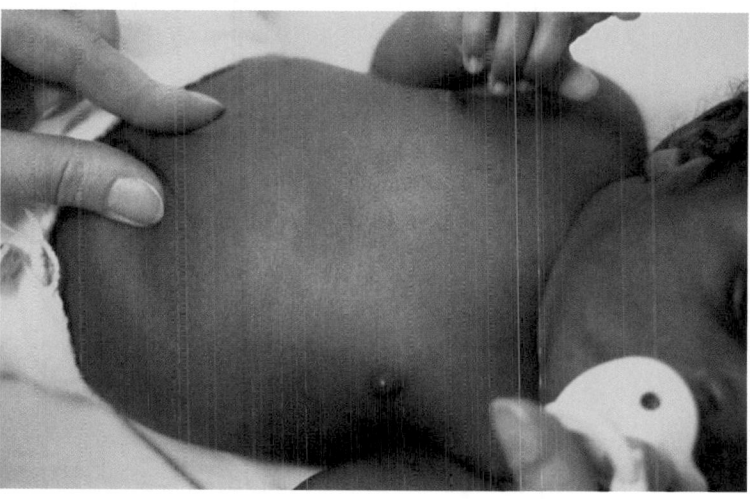

FIGURE 8-26
Testing skin turgor in an infant.

Because the normal range of skin moisture is broad, look at other factors that may suggest a problem. Excessive sweating or dryness alone rarely has pathologic significance in infants or children.

Children with atopic dermatitis or chronic skin changes involving the face will commonly rub their eyes, sufficiently sometimes to cause an extra crease or pleat of skin below the eye. This is known as the Dennie-Morgan fold; it is probably secondary to chronic rubbing and inflammation.

ADOLESCENTS

The examination of the adolescent's skin is the same as that for the adult. The adolescent's skin may have increased oiliness and perspiration, and hair oiliness may also be increased. Increased sebum production predisposes the adolescent to develop acne. Acne is a matter of deep concern to the adolescent. By all means, mention it and do not hesitate to say quite candidly that you understand how much of a problem it can be. This is a time when you might refer to your own adolescent experience.

As a reflection of maturing apocrine gland function, increased axillary perspiration occurs, and the characteristic adult body odor develops during adolescence. Hair on the extremities darkens and becomes coarser. Pubic and axillary hair in both males and females develops and assumes adult characteristics. Males develop facial and chest hair that varies in quantity and coarseness. Chapter 5 provides a more thorough discussion of the maturational changes that occur during adolescence.

PREGNANT WOMEN

Striae gravidarum (stretch marks) may appear over the abdomen, thighs, and breasts during the second trimester of pregnancy. They fade after delivery but never disappear (Fig. 8-27). There is a five-fold increase in telangiectasias (vascular spiders) which may be found on the face, neck, chest, and arms; these appear during the second to fifth month of pregnancy and usually resolve after delivery. Hemangiomas that were present before pregnancy may increase in size, or new ones may develop. Cutaneous tags (molluscum fibrosum gravidarum) are either pedunculated or sessile skin tags that are most often found on the neck and upper chest. They result from epithelial hyperplasia and are not inflammatory. Most resolve spontaneously.

An increase in pigmentation is common and is found to some extent in all pregnant women. The areas usually affected include the areolae and nipples, vulvar and perianal regions, axillae, and the linea alba. Pigmentation of the linea alba is called the linea nigra. It extends from the symphysis pubis to the top of the fundus in the midline (Fig. 8-28). Preexisting pigmented moles (nevi) and freckles may darken, with some nevi increasing in size. New nevi may form. The chloasma or "mask of pregnancy" occurs in approximately 70% of pregnant women and is found on the forehead, cheeks, bridge of the nose, and chin. It is blotchy in appearance and is usually symmetric (Fig. 8-29).

Palmar erythema is a common finding in pregnancy. A diffuse redness covers the entire palmar surface or the thenar and hypothenar eminences. The cause is unknown, and it usually disappears after delivery.

Itching over the abdomen and breasts resulting from stretching is common and not a cause for concern; however, itching accompanied by a rash may signal a pregnancy-specific der-

PHYSICAL VARIATIONS

Areolar Pigmentation

Areolar pigmentation varies by race, with blacks having the darkest areolae, whites the lightest, and Asians and Native Americans/American Indians intermediate. Despite common belief, there is no correlation between the color of the areola and nipple damage from breastfeeding.

Data from Pawson, Petrakis, 1975; Gans, 1958; Brown, Hurlock, 1975.

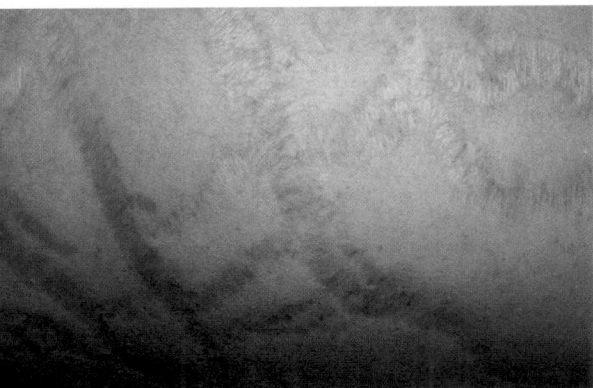

FIGURE 8-27
Striae.
Courtesy Antoinette Hood, MD, Department of Dermatology, Indiana University School of Medicine, Indianapolis.

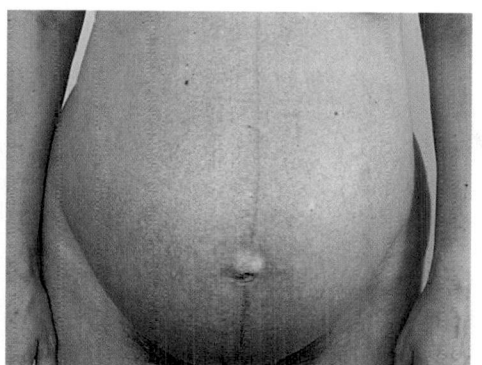

FIGURE 8-28
Linea nigra on abdomen of pregnant woman.

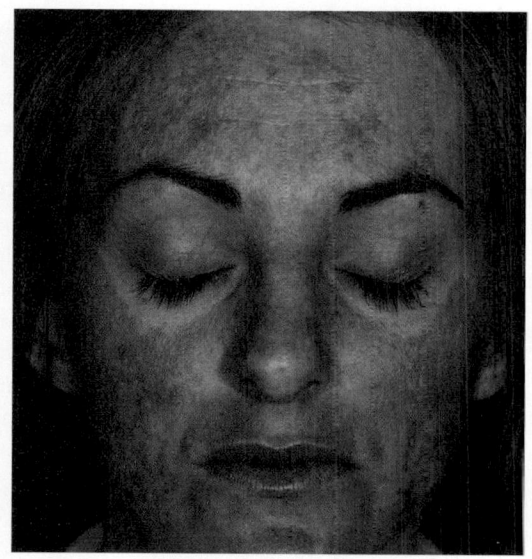

FIGURE 8-29
Facial hyperpigmentation: chloasma (melasma).
From Habif, 2004.

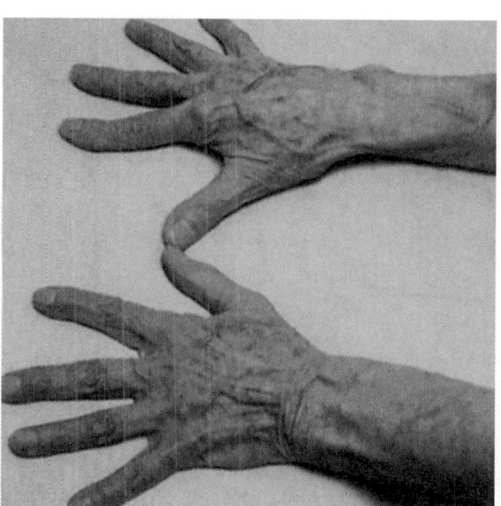

FIGURE 8-30
Hands of older adult. Note prominent veins and thin appearance of skin.

matosis, which requires further investigation. Itching during pregnancy can also be caused by impaired flow of bile from the liver, which may also produce jaundice. The itching is generalized but may be more severe on the palms and soles. Be alert to these serious manifestations of underlying pathology. Hair growth is altered in pregnancy by the circulating hormones. The growing phase of the hair is lengthened and hair loss is decreased. Two to four months after delivery, increased hair shedding occurs. Regrowth will occur in 6 to 12 months. Acne vulgaris may be aggravated during the first trimester of pregnancy but often improves in the third trimester.

OLDER ADULTS

The skin of the older adult may appear more transparent and paler in light-skinned individuals. Pigment deposits, increased freckling, and hypopigmented patches may develop, causing the skin to take on a less uniform appearance.

Flaking or scaling, associated with the drier skin that comes with aging, occurs most commonly over the extremities. The skin also becomes thinner (especially over bony prominences, the dorsal surface of hands and feet, forearms, and lower legs) and takes on a parchment-like appearance and texture (Fig. 8-30).

The skin often appears to hang loosely on the bony frame as a result of a general loss of elasticity, loss of underlying adipose tissue, and years of gravitational pull (Fig. 8-31). You may

PHYSICAL VARIATIONS
Wrinkles
Whites wrinkle sooner and their hair turns gray earlier than do other races; this can cause whites to underestimate the age of persons from other races. Conversely, persons from other races often overestimate the age of white individuals.

observe tenting of the skin when testing for turgor (Fig. 8-32). Thus in older adults turgor may not be a reliable or valid estimate of hydration status.

The immobility of some older adults, especially when combined with decreased peripheral vascular circulation, places them at risk for the development of decubitus ulcers (pressure sores). During examination, pay particular attention to bony prominences and areas subject to persistent pressure or shearing forces. Heels and the sacrum are common sites in patients who are confined to bed. Do not neglect to examine less obvious areas such as the elbows, scapulae, and back of the head. Assess the diameter and depth of the ulcer and stage it accordingly. The staging criteria are described in Box 8-7.

Increased wrinkling is evident, especially in areas exposed to sun and in expressive areas of the face. Sagging or drooping is most obvious under the chin, beneath the eyes, and in the earlobes, breasts, and scrotum. Purpura, particularly dorsal surfaces of hands and lower arm that get tapped or bumped, is commonly seen in older adults on aspirin therapy.

Several types of lesions may occur on the skin of healthy older adults. The following lesions are considered expected findings:

- Cherry angiomas are tiny, bright ruby-red, round papules that may become brown with time. They occur in virtually everyone older than 30 years of age and increase numerically with age (Fig. 8-33).
- Seborrheic keratoses are pigmented, raised, warty lesions, usually appearing on the face or trunk. These must be distinguished from actinic keratoses, which have malignant potential. Because the lesions may look similar, seek the assistance of an experienced practitioner for differential diagnosis (Fig. 8-34).

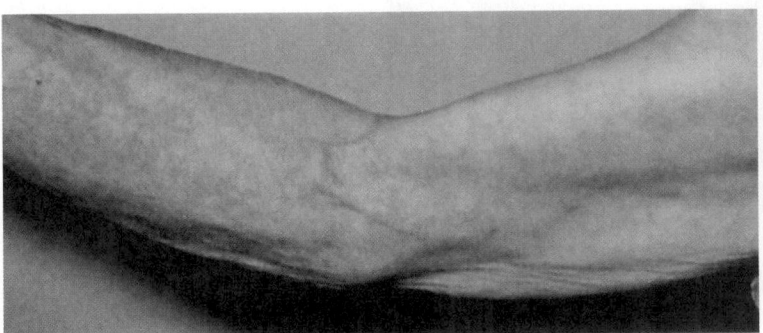

FIGURE 8-31
Skin hanging loosely, especially around bony prominences.

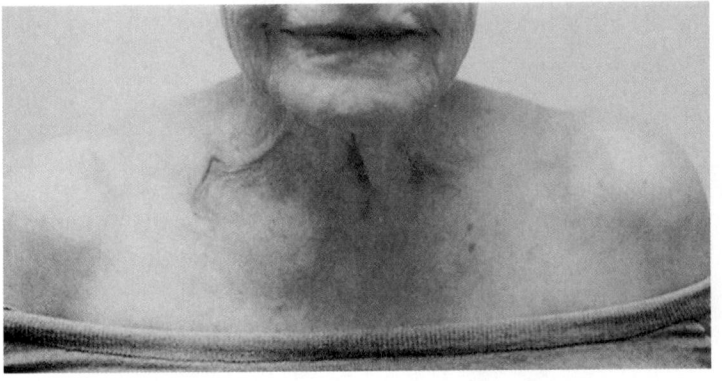

FIGURE 8-32
Skin turgor in older adult. Note tenting.

BOX 8-7

STAGING OF DECUBITUS ULCERS (PRESSURE SORES)

Stage I	Skin red but not broken
Stage II	Damage through epidermis and dermis
Stage III	Damage through to subcutaneous tissue
Stage IV	Muscle and possible bone involvement

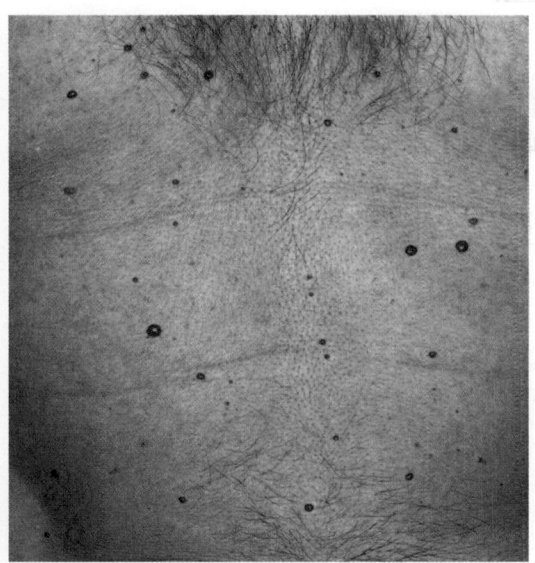

FIGURE 8-33
Cherry angioma in older adult.
From Habif, 2004.

- Sebaceous hyperplasia occurs as yellowish, flattened papules with central depressions (Fig. 8-35).
- Cutaneous tags (acrochordon) are small, soft tags of skin, usually appearing on the neck and upper chest. They are attached to the body by a narrow stalk (pedunculated) and may or may not be pigmented (Fig. 8-36).
- Cutaneous horns are small, hard projections of the epidermis, usually occurring on the forehead and face (Fig. 8-37).
- Senile lentigines are irregular, round, gray-brown lesions with a rough surface that occur in sun-exposed areas. These are often referred to as "age spots" or incorrectly as "liver spots" (Fig. 8-38).

The hair turns gray or white as melanocytes cease functioning. Head, body, pubic, and axillary hair thins and becomes sparse and drier. Men may show an increase in coarse aural, nasal, and eyebrow hair; women tend to develop coarse facial hair. Symmetric balding, usually frontal or occipital, often occurs in men.

The nails thicken, become more brittle, and may be deformed, misshapen, striated, distorted, or peeling. They can take on a yellowish color and may lose their transparency. These changes occur most often in the toenails.

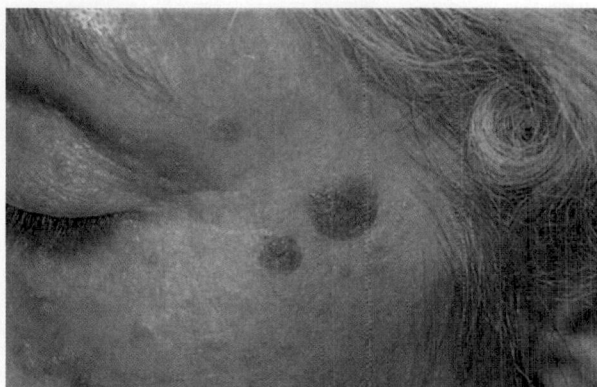

FIGURE 8-34
Seborrheic keratoses in older adult.
From Lawrence, Cox, 1993.

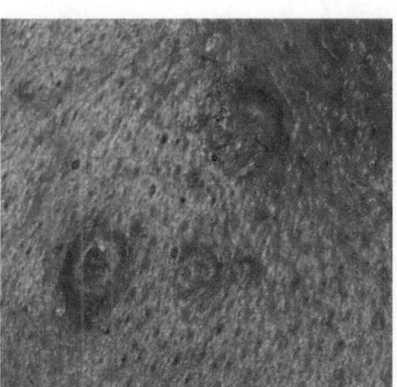

FIGURE 8-35
Sebaceous hyperplasia in older adult.
From Habif, 2004.

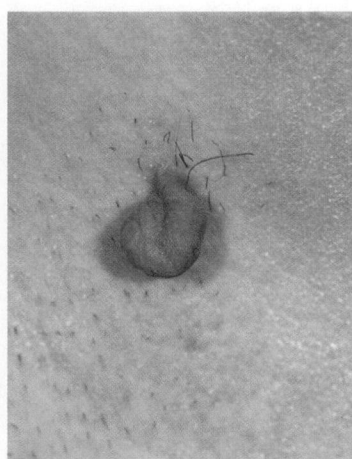

FIGURE 8-36
Cutaneous tag in older adult.
From Habif, 2004.

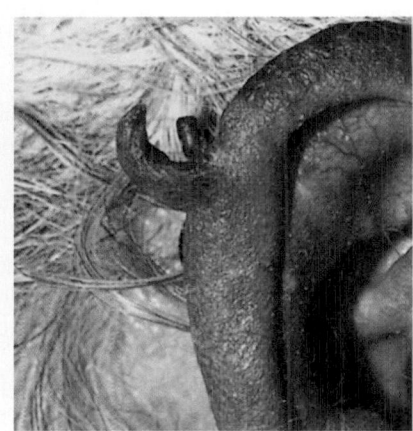

FIGURE 8-37
Cutaneous horn.
From White, 1994.

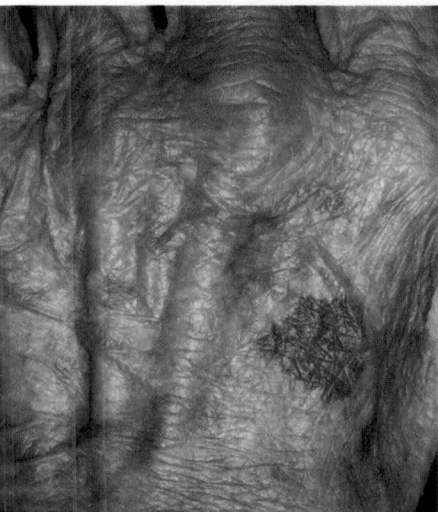

FIGURE 8-38
Lentigo, a brown macule that appears in sun-exposed areas.
From Habif, 2004.

SAMPLE DOCUMENTATION

HISTORY AND PHYSICAL EXAMINATION

Subjective

An 18-year-old female with body rash for 4 days. First noticed rash 4 days ago. Thinks it may be from drinking new citrus juice. Describes rash as red, itchy, transient bumps on face, neck, arms, legs, and torso. No known food allergies. Denies exposure to new contact irritants. No new medications; is currently taking antihistamine for allergic rhinitis. Denies respiratory difficulty, difficulty swallowing, and edema. Denies fever, cough, and malaise.

For additional sample documentation, see Chapter 26.

Objective

Skin: Dark pink macular-papular lesions on face, torso, and extremities; large urticarial wheal on right cheek. No excoriation or secondary infection. Turgor resilient. Skin uniformly warm and dry. No edema.

Hair: Curly, black, thick with female distribution pattern. Texture coarse.

Nails: Opaque, short, well-groomed, uniform and without deformities. Nail bed pink. Nail base angle 160 degrees. No redness, exudates, or swelling in the surrounding folds, and no tenderness to palpation.

SUMMARY OF EXAMINATION

SKIN, HAIR, AND NAILS

Skin

1. Perform overall inspection of entire skin surface (p. 176). During evaluation of each organ system, evaluate the overlying skin for the following characteristics:
   - Color
   - Uniformity
   - Thickness
   - Symmetry
   - Hygiene
   - Lesions (record size, shape, location, configuration, color, blanching, texture, elevation or depression, pediculation, presence of exudates, pattern of distribution, configuration) (p. 182, 189)
   - Odors
2. Palpate skin surfaces for the following (p. 181):
   - Moisture
   - Temperature
   - Texture
   - Turgor
   - Mobility

Hair

1. Inspect hair for the following (p. 191):
   - Color
   - Distribution
   - Quantity
2. Palpate hair for texture (p. 191)

Nails

1. Inspect for the following: (p. 191)
   - Pigmentation of nails and beds
   - Length
   - Symmetry
   - Ridging, beading, pitting, peeling
2. Measure nail base angle (p. 192)
3. Inspect and palpate proximal and lateral nail folds for the following (p. 192):
   - Redness
   - Swelling
   - Pain
   - Exudate
   - Warts, cysts, tumors
4. Palpate nail plate for the following (p. 192):
   - Texture
   - Firmness
   - Thickness
   - Uniformity
   - Adherence to nail bed

COMMON ABNORMALITIES

SKIN: NONMALIGNANT ABNORMALITIES

CORN

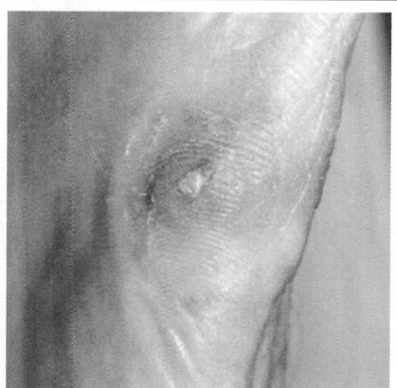

FIGURE 8-39
Corn.
From White, 1994.

Corns are flat or slightly elevated, circumscribed, painful lesions with a smooth, hard surface. "Soft" corns are caused by the pressure of a bony prominence against softer tissue; these appear as whitish thickenings, commonly between the fourth and fifth toes. "Hard" corns are sharply delineated and have a conical appearance; they occur most often over bony prominences where pressure is exerted, such as from shoes pressing on the interphalangeal joints of the toes (Fig. 8-39).

CALLUS

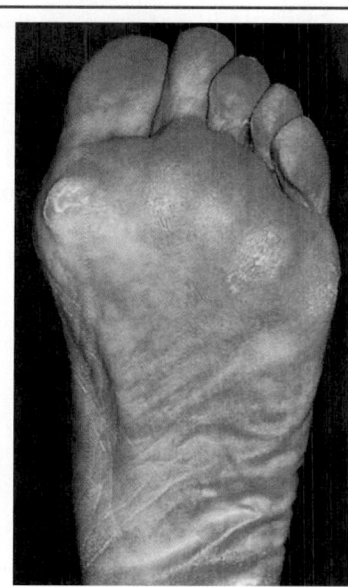

FIGURE 8-40
Calluses are common on both the sole (heels and metatarsal heads) and the dorsum of the foot (especially in women).
From Lawrence, Cox, 1993.

A superficial area of hyperkeratosis is called a callus. Calluses usually occur on the weight-bearing areas of the feet and on the palmar surface of the hands. Calluses are less well demarcated than corns and are usually not tender (Fig. 8-40).

ECZEMATOUS DERMATITIS

The most common inflammatory skin disorder is eczematous dermatitis. There are several types, including primary contact dermatitis, allergic contact dermatitis, and atopic dermatitis. The common factor of the various forms is epidermal breakdown, usually as a result of intracellular vesiculation. Eczematous dermatitis has three stages: acute, subacute, and chronic. The acute phase is characterized by erythematous, pruritic, weeping vesicles (Fig. 8-41). Excoriation from scratching predisposes to infection and causes crust formation. Subacute eczema is characterized by erythema and scaling. Itching may or may not be present. In the chronic stage, thick, lichenified, pruritic plaques are present.

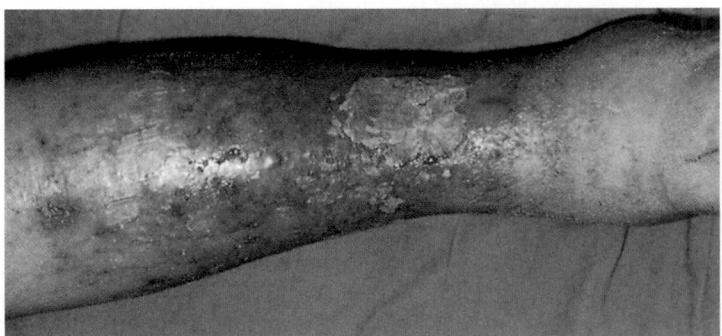

FIGURE 8-41
Contact dermatitis.
From Morison, Moffatt, 1994.

FURUNCLE

A furuncle is an acute localized staphylococcal infection. It develops initially as a small perifollicular abscess and spreads to the surrounding dermis and subcutaneous tissue. The initial nodule becomes a pustule surrounded by erythema and edema. The skin is red, hot, and tender. The center of the lesion fills with pus and forms a core that may rupture spontaneously or require surgical incision (Fig. 8-42).

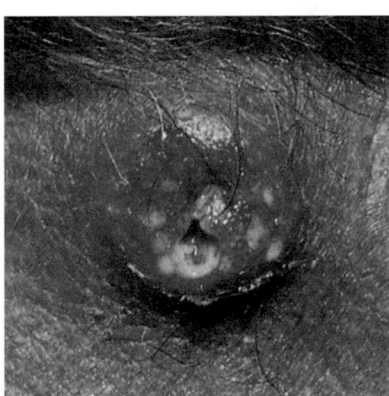

FIGURE 8-42
Furuncle.
Courtesy Jaime A. Tschen, MD, Baylor College of Medicine, Department of Dermatology, Houston; from Thompson et al, 1993.

FOLLICULITIS

Staphylococcal infection of the hair follicle and surrounding dermis produces folliculitis. The primary lesion is a small pustule 1 to 2 cm in diameter that is located over a pilosebaceous orifice and may be perforated by a hair. The pustule may be surrounded by inflammation or nodular lesions. After the pustule ruptures, a crust forms (Fig. 8-43).

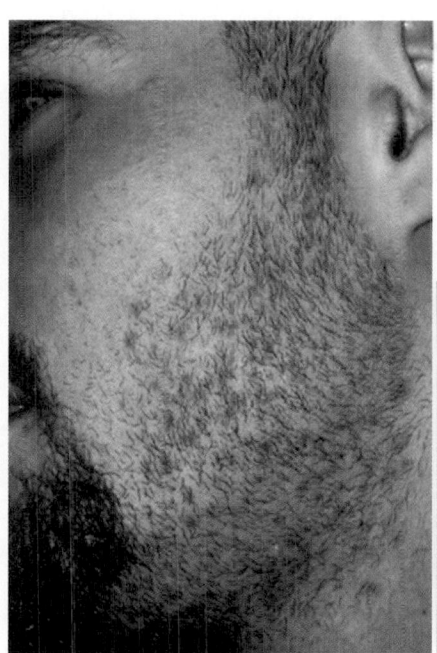
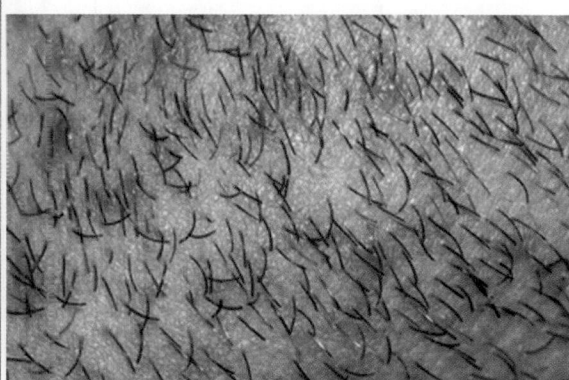

FIGURE 8-43
Beard folliculitis.
From Lemmi, Lemmi, 2000.

CELLULITIS

Diffuse, acute, streptococcal, or staphylococcal infection of the skin and subcutaneous tissue is called cellulitis. The skin is red, hot, tender, and indurated. Lymphangitic streaks and regional lymphadenopathy may be present (Fig. 8-44).

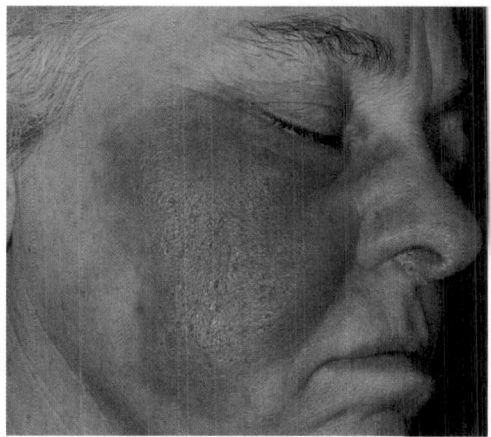

FIGURE 8-44
Streptococcal cellulitis; acute phase with intense erythema (erysipelas).
From Habif, 2004.

TINEA (DERMATOPHYTOSIS)

Tinea is a group of noncandidal fungal infections that involve the stratum corneum, nails, or hair. The lesions are usually classified according to anatomic location and can occur on non-hairy parts of the body (tinea corporis), on the groin and inner thigh (tinea cruris), on the scalp (tinea capitis), on the feet (tinea pedis), and on the nails (tinea unguium). The lesions vary in appearance and may be papular, pustular, vesicular, erythematous, or scaling. Secondary bacterial infection may be present (Fig. 8-45).

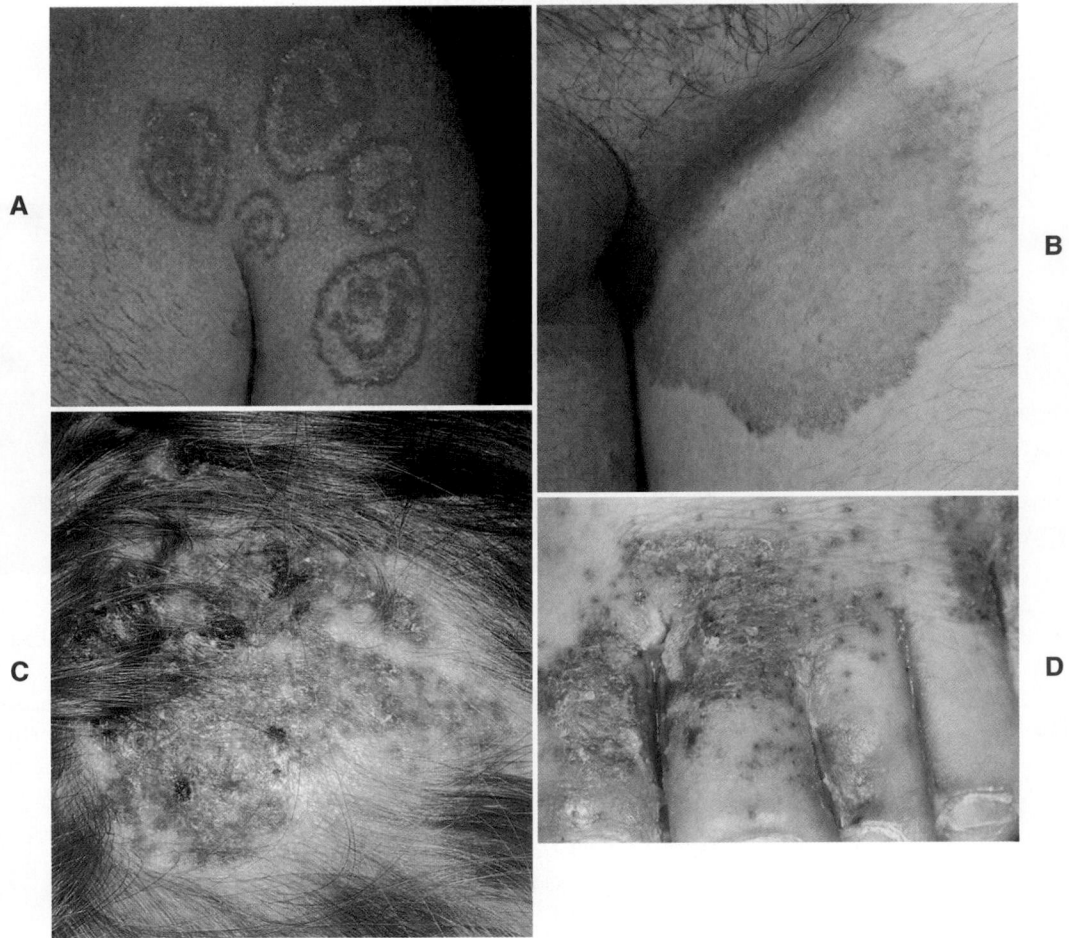

FIGURE 8-45
A, Tinea corporis. **B,** Tinea cruris. **C,** Tinea capitis. **D,** Tinea pedis.
From Habif, 2004.

PITYRIASIS ROSEA

Pityriasis rosea is a self-limiting inflammation of unknown cause. Onset is sudden with occurrence of a primary (herald) oval or round plaque with fine, superficial scaling (Fig. 8-46). A generalized eruption occurs 1 to 3 weeks later and lasts for several weeks. The lesions develop on the extremities and trunk; the palms and soles are not involved, and facial involvement is rare. The trunk lesions are characteristically distributed in parallel alignment following the direction of the ribs in a Christmas tree–like pattern. The lesions are usually pale, erythematous, and macular with fine scaling, but they may be papular or vesicular. Pruritus may be present. The condition is not infectious or contagious.

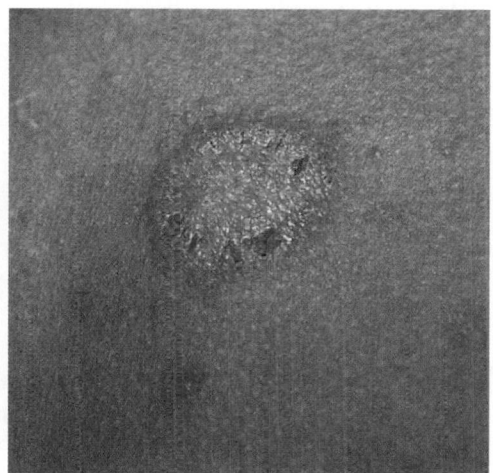

FIGURE 8-46
Pityriasis rosea herald patch.
Courtesy Walter Tunnessen, MD, University of Pennsylvania School of Medicine, Philadelphia.

PSORIASIS

Psoriasis is a chronic and recurrent disease of keratin synthesis that is characterized by well-circumscribed, dry, silvery, scaling papules and plaques. Lesions commonly occur on the back, buttocks, extensor surfaces of the extremities, and the scalp (Fig. 8-47).

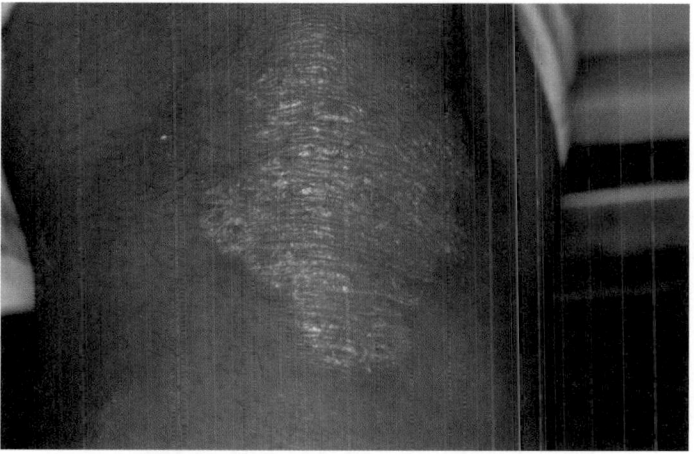

FIGURE 8-47
Psoriasis on extensor surface of knee. Note characteristic silver scaling.
From Lemmi, Lemmi, 2000.

ROSACEA

Rosacea is a chronic inflammatory skin disorder that is characterized by telangiectasia, erythema, papules, and pustules that occur particularly in the central area of the face (Fig. 8-48). Tissue hypertrophy of the nose (rhinophyma) may occur. Rhinophyma is characterized by sebaceous hyperplasia, redness, prominent vascularity, and swelling of the skin of the nose (Fig. 8-49). The cause of rosacea is unknown, but it occurs most often in persons with a fair complexion. Although rosacea resembles acne, comedones are never present. Antibiotic therapy is usually effective in treating the condition. Rhinophyma may require surgical intervention.

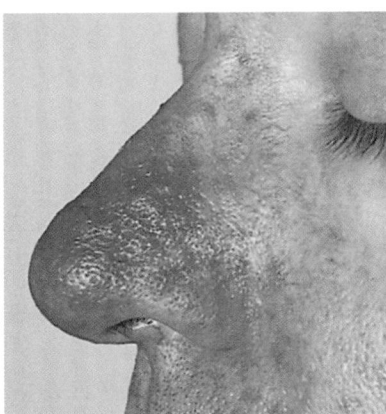

FIGURE 8-48
Rosacea.
From White, 1994.

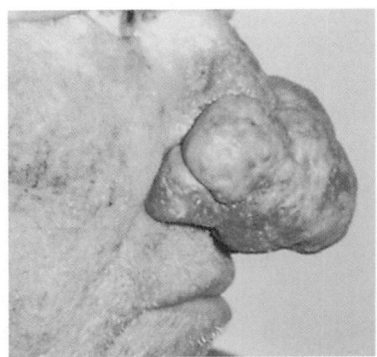

FIGURE 8-49
Rhinophyma.
Courtesy Michael O. Murphy, MD; from White, 1994.

DRUG ERUPTIONS

The most common skin reaction to a drug consists of discrete or confluent erythematous maculopapules on the trunk, face, extremities, palms, or soles of the feet. The rash appears from 1 to several days after starting the drug and fades in 1 to 3 weeks. Pruritus is characteristic (Fig. 8-50).

FIGURE 8-50
Drug eruption—hives. The most characteristic presentation is uniformly red edematous plaques surrounded by a faint white halo. These superficial lesions occur from transudation of fluid into the dermis.
From Habif, 2004.

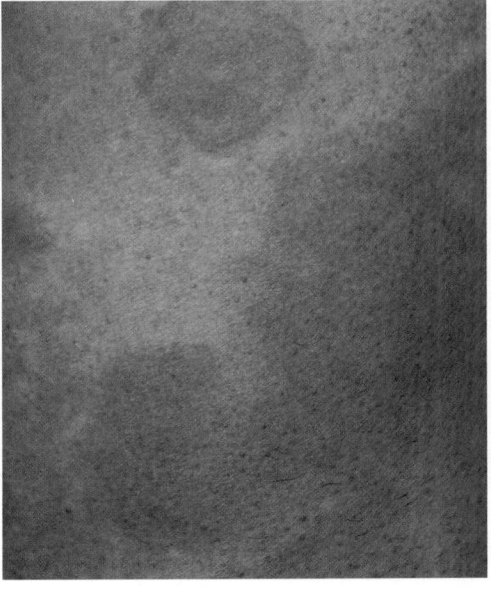

HERPES ZOSTER (SHINGLES)

Herpes zoster is a viral (varicella-zoster) infection, usually of a single dermatome, that consists of red, swollen plaques or vesicles that become filled with purulent fluid. Pain, itching, or burning of the dermatome area usually precedes eruption by 4 to 5 days (Fig. 8-51).

CLINICAL PEARL

Herpes Zoster
A reminder: Pain in the distribution of a dermatome can start many days before a rash appears with herpes zoster, an important clue when early treatment is sought.

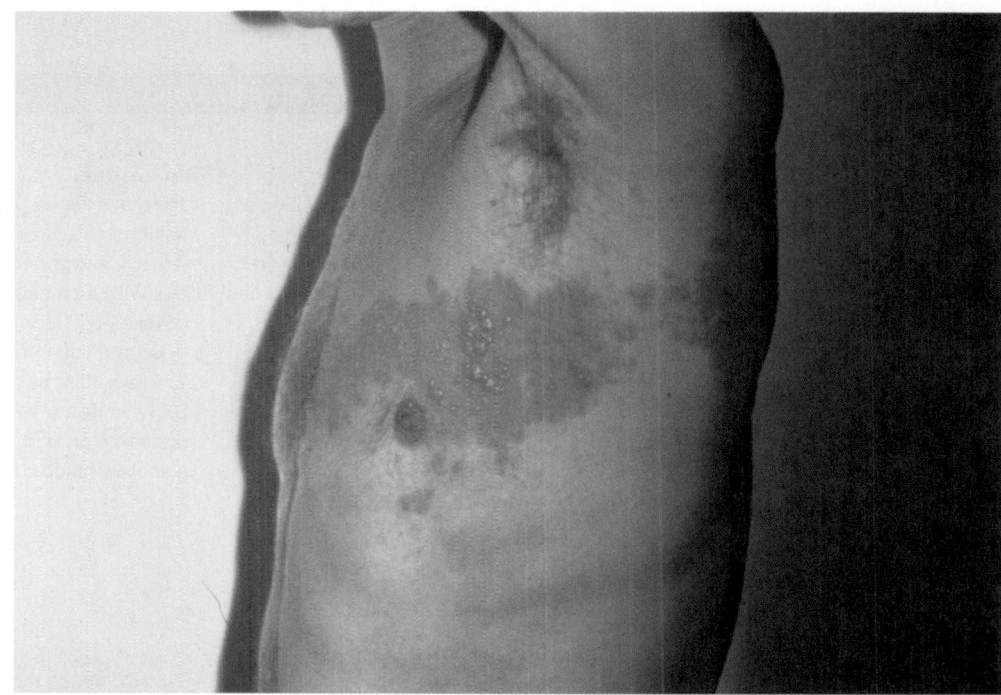

FIGURE 8-51
Herpes zoster (shingles) confined to one dermatome.
From Lemmi, Lemmi, 2000.

HERPES SIMPLEX

Viral infection by herpes simplex produces tenderness, pain, paresthesia, or mild burning at the infected site before onset of the lesions. Grouped vesicles appear on an erythematous base and then erode, forming a crust. Lesions last 2 to 6 weeks. Two different virus types cause the infection. Type 1 is usually associated with oral infection and type 2 with genital infection; however, crossover infections are becoming increasingly common (Fig. 8-52).

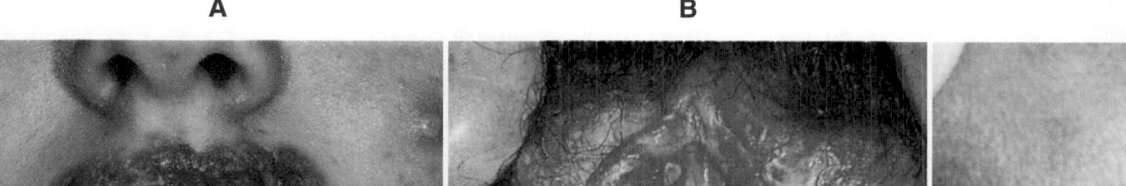

| A | B | C |

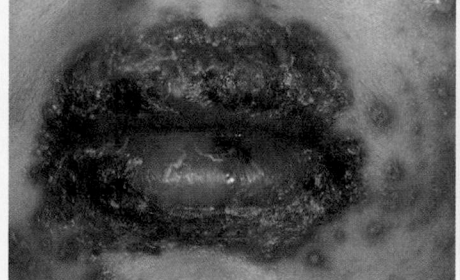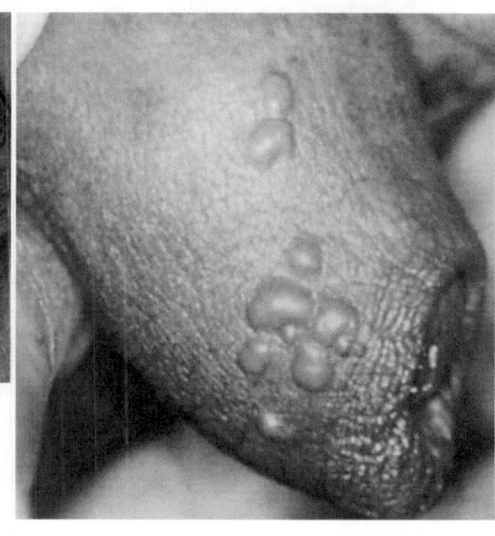

FIGURE 8-52
Herpes simplex. **A,** Oral. **B,** Female genital. **C,** Male genital.
A, B from Habif, 2004; C from Morse, Moreland, Holmes, 1996.

DISEASE CAUSED BY BIOLOGIC WARFARE

Of the numerous biologic agents that may be used as weapons, a limited number produce skin lesions. The Differential Diagnosis box below describes the cutaneous manifestations from two such pathogens.

DIFFERENTIAL DIAGNOSIS

CUTANEOUS MANIFESTATIONS OF TWO PATHOGENS THAT MAY BE USED IN BIOLOGIC WARFARE

Disease	Pathogen	Communicability	Incubation	Skin Lesions	Accompanying Symptoms
Cutaneous anthrax*	Spore-forming bacterium *Bacillus anthracis*	Direct person-to-person spread extremely unlikely	Up to 12 days following deposition of organism into skin with previous abrasion	Pruritic macule or papule that enlarges into a round ulcer by day 2. Central necrosis develops with a painless ulcer covered by black eschar, which dries and falls off in 1 to 2 weeks. May be accompanied by 1- to 3-mm vesicles that discharge clear or serosanguineous fluid.	Lymphangitis; lymphadenopathy.

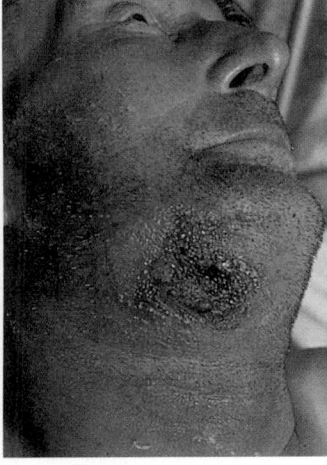

Anthrax (skin form). A Gram-stained smear of material taken from the lesion will reveal the gram-positive rods of *Bacillus anthracis*.
From Beeching, Nye, 1996.

| Smallpox | Variola virus | Direct transmission by infected saliva droplets. Most infectious during the first week of illness. However, some risk of transmission lasts until all scabs have fallen off. Contaminated clothing or bed linen could also spread the virus | 12 days (range: 7 to 17 days) following exposure | Rash appears 2 to 3 days after systemic symptoms, first on the mucosa of the mouth and pharynx, face and forearms, spreading to the trunk and legs. Starts with flat red lesions that evolve at the same rate (compared with varicella, which matures in crops). Lesions become vesicular, then pustular and begin to crust early in the second week. | Initial systemic symptoms include high fever, fatigue, headache, and backache. |

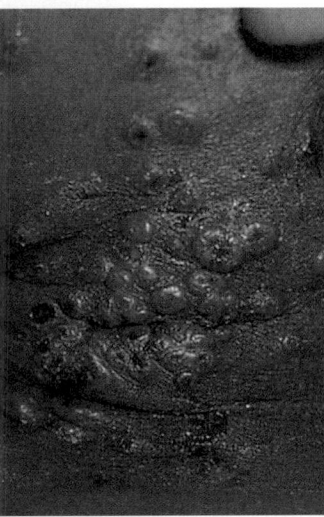

Smallpox. This archival photograph shows eczema vaccinatum acquired from a relative who had recently been vaccinated against smallpox.
From Beeching, Nye, 1996.

*Respiratory and gastrointestinal forms of anthrax also exist.

SKIN: MALIGNANT ABNORMALITIES

BASAL CELL CARCINOMA

Basal cell carcinoma is the most common form of skin cancer. It occurs most frequently on exposed parts of the body—the face, ears, neck, scalp, shoulders, and back. Persons with chronic sun exposure and fair skin are at highest risk (Box 8-8). This cancer arises in the basal layer of the epidermis. It occurs in various clinical forms including nodular, pigmented, cystic, sclerosing, and superficial (Fig. 8-53).

BOX 8-8

THE FIVE WARNING SIGNS OF BASAL CELL CARCINOMA

An open sore that bleeds, oozes, or crusts and does not heal in 3 or more weeks.

A reddish patch or irritated area, frequently occurring on the chest, shoulders, arms, or legs. The patch may crust or itch.

A shiny nodule that is pearly or translucent and is often pink, red, or white. The nodule can also be tan, black, or brown, especially in dark-haired people.

A pink growth with a slightly elevated rolled border and a crusted indentation in the center. As the growth slowly enlarges, tiny blood vessels may develop on the surface.

A scarlike area that is white, yellow or waxy, and often has poorly defined borders. The skin appears shiny and taut.

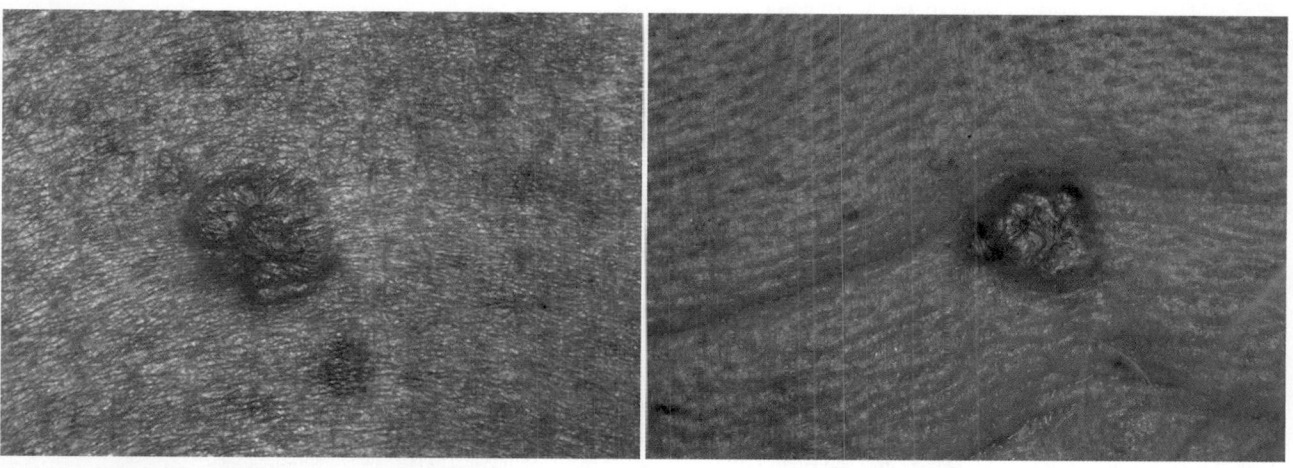

FIGURE 8-53
Two common presentations of basal cell carcinoma.
From Lemmi, Lemmi, 2000.

SQUAMOUS CELL CARCINOMA

Squamous cell carcinoma is the second most common skin cancer. This malignant tumor arises in the epithelium. It occurs most commonly in sun-exposed areas, particularly the scalp, back of hands, lower lip, and ear. The rim of the ear and the lower lip are especially vulnerable. The lesions are soft, mobile, elevated masses with a surface scale (Box 8-9). The base of the lesion may be inflamed (Fig. 8-54). See the Risk Factors box below for risk factors associated with basal cell and squamous cell carcinoma.

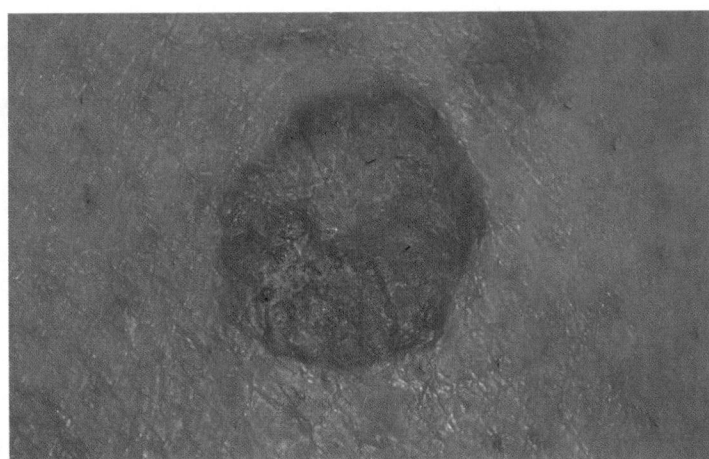

FIGURE 8-54
Squamous cell carcinoma.
From Lemmi, Lemmi, 2000.

BOX 8-9

THE WARNING SIGNS OF SQUAMOUS CELL CARCINOMA

A **wartlike growth** that crusts and occasionally bleeds.
A persistent, **scaly red patch** with irregular borders that sometimes crusts or bleeds.
An **open sore** that bleeds and crusts and persists for weeks.
An **elevated growth with a central depression** that occasionally bleeds. A growth of this type may rapidly increase in size.

RISK FACTORS

BASAL AND SQUAMOUS CELL CARCINOMA

- Age (older than 50 years of age)
- Chronic exposure to sunlight or ultraviolet radiation (UVA and UVB)
- Fair, freckled, ruddy complexion
- Light-colored hair or eyes
- Tendency to sunburn easily
- Blistering sunburns as a child
- Geographic location: near equator or at high altitudes
- Exposure to arsenic, creosote, coal tar, and/or petroleum products
- Overexposure to radium, radioisotopes, or x-rays
- Repeated trauma or irritation to skin
- Precancerous dermatoses

MALIGNANT MELANOMA

Malignant melanoma (Fig. 8-55) is a skin cancer that develops from melanocytes. These cells migrate into the skin, eye, central nervous system, and mucous membrane during fetal development. Less than half of the melanomas develop from nevi; the majority arise de novo from melanocytes. The exact cause of malignancy is not known; heredity, hormonal factors, ultraviolet light exposure, or an autoimmunologic effect may contribute to causation. The risk factors for melanoma are listed in the Risk Factors box below. Malignant melanoma is recognizable in its early stages and should be suspected in any patient with a history of change in a preexisting nevus or with a new pigmented lesion that exhibits any of the irregularities described in the ABCD Rule (Fig. 8-56).

MNEMONICS

The ABCD Rule of Melanoma

Here is a simple way to remember the characteristics that should alert you to the possibility of malignant melanoma:

A Asymmetry of lesion. One-half of a mole or birthmark does not match the other.

B Borders. Edges are irregular, ragged, notched, or blurred. Pigment may be streaming from the border.

C Color. The color is not the same all over and may have differing shades of brown or black, sometimes with patches of red, white, or blue.

D Diameter. The diameter is >6 mm (about the size of a pencil eraser) or is growing larger

RISK FACTORS

MELANOMA

Highest Risk
- Previous history melanoma
- New mole or preexisting mole that has changed or is changing
- Dysplastic nevi and family history of melanoma (first degree relative)
- Family history of melanoma (first degree relative)
- Several dysplastic or atypical nevi

Increased Risk
- >50 nondysplastic nevi
- Large congential nevus (>15 cm)
- Immune suppression
- Fair skin, light eyes
- Severe blistering sunburns as child or teen
- Sun sensitivity, relative inability to tan

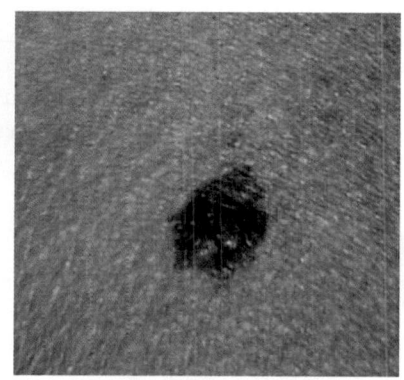

FIGURE 8-55
Malignant melanoma.
Courtesy Walter Tunnessen, MD, University of Pennsylvania, Philadelphia.

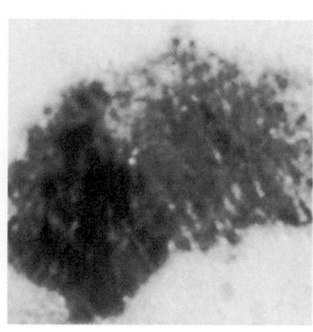
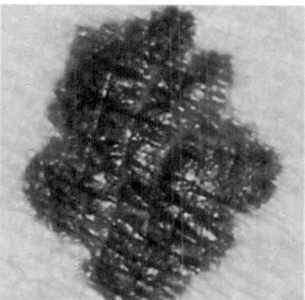
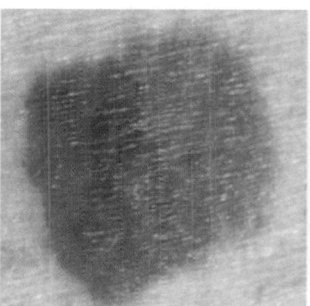
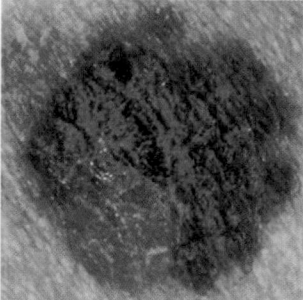

Asymmetry   Border   Color   Diameter

FIGURE 8-56
ABCD changes in moles.
From American Academy of Dermatology, 2005.

KAPOSI SARCOMA

Kaposi sarcoma (KS) is a malignant tumor of the endothelium and epithelial layer of the skin. Lesions are characteristically soft, vascular, bluish-purple, and painless. Lesions may be either macular or papular and may appear as plaques, keloids, or ecchymotic areas (Fig. 8-57). Until recently, KS was rare in the United States and was limited to a mild cutaneous form. With the spread of HIV infection, KS has become a common opportunistic infection. The form of the disease is aggressive, with cutaneous lesions as well as lesions in the gastrointestinal tract and other organs such as the lungs, liver, viscera, bones, and lymph nodes. Patients have varying degrees of cutaneous and systemic involvement. Diagnosis of KS is made by biopsy of suspect tissue or skin lesions.

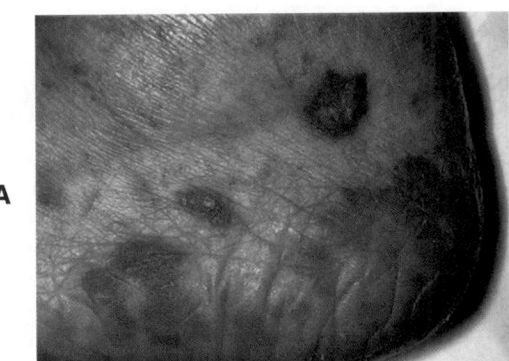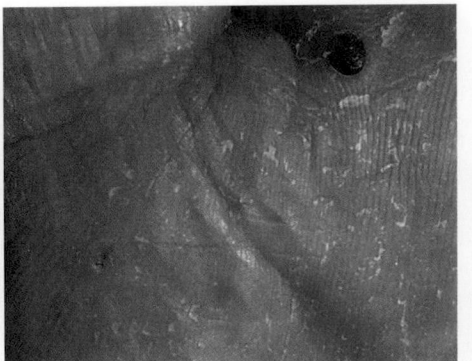

FIGURE 8-57
A, Violaceous plaques on the heel and lateral foot. **B,** Brown nodule of Kaposi sarcoma.

HAIR DISORDERS

ALOPECIA AREATA

The sudden, rapid, patchy loss of hair, usually from the scalp or face, is called *alopecia areata*. The hair shaft is poorly formed and breaks off at the skin surface. Regrowth begins in 1 to 3 months. The prognosis for total regrowth is excellent in cases with limited involvement (Fig. 8-58).

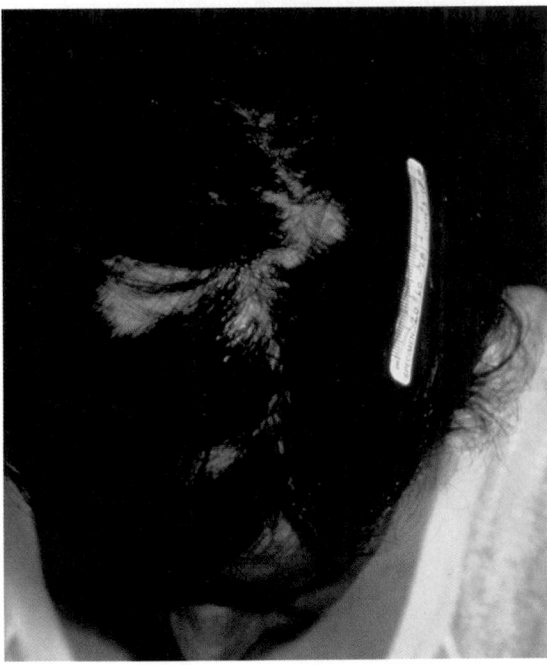

FIGURE 8-58
Alopecia areata.
From Lemmi, Lemmi, 2000.

SCARRING ALOPECIA	This type of alopecia results from skin diseases of the scalp that cause scarring and destruction of hair follicles.
TRACTION ALOPECIA	Alopecia can result from prolonged tension of the hair. It can occur from wearing certain hairstyles such as braids, or from using hair rollers and hot combs. The area of loss corresponds directly to the area of stress. The scalp may or may not be inflamed.
HIRSUTISM	Hirsutism is the growth of terminal hair in women in the male distribution pattern on the face, body, and pubic areas. Hirsutism may or may not be accompanied by other signs of virilization (Fig. 8-59).

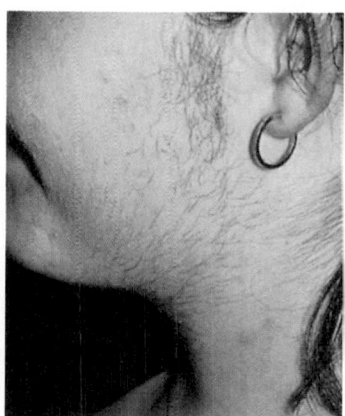

FIGURE 8-59
Facial hirsutism. Terminal hair growth is visible on the chin of this 40-year-old woman with idiopathic hirsutism.
From Lawrence, Cox, 1993.

NAILS: INFECTION

PARONYCHIA	Inflammation of the paronychium produces redness, swelling, and tenderness at the lateral and proximal nail folds. Purulent drainage often accumulates under the cuticle. It can occur as an acute or chronic process. Chronic paronychia can produce rippling of the nails (Fig. 8-60).

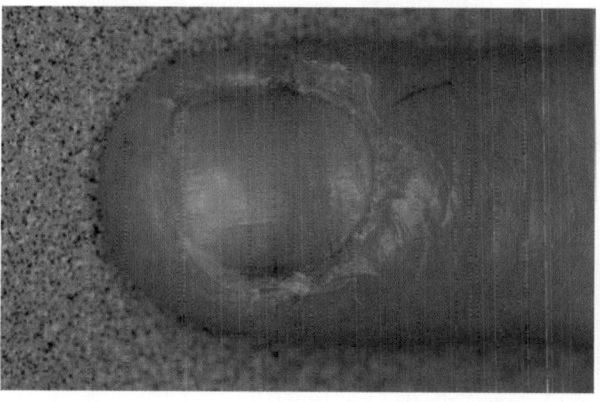

FIGURE 8-60
Paronychia.
From Lemmi, Lemmi, 2000.

TINEA UNGUIUM

Fungal infection of the nail occurs in four distinct patterns. In the most common form the distal nail plate turns yellow or white as hyperkeratotic debris accumulates, causing the nail to separate from the nail bed (onycholysis). The fungus grows in the nail plate, causing it to crumble (Fig. 8-61).

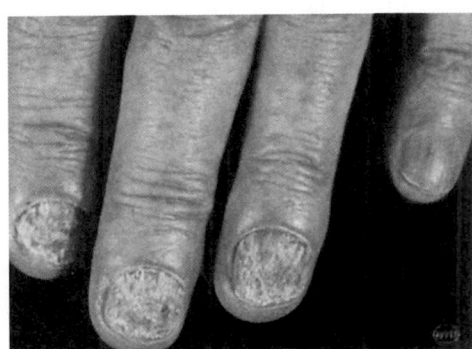

FIGURE 8-61
Tinea unguium.
Courtesy American Academy of Dermatology and Institute for Dermatologic Communication and Education, Evanston, IL.

NAILS: INJURY

INGROWN NAILS

Ingrown nails most commonly involve the large toe. The nail pierces the lateral nail fold and grows into the dermis, causing pain and swelling (Fig. 8-62).

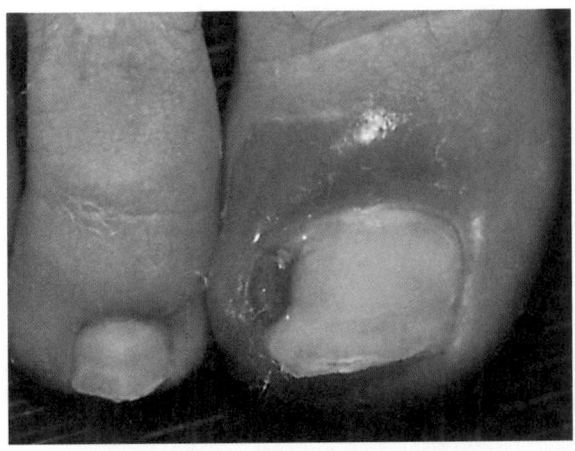

FIGURE 8-62
Ingrown toenail. Swelling and inflammation occur at lateral nail fold.
From White, 1994.

SUBUNGUAL HEMATOMA

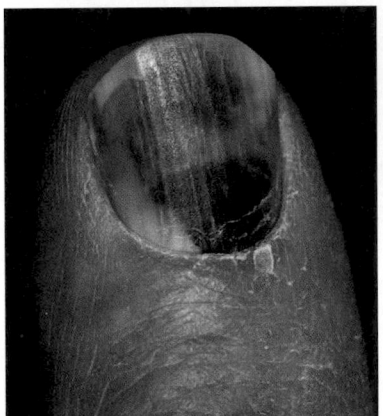

Trauma to the nail plate severe enough to cause immediate bleeding and pain produces a subungual hematoma. The amount of bleeding may be sufficient to cause separation and loss of the nail plate. Trauma to the proximal nail fold may also cause bleeding that is not apparent for several days. In either case, the hematoma remains until the nail grows out (Fig. 8-63) or is drilled to release the blood and relieve the pressure.

FIGURE 8-63
Subungual hematoma.
From Habif, 2004.

LEUKONYCHIA PUNCTATA

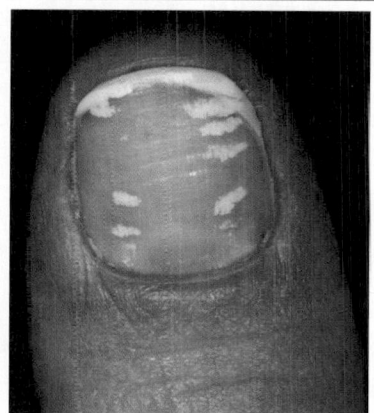

FIGURE 8-64
White spots on nail from injury (leukonychia punctata).
From Habif, 2004.

These white spots appear in the nail plate as a result of minor injury or manipulation of the cuticle. They either resolve spontaneously or grow out (Fig. 8-64).

HABIT-TIC DEFORMITY

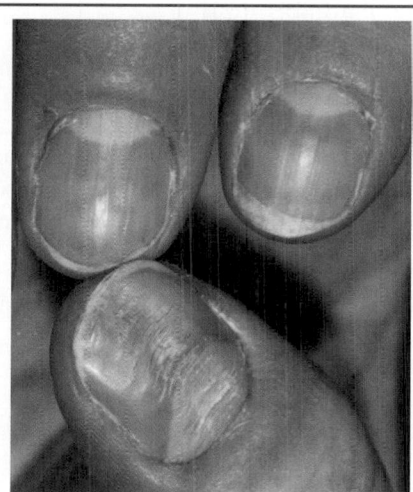

FIGURE 8-65
Habit-tic deformity.
From Habif, 2004.

This abnormality is caused by biting or picking the proximal nail fold of the thumb with the index fingernail. This results in horizontal sharp grooving in a band that extends to the tip of the nail (Fig. 8-65).

ONYCHOLYSIS

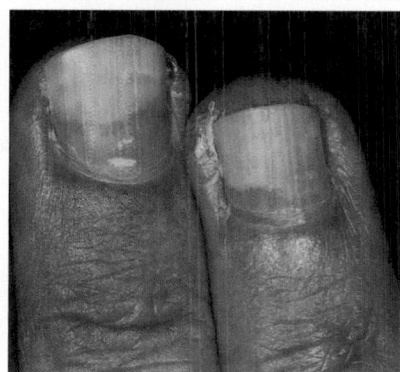

FIGURE 8-66
Onycholysis. Separation of nail plate starts at distal groove.
From Habif, 2004.

Onycholysis is loosening of the nail plate with separation from the nail bed that begins at the distal groove (Fig. 8-66). This condition is associated most commonly with minor trauma to long fingernails. Other causes include psoriasis, *Candida* or *Pseudomonas* infections, allergic contact dermatitis, and hyperthyroidism.

CURVATURE

Inward folding of the lateral edges of the nail causes the nail bed to draw up; this often becomes painful. Curvature is most common in the toenails and is thought to be caused by shoe compression (see Fig. 8-15).

NAILS: CHANGES ASSOCIATED WITH SYSTEMIC DISEASE

KOILONYCHIA (SPOON NAILS)

Central depression of the nail with lateral elevation of the nail plate produces a concave curvature and spoon appearance. This is associated with iron deficiency anemia, syphilis, fungal dermatoses, and hypothyroidism (Fig. 8-67; see also Fig. 8-15).

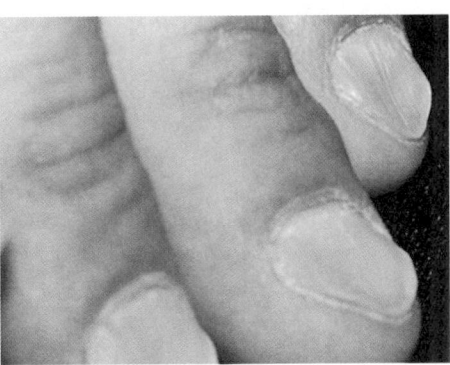

FIGURE 8-67
Koilonychia.
From White, 1994.

BEAU LINES

Weeks after a stress that temporarily interrupts nail formation, transverse depressions appear at the bases of the lunulae in all of the nails. Beau lines are associated with coronary occlusion, hypercalcemia, and skin disease. The grooves disappear when the nails grow out (Fig. 8-68).

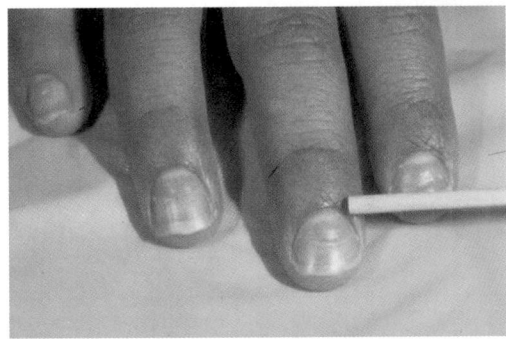

FIGURE 8-68
Beau lines following systemic disease.
From Lemmi, Lemmi, 2000.

WHITE BANDING (TERRY NAILS)

These transverse white bands cover the nail except for a narrow zone at the distal tip. The changes are associated with cirrhosis and hypoalbuminemia (Fig. 8-69).

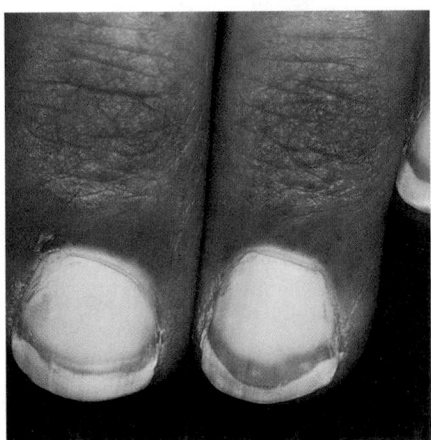

FIGURE 8-69
Terry nails; transverse white bands.
From Habif, 2004.

PSORIASIS

Psoriasis can produce pitting, onycholysis, discoloration, and subungual thickening. Yellow scaly debris often accumulates, elevating the nail plate. Severe psoriasis of the matrix and nail bed results in grossly malformed nails and splinter hemorrhages (Fig. 8-70).

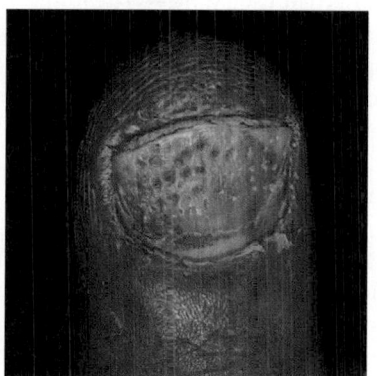

FIGURE 8-70
Nail pitting from psoriasis.
From Habif, 2004.

NAILS: PERIUNGUAL GROWTHS

WARTS

Warts are epidermal neoplasms caused by viral infection. They can occur at the nail folds and extend under the nail. A longitudinal nail groove may occur from warts located over the nail matrix (Fig. 8-71).

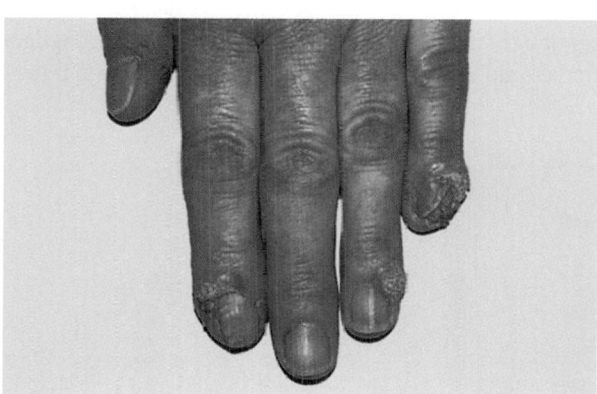

FIGURE 8-71
Periungual warts.
From Lawrence, Cox, 1993.

DIGITAL MUCOUS CYSTS

These cysts contain a clear jelly-like substance and occur on the dorsal surface of the distal phalanx. A longitudinal nail groove may occur from cysts located at the proximal nail fold (Fig. 8-72).

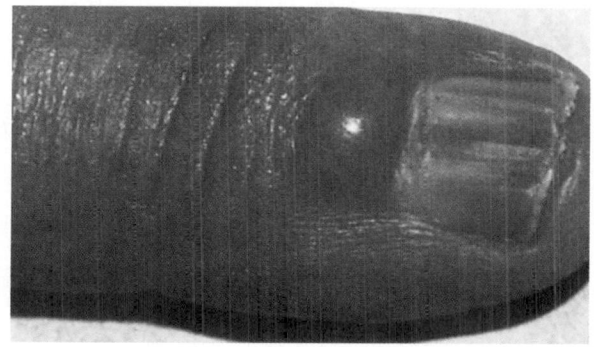

FIGURE 8-72
Digital mucous cysts causing a groove in the nail plate.
From White, 1994.

Pregnant Women

PRURITIC URTICARIAL PAPULES AND PLAQUES OF PREGNANCY (PUPPP)	PUPPP is a benign dermatosis that usually arises late in the third trimester of a first pregnancy. Intensely pruritic, erythematous, urticaria-like papules and plaques begin on the abdomen. In a few days, the eruption spreads to the thighs, buttocks, and occasionally the arms. Often halos of blanching surround the papules. The periumbilical area is spared. Small vesicles often are noted, but larger bullae do not occur and would suggest the more rare herpes gestationis. PUPPP usually does not affect the face, palms, or soles. The eruption usually resolves promptly after delivery and does not usually recur in subsequent pregnancies.
HERPES GESTATIONIS	Herpes gestationis is a rare autoimmune disorder of pregnancy. The condition is not related to the herpes virus infection; it was named on the basis of the clinical feature of herpetiform blisters. The initial clinical manifestations are erythematous urticarial patches and plaques, which typically are periumbilical. These lesions progress to tense vesicles and blisters. Palms and soles are frequently affected. Most patients present with intense unrelenting pruritus. This disease can have severe complications for the pregnant woman. The mother can develop necrosis of affected skin as well as kidney damage. Infants can be born with this rash, but it usually clears up within a few weeks of birth without treatment.

Infants and Children

CAFÉ AU LAIT PATCHES	These coffee-colored patches may be either harmless or indicative of underlying disease. The presence of more than five patches with diameters of more than 1 cm in children younger than 5 years of age suggests neurofibromatosis (von Recklinghausen disease). The beginning practitioner should consider any café au lait patches suspicious (Fig. 8-73).

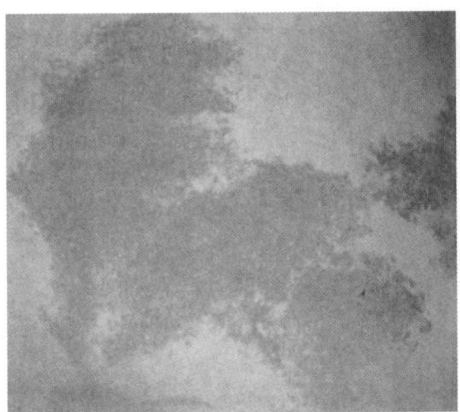

FIGURE 8-73
Café au lait patches.

SEBORRHEIC DERMATITIS

This chronic, recurrent, erythematous scaling eruption is localized in areas where sebaceous glands are concentrated (e.g., scalp, back, and intertriginous and diaper areas). The scalp lesions are scaling, adherent, thick, yellow, and crusted ("cradle cap") and can spread over the ear and down the nape of the neck. Lesions elsewhere are erythematous, scaling, and fissured (Fig. 8-74).

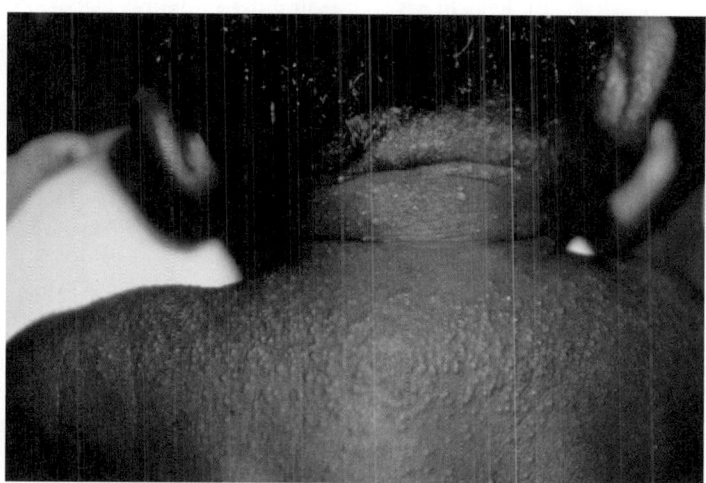

FIGURE 8-74
Pustular seborrheic dermatitis.
From Lemmi, Lemmi, 2000.

MILIARIA ("PRICKLY HEAT")

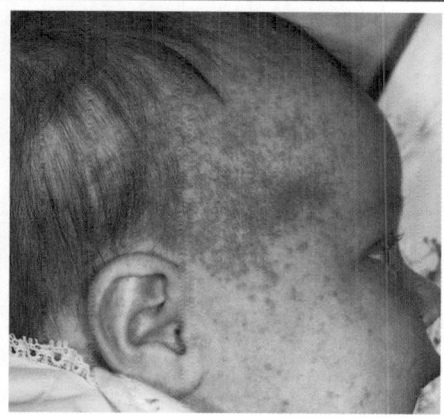

Miliaria is an irregular, red, macular rash caused by occlusion of sweat ducts during periods of heat and high humidity. Overdressed babies are susceptible to this condition in the summer (Fig. 8-75).

FIGURE 8-75
Miliaria in infant.
From Habif, 2004.

IMPETIGO

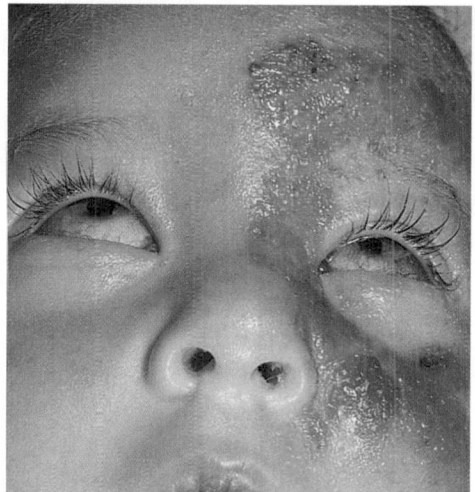

This highly contagious staphylococcal or streptococcal infection of the epidermis commonly causes pruritus, burning, and regional lymphadenopathy. The initial lesion is a small erythematous macule that changes into a vesicle or bulla with a thin roof. Crusts with a characteristic honey color form from the exudate as the vesicles or bullae rupture (Fig. 8-76).

FIGURE 8-76
Impetigo. Note characteristic crusting.
Courtesy Antoinette Hood, MD, Department of Dermatology, Indiana University School of Medicine, Indianapolis.

ACNE VULGARIS

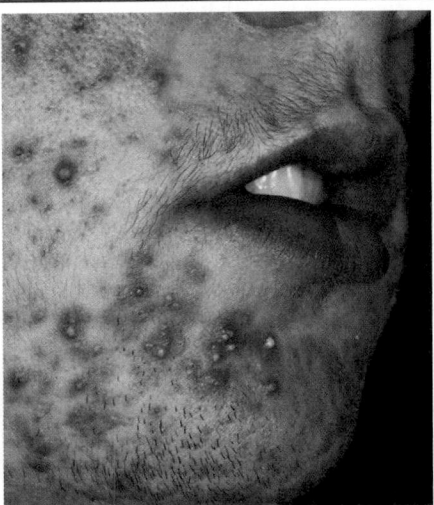

FIGURE 8-77
Acne in adolescent.
From Habif, 2004.

The inflamed lesions of acne involve stagnation of sebum and comedo formation in the pilosebaceous follicle, with bacterial invasion. Acne is seen most commonly in adolescents, though it may occur initially as an adult or continue into the adult years (Fig. 8-77).

REDDENED PATCHINESS

Irregular reddened areas that suggest a richer capillary bed can occur on the nape of the neck, upper eyelids, forehead, and upper lip. Causes of these lesions include capillary hemangioma, nevus flammeus, nevus vasculosus, and telangiectatic nevus. They usually disappear by about 1 year of age, although they may occasionally recur, even in adults (Fig. 8-78).

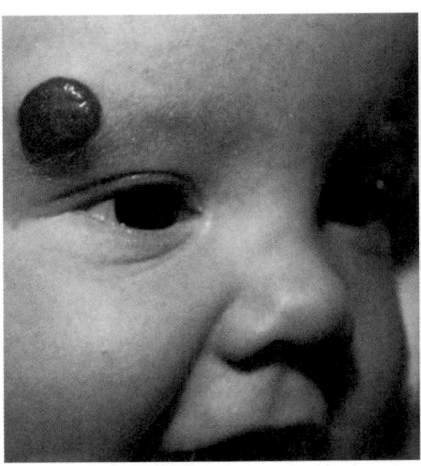
A

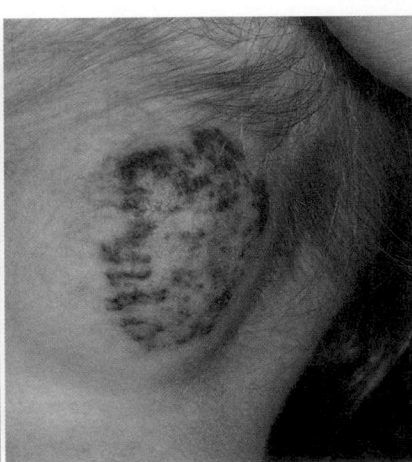
B

FIGURE 8-78
A, Strawberry hemangioma in infant. **B,** Cavernous hemangioma in infant.
From Habif, 2004.

CHICKENPOX (VARICELLA)

Chickenpox is an acute, highly communicable disease common in children and young adults, caused by the varicella-zoster virus. It is characterized by fever, mild malaise, and a pruritic maculopapular skin eruption that lasts for a few hours and then becomes vesicular. Lesions usually occur in successive outbreaks, with several stages of maturity present at one time. The lesions start on the scalp and trunk and spread centrifugally to the extremities. Lesions may also occur on the buccal mucosa, palate, or conjunctivae. The incubation period is 2 to 3 weeks; the period of communicability lasts from 1 or 2 days before onset of the rash until lesions have crusted over. Complications include conjunctival involvement, secondary bacterial infection, viral pneumonia, encephalitis, aseptic meningitis, myelitis, Guillain-Barré syndrome, and Reye syndrome. The disease is preventable by immunization (Fig. 8-79).

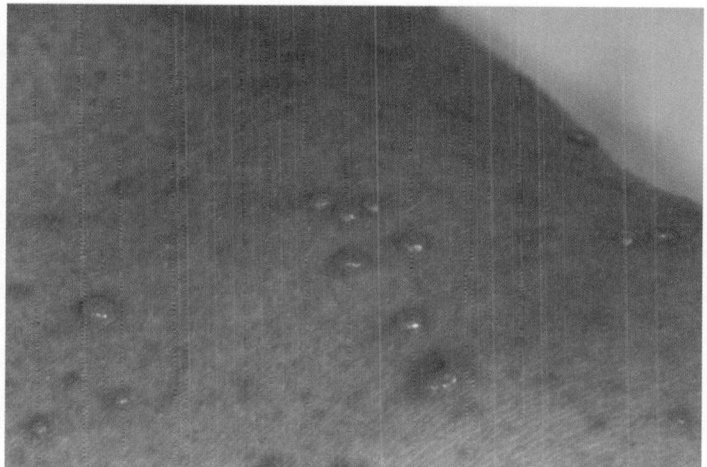

FIGURE 8-79
Varicella (chickenpox). Note vesicular lesions.
From Lemmi, Lemmi, 2000.

MEASLES (RUBEOLA)

Rubeola, also called hard measles or red measles, is a highly communicable viral disease. A characteristic prodromal fever, conjunctivitis, coryza, and bronchitis occur, followed by a red, blotchy rash. Koplik spots appear on the buccal mucosa, and a macular rash develops on the face and neck. The lesions become maculopapular and within 24 to 48 hours spread to the trunk and extremities in irregular confluent patches. The rash lasts 4 to 7 days. The incubation period is commonly 10 days; the period of communicability lasts from a few days before the fever to 4 days after appearance of the rash. Symptoms may be mild or severe. Complications involve infection of the respiratory tract and central nervous system. The disease is preventable by immunization (Fig. 8-80).

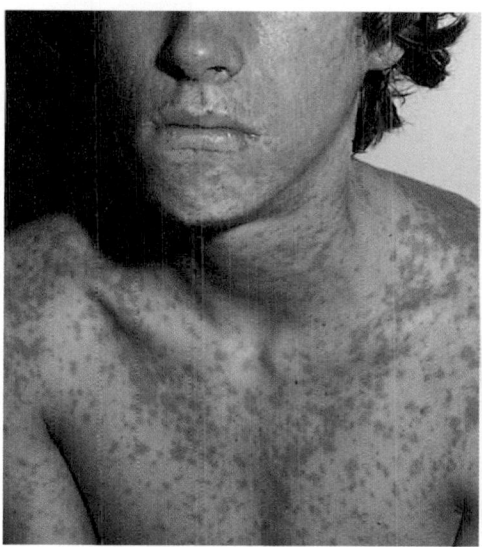

FIGURE 8-80
Rubeola.
From Zitelli, Davis, 1997.

GERMAN MEASLES (RUBELLA)

Rubella is a mild, febrile, highly communicable viral disease characterized by a generalized light pink to red maculopapular rash. During the prodromal period, low-grade fever, coryza, sore throat, and cough develop; these are followed by the appearance of a macular rash on the face and trunk that rapidly becomes papular. By the second day, the rash spreads to the upper and lower extremities; it fades within 3 days. Reddish spots occur on the soft palate during the prodrome or on the first day of the rash (Forschheimer spots). The incubation period is 14 to 23 days; the period of communicability lasts from 1 week before to 4 days after the appearance of the rash. Infection during the first trimester of pregnancy may lead to infection of the fetus and may produce a variety of congenital anomalies (congenital rubella syndrome). The disease is preventable by immunization (Fig. 8-81).

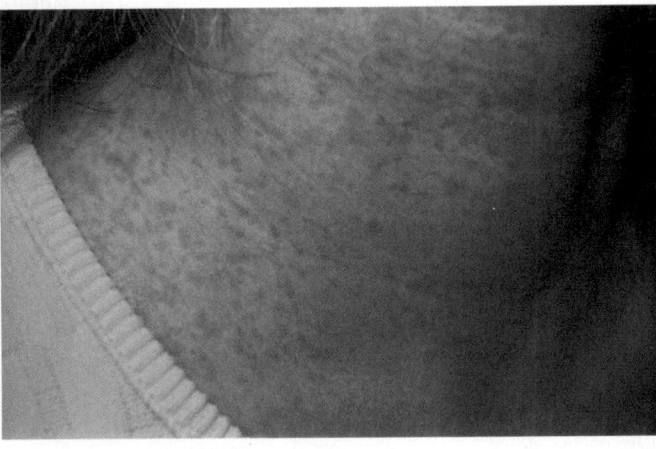
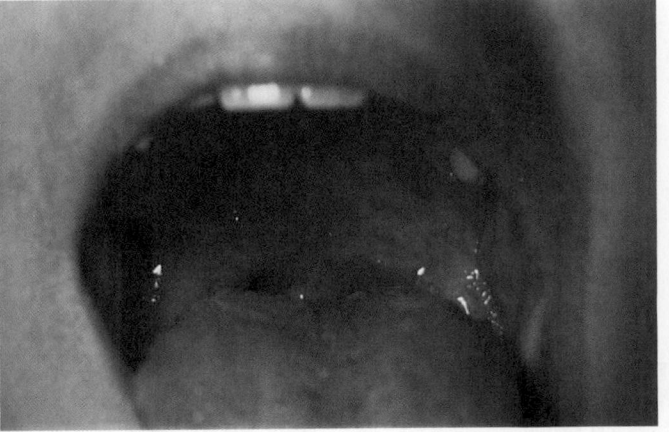

A B

FIGURE 8-81
Rubella/German measles. **A,** The exanthem of rubella usually consists of a fine, pinkish-red, maculopapular eruption that appears first at the hairline and rapidly spreads cephalocaudally. Lesions tend to remain discrete. **B,** The presence of red palatal lesions (Forschheimer spots), seen in some patients on day 1 of the rash, and occipital and posterior cervical adenopathy are findings suggestive of rubella.
Courtesy Dr. Michael Sherlock; from Zitelli, Davis, 1997.

TRICHOTILLOMANIA

Loss of scalp hair can be caused by physical manipulation. Hair is twisted around the finger and pulled or rubbed until it breaks off. The act of manipulation is usually an unconscious habit. The affected area has an irregular border, and hair density is greatly reduced, but the site is not bald (Fig. 8-82).

CLINICAL PEARL

Bald Children

Bald spots in children? Nine times out of 10, it is ringworm of the scalp, alopecia areata, or trichotillomania (a compulsive pulling out of the hair). Trichotillomania can sometimes lead to trichobezoar, a large, obstructive lump of hair in the stomach that forms after a child has swallowed a large amount of pulled-out hair.

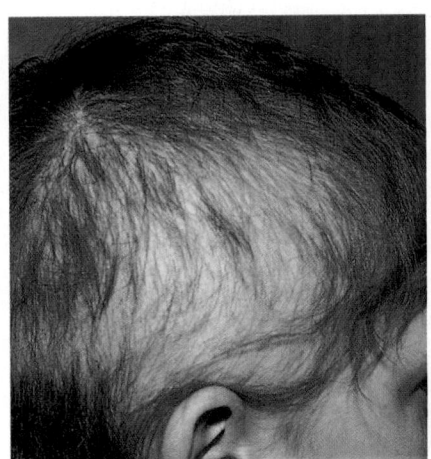

FIGURE 8-82
Trichotillomania in young child.
From Habif, 2004.

PATTERNS OF INJURY IN PHYSICAL ABUSE

Physical findings in children who are physically abused include bruises, burns, lacerations, scars, bony deformities, alopecia, retinal hemorrhages, dental trauma, and head and abdominal injuries. Skin and hair abnormalities may be the most visible clues in detecting this problem. It is important to examine the skin that is usually covered by clothing. Some skin and hair findings commonly associated with physical abuse are described in the following paragraphs.

◆ *Bruises:* These may be patterned consistent with the implement used, such as belt marks (Fig. 8-83), marks from a looped electric cord, and oval or fingertip grab marks. Bruising associated with abuse occurs over soft tissue; toddlers and older children who bruise themselves accidentally do so over bony prominences. Any bruise in an infant who is not yet developmentally able to be mobile should be cause for concern.

◆ *Lacerations:* Lacerations of the frenulum and lips are associated with forced feeding. Human bites can cause breaks in the skin and leave a characteristic bite mark.

◆ *Burns:* Patterns that are common include scald burns in stocking and glove distribution (when hands or feet are placed on hot surface or immersed); buttock burns consistent with immersion (Fig. 8-84); and cigarette burns (Fig. 8-85), a characteristic small, round burn, often on areas hidden by clothing. The absence of splash marks or a pattern consistent with spills of hot liquids may be helpful in differentiating accidental from deliberate burns.

◆ *Hair loss:* Patchy hair loss or bald spots, in the absence of a scalp disorder such as ringworm, may indicate repeated hair pulling.

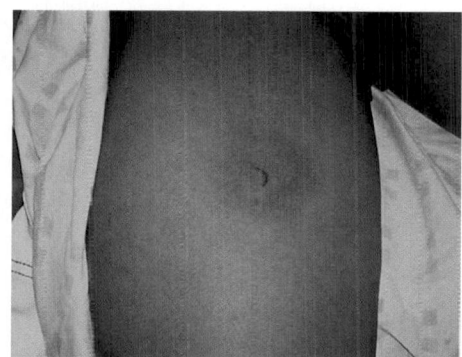

FIGURE 8-83
This contusion in the configuration of a closed horseshoe with a central linear abrasion was inflicted with a belt buckle.
From Zitelli, Davis, 1997.

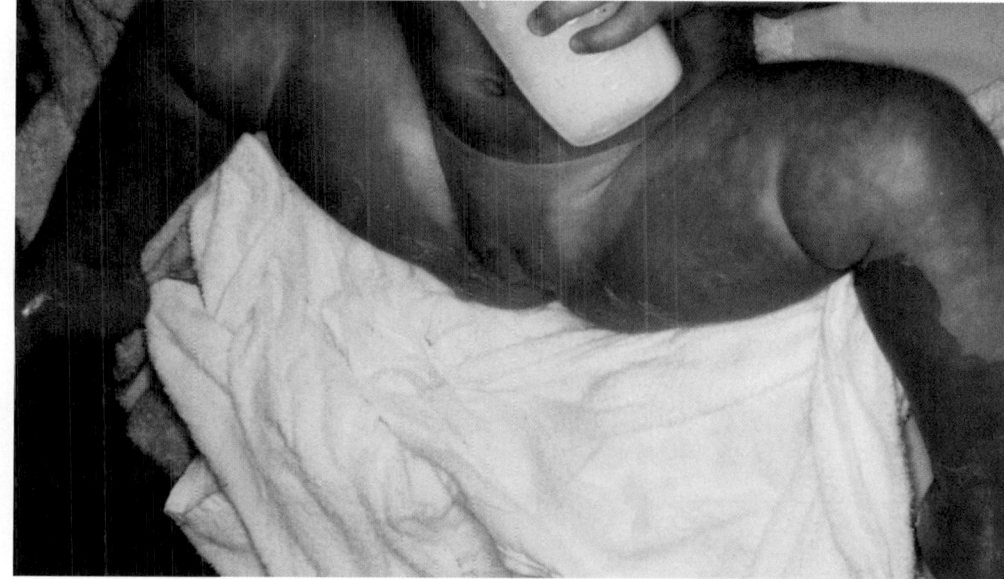

FIGURE 8-84
Burns on the perineum, thighs, legs, and feet.
Courtesy Dr. Thomas Layton, Mercy Hospital, Pittsburgh; from Zitelli, Davis, 1997.

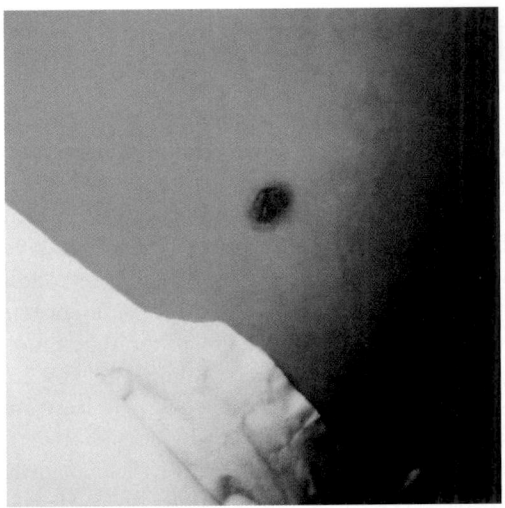

FIGURE 8-85
Cigarette burn. This older burn
has begun to granulate.
From Zitelli, Davis, 1997.

Older Adults

STASIS DERMATITIS

In this disorder, the lower legs and ankles are affected with erythematous, scaling, weeping patches. Stasis dermatitis is secondary to edema of chronic peripheral vascular disease (Fig. 8-86).

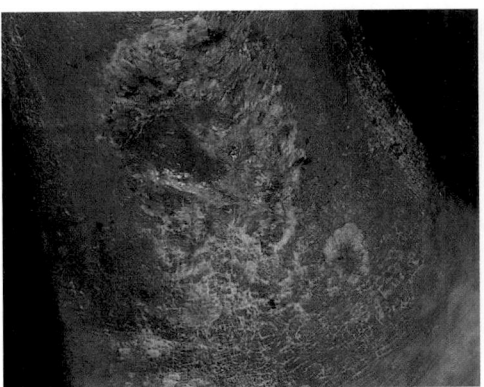

FIGURE 8-86
Stasis dermatitis in older adult
with impaired peripheral circulation.
From Habif, 2004.

SOLAR KERATOSIS (SENILE ACTINIC KERATOSIS)

This disorder produces a slightly raised erythematous lesion that is usually less than 1 cm in diameter with an irregular, rough surface. The lesion is most common on the dorsal surface of the hands, arms, neck, and face. Solar keratosis occurs secondary to chronic sun damage and has malignant potential (Fig. 8-87).

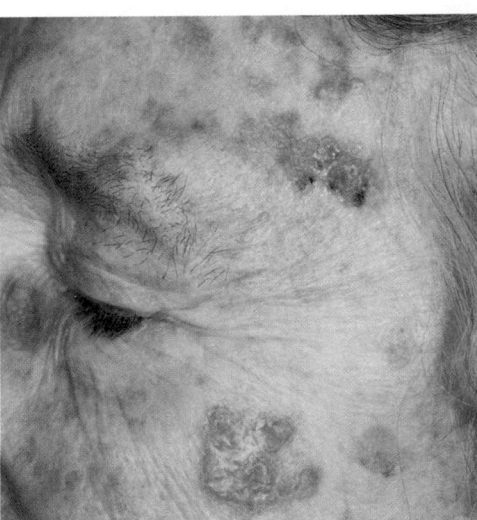

FIGURE 8-87
Actinic keratosis in older adult
in area of sun exposure.
From Habif, 2004.

PHYSICAL ABUSE IN OLDER ADULTS

Abuse in older adults can assume the form of physical abuse, neglect, sexual abuse, psychologic abuse, financial abuse, or violation of rights. Physical neglect is probably the most common type of abuse encountered by health care professionals. However, be aware that when one form of abuse is present, it is typically accompanied by other forms.

Physical abuse and neglect may present with clues that aid in detection. Assessment of general appearance may indicate poor hygiene, emaciation, healed fractures with deformity, and unexplained trauma. Carefully inspect the skin, particularly on hidden areas such as the axillae, inner thighs, soles of the feet, palms, and abdomen; look for bruising, burns, abrasions, or areas of tenderness. Bruising on extensor surfaces is common and usually occurs accidentally; bruising at various stages of resolution located on inner soft surfaces is more likely to indicate abuse.

Careful history taking is essential. When abuse is suspected, it is important to ask direct questions, such as "Is anyone hurting or harming you?" or "Have you been confined against your will?" This questioning should occur in a private setting away from accompanying family members or caregivers. Determination of mental status is also essential (see Chapter 4) because unintended self-neglect or abuse is also possible. If the patient is cognitively impaired, abuse by another may still be present but needs to be corroborated.

ELECTRONIC RESOURCES

For Weblinks and additional resources, go to

http://evolve.elsevier.com/Seidel

or to the Companion CD-ROM.

Additional information related to the content in Chapter 8 can be found on the companion website at evolve.elsevier.com/Seidel/ or on the interactive companion CD-ROM. Resources and activities for Chapter 8 include:

- Sound and Vision Theater
- Printouts for Your Practice
- Interactive Challenge
- Spanish Assessment Terms with Pronunciation Guide
- Instant Calculator

LYMPHATIC SYSTEM

ANATOMY AND PHYSIOLOGY

The lymphatic system consists of lymph fluid, the collecting ducts, and various tissues including the lymph nodes, spleen, thymus, tonsils, adenoids, and Peyer patches. Bits of lymph tissue are found in other parts of the body including the mucosa of the stomach and appendix, bone marrow, and lungs (Fig. 9-1). The entire mass of the system is no more than 3% of the total body weight. An integral part of the immune system, it supports a network of defense against the invasion of microorganisms.

The immune system protects the body from the antigenic substances of invading organisms, removes damaged cells from the circulation, and provides a partial, but often inefficient, barrier to the maturation of malignant cells within the body. When it functions well, the individual is immunocompetent. When it fails, for whatever reason, immunoincompetence can lead to a variety of illnesses: allergic, immunodeficient—either congenital or acquired (e.g., infection with human immunodeficiency virus [HIV]), or autoimmune (i.e., allergy to oneself [e.g., lupus erythematosus]). Tissue rejection of transplanted organs, on the other hand, is an unwelcome manifestation of immunocompetence.

Except for the placenta and the brain, every tissue supplied by blood vessels has lymphatic vessels. This wide-ranging presence is essential to the system's role in immunologic and metabolic processes. That role, not yet completely understood, involves the following:

- Movement of lymph fluid in a closed circuit with the cardiovascular system, a major factor in the maintenance of fluid balance
- Production of lymphocytes within the lymph nodes, tonsils, adenoids, spleen, and bone marrow
- Production of antibodies
- Phagocytosis, the ingestion and digestion by cells of solid substances such as other cells, bacteria, and bits of necrosed tissue or foreign particles; this is a specific function of cells that line the sinuses of lymph nodes
- Absorption of fat and fat-soluble substances from the intestinal tract
- Manufacture of blood when the primary sources are pathophysiologically compromised

In addition, the lymphatic system plays an undesirable role in providing at least one pathway for the spread of malignancy.

Lymph is a clear, sometimes opalescent and sometimes yellow-tinged fluid. It contains a variety of white blood cells (mostly lymphocytes) and, on occasion, red blood cells. The lymphatic and cardiovascular systems are intimately related. The fluids and proteins that consti-

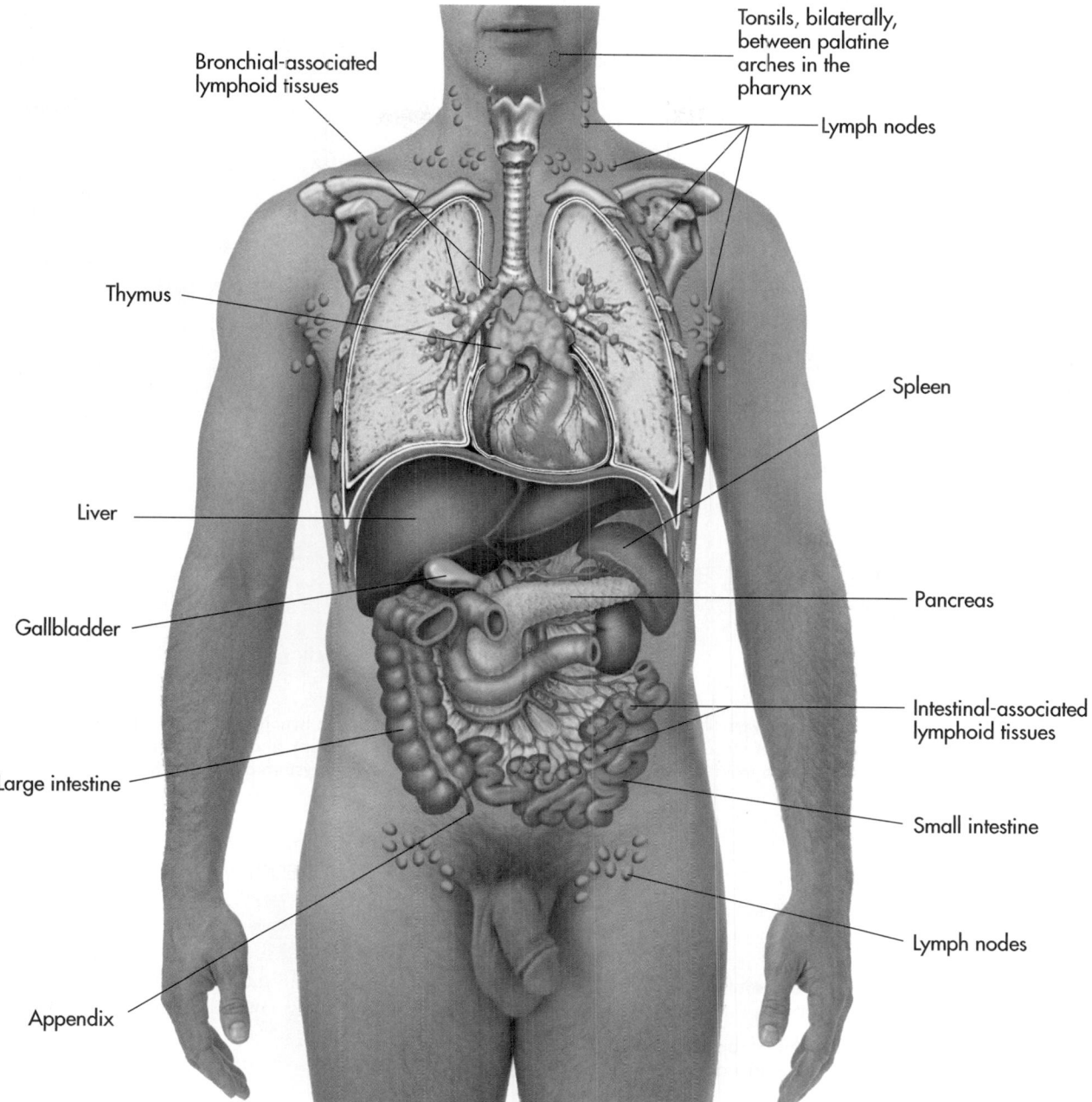

Bronchial-associated lymphoid tissues

Tonsils, bilaterally, between palatine arches in the pharynx

Lymph nodes

Thymus

Spleen

Liver

Pancreas

Gallbladder

Intestinal-associated lymphoid tissues

Large intestine

Small intestine

Lymph nodes

Appendix

FIGURE 9-1
Lymphatic system (lymphoreticular system).

tute lymphatic fluid originally move from the bloodstream into the interstitial spaces. They are then collected throughout the body by a profusion of microscopic tubules (Fig. 9-2). These tubules unite, forming larger ducts that collect lymph and carry it to the lymph nodes around the body.

The lymph nodes receive lymph from the collecting ducts in the various regions (Figs. 9-3 to 9-11), passing it on through efferent vessels. Ultimately the large ducts merge into the venous system at the subclavian veins.

The drainage point for the right upper body is a lymphatic trunk that empties into the right subclavian vein. The thoracic duct, the major vessel of the lymphatic system, drains lymph from the rest of the body into the left subclavian vein. It returns the various fluids and proteins to the cardiovascular system, forming a closed but porous circle.

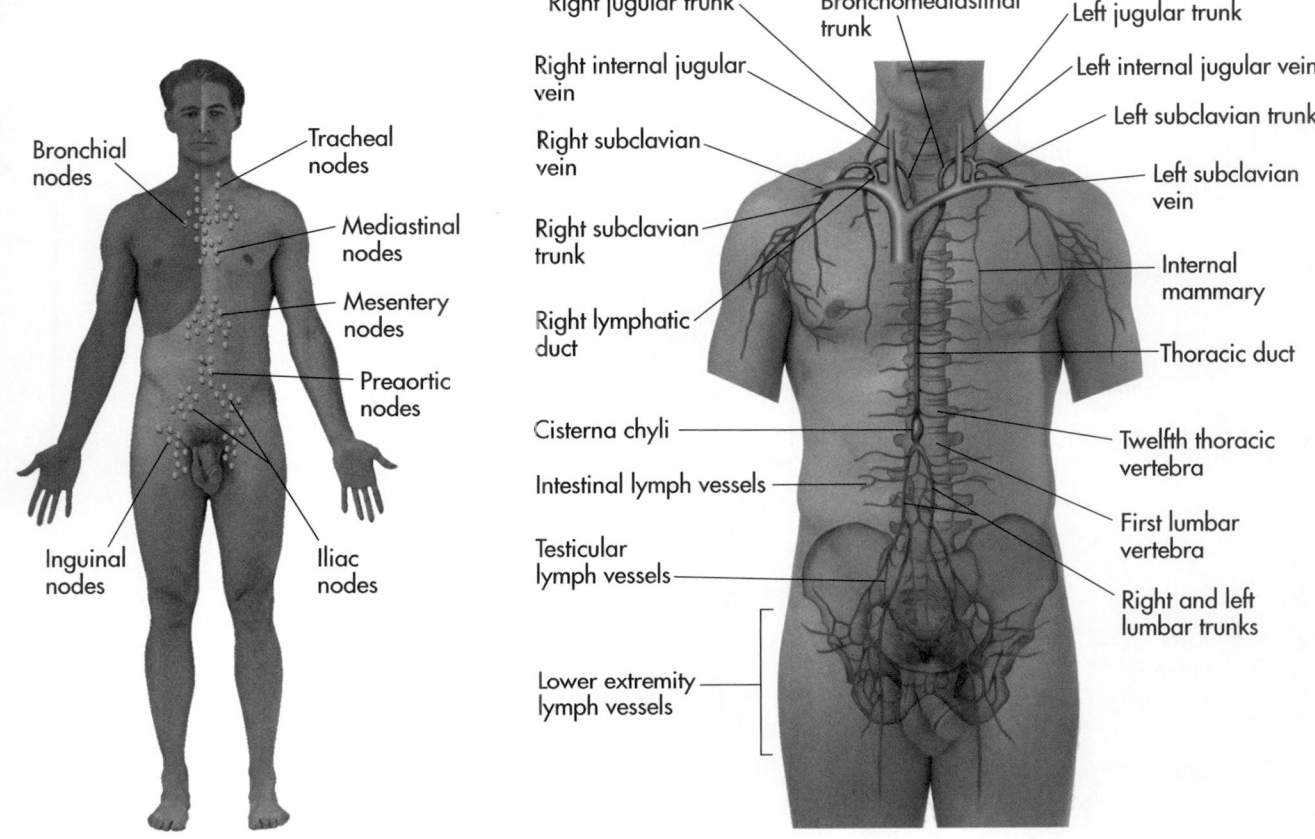

FIGURE 9-2

Lymphatic drainage pathways. Shaded area of the body is drained via the right lymphatic duct, which is formed by the union of three vessels: right jugular trunk, right subclavian trunk, and right broncho-mediastinal trunk. Lymph from the remainder of the body enters the venous system by way of the thoracic duct.

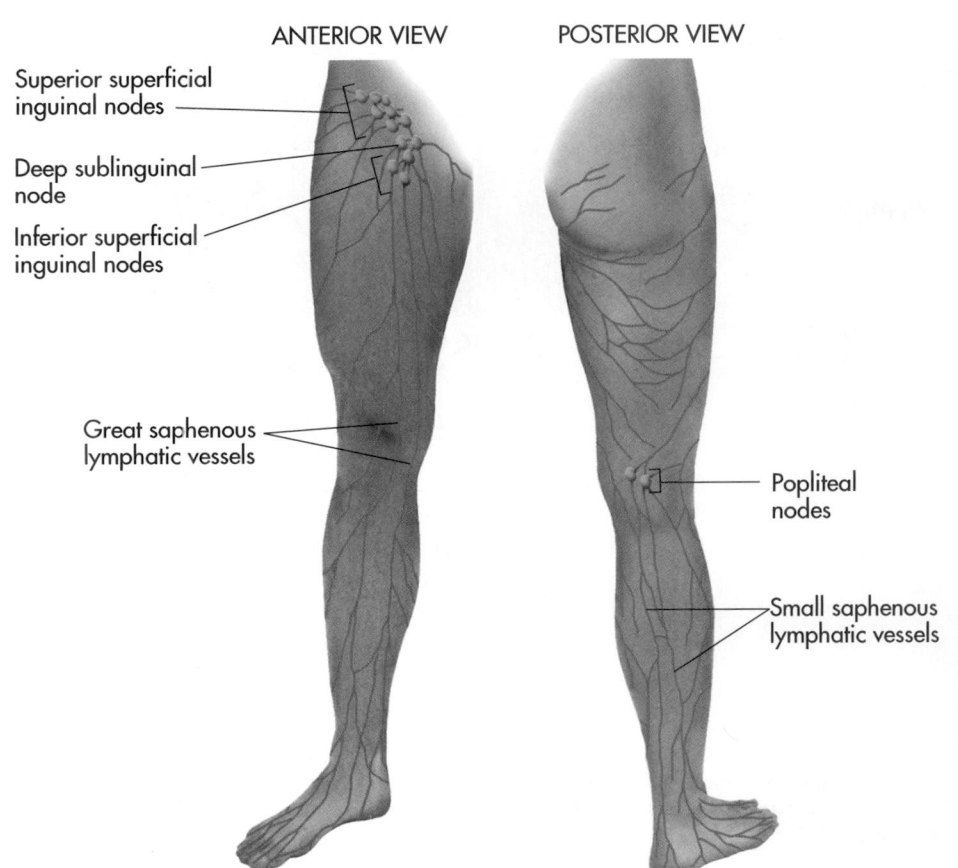

FIGURE 9-3

Lymphatic drainage of lower extremity.

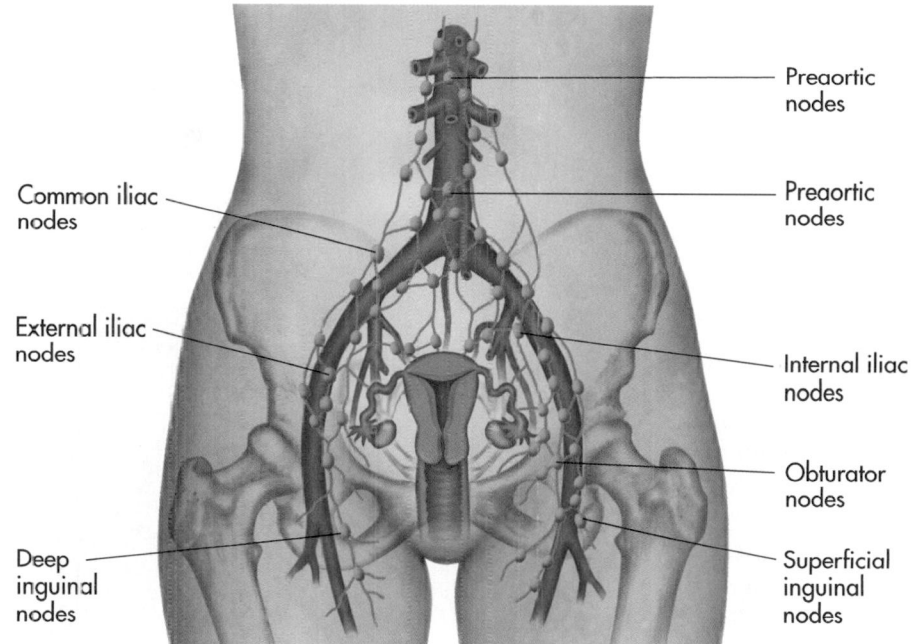

FIGURE 9-4
Lymphatic drainage of female genital tract.

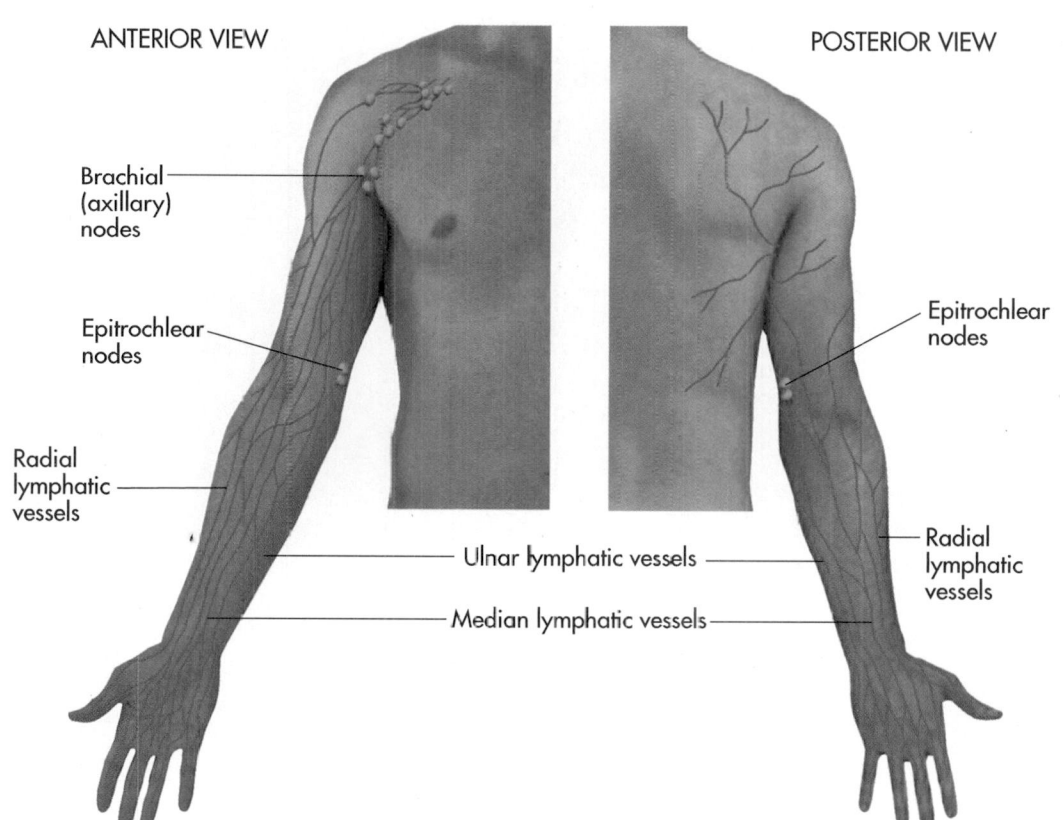

FIGURE 9-5
Systems of deep and superficial collecting ducts, carrying lymph from upper extremity to subclavian lymphatic trunk. The only peripheral lymph center is the epitrochlear, which receives some of the collecting ducts from the pathway of the ulnar and radial nerves.

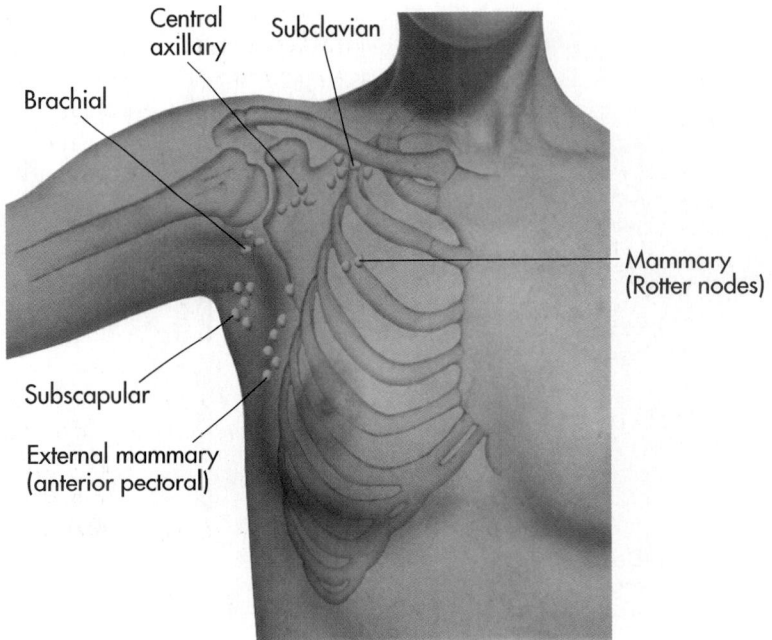

FIGURE 9-6
Six groups of lymph nodes may be distinguished in the axillary fossa.

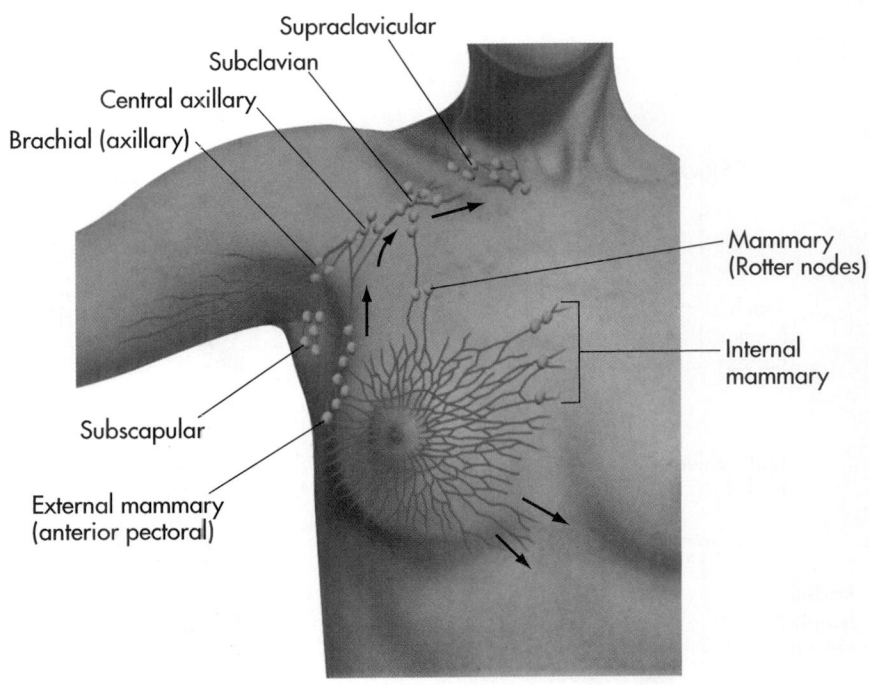

FIGURE 9-7
Lymphatic drainage of breast.

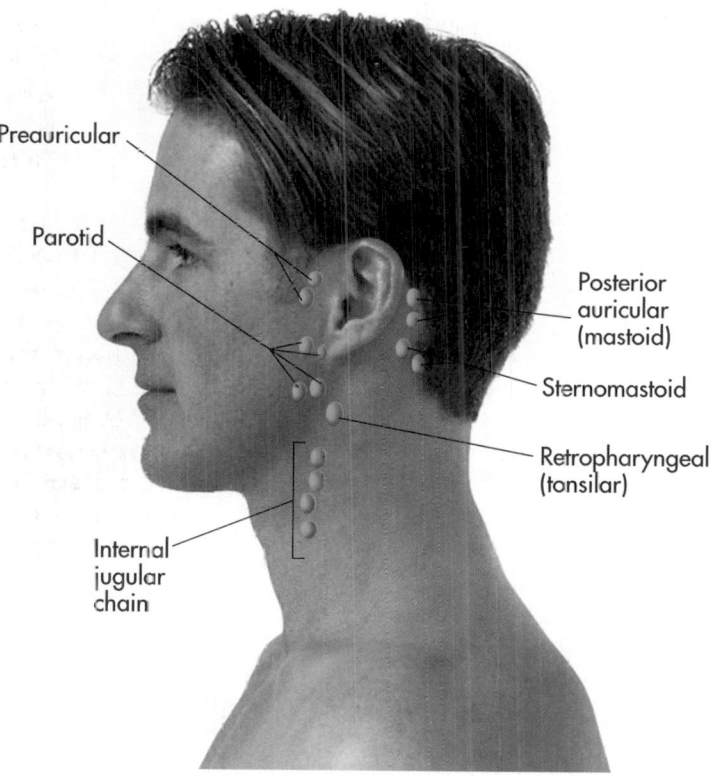

FIGURE 9-8
Lymph nodes involved with the ear.

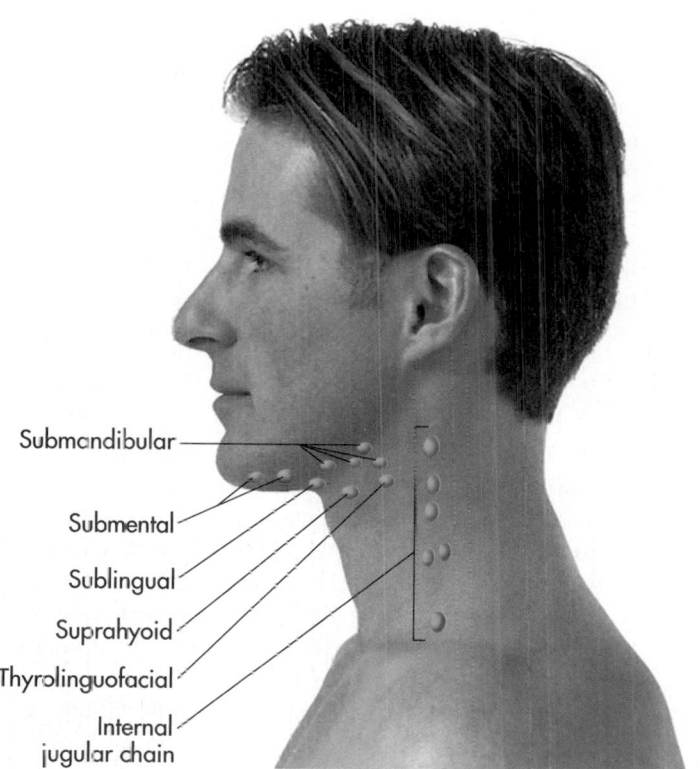

FIGURE 9-9
Lymph nodes involved with the tongue.

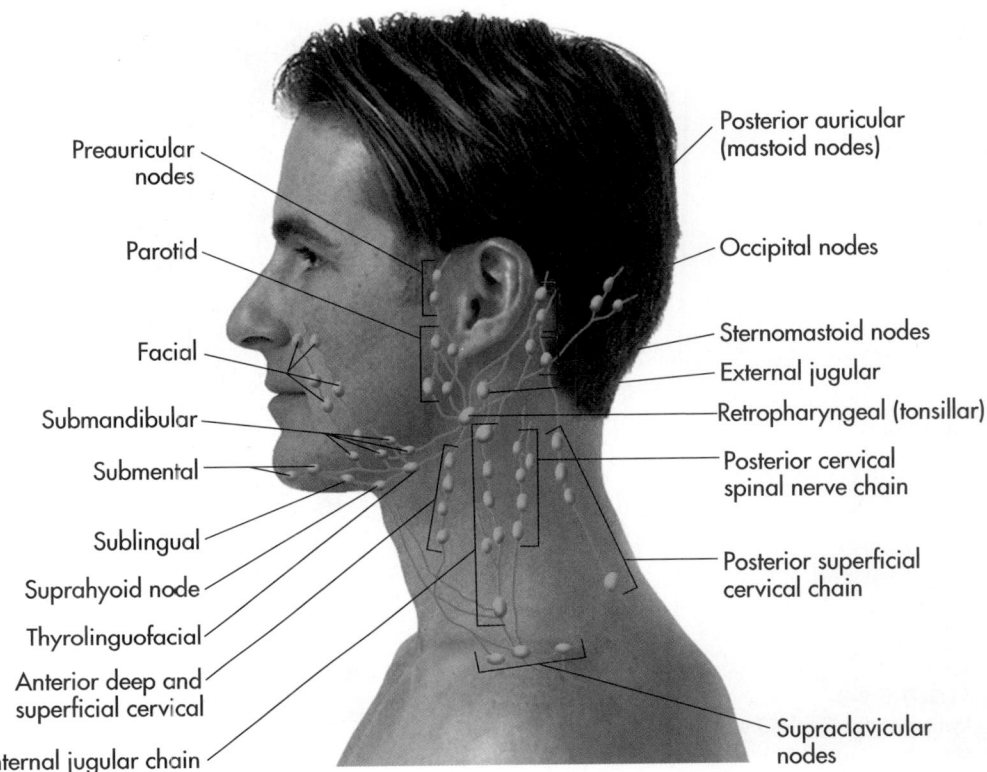

Preauricular nodes

Parotid

Facial

Submandibular

Submental

Sublingual

Suprahyoid node

Thyrolinguofacial

Anterior deep and superficial cervical

Internal jugular chain

Posterior auricular (mastoid nodes)

Occipital nodes

Sternomastoid nodes

External jugular

Retropharyngeal (tonsillar)

Posterior cervical spinal nerve chain

Posterior superficial cervical chain

Supraclavicular nodes

FIGURE 9-10
Lymphatic drainage system of head and neck. If the group of nodes is commonly referred to by another name, the second name appears in parentheses.

The lymphatic system has no built-in pumping mechanisms of its own. Because it depends on the cardiovascular system for this, the movement of lymph is sluggish compared with that of blood. As lymph fluid volume increases, it flows faster in response to mounting capillary pressure, greater permeability of the capillary walls of the cardiovascular system, increased bodily or metabolic activity, and massage. Conversely, mechanical obstruction will slow or stop the movement of lymph, dilating the system. The permeability of the lymphatic system is protective; if it is obstructed, lymph may diffuse into the vascular system, or collateral connecting channels may develop.

LYMPH NODES

Lymph nodes usually occur in groups. Superficial nodes are located in subcutaneous connective tissues, and deeper nodes lie beneath the fascia of muscles and within the various body cavities. The nodes are numerous and tiny, but some of them may have diameters as large as 0.5 to 1 cm. They defend against the invasion of microorganisms and other particles with filtration and phagocytosis, and they aid in the maturation of lymphocytes and monocytes.

The superficial lymph nodes are the gateway to assessing the health of the entire lymphatic system. Readily accessible to inspection and palpation, they provide some of the earliest clues to the presence of infection or malignancy (Box 9-1). For example, a palpable supraclavicular node should always be respected as a probable tell-tale sign of malignancy.

LYMPHOCYTES

Lymphocytes are central to the body's response to antigenic substances. They are not identical in size or function. Some are small, approximately 7 to 8 mm in diameter; others range in size to as much as five times that. They arise from a number of sites in the body, including the lymph nodes, tonsils, adenoids, and spleen; but primarily they are produced in the bone mar-

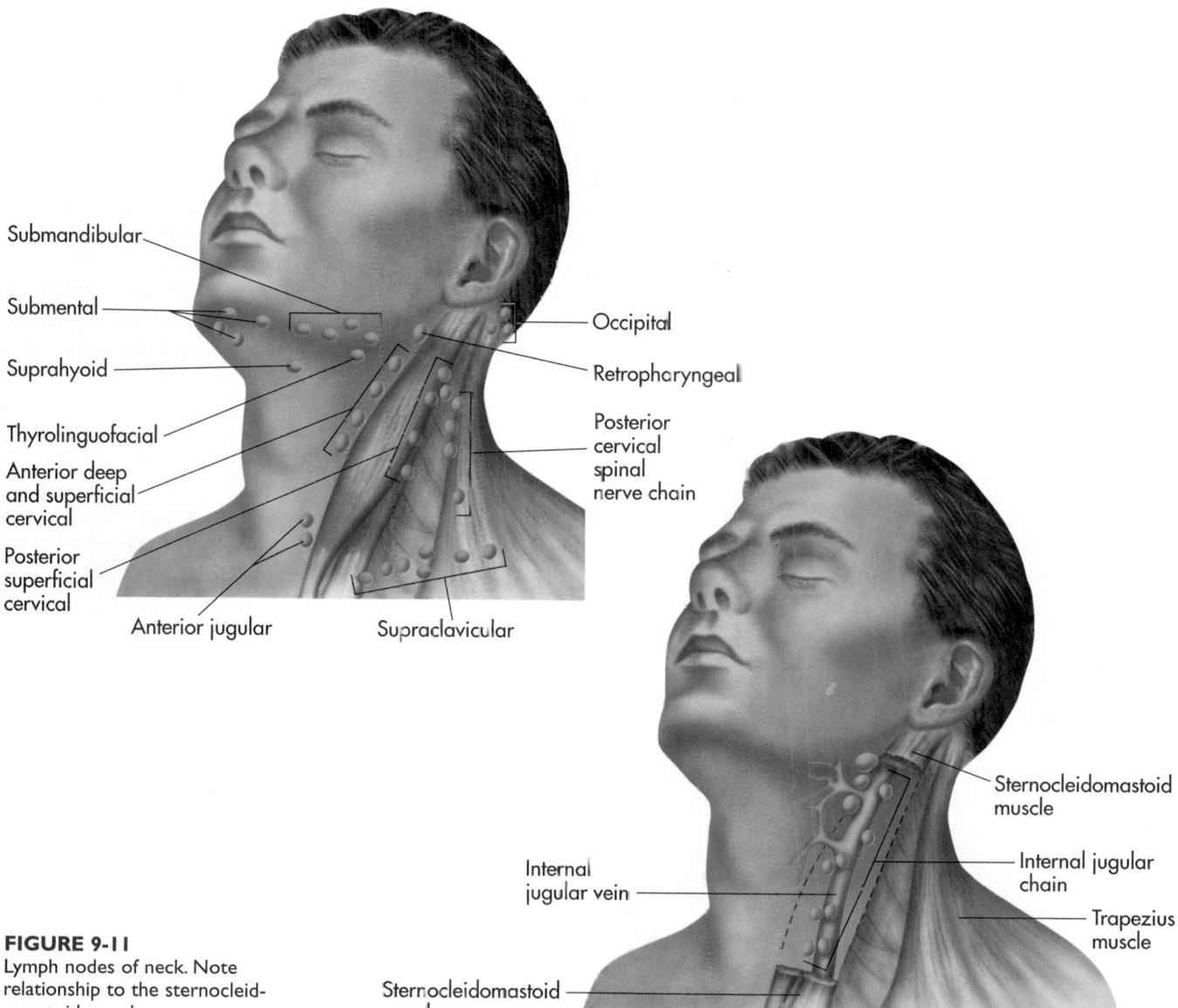

Submandibular

Submental

Suprahyoid

Thyrolinguofacial

Anterior deep and superficial cervical

Posterior superficial cervical

Anterior jugular

Supraclavicular

Occipital

Retropharyngeal

Posterior cervical spinal nerve chain

Sternocleidomastoid muscle

Internal jugular chain

Trapezius muscle

Internal jugular vein

Sternocleidomastoid muscle

FIGURE 9-11
Lymph nodes of neck. Note relationship to the sternocleidomastoid muscle.

BOX 9-1

THE LYMPH NODES MOST ACCESSIBLE TO INSPECTION AND PALPATION

The more superficial the node, the more accessible it is.

The "Necklace" of Nodes
Parotid and retropharyngeal (tonsillar)
Submandibular
Submental
Sublingual (facial)
Superficial anterior cervical
Superficial posterior cervical
Preauricular and postauricular
Sternocleidomastoid
Occipital
Supraclavicular

The Arms
Axillary
Epitrochlear (cubital)

The Legs
Superficial superior inguinal
Superficial inferior inguinal
Occasionally, popliteal

row, where early cells (i.e., stem cells) capable of developing in a variety of pathways, arise. Lymphocytes that are derived primarily from bone marrow (i.e., B-lymphocytes) produce antibodies and are characterized by the various arrangements of immunoglobulins on their surface.

Marrow-derived cells, which flow first to the thymus, can be further differentiated there as T-lymphocytes. They can sense the difference in cells of the body that have been invaded by any foreign substance (e.g., a living virus, bacterium, or parasite; some invasive chemical) or even a malignant change. Found in profusion in the centers of lymph nodes, T-lymphocytes have an important role in controlling the immune responses brought about by B-lymphocytes. There are two types of immunity: (1) humoral, involving the antibodies produced by B-cells, and (2) cellular, involving attacks on "invaders" by the cells themselves. Among lymphocytes, B-cells have a relatively short life span of 3 to 4 days. T-cells, which are four or five times as numerous as B-cells, have a life span of 100 to 200 days. An increased number of lymphocytes in the blood represents a systemic response to most viral infections and to some bacterial infections.

THYMUS

The thymus is located in the superior mediastinum, extending upward into the lower neck. In early life the thymus is essential to the development of the protective immune function (Fig. 9-12). It is the site for production of T-lymphocytes, the effector cells for cell-mediated immunity reactions and the controlling agent for the humoral immune responses generated by B-lymphocytes. In the adult, however, it has little or no demonstrated function.

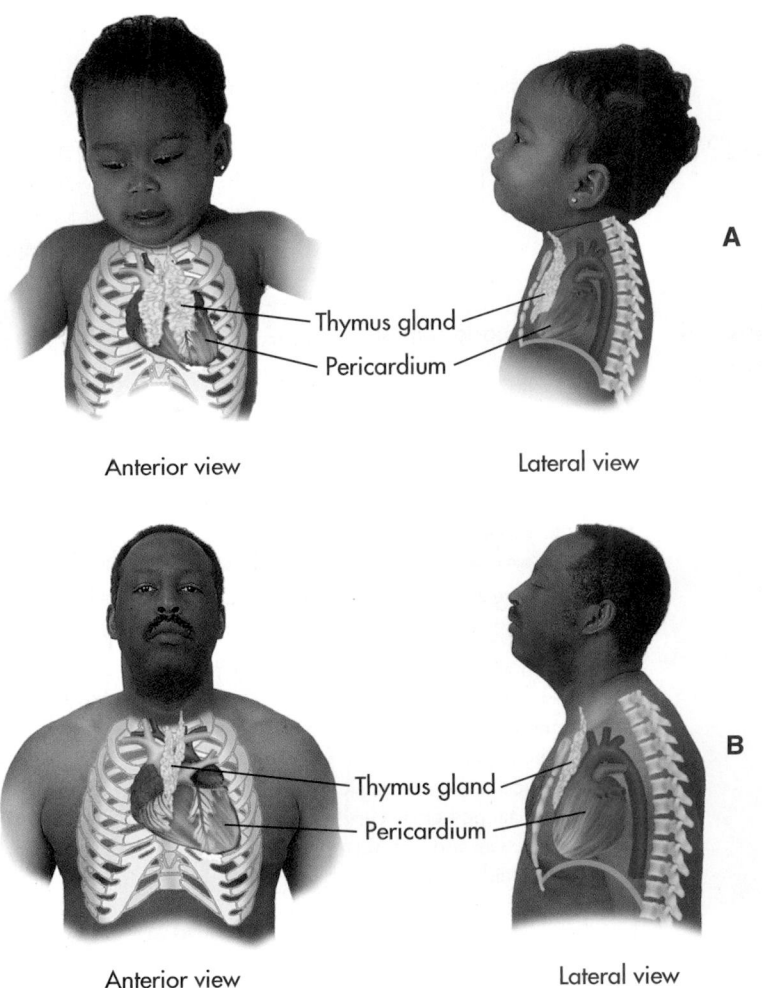

FIGURE 9-12
Location of thymus gland and its size relative to the rest of the body. **A,** During infancy. **B,** During adult life.

SPLEEN

The spleen is situated in the left upper quadrant of the abdominal cavity between the stomach and the diaphragm. A highly vascular organ, it is composed of two systems: (1) the white pulp, made up of lymphatic nodules and diffuse lymphatic tissue, and (2) the red pulp, made up of venous sinusoids. The spleen is a blood-forming organ early in life, a site for the storage of red corpuscles, and—with its plethora of blood-filtering macrophages—part of the body's defense system. The immune response to bloodborne antigens usually has its origins in the spleen. Its examination, therefore, is essential to the evaluation of the immune system (see Chapter 17).

TONSILS AND ADENOIDS

The palatine tonsils are commonly referred to as "the tonsils." Small and diamond-shaped, they are set between the palatine arches on either side of the pharynx just beyond the base of the tongue. Composed principally of lymphoid tissue, the tonsils are organized as follicles and crypts; both are covered by mucous membrane. The pharyngeal tonsils, or adenoids, are located at the nasopharyngeal border; the lingual tonsils are located near the base of the tongue. Defensive responses to inhaled and intranasal antigens are activated in these tissues. When enlarged, the adenoids and tonsils can obstruct the nasopharyngeal passageway.

PEYER PATCHES

Peyer patches are small, raised areas of lymph tissue on the mucosa of the small intestine. They consist of many clustered lymphoid nodules, and they serve the intestinal tract.

INFANTS AND CHILDREN

The immune system and the lymphoid system begin developing at about 20 weeks of gestation. The ability to produce antibodies is still immature at birth, increasing the infant's vulnerability to infection during the first few months of life. The mass of lymphoid tissue is relatively plentiful in infants; increases during childhood, especially between 6 and 9 years of age; then regresses to adult levels by puberty (see Fig. 5-3).

The thymus is at its largest relative to the rest of the body shortly after birth, but reaches its greatest absolute weight at puberty. Then it involutes, replacing much of its tissue with fat and becoming a rudimentary organ in the adult.

The palatine tonsils, like much lymphoid tissue, are much larger during early childhood than after puberty. An enlargement of the tonsils in children is not necessarily an indication of problems.

The lymph nodes have the same distribution in children that they do in adults. The finding of small 12- to 13-mm, discrete, palpable, mobile nodes in the neonate is not unusual. Before 2 years of age, inguinal, occipital, and postauricular nodes are common; after 2 years of age, they are more likely to have significance. On the other hand, cervical and submandibular nodes are uncommon during the first year and much more common in older children. Supraclavicular nodes are not usually found; their presence, associated with a high incidence of malignancy, is always a cause for concern. Circumcision does not increase the likelihood of inguinal nodes. It is possible that the infant's relatively large mass of lymphoid tissue is needed to compensate for an immature ability to produce antibodies, thus adding to the demand for filtration and phagocytosis.

The lymphatic system gradually reaches adult competency during childhood (Fig. 9-13).

CLINICAL PEARL

Umbilical Cord
The umbilical cord should drop off by 1 to 2 weeks after birth. If it hangs on much longer than that, there may be a congenital defect of the immune system.

PREGNANT WOMEN

For implantation and fetal development to occur, changes occur in the immune system during pregnancy. These complex changes are not fully understood but seem to reflect a balance between enhancement of certain immune mechanisms and suppression of others. During pregnancy, the leukocyte count increases from a usual level of about 7200 cells/mm^3 at 2

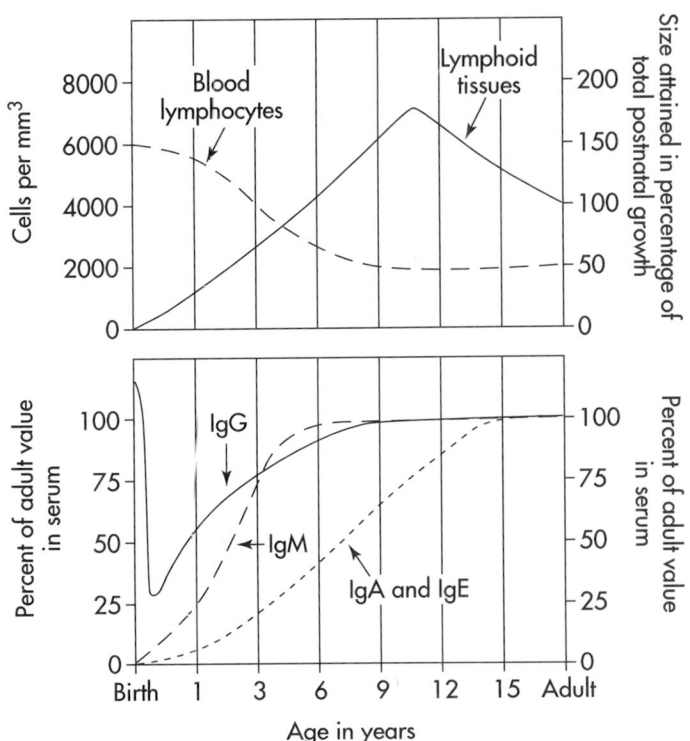

FIGURE 9-13
Relative levels of presence and function of the immune factors.

months to reach a plateau during the second and third trimesters at a mean level of 10,350/mm³, with a usual range of 5000 to 12,000/mm³. This increase is due to circulating segmented neutrophils or granulocytes, possibly due to increased estrogen and cortisol levels.

The embryo is an in utero foreign body; however, the mother's hormones and the products of the fetal trophoblast create a unique environment. Uterine contractility decreases and macrophages produce cytokines beneficial to growth of the trophoblast. A balance results. The shift from cell-mediated immunity to antibody production/humoral immunity results in increased susceptibility to certain infectious diseases. However, pregnancy can lead to remission in the mother of autoimmune/inflammatory diseases (e.g., rheumatoid arthritis) (Clark, 1999).

OLDER ADULTS

The number of lymph nodes may diminish and size may decrease with advanced age; some of the lymphoid elements are lost. The nodes of older patients are more likely to be fibrotic and fatty than those of the young, a contributing factor in an impaired ability to resist infection.

REVIEW OF RELATED HISTORY

For each of the conditions discussed in this section, targeted topics to include in the history of the present illness are listed. Responses to questions about these topics help fully assess the patient's condition and provide clues for focusing the physical examination.

HISTORY OF PRESENT ILLNESS

- Bleeding
  - Site: nose, mouth, gums, rectal (blood in stools; black, tarry stools), skin petechiae, easy bruising, blood in vomitus

RISK FACTORS
HIV INFECTION

Adolescents and Adults
Multiple and indiscriminate sexual contacts
- Prostitution
- Unprotected sexual activity with persons of known history of risk or unknown history
  Sexual contact with IV drug users
  Men with history of homosexual or bisexual activities
  Sexual contact with persons infected with HIV
  Sexual contact with homosexual or bisexual men
IV drug use
- Parenteral exposure to HIV–blood-contaminated needles and/or syringes
- Sexual contact with IV drug users
Hemophilia
- Transfusion with infected blood or blood concentrates (e.g., Factor VIII, Factor IX) particularly in the era before blood bank screening for HIV
Work related (rare)
- Rupture of the skin with needles or other sharp objects contaminated with the blood of an HIV-positive patient
Infants and Children
Mother either with or at risk for HIV infection
- During gestation
- At parturition
- During breast-feeding
Hemophilia
- Same as for adults
- Same as for adults
Sexual abuse

- Character: onset, frequency, duration, amount, color (bright red or brown to coffee-colored)
- Associated symptoms: pallor, dizziness, headache, shortness of breath
- Enlarged nodes (bumps, kernels, swollen glands)
  - Character: onset, location, duration, number, tenderness
  - Associated symptoms: pain, fever, redness, warmth, red streaks, itching (some tumors cause pruritus)
  - Predisposing factors: infection, surgery, trauma
- Swelling of extremity
  - Unilateral or bilateral, intermittent or constant, duration
  - Predisposing factors: cardiac or renal disorder, surgery, infection, trauma, venous insufficiency
  - Associated symptoms: warmth, redness or discoloration, ulceration
  - Efforts at treatment and their effect: support stockings, elevation
- Medications: chemotherapy, antibiotics
- Complementary and alternative therapies, if any

PAST MEDICAL HISTORY

- Chest x-rays
- Tuberculosis and other skin testing
- Blood transfusions, use of blood products
- Chronic illness: cardiac, renal, malignancy, HIV infection (see Risk Factors box for HIV infection above)
- Surgery: trauma to regional lymph nodes; organ transplant
- Recurrent infections
  - Autoimmune disorder

FAMILY HISTORY

- ◆ Malignancy
- ◆ Anemia
- ◆ Recent infections
- ◆ Tuberculosis
- ◆ Agammaglobulinemia, severe combined immune deficiency, other immune disorders
- ◆ Hemophilia

INFANTS AND CHILDREN

- ◆ Recurrent infections: tonsillitis, adenoiditis, bacterial infections, oral candidiasis, chronic diarrhea
- ◆ Present or recent infections, trauma distal to nodes
- ◆ Poor growth, failure to thrive
- ◆ Loss of interest in play or eating
- ◆ Immunization history
- ◆ Maternal HIV infection
- ◆ Hemophilia
- ◆ Illness in siblings

PREGNANT WOMEN

- ◆ Weeks of gestation
- ◆ Exposure to rubella and other infections
- ◆ Presence of children and pets in household

OLDER ADULTS

- ◆ Presence of an autoimmune disease
- ◆ Present or recent infection or trauma distal to nodes
- ◆ Delayed healing

EXAMINATION AND FINDINGS

EQUIPMENT

- ◆ Centimeter ruler
- ◆ Marking (skin) pencil

The lymphatic system is examined by inspection and palpation, region by region during examination of the other body systems, and by palpating the spleen, an integral part of the system (see Chapter 17). Or, sometimes you may prefer to examine the entire lymphatic system at once, exploring all the areas in which the nodes are accessible, regardless of their distribution. Individual chapters in this book discuss the lymphatic system in specific body areas. Always during this part of the examination ask whether the patient is aware of any lumps.

INSPECTION AND PALPATION

Inspect each area of the body for apparent lymph nodes, edema, erythema, red streaks, and skin lesions. Using the pads of the second, third, and fourth fingers, gently palpate for superficial lymph nodes (see Box 9-1 and Fig. 9-14). Try to detect any hidden enlargement, and note the consistency, mobility, tenderness, size, and warmth of the nodes. In areas where the skin is more mobile, move the skin over the area of the nodes. Press lightly at first, then gradually increase pressure. (Heavier pressure alone can push nodes out of the way before you have had a chance to recognize their presence.) Easily palpable lymph nodes generally are not found in

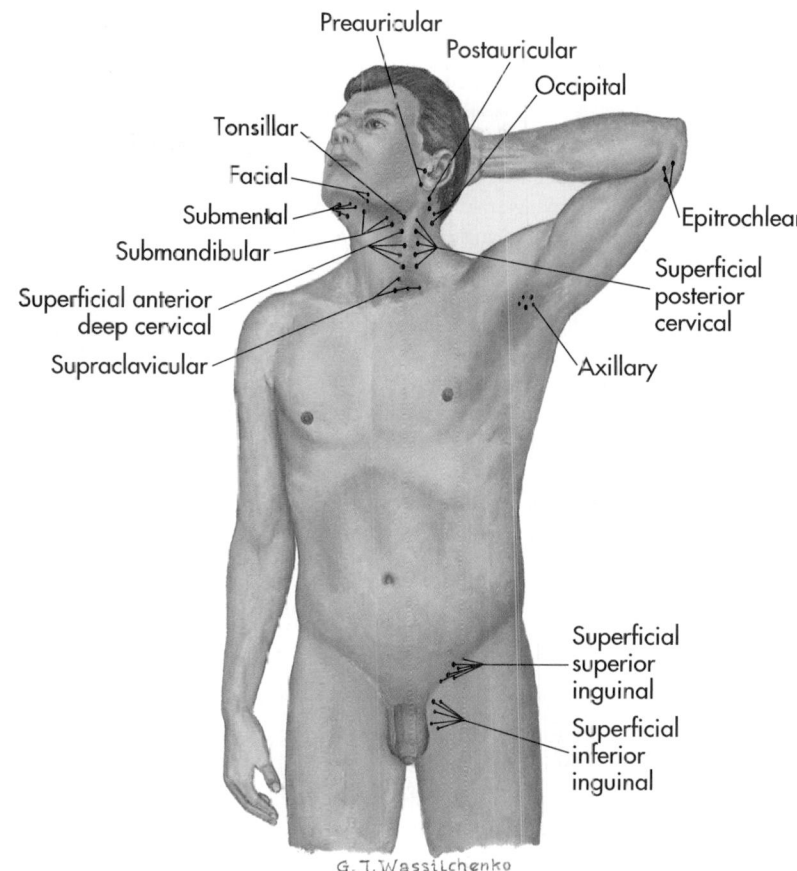

FIGURE 9-14
Some of the accessible lymph nodes.

MNEMONICS

If an Enlarged Lymph Node Is Found, Examine: PALS

P Primary site
A All associated nodes
L Liver
S Spleen

Modified from Shipman, 1984.

CLINICAL PEARL

Reminders About Nodes

- The harder the node and the more discrete, the more likely it is a malignancy.
- The more tender a node, the more likely it is an inflammation.
- Nodes do not pulsate; arteries do.
- A palpable supraclavicular node on the left is a relentless clue to thoracic or abdominal malignancy.
- Slow nodal enlargement over weeks and months suggests a benign process; rapid enlargement without inflammation suggests malignancy.

healthy adults. Superficial nodes that are accessible to palpation but not large or firm enough to be felt are common. You may detect small, movable, discrete, shotty nodes less than a centimeter in diameter that move under your fingers. When the node seems fixed in its setting, there is a greater cause for concern.

When enlarged lymph nodes are encountered, explore the accessible adjacent areas and regions drained by those nodes for signs of possible infection or malignancy. Examine other regions for enlargement. Enlarged lymph nodes in any region should be characterized according to location, size, shape, consistency, tenderness, movability or fixation to surrounding tissues, and discreteness. Lymph nodes that are enlarged and juxtaposed so that they feel like a large mass rather than discrete nodes are described as "matted." Marking with a skin pencil at the periphery of the node at the 12-, 3-, 6-, and 9-o'clock positions defines the extent of the node and helps guide the assessment of change.

Note if there is tenderness on touch or on rebound; the degree of discoloration or redness; and any unusual increase in vascularity, heat, or pulsations. (If bruits are audible with the stethoscope, it may be a blood vessel, not a lymph node.) When you are uncertain of the nature of the findings, check whether any large mass transilluminates; as a rule, nodes do not and cysts do. Lymph nodes that are large, fixed or matted, inflamed, or tender indicate a problem. Tenderness is almost always indicative of inflammation; cancerous nodes are not usually tender. With bacterial infection, nodes may become warm or tender to the touch, matted, and much less discrete, particularly if the infection persists. It is possible to infer the site of an infection from the pattern of lymph node enlargement. For example, infections of the ear usually drain to the preauricular, retropharyngeal, and deep cervical nodes (see Fig. 9-8). A child with such an infection may complain of an earache, although the pain originates in a node.

Lymph nodes to which a malignancy has spread are not usually tender. They vary greatly in size, from tiny to many centimeters in diameter. They are sometimes discrete, sometimes matted and firmly fixed to underlying tissues; they tend to be harder than expected. Involvement is often asymmetric; contralateral nodes in similar locations may not be palpable. Most of the time, masses other than nodes anterior to the sternocleidomastoid muscle are benign

MNEMONICS

Features of a Lump (Not All of Them Lymph Nodes): Nine Ss

S   Size
S   Shape
S   Surface characteristics (e.g., erythema, warmth)
S   Site
S   Symptoms (e.g., pain, pruritus)
S   Softness; fluctuation
S   Squeezability (e.g., hemangiomata)
S   Spread (e.g., lymph nodes in related areas)
S   Sensations (e.g., thrill of A-V fistula)

Modified from Shipman, 1984.

DIFFERENTIAL DIAGNOSIS
CONDITIONS SIMULATING LYMPH NODE ENLARGEMENT

- Lymphangioma (transilluminates; hemangiomas do not)
- Cystic hygroma (thin-walled, contains clear lymph fluid)
- Hemangioma (tends to feel spongy; appears reddish-blue, with color depending on size and extent of angiomatous involvement; Valsalva maneuver may enlarge the mass)
- Branchial cleft cyst (sometimes accompanied by a tiny orifice in the neck on a line extending to the ear along the sternocleidomastoid muscle; may fluctuate in size when inflamed)
- Thyroglossal duct cyst (midline in the neck; may retract when tongue is protruded)
- Granular cell tumor
- Laryngocele
- Esophageal diverticulum
- Thyroid goiter
- Graves disease
- Hashimoto thyroiditis
- Parotid swelling (e.g., from mumps or tumor)

(except for thyroid masses); those posterior may be malignant. Importantly, however, the supraclavicular node warning of malignancy lies anterior to the sternocleidomastoid muscle.

In tuberculosis, the lymph nodes, often felt in the cervical chains, are usually "cold" (actually, body temperature), soft, matted, and not tender or painful.

Features of a lump are described in the Mnemonics box.

Each of these observations suggests an aspect of the physical examination of a lump. If you keep them in mind, you can provide an accurate written description for the record by describing each of the observations in sequence. The differentiation of an enlarged lymph node from other masses depends on many variables; for example, some sites are incompatible with the distribution of nodes, and some palpable sensations (e.g., thrill, consistency) are not possible with the basic structure of nodes (see the Differential Diagnosis box above).

HEAD AND NECK

Lymphatic System:
Palpating Lymph Nodes in the Head and Neck

Lightly palpate the entire neck for nodes. The anterior border of the sternocleidomastoid muscle is the dividing line for the anterior and posterior triangles of the neck and is a useful landmark for describing location. The muscles and bones of the neck together create these "triangles" (Fig. 9-15).

Bending the patient's head slightly forward or to the side will ease taut tissues and allow better accessibility to palpation. Feel for nodes on the head in the following six-step sequence (Fig. 9-16):

1. The occipital nodes at the base of the skull
2. The postauricular nodes located superficially over the mastoid process
3. The preauricular nodes just in front of the ear (Fig. 9-17)
4. The parotid and retropharyngeal (tonsillar) nodes at the angle of the mandible
5. The submandibular nodes halfway between the angle and the tip of the mandible
6. The submental nodes in the midline behind the tip of the mandible

Then move down to the neck, palpating in the following four-step sequence:

1. The superficial cervical nodes at the sternocleidomastoid muscle
2. The posterior cervical nodes along the anterior border of the trapezius muscle (Fig. 9-18)
3. The cervical nodes deep to the sternocleidomastoid (The deep cervical nodes may be difficult to feel if you press too vigorously; probe gently with your thumb and fingers around the muscle.)

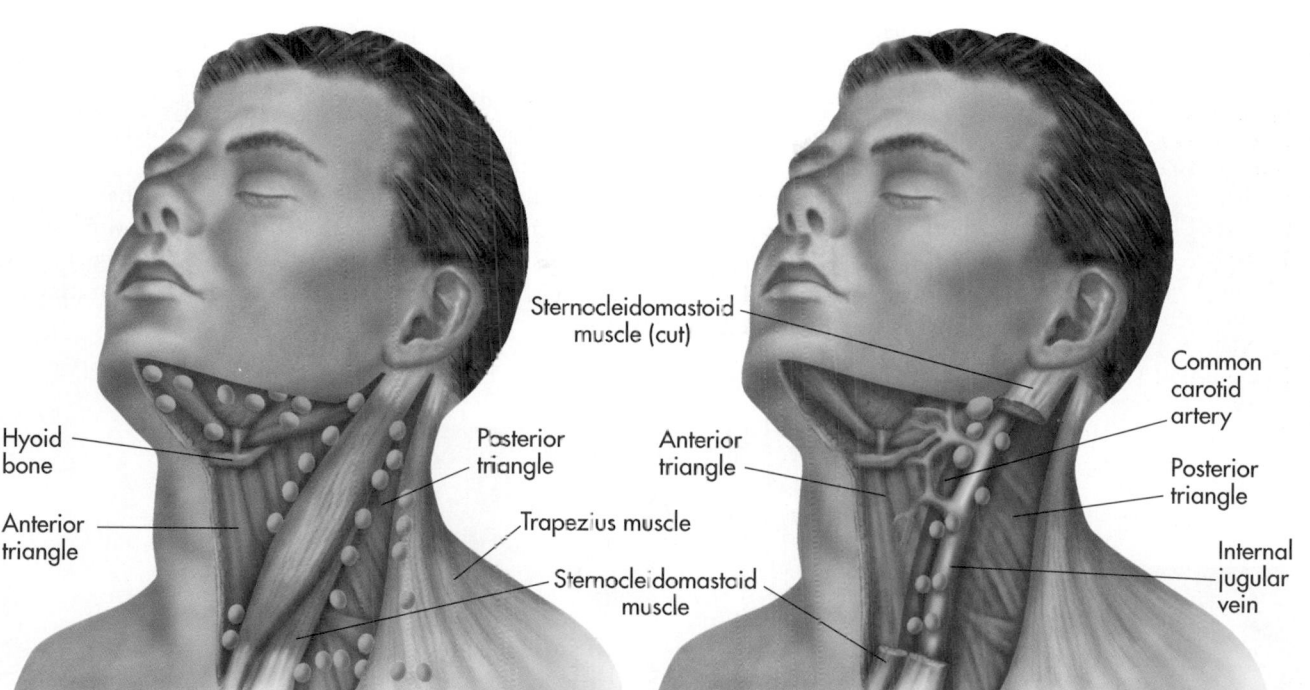

Sternocleidomastoid muscle (cut)

Hyoid bone

Anterior triangle

Posterior triangle

Trapezius muscle

Sternocleidomastoid muscle

Anterior triangle

Common carotid artery

Posterior triangle

Internal jugular vein

FIGURE 9-15
The triangles of the neck.

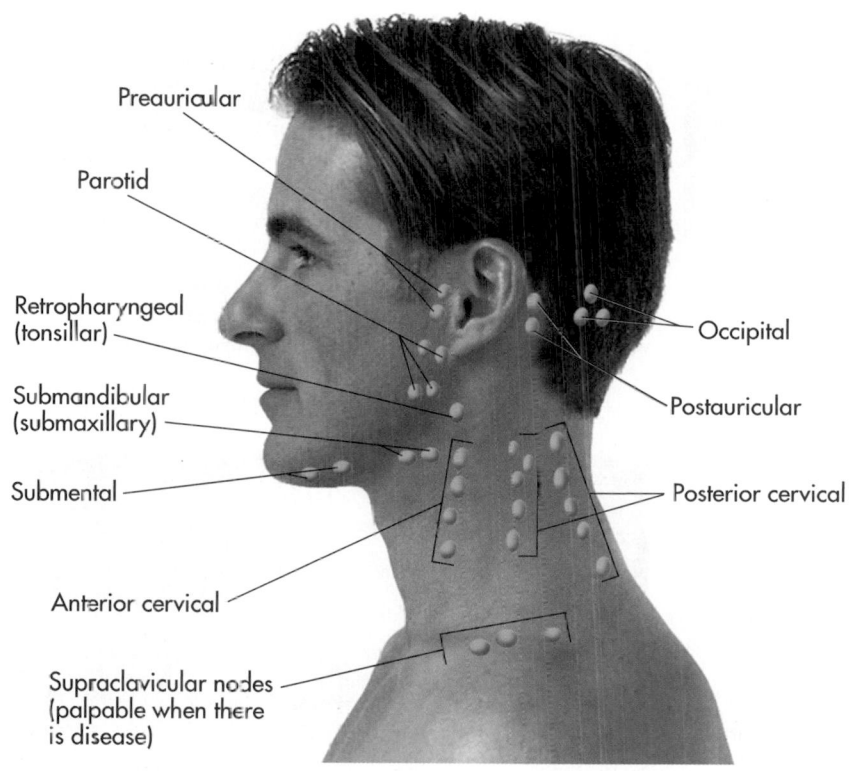

Preauricular

Parotid

Retropharyngeal (tonsillar)

Submandibular (submaxillary)

Submental

Anterior cervical

Supraclavicular nodes (palpable when there is disease)

Occipital

Postauricular

Posterior cervical

FIGURE 9-16
Palpable lymph nodes of the head and neck.

4. The supraclavicular areas, probing deeply in the angle formed by the clavicle and the sternocleidomastoid muscle, the area of Virchow nodes (Fig. 9-19) (Detection of these nodes should always be considered a cause for concern.)

On occasion, postauricular nodes affected by ear infection (particularly external otitis) may be surrounded by some cellulitis; this may cause the ears to protrude.

Supraclavicular nodes are commonly the sites of metastatic disease because they are located at the end of the thoracic duct and other associated lymphatic ducts. A Virchow node in the left supraclavicular region may be the result of either abdominal or thoracic malignancy. Mediastinal collecting ducts from the lungs go to both sides of the neck, and supraclavicular nodes may be palpated on both sides.

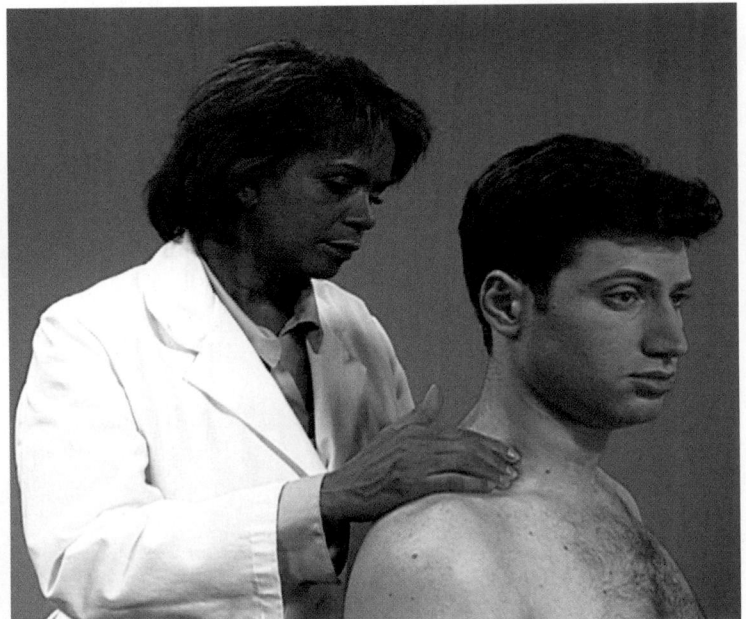

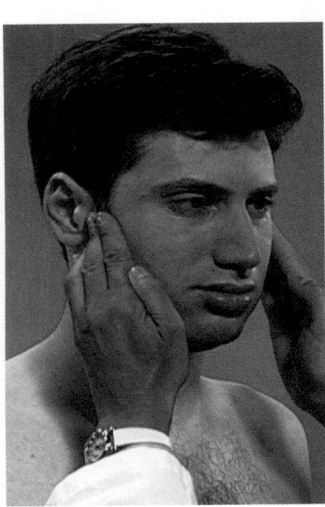

FIGURE 9-17
Palpation of preauricular lymph nodes. Compare the nodes bilaterally.

FIGURE 9-18
Palpation of posterior cervical nodes. Dorsal surfaces (pads) of the fingertips are used to palpate along the anterior surface of the trapezius muscle and then moved slowly in a circular motion toward the posterior surface of the sternocleidomastoid muscle.

FIGURE 9-19
Palpation for supraclavicular lymph nodes. The patient is encouraged to relax the musculature of the upper extremities so that the clavicles drop. The examiner's free hand is used to flex the patient's head forward to relax the soft tissues of the anterior neck. The fingers are hooked over the clavicle lateral to the sternocleidomastoid muscle.

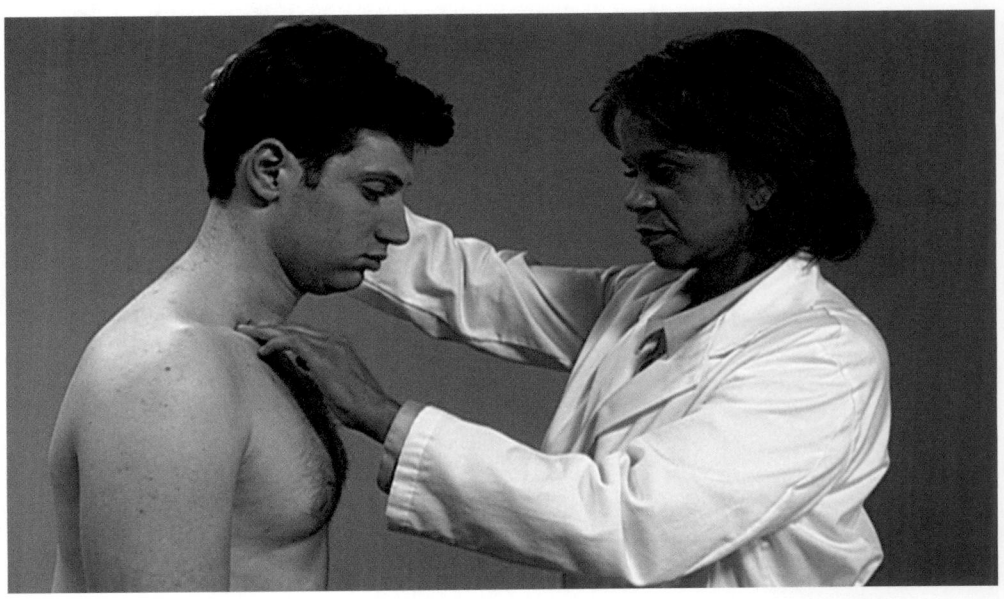

AXILLAE

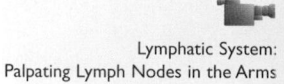

Lymphatic System:
Palpating Lymph Nodes in the Arms

Think of the axillary examination by imagining a pentagonal structure: the pectoral muscles anteriorly, the back muscles (i.e., latissimus dorsi and subscapularis) posteriorly, the rib cage medially, the upper arm laterally, and the axilla at the apex. Let the soft tissues roll between your fingers, the chest wall, and muscles as you palpate. A firm, deliberate, yet gentle touch may feel less ticklish to the patient.

On palpation of the axillary lymph nodes, support the patient's forearm with your contralateral arm and bring the palm of your examining hand flat into the axilla; alternatively, let the patient's forearm rest on that of your examining hand (Fig. 9-20). Rotate your fingertips and palm, feeling the nodes; if they are palpable, attempt to glide your fingers beneath the nodes.

A more complete examination of the breast, the axilla, and adjacent areas is described in Chapter 16.

OTHER LYMPH NODES

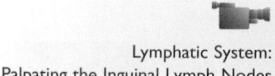

Lymphatic System:
Palpating the Inguinal Lymph Nodes

Use a systematic approach when palpating other sites of lymph node clusters. Move the hand in a circular fashion, probing gently without pressing hard. Relieve tension by flexion of the extremity. To palpate the epitrochlear nodes, support the elbow in one hand as you explore with the other (Fig. 9-21). To palpate the inguinal and popliteal area, have the patient lie supine with the knee slightly flexed (Fig. 9-22). The superior superficial inguinal (femoral) nodes are close to the surface over the inguinal canals. The inferior superficial inguinal nodes lie deeper in the groin.

CLINICAL PEARL

Vaccinations and Nodes
Immunizations given in the upper arm may cause axillary node enlargement, particularly BCG and smallpox vaccination.

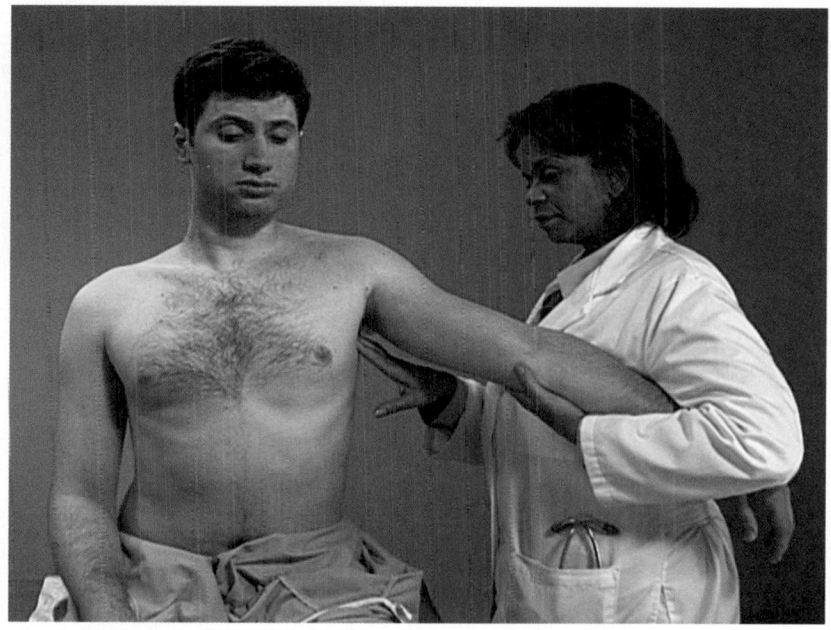

FIGURE 9-20
Soft tissues of axilla are gently rolled against the chest wall and the muscles surrounding the axilla.

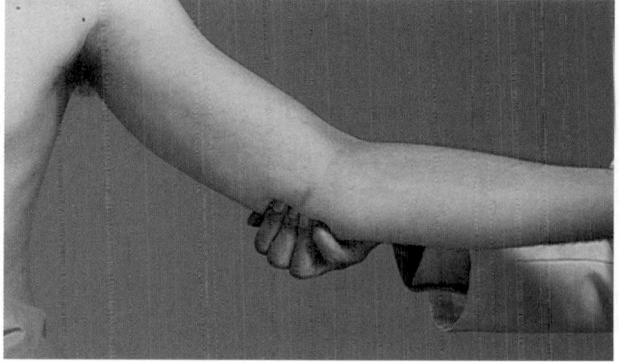

FIGURE 9-21
Palpation for epitrochlear lymph nodes is performed in the depression above and posterior to the medial condyle of the humerus.

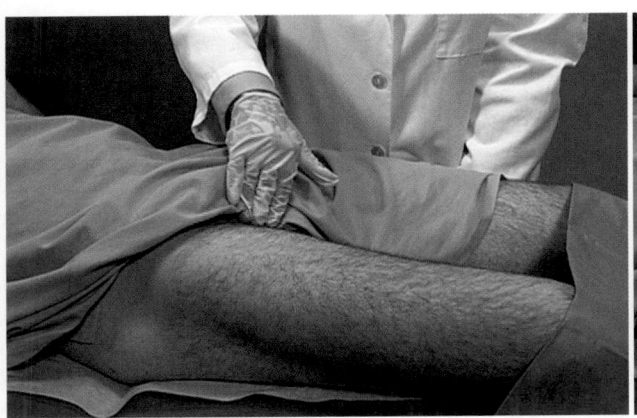
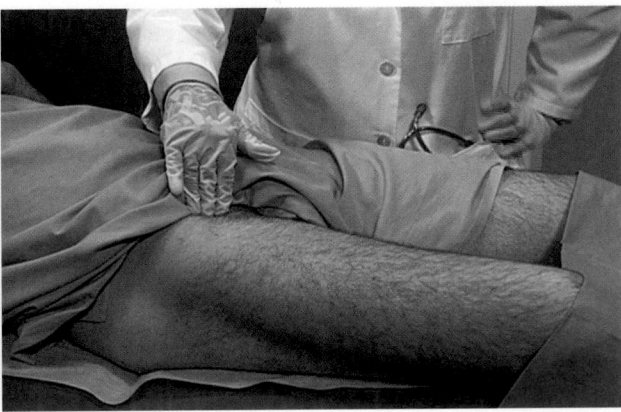

FIGURE 9-22
A, Palpation of inferior superficial inguinal (femoral) lymph nodes. **B,** Palpation of superior inguinal lymph nodes.

CLINICAL PEARL

Drugs and Nodes

Diphenylhydantoin, particularly, can cause nodal enlargement. So too, on occasion, can aspirin, barbiturates, penicillin, tetracycline, iodide, cephalosporin, sulfonamide, and mesantoin, among others.

Tunnesen, 1999.

STAYING WELL

HOLD BACK ON INVASION

One way to help patients to keep well is to limit the number of invasive tests and procedures we decide to order for them. Psychologic and physical discomfort are frequent companions to invasion. The best way to assure that we avoid the unnecessary is to perform a knowledgeable and skilled history and physical examination. There are many indications in this chapter for the biopsy of suspicious lymph nodes but just as importantly—perhaps more so—indications to resist biopsy. Every invasion thoughtfully rejected represents an effort to help patients get well and keep well.

The lymphatic drainage of the testes is into the abdomen. Enlarged nodes there are not accessible to inspection and palpation. Nodes in the inguinal area enlarge if there are lesions of the penile and scrotal surfaces.

Similarly, the internal female genitalia drain into the pelvic and paraaortic nodes and are not accessible to inspection and palpation; however, the vulva and lower one third of the vagina drain into the inguinal nodes.

INFANTS AND CHILDREN

The technique of examination is similar for all ages. You will find small, firm, discrete, and movable nodes that are neither warm nor tender located in the occipital, postauricular, cervical, and inguinal chains. The very thin child's inguinal nodes may even be readily visible. In children, such nodes are not as worrisome as in the adult. The shape is usually globular or ovoid, sometimes flatter or more cylindrical.

Lymph node enlargement in children has often been documented, much more so than in adults. In the well child, they are not warm, tender, or fluctuant; do not mat together; are not associated with erythema; and have not been demonstrated to be associated with serious illness. It is not unusual to find enlarged postauricular and occipital nodes in children younger than 2 years of age. Past that age, such enlargement is relatively uncommon and may be significant (see the Differential Diagnosis boxes on p. 249 for mumps and for immune deficiency disease in a child). Conversely, cervical and submandibular nodal enlargement is relatively less common in children younger than 1 year of age and much more common in older children. These age distributions should be considered in your decision to evaluate further lymph node enlargement (Herzog, 1983). The discovery of small lymph nodes in the inguinal, cervical, or axillary chains of neonates may not in itself require further investigation (Box 9-2). In general, laboratory tests are not indicated in otherwise well children who have cervical lymphadenopathy.

DIFFERENTIAL DIAGNOSIS
MUMPS VERSUS CERVICAL ADENITIS

Mumps, epidemic parotiditis, is characterized by a somewhat painful swelling of the parotid glands unilaterally or bilaterally and, occasionally, by swelling and tenderness of the other salivary glands along the mandible. The swelling can obscure the angle of the jaw and may appear on inspection as a cervical adenitis. On palpation, however, the two are easily distinguished. A cervical adenitis does not ordinarily obscure the angle of the jaw. Your fingers can separate the node from the angle so that you can feel the hard sharpness of the bone, a finding generally not associated with parotid swelling.

DIFFERENTIAL DIAGNOSIS
HOW TO DISCOVER AN IMMUNE DEFICIENCY DISEASE IN A CHILD

Begin with a thorough history in all regards:
- The family history
- Risk factors for HIV infection
- Illness in siblings
- Previous infections
- Previous hospitalizations
- Most important, serious recurring infections and infections that are uncommon (e.g., infection with *Pneumocystis carinii*; other infections, particularly fungal, that do not yield to therapy)

Note unusual findings on the physical examination (e.g., generalized lymphadenopathy and enlargement of the liver and/or spleen).

The child who is not doing well, who has recurrent infection, and in whom unusual findings persist could possibly have an immune deficiency. HIV infection in the young can have a long clinical latency. The least suspicion in a child at risk should lead to testing.

BOX 9-2
WHEN LYMPHADENOPATHY REQUIRES FURTHER INVESTIGATION

The detection of lymphadenopathy is common and the number of diseases associated with it is great. It is not too often necessary, however, to go beyond physical examination to resort to biopsy or other laboratory tests. Still, older patients with localized and persistent lymphadenopathy, without evidence of infection or inflammation, might be assumed to have cancer unless a biopsy proves otherwise. Young adults and children are more likely to have demonstrable infection (often Epstein-Barr virus mononucleosis); however, the young need biopsy with localized supraclavicular lymphadenopathy as much as the old. Posterior cervical lymphadenopathy also adds a risk for malignancy, more so than when lymphadenopathy occurs in the anterior cervical chain. At any age, any lump that grows rapidly and insistently should prompt a search for malignancy and, if in the midline, should be considered to have a possible relationship to the central nervous system.

Nodes smaller than 0.5 cm generally are not cause for concern, and nodes with a diameter of 1 cm or less in the cervical and inguinal chains do not always indicate a problem. If nodes have grown rapidly and are suspiciously large (i.e., more than 2 cm), mildly painful, or fixed to contiguous tissues and relatively immovable, investigate further.

The palatine tonsils may be enlarged in children; this in itself is not a problem. Excessive enlargement may obstruct the nasopharynx, increasing the risk of sleep apnea and, on rare occasions, pulmonary hypertension (see Chapter 12, Fig. 12-40).

SAMPLE DOCUMENTATION
HISTORY AND PHYSICAL EXAMINATION

Subjective
The patient reports difficulty in swallowing and a sore throat, now subsiding.
Objective
No visible enlargement in any area. On palpation, enlarged node (2 cm in diameter) in left posterior cervical triangle, firm, nontender, movable, no overlying warmth, erythema, or edema. In addition, a few shotty nodes palpable in posterior cervical triangle bilaterally and in femoral chains bilaterally.

For additional sample documentation, see Chapter 26.

SUMMARY OF EXAMINATION
LYMPHATIC SYSTEM

The lymphatic system is examined region by region during the examination of the other body systems (i.e., head and neck, breast and axillary, genitalia, and extremities).

1. Inspect the visible nodes and surrounding area for the following characteristics (p. 242):
    *   Edema
    *   Erythema
    *   Red streaks
2. Palpate the superficial lymph nodes and compare side to side for the following (pp. 242-247):
    *   Size
    *   Consistency
    *   Mobility
    *   Discrete borders or matting
    *   Tenderness
    *   Warmth

If you discover lymphadenopathy, consider the associated drainage region to suggest possible sources for a presenting problem.

COMMON ABNORMALITIES

ACUTE LYMPHANGITIS
Acute lymphangitis is an inflammation of one or more lymphatic vessels. It is characterized by pain, a feeling of malaise and illness, and possibly fever. On inspection you may find a red streak following the course of the lymphatic collecting duct. It appears as a tracing of rather fine lines streaking up the extremity. The inflammation is sometimes slightly indurated and palpable to gentle touch. Look distal to the inflammation for sites of infection, particularly interdigitally.

ACUTE SUPPURATIVE LYMPHADENITIS
Group A beta-hemolytic streptococci and coagulase-positive staphylococci cause most instances of acute lymphadenitis. The involved node is usually quite firm and tender. The overlying tissue becomes edematous, and the skin appears erythematous, usually within 72 hours. Other pathogens may play a role (e.g., actinomycotic adenitis as a result of dental disease; mycobacterial lymphadenitis in the presence of the tuberculosis organism; organisms both typical and atypical as a result of cat scratch [cat scratch disease]; or *Pasteurella multocida* infection at the site of a scratch or bite from a dog or cat). Mycobacterial adenitis is characterized by an inflammation without warmth that may or may not be slightly tender.

NON-HODGKIN LYMPHOMA
Malignant neoplasms of the lymphatic system and the reticuloendothelial tissues are usually well defined and solid. Histologically, their cells are often undifferentiated, but resemble lymphocytes, histiocytes, or plasma cells. Lymphomas occur most often in lymph nodes, the spleen, and other sites in which lymphoreticular cells are found. The nodes involved in this and other malignancies may be localized in the posterior cervical triangle or may become matted, crossing into the anterior triangle. Pain is not a prominent feature. It is often not pos-

sible or appropriate to attempt to distinguish the findings of these conditions from those in Hodgkin disease through physical examination alone.

HODGKIN DISEASE

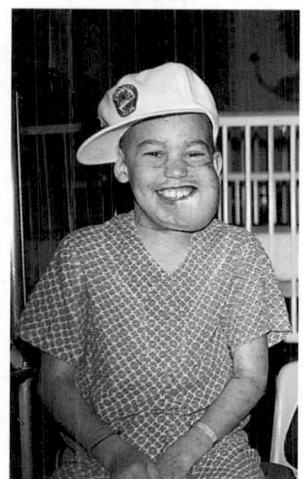

FIGURE 9-23
Hodgkin disease. Note the impressive extent of the enlargement.

Hodgkin disease is a malignant lymphoma that occurs in the young of all races, generally in late adolescence and young adulthood (Fig. 9-23), although it also occurs in people older than 50 years of age. Males are twice as likely to develop Hodgkin disease as are females. Its clinical presentation is variable. Most commonly there is a painless enlargement of the cervical lymph nodes, often in the posterior triangle, that is generally asymmetric and inexorably progressive. The nodes are sometimes matted and generally feel very firm, almost rubbery. Although asymmetry is the rule, nodes are occasionally enlarged in similar patterns on both sides of the body. The nodal size may fluctuate.

EPSTEIN-BARR VIRUS MONONUCLEOSIS

CLINICAL PEARL

Cervical Nodes
The common childhood diseases, rubella, rubeola, and varicella, often present with obvious cervical nodes, usually posterior rather than anterior. Hepatitis A or B and infectious mononucleosis have the same tendency.

Epstein-Barr virus mononucleosis (infectious mononucleosis) occurs at almost any age but is most common in adolescents and young adults. Initial symptoms include pharyngitis and, usually, fever, fatigue, and malaise. Often splenomegaly and, on occasion, hepatomegaly and/or a rash may be noted. The affected nodes may be generalized but are more commonly felt in the anterior and posterior cervical chains. They vary in firmness and are generally discrete and occasionally a bit tender. You should resist thinking of a biopsy in this illness especially if chest x-ray results are normal. The Ebstein-Barr virus has been found in the tumor cells of Burkitt lymphoma and nasopharyngeal carcinoma. This virus has a probable role in causing these malignancies. Other common viral causes of cervical adenitis include cytomegalovirus, adenovirus, varicella, and enterovirus.

TOXOPLASMOSIS

A single node, chronically enlarged and nontender, characterizes toxoplasmosis. The node is usually in the posterior cervical chain. The patient may not have other significant symptoms but there may be a history of eating raw or rare meat. A pet cat may be the source. The scalp may give evidence of seborrhea or other lesions.

ROSEOLA INFANTUM (HHV-6)

Fever—usually high grade and persistent over 3 to 4 days—is the chief presenting complaint. When the fever diminishes, a morbilliform but not particularly intense rash occurs, primarily involving the face and chest, and the patient, almost always a baby 7 to 12 months of age, begins feeling much better. The adenopathy, discrete and not noted for tenderness, involves the occipital and postauricular chains and may last a while. These should be left alone.

HERPES SIMPLEX

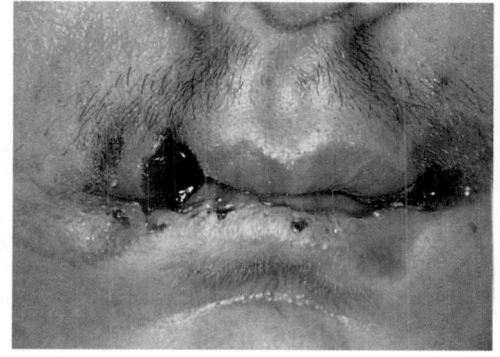

FIGURE 9-24
Herpes simplex.

Herpes simplex can cause discrete labial and gingival ulcers, high-grade fever, and enlargement of the anterior cervical and submandibular nodes (Fig. 9-24). These nodes tend to be somewhat firm, quite discrete, movable, and tender. Temperature is often high. The frequency of this condition and the symptoms are generally sufficient to establish the diagnosis. A viral culture can be obtained if necessary.

CAT SCRATCH DISEASE

Cat scratch disease is among the most common causes of subacute or chronic lymphadenitis in children. The diagnosis can be made in the presence of a nodal enlargement lasting longer than 3 weeks, accompanied by a primary lesion of the skin or eye and following an interaction with a cat, a cat scratch, or cat lick on a break in the skin. Early in the disease there may be a papule or pustule that may or may not subside over a short period of time. Tender nodes are most commonly found in the areas of the head, neck, and axillae. The accessible nodal areas in the arms and legs are less often involved. The nodes can be very large—up to several centimeters—and they may often be red and tender and occasionally suppurate. The lymphadenopathy can last for 2 to 4 months or even longer, making more serious malignant disease a common diagnostic concern.

AIDS

Acquired immune deficiency syndrome (AIDS) is characterized by the dysfunction of cell-mediated immunity. It is manifested clinically as the development of recurrent, often severe, opportunistic infections. Common life-threatening diseases associated with full-blown AIDS include Kaposi sarcoma, *Pneumocystis carinii* pneumonia, pulmonary tuberculosis, recurrent pneumonia, and invasive cervical cancer. Initial symptoms include lymphadenopathy, fatigue, fever, and weight loss. In children there may be a prolonged clinical latent period, but initial signs may include neurodevelopmental problems with loss of developmental milestones, a parotid enlargement simulating mumps, anemia and thrombocytopenia, chronic diarrhea, and recurrent infections. AIDS is caused by HIV. A CD4+ T-lymphocyte count of less than 14% is a significant marker for HIV-related immunosuppression.

HIV SEROPOSITIVITY

A person with HIV antibodies who has not yet developed the sequelae of recurrent infections and neoplastic disease is said to be HIV positive. Warning signs and symptoms may include severe fatigue, malaise, weakness, persistent unexplained weight loss, persistent lymphadenopathy, fevers, arthralgias, and persistent diarrhea.

SERUM SICKNESS

Serum sickness is an immune complex disease characterized by urticaria, other rashes, lymphadenopathy, joint pain, fever, and at times facial edema. Urticaria usually appears first. Lymphadenopathy, a common finding, is most prominent in the area draining the site of an injection of antiserum from animal sources; or, more often of late, of a variety of drugs. The nodal enlargement can be generalized. Facial edema is not unusual. These findings become apparent about 7 to 10 days following the use of the provoking substance. They subside rather more slowly, recurring at times over several weeks. The patient can react similarly to repeated exposure to the stimuli; subsequent reactions may be even more severe and even fatal.

LYMPHEDEMA

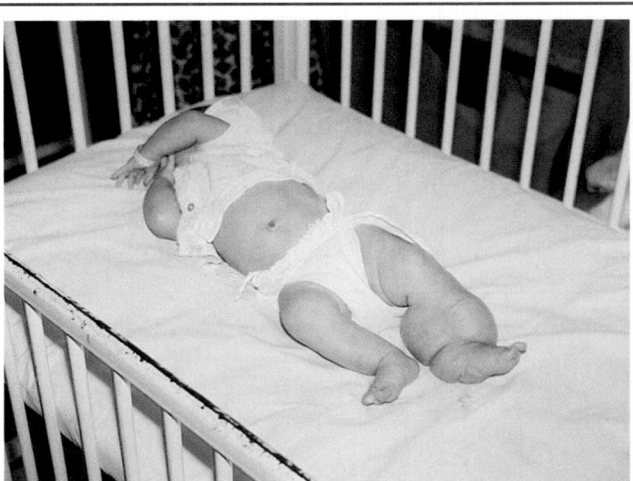

FIGURE 9-25
Lymphedema.

Congenital or "primary" lymphedema (Milroy disease), much more common in females than in males, is the hypoplasia and maldevelopment of the lymphatic system, resulting in swelling and often grotesque distortion of the extremities (Fig. 9-25). It is often apparent at birth and most often involves the legs, particularly the dorsum of the foot. A later onset, termed "praecox" in adolescence and "tarda" in patients approaching 40 years of age, is not uncommon.

The degree varies with the severity and distribution of the abnormality and may not appear until young adulthood. Acquired or "secondary" lymphedema results from trauma to the ducts of regional lymph nodes (particularly axillary and inguinal) after surgery, radiation, or metastasis. In each case, obstruction and sometimes infection block the lymphatic ducts, producing lymphedema. Lymphedema does not pit, and the overlying skin eventually thickens and feels tougher than usual.

LYMPHANGIOMA AND CYSTIC HYGROMA	Lymphangioma and cystic hygroma are the results of obstruction of developing lymphatic vessels. Most lymphangiomas are present at birth and are apparent early in life, usually in the neck or axilla, less commonly in the chest or extremities. Cystic hygromas can be so large as to distort the face and neck. They feel soft and easily compressible, and are fluid-containing. In severe circumstances, they may obstruct the airway or compromise swallowing. These malformations are generally accessible to physical examination.
ELEPHANTIASIS	Elephantiasis is a massive accumulation of lymphedema throughout the body that results from widespread inflammation and obstruction of the lymphatics by the filarial worms, *Wuchereria bancrofti* or *Brugia malayi*. Adequate drainage is prevented, and the patient becomes more susceptible to infection, cellulitis, and fibrosis. The term is often loosely used to describe the result of any obstruction, congenital or acquired (see the Differential Diagnosis box below).

DIFFERENTIAL DIAGNOSIS

WHEN THE BODY SWELLS

A significant number of pathologic processes can cause swelling of the extremities and other areas in the body. These can stem from, but are not limited to, the cardiovascular system (e.g., congestive heart failure or constrictive pericarditis), diseases of the liver (e.g., obstruction of the hepatic vein [Chiari syndrome] and portal vein thrombosis), and kidney malfunction. The most common cause, particularly of the feet and the ankles, is stasis; the result of deep venous thrombosis, this may occur in otherwise well men and women who must stand or sit for long periods. The failure to move with some regularity increases orthostatic pressure in the legs. Pregnancy is also a common contributor, even in the absence of venous abnormality in the legs. There can also be a significant disruption of lymphatic circulation in the arms after breast surgery with its disruption of lymph flow. When lymphatic disruption is at the root of swelling, the edema does not have the characteristic pitting usually seen with other causes of edema. Patients with myxedema, a finding associated with hypothyroidism that is typified by a dry, waxy swelling, share this characteristic (see Fig. 10-19). The edema in this circumstance can cause a rather typical facies, with swollen lips and a thick nose; it, too, does not pit.

ELECTRONIC RESOURCES

For Weblinks and additional resources, go to   **evolve**

http://evolve.elsevier.com/Seidel

or to the Companion CD-ROM.

Additional information related to the content in Chapter 9 can be found on the companion website at evolve.elsevier.com/Seidel/ or on the interactive companion CD-ROM. Resources and activities for Chapter 9 include:
- Sound and Vision Theater
- Printouts for Your Practice
- Interactive Challenge
- Spanish Assessment Terms with Pronunciation Guide
- Instant Calculator

HEAD AND NECK

Together the head and neck provide the bony housing and protective cover for the brain, including the special senses of vision, hearing, smell, and taste. The intrinsic musculature also permits social expression, an additional method of communication. Before examining the special senses and the neurologic system, it is important to evaluate carefully the overlying structures.

ANATOMY AND PHYSIOLOGY

The skull is composed of seven bones (two frontal, two parietal, two temporal, and one occipital) that are fused together and covered by the scalp. Bones of the skull are used to identify the site of findings referable to the head (Fig. 10-1). The facial skull has several cavities for the eyes, nose, and mouth. The bony structure of the face is formed from the fused frontal, nasal, zygomatic, ethmoid, lacrimal, sphenoid, and maxillary bones, and the movable mandible.

Major landmarks of the face are the palpebral fissures and the nasolabial folds (Fig. 10-2). Facial muscles are innervated by cranial nerve (CN) V and CN VII. The temporal artery is the major accessible artery of the face, passing just anterior to the ear, over the temporal muscle, and onto the forehead.

The parotid, submandibular, and sublingual salivary glands are paired and produce saliva, which moistens the mouth, inhibits formation of dental caries, and initiates digestion of carbohydrates. The parotid gland is located anterior to the ear and above the mandible, the submandibular gland is located medial to the mandible at the angle of the jaw, and the sublingual gland is located anteriorly in the floor of the mouth.

The neck is formed by the cervical vertebrae, ligaments, and the sternocleidomastoid and trapezius muscles, which give it support and movement (Fig. 10-3). Horizontal mobility is greatest between cervical vertebrae 4 and 5 or 5 and 6. The sternocleidomastoid muscle extends from the upper sternum and medial third of the clavicle to the mastoid process. The trapezius muscle extends from the scapula, the lateral third of the clavicle, and the vertebrae to the occipital prominence.

The relationship of these muscles to each other and to adjacent bones creates triangles used as anatomic landmarks. The posterior triangle is formed by the trapezius and sternocleidomastoid muscles and the clavicle (Fig. 10-4) and contains the posterior cervical lymph nodes (Fig. 10-5). (For a more complete description of the lymph nodes of the head and neck, see Figs. 9-8 to 9-11.)

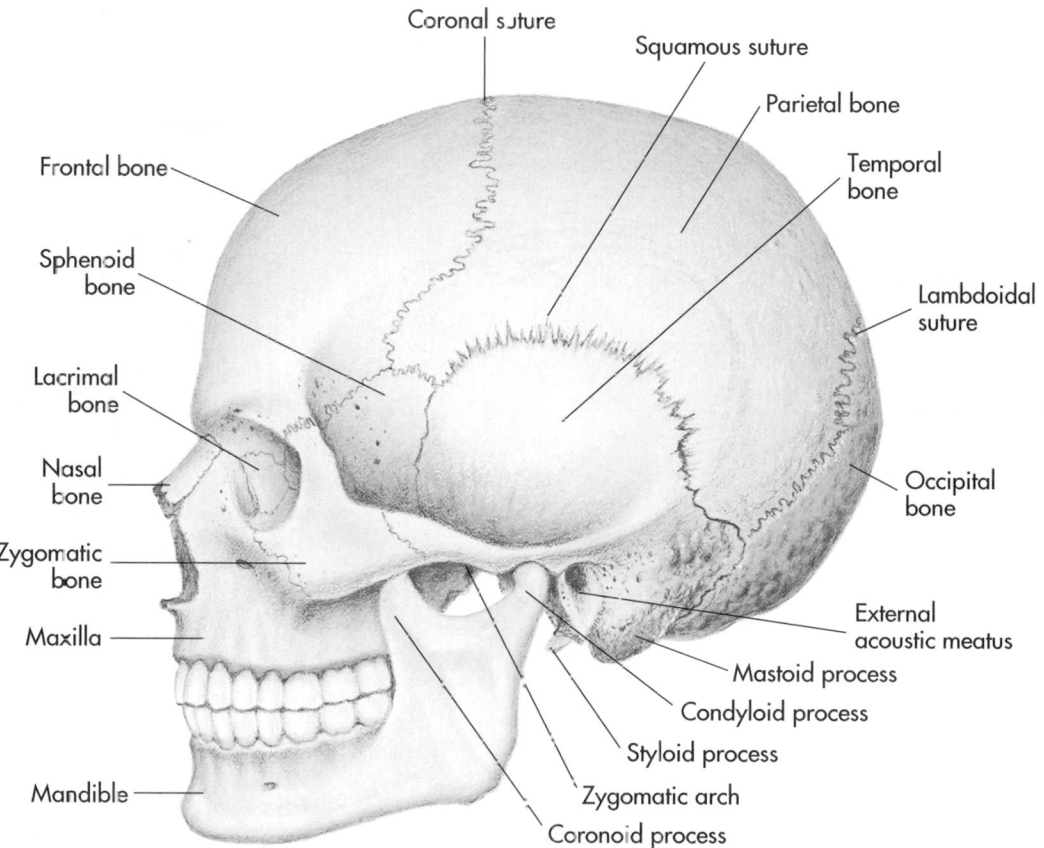

FIGURE 10-1
Bones of the skull.

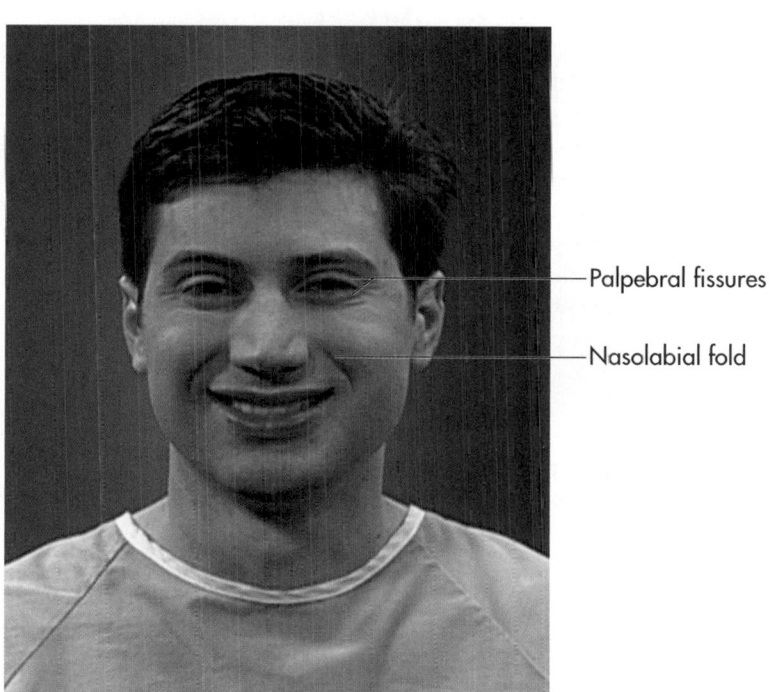

FIGURE 10-2
Landmarks of the face.

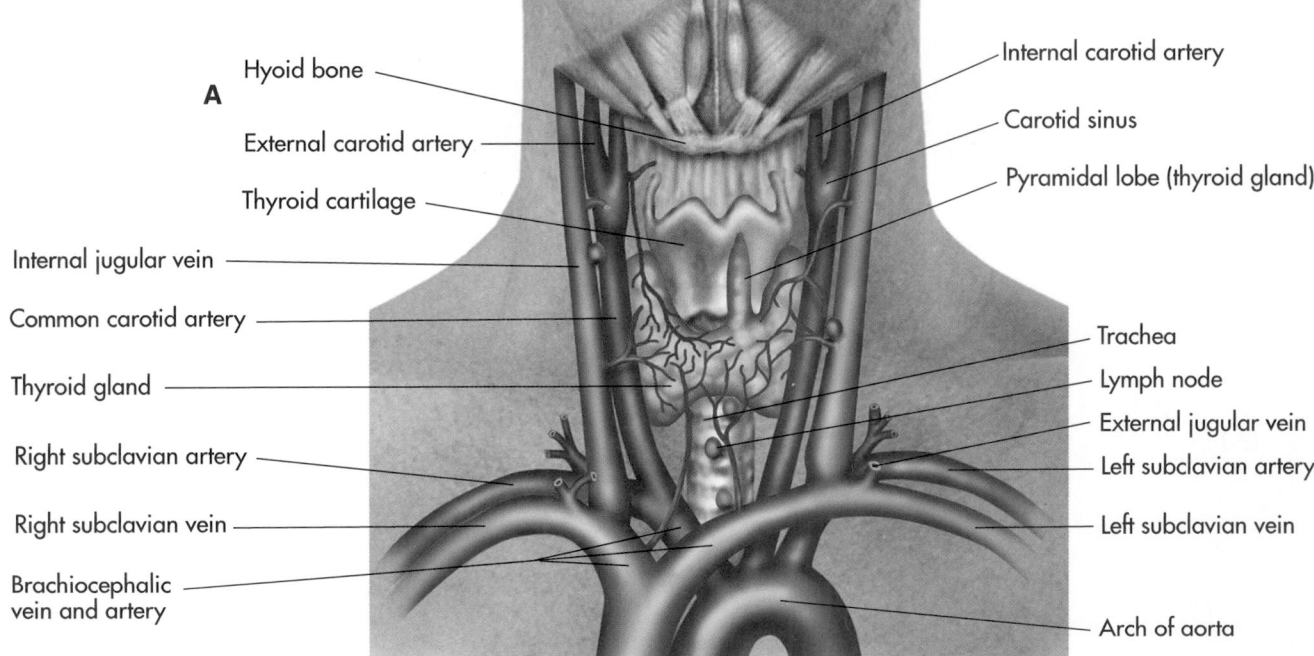

A

Hyoid bone

External carotid artery

Thyroid cartilage

Internal jugular vein

Common carotid artery

Thyroid gland

Right subclavian artery

Right subclavian vein

Brachiocephalic
vein and artery

Internal carotid artery

Carotid sinus

Pyramidal lobe (thyroid gland)

Trachea

Lymph node

External jugular vein

Left subclavian artery

Left subclavian vein

Arch of aorta

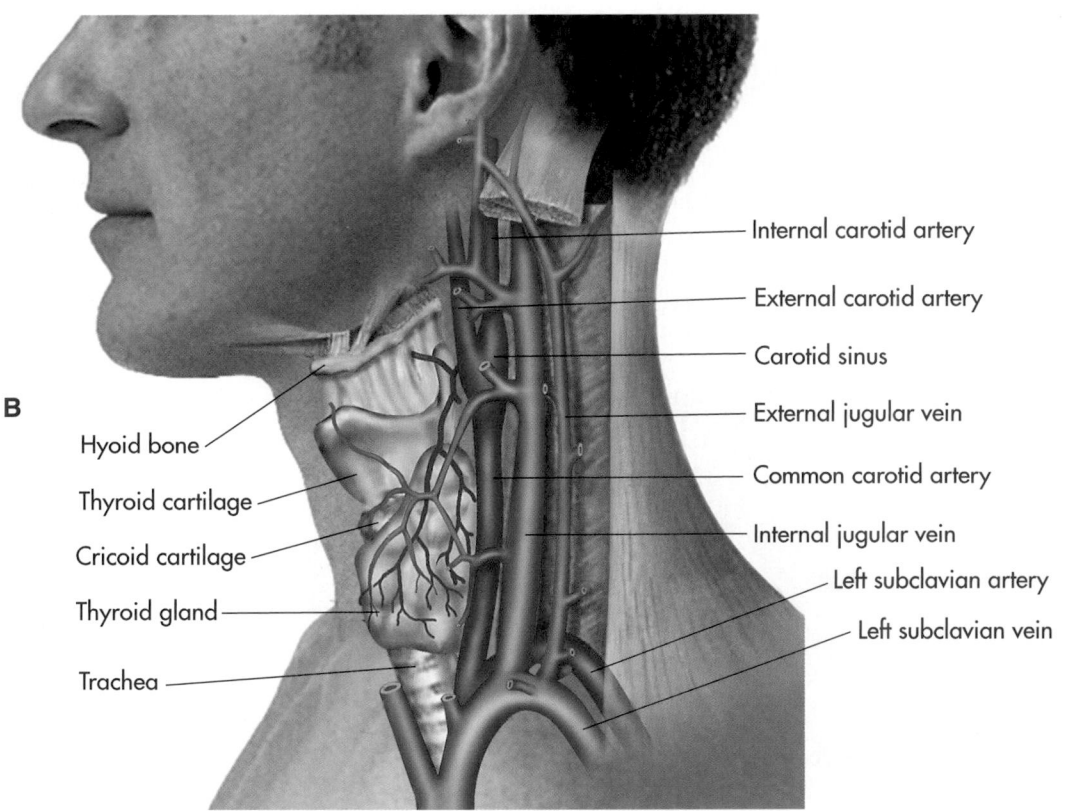

B

Hyoid bone

Thyroid cartilage

Cricoid cartilage

Thyroid gland

Trachea

Internal carotid artery

External carotid artery

Carotid sinus

External jugular vein

Common carotid artery

Internal jugular vein

Left subclavian artery

Left subclavian vein

FIGURE 10-3
Underlying structures of the neck. **A,** Anterior view. **B,** Lateral view.

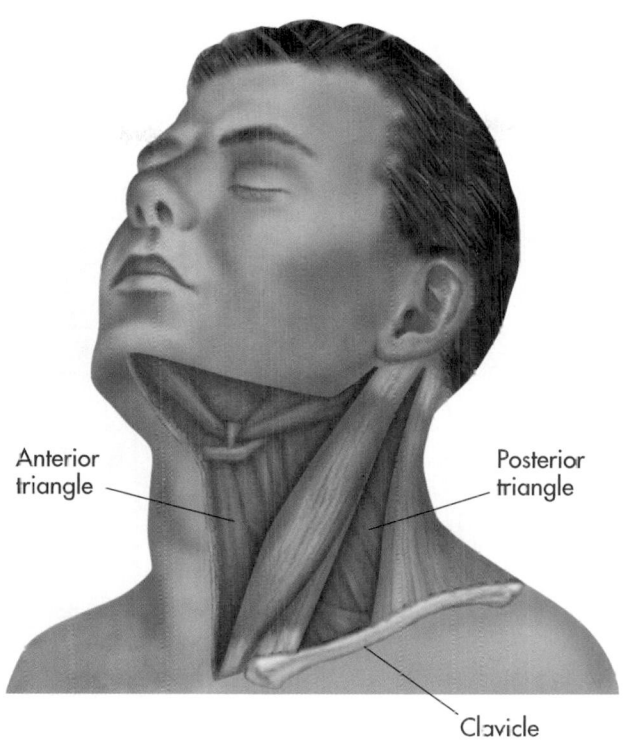

FIGURE 10-4
Anterior and posterior triangles of the neck.

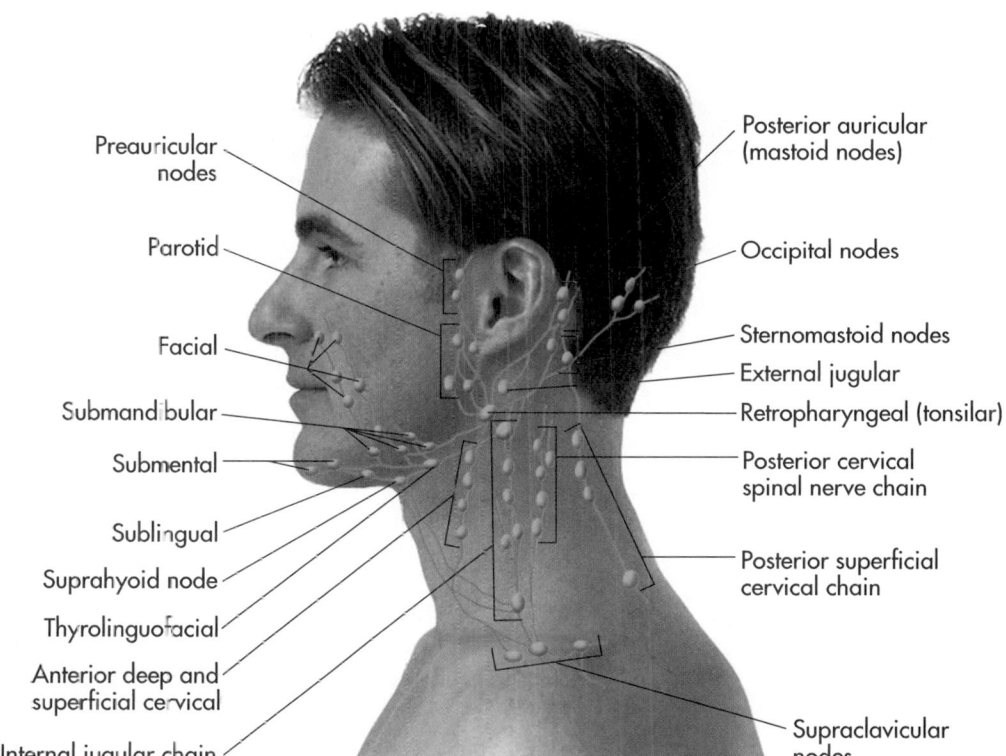

FIGURE 10-5
Lymphatic drainage system of head and neck. (If the group of nodes is often referred to by a second name, that name appears in parentheses.)

The anterior triangle is formed by the medial border of the sternocleidomastoid muscles, the mandible, and the midline. The hyoid bone, cricoid cartilage, trachea, thyroid, and anterior cervical lymph nodes lie inside these triangles. The common carotid artery and internal jugular vein lie deep and run parallel to the sternocleidomastoid muscle along its medial margin. The external jugular vein crosses the surface of the sternocleidomastoid muscle diago-

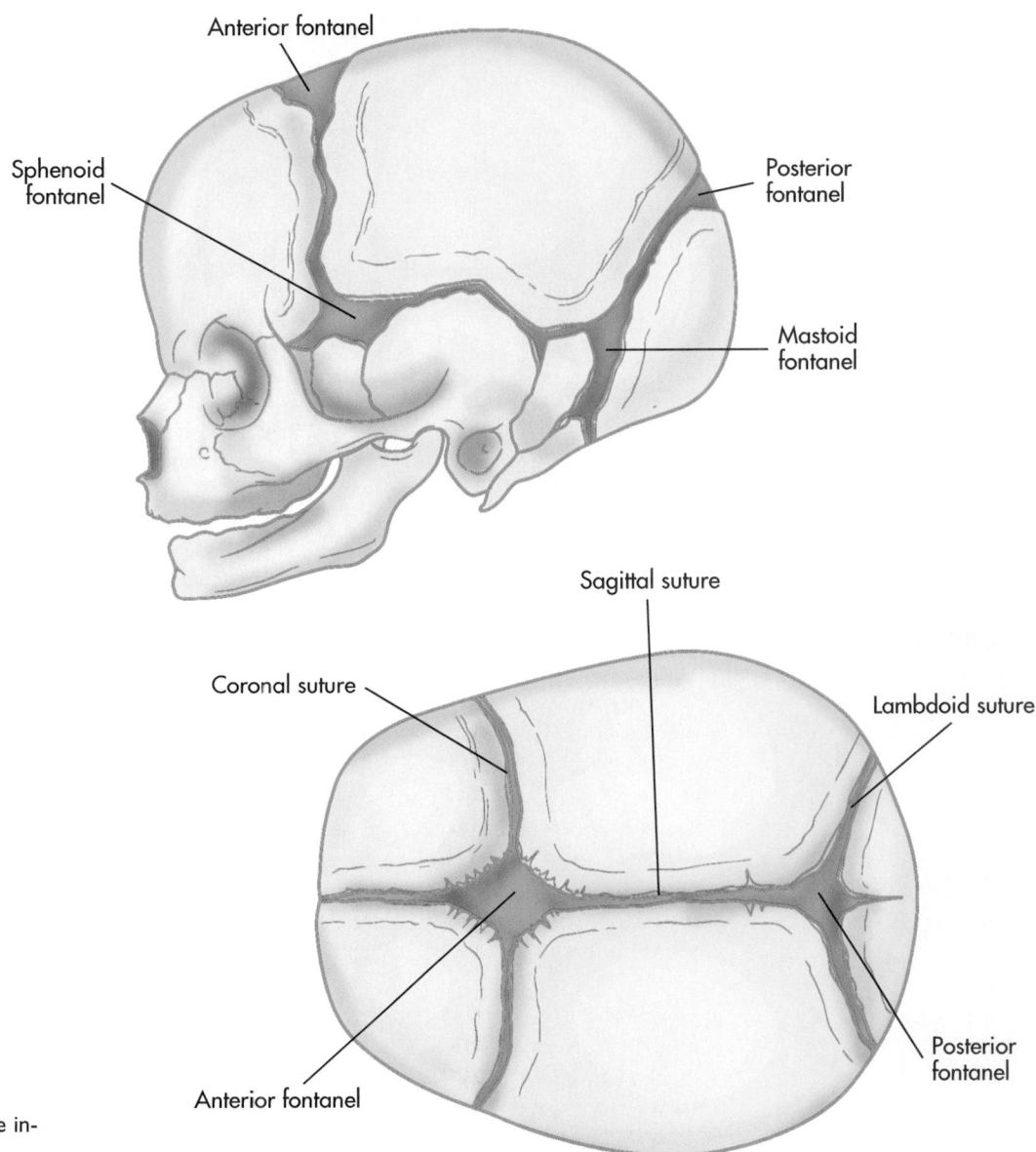

FIGURE 10-6
Fontanels and sutures on the infant's skull.

nally. The hyoid bone lies just below the mandible. The thyroid cartilage is shaped like a shield, its notch on the upper edge marking the level of bifurcation of the common carotid artery. The cricoid cartilage is the uppermost ring of the tracheal cartilages.

The thyroid is the largest endocrine gland in the body, producing two hormones: thyroxine (T_4) and triiodothyronine (T_3). Its two lateral lobes are butterfly shaped and are joined by an isthmus at their lower aspect. This isthmus lies across the trachea below the cricoid cartilage. A pyramidal lobe, extending upward from the isthmus slightly to the left of midline, is present in about one third of the population. The lobes curve posteriorly around the cartilages and are in large part covered by the sternocleidomastoid muscles.

INFANTS

In infants, the seven cranial bones are soft and separated by the sagittal, coronal, and lambdoidal sutures (Fig. 10-6). The anterior and posterior fontanels are the membranous spaces formed where four cranial bones meet and intersect. Spaces between the cranial bones permit the expansion of the skull to accommodate brain growth. Ossification of the sutures begins after completion of brain growth, at about 6 years of age, and is finished by adulthood. The fontanels ossify earlier, with the posterior fontanel usually closing by 2 months of age and the

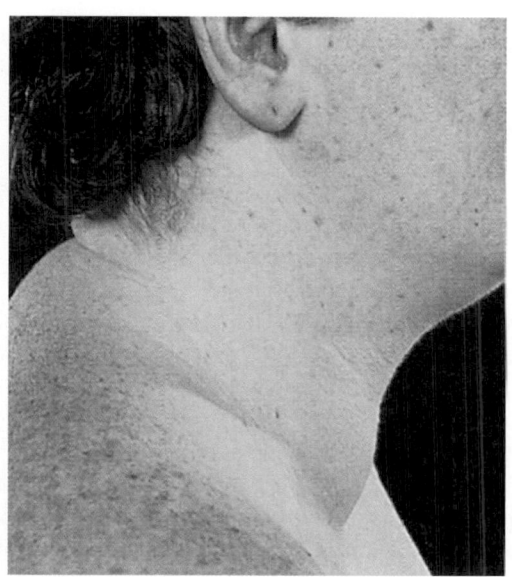

FIGURE 10-7
Thyroid enlargement (in profile) in a typical pregnancy. Some degree of goiter is physiologically normal.
From Symonds, Macpherson, 1994.

anterior fontanel closing by 24 months of age. The time of closure of the fontanel does not correlate with term or premature delivery, gender, size of the fontanel, or head circumference. Black infants tend to have somewhat larger fontanels than do whites.

The process of birth through the vaginal canal often causes molding of the newborn skull, during which the cranial bones may shift and overlap. Within days the newborn skull resumes its appropriate shape and size.

CHILDREN AND ADOLESCENTS

Subtle changes in facial appearance occur throughout childhood. In the male adolescent, the nose and thyroid cartilage enlarge, and facial hair develops, emerging first on the upper lip, then the cheeks, lower lip, and chin.

PREGNANT WOMEN

There are a number of changes that occur in the thyroid gland and in thyroid hormones during pregnancy. Pregnancy is, however, a euthyroid state. As long as adequate iodine intake is maintained (200 mcg/day), the size of the thyroid will not change by physical examination. A slight enlargement may still be detectible by ultrasound. There is an early and sustained increase in the renal clearance of iodine, and the thyroid compensates by enlarging and increasing the plasma clearance of iodine to produce sufficient thyroid hormones (Fig. 10-7). Serum bioassayable thyroid-stimulating activity is increased in the first trimester because of human chorionic gonadotropin (hCG). The hCG may cause an increase in free T_4 and T_3 levels. Thyroid-stimulating hormone levels are minimally decreased. The physical signs of weight loss, tachycardia, eye signs, and bruit over the thyroid are suggestive of hyperthyroidism. There is also an increase in thyroxine-binding globulin concentration.

OLDER ADULTS

The rate of T_4 production and degradation gradually decreases with aging, and the thyroid gland becomes more fibrotic.

REVIEW OF RELATED HISTORY

For each of the conditions discussed in this section, targeted topics to include in the history of the present illness are listed. Responses to questions about these topics help fully assess the patient's condition and provide clues for focusing the physical examination.

HISTORY OF PRESENT ILLNESS

- Head injury
  - Independent observer's description of event
  - State of consciousness after injury: immediately and 5 minutes later; duration of unconsciousness; combative, confused, alert, or dazed
  - Predisposing factors: seizure disorder, hypoglycemia, poor vision, light-headedness, syncope
  - Associated symptoms: head or neck pain, laceration, altered level of consciousness, local tenderness, change in breathing pattern, blurred or double vision, discharge from nose or ears, nausea or vomiting, urinary or fecal incontinence, ability to move all extremities (see Chapter 27)
  - Medications: prescription, nonprescription, alternative or complementary
- Headache
  - Onset: early morning, during day, during night; gradual versus abrupt
  - Duration: minutes, hours, days, weeks; relieved by medication or sleep; resolves spontaneously; occurs in clusters; headache-free periods
  - Location: entire head, unilateral, specific site (neck, sinus region, behind eyes, hatband distribution)
  - Character: throbbing, pounding, boring, shocklike, dull, nagging, constant pressure, aggravated with movement
  - Severity: same or different with each event (gradation 1-10)
  - Visual prodromal event: scotoma; hemianopia; distortion of size, shape, or location
  - Pattern: worse in morning or evening, worse or better as day progresses, occurs only during sleep
  - Episodes closer together or worsening, lasting longer
  - Change in level of consciousness as pain increases
  - Associated symptoms: nausea, vomiting, diarrhea, photophobia, visual disturbance, difficulty falling asleep, increased lacrimation, nasal discharge, tinnitus, paresthesias, mobility impairment
  - Precipitating factors: fever, fatigue, stress, food additives, prolonged fasting, alcohol, seasonal allergies, menstrual cycle, intercourse, oral contraceptives
  - Efforts to treat: sleep, pain medication
  - Medications: anticonvulsants, antiarrhythmics, beta blockers, calcium channel blockers, oral contraceptives, serotonin antagonists or agonists, uptake inhibitors, antidepressants, nonsteroidal antiinflammatory drugs, narcotics, caffeine-containing drugs, nonprescription drugs, alternative or complementary therapy
- Stiff neck
  - Neck injury or strain, head injury, swelling of neck
  - Fever, bacterial or viral illness
  - Character: limitation of movement; pain with movement, pain relieved by movement; continuous or cramping pain; radiation patterns to arms, shoulders, hands, or down the back
  - Predisposing factors: unilateral vision or hearing loss
  - Efforts to treat: heat, pain medication, physical therapy
  - Medications: prescription drugs; nonprescription drugs, alternative or complementary therapy
- Thyroid problem
  - Change in temperature preference: more or less clothing than worn by other members of the patient's family
  - Swelling in the neck; interference with swallowing; redness; pain with touch, swallowing, or hyperextension of the neck; difficulty buttoning shirt
  - Change in texture of hair, skin, or nails; increased pigmentation of skin at pressure points
  - Change in emotional stability: increased energy, irritability, nervousness, or lethargy, complaisance, disinterest

- Increased prominence of eyes; puffiness in periorbital area, blurred or double vision
- Tachycardia, palpitations
- Change in menstrual flow
- Change in bowel habits
- Medications: thyroid preparations, prescription drugs, nonprescription drugs, alternative or complementary therapy

PAST MEDICAL HISTORY

- Head trauma, subdural hematoma, recent lumbar puncture
- Radon or radium treatment around head and neck
- Headaches: migraine, vascular
- Surgery for tumor
- Seizure disorder
- Thyroid dysfunction, surgery

FAMILY HISTORY

- Headaches: type, character, similarity to patient's
- Thyroid dysfunction

PERSONAL AND SOCIAL HISTORY

- Employment: risk of head injury, use of helmet, exposure to toxins or chemicals
- Stress; tension; demands at home, work, or school
- Potential risk of injury: participation in sports, handrails available, use of seat belts, unsafe environment
- Nutrition: recent weight gain or loss, food intolerances, eating habits (e.g., skipping meals)
- Use of alcohol
- Use of street drugs

INFANTS

- Prenatal history: mother's use of drugs or alcohol, uterine abnormalities, treatment of hyperthyroidism
- Birth history: birth order (firstborn more likely to experience torticollis), vaginal or cesarean section delivery; presentation, difficulty of delivery, use of forceps (associated with caput succedaneum, cephalhematoma, Bell palsy, molding)
- Unusual head shape: bulging or flattening (congenital anomaly or positioning in utero), preterm infant, head held at angle, preferred position at rest
- Quality of head control
- Acute illness: diarrhea, vomiting, fever, stiff neck, irritability (associated with meningitis)
- Congenital anomalies: meningomyelocele, encephalocele, microcephaly, hydrocephaly
- Neonatal screening for congenital hypothyroidism

PREGNANT WOMEN

- Weeks of gestation or postpartum
- Presence of preexisting disease (e.g., hypothyroidism, hyperthyroidism), ingestion of iodine or use of antithyroid medication
- History of pregnancy-induced hypertension (PIH)
- Use of street drugs
- Medications: prescription drugs; nonprescription drugs, alternative or complementary therapy

OLDER ADULTS

- Dizziness with head or neck movement
- Weakness or impaired balance, increasing risk of falling and head injury

EXAMINATION AND FINDINGS

EQUIPMENT

- ◆ Tape measure
- ◆ Stethoscope
- ◆ Cup of water (for evaluation of thyroid gland)
- ◆ Transilluminator (electronic or flashlight attachment, for infants)

HEAD AND FACE

INSPECTION

Begin examining the head and neck with inspection of head position and facial features, making observations throughout the history and physical examination. The patient's head should be held upright and still. A horizontal jerking or bobbing motion may be associated with a tremor; a nodding movement may be associated with aortic insufficiency, especially if nodding is synchronized with the pulse. Holding the head tilted to one side to favor a good eye or ear often occurs with unilateral hearing or vision loss, but it is also associated with shortening of a sternocleidomastoid muscle (torticollis) (see Fig. 10-34).

Facial features (i.e., eyelids, eyebrows, palpebral fissures, nasolabial folds, and mouth) should be inspected for shape and symmetry with rest, movement, and expression. The integrity of cranial nerves V and VII (trigeminal and facial) has been partially tested. Complete evaluation is detailed in Chapter 22. Facial characteristics vary according to race, gender, and body build. Some slight asymmetry is common.

When facial asymmetry is present, note whether all features on one side of the face are affected or only a portion of the face, such as the forehead, lower face, or mouth. Suspect facial nerve paralysis when the entire side of the face is affected, and suspect facial nerve weakness when the lower face is affected. If only the mouth is involved, suspect a problem with the peripheral trigeminal nerve.

Tics, which are spasmodic muscular contractions of the face, head, or neck, should be noted. They may be associated with pressure on or degenerative changes of the facial nerves, or they may be psychogenic.

Note any change in the shape of the face or any unusual features, such as edema, puffiness, coarsened features, prominent eyes, hirsutism, lack of expression, excessive perspiration, pallor, or pigmentation variations. Certain disorders cause characteristic changes in facial appearance (see Common Abnormalities, p. 271).

Inspect the skull for size, shape, and symmetry. Examine the scalp by systematically parting the hair from the frontal to occipital region, noting any lesions, scabs, tenderness, parasites, nits, or scaliness (Fig. 10-8). Pay special attention to the areas behind the ears, at the hairline, and at the crown of the head. Note any hair loss pattern. In men it is common to see bitemporal recession of hair or balding over the crown of the head.

PALPATION

The skull is palpated in a gentle rotary movement progressing systematically from front to back. The skull should be symmetric and smooth. The bones should be indistinguishable because the sites of fusion are not generally palpable after 6 months of age; however, the ridge of the sagittal suture may be felt on some individuals. The scalp should move freely over the skull, and no tenderness, swelling, or depressions on palpation are expected. An indentation or depression of the skull may indicate a skull fracture.

Palpate the patient's hair, noting its texture, color, and distribution. Hair should be smooth, symmetrically distributed, and have no splitting or cracked ends. Coarse, dry, and brittle hair is associated with hypothyroidism. It is also associated with excessive cosmetic treatment. Fine, silky hair is associated with hyperthyroidism or may be familial.

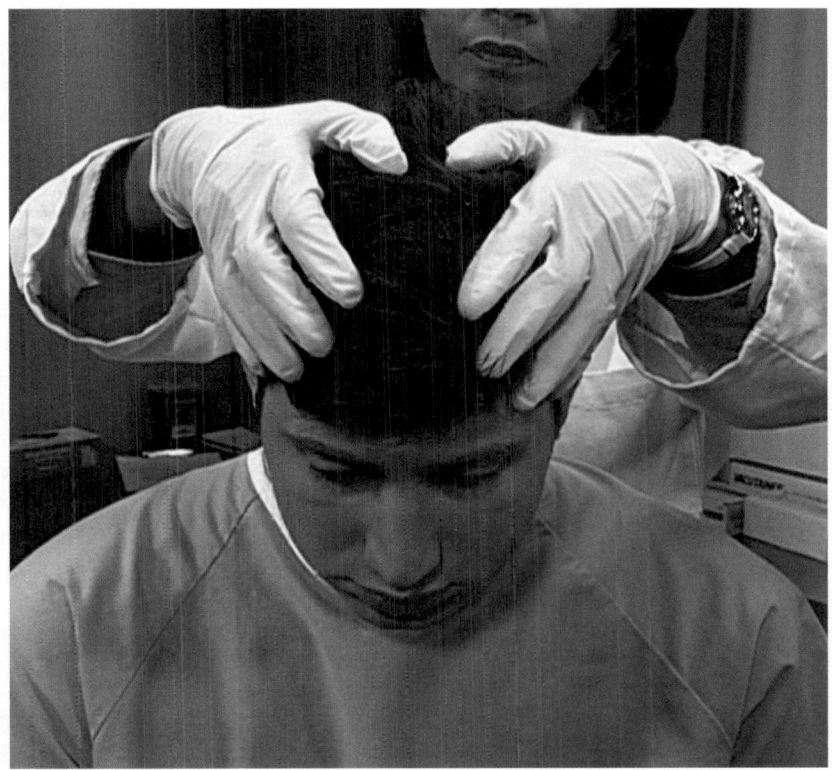

FIGURE 10-8
Inspection of the scalp.

Palpate the temporal arteries and note their course. Any thickening, hardness, or tenderness over the arteries may be associated with temporal arteritis. Palpate the temporomandibular joint space bilaterally, as described on pp. 707 and 708.

Inspect for any asymmetry or enlargement of the salivary glands. If noted, palpate for possible discrete enlargement, noting whether it is fixed or movable, soft or hard, tender or nontender. Ask the patient to open his or her mouth and try to express material through the salivary duct as you press on the gland itself. An enlarged, tender gland may suggest either viral or bacterial infection or a ductal stone preventing saliva from exiting the gland. A discrete nodule may represent a cyst or tumor, either benign or malignant.

PERCUSSION

Percussion of the head and neck is not routinely performed. However, some investigators have described a sign of hyperparathyroidism in which percussion of the skull produced a low-pitched note far different from the high-pitched crack elicited from the skull of healthy individuals.

AUSCULTATION

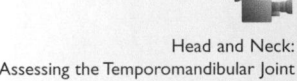

Head and Neck:
Assessing the Temporomandibular Joint

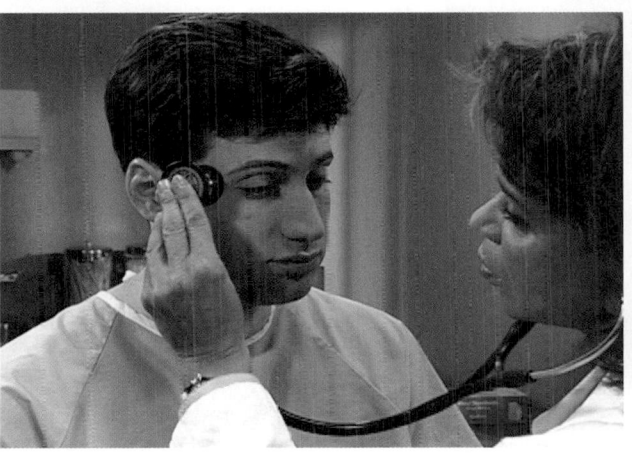

FIGURE 10-9
Auscultation for a temporal bruit.

Auscultation of the skull is not routinely performed. In individuals who have developed diplopia, a bruit or blowing sound over the orbit rarely may be heard. It suggests that an expanding cerebral aneurysm may be responsible for the diplopia. If you suspect a vascular anomaly of the brain, listen for bruits over the skull and eyes. Place the bell of the stethoscope over the temporal region, over the eyes, and below the occiput (Fig. 10-9). A bruit indicates a vascular anomaly.

NECK

INSPECTION

Inspect the neck in the usual anatomic position, in slight hyperextension, and as the patient swallows. Look for bilateral symmetry of the sternocleidomastoid and trapezius muscles, alignment of the trachea, the landmarks of the anterior and posterior triangles, and any subtle fullness at the base of the neck. Note any apparent masses, webbing, excess skinfolds, unusual shortness, or asymmetry. Observe for any distention of the jugular vein or prominence of the carotid arteries. Carotid artery and jugular vein examination is described in Chapter 15.

Webbing, excessive posterior cervical skin, or an unusually short neck may be associated with chromosomal anomalies. The transverse portion of the omohyoid muscle in the posterior triangle can sometimes be mistaken for a mass. Marked edema of the neck is associated with local infections. A mass filling the base of the neck or visible thyroid tissue that glides upward when the patient swallows may indicate an enlarged thyroid.

Evaluate range of motion by asking the patient to flex, extend, rotate, and laterally turn the head and neck (see Chapter 22). Movement should be smooth and painless and should not cause dizziness. Place your hand on the patient's cheek and jaw and ask him or her to turn toward your hand while you apply resistance. This maneuver permits evaluation of CN XI. Next ask the patient to shrug the shoulders while you apply resistance to complete evaluation of CN XI.

PALPATION

The ability to palpate and identify structures in the neck varies with the patient's habitus.

Palpate the trachea for midline position. Place a thumb along each side of the trachea in the lower portion of the neck (Fig. 10-10). Compare the space between the trachea and the sternocleidomastoid muscle on each side. An unequal space indicates displacement of the trachea from the midline and may be associated with a mass or pathologic condition in the chest.

Identify the hyoid bone and the thyroid and cricoid cartilages. They should be smooth and nontender, and they should move under your finger when the patient swallows. On palpation, the cartilaginous rings of the trachea in the lower portion of the neck should be distinct and nontender.

With the patient's neck extended, position the index finger and thumb of one hand on each side of the trachea below the thyroid isthmus (Fig. 10-11). A tugging sensation, synchronous with the pulse, is evidence of tracheal tugging, suggesting the presence of an aortic aneurysm.

> ● **CLINICAL PEARL**
> *Neck Palpation*
> It is more difficult to examine a short, thick, muscular neck than a long, slender one.

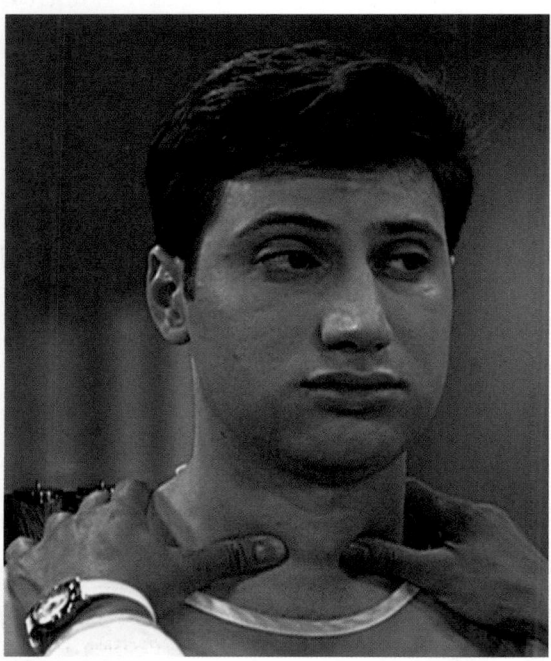

FIGURE 10-10
Position of the thumbs to evaluate the midline position of the trachea.

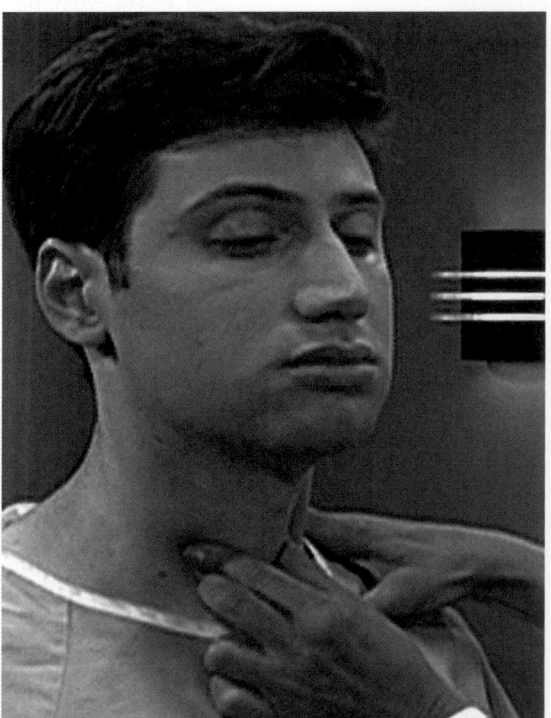

FIGURE 10-11
Position of the thumb and finger to detect tracheal tugging.

LYMPH NODES

Inspect and palpate the head and neck for lymph nodes. A description of the sequence is on pp. 244 to 246.

THYROID GLAND

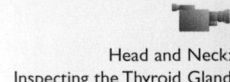

Head and Neck:
Inspecting the Thyroid Gland

Examination of the thyroid gland involves inspection, palpation, and occasionally auscultation. Begin the evaluation by asking patients to gently extend their neck. (Hyperextension can actually make the examination more difficult.) The patient should be asked to swallow, which often permits visualization of the gland's size, symmetry or asymmetry, and contour as it moves with deglutition. An enlarged thyroid gland may be visible only when observing from the lateral aspect. A glass of water is an indispensable aid for proper examination of the thyroid.

Palpation of the thyroid gland requires a gentle touch. Nodules and asymmetric position will be more difficult to detect if you press too hard. Allow your fingers to almost drift over the gland. Palpate the thyroid for size, shape, configuration, consistency, tenderness, and the presence of any nodules. Although the thyroid gland may be palpated from in front or behind the patient, facing the patient facilitates the correlation of inspection with palpation findings. It is also more convenient in most examining rooms where the table is against a wall. Choose one approach to use consistently.

For both approaches, the patient should be positioned to relax the sternocleidomastoid, with the neck flexed slightly forward and laterally toward the side being examined. Ask the patient to hold a sip of water in the mouth until you have your hands positioned, then instruct the patient to swallow.

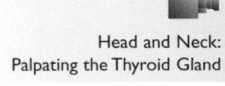

Head and Neck:
Palpating the Thyroid Gland

To palpate the thyroid using the frontal approach, have the patient sit on the examining table. First place your thumb over the trachea approximately 3 cm beneath the prominence of the thyroid cartilage. During swallowing attempt to identify the isthmus of the gland. To examine the left lobe of the thyroid, move to the left side of the patient and press the trachea toward the left with your left thumb. Such pressure helps move the lobe out of the tracheoesophageal groove for easier palpation. Then place the first three fingers of your right hand in the thyroid bed with your finger tips medial to the margin of the sternocleidomastoid muscle. Leave your fingers still while the patient again swallows, thus moving the gland beneath your fingers (Fig. 10-12). To examine the right lobe, move your hands to the reverse corresponding positions. By palpating above the cricoid cartilage, you may be able to feel the pyramidal lobe of the thyroid, if one is present.

For examining the thyroid from behind, seat the patient on a chair with the neck at a comfortable level. Using both hands, position two fingers of each hand on the sides of the trachea just beneath the cricoid cartilage. Ask the patient to swallow, feeling for movement of the isthmus. Then displace the trachea to the left, and with the first three fingers of your left hand medial to the left sternocleidomastoid, palpate the left lobe as the patient again swallows. To palpate the right lobe, again move your hands to the reverse corresponding positions (Fig. 10-13). The thyroid lobes, if felt, should be small, smooth, and free of nodules. The gland should rise freely with swallowing. The thyroid at its broadest dimension is approximately 4 cm, and the right lobe is often 25% larger than the left. The consistency of the thyroid tissue should be firm yet pliable. Coarse tissue or a gritty sensation implies that an inflammatory process has been present. If nodules are present, they need to be characterized by number, whether they are

EVIDENCE-BASED PRACTICE IN PHYSICAL EXAMINATION

THYROID EXAMINATION

Studies suggest that examination of the thyroid gland for the presence of a goiter becomes both more precise and sensitive as one gains experience in measuring the size of the thyroid gland. Estimates of size tend to be exaggerated when the gland is small and underestimated when the gland is markedly enlarged. Evaluations were made by comparing the estimated size on physical examination with the size measured by ultrasound or after surgical excision. The estimation of thyroid size by lateral inspection is the most sensitive test for determining the presence of a goiter.

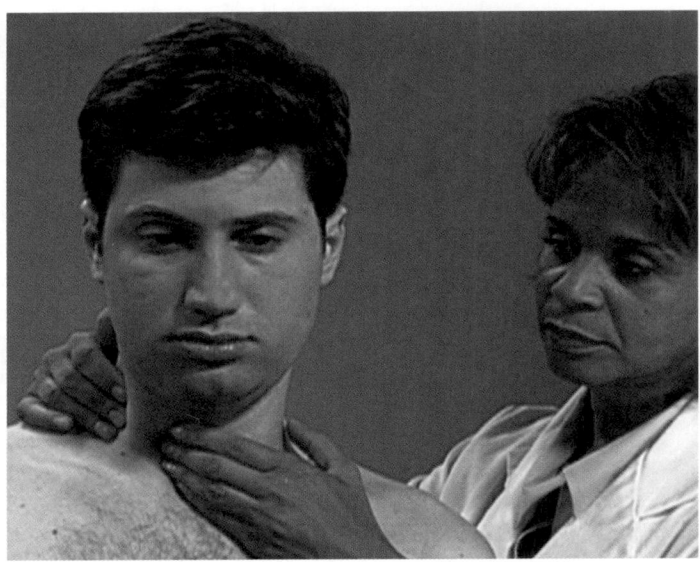

FIGURE 10-12
Palpation of the right thyroid lobe and lateral border from in front of the patient. The examiner has been moved out of proper position to better display the placement of the examining fingers.

CLINICAL PEARL

Is It the Thyroid Gland?
The thyroid gland moves with swallowing; subcutaneous fat mimicking a goiter does not.

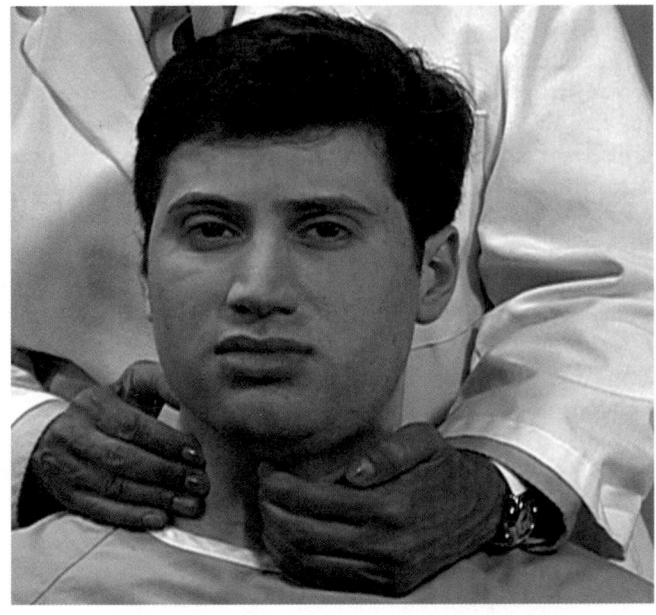

FIGURE 10-13
Palpation of the right thyroid lobe from behind the patient.

smooth or irregular, and whether they are soft or hard. An enlarged, tender thyroid may indicate thyroiditis.

If the thyroid gland is enlarged, auscultate for vascular sounds with the bell of the stethoscope. In a hypermetabolic state, the blood supply is dramatically increased and a vascular bruit, a soft, rushing sound, may be heard.

INFANTS

INSPECTION

Measure the infant's head circumference and compare it with expected size for age on a growth chart, as detailed in Chapter 5. Inspect the infant's head from all angles for symmetry of shape, noting any prominent bulges or swellings. Inspect the scalp for scaling and crusting, dilated scalp veins, the presence of excessive hair, or an unusual hairline.

You can always tell a pediatric specialist by the first movement in the examination of an infant. The hand goes almost instinctively to palpate the fontanel. Even in a social situation, you will find the pediatric specialist's fingers saying "hello" by drifting over the soft spot.

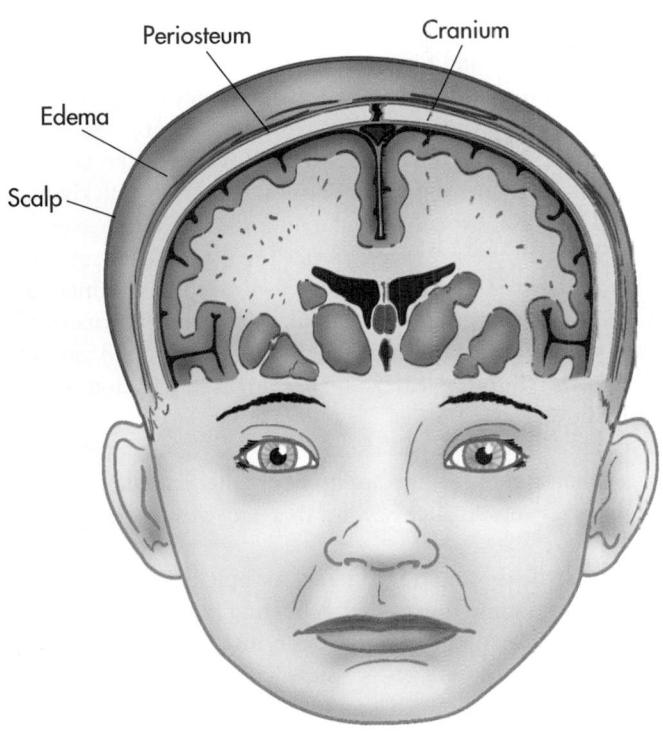

FIGURE 10-14
Caput succedaneum.

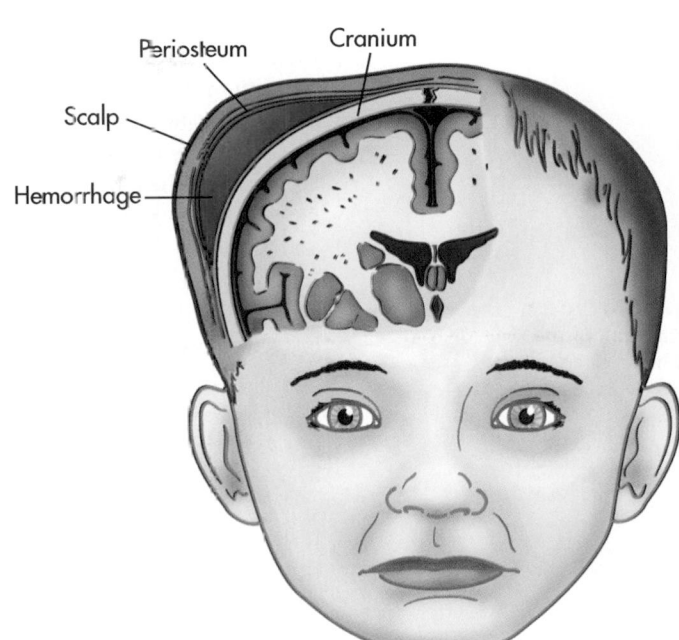

FIGURE 10-15
Cephalhematoma. Note that the swelling does not cross suture lines.

Birth trauma may cause swelling of the scalp. Caput succedaneum is subcutaneous edema over the presenting part of the head at delivery (Fig. 10-14). It is the most common form of birth trauma of the scalp and usually occurs over the occiput and crosses suture lines. The affected part of the scalp feels soft, and the margins are poorly defined. Generally the edema goes away in a few days.

Cephalhematoma is a subperiosteal collection of blood and is therefore bound by the suture lines. It is commonly found in the parietal region and, unlike caput, may not be immediately obvious at birth. A cephalhematoma is firm, and its edges are well defined; it does not cross suture lines. As it ages, the cephalhematoma may liquefy and become fluctuant on palpation (Fig. 10-15).

Head shape with an unusual contour may be related to premature or irregular closing of suture lines. Preterm infants often have long, narrow heads because their soft cranial bones become flattened with positioning and the weight of the head. Bossing (bulging of the skull) of the frontal areas is associated with prematurity and rickets. Bulging in other areas of the skull may indicate cranial defects or intracranial masses. Dilated scalp veins and a head circumference increasing faster than expected may indicate increased intracranial pressure.

Inspect the face for spacing of the features, symmetry, paralysis, skin color, and texture. Uterine positioning can cause some facial asymmetry.

Observe the infant's head control, position, and movement. Note any jerking, tremors, or inability to move the head in one direction. Chapters 21 and 22 provide further details.

Inspect the infant's neck for symmetry, size, and shape. Note the presence of edema, distended neck veins, pulsations, masses, webbing, or excessive posterior cervical skin. To observe the newborn's neck, which is usually not easily visible in the supine position, elevate the upper back of the infant and permit the head to fall back into extension. The neck appears short during infancy and lengthens by 3 to 4 years of age. Marked edema may indicate a localized infection. A cystic mass high in the neck may be a thyroglossal duct cyst or a branchial cleft cyst. A mass over the clavicle, changing size with crying or respiration, suggests a cystic hygroma. Nuchal rigidity, resistance to flexion of the neck, is associated with meningeal irritation.

PALPATION

Palpate the infant's head, identifying suture lines and fontanels. Note any tenderness over the scalp. Suture lines feel ridgelike until about 6 months of age, after which they are usually no longer palpable. Vaginally delivered newborns may have molding with prominent ridges from overriding sutures. Fontanels may be small or not palpable at birth. Molding of the head at delivery can be very distressing for parents: the football shape disappears relatively quickly, but reassurance is necessary. Drawings can help you explain that the infant's cranial bones overlap and that their relative lack of development is a protective device for the brain. Assure the parents that symmetry of the head is usually regained within 1 week of birth, with fontanels and suture line resuming their appropriate shape and size. A third fontanel (the mastoid fontanel), located between the anterior and posterior fontanels, may be an expected variant but is also common in infants with Down syndrome. Any palpable ridges in addition to the expected suture lines may indicate fractures.

Measure the size of the anterior and posterior fontanels using two dimensions (anteroposterior and lateral). In infants younger than 6 months, the anterior fontanel diameter should not exceed 4 to 5 cm. It should get progressively smaller beyond that age, closing completely by 18 to 24 months of age.

With the infant in a sitting position, palpate the anterior fontanel for bulging or depression. It should feel slightly depressed, and some pulsation is expected. A bulging fontanel feels tense, similar to the fontanel of an infant during the expiratory phase of crying. A bulging fontanel with marked pulsations may indicate increased intracranial pressure. The infant fontanel gives important clues as to what is going on inside the body. If there is infection or increased intracranial pressure, the fontanel will bulge. Interestingly, in the early months of life the fontanel may not be the sensitive indicator it becomes later in the first year. You cannot assume that an infant of 3 months whose fontanel is not bulging is free of meningitis; indeed, an infant who is symptomatic should be evaluated for meningitis even in the absence of a bulging fontanel.

Palpate the scalp firmly above and behind the ears to detect craniotabes, a softening of the outer table of the skull. A snapping sensation, similar to the bounce of a ping-pong ball, indicates craniotabes, which may be associated with rickets and hydrocephalus.

Palpate the sternocleidomastoid muscle, noting its tone and the presence of any masses. A mass in the lower third of the muscle may indicate a hematoma. Palpate the trachea. A palpatory thud felt over the trachea suggests the presence of a foreign body. The thyroid is difficult to palpate in an infant unless it is enlarged. The presence of a goiter, which may cause respiratory distress, results from intrauterine deprivation of thyroid hormone.

TRANSILLUMINATION

Transilluminate the skull of every newborn and of older infants who have a suspected intracranial lesion or a rapidly increasing head circumference. Perform the procedure in a completely darkened room, allowing a few minutes to elapse for your eyes to adjust. The transilluminator is placed firmly against the infant's scalp so that no light escapes (Fig. 10-16). Begin at the midline frontal region and inch the transilluminator over the entire head. Observe the ring of illumination through the scalp and skull around the light, noting any asymmetry. A ring of 2 cm or less beyond the rim of the transilluminator is expected on all regions of the head except the occiput, where the ring should be 1 cm or less. Illumination beyond these parameters suggests excess fluid or decreased brain tissue in the skull. Transillumination is performed less often today because examiners now place greater reliance on the computed tomography (CT) scan, but it is less expensive and still quite helpful.

STAYING WELL
METABOLIC TESTING

Because the thyroid gland is difficult to evaluate in the infant and because congenital hypothyroidism can result in cognitive impairment and much else if not discovered early, a routine metabolic screening test must be done at birth. This test is required in most states. In many states, parental consent is required.

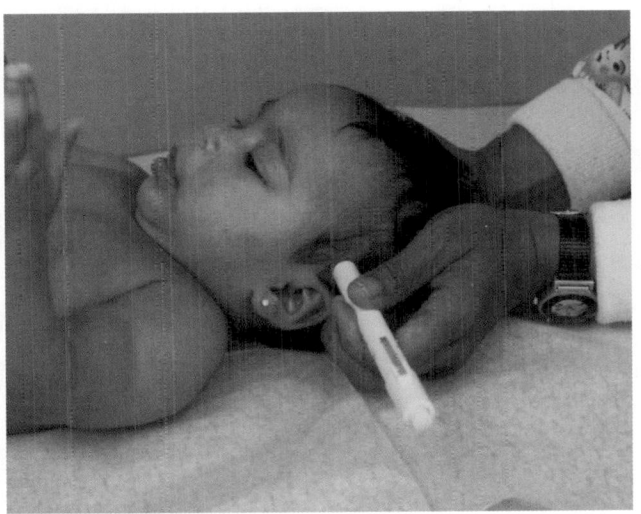

FIGURE 10-16
Transillumination of the infant's scalp.

CHILDREN

Direct percussion of the skull with one finger is useful to detect the Macewen sign, a cracked-pot sound. The sound, which is physiologic when the fontanels are open, may indicate increased intracranial pressure after fontanel closure.

Bruits are common in children up to 5 years of age or in children with anemia. After age 5 years, their presence may suggest vascular anomalies or increased intracranial pressure.

The thyroid of the young child may be palpable. Using techniques described for adults, note the size, shape, position, mobility, and any tenderness. No tenderness should be present. An enlarged, tender thyroid may indicate thyroiditis.

PREGNANT WOMEN

Beginning after 16 weeks of gestation, many pregnant women develop blotchy, brownish hyperpigmentation of the face, particularly over the malar prominences and the forehead (see Fig. 8-29). This chloasma, also called "mask of pregnancy," may further darken with sun exposure, but generally it fades after delivery. The thyroid gland hypertrophies and may become palpable. The hypertrophy is caused by hyperplasia of the glandular tissue and increased vascularity. Because of increased vascularity, a thyroid bruit may be heard. The presence of a goiter is not an expected finding.

OLDER ADULTS

The facies of older adults vary with their nutritional status. The eyes may appear sunken with soft bulges underneath, and the eyelids may appear wrinkled and hang loose.

Use caution when evaluating range of motion in the older adult's neck. Rather than have the patient perform an entire rotational maneuver, go slowly and evaluate each movement separately. Note any pain, crepitus, dizziness, jerkiness, or limitation of movement.

With aging, the thyroid becomes more fibrotic, feeling more nodular or irregular to palpation.

SAMPLE DOCUMENTATION
HISTORY AND PHYSICAL EXAMINATION

Subjective

A 32-year-old woman seeks care for a painless swelling in her throat. No difficulty swallowing or with movement of her neck. Her maternal grandmother and two maternal aunts have goiters. She has lost 5 pounds over the past 2 months without trying. She denies nervousness, palpitations, weakness, or menstrual changes.

Objective

Head: Held erect and midline; skull normocephalic, symmetrical and smooth without deformities; facial features symmetrical; salivary glands nontender; temporal artery pulsations visible bilaterally, soft and nontender to palpation; no bruits.

Neck: Trachea midline; no jugular venous distention (JVD) or carotid artery prominence; thyroid palpable, firm, gritty to palpation and symmetrically enlarged; thyroid and cartilages move with swallowing; no nodules, tenderness, or bruits; full range of motion of the neck without discomfort.

For additional sample documentation, see Chapter 26.

SUMMARY OF EXAMINATION
HEAD AND NECK

Head

1. Observe head position (p. 262).
2. Inspect skull and scalp for the following (p. 262):
   - Size
   - Shape
   - Symmetry
   - Lesions
3. Inspect facial features, including the following (p. 262):
   - Symmetry
   - Shape
   - Unusual features
   - Tics
   - Characteristic facies
4. Palpate head and scalp, noting the following (p. 262):
   - Symmetry
   - Tenderness (particularly over areas of frontal and maxillary sinuses)
   - Scalp movement
5. Palpate the temporal arteries, noting the following (p. 263):
   - Thickening
   - Hardness
   - Tenderness
6. Auscultate the temporal arteries for bruits (p. 263).
7. Inspect and palpate the salivary glands (p. 263).

Neck

1. Inspect the neck for the following (p. 264):
   - Symmetry
   - Alignment of trachea
   - Fullness
   - Masses, webbing, and skinfolds
   - Jugular vein distention
   - Carotid artery prominence
2. Palpate the neck, noting the following (p. 264):
   - Tracheal position
   - Tracheal tug
   - Movement of hyoid bone and cartilages with swallowing
3. Palpate the thyroid gland for the following (p. 265):
   - Size
   - Shape
   - Configuration
   - Consistency
   - Tenderness
   - Nodules
   - If gland is enlarged, auscultate for bruits
4. Evaluate range of motion of the neck (p. 264).

COMMON ABNORMALITIES

HEAD

HEADACHES

Headaches are one of the most common complaints and probably one of the most self-medicated. They are not always benign. A history of insistent headache, severe and recurrent, must always be given attention. Sometimes the underlying cause is life threatening, such as a brain tumor. Sometimes it is life intimidating, such as migraines. At other times it is easily confronted, such as when it is the result of drinking wine. The patient's history is fully as important as the physical examination in getting at the root of a headache. Various types of headaches are compared in the Differential Diagnosis box below.

DIFFERENTIAL DIAGNOSIS
COMPARISON OF VARIOUS TYPES OF HEADACHES

Characteristic	Classic Migraine	Common Migraine	Cluster	Hypertensive	Muscular Tension	Temporal Arteritis
Age at onset	Childhood	Childhood	Adulthood	Adulthood	Adulthood	Older adulthood
Location	Unilateral	Generalized	Unilateral	Bilateral or occipital	Unilateral or bilateral	Unilateral or bilateral
Duration	Hours to days	Hours to day	½ to 2 hours	Hours	Hours to days	Hours to days
Time of onset	Morning or night	Morning or night	Night	Morning	Anytime, commonly in afternoon or evening	Anytime
Quality of pain	Pulsating or throbbing	Pulsating or throbbing	Intense burning, boring, searing, knifelike	Throbbing	Bandlike, constricting	Throbbing
Prodromal event	Well-defined neurologic event, scotoma, aphasia, hemianopsia, aura	Vague neurologic changes, personality change, fluid retention, appetite loss	Personality changes, sleep disturbances	None	None	None
Precipitating event	Menstrual period, missing meals, birth control pills, letdown after stress	Menstrual period, missing meals, birth control pills, letdown after stress	Alcohol consumption	None	Stress, anger, bruxism	None
Frequency	Twice a week	Twice a week	Several times nightly for several nights, then none	Daily	Daily	Daily
Gender predilection	Females	Females	Males	Equal	Equal	Equal
Other symptoms	Nausea, vomiting	Nausea, vomiting	Increased lacrimation, nasal discharge	Generally remits as day progresses	None	None

Modified from Sapar, 1983.

FACIES

Facies is defined as an expression or appearance of the face and features of the head and neck that, when considered together, is characteristic of a clinical condition or syndrome. Once a facies is recognized, the examiner may be able to diagnose the condition or syndrome even before completing the examination of the patient. Facies develop slowly and should therefore not be considered a subtle diagnostic clue. As biochemical testing permits diagnosis before gross changes occur, the clinician should be more alert to early changes suggesting a developing facies. For example, a patient with early changes of acromegaly is shown among Figs. 10-17 through 10-31, which demonstrate some facies and their associated disorders.

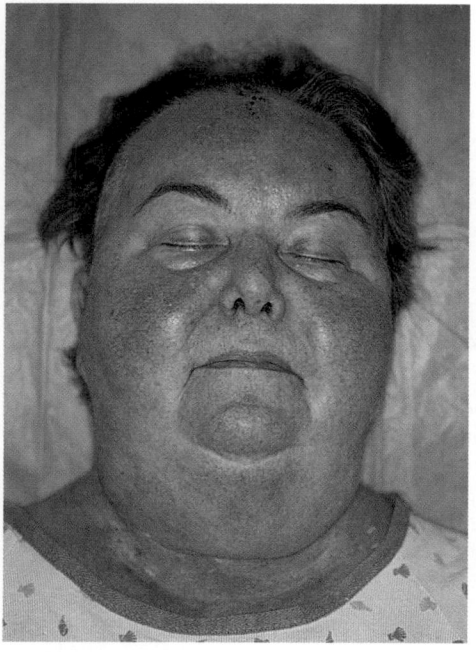

FIGURE 10-17
Cushing syndrome. Facies include a rounded or "moon-shaped" face with thin, erythematous skin. Hirsutism may also be present, especially if the condition is caused by an adrenal cancer.

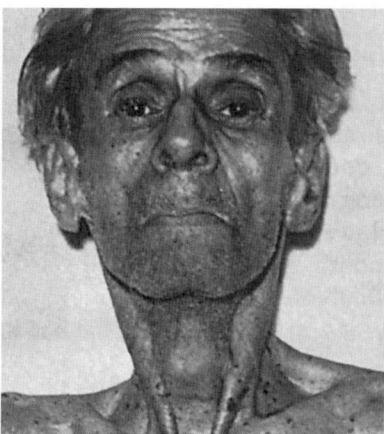

FIGURE 10-18
Hippocratic facies. Note sunken appearance of the eyes, cheeks, and temporal areas; sharp nose; and dry, rough skin, seen in the terminal stages of illness.
From Prior et al, 1981.

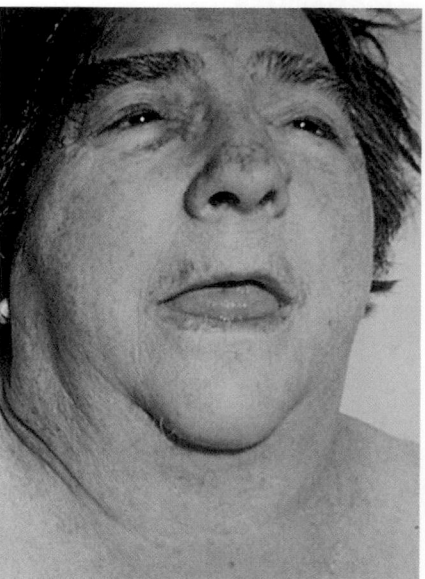

FIGURE 10-19
Myxedema facies. Note dull, puffy, yellowed skin; coarse, sparse hair; temporal loss of eyebrows; periorbital edema; and prominent tongue.
Courtesy Paul W. Ladenson, MD, The Johns Hopkins University and Hospital, Baltimore, MD.

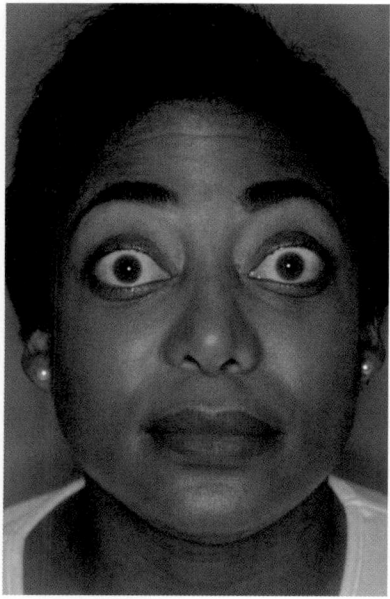

FIGURE 10-20
Hyperthyroid facies. Note fine, moist skin with fine hair, prominent eyes and lid retraction, and staring or startled expression.
From Lemmi, Lemmi, 2000.

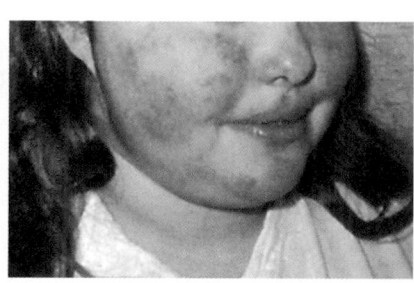

FIGURE 10-21
Butterfly rash of systemic lupus erythematosus. Note butterfly-shaped rash over malar surfaces and bridge of nose. Either a blush with swelling or scaly, red, maculopapular lesions may be present.
Courtesy Walter Tunnessen, MD, Chapel Hill, NC.

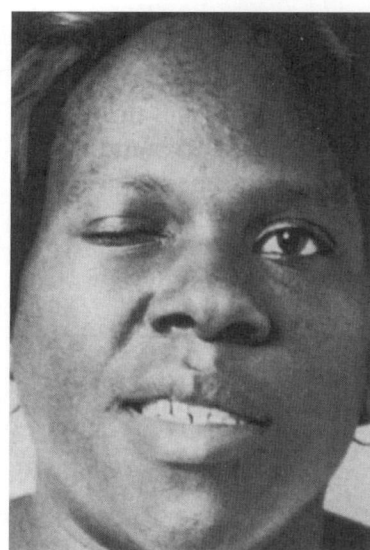

FIGURE 10-22
Left facial palsy. Facies include asymmetry of one side of the face, eyelid not closing completely, drooping lower eyelid and corner of mouth, and loss of nasolabial fold.
From Dyken, Miller, 1980.

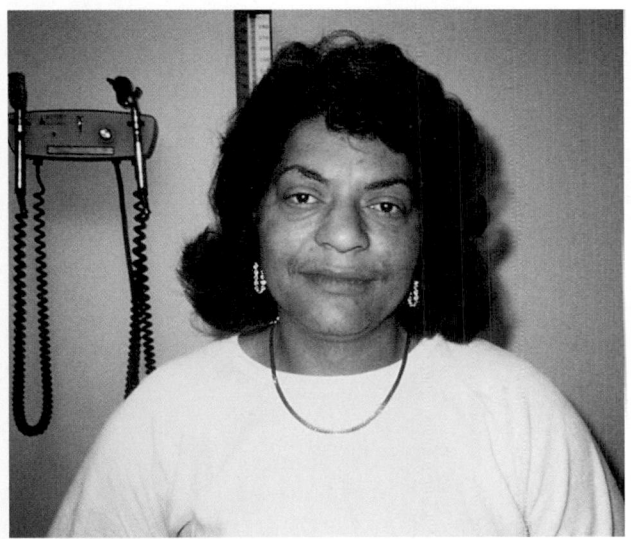

FIGURE 10-23
Early acromegaly. Note the coarsening of features with broad-ening of the nasal alae and prominence of the zygomatic arches.
Courtesy Gary Wand, MD, The Johns Hopkins University and Hospital, Baltimore.

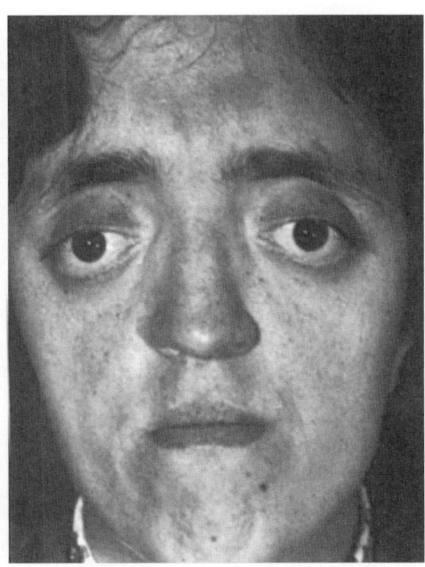

FIGURE 10-24
Craniofacial dysostosis, with characteristic mandibular prognathism, drooping lower lip and short upper lip, parrot beak nose, and proptotic eyes.
From Goodman, Gorlin, 1977.

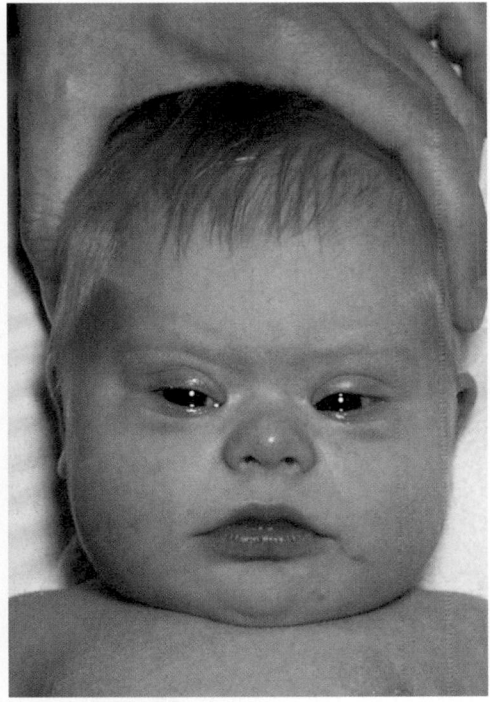

FIGURE 10-25
Down syndrome. Note depressed nasal bridge, epicanthal folds, mongoloid slant of eyes, low-set ears, and large tongue.
From Zitelli, Davis, 1997.

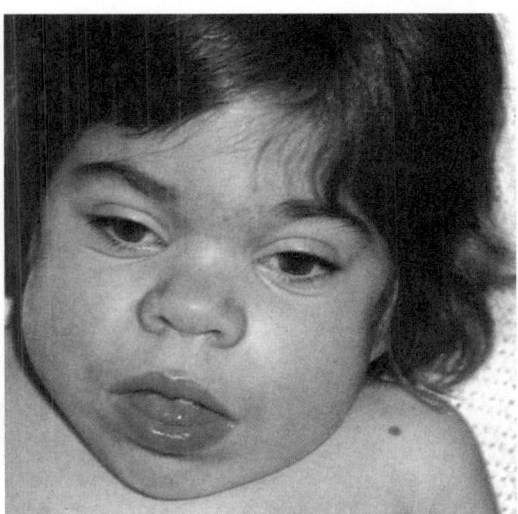

FIGURE 10-26
Hurler syndrome. Facies includes enlarged skull with low forehead, corneal clouding, and short neck.
From Ansell, Rudge, Schaller, 1992.

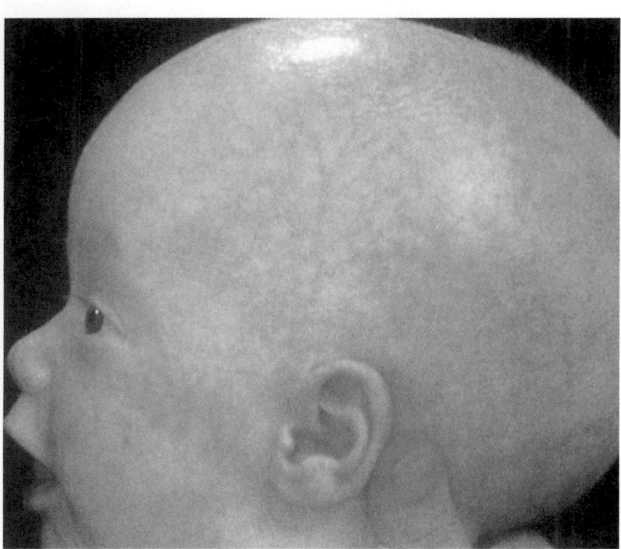

FIGURE 10-27
Hydrocephalus, with characteristic enlarged head, bulging fontanel, dilated scalp veins, bossing of the skull, and sclerae visible above the iris.
From Zitelli, Davis, 1997.

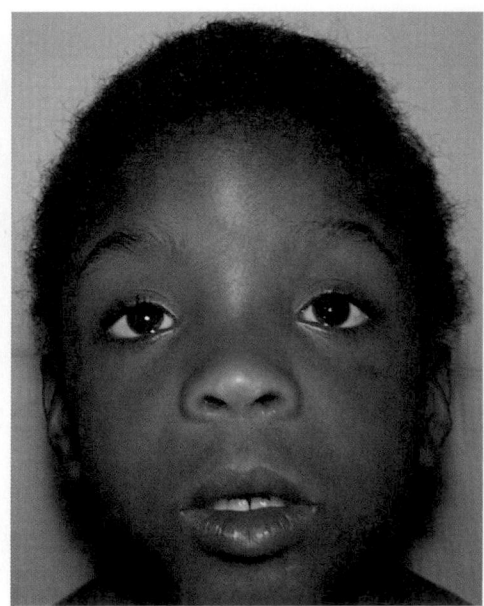

FIGURE 10-28
Fetal alcohol syndrome. This is one of the most common causes of acquired mental retardation. Note the poorly formed philtrum; widespread eyes, with inner epicanthal folds and mild ptosis; hirsute forehead; short nose; and relatively thin upper lip.
From Zitelli, Davis, 1997.

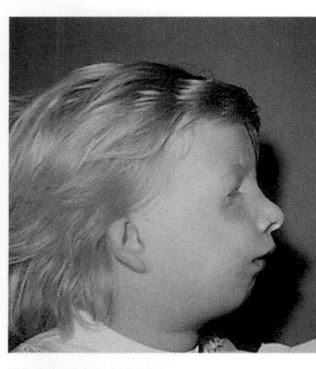

FIGURE 10-29
Treacher-Collins syndrome. Note the maxillary hypoplasia, micrognathia, and auricular deformity.
From Zitelli, Davis, 1997.

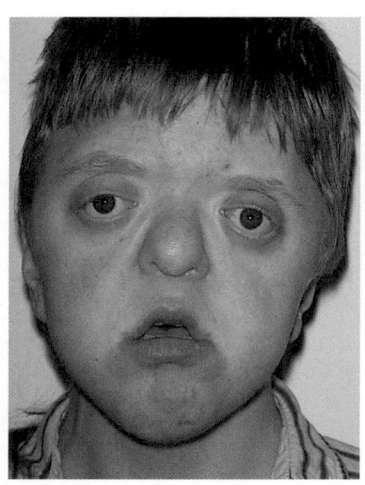

FIGURE 10-30
Apert syndrome. Note the severe maxillary and midfacial hypoplasia.
From Zitelli, Davis, 1997.

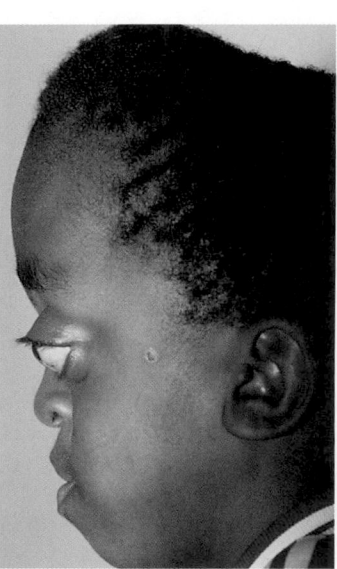

FIGURE 10-31
Crouzon syndrome. Observe the severe maxillary and midfacial hypoplasia with low-set ears.
From Zitelli, Davis, 1997.

NECK

THYROGLOSSAL DUCT CYST

This freely movable cystic mass lies high in the neck, at the midline with the duct at the base of the tongue. It is a remnant of fetal development (Fig. 10-32).

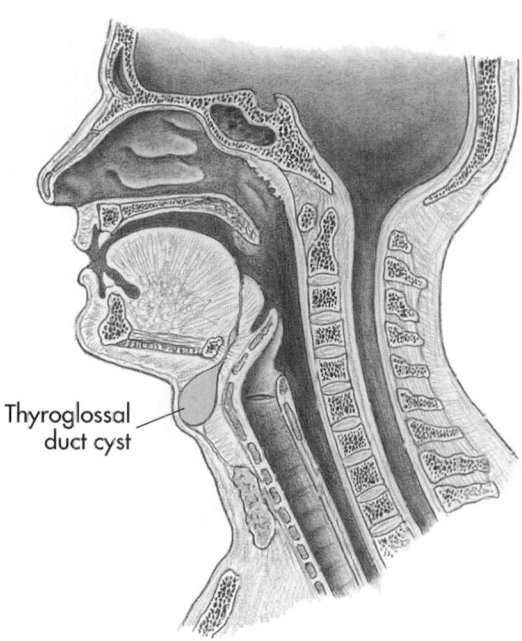

Thyroglossal duct cyst

FIGURE 10-32
Thyroglossal duct cyst location.

BRANCHIAL CLEFT CYST

This oval, moderately movable cystic mass appears near the upper third of the sternocleido-mastoid muscle and is a remnant of embryologic development. It may be associated with a fistula (Fig. 10-33).

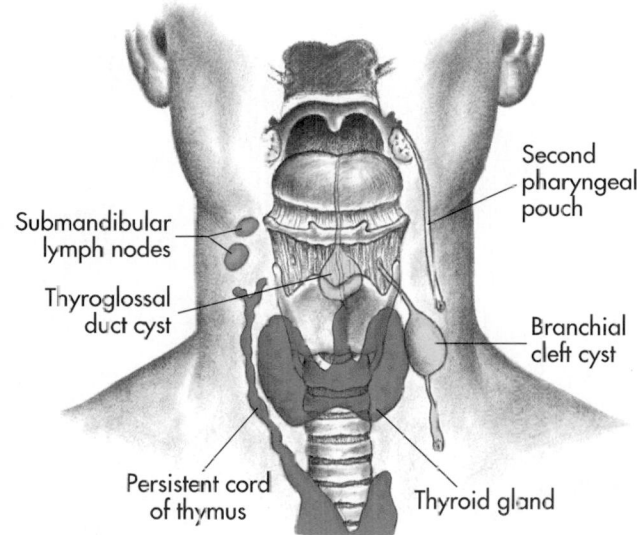

Submandibular lymph nodes

Thyroglossal duct cyst

Second pharyngeal pouch

Branchial cleft cyst

Persistent cord of thymus

Thyroid gland

FIGURE 10-33
Branchial cleft cyst location in relation to other neck masses.

TORTICOLLIS

Torticollis, or wryneck, is often the result of injury during delivery. It may also result from constraint of the infant in utero. The head is tilted and twisted toward the sternocleidomastoid muscle. A hematoma may be palpated shortly after birth, and within 2 to 3 weeks a firm, fibrous mass may be felt in the muscle (Fig. 10-34). Torticollis can also occur in older children and adults as a result of trauma, muscle spasms, viral infection, or drug ingestion.

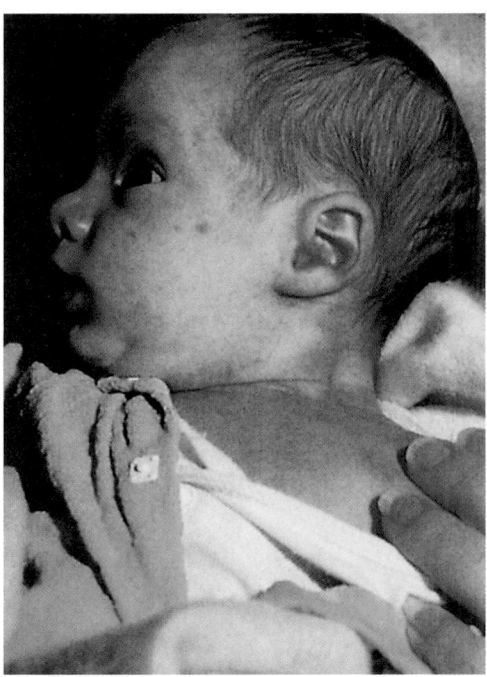

FIGURE 10-34
Torticollis, or wryneck.
From Zitelli, Davis, 1997.

SALIVARY GLAND TUMOR

Salivary gland tumors may arise in any of the salivary glands, but most commonly arise in the parotid (Fig. 10-35). These tumors are painless and may be slow-growing. Benign tumors tend to be smooth while malignant ones are often irregular and, if in the parotid, may damage the facial nerve as it passes through the gland.

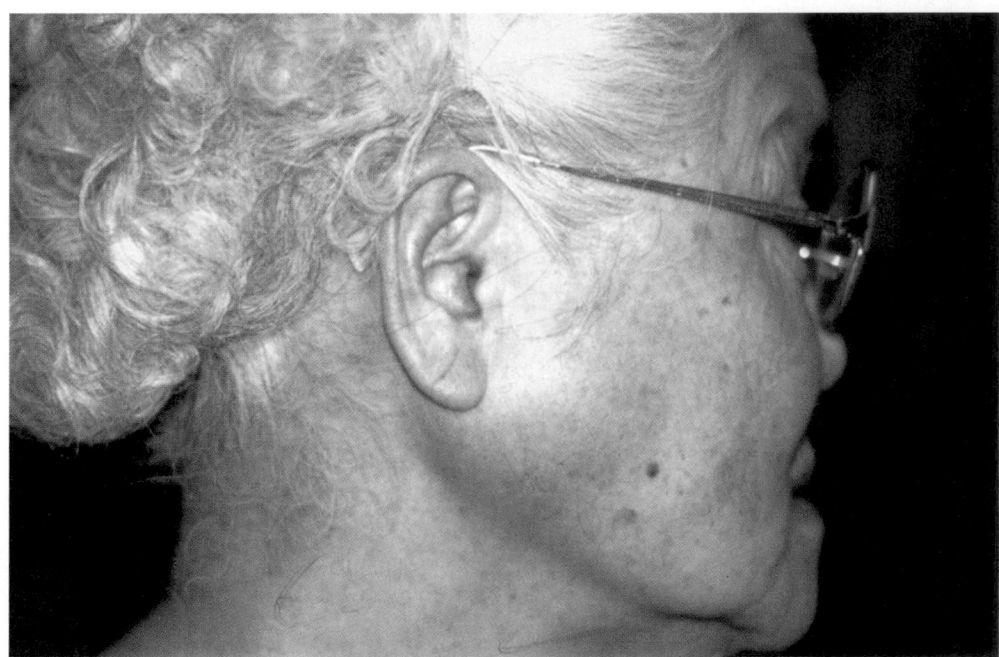

FIGURE 10-35
Malignant right parotid gland tumor.
From Lemmi, Lemmi, 2000.

TABLE 10-1	Hyperthyroidism Versus Hypothyroidism	
System or Structure Affected	**Hyperthyroidism**	**Hypothyroidism**
Constitutional		
Temperature preference	Cool climate	Warm climate
Weight	Loss	Gain
Emotional state	Nervous, easily irritated, highly energetic	Lethargic, complacent, disinterested
Hair	Fine, with hair loss; failure to hold a permanent wave	Coarse, with tendency to break
Skin	Warm, fine, hyperpigmentation at pressure points	Coarse, scaling, dry
Fingernails	Thin, with tendency to break; may show onycholysis	Thick
Eyes	Bilateral or unilateral proptosis, lid retraction, double vision	Puffiness in periorbital region
Neck	Goiter, change in shirt neck size, pain over the thyroid	No goiter
Cardiac	Tachycardia, dysrhythmia, palpitations	No change noted
Gastrointestinal	Increased frequency of bowel movements; diarrhea rare	Constipation
Menstrual	Scant flow, amenorrhea	Menorrhagia
Neuromuscular	Increasing weakness, especially of proximal muscles	Lethargic, but good muscular strength

THYROID

HYPOTHYROIDISM AND HYPERTHYROIDISM	The thyroid hormone influences the metabolism of most cells in the body. An overabundance or a paucity of the hormone can therefore cause symptoms affecting many body systems. Table 10-1 contrasts the signs and symptoms produced by hyperthyroidism and hypothyroidism.
MYXEDEMA	Adult-onset hypothyroidism associated with a decreased metabolic rate produces myxedema. The deposition of glycosaminoglycan in all organ systems leads to the characteristic mucinous edema of facial features (see Fig. 10-19). Signs and symptoms of hyperthyroidism and hypothyroidism are compared in Table 10-1.
GRAVES' DISEASE	This thyroid disorder is thought to be autoimmune. It is more common in women during the third and fourth decades of life. Multiple systems are affected, and the disease is often characterized by diffuse thyroid enlargement and hyperthyroidism with ophthalmologic, dermatologic, constitutional, menstrual, and musculoskeletal pathologic conditions (see Fig. 10-20 and Table 10-1). Pregnancy can make the diagnosis of hyperthyroidism more difficult. The presence of goiter may not be specific. The presence of weight loss, marked tachycardia, eye signs, and bruit over the thyroid are highly suggestive. Confirmation of the diagnosis is made by measuring blood levels of free T_4 and T_3.
HASHIMOTO DISEASE	Hashimoto disease is a chronic autoimmune disorder that causes symptoms of either hyperthyroidism or hypothyroidism, depending on the duration of the disease. It is common in children and in women between 30 and 50 years of age.

INFANTS

ENCEPHALOCELE

A protrusion of nervous tissue through a defect in the skull may occur any place on the scalp (Fig. 10-36).

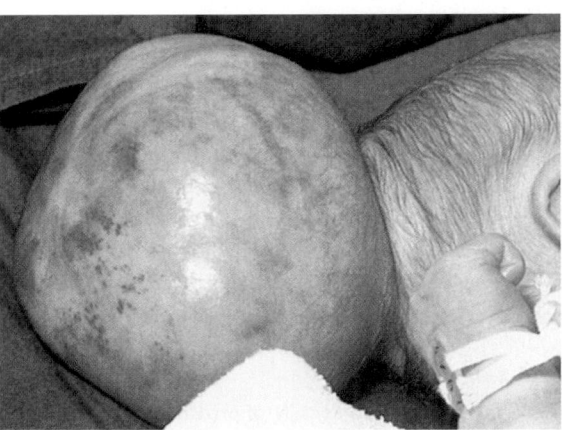

FIGURE 10-36
Encephalocele.
From Zitelli, Davis, 1997.

MICROCEPHALY

Microcephaly is evident by a congenitally small skull caused by cerebral dysgenesis or craniostenosis and is usually associated with mental retardation and failure of the brain to develop normally (Fig. 10-37).

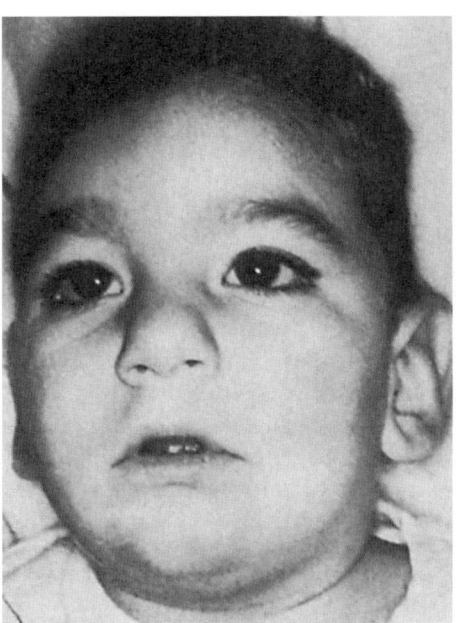

FIGURE 10-37
Primary familial microcephaly.
From Dyken, Miller, 1980.

CRANIOSYNOSTOSIS   Premature union of cranial sutures leads to a misshapen skull, usually not accompanied by mental retardation. The sutures involved determine the shape of the head (Fig. 10-38).

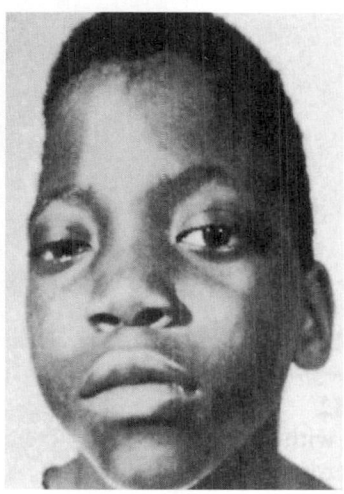

FIGURE 10-38
A 14-year-old with dolichoscaphocephaly, one of the craniosynostoses.
From Dyken, Miller, 1980.

ELECTRONIC RESOURCES

For Weblinks and additional resources, go to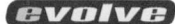

http://evolve.elsevier.com/Seidel

or to the Companion CD-ROM.

Additional information related to the content in Chapter 10 can be found on the companion website at evolve.elsevier.com/Seidel/ or on the interactive companion CD-ROM. Resources and activities for Chapter 10 include:
• Sound and Vision Theater
• Printouts for Your Practice
• Interactive Challenge
• Spanish Assessment Terms with Pronunciation Guide
• Instant Calculator

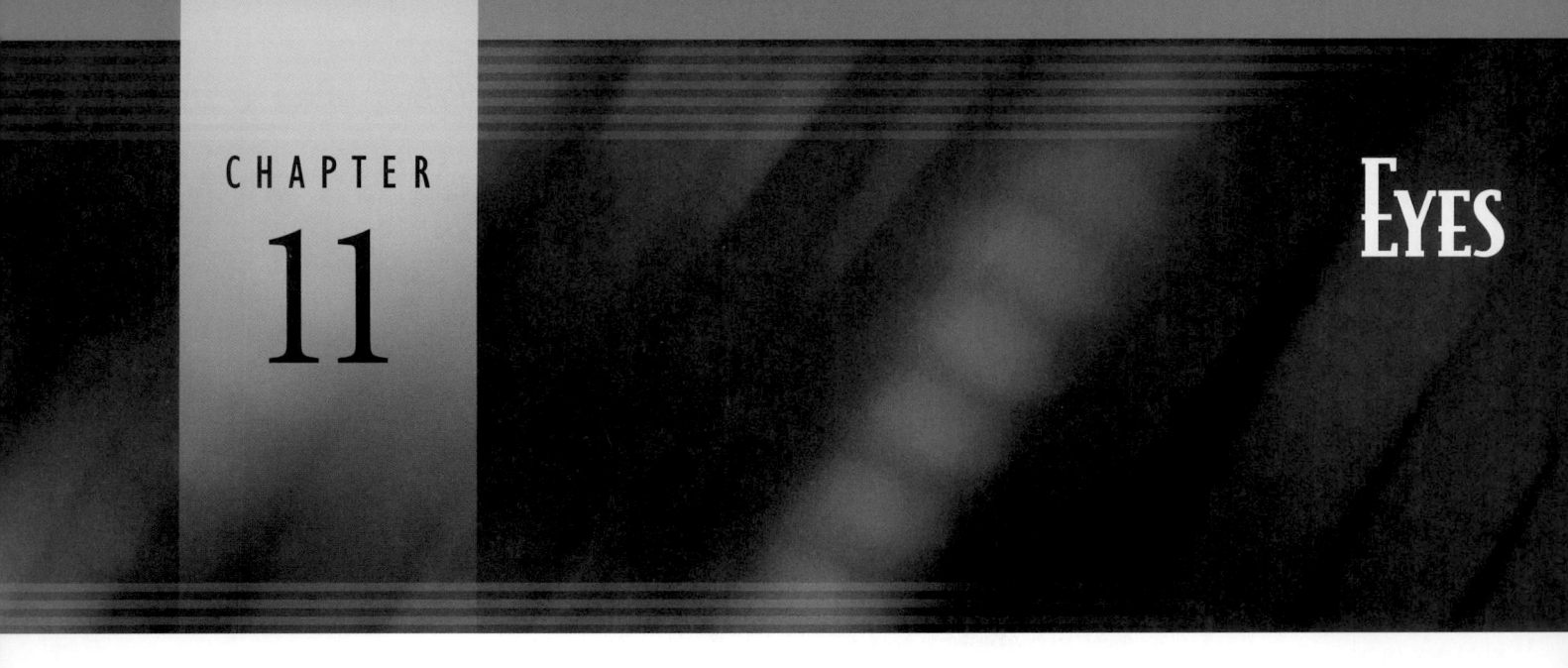

ANATOMY AND PHYSIOLOGY

The eye is the sensory organ that transmits visual stimuli to the brain for interpretation (Fig. 11-1). It occupies the orbital cavity with only its anterior aspect exposed. The four rectus and two oblique muscles attached to the eye are innervated by cranial nerves III (oculomotor), IV (trochlear), and VI (abducens) (Fig. 11-2). The eye itself is a direct embryologic extension of the brain and is connected to the brain by cranial nerve II, the optic nerve.

EXTERNAL EYE

The external eye is composed of the eyelid, conjunctiva, lacrimal gland, eye muscles, and the bony skull orbit. The orbit also contains fat, blood vessels, nerves, and connective tissue that support the eye (Fig. 11-3).

EYELID

The eyelid is composed of skin, striated muscle, the tarsal plate, and conjunctiva. The tarsus provides a skeleton to the lid and contains meibomian glands that provide oils to the tear film. The eyelid distributes tears over the surface of the eye, limits the amount of light entering it, and protects the eye from foreign bodies. Eyelashes extend from the anterior border of each lid.

CONJUNCTIVA

The conjunctiva is a thin mucous membrane covering and protecting the anterior surface of the eye with the exception of the cornea and the surface of the eyelid in contact with the globe.

LACRIMAL GLAND

The lacrimal gland is located in the temporal region of the superior eyelid and produces tears that moisten the eye (see Fig. 11-3). Tears flow over the cornea and drain via the canaliculi to the lacrimal sac and duct and then into the nasal meatus.

EYE MUSCLES

Each eye is moved by six muscles—the superior, inferior, medial, and lateral rectus muscles and the superior and inferior oblique muscles (see Fig. 11-20).

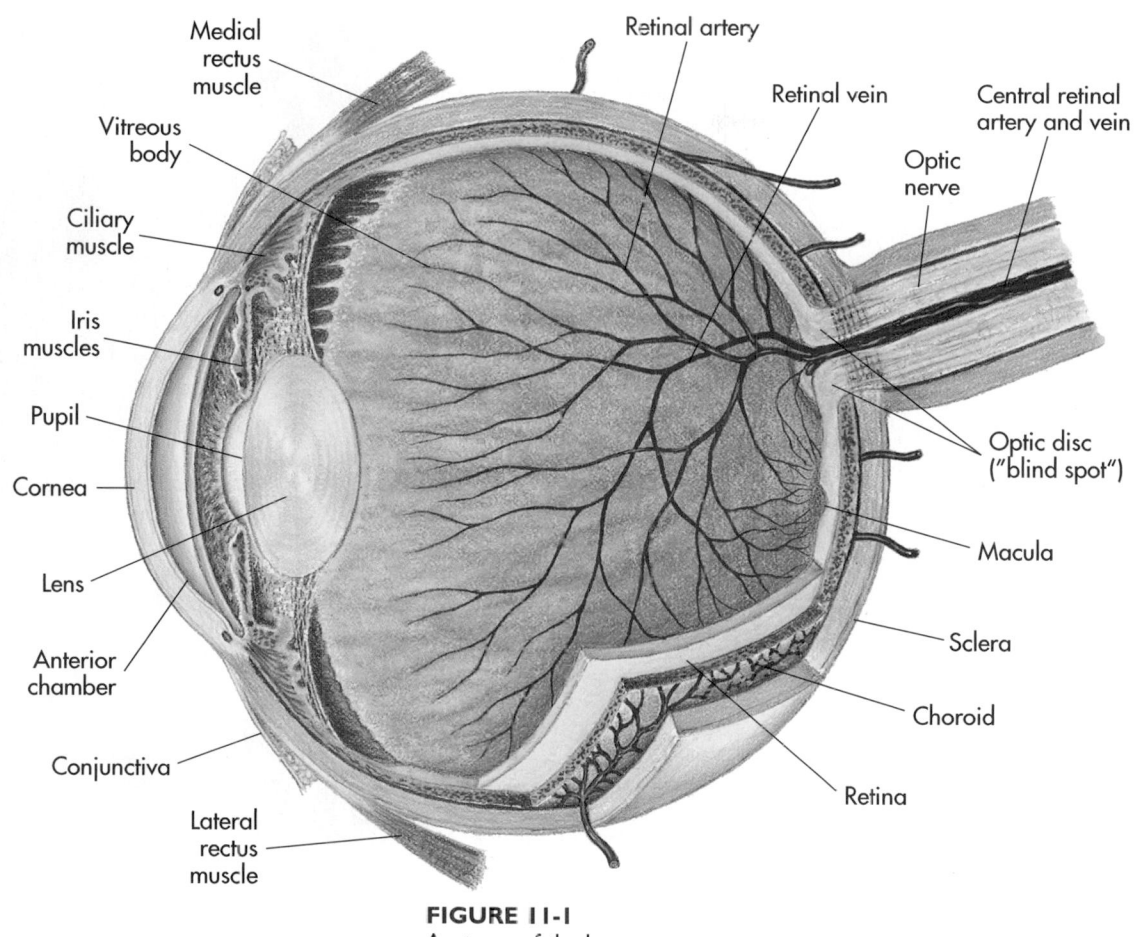

FIGURE 11-1
Anatomy of the human eye.

INTERNAL EYE

The internal structures of the eye are composed of three separate coats. The outer wall of the eye is composed of the sclera posteriorly and the cornea anteriorly. The middle layer or uvea consists of the choroid posteriorly and the ciliary body and iris anteriorly. The inner layer of nerve fibers is the retina.

SCLERA

The sclera is the dense, avascular structure that appears anteriorly as the white of the eye. It physically supports the internal structure of the eye.

CORNEA

The cornea constitutes the anterior sixth of the globe and is continuous with the sclera. It is optically clear, has rich sensory innervation, and is avascular. It is a major part of the refractive power of the eye.

UVEA

The iris, ciliary body, and choroids comprise the uveal tract. The iris is a circular, contractile muscular disk containing pigment cells that produce the color of the eye. The central aperture of the iris is the pupil, through which light travels to the retina. By dilating and contracting, the iris controls the amount of light reaching the retina. The ciliary body produces the aqueous humor and contains the muscles controlling accommodation. The choroid is a pigmented, richly vascular layer that supplies oxygen to the outer layer of the retina.

LENS

The lens is a biconvex, transparent structure located immediately behind the iris. It is supported circumferentially by fibers arising from the ciliary body. The lens is highly elastic, and contraction or relaxation of the ciliary body changes its thickness, thereby permitting images from varied distances to be focused on the retina.

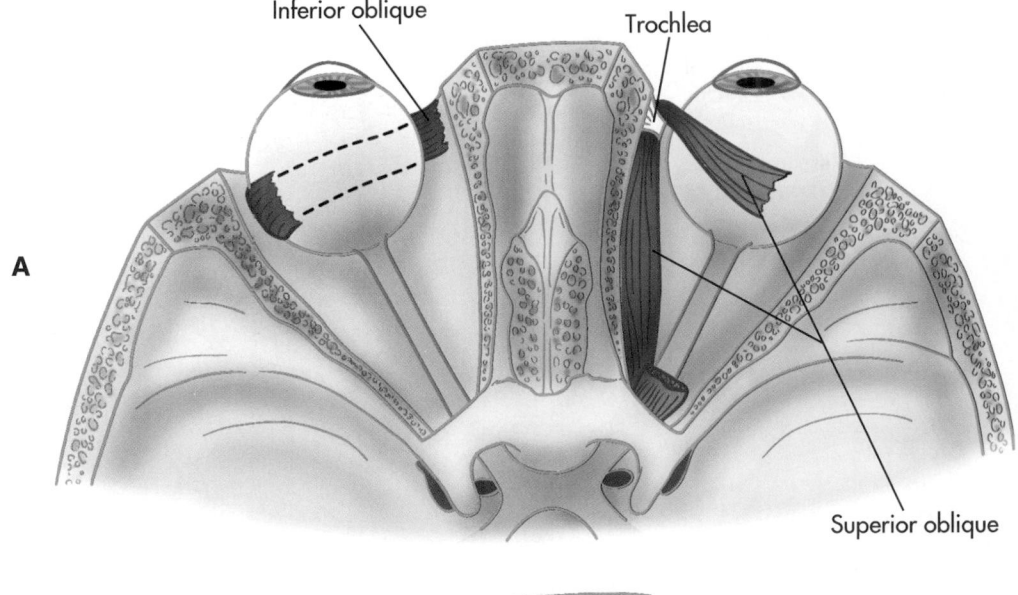

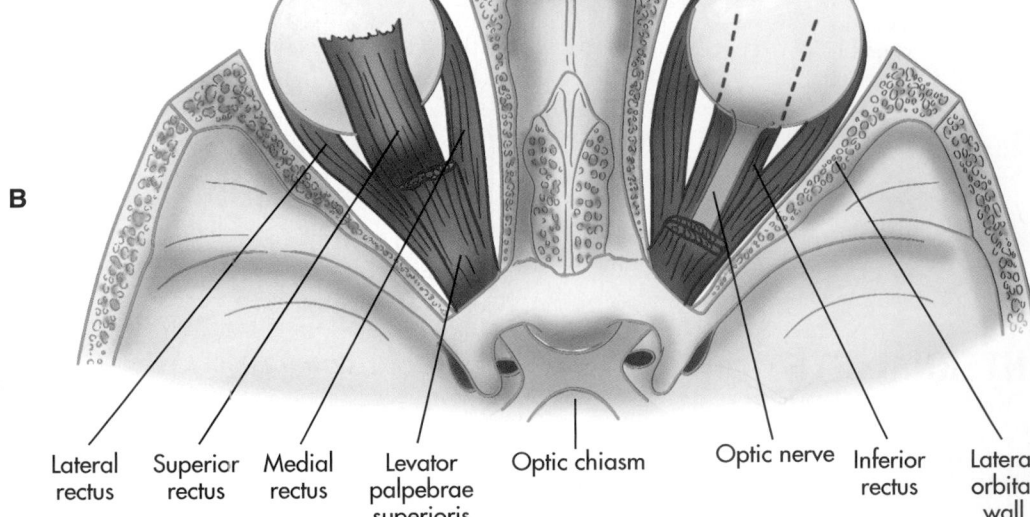

FIGURE 11-2
Extraocular muscles of the eye as viewed from above. **A,** The oblique muscles. **B,** The recti muscles.

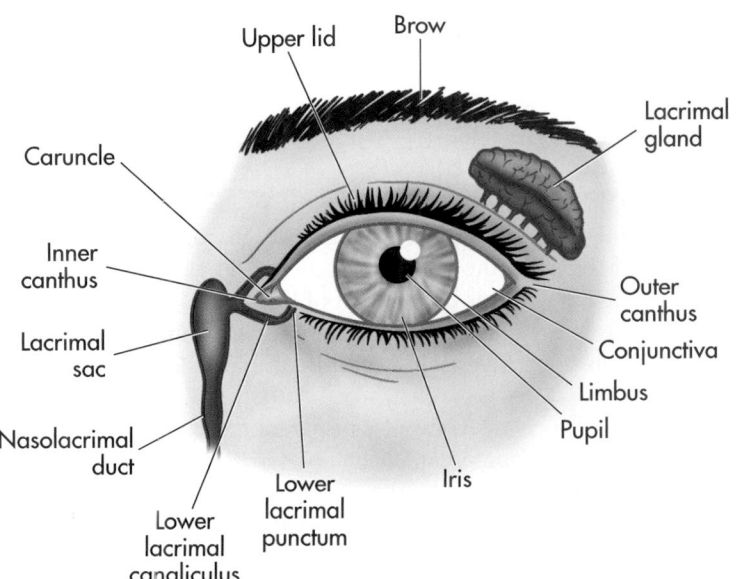

FIGURE 11-3
Important landmarks of the left external eye.
From Thompson et al, 1997.

RETINA

The retina is the sensory network of the eye. It transforms light impulses into electrical impulses, which are transmitted through the optic nerve, optic tract, and optic radiation to the visual cortex and then to consciousness in the cerebral cortex. The optic nerve communicates with the brain, passing through the optic foramen along with the ophthalmic artery and vein, and the autonomic nervous system innervation of the eye. Accurate vision is achieved by focusing an image on the retina by the cornea and the lens. An object may be perceived in each visual cortex, even when one eye is covered, if the light impulse is cast on both the temporal and the nasal retina. Fibers located on the nasal retina decussate in the optic chiasm (Fig. 11-4). Accurate binocular vision also requires the synchronous functioning of the extraocular muscles.

Major landmarks of the retina include the optic disc, from which the optic nerve originates, together with the central retinal artery and vein. The macula, or fovea, is the site of central vision. The direct ophthalmoscope is used primarily to examine these structures in the posterior pole of the eye.

INFANTS AND CHILDREN

The eye forms during the first 8 weeks of gestation and may become malformed by the insult of maternal drug ingestion or infection during this time. The development of vision, which is dependent on maturation of the nervous system, occurs over a longer period (Table 11-1). Term infants are hyperopic, with a visual acuity of less than 20/400. Although peripheral vision is fully developed at birth, central vision matures later. By 2 to 3 weeks of age, the lacrimal gland begins producing full volume of tears. The lacrimal drainage is complete at birth. By 3 to 4 months of age, binocular vision development is complete. By 6 months, vision has developed sufficiently so that the infant can differentiate colors.

Young children become less hyperopic with growth. The globe of the eye grows as the child's head and brain grow, and adult visual acuity is achieved at about 4 years of age.

PREGNANT WOMEN

The eyes undergo several changes during pregnancy because of physiologic and hormonal adaptations. These changes can result in hypersensitivity and can change the refractory power of the eye. Tears contain an increased level of lysozyme, resulting in a greasy sensation and perhaps blurred vision for contact lens wearers. The patient who wears contact lenses therefore may decide to discontinue their use during pregnancy. Because of the various changes in the eye, new lens prescriptions should not be obtained until several weeks after delivery. Dia-

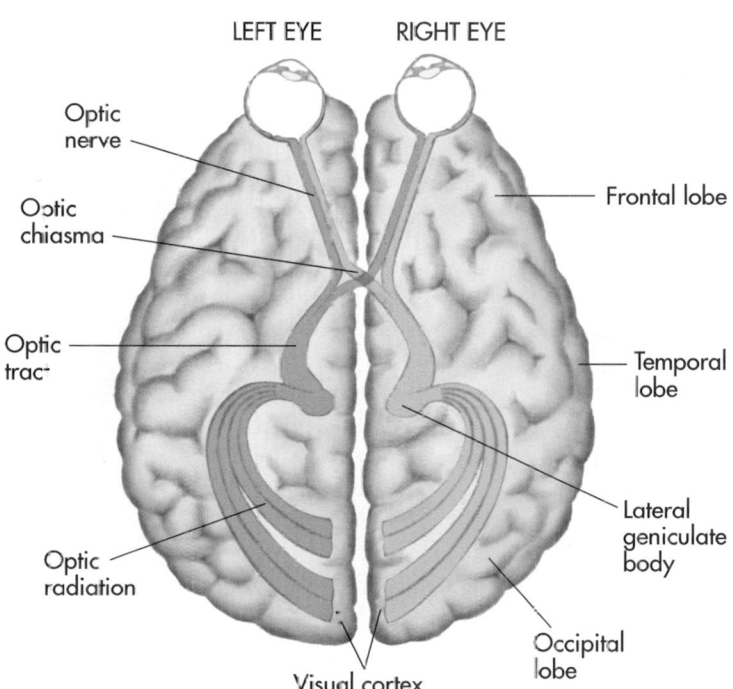

FIGURE 11-4
The visual chiasm.
Modified from Thompson et al, 1997.

betic retinopathy may worsen significantly. Mild corneal edema and thickening associated with blurred vision occur, especially in the third trimester.

Intraocular pressure falls most notably during the latter half of pregnancy. Subconjunctival hemorrhages may occur spontaneously in pregnancy or during labor; these resolve spontaneously.

OLDER ADULTS

The major physiologic eye change that occurs with aging is a progressive weakening of accommodation (focusing power) known as presbyopia. Generally by 45 years of age, the lens becomes more rigid and the ciliary muscle becomes weaker. The lens also continues to form fibers throughout life. Old fibers are compressed centrally, forming a denser central region that may cause loss of clarity of the lens and contribute to cataract formation.

TABLE 11-1	Chronology of Visual Development
Age	**Levels of Development**
Birth	Awareness of light and dark; infant closes eyelids in bright light
Neonatal	Rudimentary fixation on near objects (3 to 30 inches)
2 weeks	Transitory fixation, usually monocular at a distance of roughly 3 feet
4 weeks	Follows large, conspicuously moving objects
6 weeks	Moving objects evoke binocular fixation briefly
8 weeks	Follows moving objects with jerky eye movements Convergence beginning to appear
12 weeks	Visual following now achieved by a combination of head and eye movements Convergence improving Enjoys light objects and bright colors Beginning of depth perception Fusion of images begins to appear
16 weeks	Inspects own hands Fixates immediately on a 1-inch cube brought within 1 to 2 feet of eye Vision 20/300 to 20/200 (6/100 to 6/70)
20 weeks	Accommodative convergence reflexes all organizing Visually pursues dropped toy Shows interest in stimuli more than 3 feet away
24 weeks	Retrieves a dropped 1-inch cube Can maintain voluntary fixation of stationary object even in the presence of competing moving stimulus Hand-eye coordination appearing
26 weeks	Will fixate on a string
28 weeks	Binocular fixation clearly established
40 weeks	Marked interest in tiny objects Tilts head backward to gaze up Vision 20/200 (6/70)
52 weeks	Discriminates simple geometric forms (squares and circles) Vision 20/180 (6/60)
12-18 months	Looks at pictures with interest
18 months	Convergence well established Localization in distance crude—runs into large objects
2 years	Accommodation well developed Vision 20/30 (6/12)
3 years	Convergence smooth Fusion improving Vision 20/30 (6/9)
4 years	Vision 20/30 (6/6)

From Kemp, 1987.

REVIEW OF RELATED HISTORY

For each of the conditions discussed in this section, targeted topics to include in the history of the present illness are listed. Responses to questions about these topics help fully assess the patient's condition and provide clues for focusing the physical examination.

HISTORY OF PRESENT ILLNESS

> **CLINICAL PEARL**
>
> **Is It Blurry or Is It Double?**
> Blurred vision and diplopia are sometimes confused by the patient. Blurred vision represents a problem with visual acuity and there are many causes. Diplopia is the perception of two images and may be monocular or binocular. Monocular diplopia is an optical problem; binocular diplopia is an alignment problem.

- Eyelids: recurrent hordeola; ptosis of the lids so that they interfere with vision (unilateral or bilateral), growths or masses, itching
- Difficulty with vision: one or both eyes, corrected by lenses, involving near or distant vision, primarily central or peripheral, transient or sustained; cataracts (bilateral or unilateral, types, e.g., senile, diabetic, traumatic, surgical treatment); adequacy of color vision; presence of halos around lights, floaters, or diplopia (when one eye is covered or when both eyes are open)
- Pain: with or without loss of vision, in or around the eye, superficial or deep, insidious or abrupt in onset; burning, itching, or nonspecific uncomfortable or gritty sensation
- Secretions: color (clear or yellow), consistency (watery or purulent), duration, tears that run down the face, decreased tear formation with sensation of gritty eyes; presence of conjunctival redness
- Medications: eyedrops or ointments, antibiotics, artificial tears, mydriatics; glaucoma medications, antioxidant vitamins (to prevent macular degeneration), steroids (which cause cataract formation); prescription drugs, nonprescription drugs, complementary or alternative therapy)

PAST MEDICAL HISTORY

- Trauma: to the eye as a whole or a specific structure (e.g., cornea) or supporting structures (e.g., the floor of the orbit); events surrounding the trauma; efforts at correction and degree of success
- Eye surgery: condition requiring surgery, laser vision correction, date of surgery, outcome
- Chronic illness that may affect eyes or vision: glaucoma, diabetes, atherosclerotic cardiovascular disease (ASCVD), hypertension, thyroid dysfunction, collagen vascular diseases, human immunodeficiency virus (HIV), inflammatory bowel diseases
- Medications: steroids, Plaquenil, antihistamines, antidepressants, antipsychotics, antiarrhythmics, beta blockers

FAMILY HISTORY

- Retinoblastoma or cancer of the retina (often an autosomal dominant disorder)
- Conditions similar to the patient's such as glaucoma, macular degeneration, diabetes, hypertension, or others that may impact on vision or eye health
- Color blindness, cataract formation, retinal detachment, retinitis pigmentosa, or allergies affecting the eye
- Nearsightedness, farsightedness, strabismus, or amblyopia

RISK FACTORS

RISK FACTORS FOR CATARACT FORMATION

- Steroid medication use
- Exposure to ultraviolet light
- Cigarette smoking
- Diabetes mellitus
- Aging

PERSONAL AND SOCIAL HISTORY

- Employment: exposure to irritating gases, foreign bodies, or high-speed machinery
- Activities: participation in sporting activities that might endanger the eye (e.g., squash, racquetball, fencing, motorcycle riding)
- Allergies: type, seasonal, associated symptoms
- Corrective lenses: when last changed, how long worn, type (glasses or contact lenses), adequacy of corrected vision; methods of cleaning and storage, insertion and removal procedures of contact lenses; date of last eye examination
- Use of protective devices during work or activities that might endanger the eye
- History of cigarette smoking (a risk factor for cataract, glaucoma, macular degeneration, thyroid eye disease)

INFANTS AND CHILDREN

- Preterm: Resuscitated, ventilator or oxygen used, given diagnosis of retinopathy of prematurity, birth weight relative to gestational age, sepsis, intracranial hemorrhage, cerebral palsy
- Failure of infant to gaze at mother's face or other objects, uncertainty of mother that infant looks at her; failure of infant to blink when bright lights or threatening movements are directed at the face
- White area in the pupil on a photograph or on examination; inability of one eye to reflect light properly (may indicate retinoblastoma or other serious intraocular problem)
- Excessive tearing or discharge
- Strabismus some or all of the time; frequency; when first noted; occurring when fatigued, sick, or otherwise stressed; associated with frequent blinking or squinting, nystagmus
- Young children: Excessive rubbing of the eyes, frequent hordeola, inability to reach for and pick up small objects, night vision difficulties
- School-age children: necessity of sitting near the front of the classroom to see the board; poor progress in school not explained by intellectual ability

PREGNANT WOMEN

- Weeks gestation or postpartum
- Presence of disorders that can cause ocular complications such as pregnancy-induced hypertension or diabetes
- Use of topical eye medications (may cross the placental barrier)
- Symptoms indicative of pregnancy induced hypertension (PIH): diplopia, scotomata, blurred vision, or amaurosis

OLDER ADULTS

- Visual acuity: Decrease in central vision, distortion of central vision, use of dim or bright light to increase visual acuity, complaints of glare
- Excess tearing
- Dry eyes
- Development of scleral brown spots
- Difficulty in performing near work without lenses
- Nocturnal eye pain (a sign of subacute angle closure and a symptom of glaucoma)

EXAMINATION AND FINDINGS

EQUIPMENT

- Snellen chart or Lea Cards, Landolt C or HOTV chart
- Rosenbaum or Jaeger near vision card
- Penlight
- Cotton wisp
- Ophthalmoscope
- Eye cover, gauze, or opaque card

VISUAL TESTING

CLINICAL PEARL

Factors That Affect Visual Acuity Testing

Testing of visual acuity involves many complex factors not necessarily related to the ability to see the test object. Motivation and interest (including malingering or hysteria) as well as intelligence and attention span can modify the results of all sensory testing.

Measurement of visual acuity—the discrimination of small details—tests cranial nerve II (optic nerve) and is essentially a measurement of central vision. This is the most important test performed by the examiner who is not an ophthalmologist; it is also one that is often neglected. If possible, position the patient 20 feet (6 m) away from the Snellen chart (see Fig. 3-16), making sure it is well lighted. Alternatively special charts for use 10 feet (3 m) away from the patient are available. Test each eye individually by covering one eye with an opaque card or gauze, being careful to avoid applying pressure to the eye. If you test the patient with and without corrective lenses, record the readings separately. Always test vision without glasses first.

Ask the patient to identify all of the letters beginning at any line. Determine the smallest line in which the patient can identify all of the letters and record the visual acuity designated by that line. (If a more precise determination is needed, see p. 72.) When testing the second eye, you may want to ask the patient to read the line from right to left to reduce the chance of recall influencing the response. The test should be done rapidly enough to prevent the patient from memorizing the chart. However, one of the problems that patients confront during the vision examination is that the examiner sometimes goes too fast, asking that lines on the chart be read or that other judgments be made more quickly than feels comfortable to the patient. The patient's quick judgment may be helpful, but it is wise to pace it a bit more slowly to let the patient be comfortable and to allow time for the patient to puzzle out a response. The patient should not have to leave the examination feeling that something had been said too quickly or was not understood fully.

Visual acuity is recorded as a fraction in which the numerator indicates the distance of the patient from the chart (e.g., 20 feet or 6 m), and the denominator indicates the distance at which the average eye can read the line. Thus 20/200 (6/60) means that the patient can read at 20 feet (6 m) what the average person can read at 200 feet (6 m). The smaller the fraction, the worse the vision. Vision not correctable to better than 20/200 is considered legal blindness.

If the visual acuity is recorded at a fraction less than 20/20 (or 6/6), you can perform a pinhole test to see if the observed decrease in acuity was caused by a refractive error. Ask the patient to hold a pinhole occluder (or a piece of paper with a small hole in it) over the uncovered eye. This maneuver permits light to enter only the central portion of the lens. It should result in an improvement in visual acuity by at least one line on the chart if refractive error is responsible for the diminished acuity.

Measurement of near vision should also be tested in each eye separately with a handheld card such as the Rosenbaum Pocket Vision Screener (see Fig. 3-20). Have the patient hold the card at a comfortable distance (about 35 cm, or 14 inches) from the eyes and read the smallest line possible.

Peripheral vision can be accurately measured with sophisticated instruments, but it is generally estimated by means of the confrontation test. Sit or stand opposite the patient at eye level at a distance of about 1 m. Ask the patient to cover the right eye while you cover your left eye, so the open eyes are directly opposite each other (Fig. 11-5). Both you and the patient

EYES
Examination and Findings

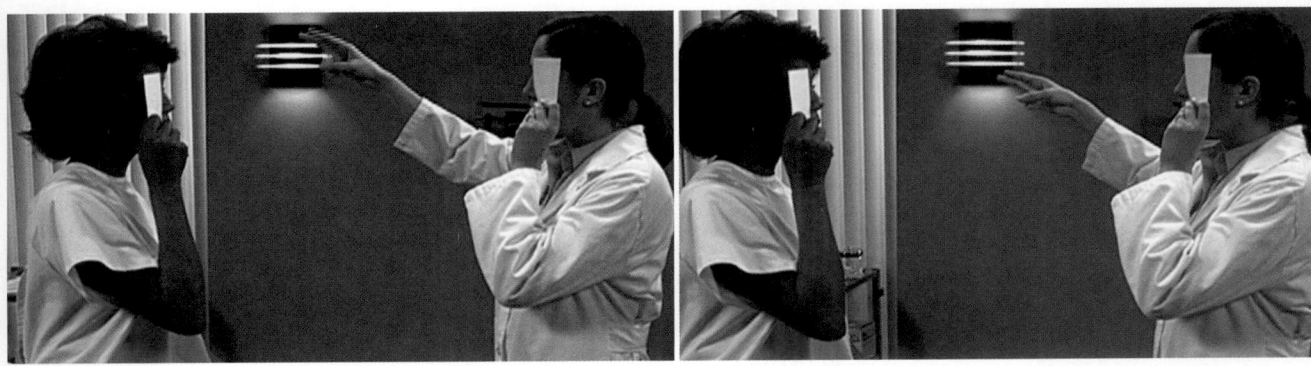

FIGURE II-5
Estimation of peripheral fields of vision. **A,** Temporal field. **B,** Nasal field.

CLINICAL PEARL

The Confrontation Test
The confrontation test is imprecise and can be considered significant only when it is abnormal. Lesions most likely to produce confrontation abnormalities include stroke, retinal detachment, optic neuropathy, pituitary tumor compression at the optic chiasm, and central retinal vascular occlusion.

should be looking at each other's eye. Fully extend your arm midway between the patient and yourself and then move it centrally with fingers moving. Have the patient tell you when the moving fingers are first seen. Compare the patient's response to the time you first note the fingers. Test the nasal, temporal, superior, and inferior fields. Remember that the nose itself interferes with the nasal portion of the visual field. Unless you are aware of a problem with your vision, you can feel comfortable that the fields are full if they correspond with yours. Actually one anticipates that the fields describe an angle of 60 degrees nasally, 90 degrees temporally, 50 degrees superiorly, and 70 degrees inferiorly.

Color vision is rarely tested in the routine physical examination. Color plates are available in which numerals are produced in primary colors and surrounded by confusing colors. The tests vary in degree of difficulty. For routine testing, check the patient's ability to appreciate primary colors. Red testing may be particularly helpful in determining subtle optic nerve disease, even when visual acuity remains nearly normal. An afferent pupillary defect (see p. 292) often coexists with a red defect.

EXTERNAL EXAMINATION

Examination of the eyes is carried out in a systematic manner, beginning with the appendages (i.e., the eyebrows and surrounding tissues) and moving inward.

SURROUNDING STRUCTURES

Inspect the eyebrows for size, extension, and texture of the hair. Note whether the eyebrows extend beyond the eye itself or end short of it. The coarseness of the hair is also important. If the patient's eyebrows are coarse or do not extend beyond the temporal canthus, the patient may have hypothyroidism. If the brows appear unusually thin, ask if the patient waxes or plucks them.

Inspect the orbital area for edema, puffiness, or sagging tissue below the orbit. Although puffiness may represent the loss of elastic tissue that occurs with aging, periorbital edema is always abnormal; the significance varies directly with the amount. It may represent the presence of thyroid eye disease, allergies, or (especially in youth) the presence of renal disease. You may see flat to slightly raised, oval irregularly shaped, yellow-tinted lesions on the periorbital tissues that represent depositions of lipids and may suggest that the patient has an abnormality of lipid metabolism. These lesions are called xanthelasma (Fig. 11-6), an elevated plaque of cholesterol deposited in macrophages most commonly in the nasal portion of the upper or lower lid.

EYELIDS

Examine the patient's lightly closed eyes for fasciculations or tremors of the lids, a sign of hyperthyroidism. Inspect the eyelids for their ability to close completely and open widely. Observe for flakiness, redness, or swelling on the eyelid margin. Eyelashes should be present on both lids and should curve away from the globe.

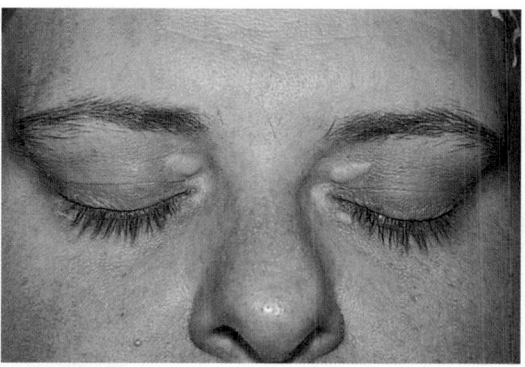

FIGURE 11-6
Xanthelasma.
Courtesy John W. Payne, MD, The Wilmer Ophthalmological Institute, The Johns Hopkins University and Hospital, Baltimore.

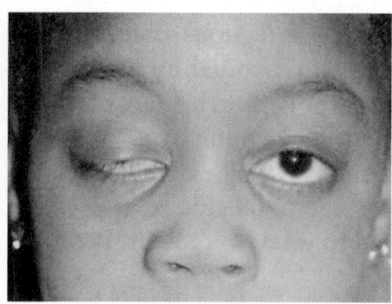

FIGURE 11-7
Ptosis, a drooping of the upper eyelid.
From Stein, Slatt, Stein, 1994.

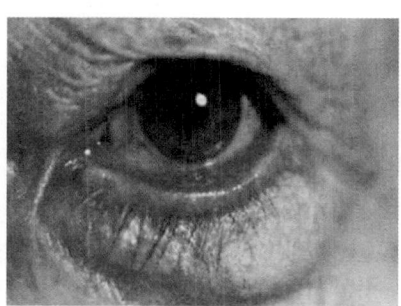

FIGURE 11-8
Ectropion.
From Stein, Slatt, Stein, 1988.

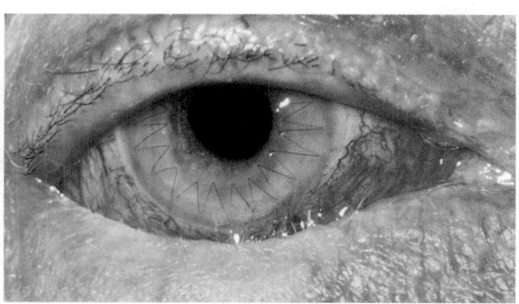

FIGURE 11-9
Entropion. Note that this patient has undergone corneal transplantation.
From Palay, Krachmer, 1997.

When the eye is open, the superior eyelid should cover a portion of the iris but not the pupil itself. If one superior eyelid covers more of the iris than the other or extends over the pupil, then ptosis of that lid is present. Ptosis indicates a congenital or acquired weakness of the levator muscle or a paresis of a branch of the third cranial nerve (Fig. 11-7). Record the difference between the two lids in millimeters. Average upper lid position is 2 mm below the limbus. Average lower lid position is at the lower limbus.

You should also note whether the lids evert or invert. When the lower lid is turned away from the eye, ectropion is present and may result in excessive tearing (Fig. 11-8). The inferior punctum, which serves as the tear-collecting system, is pulled outward and cannot collect the secretions of the lacrimal gland.

When the lid is turned inward toward the globe, a condition known as entropion (Fig. 11-9), the lid's eyelashes may cause corneal and conjunctival irritation, increasing the risk of a secondary infection. The patient often complains of a foreign body sensation.

An acute suppurative inflammation of the follicle of an eyelash can cause an erythematous or yellow lump. This hordeolum or sty is generally caused by staphylococcal organisms (Fig. 11-10).

Crusting along the eyelashes may represent blepharitis caused by bacterial infection, seborrhea, psoriasis, a manifestation of rosacea, or an allergic response (Fig. 11-11).

Ask the patient to close the eyes, and note whether the eyelids meet completely. If the closed lids do not completely cover the globe (a condition called *lagophthalmos*) the cornea may become dried and be at increased risk of infection. Thyroid eye disease, seventh nerve palsy (Bells or other causes), and overaggressive ptosis or blepharoplasty surgery are common causes.

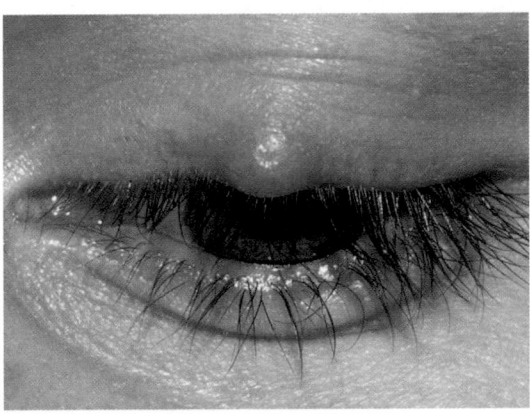

FIGURE 11-10
Acute hordeolum of upper eyelid.
From Palay, Krachmer, 1997.

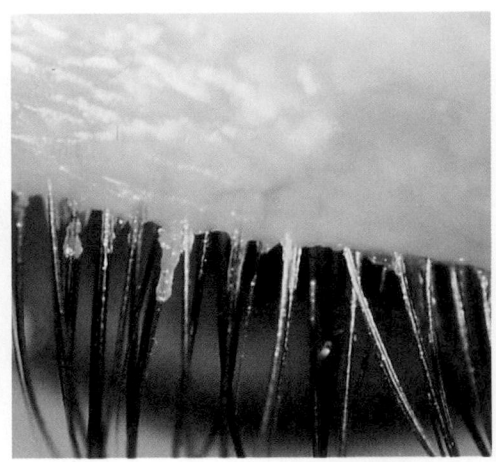

FIGURE 11-11
Blepharitis.
From Zitelli, Davis, 1997.

PALPATION

Palpate the eyelids for nodules. Next palpate the eye itself. Determine whether it feels hard or can be gently pushed into the orbit without causing discomfort. An eye that feels very firm and resists palpation may indicate glaucoma, hyperthyroidism, or the presence of a retrobulbar tumor.

CONJUNCTIVA

The conjunctivae are usually inapparent, clear, and free of erythema. Inspection of the conjunctival covering of the lower lid is easily performed by having the patient look upward while you draw the lower lid downward (Fig. 11-12).

Inspect the upper tarsal conjunctiva only when there is a suggestion that a foreign body may be present. Ask the patient to look down while you pull the eyelashes gently downward and forward to break the suction between the lid and globe (Fig. 11-13). Next evert the lid on a small cotton-covered applicator. After you inspect and remove any foreign body that may be present, return the eyelid to its regular position by asking the patient to look up while you apply downward pressure against the eyelid.

Observe the conjunctiva for increased erythema or exudate. An erythematous or cobblestone appearance, especially on the tarsal conjunctiva, may indicate an allergic or infectious conjunctivitis (Fig. 11-14). Bright red blood in a sharply defined area surrounded by healthy-appearing conjunctiva indicates subconjunctival hemorrhage (Fig. 11-15). The blood stays red because of direct diffusion of oxygen through the conjunctiva.

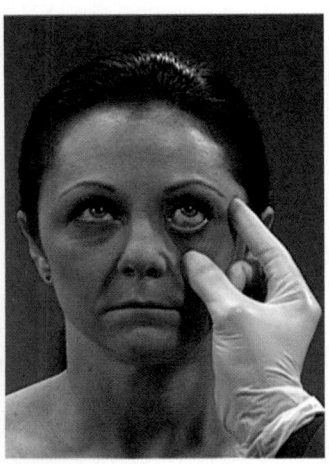

FIGURE 11-12
Pulling lower eyelid down to inspect the conjunctiva.

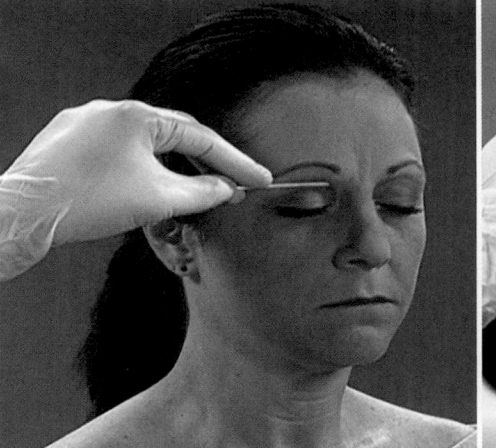

A

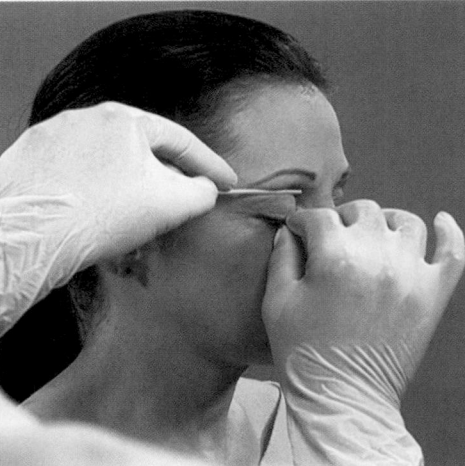

B

FIGURE 11-13
Everting upper eyelid. **A,** Placing applicator above the globe.
B, Withdrawing the lid from the globe.

A pterygium is an abnormal growth of conjunctiva that extends over the cornea from the limbus. It occurs more commonly on the nasal side (Fig. 11-16) but may arise temporally as well. A pterygium is more common in people heavily exposed to ultraviolet light. It can interfere with vision if it advances over the pupil.

CORNEA

Examine the cornea for clarity by shining a light tangentially on it. Because the cornea is normally avascular, blood vessels should not be present. Corneal sensitivity, controlled by cranial nerve V (trigeminal nerve), is tested by touching a wisp of cotton to the cornea (Fig. 11-17). The expected response is a blink, which requires intact sensory fibers of cranial nerve V and motor fibers of cranial nerve VII (facial nerve). Decreased corneal sensation is often associated with herpes simplex infection.

You may note a corneal arcus (arcus senilis), which is composed of lipids deposited in the periphery of the cornea. It may in time form a complete circle (circus senilis) (Fig. 11-18). Note the subtle clear area between the limbus and the arcus. An arcus is seen in many individuals older than 60 years of age. If present before 40 years of age, arcus senilis may indicate a lipid disorder, most commonly type II hyperlipidemia.

IRIS AND PUPIL

The iris pattern should be clearly visible. Generally the irides are the same color. Acquired heterochromia may be associated with tumors, trauma, and recently with several glaucoma medications. Note any irregularity in the shape of the pupils. They should be round, regular, and equal in size. Pupil abnormalities are described on pp. 307 and 308.

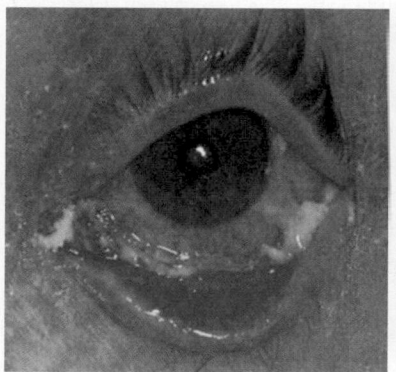

FIGURE 11-14
Acute purulent conjunctivitis.
From Newell, 1996.

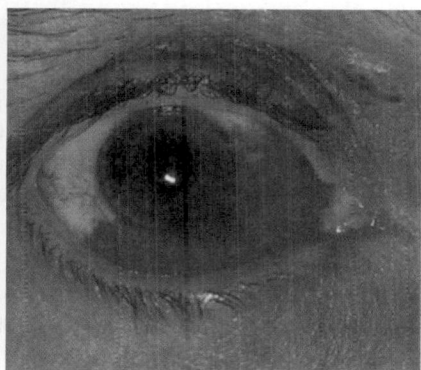

FIGURE 11-15
Subconjunctival hemorrhage.
From Newell, 1996.

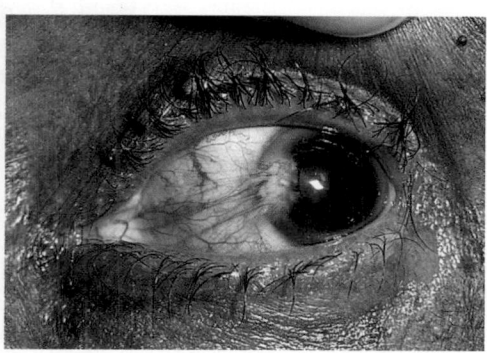

FIGURE 11-16
Pterygium.
Courtesy John W. Payne, MD, The Wilmer Ophthalmological Institute, The Johns Hopkins University and Hospital, Baltimore.

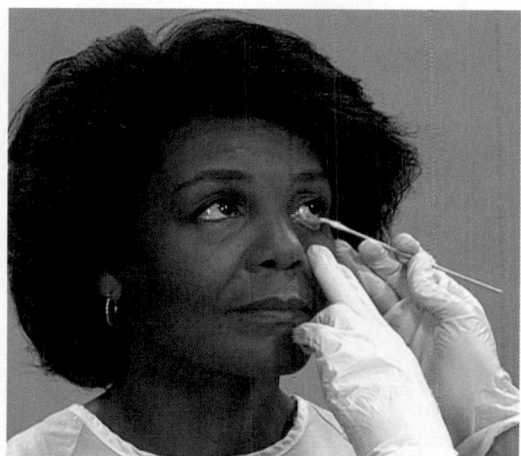

FIGURE 11-17
Testing corneal sensitivity.

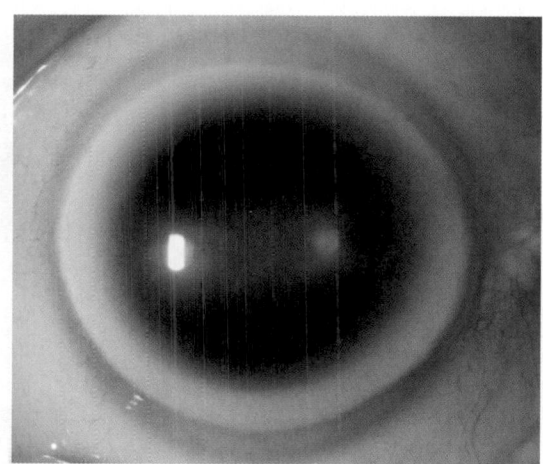

FIGURE 11-18
Corneal circus senilis.
From Palay, Krachmer, 1997.

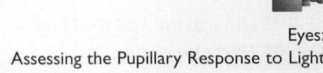

Eyes:
Assessing the Pupillary Response to Light

Test the pupils for response to light both directly and consensually. Dim the lights in the room so that the pupils dilate. Shine a penlight directly into one eye and note whether the pupil constricts. Note the consensual response of the opposite pupil constricting simultaneously with the tested pupil. Repeat the test by shining the light in the other eye.

To evaluate the health of the optic nerve, look for an afferent pupillary defect by performing the swinging flashlight test. Shine the light in one eye and then rapidly swing to the other. There should be a slight dilation in the second eye while the light is crossing the bridge of the nose but it should constrict equally to the first eye as the light enters the pupil. Repeat going in the other direction. The motion of the pupil in the second to be illuminated eye should be down. If it continues to dilate rather than constrict, an afferent pupillary defect is present. This is an important sign of optic nerve disease and can be present in any eye with poor vision from severe retinal disease. However, it is possible for an eye to have good Snellen acuity and an afferent defect. The eye, however, is not normal and the cause must be investigated.

Test the pupils for constriction to accommodation as well. Ask the patient to look at a distant object and then at a test object (either a pencil or your finger) held 10 cm from the bridge of the nose. The pupils should constrict when the eyes focus on the near object. With some patients, especially those with dark irides, it may be easier to observe pupillary dilation when the patient looks from near to far. Testing for pupillary response to accommodation is of diagnostic importance only if there is a defect in the pupillary response to light. A failure to respond to direct light but retaining constriction during accommodation is sometimes seen in patients with diabetes or syphilis.

Estimate the pupillary sizes and compare them for equality. Pupils may show size variation in a number of ways. Miosis is pupillary constriction to less than 2 mm. The miotic pupil fails to dilate in the dark. It is commonly caused by ingestion of drugs such as morphine, but drugs that control glaucoma may cause miosis as well. Pupillary dilation of more than 6 mm and failure of the pupils to constrict with light characterize mydriasis. Mydriasis is an accompaniment of coma, whether caused by diabetes, alcohol, uremia, epilepsy, or brain trauma, or may be caused by the use of some eyedrops including some glaucoma medications and atropine or similar medications used in management of amblyopia in children. Anisocoria, the inequality of pupillary size, is a common variation but may also occur in a large range of disease states.

LENS

Inspect the lens, which should be transparent. Shining a light on the lens may cause it to appear gray or yellow, but its ability to transmit light may still be great. Later examination of the lens with the ophthalmoscope will help judge the clarity.

SCLERA

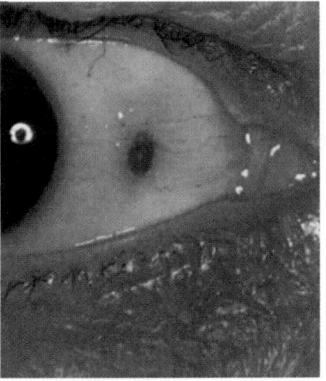

FIGURE 11-19
Senile hyaline plaque.
From Newell, 1996.

The sclera should be examined primarily to ensure that it is white. The sclera should be visible above the iris only when the eyelids are wide open. If liver disease is present, the sclerae may become pigmented and appear either yellow or green. Senile hyaline plaque appears as a dark, slate gray pigment just anterior to the insertion of the medial rectus muscle (Fig. 11-19). Its presence does not imply disease but should be noted.

LACRIMAL APPARATUS

Inspect the region of the lacrimal gland and palpate the lower orbital rim near the inner canthus. The puncta should be seen as slight elevations with a central depression on both the upper and lower lid margins nasally. If the temporal aspect of the upper lid feels full, evert the lid and inspect the gland. The lacrimal glands are rarely enlarged but may become so in some conditions such as tumors, lymphoid infiltration, sarcoid disease, and Sjögren syndrome. Despite the enlargement, the patient may complain of dry eyes because the glands produce inadequate tears.

EXTRAOCULAR MUSCLES

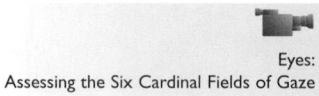

Eyes:
Assessing the Six Cardinal Fields of Gaze

Full movement of the eyes is controlled by the integrated function of the cranial nerves III (oculomotor), IV (trochlear), and VI (abducens) and the six extraocular muscles. Hold the patient's chin to prevent movement of the head and ask him or her to watch your finger as it moves through the six cardinal fields of gaze (Fig. 11-20). Then ask the patient to look to the extreme lateral (temporal) positions. Do not be surprised to observe a few horizontal rhythmic movements (nystagmic beats).

Occasionally you may note sustained nystagmus, the involuntary rhythmic movements of the eyes that can occur in a horizontal, vertical, rotary, or mixed pattern. Jerking nystagmus, characterized by faster movements in one direction, is defined by its rapid movement phase. For example, if the eye moves rapidly to the right and then slowly drifts leftward, the patient is said to have nystagmus to the right.

Finally, have the patient follow your finger in the vertical plane, going from ceiling to floor. Observe the coordinated movement of the globes and the superior lids. The movement should be accomplished smoothly and without exposure of the sclera. Full movements indicate integrity of muscle strength and cranial nerve action. Lid lag, the exposure of the sclera above the iris when the patient is asked to follow your finger as you direct the eye in a smooth movement from ceiling to floor, may indicate thyroid eye disease.

Use the corneal light reflex to test the balance of the extraocular muscles. Direct a light source at the nasal bridge from a distance of about 30 cm. Ask the patient to look at a nearby object (but not the light source). This will encourage the effort of both eyes to converge. The light should be reflected symmetrically from both eyes. When there is an imbalance found with the corneal light reflex test, perform the cover-uncover test (Fig. 11-21).

To perform the cover-uncover test, ask the patient to stare straight ahead at a near fixed point. Cover one eye and observe the uncovered eye for movement as it focuses on the designated point. Remove the cover and watch for movement of the newly uncovered eye as it fixes on the object. Repeat the process, covering the other eye. Movement of the covered or uncovered eye may indicate either esotropia or exotropia. Such a finding mandates referral to an ophthalmologist.

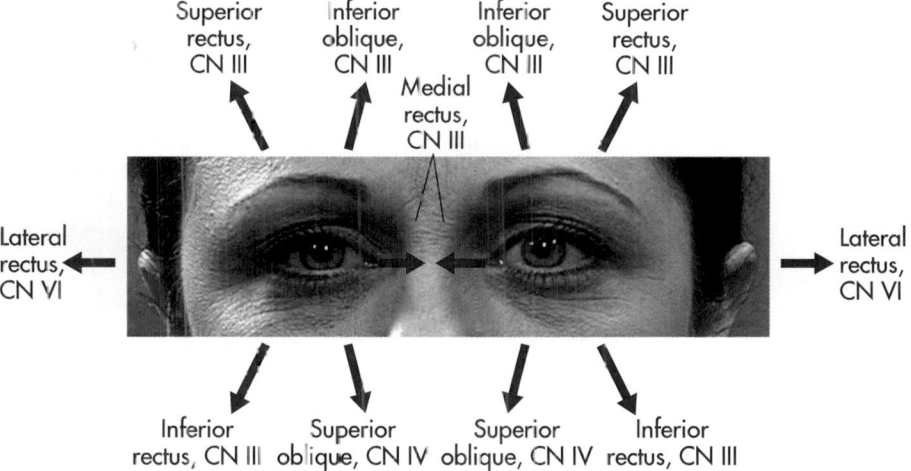

FIGURE 11-20
Cranial nerves and extraocular muscles associated with the six cardinal fields of gaze.

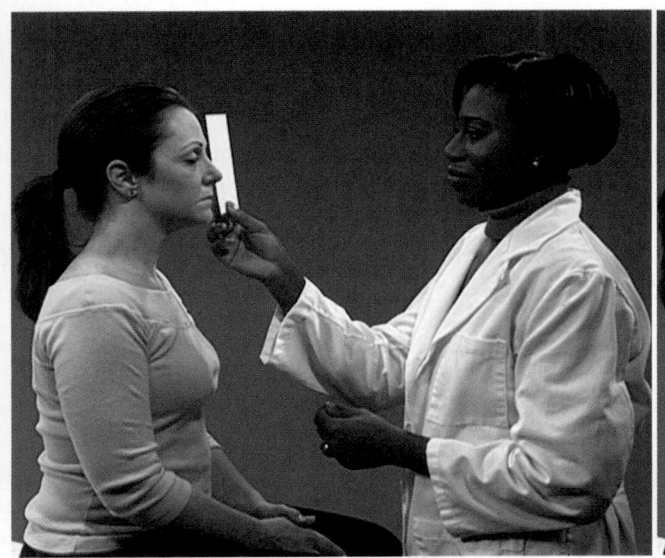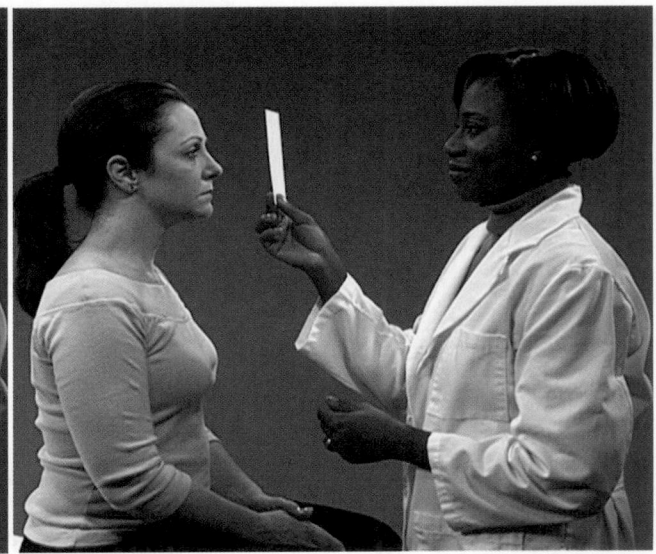

FIGURE 11-21
Evaluating eye fixation by the cover-uncover test. **A,** Patient focuses on near object. **B,** Examiner evaluates movement of covered eye as cover is removed.

OPHTHALMOSCOPIC EXAMINATION

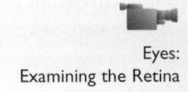

Eyes:
Examining the Retina

The ophthalmoscopic examination of the eyes is a tiring process. Avoid prolonging it by giving the patient brief intervals for rest from the bright light, a respectful consideration that reduces fatigue and improves comfort.

Inspection of the interior of the eye permits visualization of the optic disc, arteries, veins, and retina. Adequate pupillary dilation is necessary and can often be achieved by dimming the lights in the examining room. Instillation of medications that cause mydriasis is used in some cases (Box 11-1).

Examine the patient's right eye with your right eye and the patient's left eye with your left. Hold the ophthalmoscope in the hand that corresponds to the examining eye. (The structure of the ophthalmoscope is detailed in Fig 3-13.) Change the lens of the ophthalmoscope with your index finger. Start with the lens on the 0 setting, and stabilize yourself and the patient by placing your free hand on the patient's shoulder or head (Fig. 11-22).

With the patient looking at a distant fixation point, direct the light of the ophthalmoscope at the pupil from about 30 cm (12 inches) away. First visualize a red reflex, caused by the light illuminating the retina. Any opacities in the path of the light will stand out as black densities. Absence of the red reflex is often the result of an improperly positioned ophthalmoscope, but it may also indicate total opacity of the pupil by a cataract or by hemorrhage into the vitreous humor. If you locate the red reflex and then lose it as you approach the patient, simply move back and start again.

The fundus, or retina, appears as a yellow or reddish-pink background, depending on the amount of melanin in the pigment epithelium. The pigment generally varies with the complexion of the patient (Fig. 11-23). No discrete areas of lighter or darker pigmentation are expected when viewing the fundus except for crescents or dots at the disc margin, most commonly along the temporal edge.

As you approach the eye gradually, the retinal details should become apparent (Fig. 11-24). Recall that at any one time, you will see only a small portion of the retina. A blood vessel will probably be the first structure seen when you are about 3 to 5 cm from the patient. You may have to adjust the ophthalmoscope lens to be able to see the retinal details. If your patient is myopic, you will need to use a minus (red) lens; if the patient is hyperopic or lacks a lens (aphakic), you will need a plus (black) lens (see p. 70). When fundus details come into focus, you will note the branching of blood vessels. Because they always branch away from the optic disc, you can use these landmarks to find the optic disc.

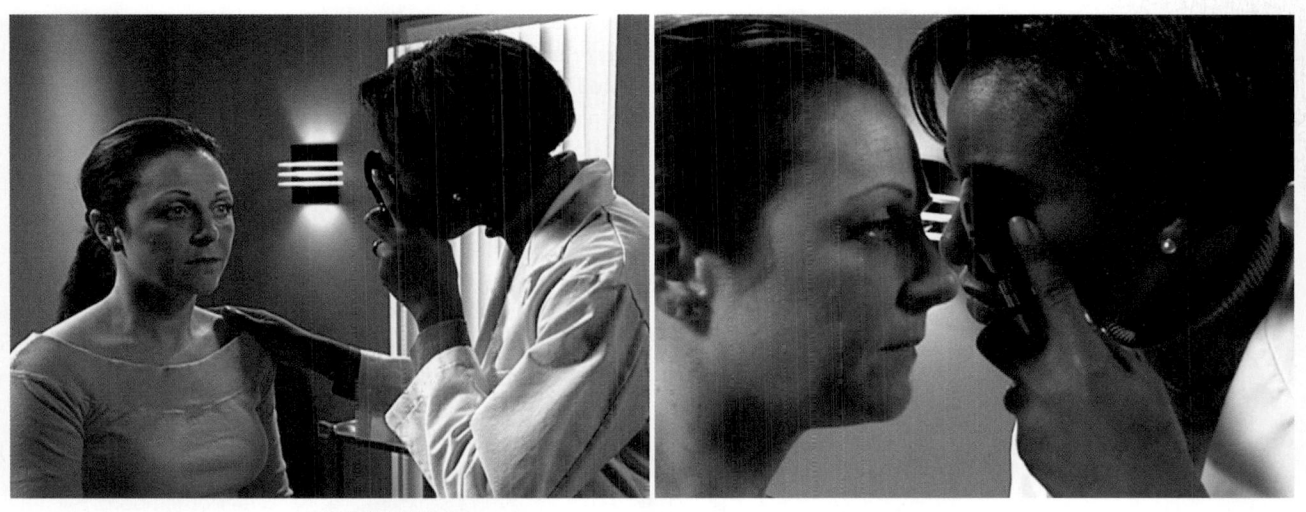

FIGURE 11-22
A, Visualization of the red reflex. **B,** Examination of the optic fundus.

BOX 11-1

TEST FOR APPLYING MYDRIATICS

Before instillation of a mydriatic, inspect the patient's anterior chamber by shining a focused light tangentially at the limbus (the union of the conjunctiva and the sclera). Note the illumination of the iris nasally. This portion of the iris is not lighted when the patient has a shallow anterior chamber, indicating a risk of acute-angle glaucoma. Mydriatics should be avoided in these patients.

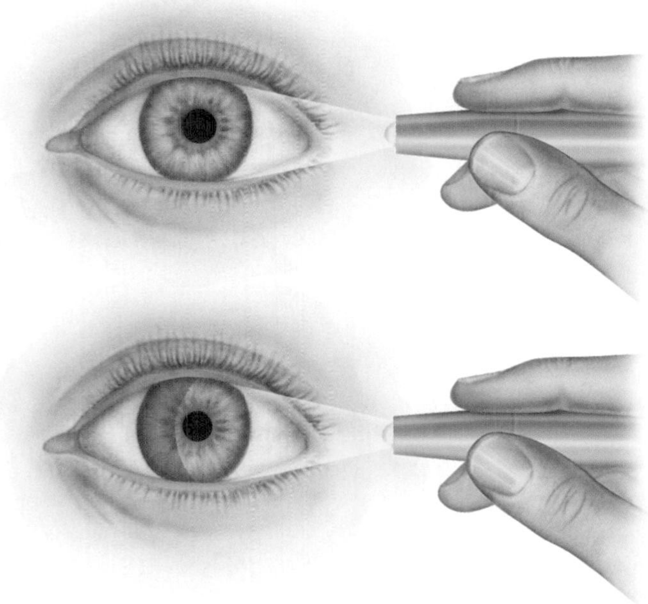

Evaluation of depth of anterior chambers. **A,** Usual anterior chamber. **B,** Shallow anterior chamber.

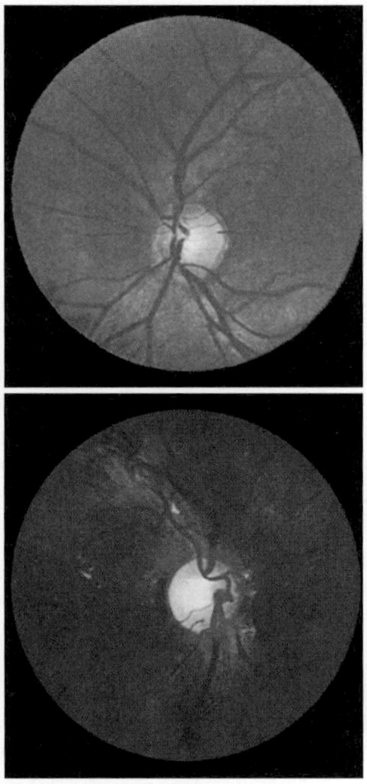

FIGURE 11-23
Fundus of a white patient **(A)** and of a black patient **(B)**.
From Medcom, 1983.

Next look at the vascular supply of the retina. The blood vessels on the disc divide into superior and inferior branches and then into nasal and temporal ones. Venous pulsation may be seen on the disc and should be noted. Arterioles are smaller than venules, generally by a ratio of 3:5 to 2:3. The light reflected from arterioles is brighter than that from venules, and the oxygenated blood is a brighter red. Follow the blood vessels distally as far as you can in each of the four quadrants. Note especially the sites of crossing of the arterioles and venules, because their characteristics may change when hypertension is present.

Finally examine the optic disc itself. The disc margin should be sharp and well defined, especially in the temporal region. The disc is generally yellow to creamy pink, but the color varies with race, being darker in individuals whose skin is dark. It is about 1.5 mm in diameter and is the unit of measurement in describing lesion size and location on the fundus. For example, an abnormality of a blood vessel may occur 2 disc diameters from the optic nerve at the 2-o'clock position (Fig. 11-25).

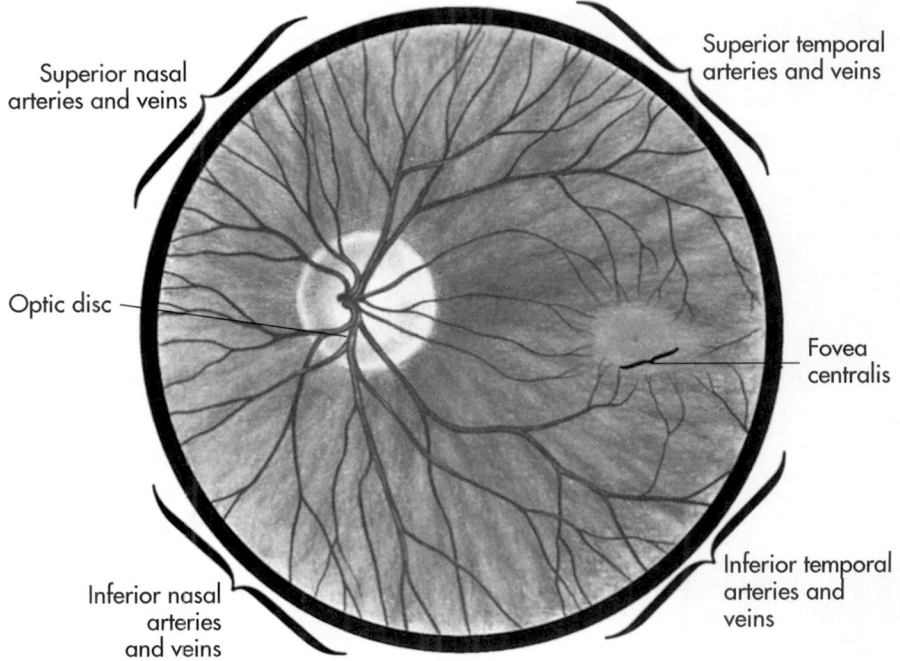

FIGURE 11-24
Retinal structures of the left eye.

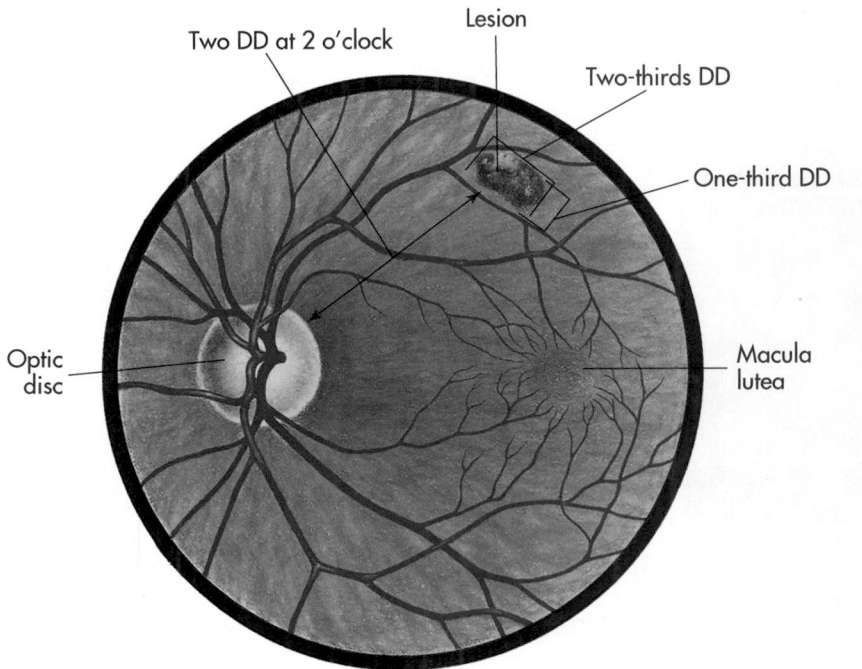

FIGURE 11-25
Method of describing the position and dimension of a lesion in terms of disc diameter. The lesion in this illustration is described as being 2 disc diameters (DD) from the optic disc at the 2-o'clock position. The lesion is two-thirds DD long and one-third DD wide.

Next examine the macula, also called the fovea centralis or macula lutea. The site of central vision, it is located approximately 2 disc diameters temporal to the optic disc. It may be impossible to examine when the pupil is not dilated, because shining light on it induces strong pupillary constriction. To bring it into your field of vision, ask the patient to look directly at the light of the ophthalmoscope. No blood vessels enter the fovea, and it appears as a lighter dot surrounded by an avascular area.

UNEXPECTED FINDINGS

Occasionally you may see unexpected findings such as myelinated nerve fibers, papilledema, glaucomatous cupping, drusen bodies, cotton wool bodies, or hemorrhages (Table 11-2).

Myelinated nerve fibers appear as a white area with soft, ill-defined peripheral margins (Fig. 11-26). The area is usually continuous with the optic disc. The nerve fiber layer is on the innermost surface of the retina. Note how the myelinated nerve fibers obscure areas of the retinal blood vessels, particularly inferiorly. This finding is due to the fact that the vessels lie deeper in the retina. The absence of pigment, feathery margins, and full visual fields help distinguish this benign condition from chorioretinitis.

TABLE II-2 Unexpected Retinal Findings

Unexpected Finding	Description	Significance
Myelinated retinal nerve fibers (see Fig. 11-26)	A white area with soft, ill-defined peripheral margins usually continuous with the optic disc The absence of pigment, feathery margins, and full visual fields help distinguish this benign condition from chorioretinitis. The nerve fiber layer is on the innermost surface of the retina and the vessels lie deeper in the retina. Note how the myelinated nerve fibers obscure areas of the retinal blood vessels, particularly inferiorly.	No physiologic significance.
Papilledema (see Fig. 11-27)	The central vessels are pushed forward, and the veins are markedly dilated. Venous pulsations are not visible and cannot be induced by pressure applied to the globe. Venous hemorrhages may occur.	Loss of definition of the optic disc margin, first obscuring superiorly and inferiorly and then nasally and temporally. Caused by increased intracranial pressure transmitted along the optic nerve. Initially vision is not altered.
Glaucomatous optic nerve head cupping (see Fig. 11-28)	The physiologic disc margins are raised with a lowered central area in which blood vessels may disappear over the edge of the disc. Look for asymmetry of the cupping between the eyes. Compare with healthy vessels as seen in Fig. 11-23.	Increased intraocular pressure leads to loss of nerve fibers with the death of ganglion cells. Impairment of the blood supply will ultimately lead to optic nerve atrophy, causing the optic disc to appear much whiter than usual.
Cotton wool spot (see Fig. 11-42)	Cotton wool spots are ill-defined, yellow areas caused by infarction of the nerve layer of the retina.	Vascular disease secondary to hypertension or diabetes mellitus are the common causes.

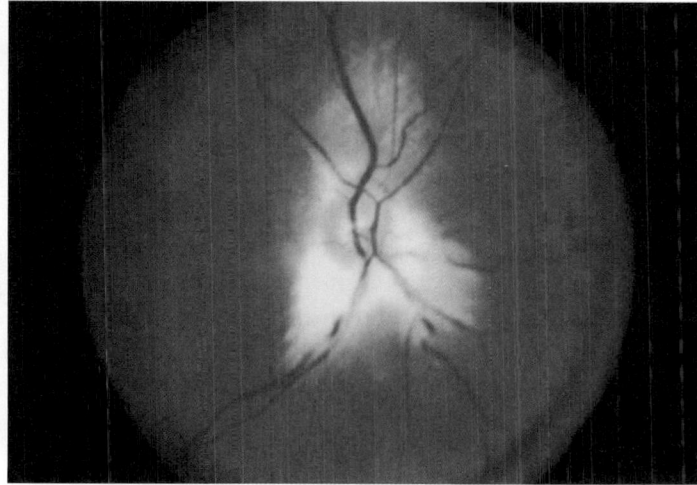

FIGURE II-26
Myelinated retinal nerve fibers. *Courtesy Andrew P. Schachat, MD, The Wilmer Ophthalmological Institute, The Johns Hopkins University and Hospital, Baltimore.*

Papilledema is characterized by loss of definition of the optic disc margin that initially occurs superiorly and inferiorly and then nasally and temporally. It is caused by increased intracranial pressure transmitted along the optic nerve. The central vessels are pushed forward, and the veins are markedly dilated. Venous pulsations are not visible and cannot be induced by pressure applied to the globe. Venous hemorrhages may occur. Initially vision is not altered (Fig. 11-27).

Glaucomatous cupping is a result of increased intraocular pressure with loss of nerve fibers and the death of ganglion cells (Fig. 11-28). Occasionally atrophy occurs unilaterally; so you should always compare the cupping on the two retinae. Blood vessels may disappear over the edge of the physiologic disc and be seen again deep within the disc. Blood vessels may also be displaced nasally. Impairment of the blood supply may lead to optic atrophy, causing the disc to appear much whiter than usual. The cup is usually not particularly enlarged in contrast to glaucomatous atrophy. Peripheral visual fields are constricted.

Drusen bodies can appear as small, discrete spots that are slightly more yellow than the retina. With time the spots enlarge. Similar appearing lesions may occur in many conditions that affect the pigment layers of the retina, but most commonly they are a consequence of the aging process and depending on size and number, are a precursor of senile macular degeneration (Fig. 11-29, *A*).

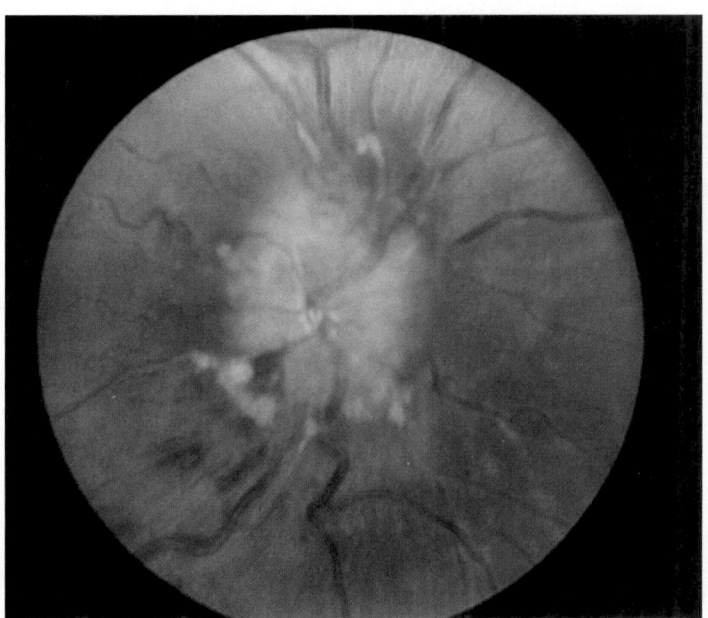

FIGURE 11-27
Severe papilledema.
Courtesy John W. Payne, MD, The Wilmer Ophthalmological Institute, The Johns Hopkins University and Hospital, Baltimore.

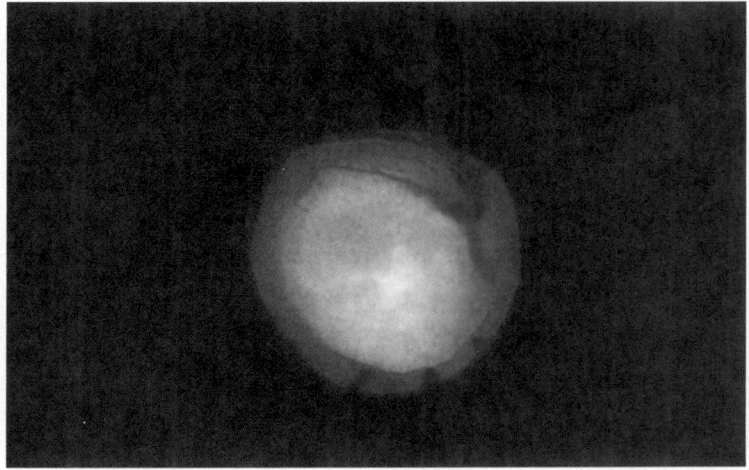

FIGURE 11-28
Marked glaucomatous optic nerve head cupping. Compare the disappearance of blood vessels here with the blood vessels of the optic disc in Fig. 11-23.
Courtesy Andrew P. Schachat, MD, The Wilmer Ophthalmological Institute, The Johns Hopkins University and Hospital, Baltimore.

When drusen bodies are noted to be increasing in number or in intensity of color, the individual should be given an Amsler grid (see Fig. 3-21). The grid is used to evaluate central vision. The patient is instructed to observe the grid with each eye, using reading glasses if needed, and to note any distortion of the grid pattern. Fig. 11-29, *B*, shows the grid of an individual with drusen bodies who has developed fluid leakage in the area of the macula.

Hemorrhages in the retina vary in color and shape, depending on the cause and location (Fig. 11-30, *A*). A hemorrhage at the disc margin often indicates poorly controlled glaucoma or undiagnosed glaucoma. Also note the loss of the vessels at the inferior margin of the disc. Flame-shaped hemorrhages occur in the nerve fiber layers, and the blood spreads parallel to the nerve fibers (Fig. 11-30, *B*). Round hemorrhages tend to occur in the deeper layers and may appear as a dark color instead of the bright red that is characteristic of flame hemorrhages. Dot hemorrhages may actually represent microaneurysms, which are common in diabetic retinopathy. The direct ophthalmoscope does not permit the distinction between dot hemorrhages and microaneurysms. Vascular changes that suggest systemic hypertension may be observed in the retina and are described in Box 11-2.

INFANTS

Infants often shut their eyes tightly when eye examination is attempted. It is difficult to separate the eyelids, and often the lids evert when too much effort is exerted. If a parent is present, have the parent hold the infant over a shoulder, and position yourself behind the parent. Even when the infant is crying, there is often a moment when the infant's eyes open. This gives you

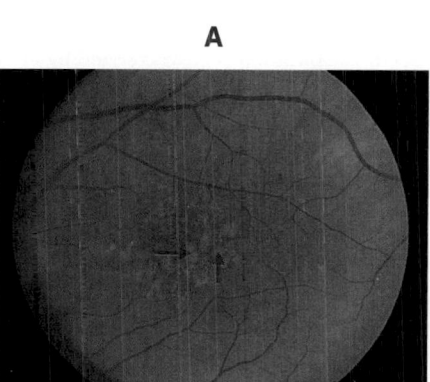

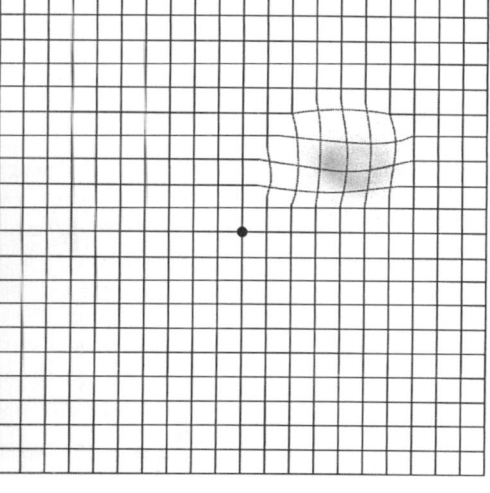

A

B

FIGURE 11-29
A, Drusen bodies. **B,** Amsler grid showing visual changes seen caused by fluid leakage under the retina.
A courtesy Robert P. Murphy, MD, Glaser Murphy Retina Treatment Center, Baltimore. B courtesy Brent A. Bauer, MFA, The Wilmer Ophthalmological Institute, The Johns Hopkins University and Hospital, Baltimore, MD.

STAYING WELL

PREVENTING MACULAR DEGENERATION

Middle-aged and older patients should be reminded that studies have now demonstrated preservation of vision with the reduction of age-related macular degeneration in individuals taking high-dose antioxidants plus zinc.

Age-related macular degeneration (see p. 298 and Fig. 11-29) is the leading cause of visual impairment and blindness in patients older than 65 years of age in the United States. Laser therapy is helpful in some cases. A clinical study undertaken in the 1990s involved more than 3600 participants from 65 to 80 years of age who were followed for more than 6 years.

Those treated with antioxidants (vitamin C, 100 mg; vitamin E, 400 International units; beta carotene, 15 mg; zinc, 80 mg, as zinc oxide; and copper, 2 mg, as cupric oxide) had a significantly better preservation of vision when compared with those treated with antioxidants, zinc and copper alone, or placebo.

Reminding your older patients to have a dilated eye examination regularly can help them determine whether they need antioxidant, zinc, and copper supplements.

Data from Age-Related Eye Disease Study Research Group, 2000.

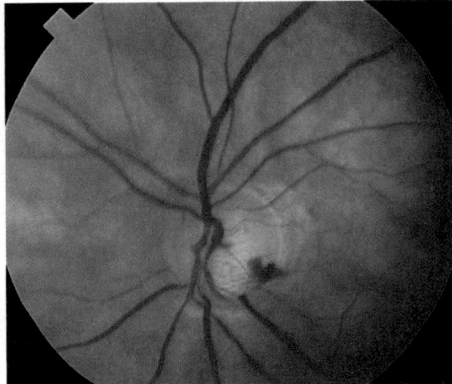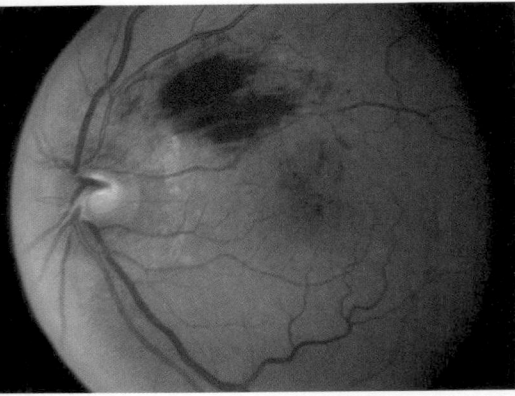

FIGURE 11-30
A, Hemorrhage at the disc margin. **B,** Flame hemorrhages.
A, Courtesy John W. Payne, MD, The Wilmer Ophthalmological Institute, The Johns Hopkins University and Hospital, Baltimore. B, Courtesy Robert P. Murphy, MD, Glaser Murphy Retina Treatment Center, Baltimore.

BOX 11-2

HYPERTENSIVE RETINOPATHY

- Retinal changes associated with hypertension are generally classified according to the Keith-Wagner-Barker (KWB) system (Keith, Wagner, Barker, 1939), which evaluates changes in the vascular supply, the retina itself, and the optic disc. For accurate rating, the changes should be present bilaterally.
- The arterial-venous size ratio is usually 3:5. That ratio decreases as arterioles become smaller because of smooth muscle contraction, hyperplasia, or fibrosis. Venules do not have a smooth muscle coat but share the adventitia of the arteriole where the arteriole and venule cross. Thickening of the arteriolar coat results in apparent nicking of the venule where the venule passes beneath the arteriole, or the venule may appear elevated when it passes over the arteriole.
- Group I of the KWB classification is characterized by increased light reflex from the arterioles. There is moderate arteriolar attenuation and focal constriction. No arterial-venous changes at crossing are noted.
- Group II is marked by the appearance of arterial-venous crossing changes. Arterioles are reduced to about one half of the usual size, and areas of localized constriction may be observed.
- Group III is characterized by a shiny retina and by the appearance of cotton wool spots, which represent ischemic infarcts of the retina. These are gray areas with poorly defined margins. Hemorrhages may also be present.
- Group IV is characterized by the appearance of papilledema.

CLINICAL PEARL

Opening an Infant's Eyes
Examining the newborn's eyes in a dimly lit room often encourages the baby to open the eyes. Holding the infant upright, suspended under its arms, or holding the baby at one's shoulder, the infant then looking behind the holder, also prompts the eyes to open.

an opportunity to learn something about the eyes, their symmetry and extraocular muscular balance, and whether there is a light reflex. The child may then start crying again, but progress has been made.

Begin by inspecting the infant's external eye structures. Note the size of the eyes, paying particular attention to small or differently sized eyes. Inspect the eyelids for swelling, epicanthal folds, and position. To detect epicanthal folds, look for a vertical fold of skin nasally that covers the lacrimal caruncle (Fig. 11-31). Prominent epicanthal folds are an expected variant in Asian infants, but they may be suggestive of Down syndrome or other genetic anomalies in children of other ethnic groups. Observe the alignment and slant of the palpebral fissures of the infant's eyes. Draw an imaginary line through the medial canthi and extend the line past the outer canthi of the eyes. The medial and lateral canthi are usually horizontal. When the outer canthi are above the line, an upward, or mongolian, slant is present. When the outer canthi are below the line, a downward, or antimongolian, slant is present (Fig. 11-32).

Inspect the level of the eyelid covering the eye. To detect the sunsetting sign, rapidly lower the infant from upright to supine position. Look for sclera above the iris (see Fig. 5-25). This sign may be an expected variant in newborns; however, it also may be observed in infants with hydrocephalus and brainstem lesions.

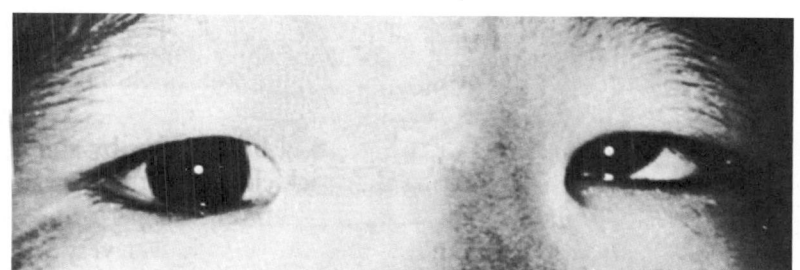

FIGURE 11-31
Epicanthal folds.
From Stein, Slatt, Stein, 1994.

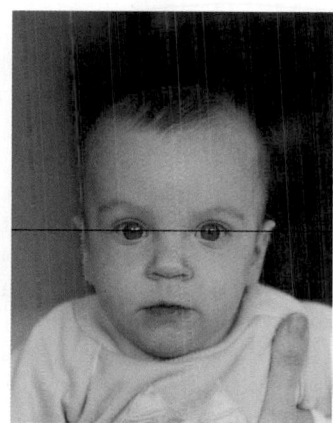

FIGURE 11-32
Drawing a line between the two medial canthi and extending it temporally to determine whether a Mongolian or anti-Mongolian slant is present.
Courtesy Matthew Watson.

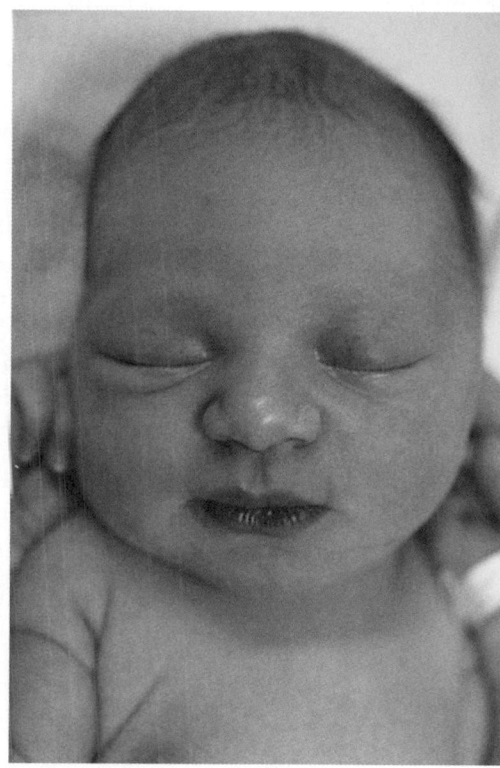

FIGURE 11-33
Swollen eyelids in a newborn.

Observe the distance between the eyes, looking for a wide spacing, or hypertelorism, which may be associated with craniofacial defects including some with mental retardation. Pseudostrabismus, the false appearance of strabismus caused by a flattened nasal bridge or epicanthal fold, is an expected variant in Asian and Native American/American Indian infants, as well as in some whites. Pseudostrabismus generally disappears by about 1 year of age. Use the corneal light reflex to distinguish pseudostrabismus from strabismus. An asymmetric light reflex may indicate a real strabismus or hypertelorism.

Inspect the sclera, conjunctiva, pupil, and iris of each eye. Inspect and compare corneal sizes. Enlarged corneas may be a sign of congenital glaucoma. The newborn's eyelids may be swollen or edematous from birth trauma (Fig. 11-33), but if accompanied by conjunctival inflammation and drainage, may represent ophthalmia neonatorum. Any redness, hemorrhages, discharge, or granular appearance beyond the newborn period may indicate infection, allergy, or trauma. Inspect each iris and pupil for any irregularity in shape. A coloboma, or keyhole pupil, is often associated with other congenital anomalies. White specks scattered in a linear pattern around the entire circumference of the iris, called *Brushfield spots*, strongly suggest Down syndrome or mental retardation.

Test the cranial nerves II, III, IV, and VI in the following manner:

♦ Vision is grossly examined by observing the infant's preference for looking at certain objects. Expect the infant to focus on and track a light or face through 60 degrees.

♦ Elicit the optical blink reflex by shining a bright light at the infant's eyes, noting the quick closure of the eyes and dorsiflexion of the head.

♦ The corneal reflex is performed as in adults.

A funduscopic examination is difficult to conduct on a newborn or young infant and is generally deferred until the infant is 2 to 6 months of age unless, as with the visual problems of prematurity, there is a compelling need. Dilation of the eyes for effective visualization of the fundi can be safely achieved in the nursery by using weak solutions of mydriatics. If an infant's irides are blue, very little of a weak solution is necessary; one drop in each eye is generally enough. With darker-colored eyes, a second drop a few seconds later is indicated. Cyclopentolate hydrochloride 0.5% is a popular mydriatic.

The red reflex should be elicited bilaterally in every newborn. Dilate the pupils if necessary. Observe for any opacities, dark spots, or white spots within the circle of red glow. Opacities or interruption of the red reflex may indicate congenital cataracts or retinoblastoma or other serious intraocular pathology (Table 11-3).

CHILDREN

Perform the inspection of the young child's external eye structures as described for the infant.

Visual acuity is tested (when the child is cooperative) with the Snellen E game, usually at about 3 years of age (see Fig. 3-16, *B*). Have one examiner point to the line on the chart and another assist the child with covering one eye. As with adults, have the child stand 20 feet (6 m) away. Allow the child to practice following the instructions before you administer the test. Instruct the child to point his or her arm or finger in the direction of the legs of the E. If the child has difficulty following these directions, a card with a large E on it can be given to the child with instructions to turn the E to match the letter indicated on the chart. Test each eye separately. If the child wears glasses, vision should be tested both with and without corrective lenses and recorded separately.

Examine visual acuity of younger children by observing their activities. Provide an opportunity for the child to play with toys in the examining room. Watch the child stacking, building, or placing objects inside of others. Children should have no visual difficulties in one eye

---

TABLE 11-3	Pediatric Eye Evaluation Screening Recommendations for Clinicians	
Recommended Age for Screening	**Screening Method**	**Criteria for Referral to an Ophthalmologist**
Newborn to 3 months	Red reflex[a] Inspection for constant strabismus	Abnormal or asymmetric Structural abnormality
6 months to 1 year	Fix and follow with each eye Alternate occlusion Corneal light reflex Red reflex[a] Inspection for strabismus	Failure to fix and follow in cooperative infant Failure to object equally to the covering of each eye Asymmetric Abnormal or asymmetric Structural abnormality
3 years (approximately)	Visual acuity[b] Corneal light reflex/cover-uncover Stereoacuity[c] Inspection	20/50 or worse, or 2 lines of difference between the eyes Asymmetric/ocular refixation movements Failure to appreciate asymmetric random dot or Titmus Stereogram Structural abnormality
Older than 5 years	Visual acuity[b] Corneal light reflex/cover-uncover Stereoacuity[c] Red reflex[a] Inspection	20/30 or worse, or 2 lines of difference between the eyes Asymmetric/ocular refixation movements Failure to appreciate stereopsis Abnormal or asymmetric Structural abnormality

NOTE: These recommendations are based on expert opinion.

Copyright American Academy of Ophthalmology: Preferred Practice Pattern: Pediatric Eye Evaluations, 2003.
[a]Physician or nurse responsibility.
[b]Figures, letters, "tumbling E," or optotypes.
[c]Optional: Random Dot E Game (RDE), Titmus Stereograms (Titmus Optical, Inc, Petersburg, VA), Randot Stereograms (Stereo Optical Company, Inc, Chicago, IL).

if these tasks are performed well. The anticipated visual acuity of young children is as follows (Sprague, 1983):

Age	Visual Acuity	Age	Visual Acuity
3 years	20/50 or better	5 years	20/30 or better
4 years	20/40 or better	6 years	20/20

When you are testing visual acuity in the child, any difference in the scores between the eyes should be noted. A two-line difference (e.g., 20/50 and 20/30) may indicate amblyopia.

Examination of extraocular movements and cranial nerves III, IV, and VI is performed as with adults. You may, however, need to hold the child's head still and use an appealing object such as a teddy bear for the child to follow through the six cardinal fields of gaze. Peripheral vision can be tested in cooperative children; the young child may prefer to sit on the parent's lap while these tests are performed.

Patience is often needed to gain the child's cooperation for the funduscopic examination. The young child is often unable to keep the eyes still and focused on a distant object. Position the young child supine on the examining table, with the head near one end. Stand at the end of the table and use your right eye to examine the child's left eye and vice versa. Do not hold the child's eyelids open forcibly because that will only lead to some resistance. Remember all retinal findings will appear upside down. Rather than move the ophthalmoscope to visualize all retinal fields, inspect the optic disc, the fovea, and the vessels as they pass by. Often the results are better when the child sits on the parent's lap. If this position is used, examine the child as you would an adult.

PREGNANT WOMEN

Retinal examination in the pregnant woman can help differentiate between chronic hypertension and PIH. Vascular tortuosity, angiosclerosis, hemorrhage, and exudates may be seen in patients with a long-standing history of hypertension. In the patient with PIH, however, there is segmental arteriolar narrowing with a wet, glistening appearance indicative of edema. This finding is not exclusive to pregnant women. Hemorrhages and exudates are rare. Detachment of the retina may occur with spontaneous reattachment after hypertension is successfully controlled.

Because of systemic absorption, cycloplegic and mydriatic agents should be avoided unless there is a need to evaluate for retinal disease. Use of nasolacrimal occlusion after instillation of topical eye medications may reduce systemic absorption.

SAMPLE DOCUMENTATION

EYES

Subjective
A 37-year-old man complains of sudden loss of vision in his right eye, no pain. Has had diabetes mellitus since age 12. Received laser therapy 2 years ago for retinopathy.
Objective
Visual acuity 20/40 left eye, by Snellen measurement; right eye, sees light only. Visual field is full by confrontation, left eye. Extraocular movements intact and full; no nystagmus. Lids and globes are symmetric. No ptosis. Eyebrows full; no edema or lesions evident. Conjunctivae pink. Sclerae white. No discharge. Cornea clear; corneal reflex intact bilaterally. Irides blue. Pupils equal and round. Both pupils constrict to light directly and consensually. Ophthalmologic examination reveals a red reflex, left eye. The left disc is well defined and cream colored. No venous pulsations evident at the disc. Arteriole-venule ratio is 3:5; no nicking or crossing changes seen. Multiple blackened laser scars in the periphery circumferentially. Dot hemorrhages and hard exudates also noted. Macula yellow and free of lesions. No red reflex or retina can be seen, right eye.

For additional sample documentation, see Chapter 26.

SUMMARY OF EXAMINATION

EYES

1. Measure visual acuity, noting the following (p. 287):
   - Near vision
   - Distant vision
   - Peripheral vision
2. Inspect the eyebrows for the following (p. 288):
   - Hair texture
   - Size
   - Extension
3. Inspect the orbital area for the following (p. 288):
   - Edema
   - Sagging tissues or puffiness
   - Lesions
4. Inspect the eyelids for the following (pp. 288 and 289):
   - Ability to open wide and close completely
   - Eyelash position
   - Ptosis
   - Fasciculations or tremors
   - Flakiness
   - Redness
   - Swelling
5. Palpate the eyelids for nodules.
6. Palpate the eye for firmness.
7. Inspect the orbits.
8. Pull down the lower lids and inspect the conjunctivae and sclerae for the following (p. 290):
   - Color
   - Discharge
   - Lacrimal gland punctum
   - Pterygium
9. Inspect the external eyes for the following (p. 291):
   - Corneal clarity
   - Corneal sensitivity
   - Corneal arcus
   - Color of irides
   - Pupillary size and shape
   - Pupillary response to light and accommodation, afferent pupillary defect, swinging flashlight test
   - Depth of anterior chamber
10. Palpate the lacrimal gland in the superior temporal orbital rim (p. 292).
11. Evaluate muscle balance and movement of eyes with the following (p. 293):
    - Corneal light reflex
    - Cover-uncover test
    - Six cardinal fields of gaze
    - Nystagmus
12. Ophthalmoscopic examination (p. 294):
    - Lens clarity
    - Red reflex
    - Retinal color and lesions
    - Characteristics of blood vessels
    - Disc characteristics
    - Macula characteristics

COMMON ABNORMALITIES

EXTERNAL EYE

EXOPHTHALMOS

Exophthalmos is an increase in the volume of the orbital content, causing a protrusion of the globes forward (Fig. 11-34). It may be bilateral or unilateral. The most common cause is Graves' disease, but when the exophthalmos is unilateral, a retro-orbital tumor must be considered, even though thyroid eye disease is the most common cause of unilateral proptosis as well. Retraction of the upper lid and exposure of the sclera above the iris may exaggerate the appearance of exophthalmos.

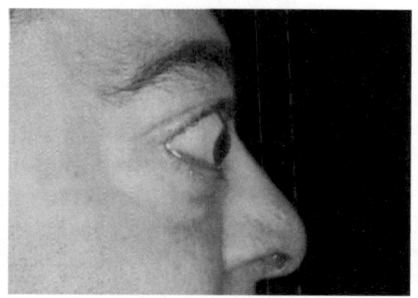

FIGURE 11-34
Thyroid exophthalmos.
From Stein, Slatt, Stein, 1994.

EPISCLERITIS

Episcleritis is an inflammation of the superficial layers of the sclera anterior to the insertion of the rectus muscles (Fig. 11-35). It is generally localized, with a purplish elevation of a few millimeters. Often the cause of the inflammation is unknown, but it is a common manifestation of Crohn's disease, rheumatoid arthritis, and other autoimmune disorders.

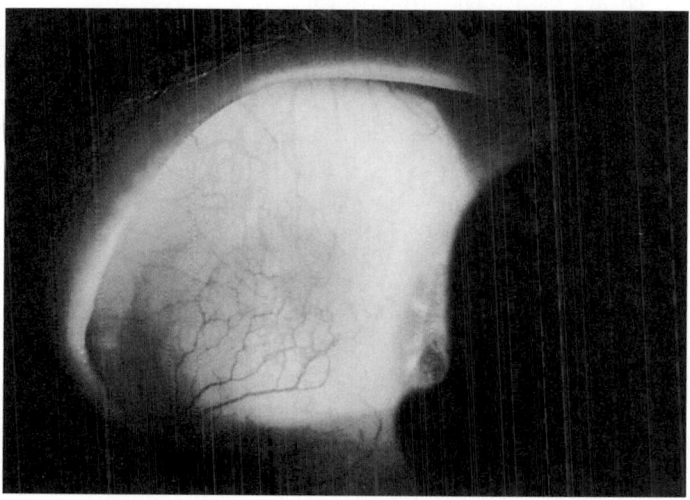

FIGURE 11-35
Episcleritis.
Courtesy Andrew P. Schachat, MD, The Wilmer Ophthalmological Institute, The Johns Hopkins University and Hospital, Baltimore.

BAND KERATOPATHY

Band keratopathy is produced by the deposition of calcium in the superficial cornea (Fig. 11-36). It appears as horizontal grayish bands interspersed with dark areas that look like holes. Band keratopathy appears as a line where the eyelids close just below the pupil; it passes over the cornea rather than around the iris as arcus senilis does. This finding is most commonly seen in patients with chronic corneal disease but may occur in patients with hyperparathyroidism and occasionally in individuals with renal failure or syphilis.

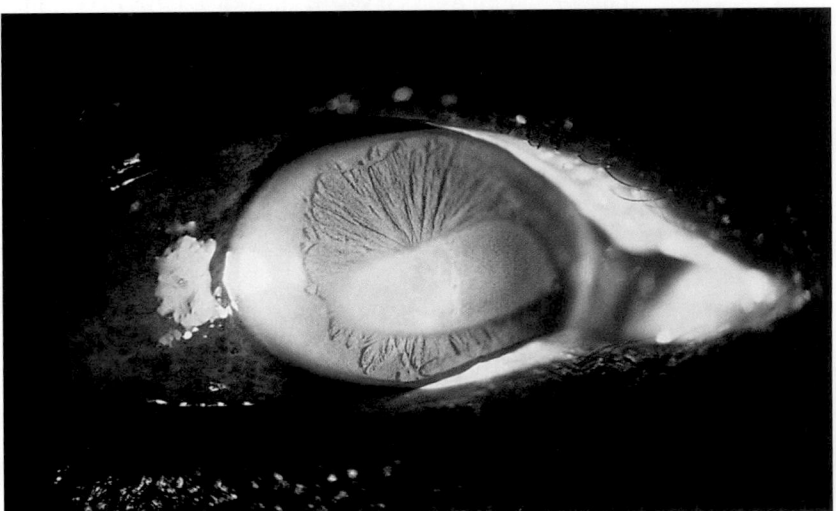

FIGURE 11-36
Band keratopathy.
Courtesy John W. Payne, MD, The Wilmer Ophthalmological Institute, The Johns Hopkins University and Hospital, Baltimore.

CORNEAL ULCER

Corneal ulcers are a disruption of the corneal epithelium and stroma caused by viral or bacterial infection, or by desiccation because of incomplete lid closure or poor lacrimal gland function. Wearing contact lenses increases the risk of developing bacterial ulceration in the otherwise healthy eye. Fig. 11-37 shows an ulcer in the lower temporal quadrant of the left cornea stained with rose Bengal.

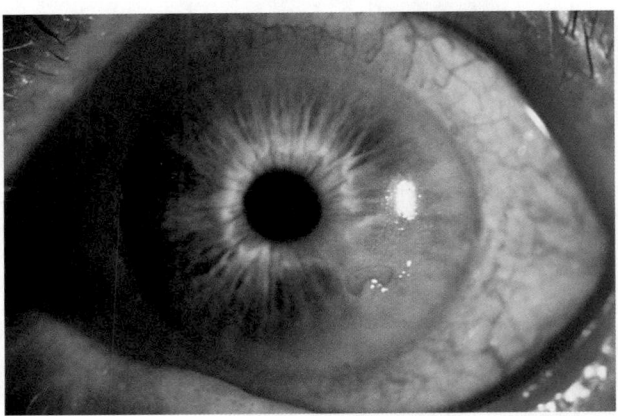

FIGURE 11-37
Corneal ulcer.
Courtesy John W. Payne, MD, The Wilmer Ophthalmological Institute, The Johns Hopkins University and Hospital, Baltimore.

EXTRAOCULAR MUSCLES

STRABISMUS (PARALYTIC AND NONPARALYTIC)

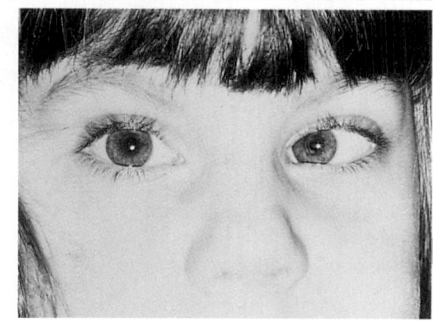

FIGURE 11-38
Right convergent strabismus.
From Stein, Slatt, Stein, 1994.

Strabismus is a condition in which both eyes do not focus on an object simultaneously. The condition may be paralytic, caused by impairment of one or more extraocular muscles or their nerve supply. If a nerve supplying an extraocular muscle has become impaired or if the muscle itself has become weakened, the eye will fail to move in the direction controlled by that muscle. For example, if the right sixth nerve is damaged, the right eye does not move temporally.

Nonparalytic strabismus has no primary muscle weakness. The patient can focus with either eye but not with both simultaneously (Fig. 11-38). It is detected by having the patient observe a near object. When one eye is covered, the other one will move to focus on the object if the covered eye was the dominant one (see Fig. 11-21). Nonparalytic strabismus can be the presenting sign of intraocular pathology producing poor vision such as an infantile cataract or a retinoblastoma.

INTERNAL EYE

Bilateral and unilateral pupil abnormalities are listed in Table 11-4.

TABLE 11-4	**Descriptions of Various Pupil Abnormalities**	
Abnormality	**Contributing Factors**	**Appearance**
BILATERAL		
Miosis (pupillary constriction; usually less than 2 mm in diameter)	Iridocyclitis; miotic eye drops (e.g., pilocarpine given for glaucoma); drug abuse	
Mydriasis (pupillary dilation; usually more than 6 mm in diameter)	Iridocyclitis; mydriatic or cycloplegic drops (e.g., atropine); midbrain (reflex arc) lesions or hypoxia; oculomotor (CN III) damage; acute angle glaucoma (slight dilation); drug abuse	
Failure to respond (constrict) with increased light stimulus	Iridocyclitis; retinal degeneration; optic nerve (CN II) destruction; midbrain synapses involving afferent pupillary fibers or oculomotor nerve (CN III) (consensual response is also lost); impairment of efferent fibers (parasympathetic) that innervate sphincter pupillae muscle, mydriatics	
Argyll Robertson pupil	Bilateral, miotic, irregularly shaped pupils that fail to constrict with light but retain constriction with convergence; pupils may or may not be equal in size; commonly caused by neurosyphilis or lesions in midbrain where afferent pupillary fibers synapse	

Modified from Thompson et al, 1997.

Continued

EYES
Common Abnormalities

TABLE 11-4	Descriptions of Various Pupil Abnormalities—cont'd	
Abnormality	**Contributing Factors**	**Appearance**
UNILATERAL Anisocoria (unequal size of pupils)	Congenital (approximately 20% of healthy people have minor or noticeable differences in pupil size, but reflexes are normal) or caused by local eye medications (constrictors or dilators), or unilateral sympathetic or parasympathetic pupillary pathway destruction (**Note:** Examiner should test whether pupils react equally to light; if response is unequal, examiner should note whether larger or smaller eye reacts more slowly [or not at all], because either pupil could represent the abnormal size.)	
Iritis constrictive response	Acute uveitis is commonly unilateral; constriction of pupil accompanied by pain and circumcorneal flush (redness)	Healthy eye Affected eye
Oculomotor nerve (CN III) damage	Pupil dilated and fixed; eye deviated laterally and downward; ptosis	Healthy eye Affected eye
Adie pupil (tonic pupil)	Affected pupil dilated and reacts slowly or fails to react to light; responds to convergence; caused by impairment of postganglionic parasympathetic innervation to sphincter pupillae muscle or ciliary malfunction; often accompanied by diminished tendon reflexes (as with diabetic neuropathy or alcoholism)	Healthy eye Affected eye

Modified from Thompson et al, 1997.

HORNER SYNDROME

Horner syndrome is caused by the interruption of the sympathetic nerve supply to the eye and results in ipsilateral miosis and mild ptosis. Because the ptosis is subtle it may be best appreciated by noting that the amount of iris seen superiorly in the opposite eye is greater. It is often caused by interruption of the cervical sympathetic trunk due to mediastinal tumors, bronchogenic carcinoma, metastatic tumors, or operative trauma. Congenital Horner syndrome has also been described (Fig. 11-39).

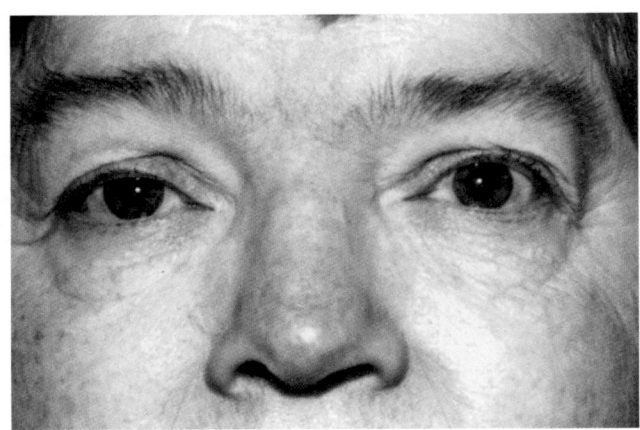

FIGURE 11-39
Horner syndrome (right eye).
Courtesy Shannath Merbs, MD, PhD, The Wilmer Ophthalmological Institute, The Johns Hopkins University and Hospital, Baltimore.

CATARACTS

The only common abnormality of the lens is cataract formation. A cataract is an opacity occurring in the lens, most commonly from denaturation of lens protein caused by aging. Almost everyone older than 65 years of age has some evidence of lens opacification. With aging, the lesion is generally central, but peripheral cataracts are common and may occur in conditions such as hypoparathyroidism. Chronic steroid use can cause significant visual disability from cataracts. Congenital cataracts can result from a number of genetic defects, maternal rubella, or other fetal insults during the first trimester of pregnancy (Fig. 11-40).

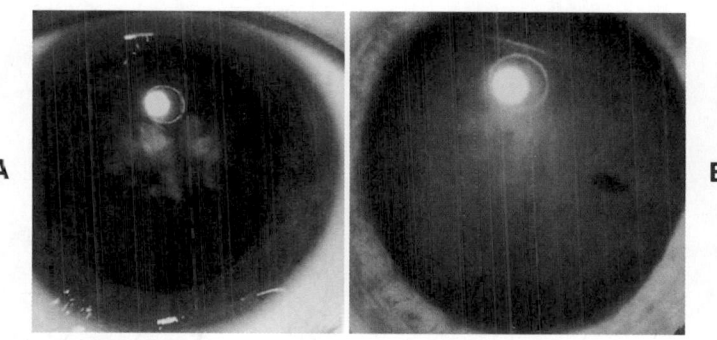

FIGURE 11-40
A, Snowflake cataract of diabetes. **B,** Senile cataract.
From Donaldson, 1976.

OPTIC ATROPHY

Optic atrophy is the result of the death of nerve fibers and myelin sheaths. The primary symptom of optic atrophy is loss of central or peripheral vision or both. The disc or a portion of it loses its yellowish-pink hue and becomes stark white. It is often helpful to compare the disc color in each eye when assessing for optic atrophy (Fig. 11-41). Cataract surgery in one eye can make the disc look somewhat paler than the non-operated eye.

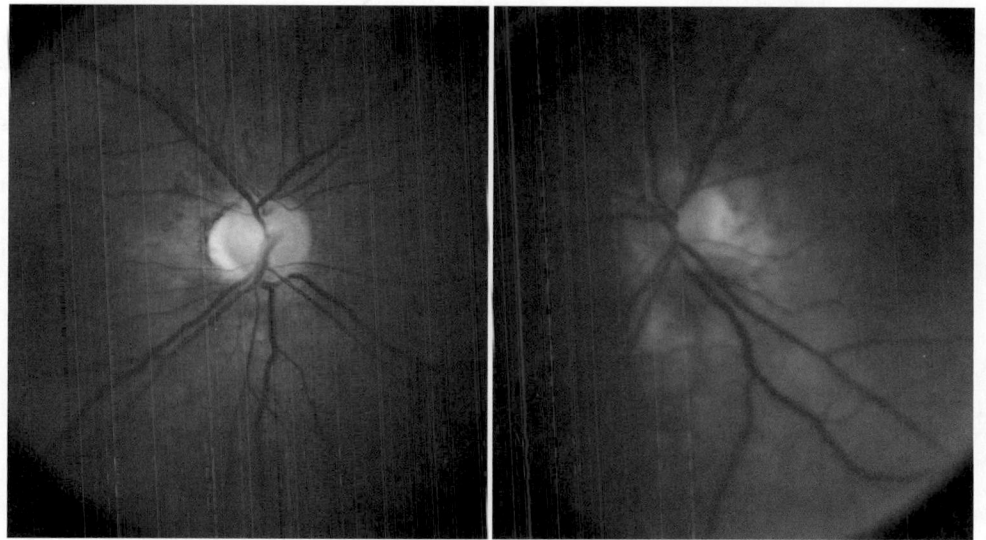

FIGURE 11-41
Optic atrophy. **A,** Patient's right eye shows atrophy. **B,** Left eye is unaffected.
Courtesy John W. Payne, MD, The Wilmer Ophthalmological Institute, The Johns Hopkins University and Hospital, Baltimore.

DIABETIC RETINOPATHY (BACKGROUND)

Diabetic retinopathy is generally divided into background and proliferative retinopathy. Background retinopathy is marked by dot hemorrhages or microaneurysms and the presence of hard and soft exudates. Hard exudates are the result of lipid transudation through incompetent capillaries; these have sharply defined borders and tend to be bright yellow. They are generally superficial in the retina and are clustered around retinal vessels. Soft exudates are caused by infarction of the nerve layer and appear as dull gray spots with poorly defined margins (Fig. 11-42).

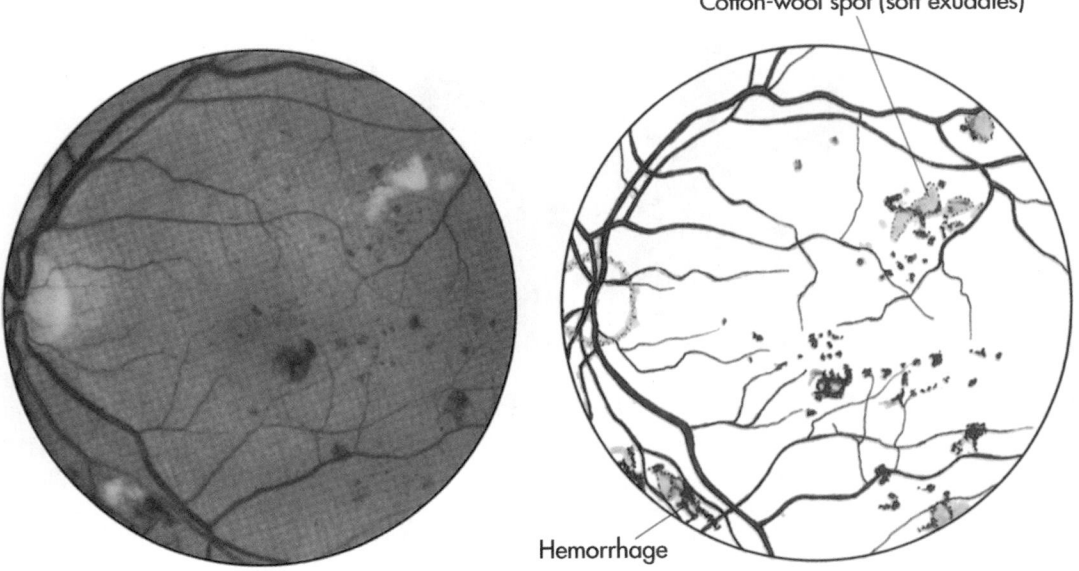

Cotton-wool spot (soft exudates)

Hemorrhage

FIGURE 11-42
Background diabetic retinopathy. Note flame-shaped and dot-blot hemorrhages, cotton-wool spots, and microaneurysms.
From Yannuzzi, Guyer, Green, 1995; courtesy of Drs. George Blankenship and Everett Ai and the Diabetes 2000 Program, St Louis.

DIABETIC RETINOPATHY (PROLIFERATIVE)

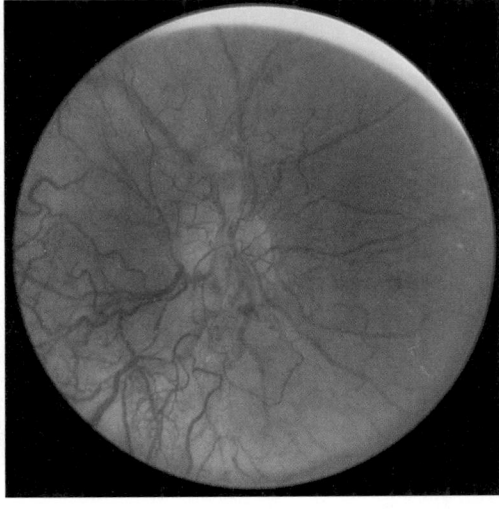

FIGURE 11-43
Proliferative diabetic retinopathy.
Courtesy John W. Payne, MD, The Wilmer Ophthalmological Institute, The Johns Hopkins University and Hospital, Baltimore.

Proliferative retinopathy is the development of new vessels as the result of anoxic stimulation (Fig. 11-43). It may occur in the peripheral retina or on the optic nerve itself. The new vessels lack the supporting structure of healthy vessels and are likely to hemorrhage. These vessels grow out of the retina toward the vitreous humor, and visualization may require change in the lens setting of the ophthalmoscope. Bleeding from these vessels is a major cause of blindness in patients with diabetes. Similar lesions may be seen in the infant born prematurely who has retinopathy of prematurity associated with oxygen therapy, but these are hard to see with the direct ophthalmoscope because they are in the far periphery. Laser therapy for diabetic retinopathy can often control this neovascularization and prevent blindness from occurring. Laser therapy in the premature infant is the current standard of care.

LIPEMIA RETINALIS

Lipemia retinalis is a dramatic condition that occurs when the serum triglyceride level exceeds 2000 mg/dL (Fig. 11-44). The blood vessels become progressively pink and then white as the triglyceride level rises. This condition may be seen in diabetic ketoacidosis and in some of the hyperlipidemic states.

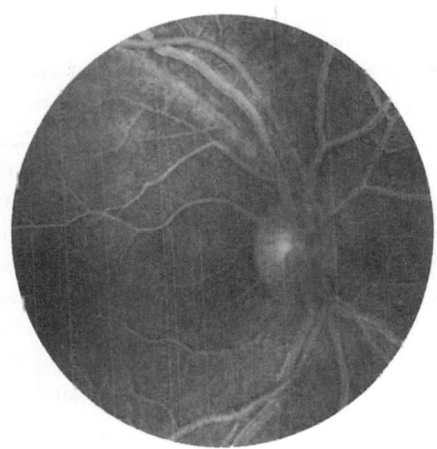

FIGURE 11-44
Lipemia retinalis.
From Newell, 1996.

RETINITIS PIGMENTOSA

Retinitis pigmentosa is an autosomal recessive condition characterized by the development of night blindness and loss of peripheral vision. Optic atrophy "waxy pallor" narrowing of the arterioles, and peripheral "bone spicule" pigmentation are hallmarks of the disease (Fig. 11-45).

A

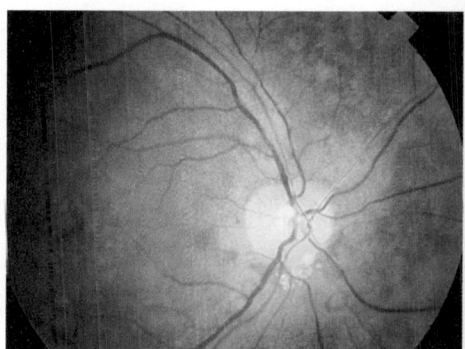

FIGURE 11-45
Retinitis pigmentosa. **A,** Optic atrophy and narrowing of the arterioles. **B,** Classic "bone spicule" pigmentation in the retinal periphery.
Courtesy John W. Payne, MD, The Wilmer Ophthalmological Institute, The Johns Hopkins University and Hospital, Baltimore.

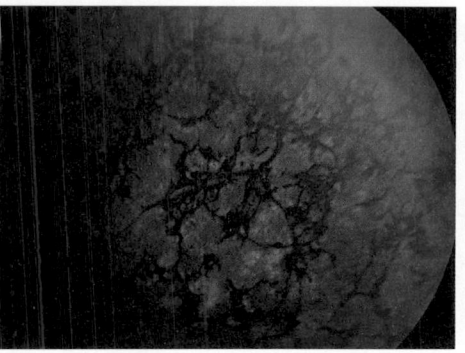

B

CYTOMEGALOVIRUS INFECTION

Cytomegalovirus (CMV) infection is a common cause of blindness in immune compromised individuals such as those with HIV. It is characterized by hemorrhage, exudates, and necrosis of the retina following the vascular pattern. CMV infection is said to create a "pizza pie" appearance in the retina (Fig. 11-46).

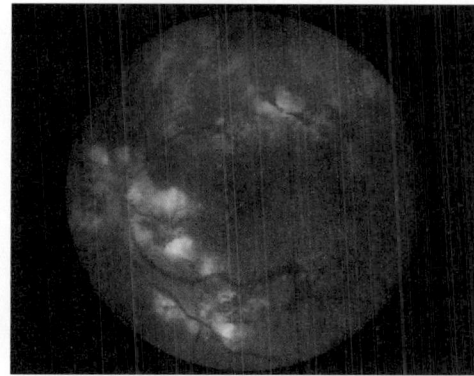

FIGURE 11-46
Cytomegalovirus retinitis.
Courtesy Douglas A. Jabs, MD, The Wilmer Ophthalmological Institute, The Johns Hopkins University and Hospital, Baltimore.

GLAUCOMA

Glaucoma is disease of the optic nerve wherein the nerve cells die, producing a characteristic appearance of the optic nerve (increased cupping). It may occur acutely with dramatically elevated intraocular pressure if the iris blocks the exit of aqueous humor from the anterior chamber. Acute glaucoma is accompanied by intense ocular pain, blurred vision, halos around lights, a red eye, and a dilated pupil. Occasionally patients complain of stomach pain, nausea, and vomiting. In chronic glaucoma, which is more common, symptoms are absent except for gradual loss of peripheral vision over a period of years (see Fig. 11-28). As many as half of the population with glaucoma is not aware of their condition.

CHORIORETINAL INFLAMMATION

Chorioretinal inflammation (Fig. 11-47) is an inflammatory process that involves both the choroid and the retina. It results in a sharply defined lesion that is generally whitish yellow and becomes stippled with dark pigment in later stages ending with a chorioretinal scar. The most common cause of these lesions today is laser therapy for diabetic retinopathy, but it may also be seen as a consequence of infectious agents such as histoplasmosis, cytomegalovirus or toxoplasmosis during fetal life. A visual field defect can be detected in individuals with a large lesion. A chorioretinal scar appears similar to the whitish pigment seen when myelin sheath persists. Myelin sheath persistence, however, causes no visual field defect (see Fig. 11-26).

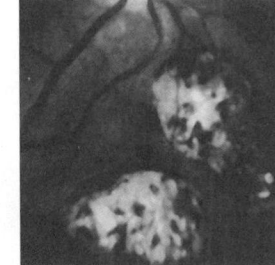

FIGURE 11-47
Patches of chorioretinitis adjacent to the optic disc.
From Stein, Slatt, Stein, 1994.

CHOROIDAL NEVUS

Choroidal nevi are pigmented lesions of the choroid (Fig. 11-48). They appear as darkened, well-defined areas of varying size beneath the retina. They should be carefully observed to detect any enlargement or elevation that would suggest malignant change (e.g., melanoma).

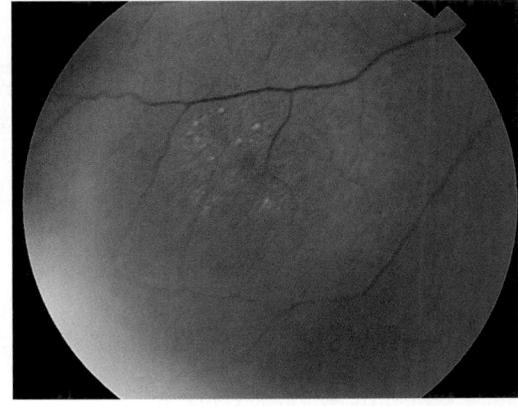

FIGURE 11-48
Choroidal nevus.
Courtesy John W. Payne, MD, The Wilmer Ophthalmological Institute, The Johns Hopkins University and Hospital, Baltimore.

VISUAL FIELDS

VISUAL FIELD DEFECTS

Defective vision or blindness in a single eye may be a consequence of degenerative changes within the eye itself (e.g., cataract) or it may stem from a lesion of the optic nerve anterior to its decussation. The most common cause is interruption of the vascular supply to the optic nerve (Fig. 11-49, *1,* and Fig. 11-50, *A*).

Bitemporal hemianopia (Fig. 11-49, *2,* and Fig. 11-50, *B*) is caused by a lesion—most commonly a pituitary tumor—interrupting the optic chiasm. Homonymous hemianopia can be caused by a lesion arising in the optic nerve radiation on either side of the brain. These lesions occur after the optic chiasm and therefore involve nerve fibers arising from the same side of each eye and are caused by the interruption of the nerve fibers as they progress to the optic cortex (Fig. 11-49, *3,* and Fig. 11-50, *C*).

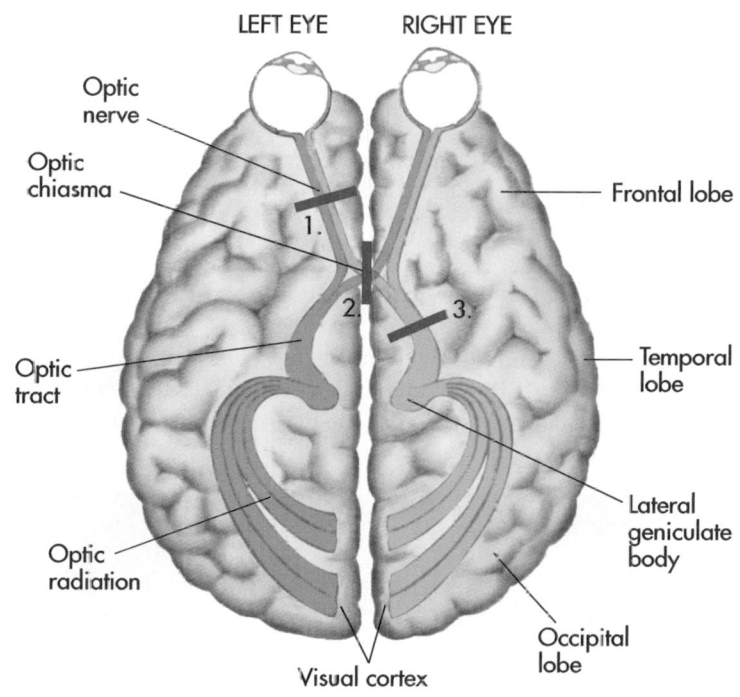

FIGURE 11-49
Site of lesions causing visual loss. *1,* Total blindness left eye. *2,* Bitemporal hemianopia. *3,* Left homonymous hemianopia.

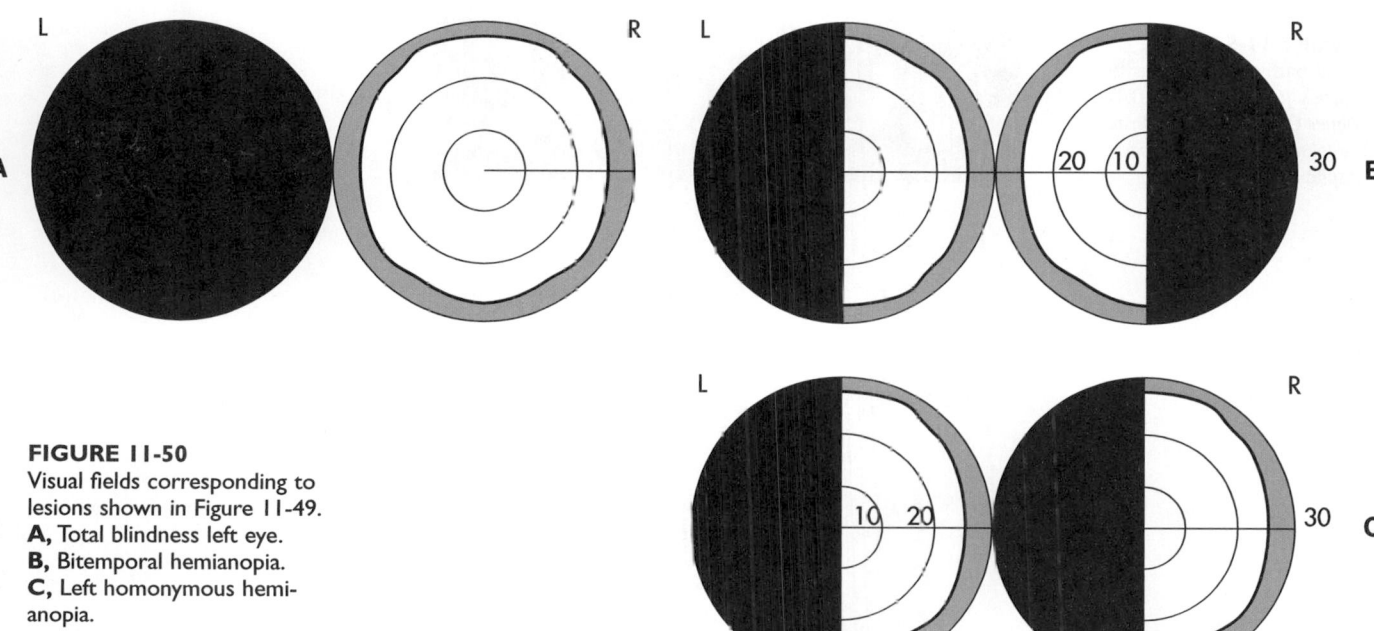

FIGURE 11-50
Visual fields corresponding to lesions shown in Figure 11-49.
A, Total blindness left eye.
B, Bitemporal hemianopia.
C, Left homonymous hemianopia.
Modified from Stein, Slatt, Stein, 1994.

CHILDREN

RETINOBLASTOMA

Retinoblastoma is an embryonal malignant tumor arising from the retina, often during the first 2 years of life. The retinoblastoma may be transmitted either by an autosomal dominant trait or by a chromosomal mutation. Initial signs are a white reflex (also called a cat's eye reflex) rather than the usual red reflex. Funduscopic examination reveals an ill-defined mass arising from the retina. Often chalky-white areas of calcification can be seen (Fig. 11-51).

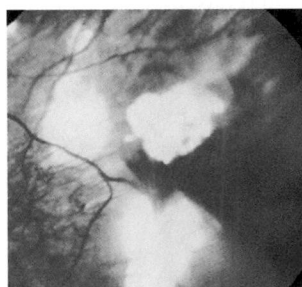

FIGURE 11-51
Retinoblastoma, the most common retinal tumor in children.
From Stein, Slatt, Stein 1994.

RETINOPATHY OF PREMATURITY (RETROLENTAL FIBROPLASIA)

Fig. 11-52 shows the changes found in the posterior pole of the left eye in the cicatricial (late) stage of the disease. Note that the blood vessels are straightened and diverted temporally. There is temporal traction on the retina in the posterior pole. Cicatricial changes may be much more severe and lead to retinal detachment, glaucoma, and blindness. Peripheral changes are seen only with the indirect ophthalmoscope.

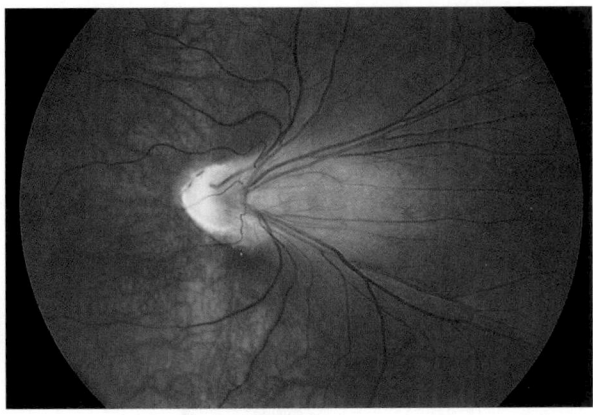

FIGURE 11-52
Retinopathy of prematurity.
Courtesy John W. Payne, MD, The Wilmer Ophthalmological Institute, The Johns Hopkins University and Hospital, Baltimore.

RETINAL HEMORRHAGES IN INFANCY

Fig. 11-53 shows multiple hemorrhages in the optic fundus of an infant who was a victim of the shaken-baby syndrome. Whenever retinal hemorrhages are seen, one must suspect infant abuse and investigate carefully.

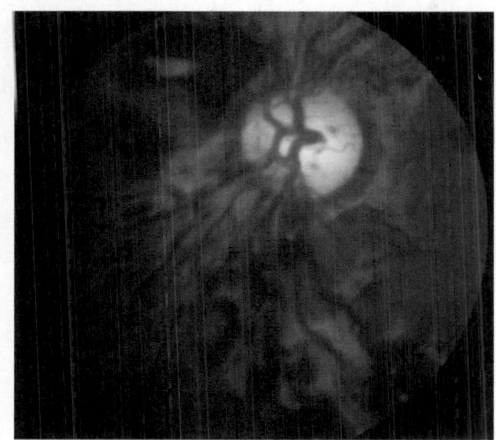

FIGURE 11-53
Multiple retinal hemorrhages are seen on funduscopic examination of this infant who was a victim of the shaken-baby syndrome.
Courtesy Daniel Garibaldi, MD, The Wilmer Ophthalmological Institute, The Johns Hopkins University and Hospital, Baltimore.

ELECTRONIC RESOURCES

For Weblinks and additional resources, go to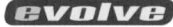

http://evolve.elsevier.com/Seidel

or to the Companion CD-ROM.

Additional information related to the content in Chapter 11 can be found on the companion website at evolve.elsevier.com/Seidel/ or on the interactive companion CD-ROM. Resources and activities for Chapter 11 include:
- Sound and Vision Theater
- Printouts for Your Practice
- Interactive Challenge
- Spanish Assessment Terms with Pronunciation Guide
- Instant Calculator

EARS, NOSE, AND THROAT

Much information about the function of the respiratory and digestive tracts can be gleaned from their accessible orifices—the ears, nose, mouth, and throat. The special senses of smell, hearing, equilibrium, and taste are also located in the ears, nose, and mouth.

ANATOMY AND PHYSIOLOGY

EARS AND HEARING

The ear is a sensory organ that functions in the identification, localization, and interpretation of sound, as well as in the maintenance of equilibrium. Anatomically, it is divided into the external, middle, and inner ear (Figs. 12-1 and 12-2).

The external ear, including the auricle (or pinna) and external auditory canal, is composed of cartilage covered with skin. The auricle, extending slightly outward from the skull, is positioned on a nearly vertical plane. Note its structural landmarks in Fig. 12-3.

The external auditory canal, an S-shaped pathway leading to the middle ear, is approximately 2.5 cm long in adults. Its skeleton of bone and cartilage is covered with very thin, sensitive skin. This canal lining is protected and lubricated with cerumen, secreted by the sebaceous glands in the distal third of the canal.

The middle ear is an air-filled cavity in the temporal bone. It contains the ossicles, three small connected bones (malleus, incus, and stapes) that transmit sound from the tympanic membrane to the oval window of the inner ear. The air-filled cells of the mastoid area of the temporal bone are continuous with the middle ear. The tympanic membrane, surrounded by a dense fibrous ring (annulus), separates the external ear from the middle ear. It is concave, being pulled in at the center (umbo) by the malleus. The tympanic membrane is translucent, permitting visualization of the middle ear cavity, including the malleus. Its oblique position to the auditory canal and conical shape account for the triangular light reflex. Most of the tympanic membrane is tense (the pars tensa), but the superior portion (pars flaccida) is more flaccid (Fig. 12-4).

The middle ear mucosa produces a small amount of mucus that is rapidly cleared by the ciliary action of the eustachian tube, a cartilaginous and bony passageway between the nasopharynx and the middle ear. This passage opens briefly to equalize the middle ear pressure with that of atmospheric pressure when swallowing, yawning, or sneezing. The equalized pressure in the middle ear permits the tympanic membrane to vibrate freely.

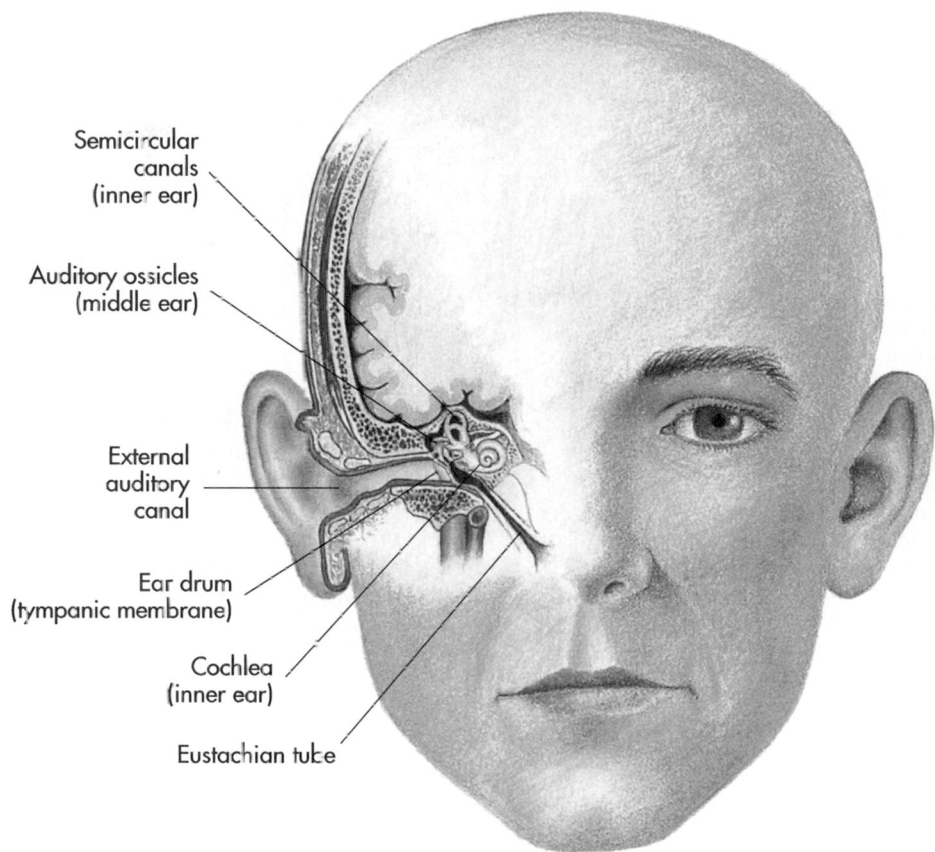

FIGURE 12-1
Cross section of the external, middle, and inner ear in relation to other structures of the head and face.

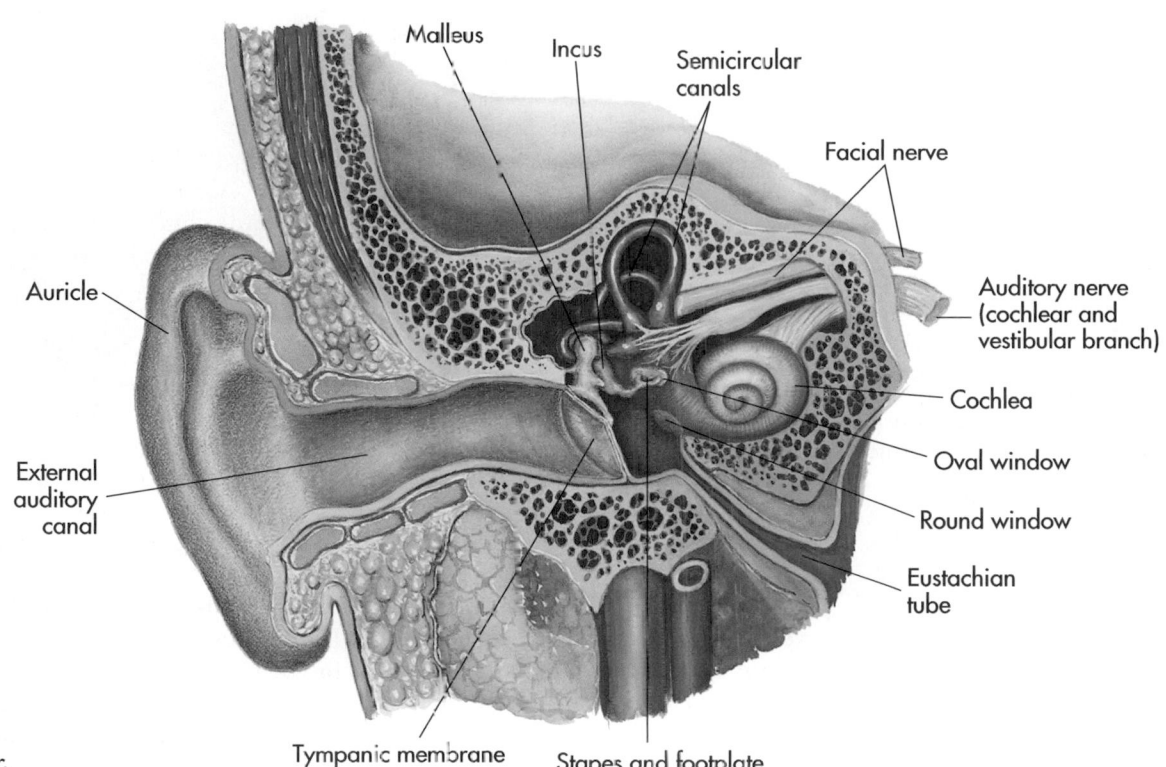

FIGURE 12-2
Anatomy of the ear.

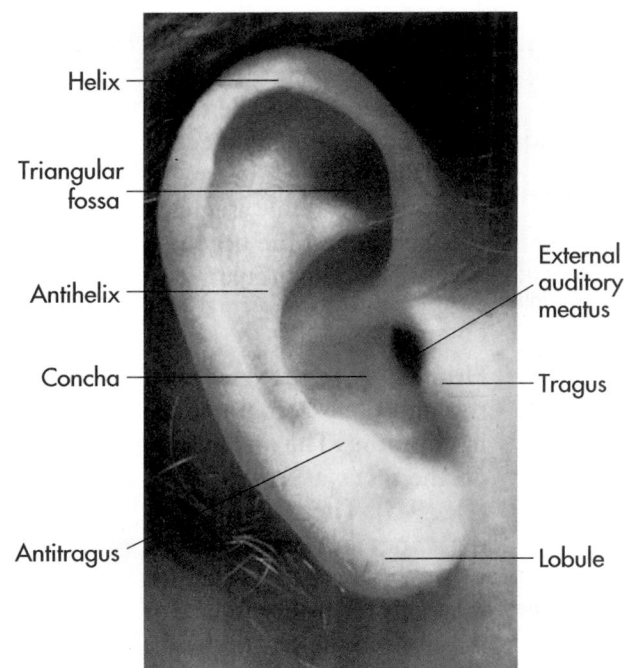

FIGURE 12-3
Anatomic structures of the auricle. The helix is the prominent outer rim, whereas the antihelix is the area parallel and anterior to the helix. The concha is the deep cavity containing the auditory canal meatus. The tragus is the protuberance lying anterior to the auditory canal meatus, and the antitragus is the protuberance on the antihelix opposite the tragus. The lobule is the soft lobe on the bottom of the auricle.

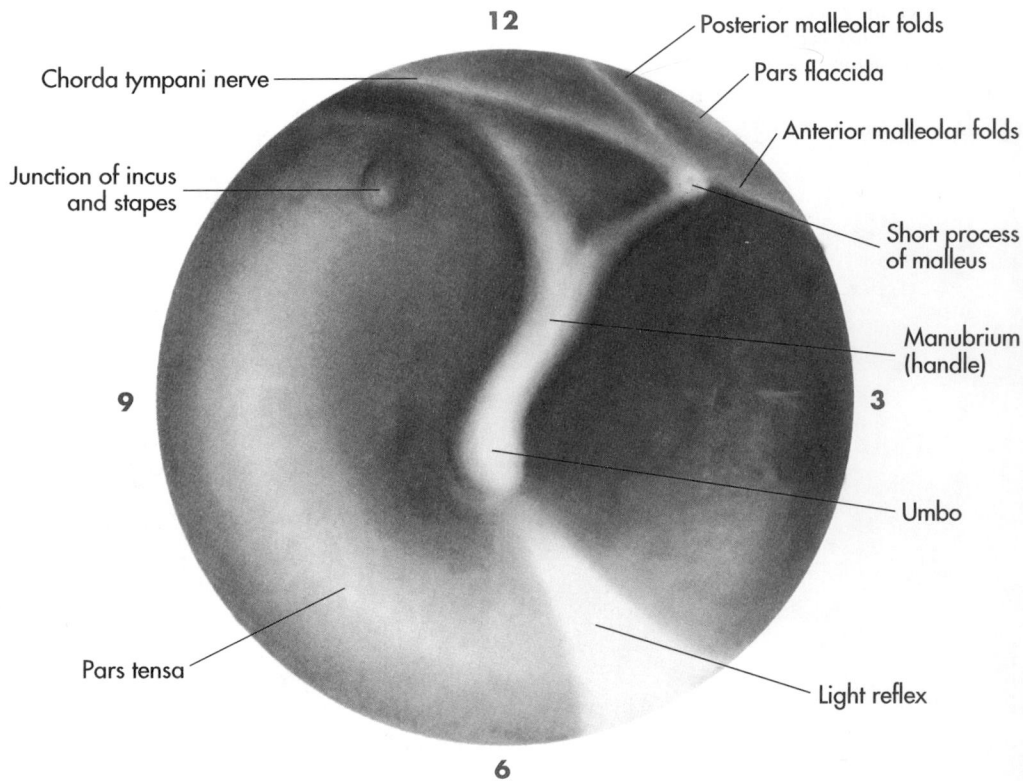

FIGURE 12-4
Structural landmarks of the right tympanic membrane in relation to a clock face.
From Barkauskas et al, 1998.

The inner ear is a membranous, curved cavity inside a bony labyrinth consisting of the vestibule, semicircular canals, and cochlea. The cochlea, a coiled structure containing the organ of Corti, transmits sound impulses to the eighth cranial nerve. The semicircular canals contain the end organs for vestibular function. Equilibrium receptors in the semicircular canals and vestibule of the inner ear respond to changes in direction of movement and send signals to the cerebellum for the maintenance of balance.

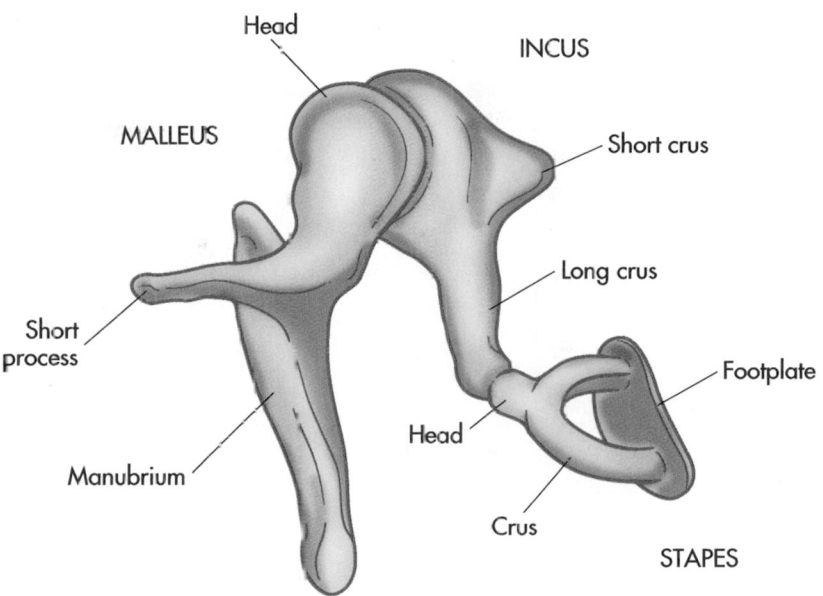

FIGURE 12-5
Ossicles of the right middle ear.

Hearing is the interpretation of sound waves by the brain. Sound waves travel through the external auditory canal and strike the tympanic membrane, setting it in vibration. The malleus, attached to the tympanic membrane, begins vibrating as do the connected incus and stapes. The vibrations are passed from the stapes to the oval window of the inner ear (Fig. 12-5). The sound waves then travel via the endolymph fluid of the cochlea to the round window where they are dissipated. Vibrations in the membrane cause the delicate hair cells of the organ of Corti to strike against the membrane of Corti, stimulating impulses in the sensory endings of the auditory division of the eighth cranial nerve. These impulses are transmitted to the temporal lobe of the brain for interpretation. Sound vibrations may also be transmitted by bone directly to the inner ear.

NOSE, NASOPHARYNX, AND SINUSES

The nose and nasopharynx have several functions:
  * Identification of odors
  * Passageway for inspired and expired air
  * Humidification, filtration, and warmth of inspired air
  * Resonance of laryngeal sound

The external nose is formed by bone and cartilage and is covered with skin. The nares, which are the anterior openings of the nose, are surrounded by the cartilaginous ala nasi and columella. The frontal and maxillary bones form the nasal bridge (Fig. 12-6).

The floor of the nose is formed by the hard and soft palate, whereas the roof is formed by the frontal and sphenoid bone. The internal nose is covered by a vascular mucous membrane thickly lined with small hairs and mucous secretions. This membrane collects and carries debris and bacteria from the inspired air to the nasopharynx for swallowing or expectoration. The mucus contains immunoglobulins and enzymes that serve as a line of defense from infection. Receptors for smell are located in the olfactory epithelium.

The internal nose is divided by the septum into two anterior cavities: the vestibules. Inspired air enters the nose through the nares and passes through the vestibules to the choanae, which are posterior openings leading to the nasopharynx. The cribriform plate, housing the sensory endings of the olfactory nerve, lies on the roof of the nose. The Kiesselbach plexus is a convergence of small fragile arteries and veins located superficially on the anterior superior portion of the septum. The adenoids lie on the posterior wall of the nasopharynx (Fig. 12-7).

The lateral walls of the nose are formed by turbinates, curved bony structures covered by vascular mucous membrane, that run horizontally and protrude into the nasal cavity. The in-

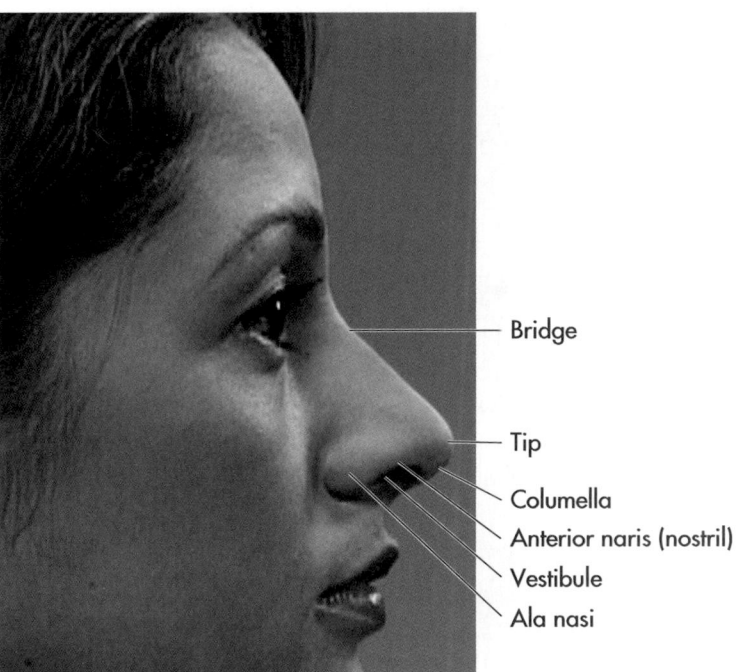

Bridge

Tip

Columella

Anterior naris (nostril)

Vestibule

Ala nasi

FIGURE 12-6
Anatomic structures of the external nose.

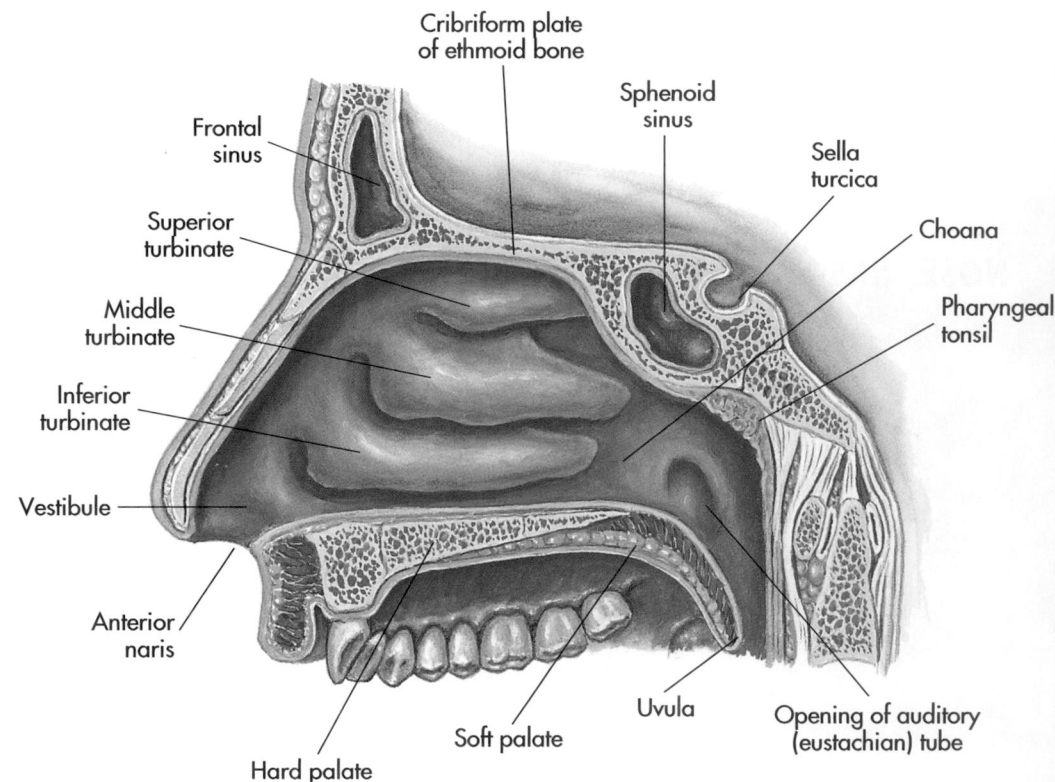

Cribriform plate
of ethmoid bone

Sphenoid
sinus

Sella
turcica

Choana

Pharyngeal
tonsil

Frontal
sinus

Superior
turbinate

Middle
turbinate

Inferior
turbinate

Vestibule

Anterior
naris

Hard palate

Soft palate

Uvula

Opening of auditory
(eustachian) tube

FIGURE 12-7
Cross-sectional view of the anatomic structures of the nose and nasopharynx.

ferior, medial, and superior turbinates increase the surface area of the nose to warm, humidify, and filter inspired air. A meatus in the area below each turbinate is named for the turbinate above it. The nasolacrimal duct drains into the inferior meatus, the paranasal sinuses drain into the medial meatus, and the posterior ethmoid sinus drains into the superior meatus.

The paranasal sinuses are air-filled, paired extensions of the nasal cavities within the bones of the skull. They are lined with mucous membranes and cilia that move secretions along excretory pathways. Their openings into the medial meatus of the nasal cavity are easily obstructed.

The maxillary sinuses lie along the lateral wall of the nasal cavity in the maxillary bone. The frontal sinuses are in the frontal bone superior to the nasal cavities. Only the maxillary and frontal sinuses are accessible for physical examination. The ethmoid sinuses lie behind the frontal sinuses and near the superior portion of the nasal cavity. The sphenoid sinuses are deep in the skull behind the ethmoid sinuses (Figs. 12-8 and 12-9).

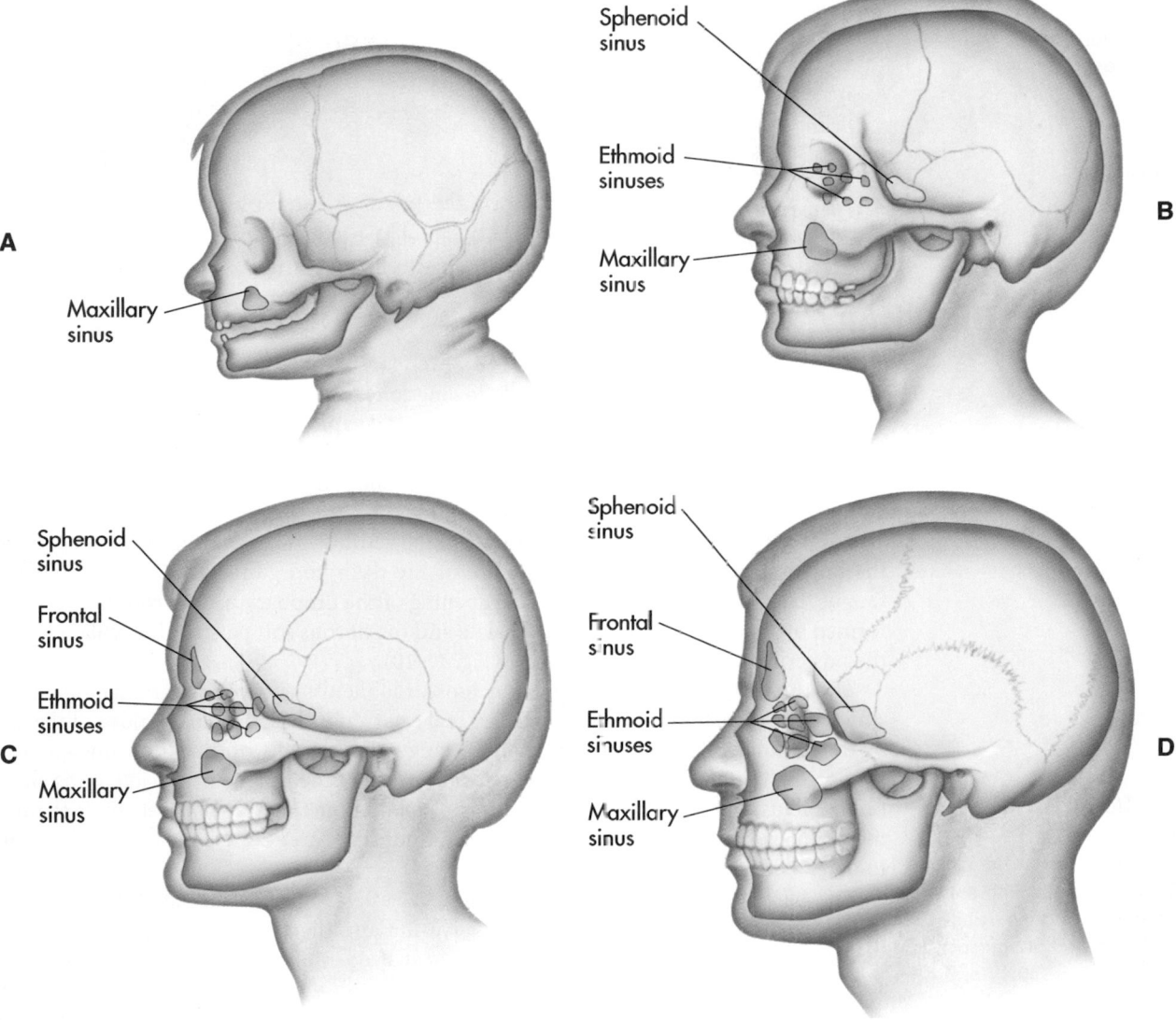

FIGURE 12-8
Location of the paranasal sinuses and comparison of their size by age. **A,** Infant, 1 year. **B,** Young child, 6 years. **C,** School-age child, 10 years. **D,** Adult, 21 years.

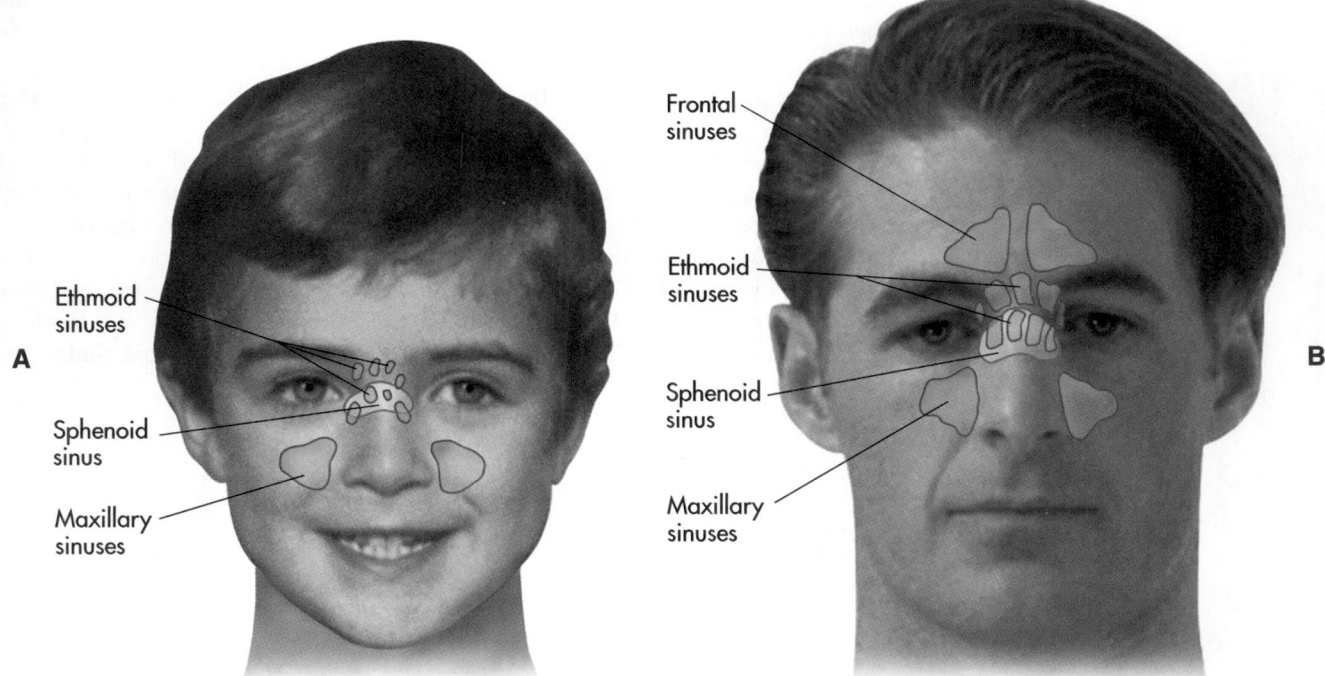

FIGURE 12-9
Anterior view of the cranial sinuses. **A,** Six-year-old child. **B,** Adult.

MOUTH AND OROPHARYNX

The mouth and oropharynx have the following functions:
- Emission of air for vocalization and non-nasal expiration
- Passageway for food, liquid, and saliva, either swallowed or vomited
- Initiation of digestion by masticating solid foods and by salivary secretion
- Identification of taste

The oral cavity is divided into the mouth and the vestibule. The vestibule is the space between the buccal mucosa and the outer surface of the teeth and gums. The mouth, housing the tongue, teeth, and gums, is the anterior opening of the oropharynx. The roof of the mouth is formed by the bony arch of the hard palate and the fibrous soft palate. The uvula hangs from the posterior margin of the soft palate (Fig. 12-10).

The floor of the mouth is formed by loose, mobile tissue covering the mandibular bone. The tongue is anchored to the back of the oral cavity at its base and to the floor of the mouth by the frenulum. The dorsal surface of the tongue is covered with thick mucous membrane, supporting the filiform papillae. The ventral surface of the tongue has visible veins and fimbriated folds, which are ridges of thin mucous membrane (Fig. 12-11). Taste buds sensitive to the primary sensations of sour, sweet, salty, and bitter are located on specific areas of the tongue.

The parotid, submandibular, and sublingual salivary glands are located in tissues surrounding the oral cavity. The secreted saliva initiates digestion and moistens the mucosa. Stensen ducts are outlets of the parotid gland that open on the buccal mucosa opposite the second molar on each side of the upper jaw. Wharton ducts, outlets of the submandibular glands, open on each side of the frenulum under the tongue. The sublingual glands have many ducts opening along the sublingual fold.

The gingivae, fibrous tissue covered by mucous membrane, are attached directly to the alveolar surface. The roots of the teeth are anchored to the alveolar ridges, and the gingivae cover the neck and roots of each tooth. Adults generally have 32 permanent teeth consisting of 4 incisors, 2 canines, 4 premolars, and 6 molars, including wisdom teeth, in each jaw (Fig. 12-12).

PHYSICAL VARIATIONS

Permanent Teeth

A common variant on 32 teeth is 28 teeth, with the wisdom teeth often being absent. This occurs most often in Asians (30%), less often in whites and Native Americans/American Indians (10% to 15%), and infrequently in blacks (1% to 2%).

Data from Brothwell, Carbonell, Goose, 1963.

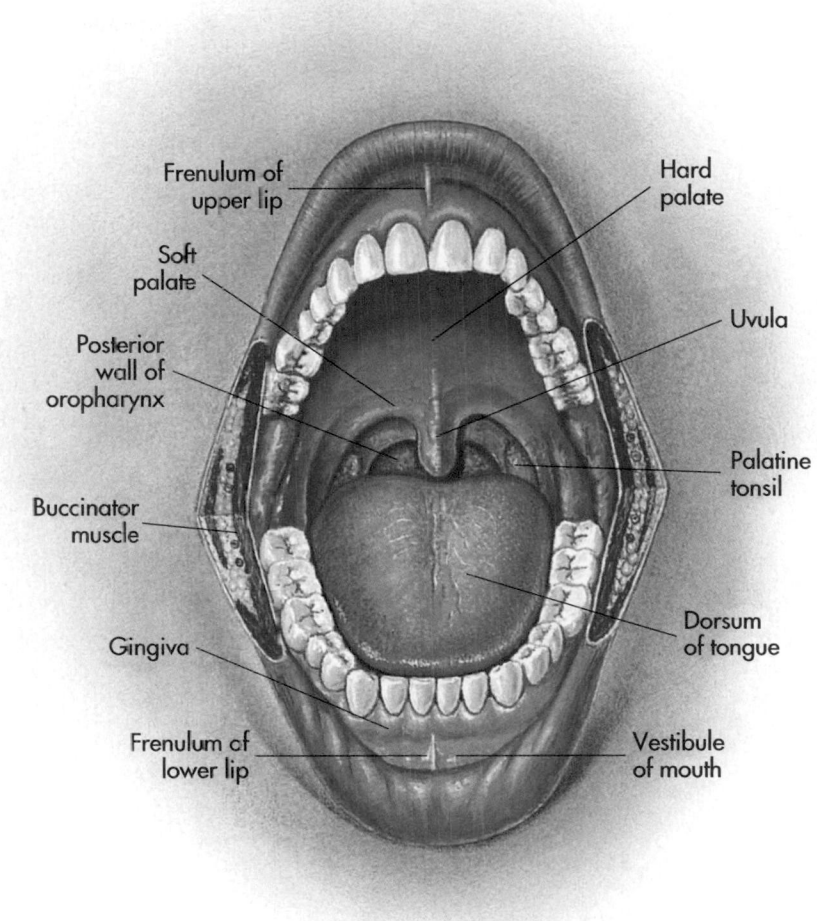

FIGURE 12-10
Anatomic structures of the oral cavity.

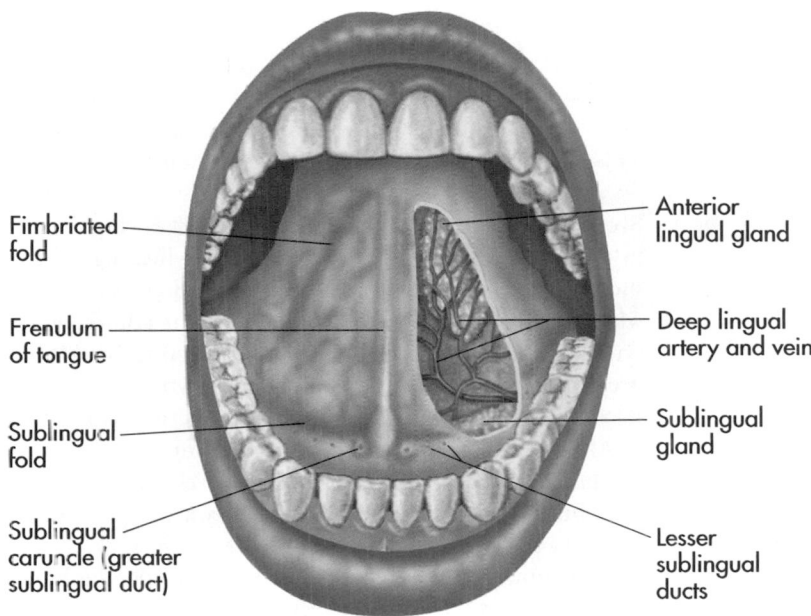

FIGURE 12-11
Landmarks of the ventral surface of the tongue.

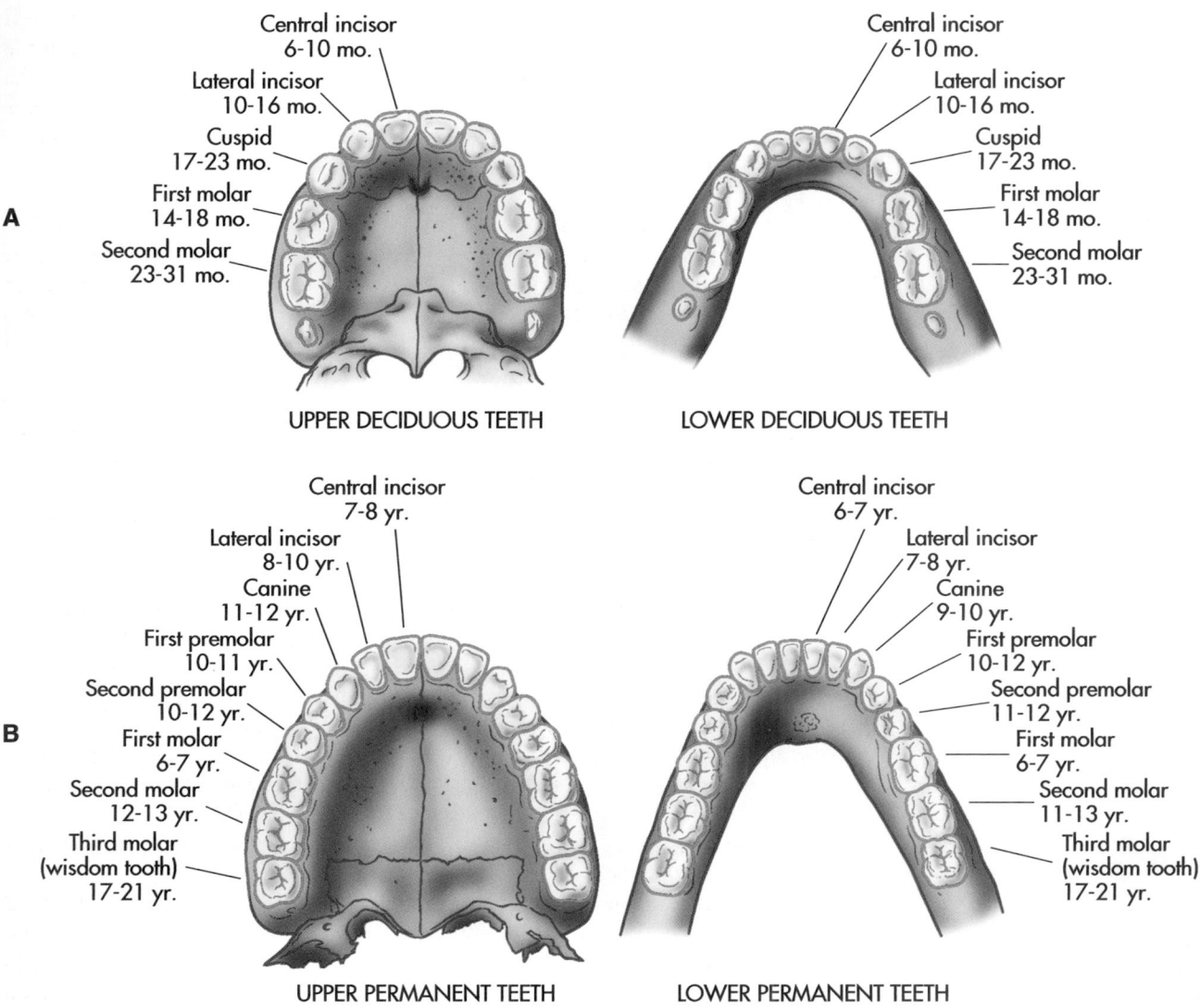

A, Dentition of deciduous teeth and their sequence of eruption. **B,** Dentition of permanent teeth and their sequence of eruption.

UPPER DECIDUOUS TEETH

Central incisor 6-10 mo.
Lateral incisor 10-16 mo.
Cuspid 17-23 mo.
First molar 14-18 mo.
Second molar 23-31 mo.

LOWER DECIDUOUS TEETH

Central incisor 6-10 mo.
Lateral incisor 10-16 mo.
Cuspid 17-23 mo.
First molar 14-18 mo.
Second molar 23-31 mo.

UPPER PERMANENT TEETH

Central incisor 7-8 yr.
Lateral incisor 8-10 yr.
Canine 11-12 yr.
First premolar 10-11 yr.
Second premolar 10-12 yr.
First molar 6-7 yr.
Second molar 12-13 yr.
Third molar (wisdom tooth) 17-21 yr.

LOWER PERMANENT TEETH

Central incisor 6-7 yr.
Lateral incisor 7-8 yr.
Canine 9-10 yr.
First premolar 10-12 yr.
Second premolar 11-12 yr.
First molar 6-7 yr.
Second molar 11-13 yr.
Third molar (wisdom tooth) 17-21 yr.

FIGURE 12-12

The oropharynx, continuous with but inferior to the nasopharynx, is separated from the mouth by the anterior and posterior tonsillar pillars on each side. The tonsils, lying in the cavity between these pillars, have crypts that collect cell debris and food particles.

INFANTS AND CHILDREN   Because development of the inner ear occurs during the first trimester of pregnancy, an insult to the fetus during that time may impair hearing. The infant's external auditory canal is shorter than the adult's and has an upward curve. The infant's eustachian tube is relatively wider, shorter, and more horizontal than the adult's, which allows easier reflux of nasopharyngeal secretions. As the child grows, the eustachian tube lengthens and its pharyngeal orifice moves inferiorly. With the growth of lymphatic tissue, specifically the adenoids, the eustachian tube may become occluded, interfering with aeration of the middle ear.

Although the maxillary and ethmoid sinuses are present at birth, they are very small. The frontal and sphenoid sinuses begin to develop at 3 years of age, but they are not fully developed until late adolescence, however, they are large enough to become infected in early childhood (Leung & Kellner, 2004).

Salivation increases by the time the infant is 3 months old, and the infant drools until swallowing is learned. Deciduous teeth begin to calcify in the third month of fetal life, each tooth erupting when it has sufficient calcification to withstand chewing. The 20 deciduous teeth usually appear between 6 and 24 months of age. The permanent teeth begin forming in the jaw by 6 months of age. Pressure from these teeth leads to the resorption of the roots of the deciduous teeth until the crown is shed. Eruption of the permanent teeth begins about 6 years of age and is completed around 14 or 15 years of age in most races. White children's third molars erupt around 18 years of age.

Pregnant Women

Elevated levels of estrogen cause increased vascularity of the upper respiratory tract. The capillaries of the nose, pharynx, and eustachian tubes become engorged, leading to symptoms of nasal stuffiness, decreased sense of smell, epistaxis, a sense of fullness in the ears, and impaired hearing. Increased vascularity and proliferation of connective tissue of the gums also may occur. Laryngeal changes are also hormonally induced so that hoarseness, deepening or cracking of the voice, vocal changes, or persistent cough may occur.

Older Adults

Hearing tends to deteriorate with degeneration of hair cells in the organ of Corti, usually after age 50. The stria vascularis, a network of capillaries that secrete endolymph and promote the sensitization of hair cells in the cochlea, may atrophy, contributing to hearing loss. Loss of cortical and organ of Corti auditory neurons interferes with the understanding of speech and localization of sound. Sensorineural hearing loss first occurs with high-frequency sounds and then progresses to tones of lower frequency.

Hearing deterioration may also result from an excess deposition of bone cells along the ossicle chain, causing fixation of the stapes in the oval window. Fewer sebaceous glands are active, and consequently the cerumen may become very dry. Cerumen may totally obstruct the external auditory canal, interfering with sound transmission. The tympanic membrane becomes more translucent and sclerotic. Conductive hearing loss occurs in each case.

Deterioration of the sense of smell results from loss of olfactory sensory neurons beginning around 60 years of age. The sense of taste begins deteriorating at about 50 years of age due to a decrease in the number of papillae on the tongue and decreased salivary gland secretion, which reduces the perception of sweet sensations (Huether & Leo, 2002). However, there may be wide variation in rate of smell and taste deterioration.

Cartilage formation continues in the ears and nose, making the auricle and nose larger and more prominent. The soft tissues of the mouth change as the granular lining on the lips and cheeks becomes more prominent. The gingival tissue is less elastic and more vulnerable to trauma. The tongue becomes more fissured. The older adult may have altered motor function of the tongue, leading to problems with swallowing.

Saliva production may decrease as a result of disease or medications taken. Lost teeth may contribute to diet changes or difficulty chewing. Sensitivity to odors and taste declines.

REVIEW OF RELATED HISTORY

For each of the conditions discussed in this section, targeted topics to include in the history of the present illness are listed. Responses to questions about these topics help fully assess the patient's condition and provide clues for focusing the physical examination.

HISTORY OF PRESENT ILLNESS

- ◆ Vertigo or dizziness
  - ◆ Time of onset, time of day, duration of attacks, circumstances of the attack, past attacks
  - ◆ Description (to and fro movement or rotary motion—room moving around patient or patient rotating), change of sensation with turning over in bed or head turning, any position better than others

- ◆ Associated symptoms: nausea, vomiting, presence or absence of tinnitus and hearing loss, double vision, sensation of fullness in ear
  - ◆ Unsteadiness, loss of balance, falling
  - ◆ Medications: ototoxic medications such as aminoglycosides, gentamicin, streptomycin, aspirin, ethacrynic acid, furosemide; salt-retaining medications such as corticosteroids; other prescription or nonprescription drugs; complementary or alternative therapies
- ◆ Earache
  - ◆ Onset, duration, pain, fever, discharge (e.g., waxy, serous, mucoid, purulent, sanguinous); association with diving or flying
  - ◆ Concurrent upper respiratory infection, frequent swimming, trauma to the head; related complaints in the mouth, teeth, sinuses, throat, or temporomandibular joint
  - ◆ Associated symptoms: reduced hearing, ringing in ear, vertigo
  - ◆ Method of ear canal cleaning; problems with impacted cerumen
  - ◆ Medications: antibiotics, ear drops (e.g., acetic acid, Auralgan, topical steroids, cerumen softeners)
- ◆ Hearing loss: one or both ears
  - ◆ Onset: instant (may indicate vascular disruption), over a few hours or days (may indicate viral infection), slow or gradual
  - ◆ Repeated history of cerumen impaction
  - ◆ Hears best: on telephone, in quiet or noisy environment; all sounds reduced or some sounds garbled; inability to discriminate words
  - ◆ Speech: soft or loud, articulation of speech sounds
  - ◆ Management: hearing aid, when worn, battery change frequency; lip reading, sign language used
  - ◆ Ototoxic medications: aminoglycosides, salicylates, furosemide, streptomycin, quinine, ethacrynic acid, cisplatin
- ◆ Nasal discharge
  - ◆ Character (e.g., watery, mucoid, purulent, crusty, bloody); odor, amount, duration, unilateral or bilateral
  - ◆ Associated symptoms: sneezing, nasal congestion, itching nasal mucosa, habitual sniffling, nasal obstruction, mouth breathing, malodorous breath, conjunctival burning or itching
  - ◆ Seasonality of symptoms; allergies or concurrent upper respiratory infection; frequency of occurrence
  - ◆ Tenderness over sinuses, postnasal drip, daytime cough, face pain, headache
  - ◆ Medications: nose drops or sprays, antihistamines, decongestants; complementary and alternative therapies

RISK FACTORS
HEARING LOSS

Adults
- Exposure to industrial or recreational noise
- Genetic disease: Ménière disease
- Neurodegenerative disorder

Infants and Children
- Prenatal factors: maternal infection, irradiation, drug abuse, syphilis
- Birth weight less than 1500 g
- Excessively high bilirubin level
- Infection: bacterial meningitis, recurrent otitis media
- Cleft palate, craniofacial abnormalities
- Ototoxic antibiotic use
- Head trauma
- Hypoxic episode

- Snoring
  - Change in snoring pattern, complaints of snoring loudness by partner, periods of apnea
  - Daytime sleepiness (associated with obstructive apnea)
  - Medications: prescription, nonprescription, complementary or alternative therapies
- Nosebleed
  - Frequency, amount of bleeding, nasal obstruction, treatment, difficulty stopping the bleeding
  - Predisposing factors: concurrent upper respiratory infection, dry heat, nose picking, forceful nose blowing, trauma, allergies
  - Site of bleeding: unilateral or bilateral, alternating sides
  - Medications: prescription, nonprescription, complementary or alternative therapies
- Dental problems
  - Pain: with chewing, localized to tooth or entire jaw, severity, interference with eating, foods no longer eaten; tooth grinding; associated with temporomandibular joint problems
  - Swollen or bleeding gums, mouth ulcers or masses, tooth loss
  - Dentures or dental appliances (e.g., braces, retainers): snugness of fit, areas of irritation, length of time dentures or appliances worn daily
  - Malocclusion: difficulty chewing, tooth extractions, previous orthodontic work
  - Medications: phenytoin, cyclosporine, calcium channel blockers, mouth rinses
- Mouth lesions
  - Intermittent or constantly present, duration, painful or painless; excessive dryness of mouth; halitosis
  - Associated with stress, foods, seasons, fatigue, tobacco use, alcohol use, dentures
  - Variations in tongue character: swelling, size change, color, coating, ulceration, difficulty moving tongue
  - Lesions any place else on the body (e.g., vagina, urethra, anus)
  - Medications: mouth rinses
- Sinus pain
  - Fever, malaise, cough, headache, maxillary toothache, eye pain
  - Nasal congestion, colored nasal discharge
  - Pain: tenderness or pressure over sinuses, pain increases when bending forward
  - Medications: change in symptoms with decongestants
- Sore throat
  - Pain with swallowing; associated with upper respiratory infection symptoms; exposure to streptococcus or gonorrhea; postnasal drip; mouth breathing; fever
  - Exposure to dry heat, smoke, or fumes
  - Hoarseness: voice overuse, infection, gastroesophageal reflux, need to clear throat frequently
  - Medications: antibiotics, nonprescription lozenges or sprays

RISK FACTORS
ORAL CANCER

- Older than 40 years of age
- Gender: men have twice the rate of women
- Ethnicity: black
- Excessive alcohol use
- Ill-fitting dentures, prior oral lesions
- Tobacco use: cigarettes, cigars, pipes, chewing tobacco, snuff; risk increases with frequency and duration of tobacco use, smoking history of more than 20 pack-years
- Occupation: textile industry, leather manufacturing
- Systemic disease: pernicious or iron-deficiency anemia, HIV infection, lichen planus, previous malignancy, human papillomavirus

- Difficulty swallowing
  - Solids, liquids, or both
  - Tightness, "catching," substernal fullness, regurgitation
  - Drooling
  - Aspiration when swallowing
  - Swallowed liquids coming out of nose

PAST MEDICAL HISTORY

- Systemic disease: hypertension, cardiovascular disease, diabetes mellitus, nephritis, bleeding disorder, gastrointestinal disease, reflux esophagitis
- Ear: frequent ear problems during childhood; surgery; labyrinthitis; antibiotic use, dosage, and duration
- Nose: trauma, surgery, chronic nosebleeds
- Sinuses: chronic postnasal drip, repeated sinusitis, allergies
- Throat: frequent documented streptococcal infections, tonsillectomy, adenoidectomy

FAMILY HISTORY

- Hearing problems or hearing loss, Ménière disease
- Allergies
- Hereditary renal disease

PERSONAL AND SOCIAL HISTORY

- Environmental hazards: exposure to loud, continuous noises (factory, airport, playing in rock band); types of protective hearing devices used (associated with hearing loss)
- Nutrition: excessive sugar intake, foods eaten (associated with caries)
- Oral care patterns: tooth brushing and flossing; last visit to dentist; current condition of teeth; braces, dentures, bridges, crowns, mouth guard use
- Tobacco use: pipe, cigarettes, cigars, smokeless; amount, number of pack-years (associated with oral cancer)
- Use of alcohol
- Intranasal use of cocaine

INFANTS AND CHILDREN

- Prenatal: maternal infection, irradiation, alcohol and drug abuse, hypertension, Rh incompatibility, diabetes
- Prematurity: birth weight less than 1500 g, anoxia, ototoxic antibiotic use
- Erythroblastosis fetalis, bilirubin greater than 20 mg/100 mL serum
- Infection: meningitis, encephalitis, recurrent or chronic otitis media, unilateral mumps, congenital syphilis
- Breast-feeding, secondary tobacco smoke exposure, childcare (associated with occurrence of otitis media)
- Congenital defect: cleft palate, craniofacial abnormality, snoring
- Playing with small objects (could place in nose or ears)
- Behaviors indicating hearing loss: no reaction to loud or strange noises, no babbling after 6 months of age, no communicative speech and reliance on gestures after 15 months of age, inattention when compared to children of the same age
- Dental care: fluoride supplementation or fluoridated water; goes to sleep with bottle of milk or juice; when first tooth erupted; number of teeth present; thumb-sucking, pacifier use

PREGNANT WOMEN

- Weeks of gestation or postpartum
- Presence of symptoms before pregnancy

- Accompanying symptoms suggestive of pathology
- Pattern of dental care
- Exposure to infection

OLDER ADULTS

- Hearing loss causing any interference with daily life
- Any physical disability: interference with oral care or denture care, problems operating hearing aid
- Deterioration of teeth, extractions, difficulty chewing
- Dry mouth (xerostomia)
- Medications decreasing salivation: anticholinergics, diuretics, antihypertensives, antihistamines, antispasmodics, antidepressants, tranquilizers; ototoxic drugs

EXAMINATION AND FINDINGS

EQUIPMENT

- Otoscope with pneumatic attachment
- Nasal speculum
- Tongue blades
- Tuning fork (500 to 1000 Hz, approximates vocal frequencies)
- Gauze
- Gloves
- Penlight, sinus transilluminator, or light from otoscope
- Vials with different odors such as mint, banana, coffee

EARS AND HEARING

EXTERNAL EAR

PHYSICAL VARIATIONS

Preauricular Pits
Preauricular pits are occasionally seen; they often occur in conjunction with lip pits, which are most common in blacks (20%) and least common in Asians (7%), with occurrence in whites being intermediate.

Data from Schaumann, Peagler, Gorlin, 1970.

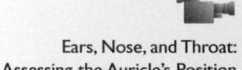

Ears, Nose, and Throat:
Assessing the Auricle's Position

Inspect the auricles for size, shape, symmetry, landmarks, color, and position on the head. Examine the lateral and medial surfaces and surrounding tissue, noting color, presence of deformities, lesions, and nodules. The auricle should have the same color as the facial skin, without moles, cysts or other lesions, deformities, or nodules. No openings or discharge should be present in the preauricular area. Darwin tubercle, a thickening along the upper ridge of the helix, is an expected variation; as are preauricular pits, which are found in front of the ear where the upper auricle originates.

The color of the auricles may vary with certain conditions. Blueness may indicate some degree of cyanosis. Pallor or excessive redness may be the result of vasomotor instability. Frostbite can cause extreme pallor.

An unusual size or shape of the auricle may be a familial trait or indicate abnormality. A cauliflower ear is the result of blunt trauma and necrosis of the underlying cartilage. Tophi—small, whitish uric acid crystals along the peripheral margins of the auricles—may indicate gout. Sebaceous cysts, which are elevations in the skin with a punctum indicating a blocked sebaceous gland, are common (Fig. 12-13).

To determine the position of the auricle, draw an imaginary line between the inner canthus of the eye and the most prominent protuberance of the occiput. The top of the auricle should touch or be above this line. Then draw another imaginary line perpendicular to the previous line just anterior to the auricle. The auricle's position should be almost vertical, with no more than a 10-degree lateral posterior angle (Fig. 12-14). An auricle with a low-set or unusual angle may indicate chromosomal aberrations or renal disorders.

Inspect the external auditory canal for discharge and note any odor. A purulent, foul-smelling discharge is associated with an otitis or foreign body. In cases of head trauma, a bloody or serous discharge is suggestive of a skull fracture.

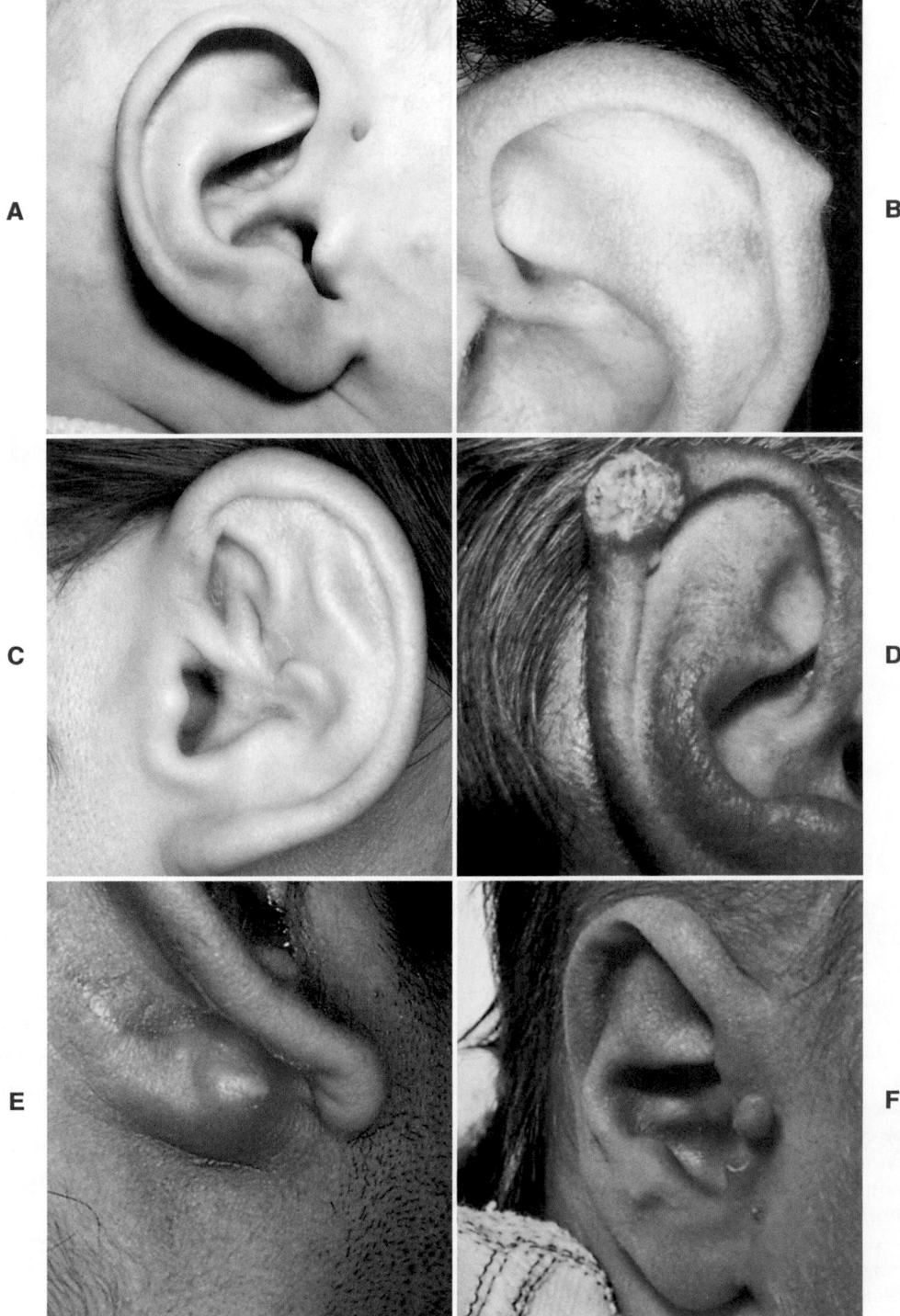

FIGURE 12-13
A, Auricular sinus. **B,** Darwin tubercle. **C,** Cauliflower ear. **D,** Tophi. **E,** Sebaceous cysts.
F, Preauricular skin tag.
A and F from Zitelli, Davis, 1997; B, C, and E from Bingham, Hawke, Kwok, 1992; D from Sigler, Schuring, 1993.

CLINICAL PEARL

Smell the Cerumen

Odor from earwax can be a clue to a problem:

- Maple syrup (maple syrup urine disease)
- Mousy (*Proteus* infection)
- Putrid (*Pseudomonas* infection)

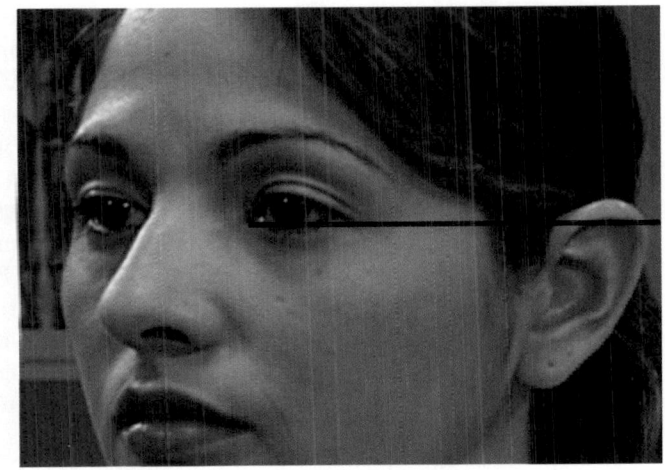

FIGURE 12-14
Assessment of auricle alignment showing expected position. Imaginary line extends from inner eye canthus to occiput.

Palpate the auricles and mastoid area for tenderness, swelling, or nodules. The consistency of the auricle should be firm, mobile, and without nodules. If folded forward it should readily recoil to its usual position. Pulling gently on the lobule should cause no pain. If pain is present, inflammation of the external auditory canal may be present. Tenderness or swelling in the mastoid area may indicate mastoiditis.

OTOSCOPIC EXAMINATION

Ears, Nose, and Throat:
Inspecting the Auditory Canal
and Tympanic Membrane

PHYSICAL VARIATIONS

Types of Cerumen

Cerumen comes in two main varieties—wet and dry. Wet cerumen is dark and sticky and occurs in whites and blacks almost 100% of the time. Dry cerumen is light brown to gray, flaky, and sparse; it can lie in the ear canal as a thin flake. Dry cerumen occurs in Asians and Native Americans/American Indians around 85% of the time. Wet cerumen is the result of a dominant gene, so individuals with dry cerumen have two dry cerumen alleles.

Data from Matsunaga, 1962; Ibraimov, 1991.

FIGURE 12-15
To examine the adult's ear with the otoscope, straighten the external auditory canal by pulling the auricle up and back.

The otoscope is used to inspect the external auditory canal and middle ear (see Fig. 3-22). Select the largest speculum that will fit comfortably in the patient's ear. Hold the handle of the otoscope between your thumb and index finger, supported on the middle finger (using the right hand for the right ear and left hand for the left ear). Depending on your preference, the bottom end of the handle may rest against the palm of the hand or space between the thumb and index finger. This leaves the ulnar side of your hand to rest against the patient's head, stabilizing the otoscope as it is inserted into the canal. Examination of the tympanic membrane with the otoscope requires that you manipulate the auricle. Be gentle: a viselike grip is not necessary, although a firm, gentle grasp is. Avoid causing discomfort to the patient. Tilt the patient's head toward the opposite shoulder and simultaneously pull the patient's auricle upward and back as the speculum is inserted, thereby straightening the auditory canal to give the best view (Fig. 12-15).

Slowly insert the speculum to a depth of 1.0 or 1.5 cm (½ inch) and inspect the auditory canal from the meatus to the tympanic membrane, noting discharge, scaling, excessive red-

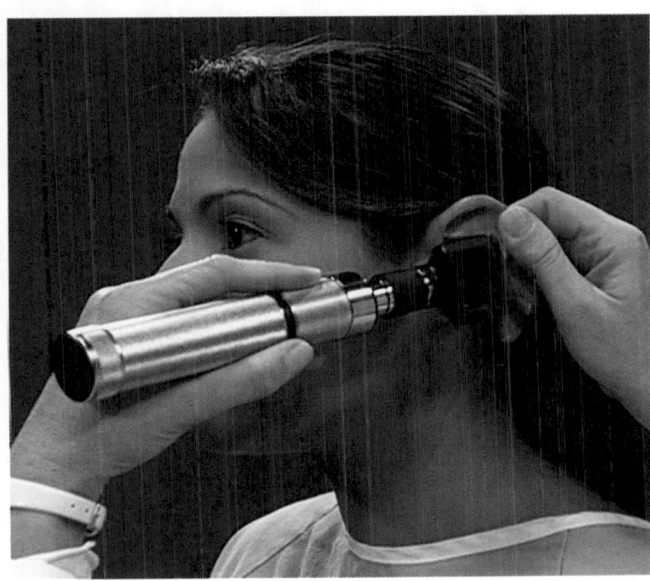

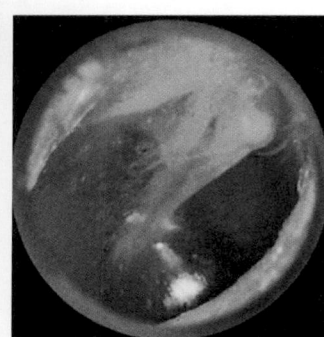

FIGURE 12-16
Healthy tympanic membrane.
*Courtesy Richard A. Buckingham,
Clinical Professor, Otolaryngology,
Abraham Lincoln School of Medicine,
University of Illinois, Chicago.*

ness, lesions, foreign bodies, and cerumen. Avoid touching the bony walls of the auditory canal (the inner two thirds) with the speculum because this will be painful for the patient. Expect to see minimal cerumen, a uniformly pink color, and hairs in the outer third of the canal. Cerumen may vary in color and texture but should have no odor. No lesions, discharge, or foreign body should be present. For suggestions to clean an obstructed auditory canal, see the Clinical Pearl.

Inspect the tympanic membrane for landmarks, color, contour, and perforations. Gently move the otoscope to see the entire tympanic membrane and the annulus. The landmarks (umbo, handle of malleus, and light reflex) should be visible (Fig. 12-16). The tympanic membrane should have no perforations and be a translucent, pearly gray color. Its contour should be slightly conical with a concavity at the umbo. A bulging tympanic membrane is more conical, usually with a loss of bony landmarks and a distorted light reflex. A retracted tympanic membrane is more concave, usually with accentuated bony landmarks and a distorted light reflex (Fig. 12-17).

The pneumatic attachment of the otoscope is used to evaluate the mobility or compliance of the tympanic membrane. Make sure the speculum inserted into the canal seals it from the outside air. If a soft-tipped speculum is not available, a piece of rubber tubing around the end of the speculum tip may help achieve a seal with the canal. Gently apply positive (squeeze) and negative (release) pressure into the canal by using the pneumatic bulb attachment. Observe

Clinical Pearl

Cleaning an Obstructed Auditory Canal

If the tympanic membrane is obscured by cerumen, the canal can be cleaned by warm water irrigation or by a cerumen spoon. Although a cerumen spoon is an acceptable tool for clearing out ear wax, the auditory canal is easily abraded and bleeds readily. When this happens, you cause pain. Irrigation with water at body temperature is the preferable approach, particularly in young patients. Water irrigation should never be performed in the presence of otitis externa, a perforated tympanic membrane, myringotomy tubes, or a mastoid cavity.

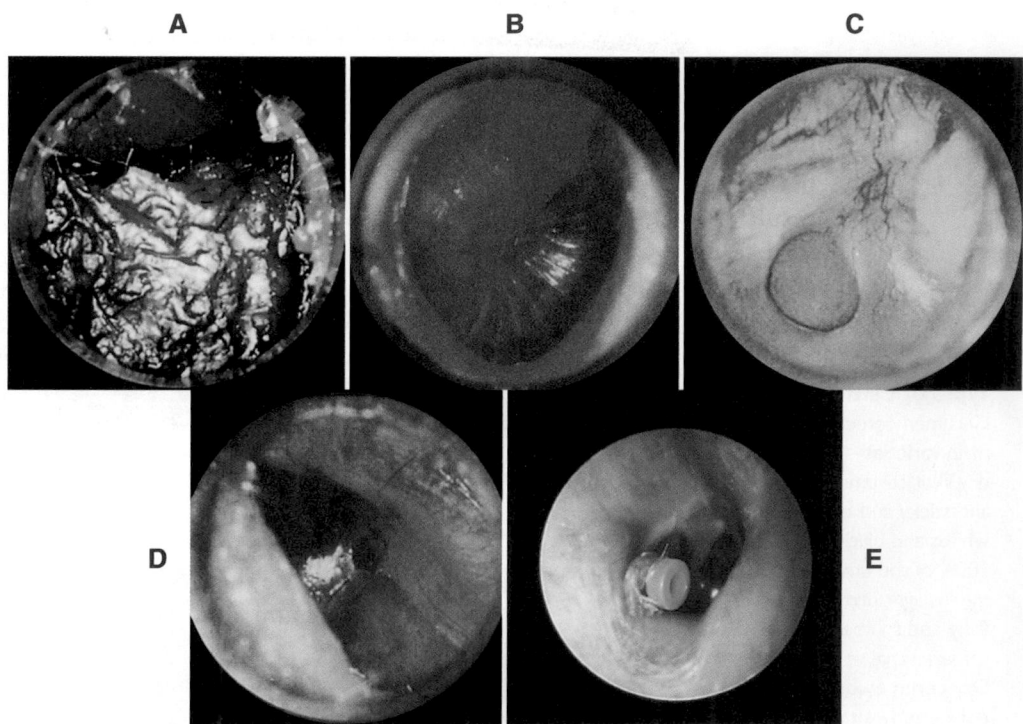

FIGURE 12-17
A, Tympanic membrane partially obscured by cerumen. **B,** Bulging tympanic membrane with loss of bony landmarks. **C,** Perforated tympanic membrane. **D,** Perforated tympanic membrane that has healed. **E,** Tympanostomy tube protruding from the right tympanic membrane.
A-D courtesy Richard A. Buckingham, MD, Clinical Professor, Otolaryngology, Abraham Lincoln School of Medicine, University of Illinois, Chicago; E from Bingham, Hawke, Kwok, 1992.

the membrane moving in and out, indicated by a change in the appearance of the cone of light. The tympanic membrane does not move when there is a perforation or a tympanostomy tube properly in place. Pathologic conditions in the middle ear may be suggested by characteristics of the tympanic membrane (Table 12-1).

Although pneumatic otoscopy has made it easier to assess the mobility of the tympanic membrane and the pressures within the middle ear, improper technique may produce misleading results. Dilation of the vessels overlying the malleus can result from applying negative pressure too slowly. The consequent redness, described as a mallear blush, may be the result of the otoscopy and can occur in the absence of infection (Bluestone and Shurin, 1974).

HEARING EVALUATION

Cranial nerve VIII is tested by evaluating hearing. Screening of auditory function begins when the patient responds to your questions and directions. The patient should respond without excessive requests for repetition. Speech with a monotonous tone and erratic volume may indicate hearing loss.

Whispered Voice. Check the patient's response to your whispered voice, one ear at a time. Mask the hearing in the other ear by having the patient place a finger in the ear canal and gently move it rapidly up and down. Stand to the side of the patient at a consistent distance best for you, about 30 to 60 cm (1 to 2 feet) away from the ear being tested, and out of the patient's line of vision. Whisper a combination of 3 letters and numbers (e.g., 3, T, 9) very softly and ask the patient to repeat the words heard. To control whisper loudness, exhale fully before whispering the sounds to produce the softest whisper. If the patient does not correctly repeat the three sounds, repeat the process with a different set of sounds. Repeat the procedure with the other ear. The patient should hear softly whispered words in each ear at a distance of 30 to 60 cm (1 to 2 feet), responding correctly more than 50% of the time (McGee, 2001).

Weber and Rinne Tests. The tuning fork is used to compare hearing by bone conduction with that by air conduction. Hold the base of the tuning fork with one hand without touching the tines, and stroke or tap the tines gently with your other hand, setting the tuning fork in vibration.

Perform the Weber test by placing the base of the vibrating tuning fork on the midline vertex of the patient's head (Fig. 12-18). Ask the patient if the sound is heard equally in both ears or is better in one ear (lateralization of sound). Avoid giving the patient a cue as to the best re-

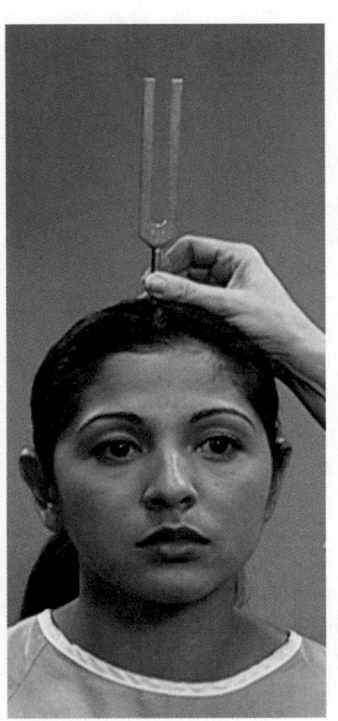

FIGURE 12-18
Weber test. Touching only the handle, place the base of the tuning fork on the midline of the skull. Avoid touching the vibrating tines.

TABLE 12-1	Tympanic Membrane Signs and Associated Conditions
Signs	**Associated Conditions/Causes**
MOBILITY	
Bulging with no mobility	Pus or fluid in middle ear
Retracted with no mobility	Obstruction of eustachian tube with or without effusion
Mobility with negative pressure only	Obstruction of eustachian tube with or without effusion
Excess mobility in small areas	Healed perforation, atrophic tympanic membrane
COLOR	
Amber or yellow	Serous fluid in middle ear
Blue or deep red	Blood in middle ear
Chalky white	Infection in middle ear
Redness	Infection in middle ear, prolonged crying
Dullness	Fibrosis
White flecks, dense white plaques	Healed inflammation
AIR BUBBLES	Serous fluid in middle ear

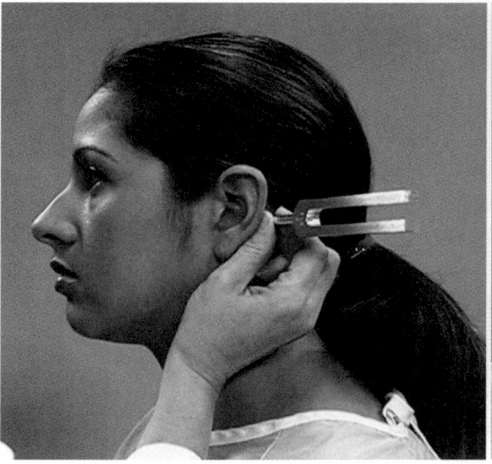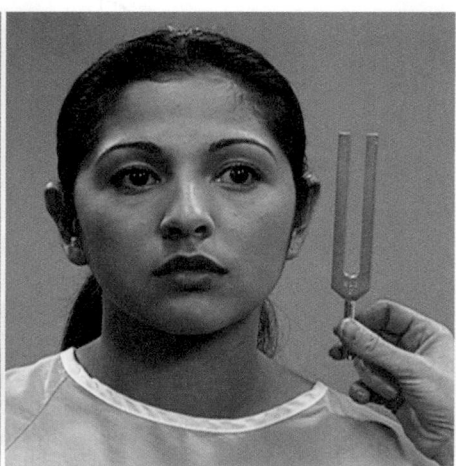

A **B**

FIGURE 12-19
Rinne test. **A,** Place the tuning fork on the mastoid bone for bone conduction. **B,** To test for air conduction hold the tuning fork 1 to 2 cm (0.5 to 1 inch) from the ear with the tines facing forward.

	TABLE 12-2	Interpretation of Tuning Fork Tests	
Test	Expected Findings	Conductive Hearing Loss	Sensorineural Hearing Loss
Weber	No lateralization, but will lateralize to ear occluded by patient	Lateralization of deaf ear unless sensorineural loss	Lateralization to better ear unless conductive loss
Rinne	Air conduction heard longer than bone conduction by 2:1 ratio (Rinne positive)	Bone conduction heard longer than air conduction in affected ear (Rinne negative)	Air conduction heard longer than bone conduction in affected ear, but less than 2:1 ratio

sponse. The patient should hear the sound equally in both ears. If the sound is lateralized, have the patient identify which ear hears the sound better. To test the reliability of the patient's response, repeat the procedure while occluding one ear, asking the patient in which ear the sound is best heard. It should be heard best in the occluded ear.

The Rinne test is performed by placing the base of the vibrating tuning fork against the patient's mastoid bone. Begin counting or timing the interval with your watch. Ask the patient to tell you when the sound is no longer heard, noting the number of seconds. Quickly position the still vibrating tines 1 to 2 cm (0.5 to 1 in) from the auditory canal, and again ask the patient to tell you when the sound is no longer heard. Continue counting or timing the interval to determine the length of time the sound is heard by air conduction (Fig. 12-19). Compare the number of seconds sound is heard by bone conduction versus air conduction. Air-conducted sound should be heard twice as long as bone-conducted sound after bone conduction stops. For example, if bone-conducted sound is heard for 15 seconds, air-conducted sound should be heard for an additional 15 seconds.

Unexpected findings from the Weber and Rinne tests must be integrated to differentiate between conductive and sensorineural hearing loss (Table 12-2). Conductive hearing loss results when sound transmission is impaired through the external or middle ear. Sensorineural hearing loss results from a defect in the inner ear that leads to distortion of sound and misinterpretation of speech. Any patient with unexpected findings should be referred for a thorough auditory evaluation.

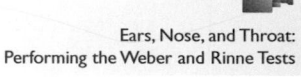

Ears, Nose, and Throat:
Performing the Weber and Rinne Tests

NOSE, NASOPHARYNX, AND SINUSES

EXTERNAL NOSE

The nose is inspected for deviations in shape, size, and color. Observe the nares for discharge and for flaring or narrowing. The skin should be smooth without swelling and conform to the color of the face. The columella should be directly midline, and its width should not ex-

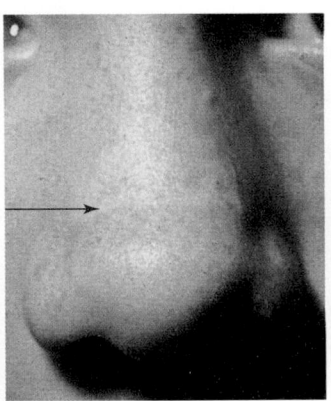

FIGURE 12-20
Transverse nasal crease.

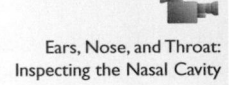

Ears, Nose, and Throat:
Inspecting the Nasal Cavity

ceed the diameter of a naris. The nares are usually oval in shape and symmetrically positioned.

If discharge is present, describe its character (e.g., watery, mucoid, purulent, crusty, or bloody); amount and color; and whether it is unilateral or bilateral. The characteristics of nasal discharge are associated with various conditions. A bilateral watery discharge, associated with sneezing and nasal congestion, is indicative of an allergy. A unilateral watery discharge occurring after head trauma may be cerebrospinal fluid and indicate a fracture of the cribriform plate. Bloody discharge usually results from epistaxis or trauma. Mucoid discharge is typical of rhinitis, and bilateral purulent discharge can occur with an upper respiratory infection. Unilateral, purulent, thick, greenish, and extremely malodorous discharge may indicate a foreign body.

A depression of the nasal bridge can result from a fractured nasal bone. Nasal flaring is associated with respiratory distress, whereas narrowing of the nares on inspiration may be indicative of chronic nasal obstruction and mouth breathing. A transverse crease at the junction between the cartilage and bone of the nose may indicate chronic nasal itching and allergies (Fig. 12-20).

Palpate the bridge and soft tissues of the nose. Note any displacement of bone and cartilage, tenderness, or masses. Place one finger on each side of the nasal arch and gently palpate, moving the fingers from the nasal bridge to the tip. The nasal structures should feel firm and stable to palpation. No tenderness or masses should be present.

Evaluate the patency of the nares. Occlude one naris by placing a finger on the side of the nose, and ask the patient to breathe in and out with mouth closed. Repeat the procedure with the other naris. Nasal breathing should be noiseless and easy through the open naris.

NASAL CAVITY

Use a nasal speculum and good light source to inspect the nasal cavity. Hold the speculum in the palm of the hand and use the index finger for stabilization. Use your other hand to change the patient's head position. The speculum should be inserted slowly and cautiously. Make sure you do not overdilate the nares or touch the nasal septum, which causes pain (Fig. 12-21). Inspect the nasal mucosa for color, discharge, masses, lesions, and swelling of the turbinates. Inspect the nasal septum for alignment, perforation, bleeding, and crusting.

Only the inferior and middle turbinates will be visible. Keep the patient's head erect to examine the vestibule and inferior nasal turbinate. Tilt the patient's head back to visualize the middle meatus and middle turbinate; then cautiously move the speculum tip toward the midline to examine the septum. Repeat the procedure in the other naris (Fig. 12-22).

The nasal mucosa should appear deep pink (pinker than the buccal mucosa) and glistening. A film of clear discharge is often apparent on the nasal septum. Hairs may be present in the vestibule. Increased redness of the mucosa may occur with an infection, whereas localized redness and swelling in the vestibule may indicate a furuncle.

The turbinates should be the same color as the surrounding area and have a firm consistency. Turbinates that appear bluish gray or pale pink with a swollen, boggy consistency may indicate allergies. A rounded, elongated mass projecting into the nasal cavity from boggy mucosa may be a polyp.

The nasal septum should be close to midline and fairly straight, appearing thicker anteriorly than posteriorly. Asymmetric size of the posterior nasal cavities may indicate deviation of the nasal septum. No perforations, bleeding, or crusting should be apparent. Crusting over the anterior portion of the nasal septum may occur at the site of epistaxis (Fig. 12-23).

The sense of smell (cranial nerve I) is often tested with recognition of different odors. This procedure is described in Chapter 22.

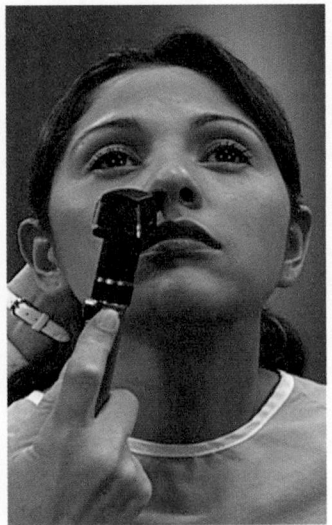

FIGURE 12-21
Use of the nasal speculum. Avoid touching the nasal septum.

SINUSES

Inspect the frontal and maxillary sinus areas for swelling. To palpate the frontal sinuses, use your thumbs to press up under the bony brow on each side of the nose. Then press up under the zygomatic processes, using either your thumbs or index and middle fingers to palpate the maxillary sinuses. No tenderness or swelling over the soft tissue should be present. Swelling, tenderness, and pain over the sinuses may indicate infection or obstruction.

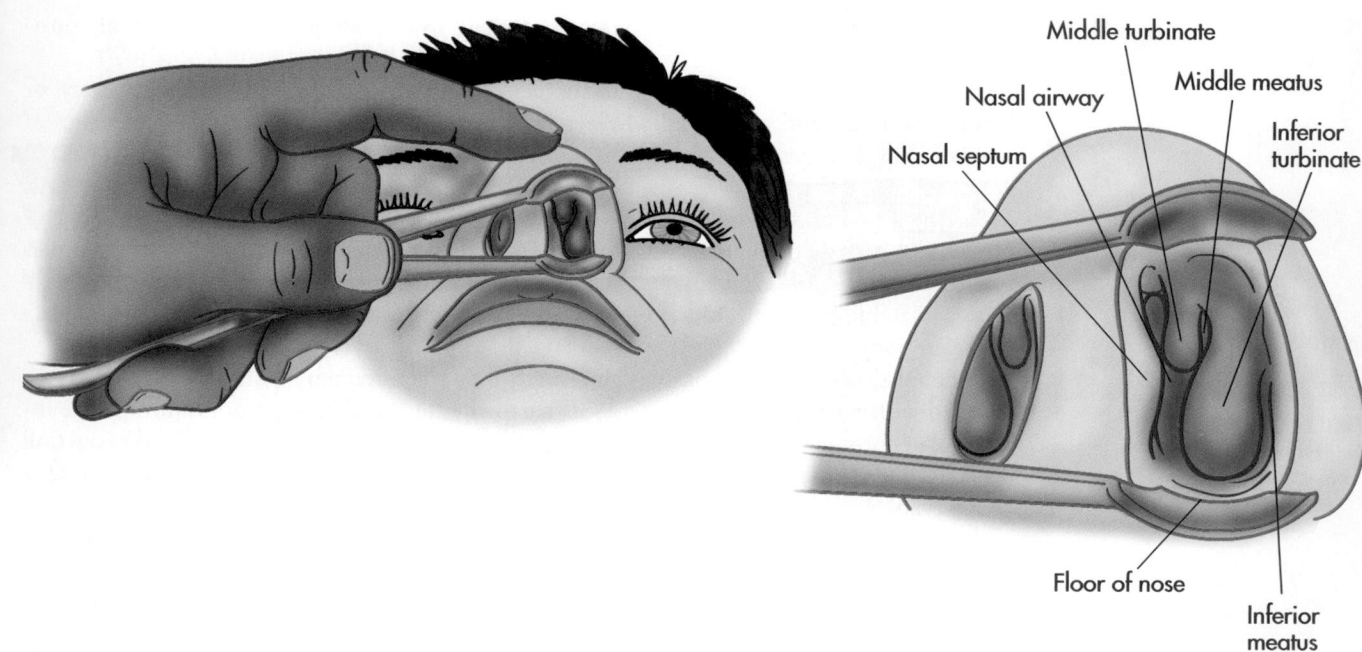

FIGURE 12-22
View of the nasal mucosa through the nasal speculum.

FIGURE 12-23
Unexpected findings on nasal examination. **A,** Nasal polyp (allergic). **B,** Purulent discharge. **C,** Deviation of the nasal septum.
C *from Bull, 1974.*

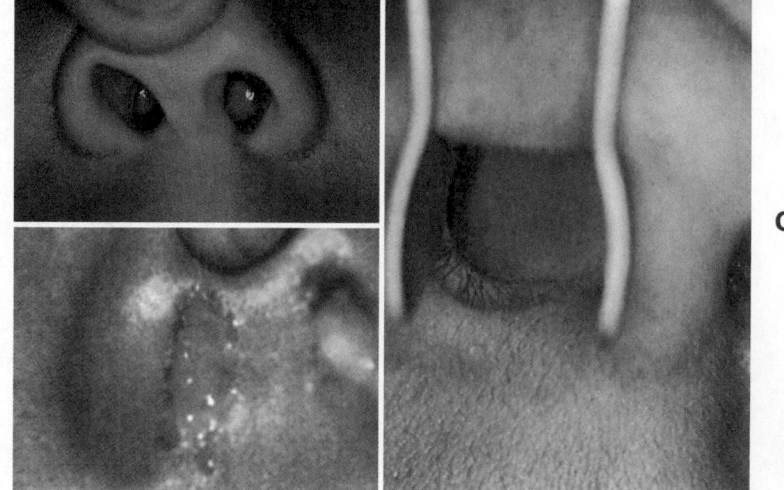

MOUTH AND OROPHARYNX

LIPS

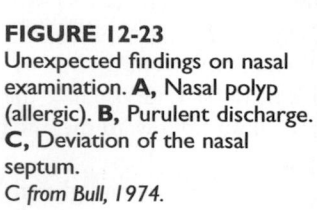

With the patient's mouth closed, inspect and palpate the lips for symmetry, color, edema, and surface abnormalities. Make sure the female patient removes her lipstick. The lips should be pink and have vertical and horizontal symmetry, both at rest and with movement. The distinct vermillion border between the lips and the facial skin should not be interrupted by lesions. The surface characteristics of the lips should be smooth and free of lesions.

Dry, cracked lips (cheilitis) may be caused by dehydration from wind chapping, dentures, braces, or excessive lip licking. Deep fissures at the corners of the mouth (cheilosis) may indicate riboflavin deficiency or overclosure of the mouth, allowing saliva to macerate the tissue. Swelling of the lips may be caused by infection, whereas angioedema may indicate allergy. Lesions, plaques, vesicles, nodules, and ulcerations may be signs of infections, irritations, or skin cancer (Fig. 12-24, *A-E*).

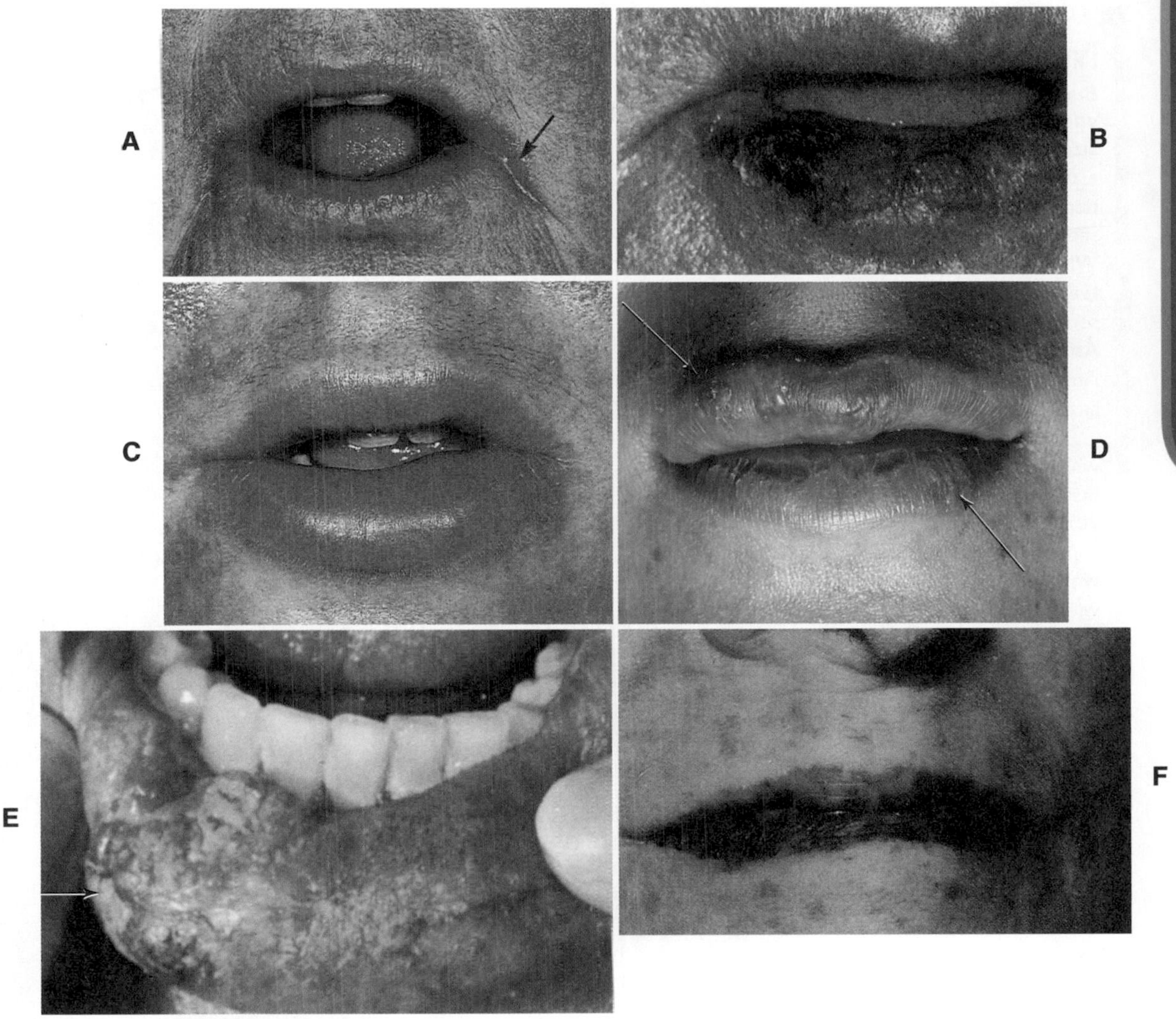

FIGURE 12-24
Unexpected findings on the lips. **A,** Angular cheilitis. **B,** Actinic cheilitis. **C,** Angioedema. **D,** Herpes labialis. **E,** Squamous cell carcinoma of the lip. **F,** Peutz-Jeghers syndrome.
A-C *from Habif, 2004;* D *courtesy Antoinette Hood, MD, University of Indiana, School of Medicine, Indianapolis;* E *from Stewart, Danto, Maddin, 1978;* F *from Chessell et al, 1984.*

PHYSICAL VARIATIONS

Lip Pits

Lip pits, slight dimpling to 4 mm deep, are sometimes found in the commissure of the lips. They are benign and often occur along with preauricular pits. Lip pits occur in approximately 20% of blacks, 12% of whites, and 7% of Asians.

Data from Schaumann, Peagler, Gorlin, 1970.

The color of the lips is influenced by various conditions. Pallor of the lips is associated with anemia, whereas circumoral pallor is associated with scarlet fever. Cyanosis from a respiratory or cardiovascular problem produces bluish purple lips. A cherry red color is associated with acidosis and carbon monoxide poisoning. Round, oval, or irregular bluish gray macules of various intensity on the lips and buccal mucosa are associated with Peutz-Jeghers syndrome (Fig. 12-24, *F*).

BUCCAL MUCOSA, TEETH, AND GUMS

Ears, Nose, and Throat: Inspecting the Buccal Mucosa, Teeth, and Gums

Ask the patient to clench his or her teeth and smile so you can observe the occlusion of the teeth. The facial nerve (cranial nerve VII) is also tested with this maneuver. Proper tooth occlusion is apparent when the upper molars interdigitate with the groove on the lower molars and the premolars and canines interdigitate fully (Fig. 12-25). Protrusion of the upper or lower incisors, failure of the upper incisors to overlap with the lower incisors, and back teeth that do not meet are indications of malocclusion and problems with the bite (Fig. 12-26). Three classes of malocclusion are listed in Table 12-3. Variations in malocclusion are defined in Box 12-1.

PHYSICAL VARIATIONS

Buccal Mucosa, Teeth, and Gums

Size differences in teeth are especially apparent if patients of several races are seen within a short time. Whites have the smallest teeth, and blacks have somewhat larger teeth; Asians and Native Americans/American Indians have the largest teeth.

Leukoedema, a grayish-white benign lesion of the buccal mucosa, occurs in 70% to 90% of blacks and approximately 40% of whites. The lesions increase with age in all races.

Oral hyperpigmentation, another common benign finding, increases with age; 10% of whites have it by 50 years of age, whereas 50% to 90% of blacks have it by the same age.

Data from Merz et al, 1991; Dahlberg, 1963; Martin, Crump, 1972; Wasserman, 1974.

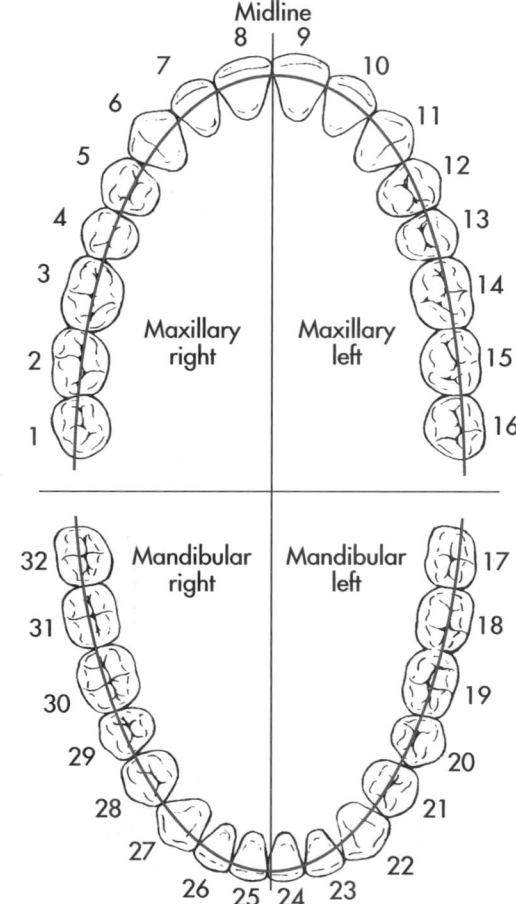

FIGURE 12-25
The line of occlusion and American Dental Association sequential tooth numbering system.
Modified from Miyasaki-Ching, 1997.

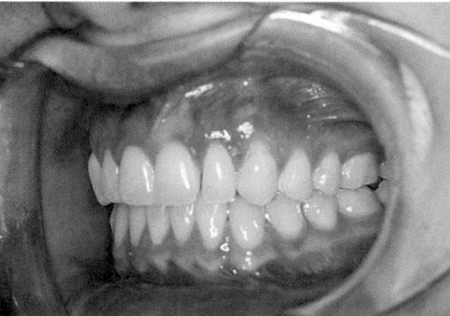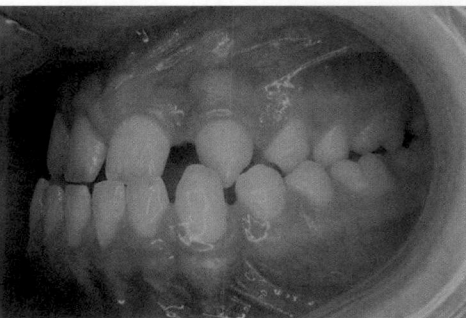

A

B

FIGURE 12-26
A, Class I malocclusion.
B, Class III malocclusion.
Courtesy Drs. Abelson and Cameron, Lutherville, MD.

TABLE 12-3	Classification of Malocclusion
Classification	**Characteristics**
Class I	Molars have customary relationship, but the line of occlusion is incorrect because of malpositioned teeth from rotation or other causes
Class II	Lower molars are distally positioned in relation to the upper molars; the line of occlusion may or may not be correct
Class III	Lower molars are medially positioned in relation to the upper molars; the line of occlusion may or may not be correct.

> **BOX 12-1**
>
> **VARIATIONS IN MALOCCLUSION**
>
> • Overbite is the amount of overlap of the maxillary incisors over the mandibular incisors.
> • Open bite occurs when the incisors do not overlap each other at all, resulting in an open space between the incisors when the molars meet.
> • Cross bite occurs when the maxilla anterior teeth are behind the mandibular anterior teeth, or the maxillary posterior teeth are lingual to their typical position or lateral to the mandibular posterior teeth.

Have the patient remove any dental appliances and open the mouth partially. Using a tongue blade and bright light, inspect the buccal mucosa, gums, and teeth. The mucous membrane should be pinkish red, smooth, and moist. The Stensen duct should appear as a whitish yellow or whitish pink protrusion in approximate alignment with the second upper molar. When swelling is noted around the Stensen duct, use gloved hands to milk the tissue toward the Stensen duct. A small amount of clear saliva is expected. Small stones or exudate coming from Stensen duct is unexpected.

Fordyce spots are ectopic sebaceous glands that appear on the buccal mucosa and lips as numerous small, yellow-white, raised lesions; they are an expected variant (Fig. 12-27, *A*). Deeply pigmented buccal mucosa may indicate an endocrine pathologic condition. Whitish or pinkish scars are a common result of trauma from poor tooth alignment. A red spot on the buccal mucosa at the opening of the Stensen duct is associated with parotitis (mumps). Aphthous ulcers on the buccal mucosa appear as white, round, or oval ulcerative lesions with a red halo (Fig. 12-27, *B*). A thickened white patch lesion that cannot be wiped away may be leukoplakia, a premalignant oral lesion.

The gingiva should have a slightly stippled, pink appearance with a clearly defined, tight margin at each tooth. The gum surface beneath dentures should be free of inflammation, swelling, or bleeding.

Using gloves, palpate the gums for any lesions, induration, thickening, or masses. No tenderness on palpation should be elicited. Epulis, a localized gingival enlargement or granuloma, is usually an inflammatory rather than neoplastic change. Enlargement of the gums occurs with pregnancy, puberty, phenytoin (Dilantin) therapy, and leukemia. A blue-black line about 1 mm from the gum margin may indicate chronic lead or bismuth poisoning. Easily bleeding, swollen gums that have enlarged crevices between the teeth and gum margins, or pockets containing debris at tooth margins, are associated with gingivitis or periodontal disease (Fig. 12-28).

Inspect and count the teeth, noting wear, notches, caries, and missing teeth. Make sure teeth are firmly anchored, probing each with a tongue blade. The teeth generally have an ivory color but may be stained yellow from tobacco or brown from coffee or tea. Loose teeth can be the result of periodontal disease or trauma. Discolorations on the crown of a tooth should raise the suspicion of caries.

ORAL CAVITY

Inspect the dorsum of the tongue, noting any swelling, variation in size or color, coating, or ulcerations. Ask the patient to extend the tongue while you inspect for deviation, tremor, and limitation of movement. The procedure also tests the hypoglossal nerve (cranial nerve XII).

FIGURE 12-27
Findings on the buccal mucosa. **A,** Fordyce spots. **B,** Aphthous ulcer.
A from Wood, Goaz, 1991; B courtesy Antoinette Hood, MD, Indiana University School of Medicine, Indianapolis.

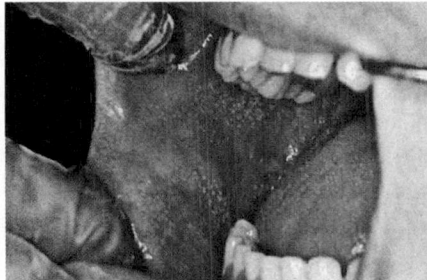 A

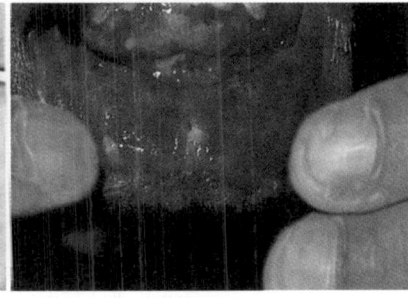 B

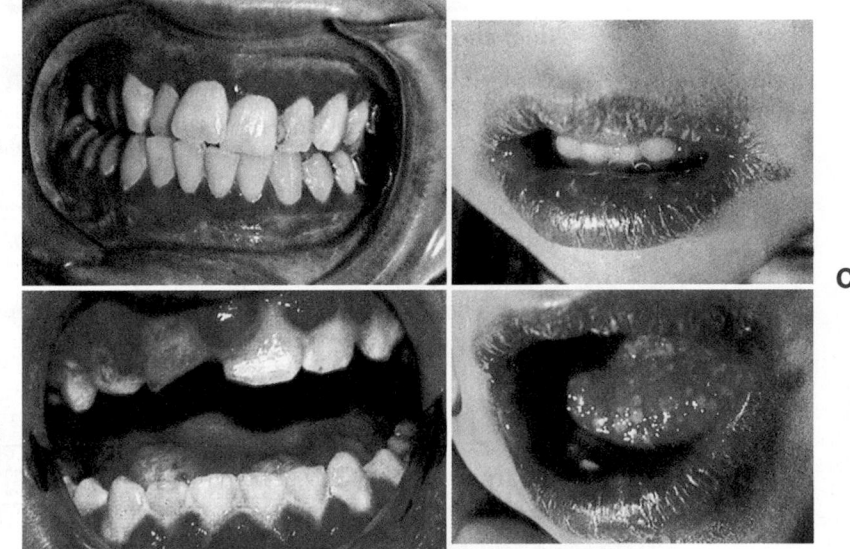

FIGURE 12-28
Unexpected findings of the gingiva. **A,** Plasma cell gingivitis. **B,** Primary herpetic gingivostomatitis. **C,** Primary gingivostomatitis showing lesions on the lips *(upper photo)* and tongue and gums *(lower photo)*.
A, B *from Wood, Goaz, 1991; C reproduced with permission of the Wellcome Foundation Ltd.*

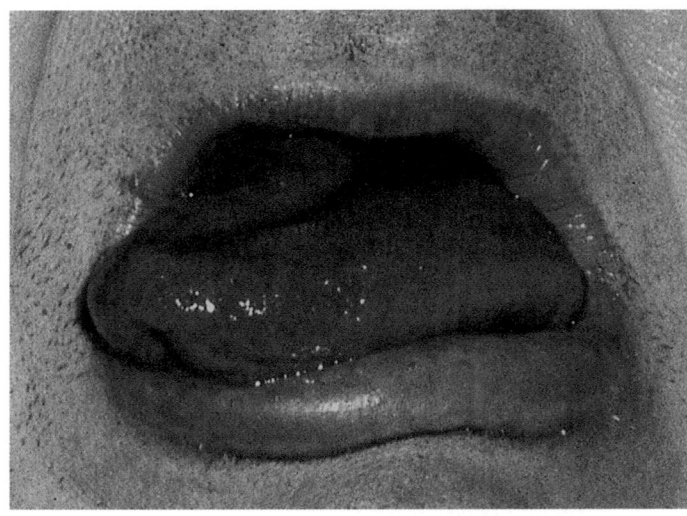

FIGURE 12-29
Left hypoglossal paralysis. The tongue deviates toward the weak side. Note atrophy on the right side of the tongue.
Courtesy Daniel M. Laskin, DDS, MS, Medical College of Virginia, Virginia Commonwealth University, Richmond, VA.

The protruded tongue should not be atrophied and should be maintained at the midline without fasciculations. Deviation to one side indicates tongue atrophy and hypoglossal nerve impairment (Fig. 12-29).

The tongue should appear dull red, moist, and glistening. Its anterior portion should have a smooth, yet roughened surface with papillae and small fissures. The posterior portion should have rugae or a smooth, slightly uneven surface with a thinner mucosa than the anterior portion. The geographic tongue, an expected variant, has superficial denuded circles or irregular areas exposing the tips of papillae. A smooth red tongue with a slick appearance may indicate a niacin or vitamin B_{12} deficiency. The hairy tongue with yellow-brown to black elongated papillae on the dorsum sometimes follows antibiotic therapy (Fig. 12-30).

Ask the patient to touch the tongue tip to the palate area directly behind the upper incisors. Inspect the floor of the mouth and the ventral surface of the tongue for swelling and varicosities, also observing the frenulum, sublingual ridge, and Wharton ducts. The tip of the tongue should have no difficulty touching the hard palate behind the upper central incisors. The ventral surface of the tongue should be pink and smooth with large veins between the frenulum and fimbriated folds. Wharton ducts should be apparent on each side of the frenulum.

Wrapping the tongue with a piece of gauze, pull the tongue to each side, inspecting its lateral borders (Fig. 12-31). Any white or red margins should be scraped to differentiate food

A   B   C

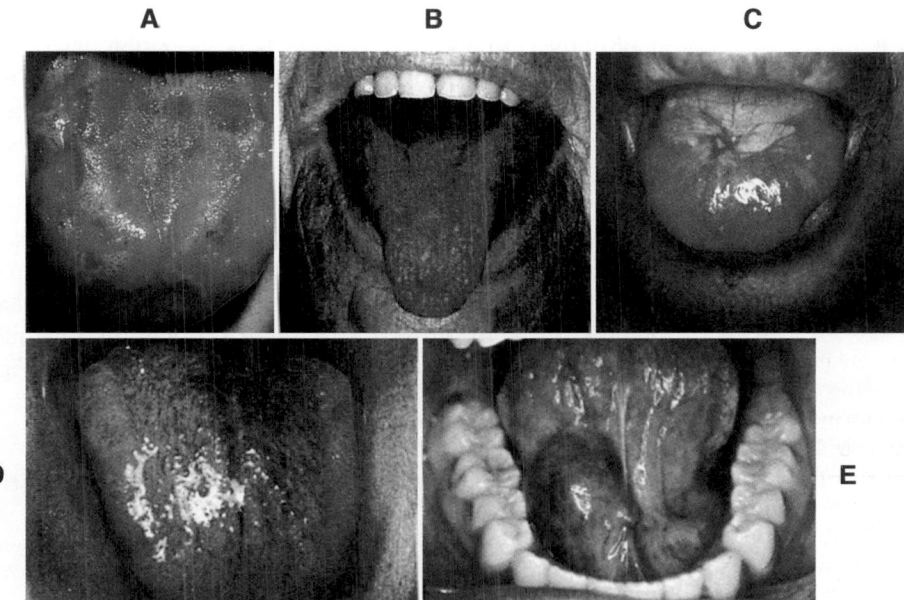

FIGURE 12-30
Findings on the tongue.
A, Geographic tongue.
B, Smooth tongue resulting from vitamin deficiency.
C, Glossitis. **D,** Black hairy tongue. **E,** Dome-shaped varicosity resembling a ranula.
A, C *courtesy Antoinette Hood, MD, Indiana University School of Medicine, Indianapolis; D from Wood, Goaz, 1991; E from Bull, 1974.*

D   E

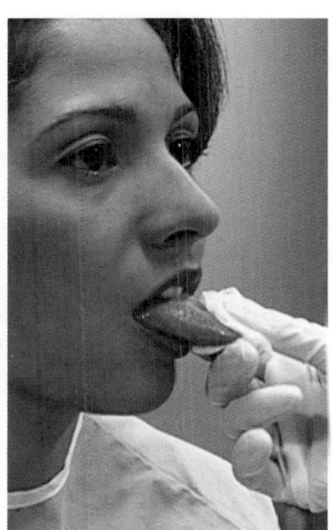

FIGURE 12-31
Inspection of lateral borders of the tongue.

STAYING WELL

SCREENING FOR ORAL CANCER

Carefully examine each of the following areas of the oral cavity, face, and neck to detect signs of oral cancer:
- Inspect the vermilion border of the lips (a high-risk site).
- Inspect the maxillary and mandibular labial mucosa, the attached gingival tissues, alveolar gingival mucosa, and vestibule by raising and lowering the lips.
- Inspect the buccal mucosa.
- Inspect the hard palate.
- Inspect the dorsal surface of the tongue, and with the tongue extended right, the left lateral and ventral surfaces of the tongue and lateral floor of the mouth. Inspect the right tongue surfaces with the tongue extended left.
- Inspect the anterior floor of the mouth.
- Palpate the floor of the mouth with a gloved finger while simultaneously using the thumb to compress tissue behind the mandible.
- Inspect and palpate the throat, neck, and temporomandibular areas.

Marder, 1998.

PHYSICAL VARIATIONS

Mandible and Uvula

A bony protuberance, the mandibular torus, occurs on the lingual surface of the mandible, near the canine and premolar teeth, and is an expected variant. Fewer than 10% of blacks and whites have mandibular tori; Asians and Native Americans/American Indians have them more commonly. The only difficulty with tori is that they cause denture fitting problems.

Sometimes the uvula is cleft into two sections. It may vary from a fishtail effect to two complete uvulas. Clefting is rare in blacks; about 2% of whites have it; around 10% of Asians have it; and some Native American/American Indian tribes have as much as an 18% incidence. Cleft uvula is a benign condition, but it is a subclinical manifestation of cleft palate.

Data from Halffman, Scott, Pedersen, 1992; Axelsson, Hedegard, 1981; Jarvis, Gorlin, 1972; Meskin, Gorlin, Isaacson, 1965; Wharton, Mowrer, 1992.

particles from leukoplakia or another fixed abnormality. Then palpate the tongue and the floor of the mouth for lumps, nodules, or ulceration.

The tongue should have a smooth, even texture without nodules, ulcerations, or areas of induration. Any ulcer, nodule, or thickened white patch on the lateral or ventral surface of the tongue may be suggestive of malignancy. Table 12-4 presents the oral manifestations of human immunodeficiency virus (HIV) infection.

Ask the patient to tilt his or her head back for you to inspect the palate and uvula. The whitish hard palate should be dome shaped with transverse rugae. The pinker soft palate should be contiguous with the hard palate. The uvula, a midline continuation of the soft palate, varies in length and thickness. The hard palate may have a bony protuberance at the midline, called torus palatinus, which has no clinical consequence (Fig. 12-32). A nodule on the palate that is not at the midline may indicate a tumor. Fig. 12-33 shows oral Kaposi sarcoma, both a moderately advanced and an advanced lesion.

TABLE 12-4	Oral Manifestations of HIV Infection
Lesion	**Characteristics**
Oral hairy leukoplakia	White, irregular lesions on lateral side of tongue or buccal mucosa; may have prominent folds or "hairy" projections
Angular cheilitis	Red, unilateral or bilateral fissures at corners of mouth
Candidiasis	Creamy white plaques on oral mucosa that bleed when scraped
Herpes simplex	Recurrent vesicular, crusting lesions on the vermilion border of the lip
Herpes zoster	Vesicular and ulcerative oral lesions in the distribution of the trigeminal nerve; may also be on gingiva
Human papillomavirus	Single or multiple, sessile or pedunculated nodules in the oral cavity
Aphthous ulcers	Recurrent circumscribed ulcers with an erythematous margin
Periodontal disease	In a mouth with little plaque or calculus, gingivitis with bone and soft tissue degeneration accompanied by severe pain
Kaposi sarcoma	In the mouth, incompletely formed blood vessels proliferate, forming lesions of various shades and size as blood extravasates in response to the malignant tumor of the epithelium

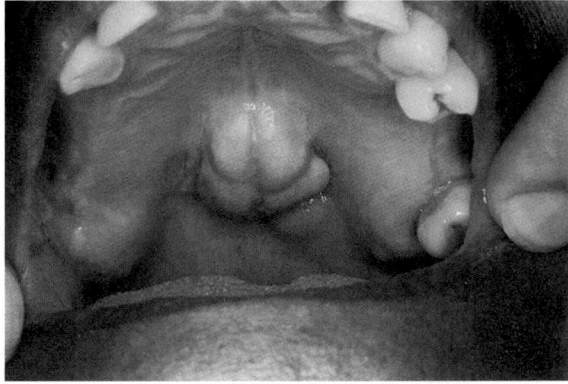

FIGURE 12-32
Torus palatinus.
Courtesy Drs. Abelson and Cameron, Lutherville, MD.

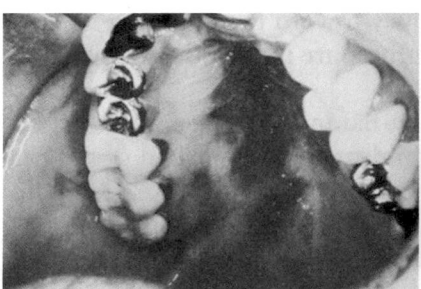 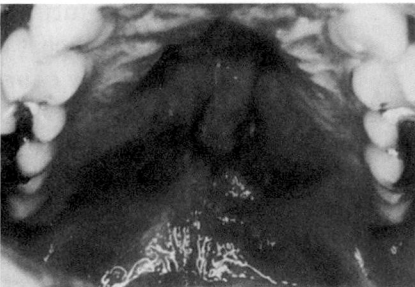

A

B

FIGURE 12-33
Oral Kaposi sarcoma.
A, Moderately advanced.
B, Advanced lesion.
From Grimes, 1991; courtesy Sol Silverman Jr., DDS, University of California, San Francisco.

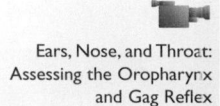

Ears, Nose, and Throat:
Assessing the Oropharynx
and Gag Reflex

Movement of the soft palate is evaluated by asking the patient to say "ah." Depressing the tongue may be necessary for this maneuver. As the patient vocalizes, observe the soft palate rise symmetrically with the uvula remaining in the midline. This maneuver also tests the glossopharyngeal and vagus nerves (cranial nerves IX and X). Failure of the soft palate to rise bilaterally with vocalization may result from paralysis of the vagus nerve. The uvula will deviate to the unaffected side.

OROPHARYNX

> ### CLINICAL PEARL
> **Use of a Tongue Blade**
> A patient of any age may anticipate the use of the tongue blade with some degree of anxiety. If the patient gags easily, there probably is little you can do to avoid setting off this reflex. Moistening the tongue blade with warm water helps reduce triggering of the gag reflex.

Inspect the oropharynx using a tongue blade to depress the tongue. Observe the tonsillar pillars, noting the size of tonsils, if present, and the integrity of the retropharyngeal wall. The tonsils usually blend into the pink color of the pharynx and should not project beyond the limits of the tonsillar pillars. Tonsils may have crypts where cellular debris and food particles collect. If the tonsils are reddened, hypertrophied, and covered with exudate, an infection may be present (Fig. 12-34).

The posterior wall of the pharynx should be smooth, glistening, pink mucosa with some small, irregular spots of lymphatic tissue and small blood vessels. A red bulge adjacent to the tonsil and extending beyond the midline may indicate a peritonsillar abscess. A yellowish mucoid film in the pharynx is typical of postnasal drip. A grayish adherent membrane is associated with diphtheria.

After preparing the patient for a gag response, touch the posterior wall of the pharynx on each side. Elicitation of the gag reflex tests the glossopharyngeal and vagus nerves (cranial nerves IX and X). Expect a bilateral response.

ADDITIONAL PROCEDURES

EQUILIBRIUM

The Romberg test, described in Chapter 22, is used to screen for equilibrium in most patients. When a vestibular function disorder is suspected by history or by a loss of balance with the Romberg test, further evaluation of the vestibular branch of the auditory nerve (cranial nerve VIII) is indicated. In most cases, the patient is referred to a specialist for the Nylen-Barany test.

For the Nylen-Barany test, the patient should be supine with the head hyperextended about 45 degrees over the end of the examining table. When the patient turns his or her head to one side, observe for nystagmus. Repeat the procedure with the patient's head turned to the other side. Nystagmus is an unexpected finding, and if it is present, note the duration and direction of eye movement (horizontal or vertical).

A   B   C

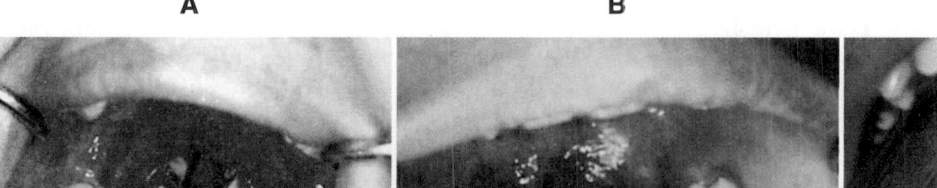
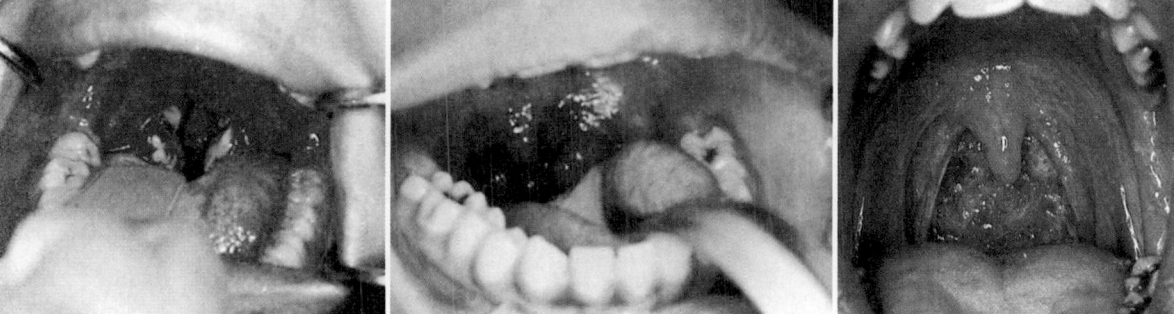

FIGURE 12-34
Findings of the oropharynx. **A,** Tonsillitis and pharyngitis. **B,** Acute viral pharyngitis. **C,** Postnasal drip.
A, B *courtesy Edward L. Applebaum, MD, Head, Department of Otolaryngology, University of Illinois Medical Center, Chicago.*

A   B

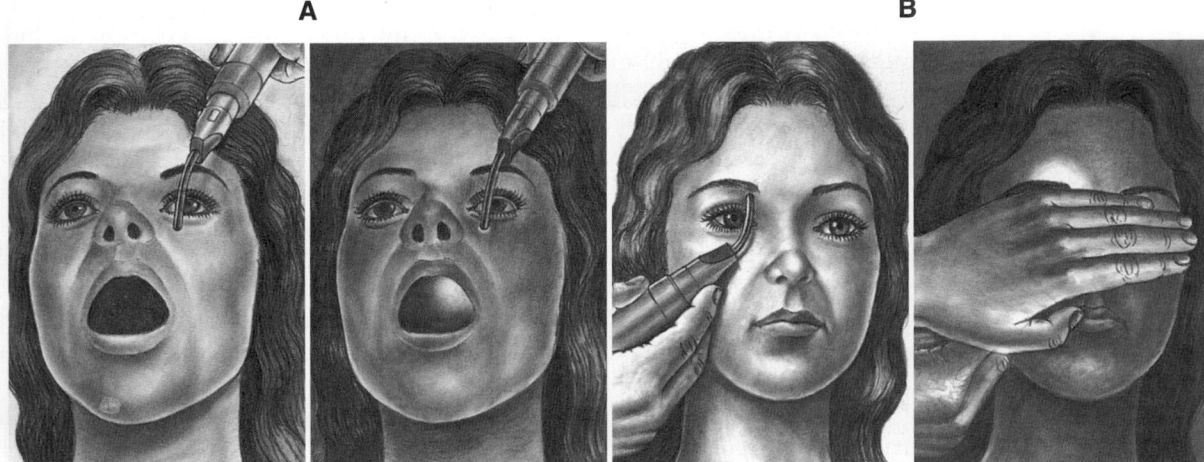

FIGURE 12-35
Transillumination of the sinuses: placement of the light source and expected area of transillumination.
A, For the maxillary sinus. **B,** For the frontal sinus.

TRANSILLUMINATION

Transillumination of the frontal and maxillary sinuses is performed if sinus tenderness is present or infection is suspected (Fig. 12-35). The examination must be performed in a completely darkened room. A sinus transilluminator or small, bright light is used.

To transilluminate the maxillary sinuses, place the light source lateral to the nose, just beneath the medial aspect of the eye. Look through the patient's open mouth for illumination of the hard palate. To transilluminate the frontal sinuses, place the light source against the medial aspect of each supraorbital rim. Look for a dim red glow as light is transmitted just above the eyebrow; however, bilateral findings may vary because the frontal sinuses develop differently. The sinuses may show differing degrees of illumination, opaque (no transillumination), dull (reduced transillumination), or a glow (expected transillumination). An opaque or dull response indicates that either the sinus is filled with secretions or it never developed. Asymmetry of transillumination is a significant finding.

INFANTS

EARS

Because the ears, nose, mouth, and throat are common sites of congenital malformations in the newborn, a thorough examination is important.

The auricle should be well formed, with all landmarks present on inspection. The tip of the auricle should cross the imaginary line between the inner canthus of the eye and the prominent portion of the occiput, varying no more than 10 degrees from vertical. Auricles either poorly shaped or positioned below the imaginary line are associated with renal disorders and congenital anomalies.

The newborn's auricle is very flexible but should have instant recoil after bending. The premature infant's auricles may appear flattened with limited incurving of the upper auricle, and ear recoil is slower.

No skin tags should be present. A small preauricular skin tag or pit is sometimes found just anterior to the tragus, indicating a remnant of the first branchial cleft.

The newborn's auditory canals are often obstructed with vernix, but they should be examined within the first few weeks of life. The tympanic membrane is usually in an extremely oblique position until the infant is 1 month old. The infant is placed in either supine or prone position so the head can be turned side to side. Hold the otoscope so that the ulnar surface of your hand rests against the infant's head, alternating the hand used (i.e.,

TABLE 12-5	The Sequence of Expected Hearing and Speech Response
Age	**Response**
Birth to 3 months	Startle reflex, crying, cessation of breathing or movement in response to sudden noise; quiets to parent's voice; makes vowel sounds "oh" or "ah"
4 to 6 months	Turns head toward source of sound but may not always recognize location of sound; responds to parent's voice; enjoys sound-producing toys; starts babbling
6 to 10 months	Responds to own name, telephone ringing, and person's voice, even if not loud; begins localizing sounds above and below, turns head 45 degrees toward sound; babbles "baba," "mama," "gaga"; begins to imitate speech sounds
10 to 12 months	Recognizes and localizes source of sound; imitates simple words and sounds; understands "no-no" and "bye-bye"; correctly uses "mama" and "dada"

Modified from Caufield, 1978, and American Academy of Audiology, 2002. Newborn hearing screening. Accessed August 7, 2005, from http://www.audiology.org/professional/tech/eihbrochure.php.

right hand for the right ear and left hand for the left ear). As the infant's head moves, the otoscope moves, preventing trauma to the auditory canal. Use your other hand to stabilize the infant's head as the thumb and index finger pull the auricle down to straighten the upward curvature of the canal. Because the tympanic membrane does not become conical for several months, the light reflex may appear diffuse. Limited mobility, dullness, and opacity of a pink or red tympanic membrane may be noted in neonates. As the middle ear matures during the infant's first months of life, the tympanic membrane takes on the expected appearance.

Audiologic evaluation is now recommended for all newborns, but hearing should continue to be evaluated at regular intervals. Knowledge of the sequence of hearing development is necessary to evaluate the infant's hearing (Table 12-5). Use a bell, your voice, or clap your hands as a sound stimulus, taking care that the infant does not respond to the air movement generated by any of these maneuvers. Remember that responses to repeated sound stimuli will diminish as the infant tunes out the stimulus.

NOSE AND SINUSES

The external nose should have a symmetric appearance and be positioned in the vertical midline of the face. Only minimal movement of the nares with breathing should be apparent. A deviation from midline of the nose may be related to fetal position. A saddle-shaped nose with a low bridge and broad base, a short small nose, or a large nose may suggest a congenital anomaly.

Inspect the internal nose by shining a light inside after gently tilting the nose tip upward with your thumb. Small amounts of clear fluid discharge may be seen in infants when crying.

Newborns are obligatory nose breathers, so nasal patency must be determined at the time of birth. With the infant's mouth closed, occlude one naris and then the other, observing the respiratory pattern. With total obstruction, the infant will not be able to inspire or expire through the noncompressed naris. With any breathing difficulty, a small catheter is passed through each naris to the choana, the posterior nasal opening to assess patency. An obstruction may indicate choanal atresia or septal deviation from delivery trauma.

Because the maxillary and ethmoid sinuses are small during infancy, few problems arise in these areas, and examination is generally unnecessary.

MOUTH

The lips should be well formed with no cleft. The newborn may have sucking calluses on the upper lips for the first few weeks of life; these appear as plaques or crusts. Healthy newborns may have circumoral cyanosis at birth and for a short while afterward.

The crying infant provides an opportunity to examine the mouth. Avoid depressing the tongue because this stimulates a strong reflex protrusion, making visualization of the mouth difficult.

The buccal mucosa should be pink and moist with sucking pads but have no other lesions. Scrape any white patches on the tongue or buccal mucosa with a tongue blade. Nonadherent patches are usually milk deposits, whereas adherent patches may indicate candidiasis (thrush) (Fig. 12-36, *A*). Secretions that accumulate in the newborn's mouth requiring frequent suctioning may indicate esophageal atresia.

Drooling is common in infants between 6 weeks and 6 months of age; however, it may be indicative of a neurologic disorder in infants older than 12 months of age.

The newborn's gums should be edentulous, smooth with a serrated edge of tissue along the buccal margins. Occasionally you will find a tooth or tooth buds in a newborn (Fig. 12-36, *B*). Determine whether natal teeth are loose and whether there is potential for aspiration. Such teeth are not usually firmly fixed and it is probably wisest, in most instances, to remove them. Consult the parents first, however. In older infants, count the deciduous teeth, noting any unusual sequence of eruption. Pearl-like retention cysts that sometimes appear along the buccal margin disappear in 1 to 2 months.

The tongue should fit well in the floor of the mouth. The frenulum of the tongue usually attaches at a point midway between the ventral surface of the tongue and its tip (Fig. 12-36, *C*). If the tongue protrudes beyond the alveolar ridge, no feeding difficulties should occur. Macroglossia is associated with congenital anomalies such as congenital hypothyroidism—another reminder that external clues to pathophysiologically severe problems abound (Fig. 12-36, *D*). The palatal arch should be dome shaped with no clefts in either the hard or soft

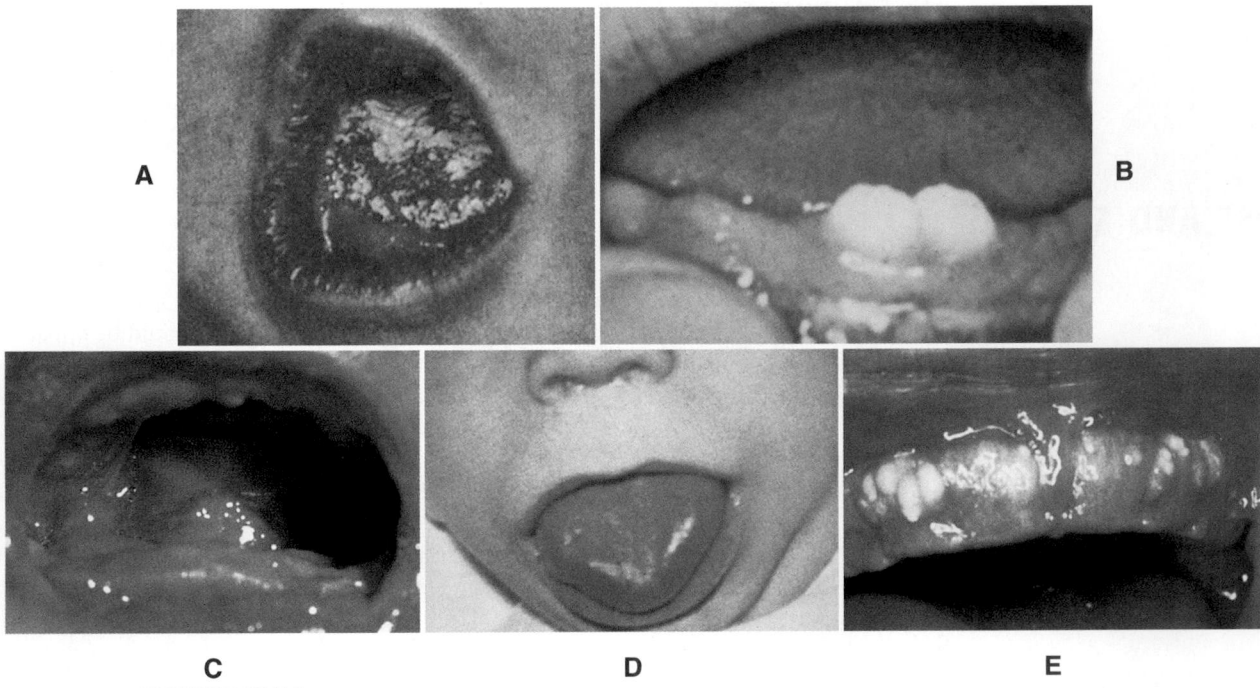

FIGURE 12-36
Findings in the infant's mouth. **A,** Thrush. **B,** Natal teeth. **C,** Short frenulum. **D,** Macroglossia. **E,** Epstein pearls.
Courtesy Mead Johnson & Co., Evansville, IN.

palate. A narrow, flat palate roof or a high, arched palate (associated with congenital anomalies) will affect the tongue's placement and lead to feeding and speech problems. The soft palate should rise symmetrically when the infant cries. Petechiae are often seen on the newborn's soft palate. Epstein pearls—small, whitish-yellow masses at the juncture between the hard and soft palate—are common and disappear within a few weeks after birth (Fig. 12-36, *E*).

Insert your gloved index finger into the infant's mouth, with the fingerpad to the roof of the mouth. Simultaneously evaluate the infant's suck and palpate the hard and soft palates. (This maneuver may be performed when quieting the infant to auscultate the heart and lungs.) The infant should have a strong suck, the tongue pushing vigorously upward against the finger. Neither the hard nor soft palate should have palpable clefts. Stimulate the gag reflex by touching the tonsillar pillars. A bilateral gag reflex should be present.

CHILDREN

Because the young child often resists otoscopic and oral examination, it may be wise to postpone these procedures until the end. Be prepared to immobilize if encouraging the child to cooperate fails. Another person, usually the parent, may be needed to effectively hold the child.

Children of any age who are not too big to sit on their parent's lap are better examined there rather than in a prone or supine position on the examining table. If the baby or toddler is comfortably seated in the parent's lap, with the back to the parent's chest and legs between the adult's legs, the parent can then reach comfortably around to restrain the child's arms with one arm and control the child's head with the other. The otoscopic and oral examinations can usually be accomplished without forcing, avoiding extra stress for the child, the parent, and you (Fig. 12-37, *A*).

To perform the otoscopic examination on an older toddler, face the child sideways with one arm placed around the parent's waist. The parent holds the child firmly against his or her trunk, using one arm to restrain the child's head and the other arm to restrain the child's body. You further stabilize the child's head as you insert the otoscope. For the oral examination, face the child forward.

When the child actively resists your efforts to examine the ears and mouth, place him or her in supine position on the examining table. The parent holds the child's arms extended above the head and assists in immobilizing the head. You lie across the child's trunk and stabilize the child's head with your hands as you insert the otoscope or tongue blade. A third person may hold the child's legs, if necessary (Fig. 12-37, *B*).

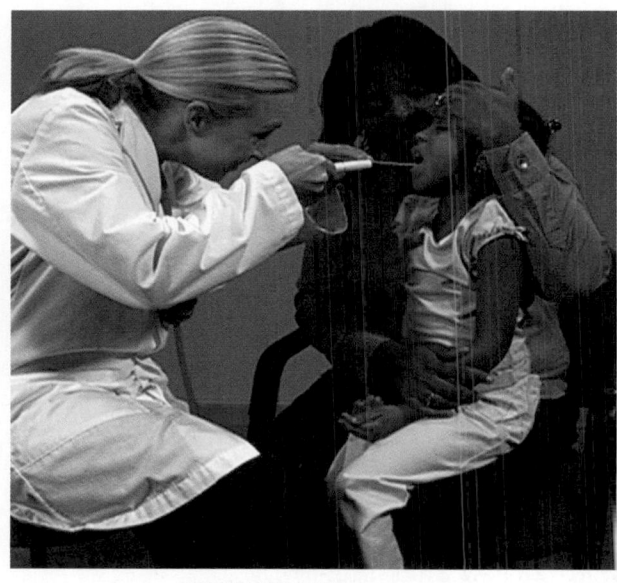

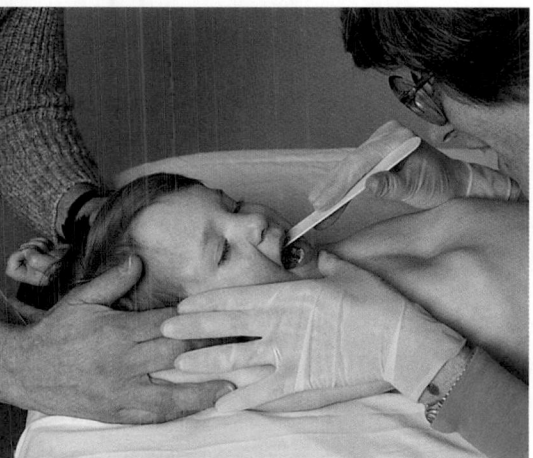

FIGURE 12-37
Positioning of toddler for oral examination. **A,** Sitting position. **B,** Supine position.

EARS

When performing the otoscopic examination, pull the auricle either downward and back or upward and back to gain the best view of the tympanic membrane. As the child grows, the shape of the auditory canal changes to the S-shaped curve of the adult. If the child is crying or has recently cried vigorously, dilation of blood vessels in the tympanic membrane can cause redness. Thus you cannot assume that redness of the membrane alone is a hallmark of acute otitis media. The pneumatic otoscope is especially important for differentiating a red tympanic membrane caused by crying (the membrane is mobile) from that resulting from disease (no mobility). Tympanometry provides an accurate way to identify middle ear effusion (Fig. 12-38). Make sure the earpiece is sealed in the canal.

Evaluate the toddler's hearing by observing the response to a whispered voice and various noisemakers (e.g., rattle, bell, or tissue paper). Position yourself behind the child while the parent distracts the child. Whisper or use noisemakers outside of the child's field of vision. The child should turn toward the sound consistently. Development of speech provides another indication of hearing acuity. When whispering, particularly to children, use words that will have more meaning for them, such as the name of a popular television personality or a comic strip character (e.g., Big Bird, Mickey Mouse, Spider Man).

In addition to these procedures, evaluate the young child's hearing by asking the child to perform tasks, using a soft voice. Avoid giving visual cues. The Weber and Rinne tests are used when the child understands directions and can cooperate with the examiner, usually between 3 and 4 years of age. Audiometric evaluation should be performed in all young children.

NOSE AND SINUSES

As with infants, when inspecting the internal nose, it is usually adequate to tilt the nose tip upward with your thumb; however, if visualization of a larger area is needed, the largest otoscope speculum may be used.

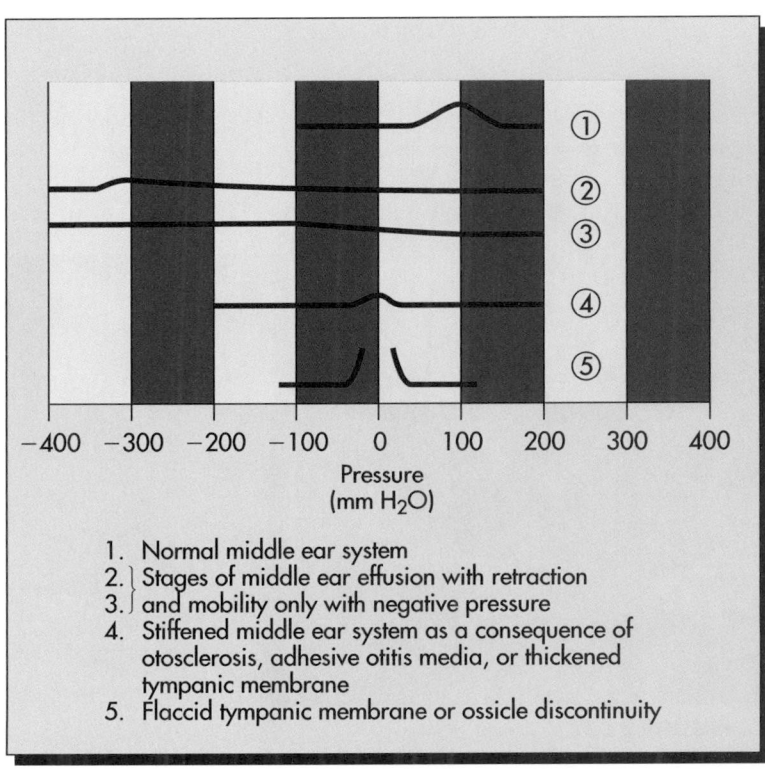

FIGURE 12-38
Tympanometric configuration for middle ear conditions.

1. Normal middle ear system
2. } Stages of middle ear effusion with retraction
3. } and mobility only with negative pressure
4. Stiffened middle ear system as a consequence of otosclerosis, adhesive otitis media, or thickened tympanic membrane
5. Flaccid tympanic membrane or ossicle discontinuity

The transverse crease at the juncture between the cartilage and the bone of the nose is often the result of the "adenoidal" or "allergic salute." Children are particularly prone to wipe their noses with an upward sweep of the palm of the hand, which if repeated often enough, causes the crease (see Figure 12-20).

The maxillary sinuses may be palpated as they are developed by 4 years of age. The frontal sinuses may be palpated by 5 to 6 years of age when they are developed. Note any tenderness indicating a potential sinus infection in the child with an upper respiratory infection that has not improved after 10 days (Leung & Kellner, 2004).

MOUTH

Encourage the child to cooperate with the oral examination. Letting the child hold and manipulate the tongue blade and light may reduce the fear of the procedure. Begin by asking the child to show you his or her teeth, usually not a threatening request. Flattened edges on the teeth may indicate bruxism, unconscious grinding of the teeth. Multiple brown areas or caries on the upper and lower incisors may be the result of a bedtime bottle of juice or milk, commonly called "baby bottle syndrome" (Fig. 12-39). Teeth with a black or gray color may indicate pulp decay or oral iron therapy. Mottled or pitted teeth are often the result of tetracycline treatment during tooth development or enamel dysplasia. Chalky white lines or speckles on the cutting edges of permanent incisors may result from excessive fluoride intake.

If the child will protrude the tongue and say "ah," the tongue blade is often unnecessary for the oral examination. Ask the child to "pant like a puppy" to raise the palate. When the child refuses to open the mouth, insert a tongue blade through the lips to the back molars. Gently but firmly insert the tongue blade between the back molars and press the tongue blade to the tongue. This maneuver should stimulate the gag reflex and give you a brief view of the mouth and oropharynx.

Koplik spots, white specks with a red base on the buccal mucosa opposite the first and second molars, occur with rubeola in a child with fever, coryza, and cough. A highly arched palate may be observed in children who are chronic mouth breathers.

The tonsils, lying deep in the oral cavity, should blend with the color of the pharynx. They gradually enlarge to their peak size between 2 and 6 years of age, but the oropharynx should retain an unobstructed passage. Enlarged tonsils are graded to describe their size (Fig. 12-40).

If the tonsils appear pushed backward or forward, possibly displacing the uvula, consider a peritonsillar abscess.

When the tongue is depressed, the epiglottis is visible as a glistening pink structure behind the base of the tongue.

PREGNANT WOMEN

Edema and erythema in the nose and pharynx of the pregnant woman result from the increased vascularization of the respiratory tract with increased secretion of mucus due to increased estrogen production. Nosebleeds may occur. Tympanic membranes may have increased vascularity and be retracted or bulging with serous fluid. The gums may appear red-

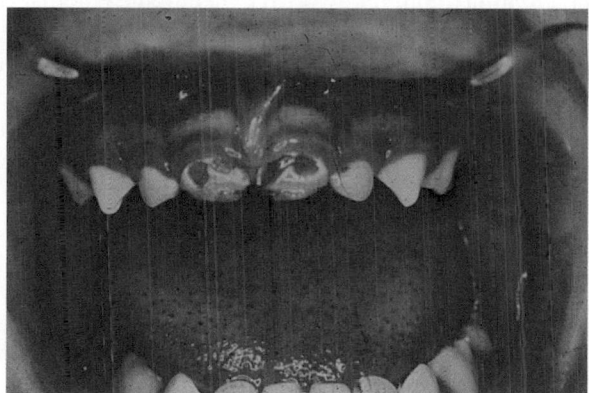

FIGURE 12-39
Baby bottle syndrome.
Courtesy Drs. Abelson and Cameron, Lutherville, MD.

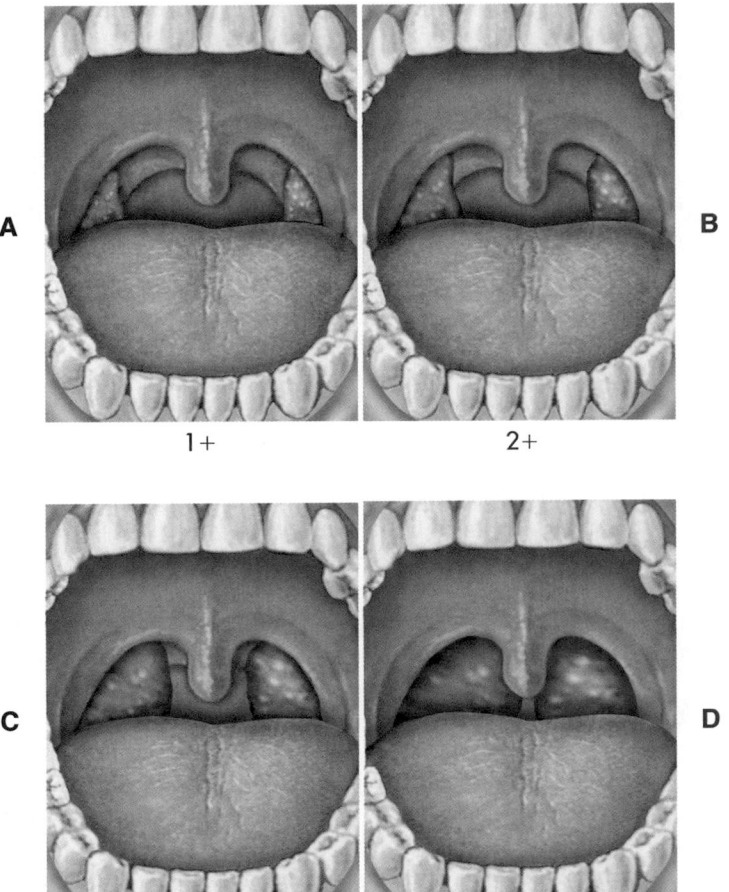

1+

2+

3+

4+

FIGURE 12-40
Enlarged tonsils are graded to describe their size: **A,** 1+, visible; **B,** 2+, halfway between tonsillar pillars and the uvula; **C,** 3+, nearly touching the uvula; **D,** 4+, touching each other.

dened, swollen, and spongy, with the hypertrophy resolving within 2 months of delivery. Often there is an increased incidence of nasal congestion and sinusitis or cold symptoms throughout the pregnancy (Gordon, 2002).

OLDER ADULTS

EARS AND HEARING

Inspect the auditory canal of the patient who wears a hearing aid for areas of irritation from the ear mold. Coarse, wirelike hairs are often present along the periphery of the auricle. On otoscopic examination, the tympanic membrane landmarks may appear slightly more pronounced from sclerotic changes.

Some degree of sensorineural hearing deterioration with advancing age (presbycusis) may be noted. This is marked by greater difficulty understanding speech, particularly consonants, rather than a reduction in all sounds heard. Problems are most prominent when the patient is in a room with considerable background noise. Conductive hearing loss from otosclerosis and cerumen impaction may also occur.

NOSE

The nasal mucosa may appear dryer, less glistening. An increased number of bristly hairs in the vestibule are common, especially in men.

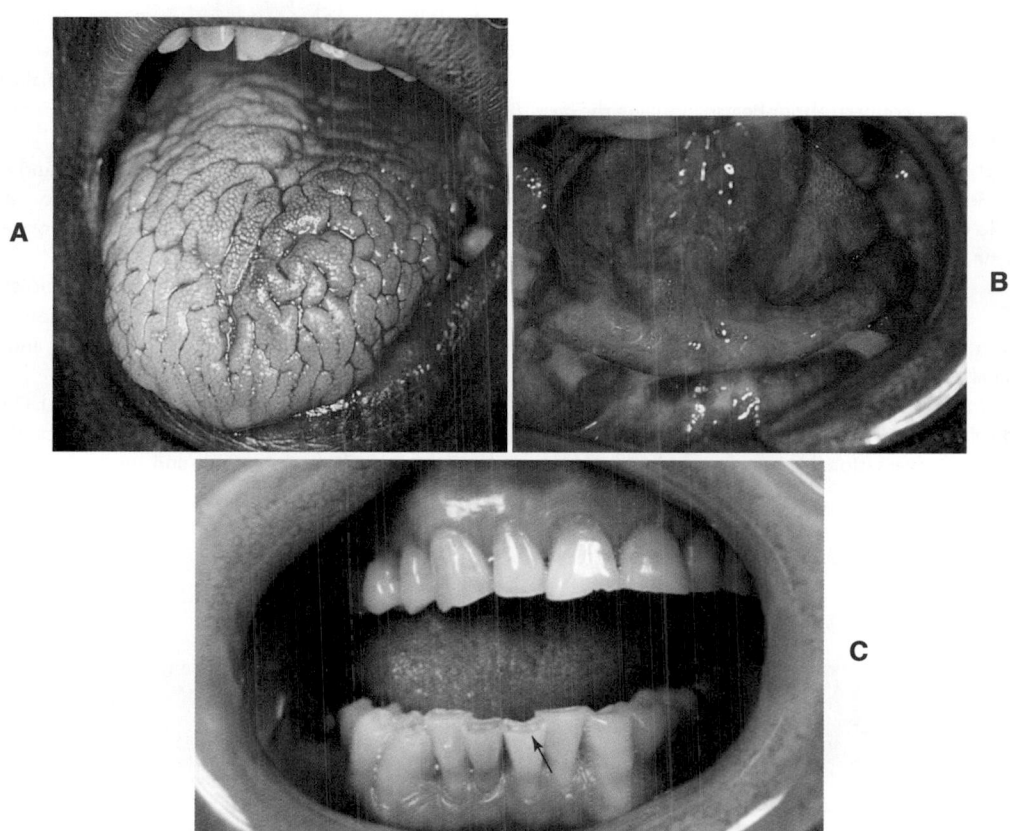

FIGURE 12-41
Common findings in the older adult's mouth. **A,** Fissured tongue. **B,** Varicose veins on tongue. **C,** Attrition of teeth and resorption of gums.
A, B *courtesy Drs. Abelson and Cameron, Lutherville, MD; C courtesy Daniel M. Laskin, DDS, MS, Medical College of Virginia, Virginia Commonwealth University, Richmond, VA.*

Functional Assessment

Ears, Nose, and Throat

The ability to perform activities of daily living is often dependent on the person's ability to hear, speak, chew food, and swallow. Hearing and speech are important for the personal social components of the functional assessment. The ability to chew and swallow food is important for adequate nutrition. When the patient has dentures, a hearing aid, or other assistive device, evaluate how effectively the patient uses these devices and is able to care for them.

MOUTH

The lips have increased vertical markings and appear dryer when salivary flow is reduced. The buccal mucosa is thinner, less vascular, and less shiny than that of the younger adult. The tongue may appear more fissured, and veins on its ventral surface may appear varicose (Fig. 12-41).

Many adults older than 65 years of age are edentulous. Natural teeth may be worn down, and dental restorations may have deteriorated. The teeth often appear longer as resorption of the gum and bone progresses. Dental malocclusion is commonly caused by the migration of remaining teeth after extractions. The lower jaw may protrude in patients with a stooping and head-thrusting posture.

SAMPLE DOCUMENTATION

HISTORY AND PHYSICAL EXAMINATION

Subjective

A 55-year-old man with concern about hearing loss for the past few months, particularly with high-pitched tones. Has difficulty hearing on the phone and in conversations when multiple people are talking. Hears noise in both ears when trying to go to sleep at night. No ear pain. No nasal discharge or sinus pain. No mouth lesions or masses, no recent dental problems, no sore throat.

Objective

Ears: Auricles in alignment, lobes without masses, lesions, or tenderness. Canals totally obstructed by cerumen. After irrigation, tympanic membranes are pearly gray, intact, with bony landmarks and light reflex visualized bilaterally. No evidence of fluid or retraction. Conversational hearing appropriate. Able to

hear whispered voice. Weber—lateralizes equally to both ears; Rinne—air conduction greater than bone conduction bilaterally (30 sec/15 sec).

Nose: No discharge or polyps, mucosa pink and moist, septum midline, patent bilaterally. No edema over frontal or maxillary sinuses. No sinus tenderness to palpation. Correctly identifies mint, banana, and ammonia odors.

Mouth: Buccal mucosa pink and moist without lesions. Twenty-six teeth present in various states of repair. Lower second molars (18, 30) absent bilaterally. Gingiva pink and firm. Tongue midline with no tremors or fasciculation.

Pharynx: Clear without erythema, tonsils 1+ without exudate. Uvula rises evenly and gag reflex is intact. No hoarseness. Patient identifies tastes of salt and sugar.

For additional sample documentation, see Chapter 26.

SUMMARY OF EXAMINATION

ABDOMEN

Ears, Nose, and Throat

The following steps should be performed with the patient sitting.

Ears

1. Inspect the auricles and mastoid area for the following (see p. 329):
   - Size
   - Shape
   - Symmetry
   - Landmarks
   - Color
   - Position
   - Deformities or lesions
2. Palpate the auricles and mastoid area for the following (see p. 331):
   - Tenderness
   - Swelling
   - Nodules
3. Inspect the auditory canal with an otoscope, noting the following (see pp. 331-332):
   - Cerumen
   - Color
   - Lesions
   - Discharge, or foreign bodies
4. Inspect the tympanic membrane for the following (see pp. 332-333):
   - Landmarks
   - Color
   - Contour
   - Perforations
   - Mobility
5. Assess hearing through the following (see pp. 333-334):
   - Response to questions during history

- Response to a whispered voice
- Response to tuning fork for air and bone conduction

Nose and Sinuses

1. Inspect the external nose for the following (see pp. 334-335):
   - Shape
   - Size
   - Color
   - Nares
2. Palpate the ridge and soft tissues of the nose for the following (see p. 335):
   - Tenderness
   - Displacement of cartilage and bone
   - Masses
3. Evaluate the patency of the nares (see p. 335):
4. Inspect the nasal mucosa and nasal septum for the following (see p. 335):
   - Color
   - Alignment
   - Discharge
   - Swelling of turbinates
   - Perforation
5. Inspect the frontal and maxillary sinus area for swelling (see p. 335):
6. Palpate the frontal and maxillary sinuses for the following (see p. 335):
   - Tenderness or pain
   - Swelling

Mouth

1. Inspect and palpate the lips for the following (see pp. 336-337):
   - Symmetry
   - Color
   - Edema
2. Inspect the teeth for the following (see pp. 337-339):
   - Occlusion
   - Caries
   - Loose or missing teeth
   - Surface abnormalities
3. Inspect and palpate the gingivae for the following (see p. 339):
   - Color
   - Lesions
   - Tenderness
4. Inspect the tongue and buccal mucosa for the following (see pp. 339-342):
   - Color
   - Symmetry
   - Swelling
   - Ulcerations
   - Cranial nerve XII (hypoglossal)
5. Palpate the tongue (see p. 342).
6. Inspect the palate and uvula (see p. 342).
7. Inspect the following oropharyngeal characteristics (see p. 343):
   - Tonsils
   - Posterior wall of pharynx
8. Elicit gag reflex (cranial nerves IX and X) (see p. 343).

COMMON ABNORMALITIES

EAR

OTITIS EXTERNA (SWIMMER'S EAR)	Otitis externa is an infection of the auditory canal resulting when trauma or a moist environment favors bacterial or fungal growth (Table 12-6).
MIDDLE EAR EFFUSION	This is an inflammation of the middle ear resulting in the collection of serous, mucoid, or purulent fluid (effusion) in the middle ear when the tympanic membrane is intact. Signs of middle ear effusion include bulging of the tympanic membrane, limited or absent mobility of the tympanic membrane, air fluid level behind the tympanic membrane, and otorrhea (American Academy of Pediatrics, 2004). Conductive hearing loss often results. Causes of this disorder include an obstructed or dysfunctional eustachian tube, allergies, and enlarged lymphoid tissue in the nasopharynx. Once the obstruction occurs, the middle ear absorbs the air, creating a vacuum, and the mucosa secretes a transudate into the middle ear (Fig. 12-42; see Table 12-6).

TABLE 12-6	Differentiating Between Otitis Externa, Acute Otitis Media, and Middle Ear Effusion		
Signs and Symptoms	**Otitis Externa**	**Acute Otitis Media**	**Middle Ear Effusion**
Initial symptoms	Itching in ear canal	Abrupt onset, fever, feeling of blockage, anorexia, irritability, dizziness, vomiting and diarrhea	Sticking or cracking sound on yawning or swallowing; no signs of acute infection
Pain	Intense with movement of pinna, chewing	Deep-seated earache that interferes with activity or sleep, pulling at ear	Discomfort, feeling of fullness
Discharge	Watery, then purulent and thick, mixed with pus and epithelial cells; musty, foul-smelling	Only if tympanic membrane ruptures or through tympanostomy tubes; foul-smelling	Uncommon
Hearing	Conductive loss caused by exudate and swelling of ear canal	Conductive loss as middle ear fills with pus	Conductive loss as middle ear fills with fluid
Inspection	Canal is red, edematous; tympanic membrane obscured	Tympanic membrane with distinct erythema thickened, or clouding; bulging; limited or absent movement to positive or negative pressure, air-fluid level and/or bubbles	Tympanic membrane retracted or bulging, impaired mobility, yellowish; air-fluid level and/or bubbles

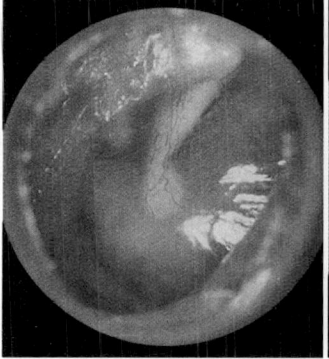 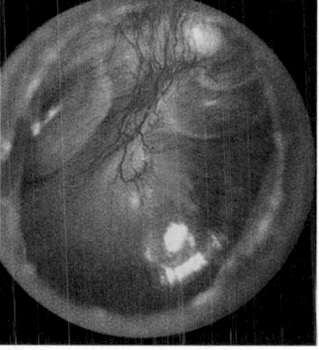

A   B

FIGURE 12-42
Middle ear effusion. **A,** Middle ear filled with serous fluid. **B,** Air-fluid levels in upper middle ear.
Courtesy Richard A. Buckingham, MD, Clinical Professor, Otolaryngology, Abraham Lincoln School of Medicine, University of Illinois, Chicago.

ACUTE OTITIS MEDIA

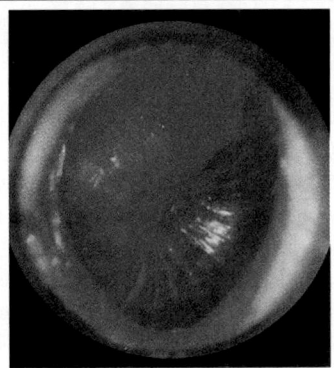

FIGURE 12-43
Acute otitis media.
Courtesy Richard A. Buckingham, MD, Clinical Professor, Otolaryngology, Abraham Lincoln School of Medicine, University of Illinois, Chicago.

This is an abrupt onset of symptoms and signs of middle ear inflammation and middle ear effusion (American Academy of Pediatrics, 2004). Signs of middle ear inflammation include distinct erythema of the tympanic membrane or distinct otalgia (ear pain) in the affected ear that interferes with normal activity and sleep. Signs of middle ear effusion are listed in the previous paragraph. Causes of the disorder may include bacterial infections (Fig. 12-43; see Table 12-6).

CHOLESTEATOMA

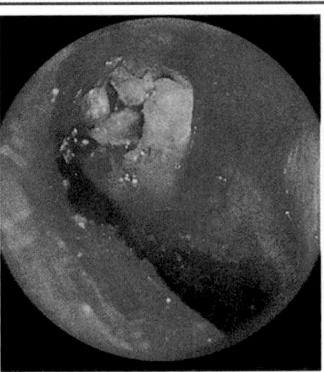

FIGURE 12-44
Cholesteatoma.
Courtesy Richard A. Buckingham, MD, Clinical Professor, Otolaryngology, Abraham Lincoln School of Medicine, University of Illinois, Chicago.

An epithelial growth that migrates through a perforation in the tympanic membrane often results in a cholesteatoma. White, shiny, greasy flecks of debris are visualized in the posterior-superior section of the middle ear through the tympanic membrane or through a perforation. A foul-smelling discharge may be found when a perforation is present. Symptoms include progressive hearing loss, fullness in the ear, tinnitus, and mild vertigo. If untreated, the cholesteatoma can lead to intracranial complications by eroding the temporal bone (Fig. 12-44).

OTOSCLEROSIS

Otosclerosis is a hereditary condition that is more common in women. Irregular ossification occurs within the bony labyrinth or otic capsule, resulting in fixation of the stapes. Symptoms include tinnitus and slowly progressive low- to medium-pitch conductive hearing loss, usually noticed between late teens and 30 years of age. Sensorineural hearing loss may also develop, causing a mixed hearing loss.

MÉNIÈRE DISEASE

Ménière disease affects the vestibular labyrinth, leading to profound sensorineural hearing loss. Symptoms include abrupt and recurrent attacks of severe vertigo, tinnitus, and progressive hearing loss, initially of low tones. The patient may complain of fullness in the ears. The disorder may be unilateral at first and then may involve the other ear.

LABYRINTHITIS

Inflammation of the labyrinthine canal of the inner ear occurs as a complication of an acute upper respiratory viral or bacterial infection. Symptoms of severe vertigo, which are associated with nystagmus and which are increased in severity with head movement, may last for several days. Labyrinthitis may be a complication of otitis media or meningitis.

NOSE AND SINUSES

SINUSITIS

An infection of one or more of the paranasal sinuses may be a complication of a viral upper respiratory infection, dental infection, allergies, or a structural defect of the nose. Sinusitis may be caused by a blockage of the sinus meatus that prevents drainage of secretions from the sinus cavity, by malfunction of the cilia that help move mucus, or by an overproduction of mucus as a result of inflammation. Acute sinusitis is characterized by an upper respiratory infection that worsens after 5 days, persists longer than 10 days, and has more severe symptoms than a typical upper respiratory infection (Pletcher, Goldberg, 2003). Symptoms include purulent nasal or postnasal drainage, nasal congestion, facial pain or pressure. There may be swelling of the skin overlying the involved sinus. Signs in children may include rhinorrhea, cough, fever, halitosis, hyponasal speech, pain or headache, periorbital swelling, sinus tenderness, postnasal drip, and absent transillumination.

EVIDENCE-BASED PRACTICE IN PHYSICAL EXAMINATION
PREDICTORS OF SINUSITIS

The strongest predictor of sinusitis is a combination of four or more of the following signs and symptoms: (1) maxillary toothache, (2) purulent nasal secretions, (3) dull or opaque sinus transillumination, (4) poor response to decongestants, and (5) colored nasal discharge (Williams et al, 1992).

COCAINE ABUSE

Nasal insufflation (snorting) of cocaine, a currently favored substance for abuse, must be considered when examining all adolescents and adults. Commonly, patients complain of such chronic nasal symptoms as sniffling, nasal congestion, recurrent nosebleeds, and sinus problems. Signs of very recent insufflation include hyperemia and edema of the nasal mucosa and rhinorrhea. White powder may still be present on the nasal hairs and mustache. Signs of chronic cocaine insufflation include scabs on the nasal mucosa, decreased perception of taste and smell, and perforation of the nasal septum due to ischemic necrosis of the septal cartilage resulting from chronic irritation.

MOUTH AND OROPHARYNX

TONSILLITIS

Inflammation or infection of the tonsils is commonly caused by streptococci. Symptoms include sore throat, referred pain to the ears, dysphagia, fever, fetid breath, and malaise. The tonsils appear red and swollen, and tonsillar crypts are filled with purulent exudate (Fig. 12-45). Tonsils studded with yellow follicles are associated with streptococcal infections. Anterior cervical lymph nodes are enlarged.

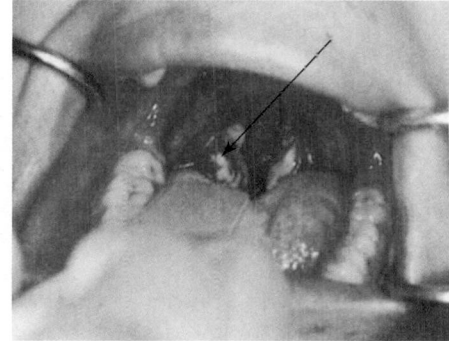

FIGURE 12-45
Tonsillitis and pharyngitis.
Courtesy Edward L. Applebaum, MD, Head, Department of Otolaryngology, University of Illinois Medical Center, Chicago.

EVIDENCE-BASED PRACTICE IN PHYSICAL EXAMINATION
PREDICTORS OF BETA STREP INFECTION

Clinical signs most predictive of group A beta-hemolytic *Streptococcus* (GABHS) include tonsillar enlargement and exudates, tender and enlarged cervical nodes, and pharyngeal erythema. However, even when all these signs are present, they provide no assurance of diagnosis with only a 71% sensitivity and 77% specificity. A throat culture is still vitally important for an accurate diagnosis (Nawaz et al, 2000).

Nevertheless, in a study by Attia and colleagues (Attia et al, 2001), a simple scale was found to be more accurate than simple observation in predicting the presence of beta strep infection:

	Present	Absent
Moderate to severe tonsillar swelling	1	0
Moderate to severe cervical lymphadenopathy	1	0
Scarlatiniform rash	2	0
No coryza	1	0
Total score	5	0

When the patient's score was 3 (without rash), the agreement with throat culture results was 65%; when rash was present (for a total score of 5) the agreement was 95%. The scale was more accurate than observers making a judgment without the discipline of the scale. Bottom line: The laboratory culture is still better than just looking, but the scale can certainly be a help when the laboratory is not handy.

PERITONSILLAR ABSCESS

Infection of the tissue between the tonsil and tonsillar pillar occurs as a complication of tonsillitis. Symptoms include dysphagia, drooling, severe sore throat with pain radiating to the ear, muffled voice, malaise, and fever. The tonsil, tonsillar pillar, and adjacent soft palate become red and swollen (Fig. 12-46). The tonsil may appear pushed forward or backward, possibly displacing the uvula. Cervical lymphadenopathy is present.

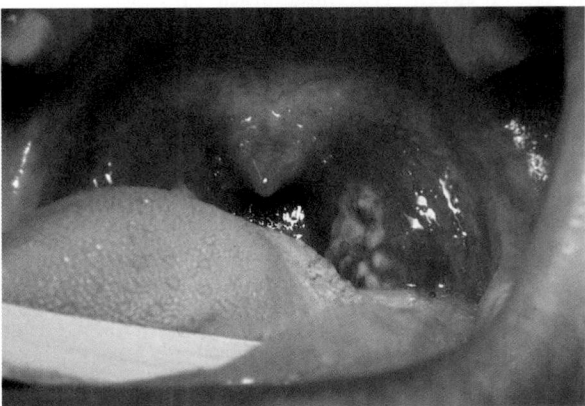

FIGURE 12-46
Swelling of peritonsillar abscess.
Courtesy Daniel M. Laskin, DDS, MS, Medical College of Virginia, Virginia Commonwealth University, Richmond, VA.

ORAL CANCER

Oral cancer may appear as an ulcerative lesion that may be erythematous, white, or pigmented, appearing as piled up edges around a core that often appears on the lateral border or floor of the mouth. Other locations are the hard and soft palate and the alveolar ridges. Signs include a sore in the mouth that will not heal, a white or red patch on the gums, tongue, tonsil, or buccal mucosa, bleeding, ulceration, and a lump or thickening in the cheek. Early lesions are usually painless, but advanced lesions become painful with erosion of tissue. Cervical adenopathy is usually present (Fig. 12-47).

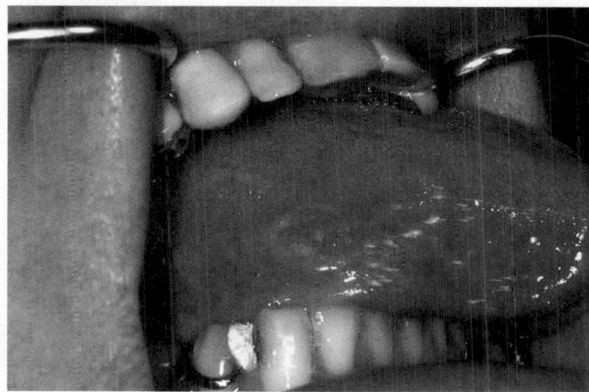

FIGURE 12-47
Squamous cell cancer on the tongue.
Courtesy Daniel M. Laskin, DDS, MS, Medical College of Virginia, Virginia Commonwealth University, Richmond, VA.

SLEEP APNEA

Sleep apnea is a periodic cessation of breathing during sleep that is associated with either an obstruction to airflow or with failure of the central nervous system to stimulate the respiratory effort to breathe. In obstructive sleep apnea, muscles in the nasopharynx, hypopharynx, and pharynx relax during sleep, resulting in loud snoring, restless sleep, and a pause in nasal and oral airflow with respiratory effort. This can result in progressive hypercapnia, hypoxemia, increased pulmonary arterial pressures, and possibly life-threatening cardiac arrhythmias. Patients are typically overweight, middle-aged men who complain of excessive daytime sleepiness and morning headaches. This can occur in preschool children when enlarged tonsils and adenoids obstruct the airway.

INFANTS AND CHILDREN

CLEFT LIP AND PALATE

This congenital malformation of the face appears as a fissure of the upper lip or palate. Each may occur without the other; however, they often occur together. There may be a complete cleft extending through the lip and hard and soft palates to the nasal cavity, or there may be a partial cleft in any of these tissues. Long-term problems for the affected child include hearing loss, chronic otitis media, speech difficulties, feeding problems, and improper tooth development and alignment (Fig. 12-48).

PHYSICAL VARIATIONS
Cleft Lip and Palate
The incidence of cleft lip and palate is higher in whites and Japanese, and lower in blacks.

From Bluestone, Klein, 2001.

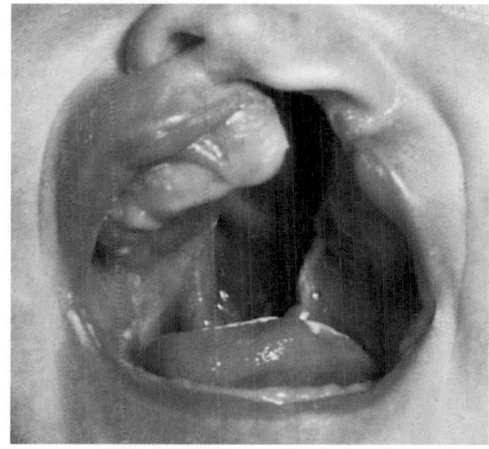

FIGURE 12-48
Unilateral cleft lip and palate.
From Zitelli, Davis, 1997.

RETROPHARYNGEAL ABSCESS

Retropharyngeal abscess is a pediatric emergency because it occludes the airway. The condition may result from trauma to the posterior pharyngeal wall or a dental infection that leads to infection in the retropharyngeal lymph nodes. Because these nodes communicate with each other, bacteria spread to other nodes and extend the infection. Group A *Streptococcus* and *Staphylococcus* are common causative organisms. The child is usually acutely ill, febrile, drooling, anorexic, and restless. Respiratory distress is often present along with a muffled voice and stridor. The child may refuse to move the neck. This condition is most common in children younger than 3 to 4 years because the retropharyngeal lymph nodes tend to atrophy by 5 or 6 years of age (Fig. 12-49).

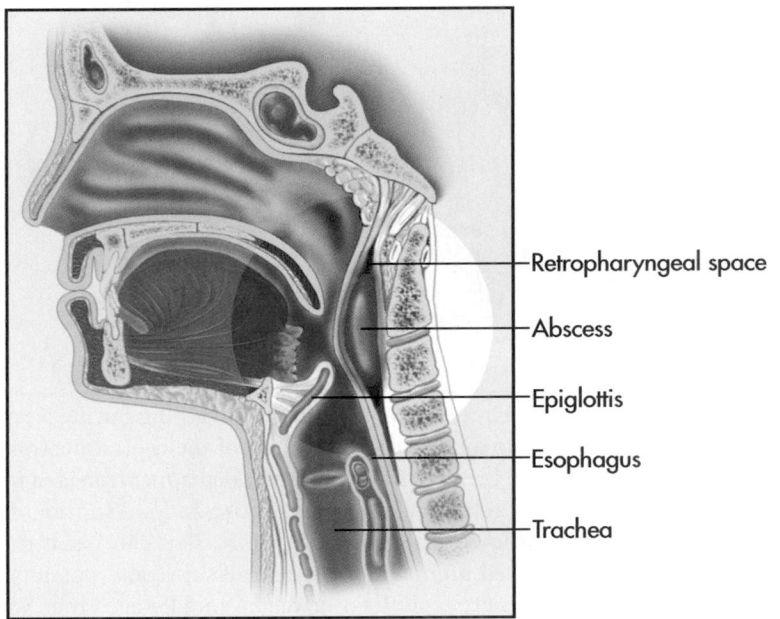

Retropharyngeal space
Abscess
Epiglottis
Esophagus
Trachea

FIGURE 12-49
Retropharyngeal abscess.

OLDER ADULTS

PRESBYCUSIS

Presbycusis is a common auditory disorder in which there is bilateral sensorineural hearing loss associated with aging. It is caused by degenerative changes in the inner ear or auditory nerve. There is a loss in the perception of auditory stimuli—initially of high-frequency sounds—and tinnitus. Speech may be poorly understood when spoken quickly or when background noise is present.

XEROSTOMIA

Xerostomia is a dry mouth caused by the ingestion of anticholinergic or antidepressant drugs that interfere with the production of saliva. Xerostomia is also caused by systemic disease such as rheumatoid arthritis, scleroderma, polymyositis, and Sjögren syndrome. The condition is also found in patients who are heavy smokers or those who have received radiation to the head and neck.

ELECTRONIC RESOURCES

For Weblinks and additional resources, go to

http://evolve.elsevier.com/Seidel

or to the Companion CD-ROM.

Additional information related to the content in Chapter 12 can be found on the companion website at evolve.elsevier.com/Seidel/ or on the interactive companion CD-ROM. Resources and activities for Chapter 12 include:
- Sound and Vision Theater
- Printouts for Your Practice
- Interactive Challenge
- Spanish Assessment Terms with Pronunciation Guide
- Instant Calculator

CHEST AND LUNGS

ANATOMY AND PHYSIOLOGY

The chest, or thorax, is a cage of bone, cartilage, and muscle capable of movement as the lungs expand. It consists anteriorly of the sternum, manubrium, xiphoid process, and costal cartilages; laterally, of the 12 pairs of ribs; and posteriorly, of the 12 thoracic vertebrae (Figs. 13-1 and 13-2). All the ribs are connected to the thoracic vertebrae; the upper seven are attached anteriorly to the sternum by the costal cartilages, and ribs 8, 9, and 10 join with the costal cartilages just above them. The transverse diameter of the chest generally exceeds the anteroposterior (AP) diameter in adults.

The primary muscles of respiration are the diaphragm and the intercostal muscles. The diaphragm, the dominant muscle, contracts and moves downward during inspiration, lowering the abdominal contents to increase the intrathoracic space. The external intercostal muscles increase the AP chest diameter during inspiration, and the internal intercostals decrease the transverse diameter during expiration. The sternocleidomastoid and trapezius muscles may also contribute to respiratory movements but these "accessory" muscles are usually brought into play only when there are pulmonary problems and compromise (Fig. 13-3).

The interior of the chest is divided into three major spaces: the right and left pleural cavities and the mediastinum. The mediastinum, situated between the lungs, contains all of the thoracic viscera except the lungs. The pleural cavities are lined with the parietal and visceral pleurae, serous membranes that enclose the lungs. The spongy and highly elastic lungs are paired but not symmetric, the right having three lobes and the left two (Fig. 13-4). The left upper lobe has an inferior tonguelike projection, the lingula, which is a counterpart of the right middle lobe. Each lung has a major fissure—the oblique—that divides the upper and lower portions. In addition, a lesser horizontal fissure divides the upper portion of the right lung into the upper and middle lobes at the level of the fifth rib in the axilla and the fourth rib anteriorly. Each lobe consists of blood vessels, lymphatics, nerves, and an alveolar duct connecting with the alveoli (as many as 300 million in an adult). The entire lung parenchyma is shaped by an elastic subpleural tissue that limits its expansion. Each lung is conical; the apex is rounded and extends anteriorly about 4 cm above the first rib into the base of the neck in adults. Posteriorly, the apexes of the lungs rise to about the level of T1. The lower borders descend on deep inspiration to about T12 and rise on forced expiration to about T9. The base of each lung is broad and concave, resting on the convex surface of

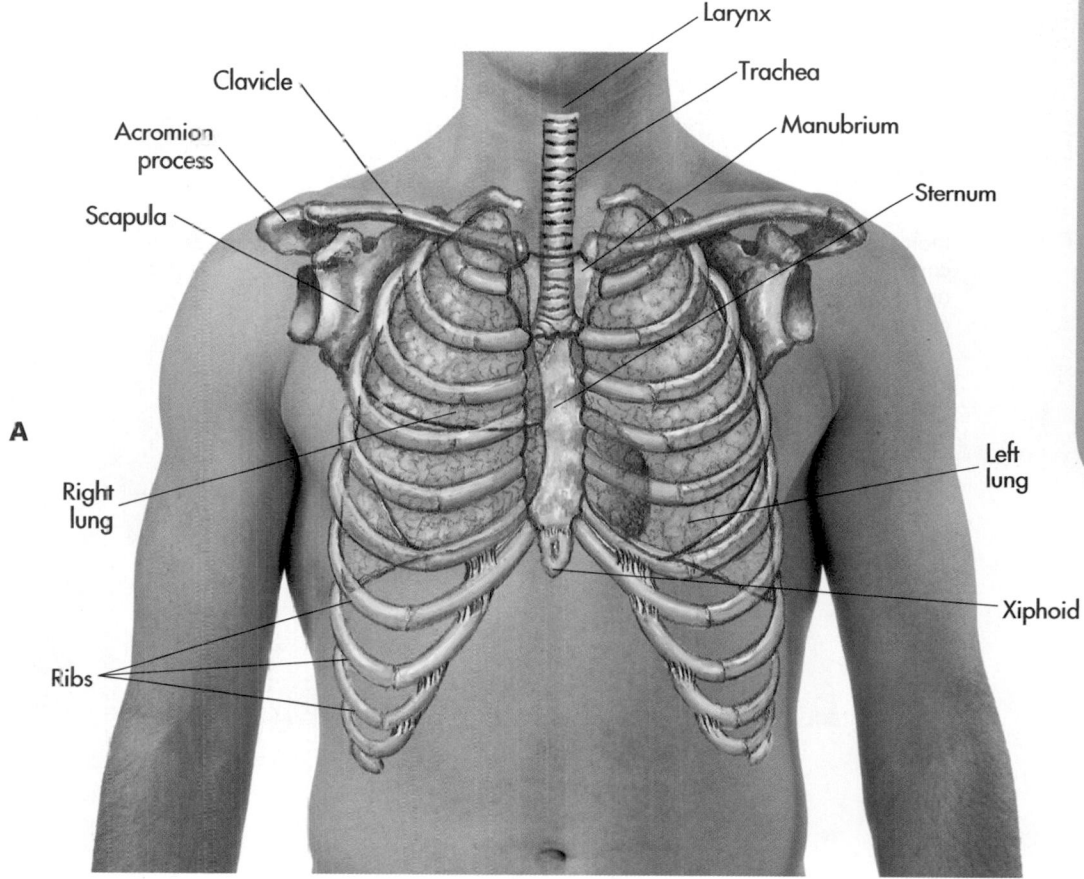

A

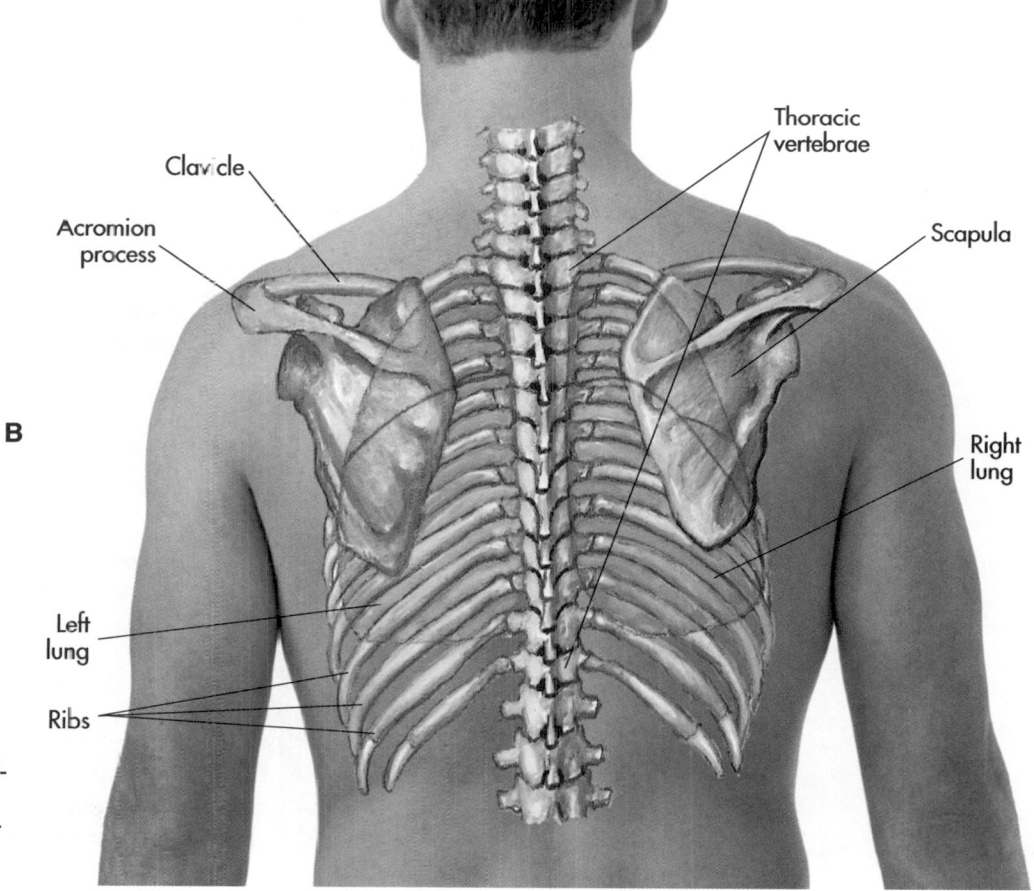

B

FIGURE 13-1
The bony structures of the chest form a protective expandable cage around the lungs and heart. **A,** Anterior view. **B,** Posterior view.
From Thompson, Wilson, 1996.

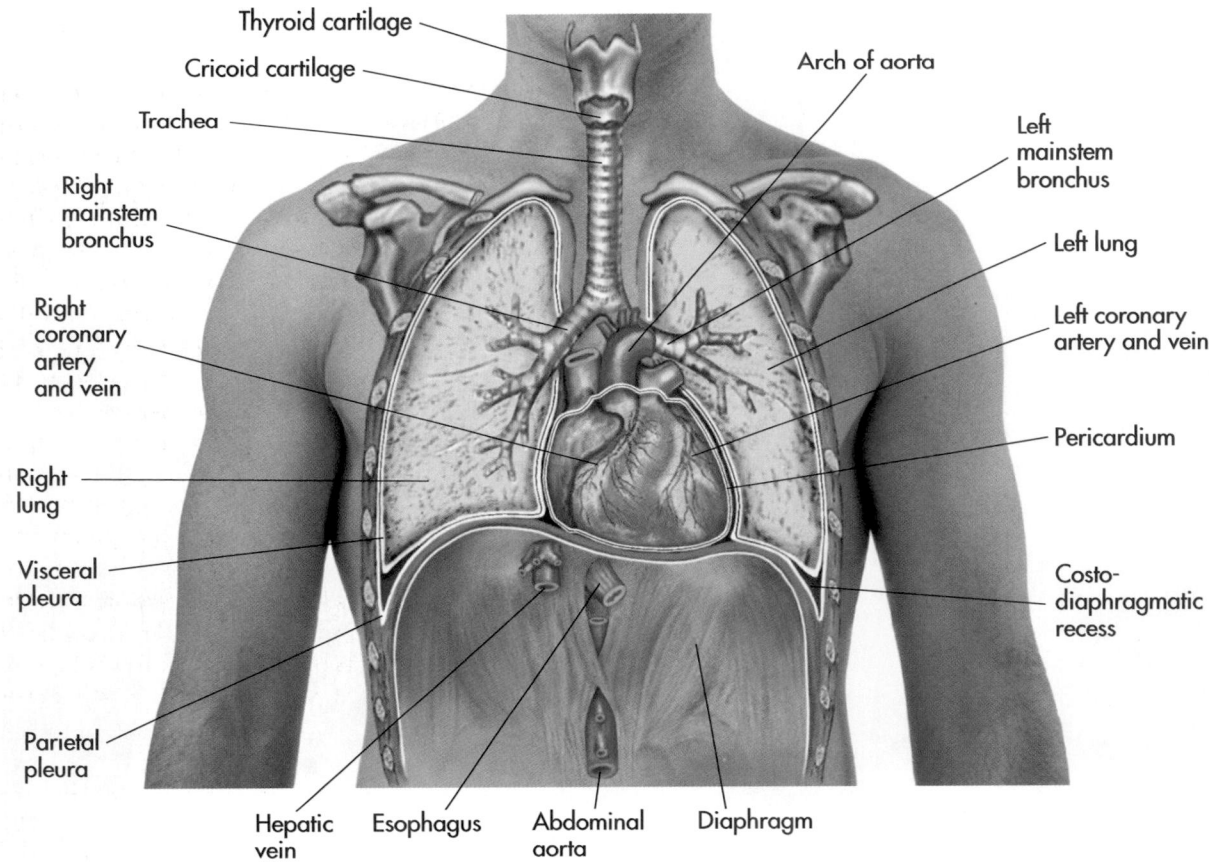

Thyroid cartilage

Cricoid cartilage

Trachea

Right mainstem bronchus

Right coronary artery and vein

Right lung

Visceral pleura

Parietal pleura

Arch of aorta

Left mainstem bronchus

Left lung

Left coronary artery and vein

Pericardium

Costo-diaphragmatic recess

Hepatic vein

Esophagus

Abdominal aorta

Diaphragm

FIGURE 13-2
Chest cavity and related anatomic structures.

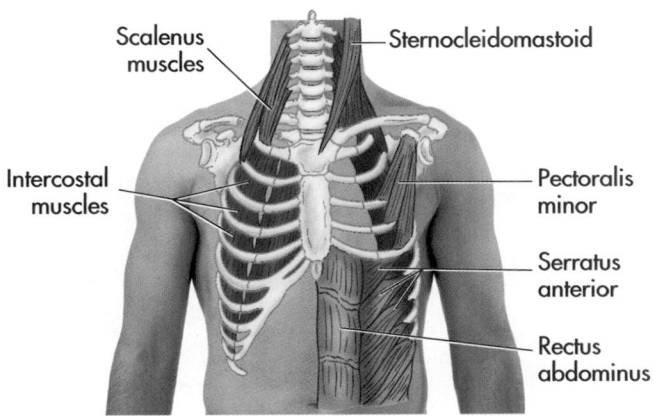

Scalenus muscles

Sternocleidomastoid

Intercostal muscles

Pectoralis minor

Serratus anterior

Rectus abdominus

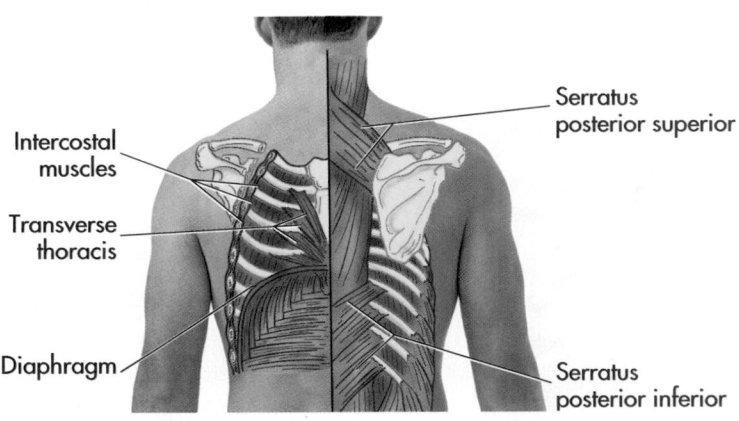

Intercostal muscles

Transverse thoracis

Diaphragm

Serratus posterior superior

Serratus posterior inferior

FIGURE 13-3
Muscles of ventilation. **A,** Anterior view. **B,** Posterior view.

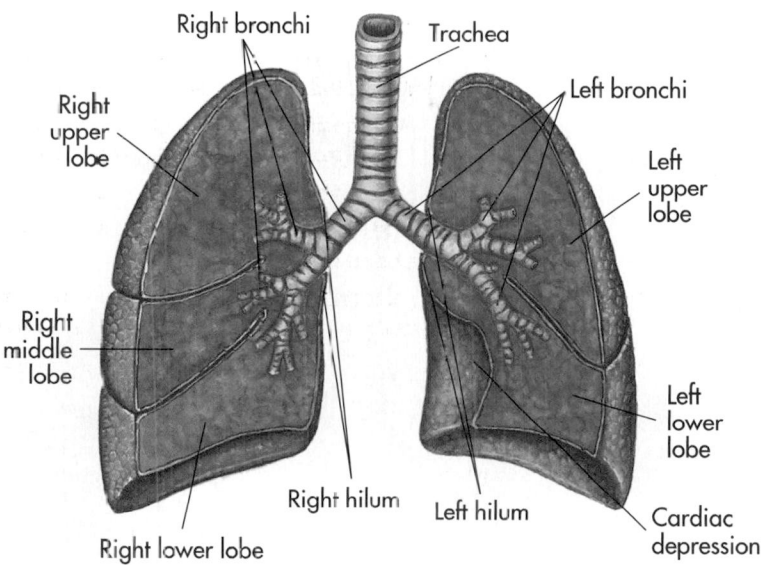

FIGURE 13-4
The lobes of the lungs.
From Wilson, Thompson, 1990.

the diaphragm. The medial surfaces of the lung are to some extent concave, providing a cradle for the heart.

The tracheobronchial tree is a tubular system that provides a pathway along which air is filtered, humidified, and warmed as it moves from the upper airway to the farthest alveolar reaches. The trachea is 10 to 11 cm long and about 2 cm in diameter. It lies anterior to the esophagus and posterior to the isthmus of the thyroid. The trachea divides into the right and left main bronchi at about the level of T4 or T5 and just below the manubriosternal joint.

The right bronchus is wider, shorter, and more vertically placed than the left bronchus (and therefore more susceptible to aspiration of foreign bodies). The main bronchi are divided into three branches on the right and two on the left, each branch supplying one lobe of the lungs. The branches then begin to subdivide into terminal bronchioles and ultimately into respiratory bronchioles so small that each is associated with but one acinus, or terminal respiratory unit. The acini consist of the respiratory bronchioles, alveolar ducts, alveolar sacs, and alveoli. The bronchi transport air and, to some extent, trap noxious foreign particles in the mucus of their cavities and sweep them toward the pharynx with their cilia.

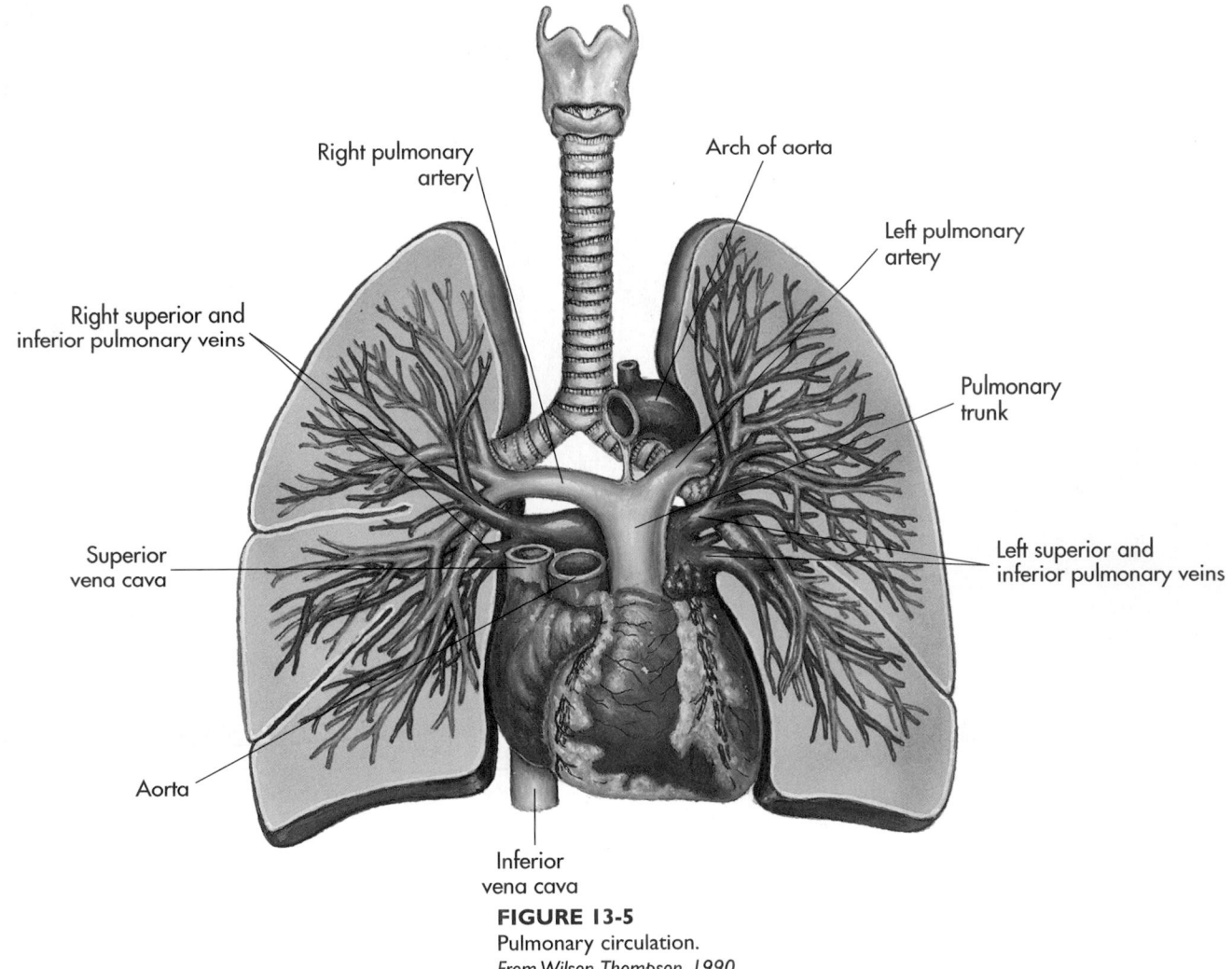

FIGURE 13-5
Pulmonary circulation.
From Wilson, Thompson, 1990.

The bronchial arteries branch from the anterior thoracic aorta and the intercostal arteries, supplying blood to the lung parenchyma and stroma. The bronchial vein is formed at the hilum of the lung, but most of the blood supplied by the bronchial arteries is returned by the pulmonary veins (Fig. 13-5 and Box 13-1).

CHEMICAL AND NEUROLOGIC CONTROL OF RESPIRATION

The purpose of respiration is to keep the body adequately supplied with oxygen and protected from excess accumulation of carbon dioxide. It involves the movement of air back and forth from the deepest reaches of the alveoli to the outside (ventilation); gas exchange across the alveolar-pulmonary capillary membranes (diffusion and perfusion); and circulatory system transport of oxygen to, and carbon dioxide from, the peripheral tissues. Control of this complex process is as yet only partially understood. Chemoreceptors in the medulla oblongata are exquisitely sensitive and respond quickly to changes in hydrogen ion concentration in the blood and spinal fluid. Peripherally, chemoreceptors in the carotid body at the bifurcation of the common carotid arteries also respond to changes in arterial oxygen and carbon dioxide levels. Both types of chemoreceptors respond by sending signals to the respiratory center in the medulla oblongata. Nerve impulses from here are transmitted to two subcenters in the pons, which regulate the respiratory muscles. Excess levels of carbon dioxide stimulate the rate and depth of respiration.

BOX 13-1

VISUALIZING THE LUNGS FROM THE SURFACE

Anteriorly

The right lung may ride higher because of the fullness of the dome of the liver. Except for an inferior lateral triangle, the anterior view on the right is primarily the upper and middle lobes, separated by the horizontal fissure at about the fifth rib in the midaxilla to about the fourth at the sternum; on the left as on the right, the lower lobe is set off by a diagonal fissure stretching from the fifth rib at the axilla to the sixth at the midclavicular line.

Posteriorly

Except for the apices, the posterior view is primarily the lower lobe, which extends from about T3 to T10 or T12 during the respiratory cycle.

Right Lateral

The lung underlies the area extending from the peak of the axilla to the seventh or eighth rib. The upper lobe is demarcated at about the level of the fifth rib in the midaxillary line and the sixth rib more anteriorly.

Left Lateral

The lung underlies the area extending from the peak of the axilla to the seventh or eighth rib. The entire expanse is virtually bisected by the oblique fissure from about the level of the third rib medially to the sixth rib anteriorly.

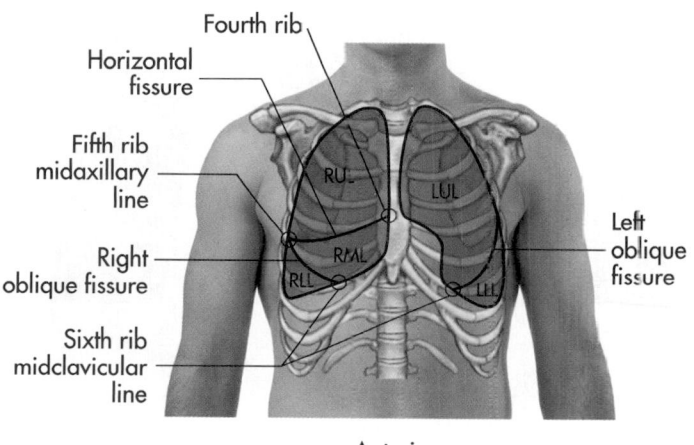

Anterior

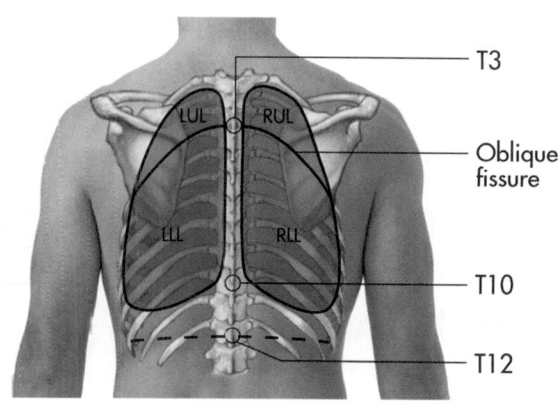

Posterior

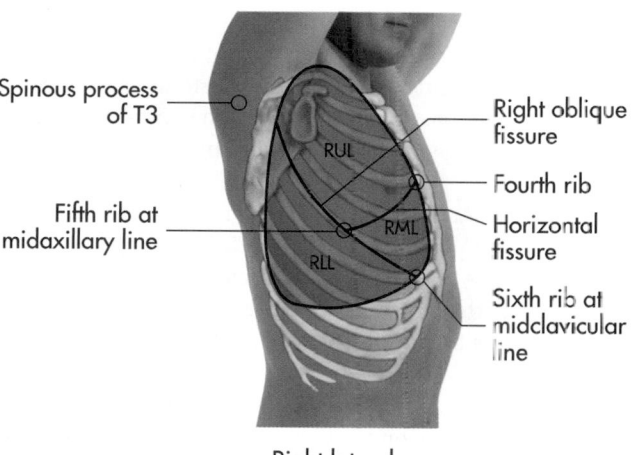

Right lateral

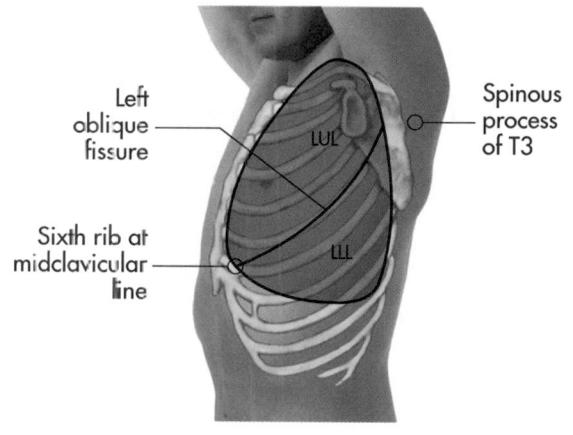

Left lateral

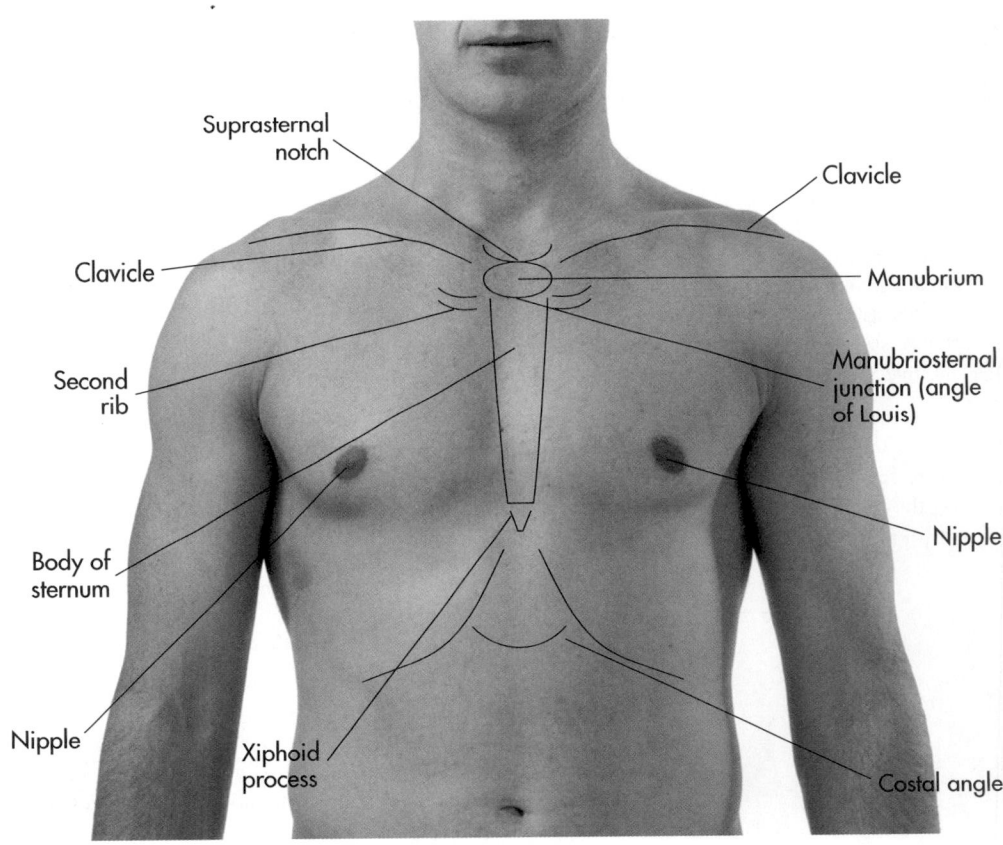

FIGURE 13-6
Topographic landmarks of the chest.
From Thompson, Wilson, 1996.

ANATOMIC LANDMARKS

The following topographic markers on the chest are used to describe findings (Fig. 13-6):

1. The nipples.
2. The manubriosternal junction (angle of Louis). A visible and palpable angulation of the sternum and the point at which the second rib articulates with the sternum. One can count the ribs and intercostal spaces from this point. The number of each intercostal space corresponds to that of the rib immediately above it.
3. The suprasternal notch. A depression, easily palpable and most often visible at the base of the ventral aspect of the neck, just superior to the manubriosternal junction.
4. Costal angle. The angle formed by the blending together of the costal margins at the sternum. It is usually no more than 90 degrees, with the ribs inserted at approximately 45-degree angles.
5. Vertebra prominens. The spinous process of C7. It can be more readily seen and felt with the patient's head bent forward. If two prominences are felt, the upper is that of the spinous process of C7, and the lower is that of T1. It is difficult to use this as a guide to counting ribs posteriorly because the spinous processes from T4 down project obliquely, thus overlying the rib below the number of its vertebra.
6. The clavicles

INFANTS AND CHILDREN

At about 4 weeks of gestation, the lung is a groove on the ventral wall of the gut. It evolves ultimately from a simple sac to an involuted structure of tubules and spaces. The lungs contain no air, and the alveoli are collapsed. Relatively passive respiratory movements occur throughout much of gestation; they do not open the alveoli or move the lung fields. Rather, they prepare the term infant to respond to postnatal chemical and neurologic respiratory stimuli. Fetal gas exchange is mediated by the placenta.

At birth the change in respiratory function is rapid and dramatic. After the cord is cut, the lungs fill with air for the first time; this first respiratory effort is great. No longer coursing through the placenta, blood flows through the lungs more vigorously. The pulmonary arteries expand and relax, offering much less resistance than the systemic circulation. This relative

CLINICAL PEARL

First Breath
The first breath an infant takes provides a moment of drama as intense as any in later life—and is far more often accompanied by joy.

decrease in pulmonary pressure most often leads to closure of the foramen ovale within minutes after birth, and the increased oxygen tension in the arterial blood usually stimulates contraction and closure of the ductus arteriosus. (Reminder: the foramen ovale and the ductus arteriosus do not always close so readily.) The pulmonary and systemic circulations adopt their mature configurations, and the lungs are fully integrated for postnatal function. The entire process is facilitated by pulmonary surfactant, a complex of proteins and phospholipids and a lubricant that stabilizes the alveoli by lessening surface tension at the air-liquid interface.

The chest of the newborn is generally round, the AP diameter approximating the transverse, and the circumference is roughly equal to that of the head until the child is about 2 years old (Fig. 13-7). With growth, the chest assumes adult proportions, with the lateral diameter exceeding the AP diameter.

The relatively thin chest wall of the infant and young child makes the bony structure more prominent than in the adult. It is more cartilaginous and yielding, and the xiphoid process is often more prominent and a bit more movable.

CLINICAL PEARL

Lung Development

The lung is not fully grown at birth: That is why infants are so pneumonically challenged. The number of alveoli increase at a very rapid rate in the first 2 years of life. This slows down, becoming a barely noticeable trickle by the age of 8 years.

PREGNANT WOMEN

Mechanical and biochemical factors, including the enlarged uterus and an increased level of circulating progesterone, interact to create changes in the respiratory function of the pregnant woman. Anatomic changes that occur in the chest as the lower ribs flare include an increase in the transverse diameter of about 2 cm and an increase in the circumference of 5 to 7 cm. The subcostal angle progressively increases from about 68.5 degrees to approximately 103.5 degrees in later pregnancy. In addition, the diaphragm at rest rises as much as 4 cm above its usual resting position, yet diaphragmatic movement increases so that the major work of breathing is done by the diaphragm. Minute ventilation increases 30% to 50% with a corresponding 50% to 70% increase in alveolar ventilation. Increased tidal volume appears to account for the increase in minute ventilation. The respiratory rate remains unchanged (Weinberger, Weiss, 1999).

OLDER ADULTS

The barrel chest that is characteristic of many older adults results from loss of muscle strength in the thorax and diaphragm (see Fig. 13-9), coupled with the loss of lung resiliency. In addition, skeletal changes of aging tend to emphasize the dorsal curve of the thoracic spine, resulting in an increased AP chest diameter. There may also be stiffening and decreased expansion of the chest wall.

The alveoli become less elastic and relatively more fibrous. The associated loss of some of the interalveolar folds decreases the alveolar surface available for gas exchange. This and the loss of some tensile strength in the muscles of respiration result in underventilation of the alveoli in the lower lung fields and a decreased tolerance for exertion. The net result of these changes is a decrease in vital capacity and an increase in residual volume. Dyspnea can occur when older persons exceed their customary light or moderate exertional demands.

Aging mucous membranes tend to become drier and less able to rid themselves of mucus. Retained mucus encourages bacterial growth and predisposes the older adult to respiratory infection.

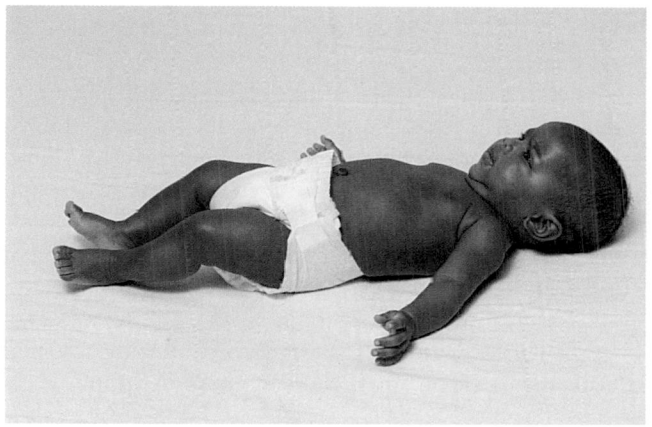
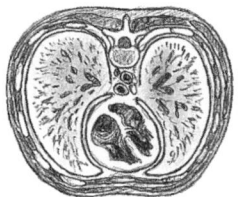

FIGURE 13-7
Chest of healthy infant. Note that the anteroposterior diameter is approximately the same as transverse diameter.

REVIEW OF RELATED HISTORY

For each of the conditions discussed in this section, targeted topics to include in the history of the present illness are listed. Responses to questions about these topics help fully assess the patient's condition and provide clues for focusing the physical examination.

HISTORY OF PRESENT ILLNESS

CLINICAL PEARL

Chest Pain

Chest pain does not generally originate in the heart when

- There is a constant achiness that lasts all day;
- It stays in one position;
- It is made worse by pressing on the precordium
- It is a fleeting, needle-like jab that lasts only a second or two;
- It is situated in the shoulders or between the shoulder blades in the back.

Think of the heart but, importantly, also in such circumstances of other possibilities in the chest and its environs.

From Harvey, 1943.

- Coughing
  - Onset: sudden, gradual; duration
  - Nature of cough: dry, moist, wet, hacking, hoarse, barking, whooping, bubbling, productive, nonproductive
  - Sputum production: duration, frequency, with activity, at certain times of day
  - Sputum characteristics: amount, color (clear, mucoid, purulent, blood-tinged, mostly blood), foul odor
  - Pattern: occasional, regular, paroxysmal; related to time of day, weather, activities, (e.g., exercise), talking, deep breaths; change over time
  - Severity: tires patient, disrupts sleep or conversation, causes chest pain
  - Associated symptoms: shortness of breath, chest pain or tightness with breathing, fever, coryza, stuffy nose, noisy respirations, hoarseness, gagging, choking, stress
  - Efforts to treat: prescription or nonprescription drugs, vaporizers; effectiveness
  - Other medications: prescription or nonprescription
- Shortness of breath
  - Onset: sudden or gradual; duration; gagging or choking event few days before onset
  - Pattern
  - Position most comfortable, number of pillows used
  - Related to extent of exercise, certain activities, time of day, eating
  - Harder to inhale or exhale
  - Severity: extent of activity limitation, fatigue with breathing, anxiety about getting air
  - Associated symptoms: pain or discomfort (relationship to specific point in respiratory exertion, location), cough, diaphoresis, ankle edema
  - Efforts to treat: prescription or nonprescription drugs, oxygen use
- Chest pain
  - Onset and duration; associated with trauma, coughing, lower respiratory infection, recent anesthesia longer than 30 minutes, history of thrombophlebitis
  - Associated symptoms: shallow breathing, fever, coughing, anxiety about getting air, radiation of pain to neck or arms
  - Efforts to treat: heat, splinting, pain medication
  - Other medications: prescription or nonprescription, street drugs (e.g., cocaine)

PAST MEDICAL HISTORY

- Thoracic, nasal and/or pharyngotracheal trauma or surgery, hospitalizations for pulmonary disorders, dates
- Use of oxygen or ventilation-assisting devices
- Chronic pulmonary diseases: tuberculosis (date, treatment, compliance), bronchitis, emphysema, bronchiectasis, asthma, cystic fibrosis
- Other chronic disorders: cardiac, cancer, blood clotting disorders
- Testing: allergy, pulmonary function tests, tuberculin and fungal skin tests, chest x-ray examinations
- Immunization against pneumonia, influenza
- Daily medications, prescribed and nonprescription

FAMILY HISTORY

- Tuberculosis
- Cystic fibrosis
- Emphysema
- Allergy, asthma, atopic dermatitis
- Malignancy
- Bronchiectasis
- Bronchitis
- Clotting disorders (risk of pulmonary embolism)

PERSONAL AND SOCIAL HISTORY

CLINICAL PEARL

Pain from Cocaine

If an adult—especially a young adult—or an adolescent complains of severe, acute chest pain, ask about drug use, particularly cocaine. This situation will not occur often, but the possibility exists that drug use is causing the pain. Cocaine can cause tachycardia, hypertension, coronary arterial spasm (with infarction), and pneumothorax with severe acute chest pain being the common result.

- Employment: nature of work, extent of physical and emotional effort and stress, environmental hazards, exposure to chemicals, animals, vapors, dust, pulmonary irritants (e.g., asbestos), allergens, use of protective devices
- Home environment: location, possible allergens, type of heating, use of air conditioning, humidifier, ventilation
- Tobacco use: type of tobacco (cigarettes, cigars, pipe, smokeless), duration and amount (Pack years = Number of years of smoking × Number of packs smoked per day), age started, efforts to quit smoking with factors influencing success or failure, the extent of smoking by others at home or at work (passive smoking)
- Exposure to respiratory infections, influenza, tuberculosis
- Nutritional status: weight loss or obesity
- Use of herbal or other remedies, consistent with complementary/alternative therapies
- Regional or travel exposures (e.g., human immunodeficiency virus [HIV] infection in central Africa, the Caribbean; histoplasmosis in Southeastern and Midwestern United States; schistosomiasis in the Orient, Africa, Caribbean, Southwest Asia)
- Hobbies: owning pigeons, parrots, or other animals, woodworking, welding; other possibilities of noxious exposure (e.g., with employment)
- Use of alcohol
- Use of illegal drugs
- Exercise tolerance: diminished ability to perform up to expectations

INFANTS AND CHILDREN

- Low birth weight: premature, duration of ventilation assistance if any, respiratory distress syndrome, bronchopulmonary dysplasia, transient tachypnea of the newborn
- Coughing or difficulty breathing of sudden onset
- Possible aspiration of small object, toy, or food
- Possible ingestion of kerosene or other hydrocarbon
- Difficulty feeding: increased perspiration, cyanosis, tiring quickly, disinterest in feeding, inadequate weight gain (good indication of exercise intolerance)
- Apneic episodes: use of apnea monitor, sudden infant death in sibling
- Recurrent spitting up and choking, recurrent pneumonia (possible gastroesophageal reflux)
- History of pneumococcal vaccination (in particular, sickle cell disease, cystic fibrosis, other chronic problems)

PREGNANT WOMEN

- Weeks of gestation or estimated date of conception (EDC)
- Presence of multiple fetuses, polyhydramnios, or other conditions in which a larger uterus displaces the diaphragm upward
- Exercise type and energy expenditure
- Exposure to and frequency of respiratory infections, history of annual influenza immunization, history of pneumococcal vaccination

OLDER ADULTS

- Exposure to and frequency of respiratory infections, history of pneumococcal vaccination and annual influenza immunization
- Effects of weather on respiratory efforts and occurrence of infections
- Immobilization or marked sedentary habits
- Difficulty swallowing
- Alteration in daily living habits or activities as a result of respiratory symptoms
- Because older adults are at risk for chronic respiratory diseases (lung cancer, chronic bronchitis, emphysema, and tuberculosis), reemphasize the following:
  - Smoking history
  - Cough, dyspnea on exertion, or breathlessness
  - Blood-tinged or yellowish/greenish sputum
  - Fatigue
  - Significant weight changes
  - Fever, night sweats

EXAMINATION AND FINDINGS

EQUIPMENT

- Marking pencil or eyeliner (silver is good for dark skin)
- Centimeter ruler and tape measure
- Stethoscope with bell and diaphragm (for children, the diaphragm may but does not necessarily need to have a smaller diameter)
- Drapes

The sequence of steps in examination of the chest and lungs is traditional: inspection, palpation, percussion, and auscultation. None of these techniques alone will provide adequate information for the accurate definition of a pathologic process; the integration of all four, together with the history, often will. Listening to the lungs without also inspecting and palpating the chest will deny you the chance to interpret your findings in the most accurate way. Dullness on percussion, for example, is present in both pleural effusion and lobar pneumonia. Breath sounds are absent in the former and may be bronchial in the latter. On palpation you will often find that tactile fremitus is absent when an effusion exists and is increased with lo-

RISK FACTORS

RESPIRATORY DISABILITY: BARRIERS TO COMPETENT FUNCTION

- Gender: greater in men, but the difference between the genders diminishes with advancing age
- Age: increases inexorably with advancing age
- Family history of asthma, cystic fibrosis, tuberculosis and other contagious disease, neurofibromatosis
- Smoking
- Sedentary lifestyle or forced immobilization
- Occupational exposure to asbestos, dust, or other pulmonary irritants and toxic inhalants
- Extreme obesity
- Difficulty swallowing for any reason
- Weakened chest muscles for any reason
- History of frequent respiratory infections

bar pneumonia. The differentiation of these conditions may well be established on a complete physical examination.

INSPECTION

Have the patient sit upright, if possible without support, naked to the waist. Clothing of any kind is a barrier. A drape should cover the patient when full exposure is not necessary. The room and stethoscope should be comfortably warm, and a bright tangential light is needed to highlight chest movement. Positioning the patient so that the light source comes at different angles may accentuate findings that are more subtle and otherwise difficult to detect, such as minimal pulsations or retractions, or the presence of deformity (e.g., minimal pectus excavatum). If the patient is in bed and mobility is limited, you should have access to both sides of the bed. Do not hesitate to raise and lower the bed as needed.

Note the shape and symmetry of the chest from both the back and the front, the costal angle, the angle of the ribs, and the intercostal spaces. The bony framework is obvious, the clavicles prominent superiorly, the sternum usually rather flat and free of an abundance of overlying tissue. (Box 13-2 lists thoracic landmarks to use as you record findings.) The chest will not be absolutely symmetric, but one side can be used as a comparison for the other. The AP diameter of the chest is ordinarily less than the transverse diameter, at times by as much as half (Fig. 13-8).

Barrel chest (Fig. 13-9) results from compromised respiration as in, for example, chronic asthma, emphysema, or cystic fibrosis. The ribs are more horizontal, the spine at least some-

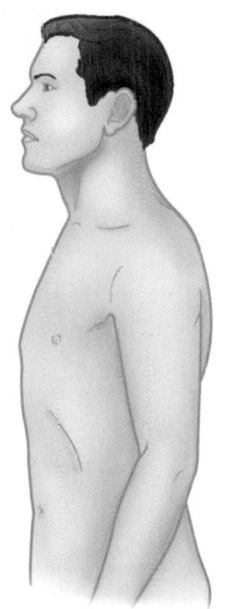
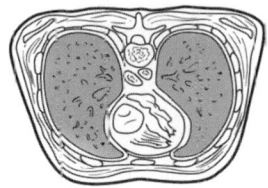

FIGURE 13-8
Thorax of healthy adult male. Note that the anteroposterior diameter is less than transverse diameter.

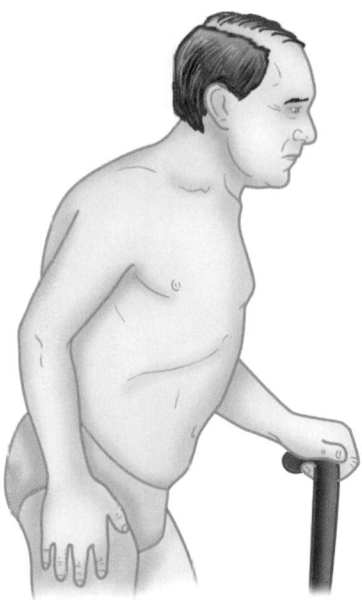
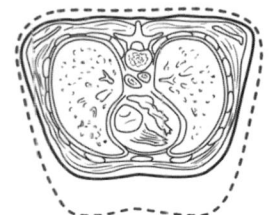

FIGURE 13-9
Barrel chest. Note increase in the anteroposterior diameter.

BOX 13-2

THORACIC LANDMARKS

In conjunction with the anatomic landmarks of the chest, the following imaginary lines on the surface will help localize the findings on physical examination (Fig. 13-10):

1. Midsternal line: vertically down the midline of the sternum
2. Right and left midclavicular lines: parallel to the midsternal line, beginning at midclavicle; the inferior borders of the lungs generally cross the sixth rib at the midclavicular line
3. Right and left anterior axillary lines: parallel to the midsternal line, beginning at the anterior axillary folds
4. Right and left midaxillary lines: parallel to the midsternal line, beginning at the midaxilla
5. Right and left posterior axillary lines: parallel to the midsternal line, beginning at the posterior axillary folds
6. Vertebral line: vertically down the spinal processes
7. Right and left scapular lines: parallel to the vertebral line, through the inferior angle of the scapula when the patient is erect

The spinous process of the seventh cervical vertebra is readily palpated. The thoracic vertebrae can then be counted down from that point (Fig. 13-11). Although the head of each rib articulates with its corresponding vertebra, remember that the spinous process of that vertebra is the palpable portion. It extends caudally and is dorsal to the next vertebral body. Thus the rib you feel in apparent association with the spinous process is really the number of that process plus one.

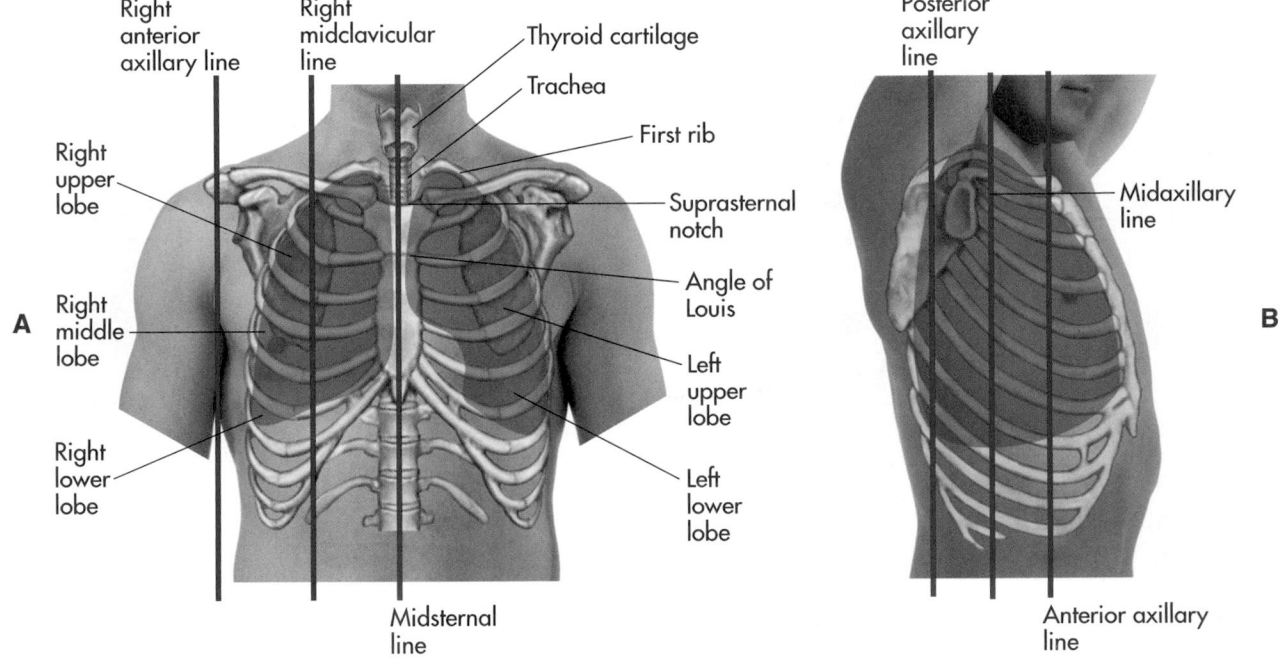

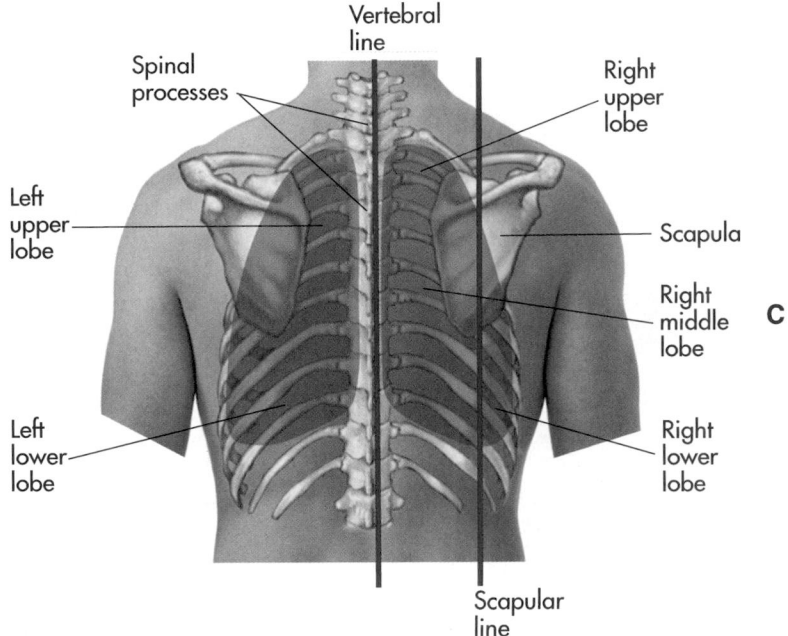

FIGURE 13-10

Thoracic landmarks. **A,** Anterior thorax. **B,** Right lateral thorax. **C,** Posterior thorax.

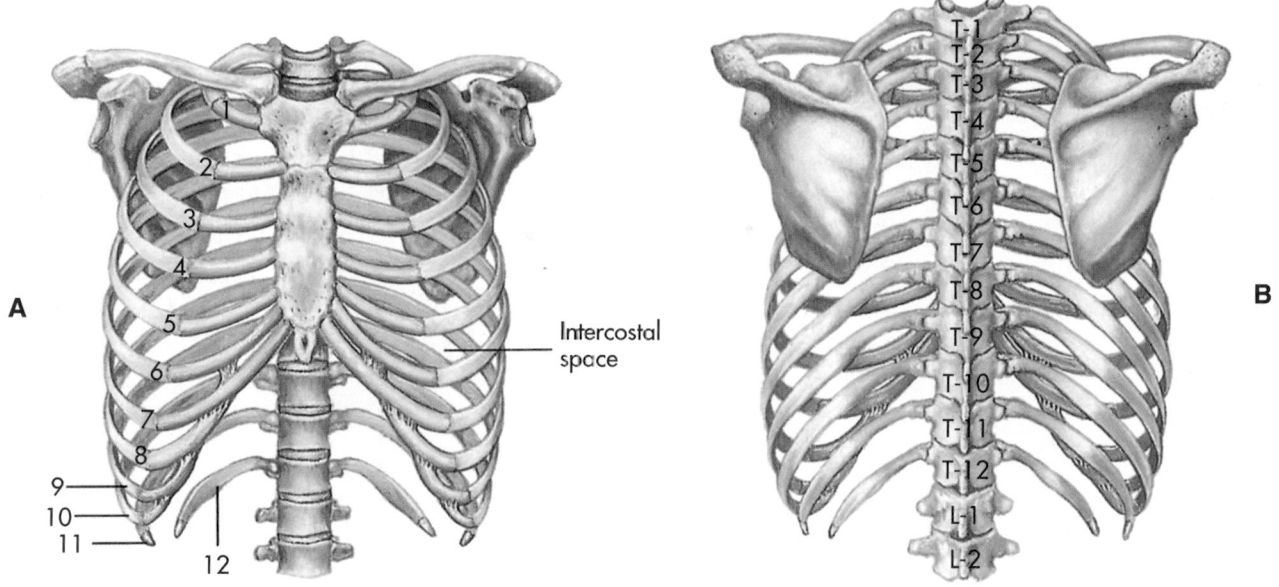

FIGURE 13-11
Rib cage. **A,** Anterior view. **B,** Posterior view.

what kyphotic, and the sternal angle more prominent. The trachea may be posteriorly displaced. Ordinarily, the AP diameter should be less than the lateral diameter. The relationship is expressed as the "thoracic ratio" and is expected to be about 0.70 to 0.75. It does increase with age; however, when the AP diameter approaches or equals the transverse diameter (a ratio of 1.0 or even more), there is most often a problem.

Other changes in chest wall contour may be the result of structural problems in the spine, rib cage, or sternum. The spine may be deviated either posteriorly (kyphosis) or laterally (scoliosis) (see Fig. 21-20, *B*, and Fig. 21-77). Two common structural problems are pigeon chest (pectus carinatum), which is a prominent sternal protrusion; and funnel chest (pectus excavatum), which is an indentation of the lower sternum above the xiphoid process (Fig. 13-12).

Inspect the skin, nails, lips, and nipples, noting whether cyanosis or pallor is present. These may be clues to respiratory or cardiac disorder. Smell the breath; intrathoracic infection may make it malodorous. Note whether there are supernumerary nipples; these are often a clue to other congenital abnormalities, particularly in white patients. Look for any superficial venous patterns over the chest, which may be a sign of heart disorders or vascular obstruction or disease. The underlying fat and relative prominence of the ribs give some clue to general nutrition.

RESPIRATION

Determine the respiratory rate. The rate should be 12 to 20 respirations per minute; the ratio of respirations to heartbeats is approximately 1:4. You need not tell the patient that you are counting respirations. Often the patient will have a self-conscious response that may be misleading; therefore, make your count as you are palpating the pulse. Check each of the rates in sequence without the patient being precisely aware of what you are doing. Respiratory rates can vary in the different waking and sleep states. Noting the behavior of the patient relative to the rate is often helpful.

Note the pattern (or rhythm) of respiration and the way in which the chest moves (Fig. 13-13). Expansion of the chest should be bilaterally symmetric. Expect the patient to breathe easily, regularly, and without apparent distress. The pattern of breathing should be even, neither too shallow nor too deep. Note any variations in respiratory rate.

DESCRIPTORS OF RESPIRATION

Dyspnea, difficult and labored breathing with shortness of breath, is commonly observed with pulmonary or cardiac compromise. A sedentary lifestyle and obesity can cause it in an otherwise well person. In general, dyspnea increases with the severity of the underlying condition. It is important to establish the amount and kind of effort that produces dyspnea:

♦ Is it present even when the patient is resting?

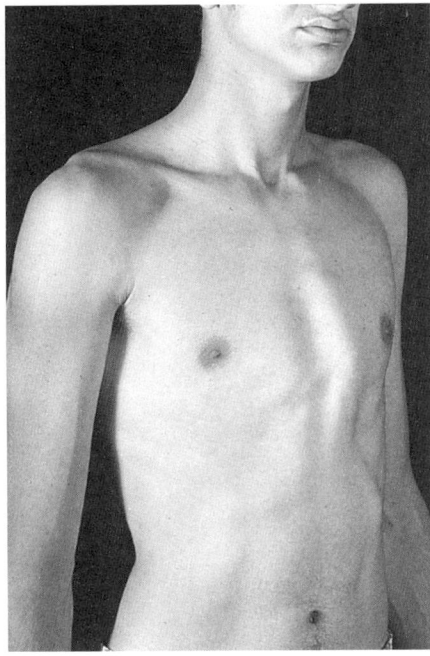
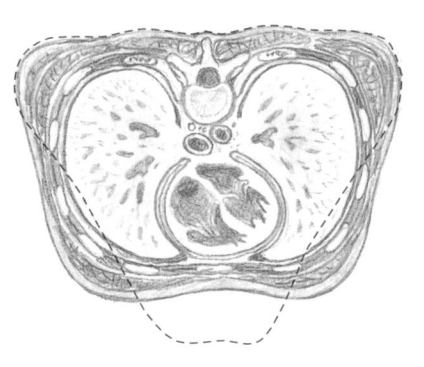

A

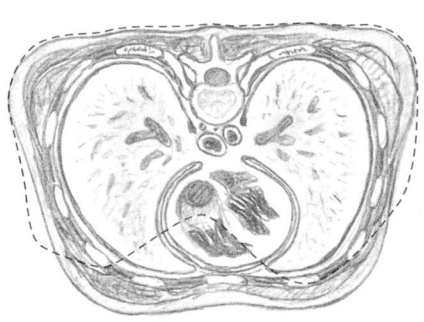
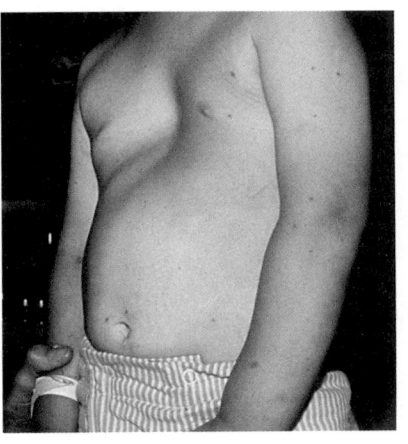

B

FIGURE 13-12
A, Unilateral pectus carinatum (pigeon chest) in an 18-year-old. **B,** Pectus excavatum (funnel chest) in a young child. Note the child's poor posture, potbelly, and sunken chest.

> **MNEMONICS**
>
> ***Dyspnea of Rapid Onset:
> 10 Ps***
>
> **P** Pneumonia
> **P** Pneumothorax
> **P** Pulmonary constriction/
>   asthma
> **P** Peanut (or other for-
>   eign body)
> **P** Pulmonary embolus
> **P** Pericardial tamponade
> **P** Pump failure (heart
>   failure)
> **P** Peak seekers (high alti-
>   tudes)
> **P** Psychogenic
> **P** Poisons
>
> Modified from Shipman, 1984.

- How much walking? On a level surface? Up stairs?
- Is it necessary to stop and rest when climbing stairs?
- With what other activities of daily life does dyspnea begin? With what level of physical demand?

Other manifestations of respiratory difficulty include the following:

- *Orthopnea*—shortness of breath that begins or increases when the patient lies down; ask whether the patient needs to sleep on more than one pillow and whether that helps.
- *Paroxysmal nocturnal dyspnea*—a sudden onset of shortness of breath after a period of sleep; sitting upright is helpful.
- *Platypnea*—dyspnea increases in the upright posture.

Tachypnea is a persistent respiratory rate approaching 25 respirations per minute. Double check to be sure that the respiratory rate is persistent. Rapid, shallow breathing may occur during hyperventilation or simply as a self-conscious response to your observation. It is often a symptom of protective splinting from pain of a broken rib or pleurisy. Massive liver enlargement or abdominal ascites may prevent descent of the diaphragm and produce a similar pattern. *Bradypnea,* a rate slower than 12 respirations per minute, may indicate neurologic or electrolyte disturbance, infection, or a sensible response to protect against the pain of pleurisy or other irritative phenomena. It may also indicate a splendid level of cardiorespiratory fitness.

Note any variations in respiratory rhythm. It may be difficult to discern abnormalities unless they are quite obvious (Box 13-3). If the patient is breathing laboriously, as if forced, and

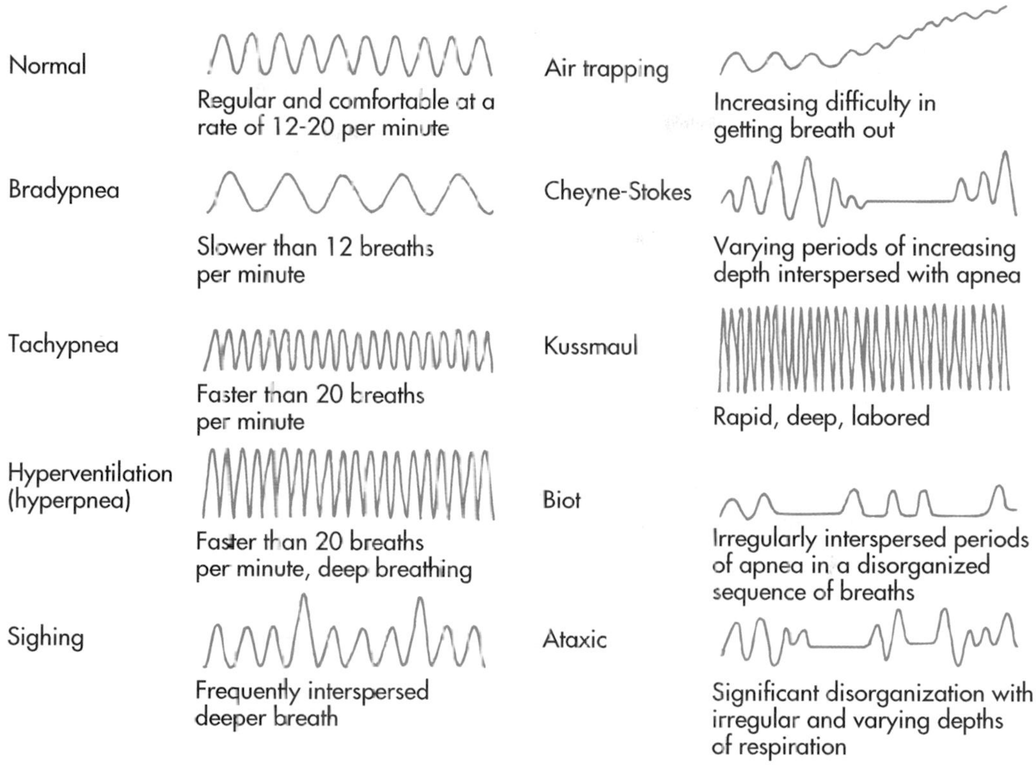

Normal		Air trapping	
	Regular and comfortable at a rate of 12-20 per minute		Increasing difficulty in getting breath out
Bradypnea		Cheyne-Stokes	
	Slower than 12 breaths per minute		Varying periods of increasing depth interspersed with apnea
Tachypnea		Kussmaul	
	Faster than 20 breaths per minute		Rapid, deep, labored
Hyperventilation (hyperpnea)		Biot	
	Faster than 20 breaths per minute, deep breathing		Irregularly interspersed periods of apnea in a disorganized sequence of breaths
Sighing		Ataxic	
	Frequently interspersed deeper breath		Significant disorganization with irregular and varying depths of respiration

FIGURE 13-13
Patterns of respiration. The horizontal axis indicates the relative rates of these patterns. The vertical swings of the lines indicate the relative depth of respiration.

BOX 13-3

INFLUENCES ON THE RATE AND DEPTH OF BREATHING

The rate and depth of breathing will:

Increase With	Decrease With
Acidosis (metabolic)	Alkalosis (metabolic)
Central nervous system lesions (pons)	Central nervous system lesions (cerebrum)
Anxiety	Myasthenia gravis
Aspirin poisoning	Narcotic overdoses
Oxygen need (hypoxemia)	Obesity (extreme)
Pain	

---

deeply *(hyperpnea)*, hyperventilation results, particularly when respirations are also rapid. Exercise and anxiety can cause hyperpnea, but so can central nervous system and metabolic disease. *Kussmaul breathing*, always deep and most often rapid, is the eponym applied to the respiratory effort associated with metabolic acidosis. *Hypopnea*, on the other hand, refers to abnormally shallow respirations (e.g., when pleuritic pain limits excursion).

A regular periodic pattern of breathing, with intervals of apnea followed by a crescendo/decrescendo sequence of respiration, is called *periodic breathing* or *Cheyne-Stokes* respiration. Children and older adults may breathe in this pattern during sleep, but otherwise it occurs in patients who are seriously ill, particularly those with brain damage at the cerebral level or with drug-caused respiratory compromise (Box 13-4).

An occasional deep, audible sigh that punctuates an otherwise regular respiratory pattern is associated with emotional distress or an incipient episode of more severe hyperventilation. Sighs are significant only if they exceed the infrequent and relatively inconsequential sighs of daily life.

If the pulmonary tree is seriously obstructed for any reason, inspired air has difficulty overcoming the resistance and getting out. *Air trapping* is the result of a prolonged but inefficient

BOX 13-4

APNEA

Apnea, the absence of spontaneous respiration, may have its origin in the respiratory system and, as well, in a variety of central nervous system and cardiac abnormalities. Common contributors include seizures, central nervous system trauma or hypoperfusion, a variety of infections of the respiratory passageway, drug ingestions, and obstructive sleep disorders. *Cheyne-Stokes respiration* has characteristic moments of apnea. There is the universal expectation of the absence of breathing when one is swallowing (deglutition apnea). *Primary apnea* is a self-limited condition, and not uncommon after a blow to the head. It is especially noted immediately after the birth of a newborn, who will breathe spontaneously when sufficient carbon dioxide accumulates in the circulation. If irritating and nausea-provoking vapors or gases are inhaled, there can be an involuntary, obviously temporary halt to respiration (reflex apnea). *Secondary apnea* is grave. The breathing stops and it will not begin spontaneously unless resuscitative measures

are immediately instituted. Any event that severely limits the absorption of oxygen into the bloodstream will lead to secondary apnea. *Sleep apnea*, characterized by periods of an absence of breathing effort during sleep, can be very disturbing; the respiratory muscles do not function and airflow is not maintained through the nose and mouth. *Selective apnea* affects only a part of the breathing cycle. *Apneustic breathing* is characterized by a long inspiration and what amounts to expiration apnea. The neural center for control is in the pons. When it is affected, breathing can become gasping, because inspirations are prolonged and expiration constrained. The *apnea of prematurity* is a more intense version of *periodic apnea of the newborn*, a normal condition characterized by an irregular pattern of rapid breathing interspersed with brief periods of apnea that one usually associates with rapid eye movement sleep.

---

expiratory effort. The rate of respiration increases in order to compensate; as this happens, the effort becomes more shallow, the amount of trapped air increases, and the lungs inflate.

Biot respiration consists of somewhat irregular respirations varying in depth and interrupted by intervals of apnea, but lacking the repetitive pattern of periodic respiration. On occasion, the respirations may be regular, but the apneic periods may occur in an irregular pattern. Biot respiration usually is associated with severe and persistent increased intracranial pressure, respiratory compromise resulting from drug poisoning, or brain damage at the level of the medulla. It may be referred to as ataxic in its more extreme expression. Changes in breathing pattern are usually significant. When breathing is labored or respirations are deeper than usual, the accessory muscles of respiration, the sternocleidomastoid and trapezius muscles, may be used.

OBSERVING RESPIRATION

Inspect the chest wall movement during respiration. Again, different angles of illumination will aid inspection and help delineate chest wall deformities. Expansion should be symmetric, without apparent use of accessory muscles. Thoracic (costal) respiration is primarily the result of the use of intercostal muscles. Diaphragmatic respiration, on the other hand, is primarily the result of the movement of the diaphragm responding to intrathoracic pressure. Abdominal respiration involves contraction of the diaphragm and the interplay of the abdominal muscles, resulting in the expansion and recoil of the abdominal walls. It is not unusual to see abdominal respiration, particularly in very young infants. Thoracic respiration, however, is the rule at most ages unless the intercostal and other thoracic muscles are compromised or the person has a pathophysiologic need to use every respiratory resource. Men are more likely to use diaphragmatic respiration and women, particularly when they are pregnant, are more likely to use thoracic.

Chest asymmetry can be associated with unequal expansion and respiratory compromise caused by a collapsed lung or limitation of expansion by extrapleural air, fluid, or a mass. Unilateral or bilateral bulging can be a reaction of the ribs and interspaces to respiratory obstruction. A prolonged expiration and bulging on expiration are probably caused by outflow obstruction or the valvelike action of compression by a tumor, aneurysm, or enlarged heart. When this happens, the costal angle widens beyond 90 degrees.

Retractions suggest an obstruction to inspiration at any point in the respiratory tract. As intrapleural pressure becomes increasingly negative, the musculature "pulls back" in an effort to overcome blockage. Any significant obstruction makes the retraction observable with each inspiratory effort. The degree and level of retraction depend on the extent and level of ob-

---

BOX 13-5

IS THE AIRWAY PATENT OR OBSTRUCTED?

Determining the patency of the upper airway is essential to a complete evaluation of pulmonary status. When is the upper airway obstructed?

- When there is:
  - Inspiratory stridor (with a ratio with expiration of more than 2:1)
  - A hoarse cough or cry
  - Flaring of the alae nasi
  - Retraction at the suprasternal notch
- Severely so, when:
  - Stridor is inspiratory and expiratory
  - Cough is barking
  - Retractions also involve the subcostal and intercostal spaces
  - Cyanosis is obvious even with blow-by oxygen
- When the obstruction is above the glottis:
  - Stridor tends to be quieter
  - The voice is muffled, as if there is a "hot potato" in the mouth
  - Swallowing is more difficult
  - Cough is not a factor
  - The head and neck may be awkwardly positioned to preserve the airway (e.g., extended with retropharyngeal abscess; head to the affected side with peritonsillar abscess)
- When the obstruction is below the glottis:
  - Stridor tends to be louder, more rasping
  - The voice is hoarse
  - Swallowing is not affected
  - Cough is harsh, barking
  - Positioning of the head is not a factor

● **CLINICAL PEARL**

Clubbing

Clubbing is usually symmetric and painless. While it ordinarily suggests significant disease, it may be hereditary.

struction (Box 13-5). When the obstruction is high in the respiratory tree (e.g., with tracheal or laryngeal involvement), breathing is characterized by stridor, and the chest wall seems to cave in at the sternum, between the ribs, at the suprasternal notch, above the clavicles, and at the lowest costal margins. Paradoxic breathing occurs when a negative intrathoracic pressure is transmitted to the abdomen by a weakened, poorly functioning diaphragm; obstructive airway disease; or during sleep, in the event of upper airway obstruction. Thus, on inspiration, the lower thorax is drawn in, and on expiration, the opposite occurs.

A foreign body in one or the other of the bronchi (usually the right because of its broader bore and more vertical placement) causes unilateral retraction, but the suprasternal notch is not involved. Retraction of the lower chest occurs with asthma and bronchiolitis.

LOOKING FOR CLUES AT THE PERIPHERY

Observe the lips and nails for cyanosis, the lips for pursing, the fingers for clubbing, and the alae nasi for flaring. Any of these peripheral clues suggests pulmonary or cardiac difficulty. Pursing of the lips is an accompaniment of increased expiratory effort. Patients learn without being taught that it reduces the effort of dyspnea. Clubbing, enlargement of the terminal phalanges of the fingers and/or toes is associated, for example, with chronic fibrotic changes within the lung, the chronic cyanosis of congenital heart disease, or cystic fibrosis. (Note that other chronic problems involving the lungs [e.g., asthma and emphysema] are not associated with clubbing.) Flaring of the alae nasi during inspiration is a common sign of air hunger, particularly when the alveoli are considerably involved.

PALPATION

Palpate the thoracic muscles and skeleton, feeling for pulsations, areas of tenderness, bulges, depressions, masses, unusual movement, and unusual positions. There should be bilateral symmetry and some elasticity of the rib cage, but the sternum and xiphoid should be relatively inflexible and the thoracic spine rigid.

Crepitus, a crackly or crinkly sensation, can be both palpated and heard—a gentle, bubbly feeling. It indicates air in the subcutaneous tissue from a rupture somewhere in the respiratory system or by infection with a gas-producing organism. It may be localized (e.g., over the suprasternal notch and base of the neck) or cover a wider area of the thorax, usually anteriorly and toward the axilla. Crepitus is always a sign requiring attention.

A palpable, coarse, grating vibration, usually on inspiration, suggests a *pleural friction rub* caused by inflammation of the pleural surfaces. Think of it as the feel of leather rubbing on leather.

Chest and Lungs:
Palpating for Thoracic Expansion

To evaluate thoracic expansion during respiration, stand behind the patient and place your thumbs along the spinal processes at the level of the tenth rib, with your palms lightly in contact with the posterolateral surfaces (Fig. 13-14). Watch your thumbs diverge during quiet and deep breathing. A loss of symmetry in the movement of the thumbs suggests a problem on one or both sides. Then face the patient and place your thumbs along the costal margin and the xiphoid process, with your palms touching the anterolateral chest. Again, watch your thumbs diverge as the patient breathes. A barrel-chested patient with chronic obstructive pulmonary disease may not demonstrate this. The chest is so inflated that it cannot expand further and your hands may even come together a bit.

Note the quality of the *tactile fremitus*, the palpable vibration of the chest wall that results from speech or other verbalizations. Fremitus is best felt parasternally at the second intercostal space at the level of the bifurcation of the bronchi. There is great variability depending on the intensity and pitch of the voice and the structure and thickness of the chest wall. In addition, the scapulae obscure fremitus.

Ask the patient to recite a few numbers or say a few words ("99" is a favorite, as is "Mickey Mouse," depending perhaps on the age) while you systematically palpate the chest with the palmar surfaces of the fingers or with the ulnar aspects of the hand. Use a firm, light touch, establishing even contact. For comparison, palpate both sides simultaneously and symmetrically; or use one hand, quickly alternating between the two sides. Move about the patient, palpating each area carefully: front to back, right side to left side, the lung apices (Fig. 13-15). Other examiners prefer to use what they determine is their dominant hand, the one their experience tells them is best suited for the assessment, moving it back and forth to make comparisons. As always, you must decide what better suits your need.

Decreased or absent fremitus may be caused by excess air in the lungs or may indicate emphysema, pleural thickening or effusion, massive pulmonary edema, or bronchial obstruction. Increased fremitus, often coarser or rougher in feel, occurs in the presence of fluids or a solid

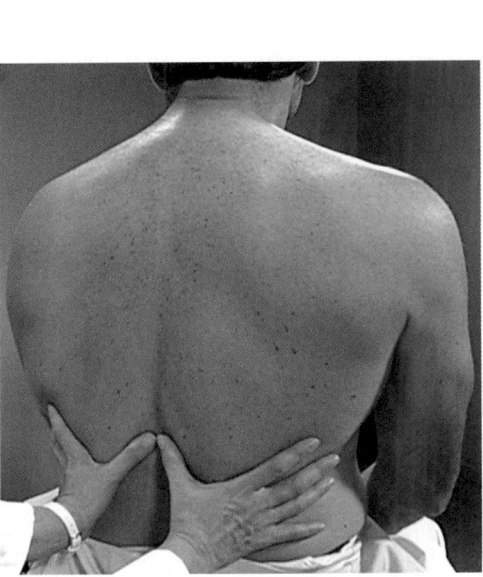

FIGURE 13-14
Palpating thoracic expansion. The thumbs are at the level of the tenth rib.

mass within the lungs and may be caused by lung consolidation, heavy but nonobstructive bronchial secretions, compressed lung, or tumor. Gentle, more tremulous fremitus than expected occurs with some lung consolidations and some inflammatory and infectious processes.

EXAMINING THE TRACHEA

Note the position of the trachea. Place an index finger in the suprasternal notch and move it gently, side to side, along the upper edges of each clavicle and in the spaces above to the inner borders of the sternocleidomastoid muscles. These spaces should be equal on both sides, and the trachea should be in the midline directly above the suprasternal notch. This can also be determined by palpating with both thumbs simultaneously (Fig. 13-16). A slight, barely noticeable deviation to the right is not unusual.

The trachea may be deviated because of problems within the chest and may, on occasion, seem to pulsate. It may be displaced by atelectasis, thyroid enlargement, significant parenchymal and/or pleural fibrosis, or pleural effusion; it may be pushed to one side by tension pneumothorax, a tumor, or nodal enlargements on the contralateral side; or it may be pulled by a tumor on the side to which it deviates. Anterior mediastinal tumors may push it posteriorly; with mediastinitis, the trachea may be pushed forward. A palpable pull out of midline with respiration is called a "tug."

Reminder: The examination of a woman's chest may be obscured by the breasts. It is permissible, when necessary, to move the breast gently or to ask the patient to do this for you. For example, when percussing you may shift the breast slightly with the pleximeter hand and, keeping it in place, strike the finger of that hand with the plexor of your free hand.

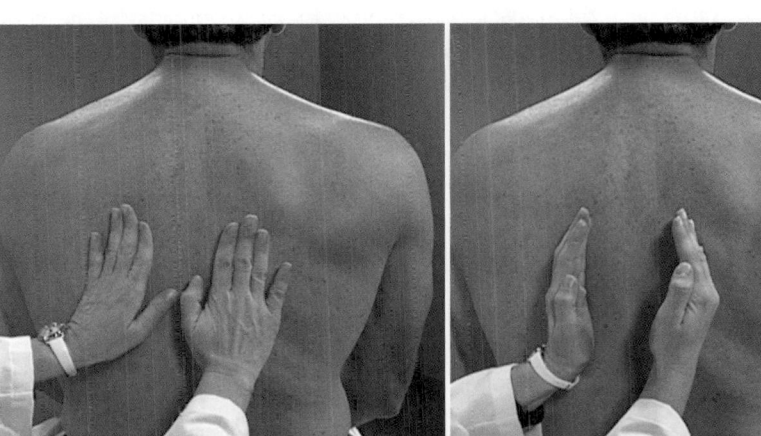

FIGURE 13-15
Two methods for evaluating tactile fremitus. **A,** With palmar surface of both hands. **B,** With ulnar aspect.

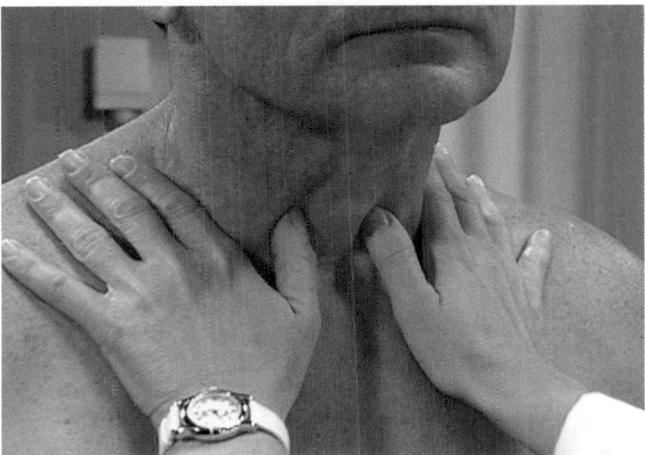

FIGURE 13-16
Palpating to evaluate midline position of the trachea.

PERCUSSION

Percussion tones heard over the chest, as elsewhere, are described in Chapter 3 and summarized in Fig. 13-17 and Table 13-1. You can percuss directly or indirectly, as described in Chapter 3. Remember that the heavier the stroke you use, the more likely you are to miss a transitional area from resonance to dullness. Tap sharply and consistently from the wrist but do not bang on your finger.

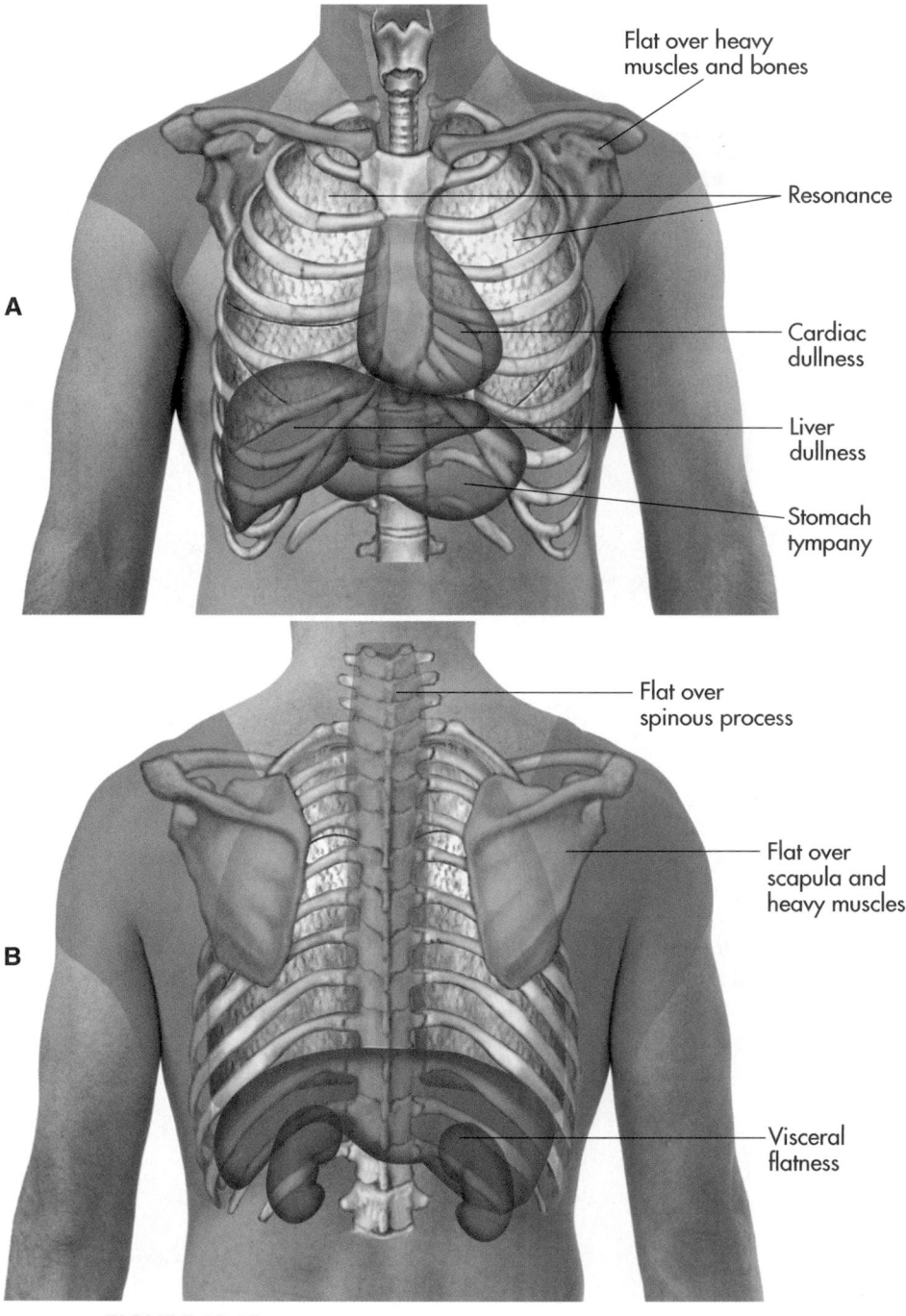

A

Flat over heavy
muscles and bones

Resonance

Cardiac
dullness

Liver
dullness

Stomach
tympany

B

Flat over
spinous process

Flat over
scapula and
heavy muscles

Visceral
flatness

FIGURE 13-17
Percussion tones throughout chest. **A,** Anterior view. **B,** Posterior view.

TABLE 13-1	Percussion Tones Heard over the Chest			
Type of Tone	**Intensity**	**Pitch**	**Duration**	**Quality**
Resonant	Loud	Low	Long	Hollow
Flat	Soft	High	Short	Very dull
Dull	Medium	Medium to high	Medium	Dull thud
Tympanic	Loud	High	Medium	Drumlike
Hyperresonant*	Very loud	Very low	Longer	Booming

See Chapter 3 for definitions and a more complete discussion of these tones.
*Hyperresonance is an abnormal sound, the result of air trapping (e.g., in obstructive lung disease).

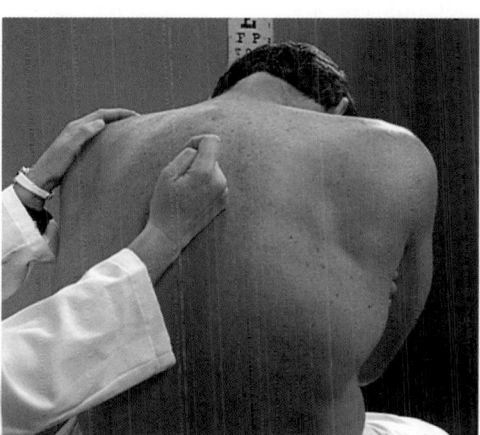
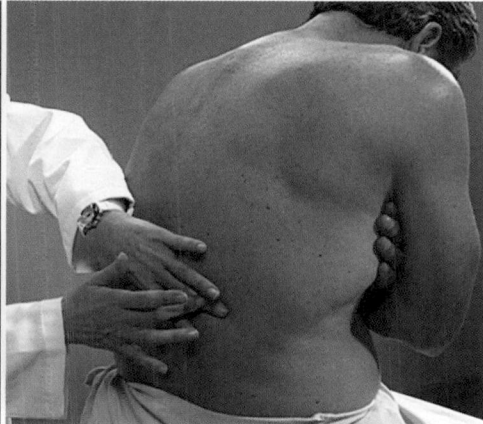

FIGURE 13-18
A, Direct percussion using ulnar aspect of fist. **B,** Indirect percussion.

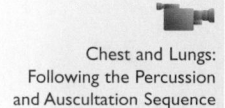

Chest and Lungs:
Following the Percussion
and Auscultation Sequence

Compare all areas bilaterally, using one side as a control for the other. The following sequence serves as one model. First, examine the back with the patient sitting with head bent forward and arms folded in front. This moves the scapulae laterally, exposing more of the lung. Then ask the patient to raise the arms overhead while you percuss the lateral and anterior chest. For all positions, percuss at 4- to 5-cm intervals over the intercostal spaces, moving systematically from superior to inferior and medial to lateral (Figs. 13-18 and 13-19). This sequence is one of many that you may follow. Adopt the one most comfortable for you and use it consistently. Resonance, the expected sound, can usually be heard over all areas of the lungs. Hyperresonance associated with hyperinflation may indicate emphysema, pneumothorax, or asthma. Dullness or flatness suggests atelectasis, pleural effusion, pneumothorax, or asthma. Tympany is the sound usually associated with percussion over the abdomen.

DIAPHRAGMATIC EXCURSION

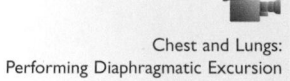

Chest and Lungs:
Performing Diaphragmatic Excursion

Measure the diaphragmatic excursion. Its descent may be limited by several types of lesions: pulmonary (e.g., as a result of emphysema), abdominal (e.g., massive ascites, tumor), or superficial painful (e.g., fractured rib). The diaphragm is usually higher on the right than on the left because it sits over the bulk of the liver.

The following steps suggest one approach to measuring the diaphragmatic excursion:
◆ Ask the patient to take a deep breath and hold it.
◆ Percuss along the scapular line until you locate the lower border, the point marked by a change in note from resonance to dullness.
◆ Mark the point with a skin pencil at the scapular line. Allow the patient to breathe, and then repeat the procedure on the other side.
◆ Ask the patient to take several breaths, to exhale as much as possible, and then to hold (Box 13-6).
◆ Percuss up from the marked point and make a mark at the change from dullness to resonance. Remind the patient to start breathing. Repeat on the other side.

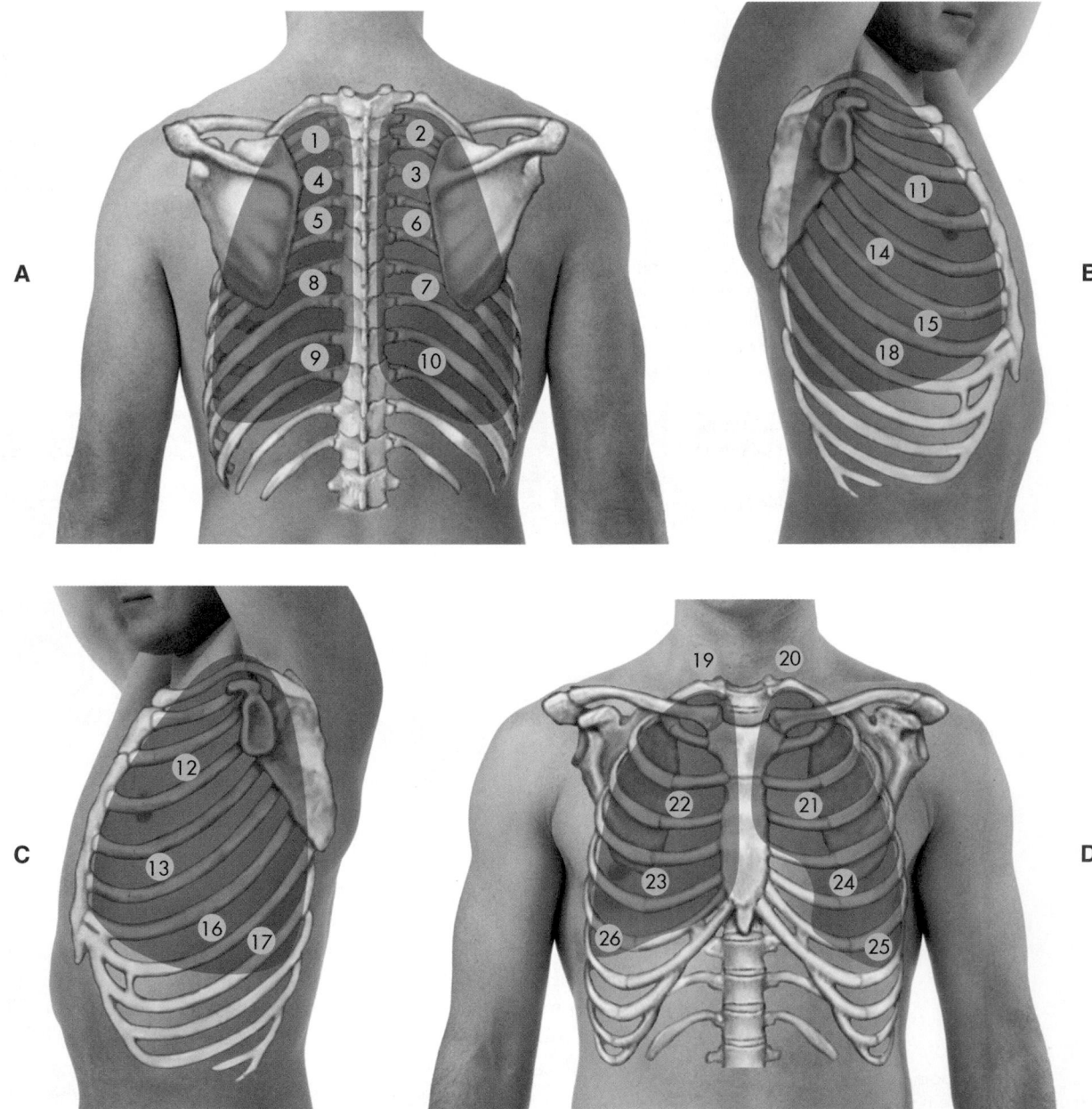

FIGURE 13-19
Suggested sequence for systematic percussion and auscultation of the thorax. **A,** Posterior thorax.
B, Right lateral thorax. **C,** Left lateral thorax. **D,** Anterior thorax. The pleximeter finger or the
stethoscope is moved in the numeric sequence suggested; however, other sequences are possible. It
is beneficial to be systematic.

◆ Measure and record the distance in centimeters between the marks on each side. The excursion distance is usually 3 to 5 or 6 cm (Fig. 13-20).

Some examiners object to the use of marking pencils and writing on the back. Alternatively, you might (a bit awkwardly) use strips of tape, or use one hand as a stationary landmark, percussing directly with the other and estimating the distance. It must be noted, however, that such estimates are not always consistent with radiologic confirmation.

> **BOX 13-6**
>
> **BAD BREATH: A POSSIBLE SIGN OF INFECTION**
>
> **Smell the Breath**
>
> Auscultation of the lungs makes it possible (occasionally, even uncomfortably so) to become aware of a patient's breath odor. Bad breath, even when it is not too distinct, is rather easily noticed. Infection, either acute or chronic, somewhere in the nasal or oral cavity or deep in the lung, can be the source. An especially foul or putrid odor of breath and/or sputum suggests anaerobic respiratory infections, empyema, bronchiectasis, lung abscess, or a particularly insistent bronchitis. Your nose may provide a significant clue:
>
> | | |
> |---|---|
> | Sweet, fruity | Diabetic ketoacidosis; starvation ketosis |
> | Fishy, stale | Uremia (trimethylamines) |
> | Ammonia-like | Uremia (ammonia) |
> | Musty fish, clover | Fetor hepaticus: hepatic failure, portal vein thrombosis, portacaval shunts |
> | Foul, feculent | Intestinal obstruction/diverticulum |
> | Foul, putrid | Nasal/sinus pathology: infection, foreign body, cancer; respiratory infections: empyema, lung abscess, bronchiectasis |
> | Halitosis | Tonsillitis, gingivitis, respiratory infections, Vincent angina, gastroesophageal reflux |
> | Cinnamon | Pulmonary tuberculosis |
>
> Data from Wilson, 1997; McMillan, Stockman, Oski, 1982.

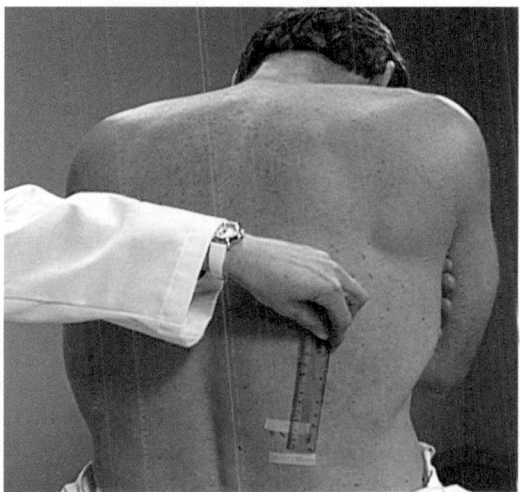

FIGURE 13-20
Measuring diaphragmatic excursion. Excursion distance is usually 3 to 5 cm.

AUSCULTATION

Auscultation with a stethoscope provides important clues to the condition of the lungs and pleura. (On relatively rare occasions, a sound is apparent to the ear directly that might be lost via the stethoscope, for example, the click of an aspirated foreign body.) All sounds can be characterized in the same manner as the percussion notes: intensity, pitch, quality, and duration (Table 13-2).

Have the patient sit upright, if possible, and breathe slowly and deeply through the mouth, exaggerating normal respiration. Demonstrate this yourself. Caution the patient to keep a pace consistent with comfort; hyperventilation, which occurs more easily than one might think, may cause faintness, and exaggerated breathing can be tiring, especially for older or ill patients. Because most pulmonary pathologic conditions in older patients occur at the lung bases, it is a good idea to examine these first, before fatigue sets in.

TABLE 13-2	Characteristics of Normal Breath Sounds	
Sound	**Characteristics**	**Findings**
Vesicular	Heard over most of lung fields; low pitch; soft and short expirations (see Figs. 13-22 and 13-23); more prominent in a thin person or a child, diminished in the overweight or very muscular patient	
Bronchovesicular	Heard over main bronchus area and over upper right posterior lung field; medium pitch; expiration equals inspiration	
Bronchial/tracheal (tubular)	Heard only over trachea; high pitch; loud and long expirations, sometimes a bit longer than inspiration	

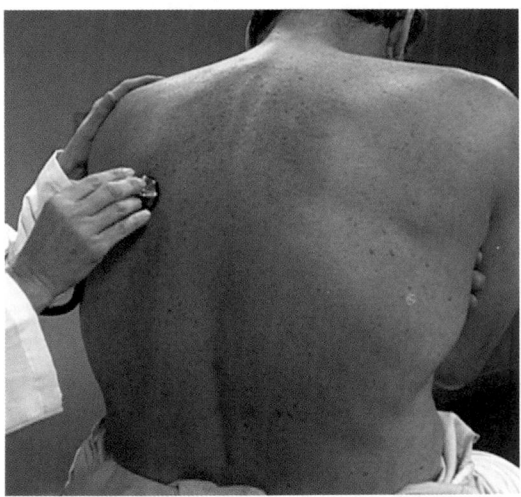

FIGURE 13-21
Auscultation with a stethoscope.

The diaphragm of the stethoscope is usually preferable to the bell for listening to the lungs because it transmits the ordinarily high-pitched sounds better and because it provides a broader area of sound. Place the stethoscope firmly on the skin (Fig. 13-21). When the individual breath sound is being evaluated, there should be no movement of patient or stethoscope except for the respiratory excursion.

To auscultate the back, ask the patient to sit as for percussion, with head bent forward and arms folded in front to enlarge the listening area (see Fig. 13-21). Then have the patient sit more erect with arms overhead for auscultating the lateral chest. Finally, ask the patient to sit erect with the shoulders back for auscultation of the anterior chest. As with so much else, the exact sequence you adopt is not as important as using the same sequence each time to ensure that the examination is thorough.

Listen systematically at each position throughout inspiration and expiration, taking advantage of a side-to-side comparison as you move downward from apex to base at intervals of several centimeters. The sounds of the middle lobe of the right lung and the lingula on the left are best heard in the respective axillae.

CLINICAL PEARL

Congestive Heart Failure
If the patient may have congestive heart failure, you should begin auscultation at the base of the lungs to detect crackles that may disappear with continued exaggerated respiration.

BREATH SOUNDS

Breath sounds are made by the flow of air through the respiratory tree. They are characterized by pitch, intensity, quality, and relative duration of their inspiratory and expiratory phases, and are classified as vesicular, bronchovesicular, and bronchial (tubular) (Fig. 13-22; see Table 13-2).

Vesicular breath sounds are low-pitched, low-intensity sounds heard over healthy lung tissue. *Bronchovesicular* sounds are heard over the major bronchi and are typically moderate in

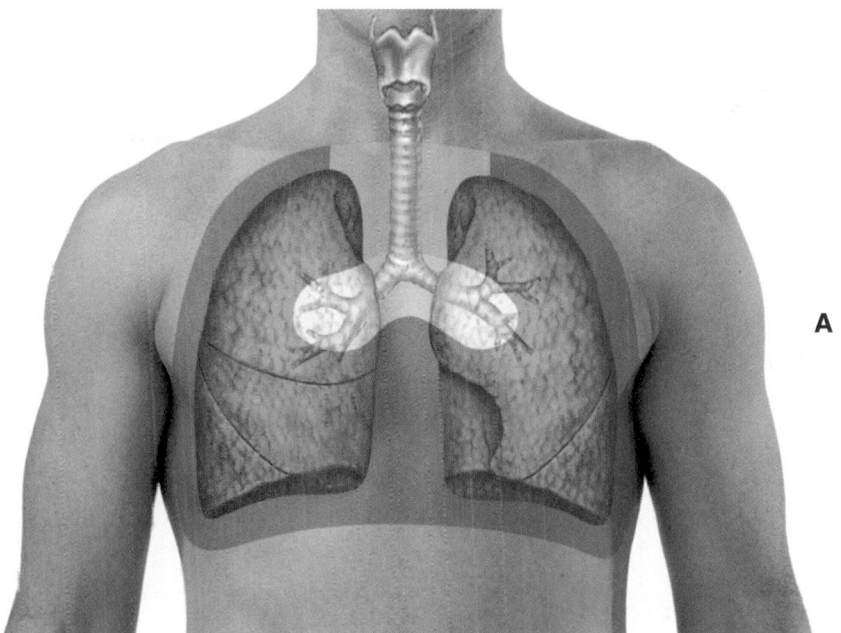

A

KEY:

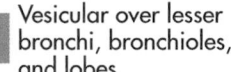 Bronchovesicular
over main bronchi

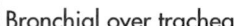 Vesicular over lesser
bronchi, bronchioles,
and lobes

Bronchial over trachea

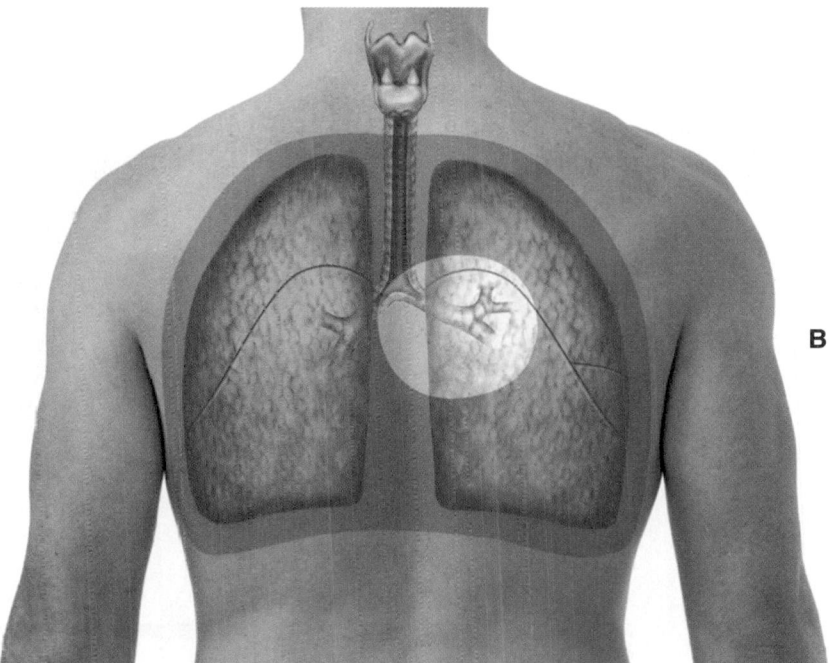

B

FIGURE 13-22
Expected auscultatory sounds.
A, Anterior view. **B,** Posterior
view.

pitch and intensity. The sounds highest in pitch and intensity are the *bronchial* breath sounds, which are ordinarily heard only over the trachea. Both bronchovesicular and bronchial breath sounds are abnormal if they are heard over the peripheral lung tissue.

Breathing that resembles the noise made by blowing across the mouth of a bottle is defined as *amphoric* and is most often heard with a large, relatively stiff-walled pulmonary cavity or a tension pneumothorax with bronchopleural fistula. *Cavernous breathing,* sounding as if coming from a cavern, is commonly heard over a pulmonary cavity in which the wall is rigid.

Breath sounds, dependent in large part for their intensity or the speed with which air enters and leaves the mouth, are relatively more difficult to hear or are absent if fluid or pus has accumulated in the pleural space, if secretions or a foreign body obstructs the bronchi, if the lungs are hyperinflated, or if breathing is shallow from splinting because of pain. Breath sounds are easier to hear when the lungs are consolidated; the mass surrounding the tube of the respiratory tree promotes sound transmission better than do air-filled alveoli.

Most of the unexpected sounds heard during lung auscultation are superimposed on the breath sounds. Extraneous sounds such as the crinkling of chest or back hair must be carefully distinguished from far more significant adventitious sounds. Sometimes it helps to moisten chest hair to minimize this problem. The common terms used to describe adventitious sounds are *crackles* (formerly called *rales*), *rhonchi, wheezes,* and *friction rub* (Fig. 13-23 and Box 13-7). Crackles are discontinuous; rhonchi and wheezes are continuous. Box 13-8 gives a detailed description of adventitious breath sounds. Table 13-3 summarizes nomenclature for adventitious breath sounds in several languages.

Crackles. A crackle is an abnormal respiratory sound heard more often during inspiration and characterized by discrete discontinuous sounds, each lasting just a few milliseconds. The individual noise tends to be brief and the interval to the next one similarly brief.

Crackles may be fine, high pitched, and relatively short in duration; or coarse, low pitched, and relatively longer in duration. They are caused by the disruptive passage of air through the small airways in the respiratory tree. High-pitched crackles are described as *sibilant;* the more low pitched are termed *sonorous.* Crackles with a dry quality, more crisp than gurgling, are apt

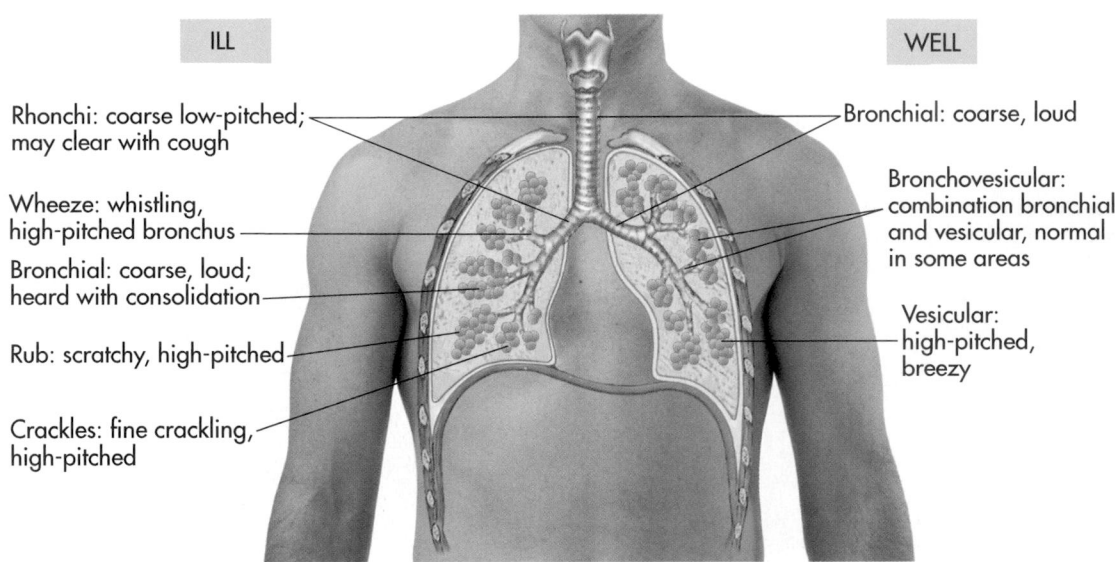

ILL

Rhonchi: coarse low-pitched; may clear with cough

Wheeze: whistling, high-pitched bronchus

Bronchial: coarse, loud; heard with consolidation

Rub: scratchy, high-pitched

Crackles: fine crackling, high-pitched

WELL

Bronchial: coarse, loud

Bronchovesicular: combination bronchial and vesicular, normal in some areas

Vesicular: high-pitched, breezy

FIGURE 13-23
Schema of breath sounds in the ill and well patient.

BOX 13-7

THE TERMINOLOGY OF BREATH SOUNDS

Breath sounds are easier to recognize than to describe. Perhaps that is why the traditional use of the word *rales* has yielded to *crackles.* The terminology we use follows the suggestion of the American Thoracic Society; it is reflected in Table 13-3 (in several languages). However, terms cannot be rigid because the airway is continuous and there may be overlapping noises which, while obvious to the ear, may not lend themselves to precise description. Terminology, however, attempts to follow a common understanding in the sometimes frustrating effort to be exact. For example, you may hear expiratory wheezing without the stethoscope or, on inspiration in patients with chronic bronchitis or asthma, a radio static-like sound lacking a musical pitch. This, perhaps without a common understanding, is termed "white noise" and is caused by a narrowed central airway.

Data from McGee, 2001.

to occur higher in the respiratory tree. You might listen for crackles at the open mouth. If their origin is in the upper airways, they will be easily heard; if in the lower, not so easily.

Rhonchi. *Rhonchi (sonorous wheezes)* are deeper, more rumbling, more pronounced during expiration, more likely to be prolonged and continuous, and less discrete than crackles. They are caused by the passage of air through an airway obstructed by thick secretions, muscular

---

BOX 13-8

ADVENTITIOUS BREATH SOUNDS

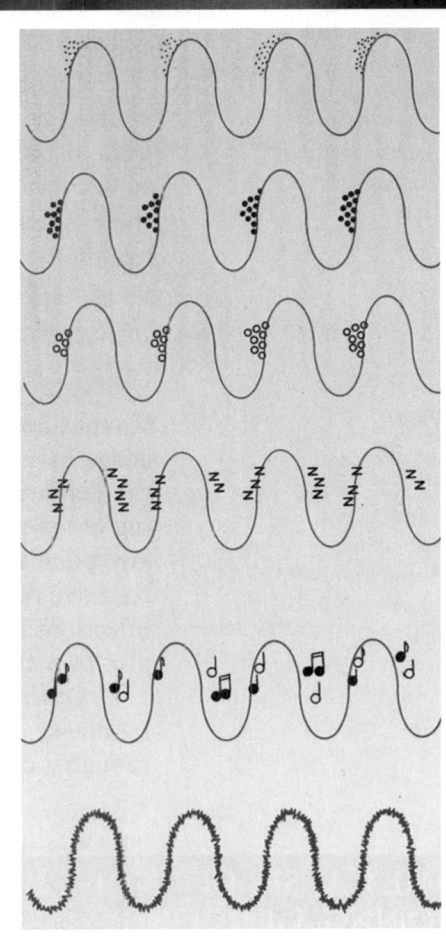

Fine crackles: high-pitched, discrete, discontinuous crackling sounds heard during the end of inspiration; not cleared by a cough

Medium crackles: lower, more moist sound heard during the midstage of inspiration; not cleared by a cough

Coarse crackles: loud, bubbly noise heard during inspiration; not cleared by a cough

Rhonchi (sonorous wheeze): loud, low, coarse sounds like a snore most often heard continuously during inspiration or expiration; coughing may clear sound (usually means mucus accumulation in trachea or large bronchi)

Wheeze (sibilant wheeze): musical noise sounding like a squeak; most often heard continuously during inspiration or expiration; usually louder during expiration

Pleural friction rub: dry, rubbing, or grating sound, usually caused by inflammation of pleural surfaces; heard during inspiration or expiration; loudest over lower lateral anterior surface

Modified from Thompson et al, 1997.

TABLE 13-3	Nomenclature for Adventitious Breath Sounds				
Lung Sound	**English**	**French**	**German**	**Spanish**	**Portuguese**
Discontinuous					
Fine (high pitched, low amplitude, short duration)	Fine crackles	Râles crepitants	Feines Rassein	Esterfores finos	Estertores finos
Coarse (low pitched, high amplitude, long duration)	Coarse crackles	Râles bulleux ou Sous-crepitants	Grobes Rassein	Estertore grossos	Estertores gruesos
Continuous					
High pitched	Wheezes	Râles sibilants	Pfeifen	Sibilancias	Sibilos
Low pitched	Rhonchus	Râles ronflants	Brummen	Roncus	Roncos

From Cugell, 1987.

VOCAL RESONANCE

spasm, new growth, or external pressure. The more sibilant, higher-pitched rhonchi arise from the smaller bronchi, as in asthma; the more sonorous, lower-pitched rhonchi arise from larger bronchi, as in tracheobronchitis. All rhonchi may at times be palpable.

It may be difficult to distinguish between crackles and rhonchi. In general, rhonchi tend to disappear after coughing, whereas crackles do not. If such sounds are present, listen to several respiratory excursions: a few with the patient's accustomed effort, a few with deeper breathing, a few before coughing, and a few after.

Wheezes. A *wheeze (sibilant wheeze)* is sometimes thought of as a form of rhonchus. It is a continuous, high-pitched, musical sound (almost a whistle) heard during inspiration or expiration. It is caused by a relatively high-velocity air flow through a narrowed or obstructed airway. The longer the wheeze and the higher the pitch, the worse the obstruction. Wheezes may be composed of complex combinations of a variety of pitches or of a single pitch, and they may vary from area to area and minute to minute. If a wheeze is heard bilaterally, it may be caused by the bronchospasm of asthma (reactive airway disease) or acute or chronic bronchitis. Unilateral or more sharply localized wheezing or stridor may occur with a foreign body. A tumor compressing a part of the bronchial tree can create a consistent wheeze or whistle of single pitch at the site of compression. If infection is the source of wheezing, the organism is usually a virus, not a bacterium. The Differential Diagnosis box on p. 389 discusses anthrax and selected elements of bioterrorism and list other possible causes of wheezing and of noisy breathing in general.

Other Sounds. A *friction rub* occurs outside the respiratory tree. It has a dry, crackly, grating, low-pitched sound and is heard in both expiration and inspiration. It may have a machine-like quality. It may have no significance if heard over the liver or spleen; however, a friction rub heard over the heart or lungs is caused by inflamed, roughened surfaces rubbing together. Over the pericardium, this sound suggests pericarditis; over the lungs, pleurisy. The respiratory rub disappears when the breath is held; the cardiac rub does not.

Mediastinal crunch (Hamman sign) is found with mediastinal emphysema. There is a great variety of noise—loud crackles and clicking and gurgling sounds. These are synchronous with the heartbeat and not particularly so with respiration, but the sounds can be more pronounced toward the end of expiration. They are easiest to hear when the patient leans to the left or lies down on the left side.

Air and fluid simultaneously present in the pleural cavity or in large cavities within the lungs can be heard if one listens over the possibly involved area while gently shaking the patient. With the patient sitting, place a hand on the patient's shoulder and then move the patient from side to side, not brusquely but with a bit of vigor. The fluid will splash, and in the presence of air, a *succussion splash* will be heard.

The spoken voice vibrates and transmits sounds through the lung fields that may be judged with the stethoscope with reasonable ease. Ask the patient to recite numbers, names, or other words. These transmitted sounds are usually muffled and indistinct, and are best heard medially. Pay particular attention to vocal resonance if there are other unexpected findings during any part of the examination of the lungs, such as dullness on percussion or changes in tactile fremitus. The factors that influence tactile fremitus similarly influence vocal resonance.

Greater clarity and increased loudness of spoken sounds are defined as *bronchophony*. If bronchophony is extreme (e.g., in the presence of consolidation of the lungs), even a whisper can be heard clearly and intelligibly through the stethoscope *(whispered pectoriloquy)*. When the intensity of the spoken voice is increased and there is a nasal quality (e.g., *e*'s become stuffy broad *a*'s), the auditory quality is called *egophony*. These auditory changes may be present in any condition that consolidates lung tissue. Conversely, vocal resonance diminishes and loses intensity when there is blockage of the respiratory tree for any reason (e.g., with emphysema).

DIFFERENTIAL DIAGNOSIS
ANTHRAX IN A TIME OF TERROR

Anthrax is tough. It must be suspected early and treated early—often merely on the basis of suspicion and without waiting for laboratory confirmation—and it does not announce itself as other devastating and potentially terror-borne diseases might (e.g., smallpox and plague). Your patients might come in with flu-like fever, achiness, sniffles, and little else; this is how the disease process starts when spores of *Bacillus anthracis* are inhaled. (The more common skin manifestations of the disease are another matter [see p. 212]). Once the inhaled bacilli have taken hold, progression can be rapid and irreversible. An early detectable finding might be pleural effusion; then progressive respiratory distress; and, ultimately, cyanosis, shock, and coma. Clearly, there is little specific in the presenting symptoms or your early physical examination that might arouse suspicion. Inhalation anthrax is not announced by a skin lesion or other specific herald. The history is essential.

What is the patient's occupation? What are the problems we confront as a community? In the past, the pulmonary form of anthrax was called "woolsorter's disease" after people who handle wool contaminated with the bacillus. The disease was rare and generally limited to those who work with cattle, sheep, horses, and goats and in that way have contact with animal hides, hair, and waste. Terror-borne anthrax, however, can infect postal workers and any of those who come in contact with a contaminated powder sent in the mail (or, for that matter, in any number of potential delivery possibilities available to the terrorist). The tenor of these times mandates an easily aroused suspicion and treatment without waiting for final laboratory confirmation.

Other diseases thought to be available to terrorists do announce themselves in more specific ways:

- Smallpox, caused by the variola virus, is generally transmitted patient to patient and presents with a prodrome lasting 3 to 4 days characterized by nonspecific headache, chills, fever, and generalized aches and pains. Temperature drops and then skin lesions begin to appear, at first primarily on the face and upper extremities (see p. 212). Those lesions announce the disease. Be alert then to the common complication of pneumonia.
- Plague, caused by *Yersinia pestis,* is harbored in rats and other rodents and spread by droplet infection from patient to patient. It also begins with nonspecific fever and malaise, and even mental confusion and a possible staggering gait. It has a more specific herald, the appearance of acutely inflamed, tender, enlarged lymph nodes in the groin and elsewhere (buboes), easily accessible to physical examination (see figure). Pulmonary disease with symptoms of respiratory distress usually follows the appearance of nodal enlargement—but not always! Pulmonary plague may occur without buboes, and, at times, plague may be septicemic without nodal or pulmonary involvement.
- Anthrax, smallpox, and plague are nasty diseases that may be seen in nasty times. Anthrax is probably the toughest to diagnose, but none of them is easy. The problem is complicated by a widespread lack of experience with these illnesses among health care professionals who must be alert and suspicious. We have a lot to learn.

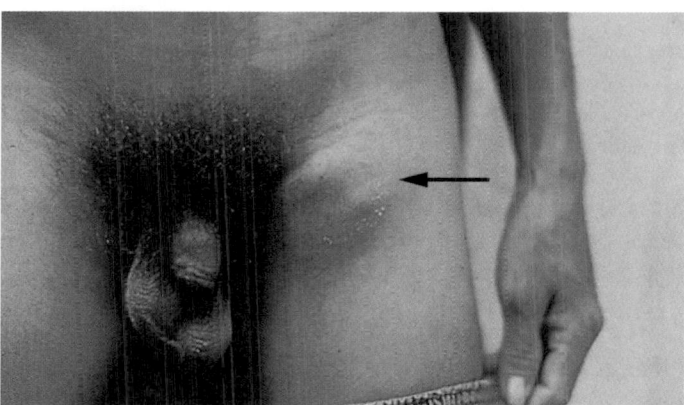

Bubonic plague. Fluid is aspirated from the bubo for gram staining and culture for *Yersinia pestis.*
From Beeching, Nye, 1996.

COUGHS

Coughs are a common symptom of a respiratory problem. They are usually preceded by a deep inspiration; this is followed by closure of the glottis and contraction of the chest, abdominal, and even the pelvic muscles, and then a sudden, spasmodic expiration, forcing a sudden opening of the glottis. Air and secretions are exhaled. The causes may be related to localized or more general insults at any point in the respiratory tract. Coughs may be voluntary, but they are usually reflexive responses to an irritant such as a foreign body (microscopic or

DIFFERENTIAL DIAGNOSIS

SOME CAUSES OF NOISY BREATHING: STRIDOR, HOARSENESS, WHEEZING, SNORING, GURGLING

Infection
- Upper respiratory infection*
- Peritonsillar abscess*
- Retropharyngeal abscess*
- Epiglottitis
- Laryngitis*
- Tracheitis*
- Bronchitis*
- Bronchiolitis*
- Viral croup*

Irritants and allergens
- Hyperactive airway*
- Asthma (reactive airway disease)*
- Rhinitis*
- Angioneurotic edema

Compression (from the outside of the airway)
- Esophageal cysts or foreign body
- A variety of tumors
- Lymphadenopathy

Congenital malformation and abnormality
- Vascular rings
- Laryngeal webs
- Laryngomalacia
- Tracheomalacia
- Hemangiomas within the upper airway
- Stenoses within the upper airway*
- Cystic fibrosis*

Acquired abnormality (at every level of the airway)
- Excessive talking*, yelling*, screaming*
- Nasal polyps
- Hypertrophied adenoids and/or tonsils
- Foreign body, corrosive ingestion*
- Intraluminal tumors
- Bronchiectasis
- Burns, thermal injury, smoke inhalation
- Post-intubation (e.g., nasogastric tube)

Neurogenic disorder
- Vocal cord paralysis (also, postsurgical)

The exact nature and location of the stimulus to noisy breathing will determine the type of noise. Snoring and gurgling tend to arise in the nasopharynx; stridor, in the area of the glottis; and wheezing, much lower in the respiratory tree.

*Common causes.

---

larger), an infectious agent, or a mass of any sort compressing the respiratory tree. They may also be a clue to an anxiety state.

Describe a cough according to its moisture, frequency, regularity, pitch and loudness, and quality. The type of cough may offer some clue to the cause. Although a cough may not have a serious cause, do not ignore it.

Dry or Moist. A moist cough may be caused by infection and can be accompanied by sputum production. A dry cough can have a variety of causes (e.g., cardiac problems, allergies, HIV infection), which may be indicated by the quality of its sound.

Onset. An acute onset, particularly with fever, suggests infection; in the absence of fever, a foreign body or inhaled irritants are additional possible causes.

Frequency of Occurrence. Note whether the cough is seldom or often present. An infrequent cough may result from allergens or environmental insults.

Regularity. A regular, paroxysmal cough is heard in pertussis. An irregularly occurring cough may have a variety of causes (e.g., smoking, early congestive heart failure, an inspired foreign body or irritant, or a tumor within or compressing the bronchial tree).

Pitch and Loudness. A cough may be loud and high-pitched or quiet and relatively low-pitched.

Postural Influences. A cough may occur soon after a person has reclined or assumed an erect position (e.g., with a nasal drip or pooling of secretions in the upper airway).

Quality. A dry cough may sound brassy if it is caused by compression of the respiratory tree (as by a tumor) or hoarse if it is caused by croup. Pertussis produces an inspiratory whoop at the end of a paroxysm of coughing.

See Box 13-9 for a summary of expected findings of a healthy chest and lungs.

BOX 13-9

SUMMARY OF EXPECTED FINDINGS OF CHEST AND LUNGS

When the lungs are healthy, the respiratory tree clear, the pleurae unaffected by disease, and the chest wall symmetrically and appropriately structured and mobile, the following characteristics will be found:

On inspection
  - Symmetry of movement on expansion
  - Absence of retractions
On palpation
  - Midline trachea without a tug
  - Symmetric, unaccentuated tactile fremitus
On percussion
  - Range of 3 to 5 cm in the descent of diaphragm
  - Resonant and symmetric percussion notes
On auscultation
  - Absence of adventitious sounds
  - Vesicular breath sounds, except for bronchovesicular sounds beside the sternum and the more prominent bronchial components in the area of the larger bronchi

---

FUNCTIONAL ASSESSMENT

JUDGING PULMONARY CAPABILITY AT HOME?

McGee writes of the "Blow-Out-the-Match Test," confirming that it is a handy method for providing a valid indicator of reduced pulmonary function. The technique is simple. A match is lit and held about 10 to 15 cm in front of a sitting patient, not too close, of course. The patient is asked to blow out the match as hard as possible but with the mouth open and the lips not pursed. There is a problem compromising pulmonary function if it cannot be done, perhaps chronic obstructive pulmonary disease or some other limiting factor. Importantly, many patients, not asked to do so, pick up on this test quickly, do it at home, and provide a guide for their activities of daily living. McGee does not mention this nor have we suggested it. Still, it happens. The evidence to support it is only anecdotal.

Modified from McGee, 2001.

MEASURES OF PULMONARY FUNCTION

The ability of the lungs to do their work can be quantified. Essentially, the need is to know how much of the air they exchange is of functional use and how easily it can be moved to and fro. The vital capacity (VC) is a valuable indicator of the amount of air that is expelled after the patient takes a maximal inspiration and follows that with a maximal expiration. The physical dimensions of the chest cage, posture, gender (the volume in males is greater than that in females), age, height, and the degree of physical fitness are among the variables that influence VC. When VC is impaired, a variety of disease processes can be suspect (e.g., loss of lung tissue, airway obstruction, loss of muscle strength, chest deformity, pneumothorax). The VC cannot differentiate among these.

The peak expiratory flow rate (PEFR), a measure of the maximum flow of air that can be achieved during forced expiration, is a useful surrogate for the VC in children as well as adults. It provides an easily reproducible number obtained by using inexpensive, handheld, peak flow meters. The reliability of the PEFR is limited by the patient's ability to cooperate, and it is useful as a measure only for large airway function; however, it does suggest the extent of impairment and it can be used as a guide to measure the success (or lack of it) of treatment. It is best to compare a patient's PEFR to a previous "personal best," if possible, rather than to an expected predicted value attainable from a nomogram geared to the patient's height and based on the generalization that lung volume parallels height, age, and gender.

If there is no measuring tool available, forced vital capacity (FVC) can be roughly estimated by asking the patient to exhale to the limit and then to hold the breath. Count the seconds until a breath must be taken and multiply that number by 50 to get the number of cc's of FVC. Again, personal best should be the continuing guide.

SPUTUM

The production of sputum is generally associated with cough. Sputum in more than small amounts and with any degree of consistency always suggests the presence of disease. If the onset is acute, infection is most probable. Once there is some chronicity, the possibility of a significant anatomic change (e.g., tumor, cavitation, or bronchiectasis) becomes apparent. The Differential Diagnosis box below delineates possible pathologic conditions and their accompanying sputum findings.

DIFFERENTIAL DIAGNOSIS
SOME CAUSES OF SPUTUM

Cause	Possible Sputum Characteristics
Bacterial infection	Yellow, green, rust (blood mixed with yellow sputum), clear, or transparent; purulent; blood streaked; mucoid, viscid
Viral infection	Mucoid, viscid; blood streaked (not common)
Chronic infectious disease	All of the above; particularly abundant in the early morning; slight, intermittent blood streaking; occasionally, large amounts of blood*
Carcinoma	Slight, persistent blood streaking
Infarction	Blood clotted; large amounts of blood
Tuberculous cavity	Large amounts of blood*

*Remember to ascertain that the blood is not swallowed from a nosebleed.
Modified from Harvey et al, 1988.

EVIDENCE-BASED PRACTICE IN PHYSICAL EXAMINATION
EXAMINATION OF THE INFANT'S CHEST AND LUNGS

Sometimes a technologic advancement, even one as simple to use as pulse oximetry, can complicate care when observation and the skills of physical examination will serve the patient better. Schroeder and colleagues observed 62 infants with bronchiolitis. Sixteen of these babies had their stay in hospital prolonged by an average of 1.6 days per hospitalization, or 0.4 day per hospitalization for all 62 patients. This greater separation from home, continued exposure to the risk of being in a hospital, and the additional cost were imposed by a perceived need for supplemental oxygen based on pulse oximetry readings alone. Examination of the babies did not suggest the continued need. Bergman cites the study of Mallory's group, which suggests that reliance on pulse oximetry by 118 pediatric emergency physicians might be responsible for the 250% increase in bronchiolitis hospitalization rates over the past 20 years. Many have termed pulse oximetry the *fifth vital sign*. We should question that inappropriate application of a technology that does, of course, have its proper uses.

Were the babies better off? There is no evidence to suggest that they were. Bergman quotes the work of Shay and colleagues that shows that mortality rates for bronchiolitis have remained relatively constant for the past 2 decades. There is, then, considerable evidence that oximetry data are used uncritically and, as Bergman also suggests, their use indicates a certain worship at the shrine of numbers by many caregivers that, in our view, erodes the very necessary development of the skills of physical examination if our patients are to be cared for appropriately.

Data from Schroeder et al, 2004; Bergman, 2004; Mallory et al, 2003; Shay et al, 2001.

INFANTS

The examination of the chest and lungs of the newborn follows a sequence similar to that for adults. Inspecting without disturbing the baby is key. Percussion, however, may be unreliable. The examiner's fingers may be too large for a baby's chest, and particularly so for the premature infant.

A newborn's Apgar scores at 1 and 5 minutes after birth tell you a great deal about the infant's respiratory efforts. An infant whose respirations are inadequate but who is otherwise normal may initially score 1 or even 0 on heart rate, muscle tone, response to a catheter, or color. Depressed respiration often has its origins in the maternal environment during labor, such as sedatives or compromised blood supply to the child; or it may result from mechanical obstruction by mucus. Table 13-4 explains the Apgar scoring system. This score requires some subjective judgment and cannot be considered absolute.

Inspect the thoracic cage, noting size and shape; measure the chest circumference, which in the healthy full-term infant is usually about 30 to 36 cm, sometimes 2 to 3 cm smaller than the head circumference. This difference between the two increases with prematurity. An infant with intrauterine growth retardation will have a relatively smaller chest circumference compared to the head, whereas the infant of a poorly controlled diabetic mother will have a relatively larger chest circumference. As a rough measure, the distance between the nipples is about one-fourth the circumference of the chest.

Observe the nipples for symmetry in size and for the presence of swelling and discharge, as detailed in Chapter 16. On occasion you will see supernumerary nipples, ordinarily not fully developed, along a line drawn caudad from the primary nipple. In white children, but not as often in blacks, they may be associated with a variety of congenital abnormalities.

The newborn's lung function is particularly susceptible to a number of environmental factors. The pattern of respirations will vary with room temperature, feeding, and sleep. In the first few hours after birth, the respiratory effort can be depressed by the passive transfer of drugs given to the mother before delivery.

Cyanosis of the hands and feet (acrocyanosis) is common in the newborn and can persist for several days in a cool environment without causing concern (see Fig. 8-23).

Count the respiratory rate for 1 minute. The expected rate varies from 40 to 60 respirations per minute, although a rate of 80 is not uncommon. Babies delivered by cesarean section generally have a more rapid rate than do babies delivered vaginally. If the room temperature is very warm or cool, a noticeable variation in the rate occurs, most often tachypnea but sometimes bradypnea.

Note the regularity of respiration. Babies are obligate nose breathers and, at this age, nasal flaring is common. It sometimes seems that they would prefer respiratory distress to opening their mouths to breathe. The more premature an infant at birth, the more likely some irregularity in the respiratory pattern will be present. *Periodic breathing,* a sequence of relatively vigorous respiratory efforts followed by apnea of as long as 10 to 15 seconds, is common. It is cause for concern if the apneic episodes tend to be prolonged and the baby becomes centrally cyanotic (i.e., cyanotic about the mouth, face, and torso). The persistence of periodic breathing episodes in preterm infants is relative to the gestational age of the baby, with the apneic

PHYSICAL VARIATIONS
Supernumerary Nipples
The incidence of supernumerary nipples in blacks is 11.4 in 1000; in whites it is 0.9 in 1000.

Data from Christianson et al, 1981.

TABLE 13-4	Infant Evaluation at Birth—Apgar Scoring System		
	0	**1**	**2**
Heart rate	Absent	Slow (below 100 beats/min)	Over 100 beats/min
Respiratory effort	Absent	Slow or irregular	Good crying
Muscle tone	Limp	Some flexion of extremities	Active motion
Response to catheter in nostril (tested after oropharynx is clear)	No response	Grimace	Cough or sneeze
Color	Blue or pale	Body pink, extremities blue	Completely pink

Add the scores of the five individual observations to get the full Apgar score. The lower the total, the more likely a problem.

CLINICAL PEARL

A Diaphragmatic Hernia

A diaphragmatic hernia (see Fig. 13-24), the result of an imperfectly structured diaphragm, occurs once in slightly more than 2000 live births. It is on the left side at least 90% of the time; the liver is not there to get in the way. The degree of respiratory distress can be slight or very severe and accompanied by intense cyanosis, depending on the extent to which the bowel has invaded the chest through the defect. Although prenatal ultrasonography can identify as many as 75% of the cases, physical examination remains essential for the rest. Bowel sounds heard in the chest and a flat or scaphoid abdomen are significant clues. The heart is usually displaced to the right. This abnormal development of the diaphragm can be associated with significant defects in one or both lungs.

period diminishing in frequency as the baby approaches term status. In the term infant, periodic breathing should wane a few hours after birth.

Coughing is rare in the newborn and should be considered a problem. Sneezing, on the other hand, is frequent and expected—it clears the nose. Hiccups are also frequent, though usually silent, particularly after meals. Frequent hiccupping, however, may suggest seizures, drug withdrawal, or encephalopathy, among other possibilities.

Newborns rely primarily on the diaphragm for their respiratory effort, only gradually adding the intercostal muscles. Infants quite commonly also use the abdominal muscles. Paradoxic breathing (the chest wall collapses as the abdomen distends on inspiration) is common, particularly during sleep.

If the chest expansion is asymmetric, suspect some compromise of the baby's ability to fill one of the lungs (e.g., pneumothorax or diaphragmatic hernia) (Fig. 13-24).

Palpate the rib cage and sternum, noting loss of symmetry, unusual masses, or crepitus. Crepitus around a fractured clavicle (with no evidence of pain) is common after a difficult forceps delivery. The newborn's xiphoid process is more mobile and prominent than that of the older child or adult. It has a sharp inferior tip that moves slightly back and forth under your finger.

Listen to the chest. If the baby is crying and restless, it pays to wait for a more quiet moment. Localization of breath sounds is difficult, particularly in the very small chest of the preterm infant. Breath sounds are easily transmitted from one segment of the auscultatory area to another; therefore the absence of sounds in any given area may be difficult to detect. Sometimes it helps to listen to both sides of the chest simultaneously. Some neonatologists use a double-belled stethoscope for this purpose (Box 13-10).

It is not uncommon to hear crackles and rhonchi immediately after birth because fetal fluid has not been completely cleared. Whenever auscultatory findings are asymmetric, a problem should be suspected as, for example, with the aspiration of meconium. Gurgling from the intestinal tract, slight movement, and mucus in the upper airway may all contribute to adventitious sounds, making evaluation difficult. If gastrointestinal gurgling sounds are persistently heard in the chest, one must suspect diaphragmatic hernia, but wide transmission of these sounds can sometimes be deceptive.

Stridor is a high-pitched, piercing sound most often heard during inspiration. It is the result of an obstruction high in the respiratory tree. A compelling sound at any age, it cannot be dismissed as inconsequential, particularly when inspiration (I) may be three to four times longer than expiration (E), giving an I/E ratio of 3:1 or 4:1. If it is accompanied by a cough,

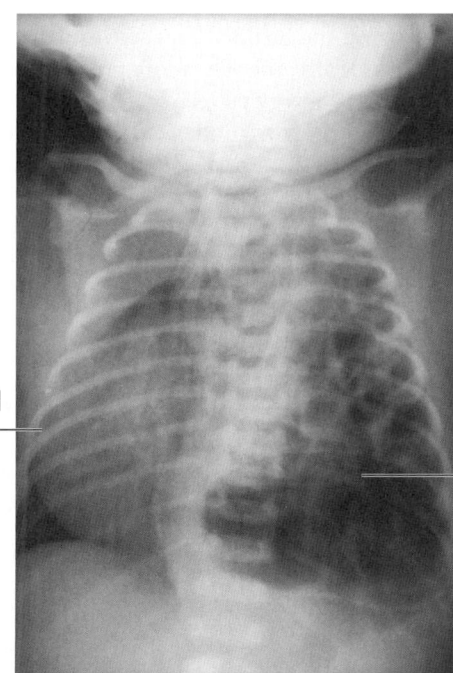

Heart pushed into right chest

Diaphragmatic hernia in chest; stomach and intestinal gas in chest

FIGURE 13-24
X-ray film showing diaphragmatic hernia.

BOX 13-10

COMPARING VENTILATION REGIONALLY

It is sometimes helpful to compare two areas in the lungs fields simultaneously. This is accomplished with a stethoscope that has a double-bell or double-diaphragm and is modified so that the chest pieces are connected as illustrated. This procedure, not commonly used by many examiners, is useful in emergent or other stressful situations, particularly with preterm infants. Atelectasis and pneumothorax, for example, can be differentiated and their sites localized.

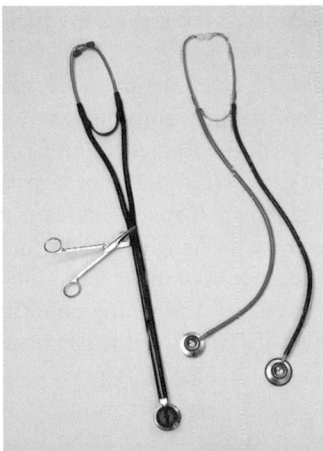

Two conventional single-tube stethoscopes are cut and re-assembled into a double-headed stethoscope.

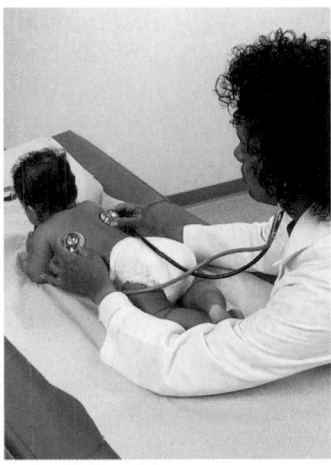

Lateral placement of the stethoscope heads allows the best appreciation of differences in breath sounds.

---

hoarseness, and retraction, stridor signifies a serious problem in the trachea or larynx (e.g., a floppy epiglottis; congenital defects; croup; or an edematous response to an infection, allergen, smoke, chemicals, or aspirated foreign body). Infants who have a narrow tracheal lumen readily respond with stridor to its compression by a tumor, abscess, or double aortic arch. Retraction at the supraclavicular notch and contraction of the sternocleidomastoid muscles should be considered significant. Vigorous contraction, when the infant is supine and the head given suboccipital support, might make the head bob.

Respiratory grunting is a mechanism by which the infant tries to expel trapped air or fetal lung fluid while trying to retain air and increase oxygen levels. When persistent, it is cause for concern. *Flaring of the alae nasi* is another indicator of respiratory distress at this, or any, age.

CHILDREN

Children use the thoracic (intercostal) musculature for respiration by the age of 6 or 7 years. In young children, obvious intercostal exertion (retractions) on breathing suggests an airway problem (e.g., asthma). Usual respiratory rates for children are listed below. Rates decrease with age with a greater variation in the first 2 years of life and without significant gender difference. Sustained rates that exceed the indicated limits should suggest difficulty (Box 13-11):

Age	Respirations per Minute
Newborn	30 to 80
1 year	20 to 40
3 years	20 to 30
6 years	16 to 22
10 years	16 to 20
17 years	12 to 20

If the roundness of the young child's chest persists past the second year of life, be concerned about the possibility of a chronic obstructive pulmonary problem such as cystic fibrosis. The persistence of a barrel chest at the age of 5 or 6 years can be ominous.

Seize the opportunity that a crying child presents. A sob is often followed by a deep breath. The sob itself allows the evaluation of vocal resonance and the feel for tactile fremitus; gently use the whole hand, palm and fingers. The crying child may pause occasionally, and the heart sounds may be heard. These pauses may be a bit prolonged as the breath is held, giving the chance to distinguish a murmur from a breath sound. In any event, your ear can suppress ambient noise to some extent, much as at a noisy restaurant, allowing you to concentrate on the matter at hand.

Children younger than 5 or 6 years may not be able to give enough of an expiration to satisfy you, particularly when you suspect subtle wheezing. Asking them to "blow out" your flashlight or to blow away a bit of tissue in your hand may help bring out otherwise difficult-to-hear end expiratory sounds. It is also easier to hear the breath sounds when the child breathes more deeply after running up and down the hallway.

The child's chest is thinner and ordinarily more resonant than the adult's chest; the intrathoracic sounds are easier to hear, and hyperresonance is common in the young child. With either direct or indirect percussion, it is easy to miss the dullness of an underlying consolidation. If you sense some loss of resonance, give it as much importance as you would give frank dullness in the adolescent or adult. Also, your pleximeter finger can learn to feel the dull areas, a tactile sense that comes in handy at times with a crying child. The dull areas are sensed as having more resistance than resonant areas because they move less.

Because of the thin chest wall, the breath sounds of the young child may sound louder, harsher, and more bronchial than those of the adult. Bronchovesicular breath sounds may be heard throughout the chest.

BOX 13-11

ASSESSMENT OF RESPIRATORY DISTRESS

Important observations to be made of the respiratory effort include the following:
- Does a loss of synchrony between left and right occur during the respiratory effort? Is there a lag in movement of the chest on one side? Atelectasis? Diaphragmatic hernia?
- Is there stridor? Croup? Epiglottitis?
- Is there retraction at the suprasternal notch? Intercostally? At the xiphoid process?
- Do the nares dilate and flare with respiratory effort? Is pneumonia present?
- Is there an audible expiratory grunt? Is it audible with the stethoscope only or without the stethoscope? Is there lower airway obstruction? Focal atelectasis?
- Is there paradoxic breathing?

STAYING WELL

THE TEEN AND NICOTINE

A major risk to the preservation of pulmonary health during late childhood and adolescence is the first experiment with a cigarette. However, the influence of peers and omnipresent advertising are powerful pressures that recent studies suggest can be frustrated. Programs in high schools that formally engage students in community-advocacy activities that deal with the adverse environmental influences of cigarette smoking have demonstrated that the behavioral change is possible and that there can be a decrease in the use of cigarettes and even a refusal to try the first one. The important concept underlying such programs is involvement of the participants in defining the social context and in the planning of implementation. Specific to the adolescent and based in the school, this promises more favorable results than nicotine replacement therapy—an undesirable first-line treatment for adolescent smoking habituation.

Adelman, 2004; Winkleby et al, 2004

PREGNANT WOMEN

Pregnant women experience both structural and ventilatory changes. Dyspnea is common in pregnancy and is usually a result of normal physiologic changes. The most apparent change in lung volume is a decrease in functional residual capacity (FRC), which is the volume of air in the lungs at the end of quiet exhalation (Thompson, Cohen, 1938). There is an increase of 100 to 200 mL in vital capacity, the amount of air that can be expelled at the normal rate of exhalation after a maximum inspiration. The tidal volume, the amount of air inhaled and exhaled during normal breathing, increases 40% along with minute ventilation. Overall, the pregnant woman increases her ventilation by breathing more deeply, not more frequently. There are changes in arterial pO_2 that have little clinical significance in those without pulmonary disease. In late pregnancy the supine position can further decrease pO_2. Asthma can have a varied course, getting worse, getting better, or being unaffected by the pregnancy with about equal frequency.

OLDER ADULTS

The examination procedure for older adults is the same as that for younger adults, although there may be variations in some expected findings. Chest expansion is often decreased. The patient may be less able to use the respiratory muscles because of muscle weakness, general physical disability, or a sedentary lifestyle. Calcification of rib articulations may also interfere with chest expansion, requiring use of accessory muscles. Bony prominences are marked, and there is loss of subcutaneous tissue. The dorsal curve of the thoracic spine is prominent (kyphosis) with flattening of the lumbar curve (Fig. 13-25). The AP diameter of the chest is increased in relation to the lateral diameter.

Older patients may have more difficulty breathing deeply and holding their breath than younger patients, and they may tire more quickly even when well. The pace and demands of examination should therefore be adapted to individual need.

Some older patients may display hyperresonance as a result of increased distensibility of the lungs. This finding must be evaluated in the context of the presence or absence of other symptoms.

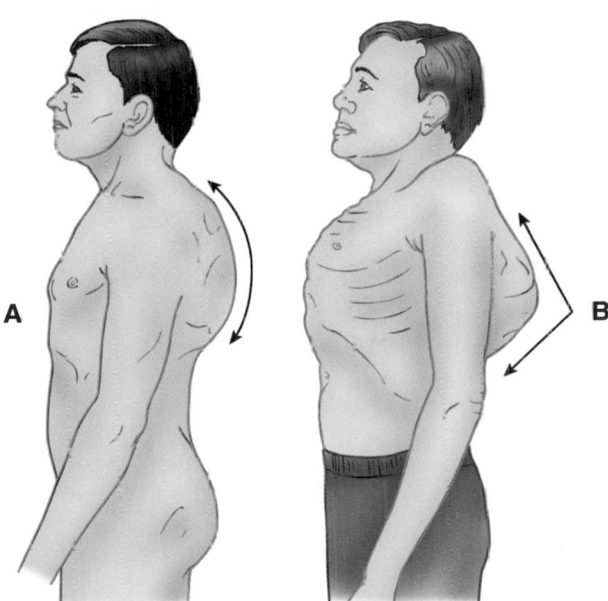

FIGURE 13-25
Pronounced dorsal curvature in older adult. **A,** Kyphosis. **B,** Gibbus (extreme kyphosis).

SAMPLE DOCUMENTATION

HISTORY AND PHYSICAL EXAMINATION

Subjective

Chief complaint: Cough and fever

History of present illness: Nonproductive cough for past several days. Persistent, worse when lies down. Feels ill. Chest feels "heavy." Feels short of breath. Fever up to 101° F. Taking a nonprescription cough syrup without relief.

Objective

Minimal increase in the AP diameter of chest, without kyphosis or other distortion. Thoracic expansion symmetric. Respirations rapid and somewhat labored, not accompanied by retractions or stridor. On palpation, trachea in midline without tug; no friction rubs or tenderness over the ribs or other bony prominences. Over the left base posteriorly, tactile fremitus diminished; percussion note dull; on auscultation, crackles were heard and did not clear with cough; breath sounds diminished. Remainder of lung fields clear and free of adventitious sounds, with resonant percussion tones. Diaphragmatic excursion 3 cm bilaterally.

For additional sample documentation, see Chapter 26.

SUMMARY OF EXAMINATION

CHEST AND LUNGS

The following steps are performed with the patient sitting.

1. Inspect the chest, front and back, noting thoracic landmarks, for the following (see p. 371):
   - Size and shape (anteroposterior diameter compared with transverse diameter)
   - Symmetry
   - Color
   - Superficial venous patterns
   - Prominence of ribs
2. Evaluate respirations for the following (see p. 373):
   - Rate
   - Rhythm or pattern
3. Inspect chest movement with breathing for the following (see p. 376):
   - Symmetry
   - Bulging
   - Use of accessory muscles
4. Note any audible sounds with respiration (i.e., stridor or wheezes) (see p. 377).
5. Palpate the chest for the following (see p. 377):
   - Symmetry
   - Thoracic expansion
   - Pulsations
   - Sensations such as crepitus, grating vibrations
   - Tactile fremitus
6. Perform direct or indirect percussion on the chest, comparing sides, for the following (see p. 380):
   - Diaphragmatic excursion
   - Percussion tone intensity, pitch, duration, and quality
7. Auscultate the chest with the stethoscope diaphragm, from apex to base, comparing sides for the following (see p. 383):
   - Intensity, pitch, duration, and quality of expected breath sounds
   - Unexpected breath sounds (crackles, rhonchi, wheezes, friction rubs)
   - Vocal resonance

COMMON ABNORMALITIES

Physical findings associated with many common conditions are listed in Table 13-5; some causes of persistent cough are listed in Table 13-6.

TABLE 13-5	Physical Findings Associated with Common Respiratory Conditions*			
Condition	**Inspection**	**Palpation**	**Percussion**	**Auscultation**
Asthma	Tachypnea Dyspnea	Tachycardia Diminished fremitus	Occasional hyper-resonance Occasional limited diaphragmatic descent; diaphragmatic level lower	Prolonged expiration Wheezes Diminished lung sounds
Atelectasis	Delayed and/or diminished chest wall movement (respiratory lag), narrowed intercostals spaces on affected side Tachypnea	Diminished fremitus Apical cardiac impulse deviated ipsilaterally Trachea deviated ipsilaterally	Dullness over affected lung	In upper lobe, bronchial breathing, egophony, whispered pectoriloquy In lower lobe, diminished or absent breath sounds Wheezes, rhonchi, and crackles in varying amounts depending on extent of collapse
Bronchiectasis	Tachypnea Respiratory distress Hyperinflation	Few, if any, consistent findings	No unusual findings if there are no accompanying pulmonary disorders	A variety of crackles, usually coarse; and rhonchi, sometimes disappearing after cough
Bronchitis	Occasional tachypnea Occasional shallow breathing Often no deviation from expected findings	Tactile fremitus undiminished	Resonance	Breath sounds may be prolonged Occasional crackles Occasional expiratory wheezes
Chronic obstructive pulmonary disease	Respiratory distress Audible wheezing Cyanosis Distention of neck veins, peripheral edema, and—rarely—finger clubbing (in presence of right-sided heart failure)	Somewhat limited mobility of diaphragm Somewhat diminished vocal fremitus	Occasional hyper-resonance	Postpertussive rhonchi (sonorous wheezes) and sibilant wheezing Inspirational crackles (best heard with stethoscope held over open mouth) Breath sounds somewhat diminished
Emphysema	Tachypnea Deep breathing Pursed lips Barrel chest Thin, underweight	Apical impulse may not be felt Liver edge displaced downward Diminished fremitus	Hyperresonance Limited descent of diaphragm on inspiration Upper border of liver dullness pushed downward	Diminished breath and voice sounds with occasional prolonged expiration Diminished audibility of heart sounds Only occasional adventitious sounds
Pleural effusion and/or thickening	Diminished and delayed respiratory movement (lag) on affected side	Diminished and delayed respiratory movement on affected side Cardiac apical impulse shifted contralaterally Trachea shifted contralaterally Diminished fremitus Tachycardia	Dullness to flatness Hyperresonant note in area superior to effusion	Diminished to absent breath sounds Bronchophony, whispered pectoriloquy Egophony in area superior to effusion Occasional friction rub

*Physical findings will vary in intensity depending on the severity of the underlying problem and on occasion may not be present in the early stages.

Continued

TABLE 13-5	Physical Findings Associated with Common Respiratory Conditions—cont'd			
Condition	Inspection	Palpation	Percussion	Auscultation
Pneumonia consolidation	Tachypnea Shallow breathing Flaring of alae nasi Occasional cyanosis Limited movement at times on involved side; splinting	Increased fremitus in presence of consolidation Decreased fremitus in presence of a concomitant empyema or pleural effusion Tachypnea	Dullness if consolidation is great	A variety of crackles with lobar and occasional rhonchi Bronchial breath sounds Egophony, bronchophony, whispered pectoriloquy
Pneumothorax	Tachycardia Cyanosis Respiratory distress Bulging intercostal spaces Respiratory lag on affected side Tracheal deviation	Diminished to absent fremitus Cardiac apical impulse, trachea, and mediastinum shifted contralaterally Diminished to absent tactile fremitus Tachycardia	Hyperresonance	Diminished to absent breath sounds Succussion splash audible if air and fluid mix Sternal and precordial clicks and crackling (Hamman sign) if air underlies that area Diminished to absent whispered voice sounds

TABLE 13-6	Some Causes of Persistent Cough

ALLERGY
Allergic rhinitis
Classic asthma
Cough-variant asthma

ANATOMIC DISRUPTION
Bronchiectasis
Bronchogenic cyst
Chronic obstructive pulmonary disease
Pulmonary sequestration
Tumors (benign, malignant, pulmonary, mediastinal)

BEHAVIORAL
Habit cough

CONGENITAL PROBLEMS
Anatomic abnormalities
  Adductor vocal cord paralysis
  Laryngeal cleft
  Tracheobronchomalacia
  Tracheoesophageal fistula
Ciliary dyskinesia
Cystic fibrosis
Gastroesophageal reflux
Immunodeficiency syndromes
Neurodevelopmental delay with aspiration
Swallowing dysfunction (acquired as well as congenital)

EXTRINSIC SOURCES
Foreign body aspiration
Irritating vapors
  Air pollution, e.g., smog
  Glue sniffing
  Tobacco smoke
  Wood smoke
  Volatile chemicals

RESPIRATORY INFECTION (ACUTE OR CHRONIC, NASOPHARYNX TO ALVEOLI)
Adenovirus
Chlamydia
Fungi
HIV infection
Influenza
Mycobacterium tuberculosis
Parainfluenza
Pertussis
Respiratory syncytial virus

SINUS INFECTION
Haemophilus influenzae (nontypeable)
Moraxella catarrhalis
Streptococcus pneumoniae

SYSTEMIC CAUSES
Congestive heart failure

Modified from Guilbert, Taussig, 1998.

ASTHMA (REACTIVE AIRWAY DISEASE)

Asthma is a chronic obstructive pulmonary disease (COPD) characterized by airway inflammation and generally resulting from airway hyperreactivity triggered by allergens, anxiety, upper respiratory infections, cigarette smoke or other environmental poisons, or exercise. Cold air aggravates asthma; warm, humid air less so. The result is mucosal edema, increased secretions, and bronchoconstriction. Airway resistance increases and respiratory flow is impeded.

Episodes are characterized by paroxysmal dyspnea; tachypnea; cough; wheezing on expiration and inspiration; and, as airway resistance increases, more prolonged expiration. Chest pain is common and, with it, a feeling of tightness. The episodes may last for minutes or hours, or may be prolonged over days. Unlike other forms of COPD in older adults, the obstruction of asthma is reversible either spontaneously or in response to therapy. Between episodes, the patient may be asymptomatic. However, at times, chronic bronchitis and/or emphysema may complicate the picture.

Asthma varies in intensity, even from moment to moment and often from one area of the lungs to another, but it is always acutely anxiety provoking. It is an increasingly common disorder that all too often begins in childhood and that can be life-threatening if not treated promptly and adequately. Allergic skin conditions may coexist. A wheezing patient with generalized pulmonary findings may have asthma or a viral infection but rarely, if ever, a bacterial infection. Occasionally, a persistent cough may be the only manifestation.

CLINICAL PEARL

Foreign Body
Think about the possibility of a foreign body when a patient, particularly a youngster, presents with wheezing for the first time. The history may not at first offer a clue.

ATELECTASIS

Atelectasis is the incomplete expansion of the lung at birth or the collapse of the lung at any age (Fig. 13-26). Collapse can be caused by compression from outside (e.g., exudates, tumors) or resorption of gas from the alveoli in the presence of complete internal obstruction (the loss of elastic recoil of the lung for any reason [e.g., thoracic or abdominal surgery, plugging, exudates, foreign body]). The affected area of the lung is airless. The overall effect is to dampen or mute the sounds in the involved area.

EVIDENCE-BASED PRACTICE IN PHYSICAL EXAMINATION
OBESITY AND ASTHMA

A high (more than 4.5 kg), but not low (less than 2.5 kg), birthweight predisposes to increased incidence of asthma in childhood. The risk increases linearly beyond a birthweight of 4.5 kilograms. Obesity is proinflammatory. At 4.5 kg, the risk is 20% greater than for babies with a birthweight of 2.5 to 4.5 kg, and it increases by about 10% for every 0.10-kg increase over 4.5 kg. Clearly, the effort to achieve wellness requires attention to weight from the earliest days of life.

Modified from Sin et al, 2004.

EVIDENCE-BASED PRACTICE IN PHYSICAL EXAMINATION
ETHNIC DIFFERENCES IN DESCRIBING ASTHMA SYMPTOMS

Do blacks with asthma report their symptoms differently than do whites?

Blacks are generally more severely afflicted with asthma than whites. Could it be in part because they report their symptoms differently from whites and that their problems are then not so readily diagnosed? There is evidence that that is so. A recent study (Hardie et al, 2000) found that two groups of patients, carefully matched except for race, reported the experience of asthma (breathlessness) differently when bronchoconstriction was experimentally induced. Whites used lower airway descriptors (e.g., "out of breath," "hurts to breathe," "aware of breathing"). Blacks tended to use upper airway terms (e.g., "itchy throat," "tight throat," "voice tight"). The probability is that upper airway terms may not reflect the source of breathlessness. This study is limited in its power but it does help stimulate our thinking about the way patients report their symptoms and the relevance of the terms used to the source of difficulty.

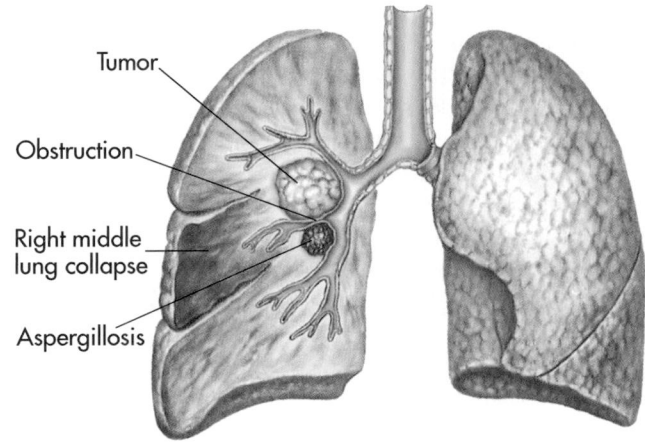

FIGURE 13-26
Atelectasis.
*Modified from Wilson, Thompson,
1990.*

BRONCHITIS

Bronchitis is an inflammation of the mucous membranes of the bronchial tubes. Acute bronchitis may be more severe or less severe than chronic bronchitis, and it may be accompanied by fever and chest pain (Fig. 13-27). Chronic bronchitis has a variety of causes and physical manifestations, including excessive secretion of mucus in the bronchial tree. In either type, the initial stimulus is irritation by an internal or external noxious influence. Either an acute or chronic condition can show varying degrees of involvement, with the possibility of obstructive phenomena and even atelectasis, but bronchitis is most often quite mild.

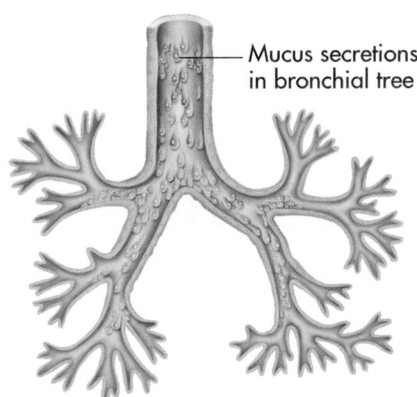

FIGURE 13-27
Acute bronchitis.
From Wilson, Thompson, 1990.

PLEURISY

Pleurisy is an inflammatory process involving the visceral and parietal pleura, often the result of pulmonary infections, bacterial or viral, and sometimes associated with neoplasm or asbestosis. The onset is usually sudden and the typical pleuritic pain is acute. The pleura becomes "dry," actually edematous and fibrinous, making breathing difficult (Fig. 13-28). The resultant rubbing can be felt and heard. The respirations are rapid and shallow, with diminished breath sounds. The symptoms vary considerably with the area of involvement. If it is close to the diaphragm, the pain can be referred to the ipsilateral shoulder. As the process continues, and if pleural effusion results, the pain and rub may disappear; but the fever, tachypnea, and malaise will not.

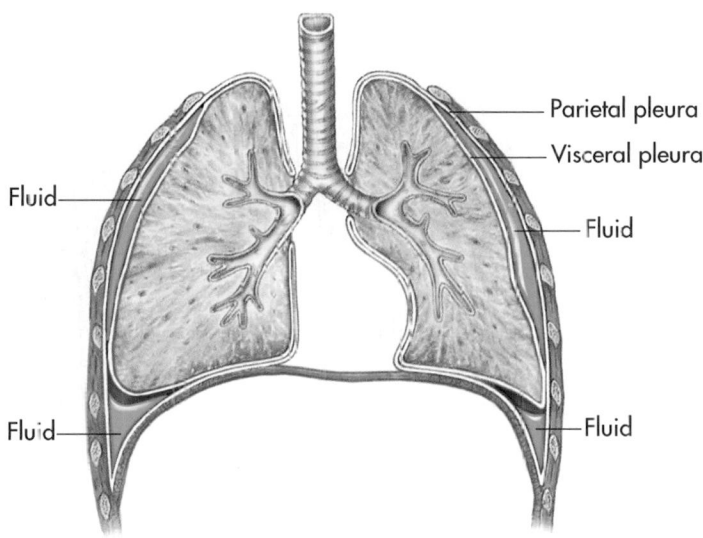

FIGURE 13-28
Pleurisy.
Modified from Wilson, Thompson, 1990.

PLEURAL EFFUSION

Excessive nonpurulent fluid in the pleural space can result in permanent fibrotic thickening. The sources of fluid vary: infection, neoplasm, and trauma are all possible causes. The extent of embarrassment varies with the amount of fluid, and the degree of fibrosis varies with the chronicity of the condition. The findings vary with severity and also with the position of the patient. Fluid is mobile; it will gravitate to the most dependent position. In the affected areas, the breath sounds are muted (Fig. 13-29). Grocco's triangle is a right-angled area of dullness over the posterior chest, which can sometimes be percussed opposite a large pleural effusion,

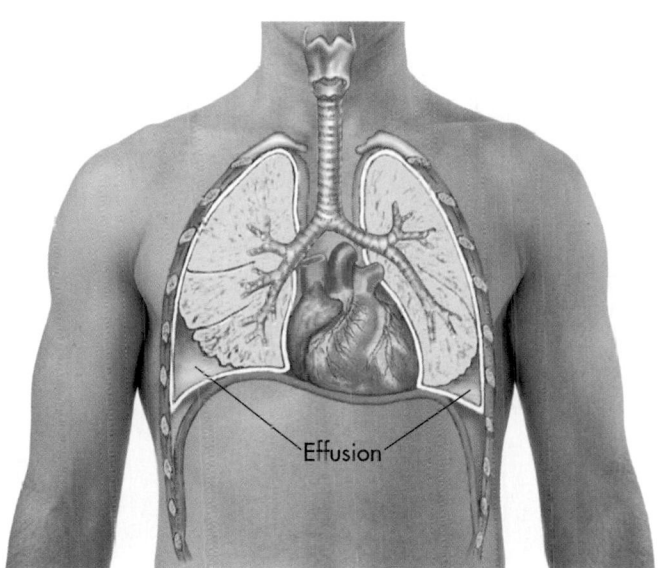

FIGURE 13-29
Pleural effusion.
Modified from Wilson, Thompson, 1990.

the diaphragm on the horizontal of the triangle, the spinous processes, the vertical. Also, the percussion note is often hyperresonant (Skodaic resonance) in the area above the perfusion (McGee, 2001).

EMPYEMA

Empyema is said to occur when fluid collected in the pleural spaces is a purulent exudate, arising most commonly from adjacent infected, sometimes traumatized, tissues (Fig. 13-30). It may be complicated by pneumonia, a penetrating injury, simultaneous pneumothorax, or bronchopleural fistulae. Breath sounds are distant or absent in the affected area, the percussion note is dull, vocal fremitus is absent, and the patient is often febrile and tachypneic and appears ill.

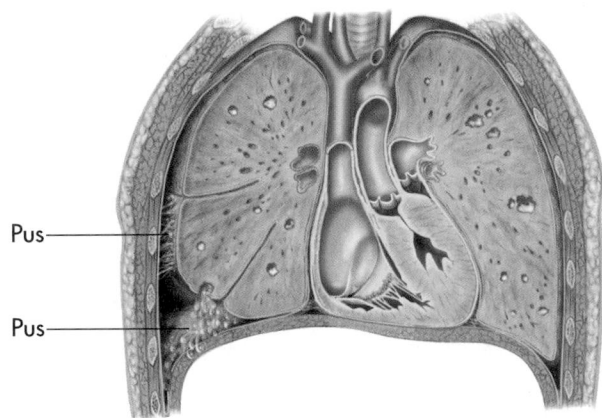

Pus

Pus

FIGURE 13-30
Empyema.
Modified from Wilson, Thompson, 1990.

LUNG ABSCESS

A lung abscess is a well-defined, circumscribed mass defined by inflammation, suppuration, and subsequent central necrosis (Fig. 13-31). It may at first appear to be a localized pneumonia, and it may elude diagnosis for a long time unless it invades a bronchus so that resulting drainage will allow detection of an air-fluid level. The causes are many. Aspiration of food or infected material from upper respiratory or dental sources of infection are perhaps most common, given an inoculum of sufficient size in a patient whose immunologic defenses may be down for any reason. The percussion note is dull and the breath sounds distant or absent over the affected area. There may be a pleural friction rub, and cough may produce a purulent, foul-smelling sputum. The patient is usually obviously ill and febrile, sometimes tachypneic. The breath commonly has a foul odor.

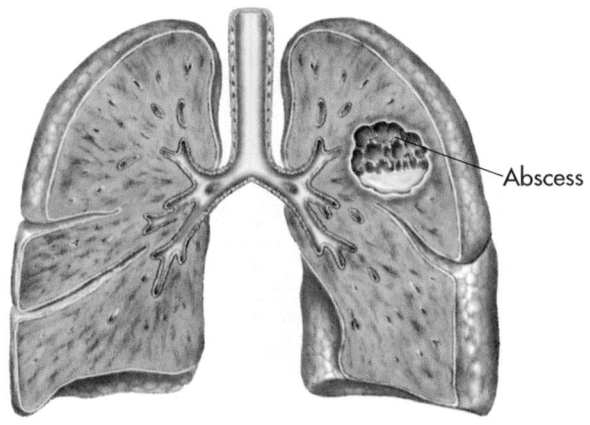

Abscess

FIGURE 13-31
Lung abscess.
Modified from Wilson, Thompson, 1990.

PNEUMONIA

Pneumonia is an inflammatory response of the bronchioles and alveolar spaces to an infective agent (bacterial, fungal, or viral) (Fig. 13-32). Exudates lead to lung consolidation, resulting in dyspnea, tachypnea, and crackles. Diminished breath sounds and dullness to percussion occur over the area of consolidation. Involvement of the right lower lobe can stimulate the tenth and eleventh thoracic nerves to cause right lower quadrant pain and simulate an abdominal process.

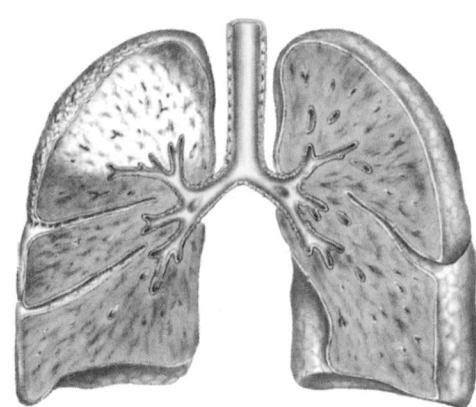

FIGURE 13-32
Lobar pneumonia (right upper lobe).
Modified from Wilson, Thompson, 1990.

CLINICAL PEARL

Pneumonia
In children particularly, but also in adults, audible crackles are not necessary to give evidence of pneumonia. Flaring of the alae nasi, tachypnea, and a possibly productive cough in the absence of crackles and out of proportion to other clinical findings should alert you to the possibility of acute bacterial pneumonia.

EVIDENCE-BASED PRACTICE IN PHYSICAL EXAMINATION
CHILDREN WITH PNEUMONIA

Many caregivers worry that children treated on an outpatient basis for pneumonia carry with them the serious risk of bacteremia. The evidence suggests otherwise. Five hundred and eighty children with an average age just beyond 14 months were studied. Only nine had a proven septicemia. None of them required hospitalization. The evidence supports the conclusion that this particular fear should not tip the primary caregiver toward seeking hospitalization for such a patient.

Shah et al, 2003.

INFLUENZA

A host of viruses, many frequently mutating, some as yet undiscovered or uncharacterized, cause this acute, generalized, febrile illness. In varying degree, it is characterized by cough, fever, malaise, headache, and the coryza and mild sore throat typical of the common cold. When it is mild, it may seem to be just a cold; however, the aged, the very young, and the chronically ill are particularly susceptible. In these persons, influenza may be fatal, although yearly immunization is often preventive. The entire respiratory tract may be overwhelmed by interstitial inflammation and necrosis extending throughout the bronchiolar and alveolar tissue (Fig. 13-33). There may be a variety of respiratory findings: crackles, rhonchi, and tachypnea, as well as cough (generally nonproductive) and substernal pain.

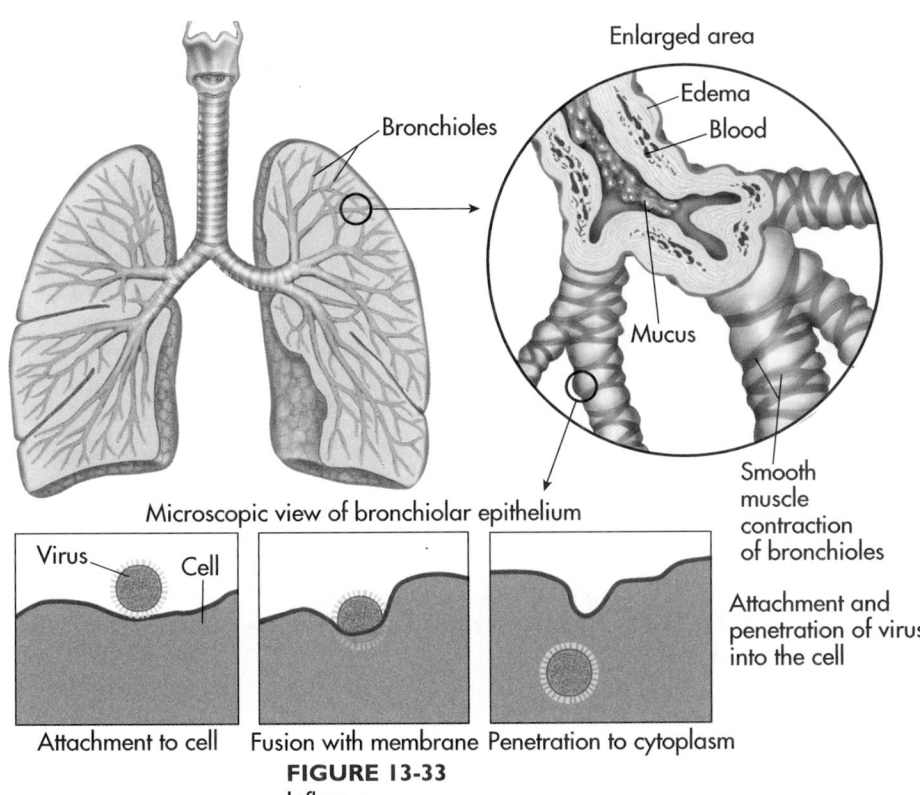

Enlarged area
Edema
Blood
Bronchioles
Mucus
Smooth muscle contraction of bronchioles
Attachment and penetration of virus into the cell

Microscopic view of bronchiolar epithelium

Virus   Cell

Attachment to cell   Fusion with membrane   Penetration to cytoplasm

FIGURE 13-33
Influenza.
Modified from Wilson, Thompson, 1990.

TUBERCULOSIS

Tuberculosis is a chronic infectious disease that most often begins in the lung but may then have widespread manifestations in many organs and systems. Most often, at the start, the tubercle bacillus (usually *Mycobacterium tuberculosis;* occasionally *Mycobacterium bovis* or an atypical mycobacterium) is inhaled from the airborne moisture of the coughs and sneezes of infected persons and given the opportunity to settle in the furthest reaches of the lung (Fig. 13-34). There is then a latent period as the organism entrenches itself. The patient may not be ill, and only a bit of lung and some regional lymph nodes may be involved. There is always the potential for a postprimary spread locally or throughout the body. Although treatment for tuberculosis has been effective in recent decades, the compromise caused by the HIV and the increasing incidence of HIV infection has been paralleled by an increasing incidence of tuberculosis and of mycobacteria that are resistant to treatment, in part because of a common failure to comply with drug regimens.

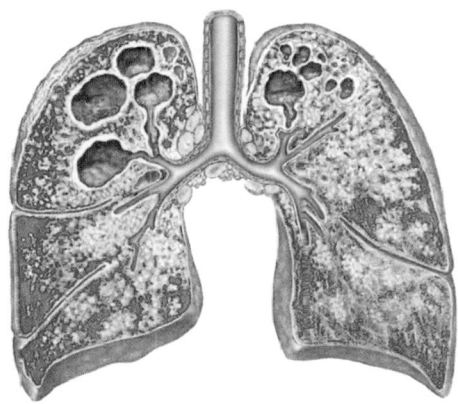

FIGURE 13-34
Tuberculosis.
Modified from Wilson, Thompson, 1990.

PNEUMOTHORAX

CLINICAL PEARL

Minimal Pneumothorax
An unexplained but persistent tachycardia may be a clue to a minimal pneumothorax that will not otherwise be detected on physical examination.

The presence of air or gas in the pleural cavity may be the result of trauma or may occur spontaneously, perhaps because of rupture of a congenital bleb. The air in the pleural space may not communicate with that in the lung; but in tension pneumothorax, air leaks continually into the pleural space, becoming trapped on expiration and resulting in increasing pressure in the pleural space (Fig. 13-35). Minimal collections of air without the presence of associated inflammatory lesions may easily escape detection at first, particularly because spontaneous pneumothorax paradoxically has its onset most often when the patient is at rest and not vigorously engaged. Larger collections cause varying degrees of the possible findings. Overall, the breath sounds are distant but the percussion note may boom.

A positive "coin click" can help. Place a coin over the suspicious area in the chest (e.g., posteriorly) and, while listening to the opposite side (anteriorly), have someone strike the coin with the edge of another. A clear click will be heard only in the event of a pronounced pneumothorax.

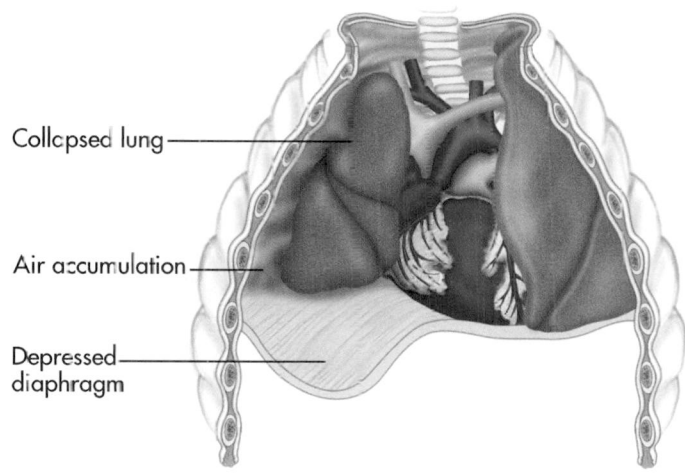

Collapsed lung

Air accumulation

Depressed diaphragm

FIGURE 13-35
Pneumothorax.

HEMOTHORAX

The presence of blood in the pleural cavity, *hemothorax* (Fig. 13-36), may be the result of trauma or invasive medical procedures (e.g., thoracentesis, pleural biopsy). Sometimes air may be present with the blood; this is called a *hemopneumothorax*. If there is no air, or if blood predominates, the breath sounds will be distant or absent, the percussion note will be dull, and the "coin click" will be absent.

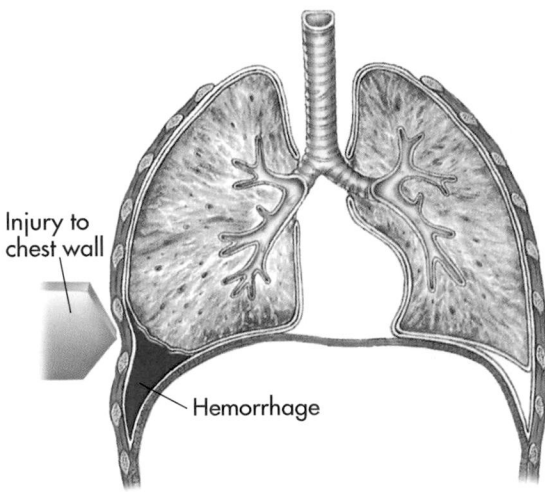

Injury to
chest wall

Hemorrhage

FIGURE 13-36
Hemothorax.
*Modified from Wilson, Thompson,
1990.*

LUNG CANCER

Lung cancer generally refers to bronchogenic carcinoma, a malignant tumor that evolves from bronchial epithelial structures. Etiologic agents include tobacco smoke, asbestos, ionizing radiation, and other inhaled chemicals and noxious agents. It may cause cough, wheezing, a variety of patterns of emphysema and atelectasis, pneumonitis, and hemoptysis. The extent of the tumor and the patterns of its invasion and metastasis are often determined by its histologic nature (Fig. 13-37). There are many other less common examples of uncontrolled growth primary in the lung, and numerous examples of metastasis from distant sites.

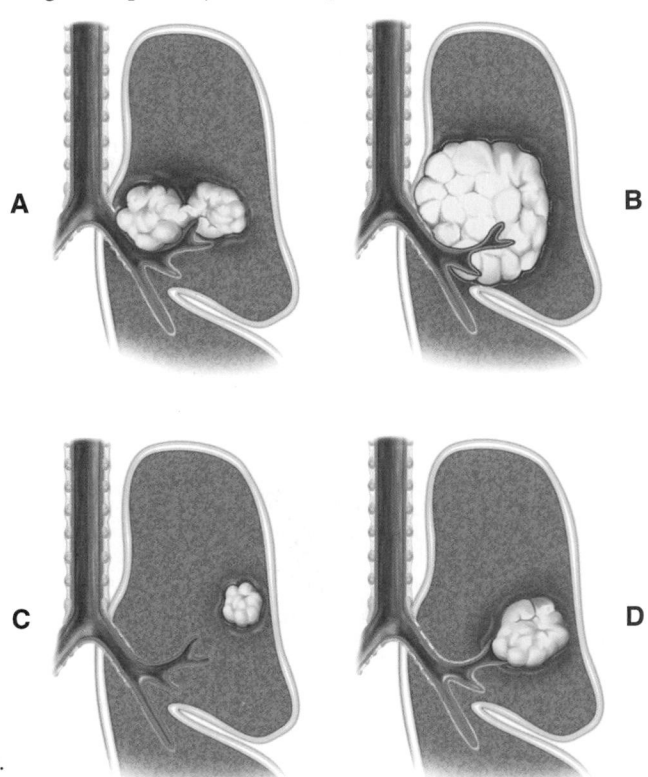

A

B

C

D

FIGURE 13-37
Cancer of the lung. **A,** Squamous (epidermoid) cell carcinoma. **B,** Small cell (oat cell) carcinoma. **C,** Adenocarcinoma. **D,** Large cell carcinoma.

COR PULMONALE

Cor pulmonale is an acute or chronic condition involving right-sided heart failure. In the acute phase, the right side of the heart is dilated and fails, most often as a direct result of pulmonary embolism. In chronic cor pulmonale, a chronic, massive disease of the lungs causes gradual obstruction that produces a more gradual hypertrophy of the right ventricle, increasing stress, and ultimate heart failure (Fig. 13-38). An isolated failure of the right side of the heart is rare except in the circumstance of pulmonary obstruction caused by emboli, primary pulmonary hypertension, or extensive infection and noxious involvement of the lung.

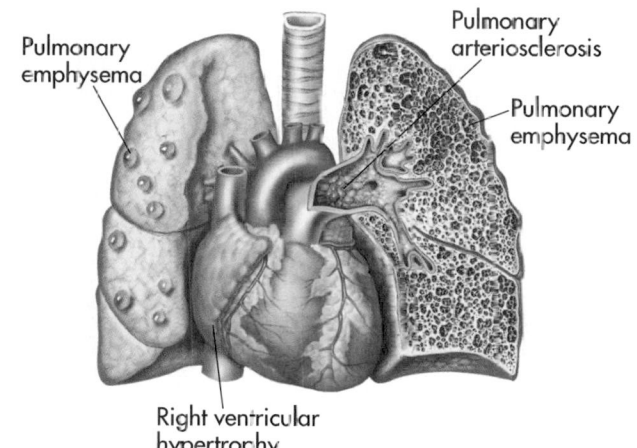

Pulmonary emphysema

Pulmonary arteriosclerosis

Pulmonary emphysema

Right ventricular hypertrophy

FIGURE 13-38
Cor pulmonale. Notice extensive pulmonary emphysema, pulmonary arteriosclerosis, and right ventricular hypertrophy. *Modified from Wilson, Thompson, 1990.*

PULMONARY EMBOLISM

Pulmonary embolism is a relatively common condition that is very difficult to diagnose. Of every six patients with the problem, one to two die of it. There is no finding in the history, on physical examination, or in any noninvasive diagnostic test that is sufficiently sensitive or specific to assure correct diagnosis. In fact, the diagnosis, too frequently obscured by a coexisting disease or operative procedure, is often not even considered. Risk factors include, among others, age older than 40 years, a history of venous thromboembolism, surgery with anesthesia longer than 30 minutes, heart disease, cancer, fracture of the pelvis and leg bones, obesity, and acquired or genetic thrombophilia. Pleuritic chest pain in the absence of dyspnea is a major clue to embolism. There may be a low-grade fever. (The degree of the fever does not necessarily suggest the severity of the problem.) You should be alert to the possibility of the disease and its potential severity, which should quicken the search for further diagnostic help (Fedullo, Tapson, 2003).

CHILDREN AND ADOLESCENTS

CYSTIC FIBROSIS

Cystic fibrosis (CF) is an autosomal recessive disorder of exocrine glands involving the lungs, pancreas, and sweat glands. Cough with sputum is a hallmark in children younger than 5 years. Salt loss in sweat is distinctive; a parent may notice that the child's skin tastes unusually salty. Abnormally thick mucus may cause progressive clogging of the bronchi and bronchioles, and subsequent pulmonary infections (Fig. 13-39). Initially, areas of hyperinflation and atelectasis are evident. As pulmonary dysfunction progresses, the tolerance for exercise diminishes and pulmonary hypertension and cor pulmonale often occur. Recent advances in treatment have extended life expectancy. In adults, apparently mild disease may be manifested by nasal polyps, cough, and male sterility. Approximately 10% of the diagnoses of CF are made in adults.

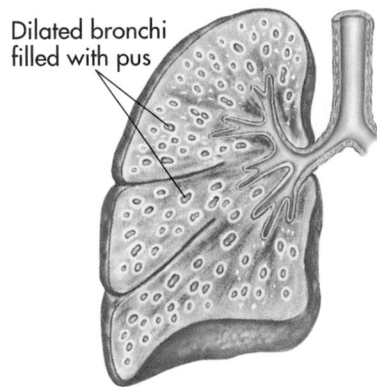

Dilated bronchi filled with pus

FIGURE 13-39
Cystic fibrosis.
Modified from Wilson, Thompson, 1990.

EPIGLOTTITIS

Epiglottitis is an acute, life-threatening disease almost always caused by *Haemophilus influenzae* type B. It begins suddenly and progresses rapidly, often to full obstruction of the airway (Fig. 13-40, *A*) and resulting in death. It may occur at any age but occurs most often in children between the ages of 3 and 7. The child sits straight up with neck extended and head held forward, appears very anxious and ill, is unable to swallow, and is drooling from an open mouth; cough is not common. The fever may be high. The epiglottis appears beefy red. It is vital to note that no attempt should be made to visualize the epiglottis, and that any suspicion of epiglottitis should be treated as a medical emergency. Immediate attention is required with the help of an anesthesiologist and/or otolaryngologist and radiologist in an emergency department. The tentative diagnosis should be based on the history and clinical appearance of the child before physical examination. Any attempt to visualize the epiglottis without skilled assistance and appropriate equipment for establishing an artificial airway is not justified. Direct examination of the throat, with or without a tongue blade, is to be avoided. While immunization has greatly reduced the incidence in this country, its gravity and its occurrence worldwide mandates the attention we give it.

CROUP

Croup is a syndrome that generally results from infection with a variety of viral agents, particularly the parainfluenza viruses. It occurs most often in very young children, generally from about 1½ to 3 years of age. Boys are more commonly affected than girls, and for reasons unknown, some children are susceptible to recurrent episodes. It is not unusual to have an episode begin in the evening, often after the child has gone to sleep. The child awakens sud-

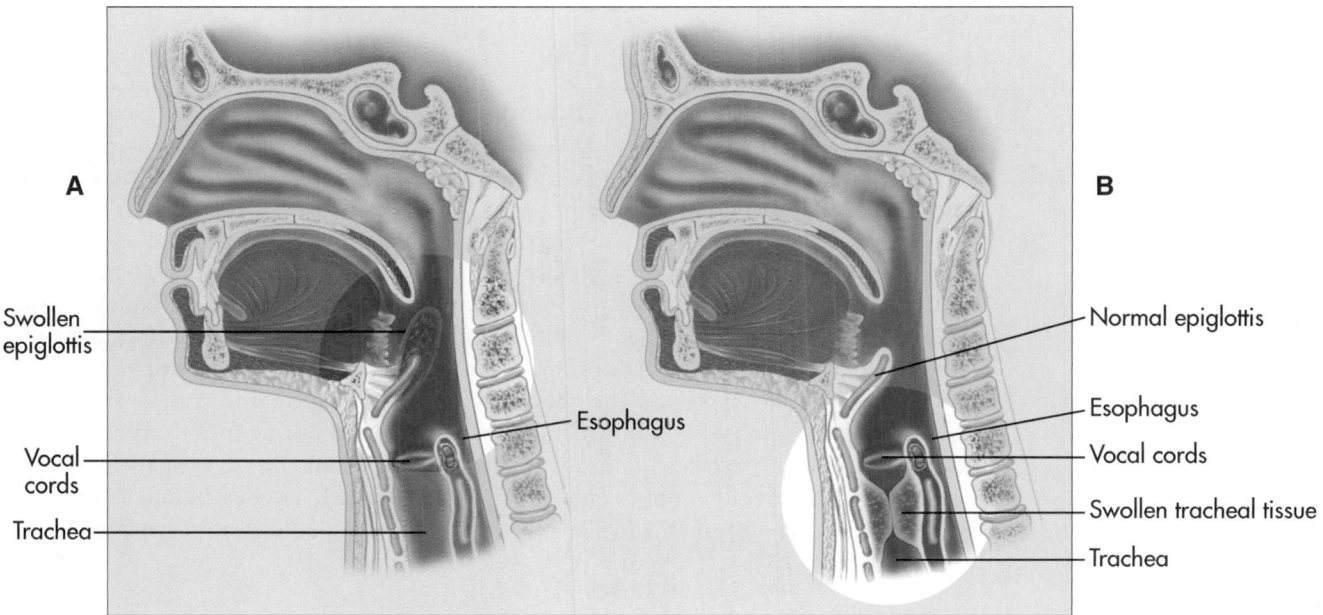

FIGURE 13-40
Croup syndrome. **A,** Acute epiglottitis. **B,** Laryngotracheobronchitis.

denly, often very frightened, with a harsh, bark-like cough. Labored breathing, retraction, hoarseness, and inspiratory stridor are characteristic. Fever does not always accompany croup. The inflammation is subglottic and may involve areas beyond the larynx (laryngotracheobronchitis) (see Fig. 13-40, *B*). Children with croup may be frightened, but they do not have the toxic, drooling facies of persons with epiglottitis. An aspirated foreign body may mimic croup on occasion.

RESPIRATORY DISTRESS SYNDROME	The term respiratory distress syndrome (RDS) is self-descriptive: The infant has trouble breathing. RDS characteristically occurs in preterm infants because of surfactant deficiency. The risk increases with decreasing gestational age, maternal diabetes, acute asphyxia, and with a family history of the problem. White males and the second of twins are also at greater risk. Tachypnea, retractions, grunting, and cyanosis are all part of the clinical picture. Early diagnosis and exogenous surfactant therapy are essential. Full-term infants have on occasion suffered adult respiratory distress syndrome (ARDS), a harrowing problem because of the complications of shock, asphyxia, and aspiration.
TRACHEOMALACIA	"Noisy breathing" in infancy, sometimes described as wheezing, is often inspiratory stridor. It can often be attributed to a floppiness of the trachea or airway, a lack of rigidity termed tracheomalacia. This condition causes the trachea to change in response to the varying pressures of inspiration and expiration. Although tracheomalacia tends to be benign and self-limited with increasing age, it is necessary to eliminate the possibilities of fixed lesions (e.g., a vascular lesion), tracheal stenosis, or even a foreign body. At times, the larynx may also have the same yielding characteristic (*laryngomalacia;* if the entire large airway is involved, the condition is called *laryngotracheomalacia*).
BRONCHIOLITIS	Bronchiolitis occurs most often in infants younger than 6 months old. The principal characteristic is hyperinflation of the lungs. The cause is viral, usually the respiratory syncytial virus. Expiration becomes difficult, and the infant appears anxious and tachypneic. Generalized retraction and perioral cyanosis are common. Because of lung hyperinflation, the AP diameter of the thoracic cage may be increased and percussion hyperresonant. Wheezing may or may not be apparent. In the presence of severe tachypnea, air exchange is poor and the breaths are rapid and short, with the expiratory phase prolonged. Crackles may or may not be heard. The abdomen appears distended from swallowed air.

OLDER ADULTS

CHRONIC OBSTRUCTIVE PULMONARY DISEASE

COPD is a nonspecific designation that includes a group of respiratory problems in which coughs, chronic and often excessive sputum production, and dyspnea are prominent features. Ultimately, an irreversible expiratory airflow obstruction occurs. Chronic bronchitis, emphysema (Fig. 13-41), asthmatic bronchitis, bronchiectasis, and even cystic fibrosis may be included in that group. One need not be an older adult, of course, to have one of these problems. Most patients, however, are certainly not young, and most patients have been smokers. A careful history will reveal a legacy of episodes of coughs and sputum and limited tolerance for exercise. The patient will often breathe through pursed lips to ease the effort of dyspnea. (We do not really know why this works.) Dyspnea can also be eased by leaning forward and resting the arms on the knees. The chest may be barrel shaped, and scattered crackles or wheezes may be heard. Airway obstruction can be evaluated during forced maximal expiration. Listen over the trachea with the diaphragm of your stethoscope as the patient inhales to the limit and then breathes out as quickly as possible through an open mouth. If this forced expiration time is longer than 4 to 5 seconds, you should suspect airway obstruction.

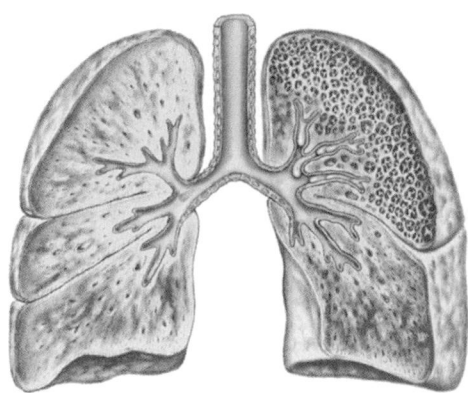

FIGURE 13-41
Chronic obstructive pulmonary disease with lobar emphysema.
Modified from Wilson, Thompson, 1990.

STAYING WELL

NEVER SMOKE/STOP SMOKING

COPD is, at the moment, the fourth leading cause of death in the United States and this will likely get worse by 2020. The major risk factor is cigarette smoking. Although as many as 20% of people who die from the disease have never smoked, the vital key to prevention is the cessation of smoking or, better yet, never tasting a cigarette. It is our responsibility as care providers to be persistent in our attention to patient education in this regard, not once, not twice, but constantly.

Data from Rennard, 2004.

EMPHYSEMA

Emphysema, perhaps the most severe chronic obstructive pulmonary disorder, is a condition in which air may take over and dominate a space in a way that disrupts function. The air spaces beyond the terminal bronchioles dilate, rupturing alveolar walls, permanently destroying them, reducing their number, and permanently hyperinflating the lung. Alveolar gas is trapped, essentially in expiration, and gas exchange is seriously compromised. Chronic bronchitis is a common precursor. Involutionary changes as the lungs lose elasticity because of aging, smoking, or impairment of the defenses mediated by α-antitrypsin are also contributors. The overinflated lungs tend to be hyperresonant on percussion. Further expansion on inspiration is limited; occasionally there is a prolonged expiratory effort (i.e., longer than 4 or 5 seconds) to expel air. Dyspnea is common even at rest. Cough is infrequent without much production of sputum. The patient is often thin and barrel-chested, even cachectic.

BRONCHIECTASIS

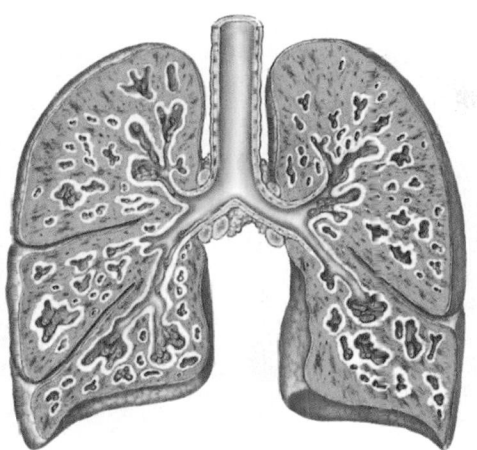

FIGURE 13-42
Bronchiectasis.
Modified from Wilson, Thompson, 1990.

Chronic dilation of the bronchi or bronchioles is caused by repeated pulmonary infections and bronchial obstruction (Fig. 13-42). The dilations may involve the tube uniformly (cylindric) or irregularly (saccular); at the terminal ends, the enlargement may be bulbous. Bronchiectasis may lead to malfunction of bronchial muscle tone and loss of elasticity. The extent of findings on physical examination is governed by the degree of "wetness." The cough and expectoration are most often the major clues. Kartagener syndrome, an autosomal recessive condition, is characterized by bronchiectasis, sinusitis, dextrocardia, and male infertility.

CHRONIC BRONCHITIS

This condition may occur at any age but is commonly a problem for patients older than 40. The mucus of the bronchi is chronically inflamed, recurrent bacterial infections are common, dyspnea may be present although not severe, and cough and sputum are impressive. Smoking is prominent in the history; many of these patients are emphysematous. These conditions are all clearly correlated. Severe chronic bronchitis may result in right ventricular failure with dependent edema.

ELECTRONIC RESOURCES

For Weblinks and additional resources, go to   *evolve*

http://evolve.elsevier.com/Seidel

or to the Companion CD-ROM.

Additional information related to the content in Chapter 13 can be found on the companion website at evolve.elsevier.com/Seidel/ or on the interactive companion CD-ROM. Resources and activities for Chapter 13 include:

- Sound and Vision Theater
- Printouts for Your Practice
- Interactive Challenge
- Spanish Assessment Terms with Pronunciation Guide
- Instant Calculators

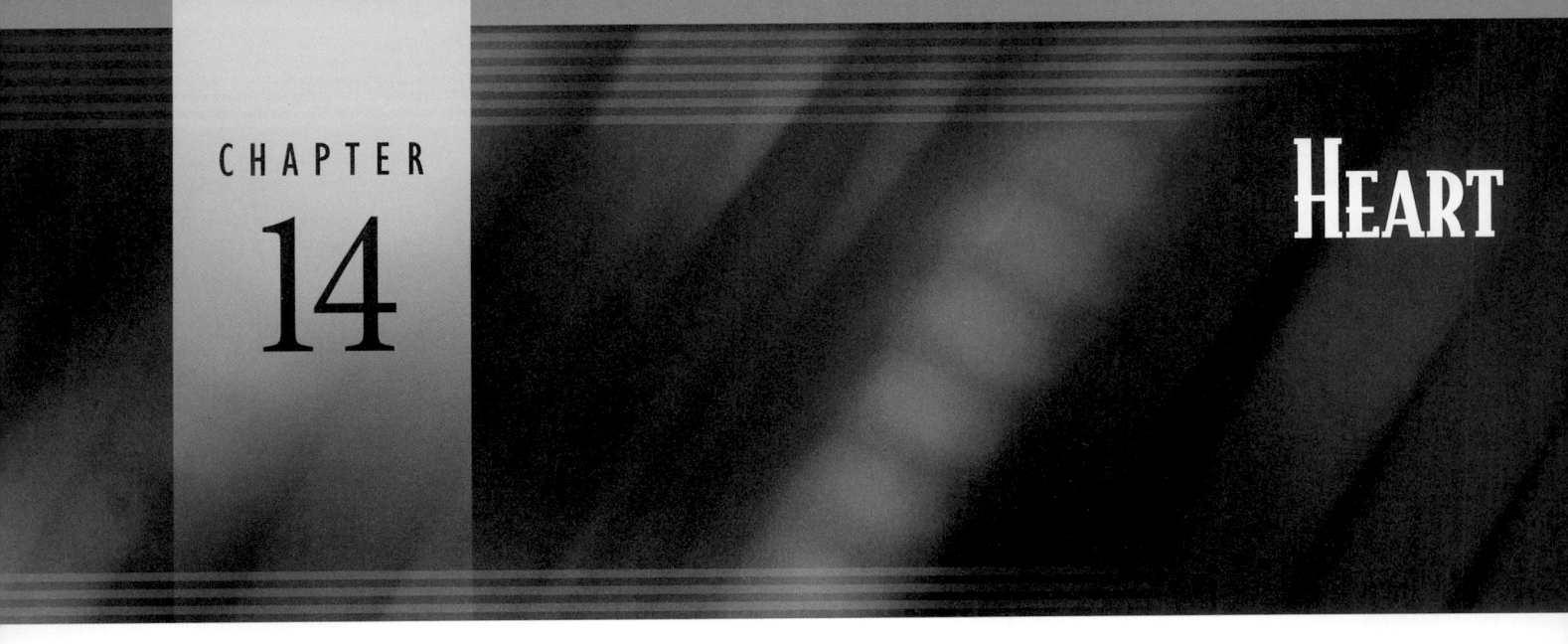

ANATOMY AND PHYSIOLOGY

The heart lies in the mediastinum, to the left of the midline, just above the diaphragm, and is cradled between the medial and lower borders of the lungs. It is positioned behind the sternum and the contiguous parts of the third to the sixth costal cartilages. The area of the chest overlying the heart is the precordium. Because of the heart's conelike shape, the broader upper portion is called the base, and the narrower lower tip of the heart is the apex (Fig. 14-1).

The position of the heart can vary considerably depending on body build, configuration of the chest, and level of the diaphragm. In a tall, slender person, the heart tends to hang vertically and to be positioned centrally. With increasing stockiness and shortness, it tends to lie more to the left and more horizontally. On occasion, the heart may be positioned to the right, either rotated or displaced, or as a complete mirror image of the expected. Such a circumstance is called *dextrocardia*. If the heart and stomach are placed to the right and the liver to the left, this habitus is termed *situs inversus*.

STRUCTURE

The pericardium is a tough, double-walled, fibrous sac encasing and protecting the heart. Several milliliters of fluid are present between the inner and outer layers of the pericardium, providing for easy, low-friction movement (Fig. 14-2).

The epicardium, the thin outermost muscle layer, covers the surface of the heart and extends onto the great vessels. The myocardium, the thick muscular middle layer, is responsible for the pumping action of the heart. The endocardium, the innermost layer, lines the chambers of the heart and covers the heart valves and the small muscles associated with the opening and closing of these valves (Fig. 14-3).

The heart is divided into four chambers. The two upper chambers are the right and left atria (or auricles, because of their earlike shape), and the bottom chambers are the right and left ventricles. The left atrium and left ventricle together are referred to as the *left heart*; the right atrium and right ventricle together are referred to as the *right heart*. The left heart and right heart are divided by a blood-tight partition called the *cardiac septum*.

The atria are small, thin-walled structures that act primarily as reservoirs for the blood returning to the heart from the veins throughout the body. The ventricles are large, thick-walled chambers that pump blood to the lungs and throughout the body. The right and left ventricles together form the primary muscle mass of the heart.

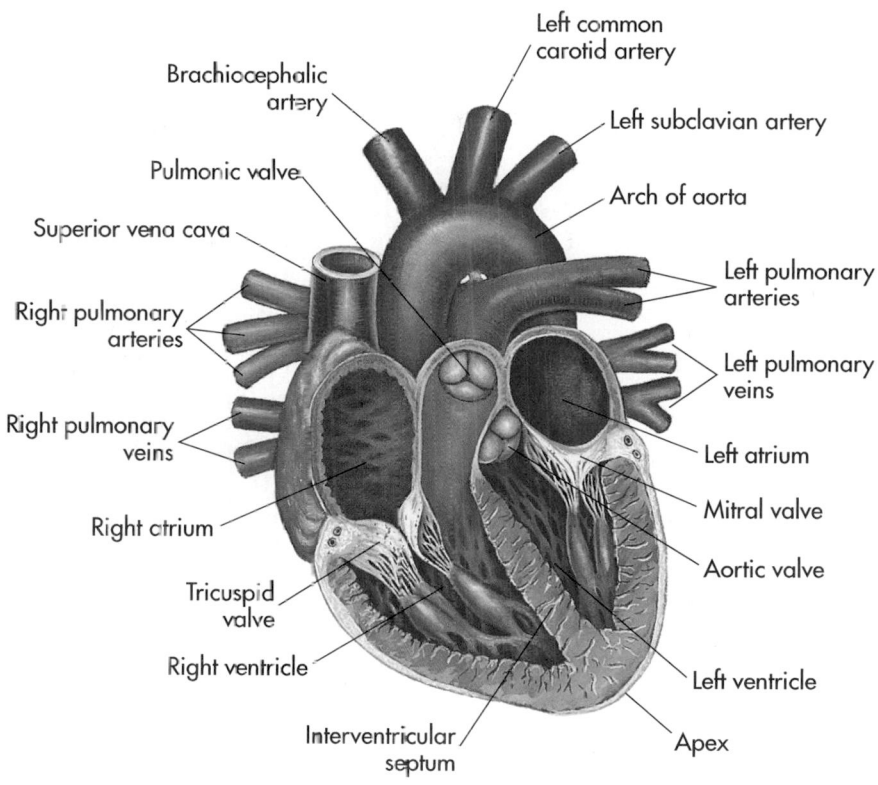

FIGURE 14-1
Frontal section of the heart.

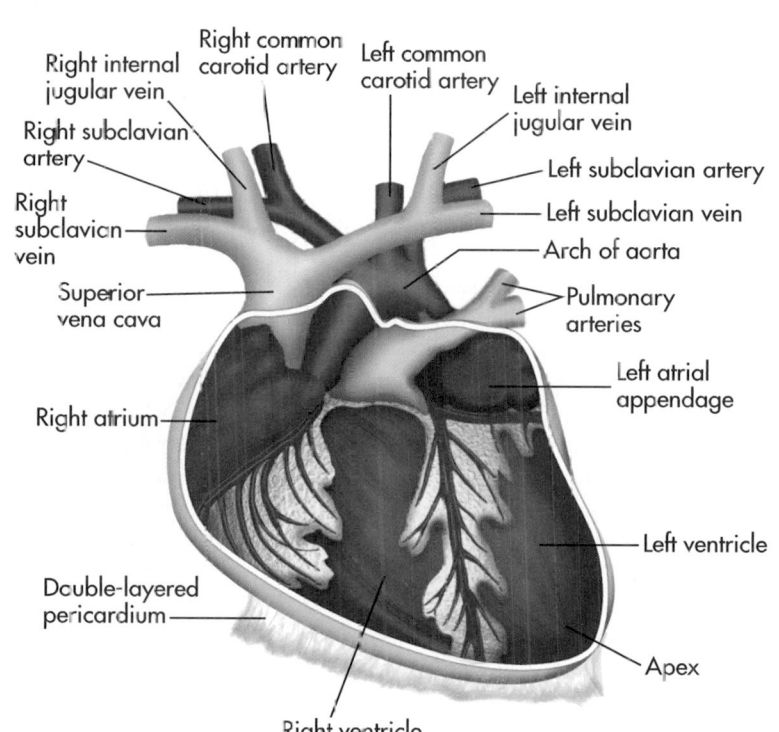

FIGURE 14-2
Heart within the pericardium.

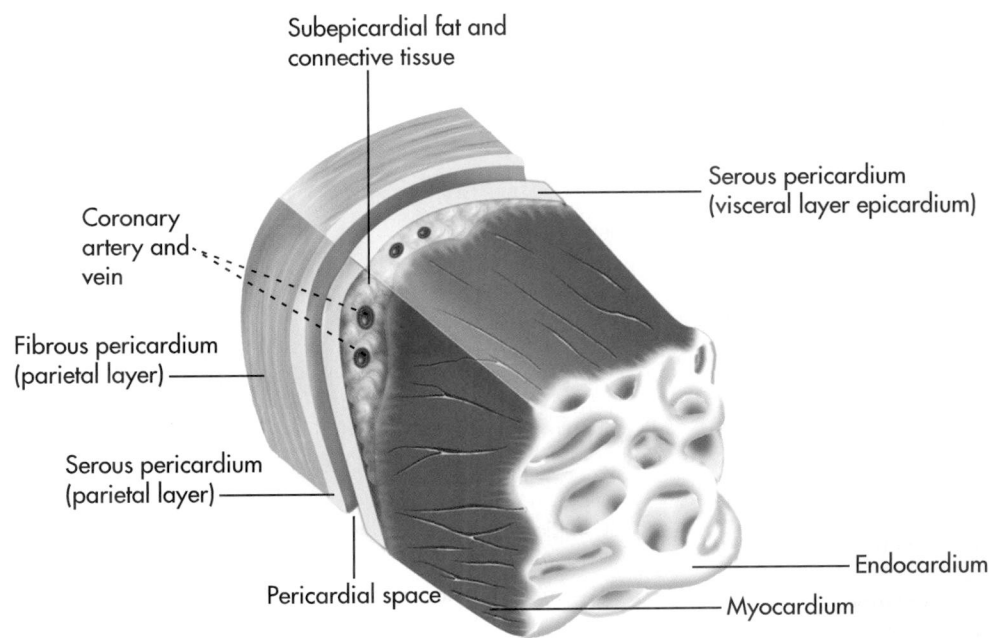

Subepicardial fat and
connective tissue

Serous pericardium
(visceral layer epicardium)

Coronary
artery and
vein

Fibrous pericardium
(parietal layer)

Serous pericardium
(parietal layer)

Endocardium

Pericardial space

Myocardium

FIGURE 14-3
Cross section of the cardiac
muscle.

Most of the anterior surface of the heart is formed by the right ventricle. The left ventricle is positioned behind the right but extends anteriorly, forming the left border of the heart. Its contraction and thrust are responsible for the apical impulse usually felt in the fifth left intercostal space at the midclavicular line. The right atrium lies above and slightly to the right of the right ventricle, participating in the formation of the right border of the heart. The left atrium is above the left ventricle, forming the more posterior aspect of the heart. The heart is, in effect, turned ventrally on its axis, putting its right side more forward. The adult heart is about 12 cm long, 8 cm wide at the widest point, and 6 cm in its anteroposterior diameter (Fig. 14-4).

The four chambers of the heart are connected by two sets of valves: the atrioventricular and semilunar valves. In the fully formed heart that is free of defect, these are the only intracardiac pathways (Fig. 14-5). They permit the flow of blood in only one direction.

The atrioventricular valves, situated between the atria and the ventricles, include the tricuspid and mitral valves. The tricuspid valve, which has three cusps (or leaflets), separates the right atrium from the right ventricle. The mitral valve, which has two cusps, separates the left atrium from the left ventricle. When the atria contract, the atrioventricular valves open, allowing blood to flow into the ventricles. When the ventricles contract, these valves snap shut, preventing blood from flowing back into the atria.

The two semilunar valves each have three cusps. The pulmonic valve separates the right ventricle from the pulmonary artery. The aortic valve lies between the left ventricle and the aorta. Contraction of the ventricles opens the semilunar valves, causing blood to rush into the pulmonary artery and aorta. When the ventricles relax, the valves close, shutting off any backward flow into the ventricles.

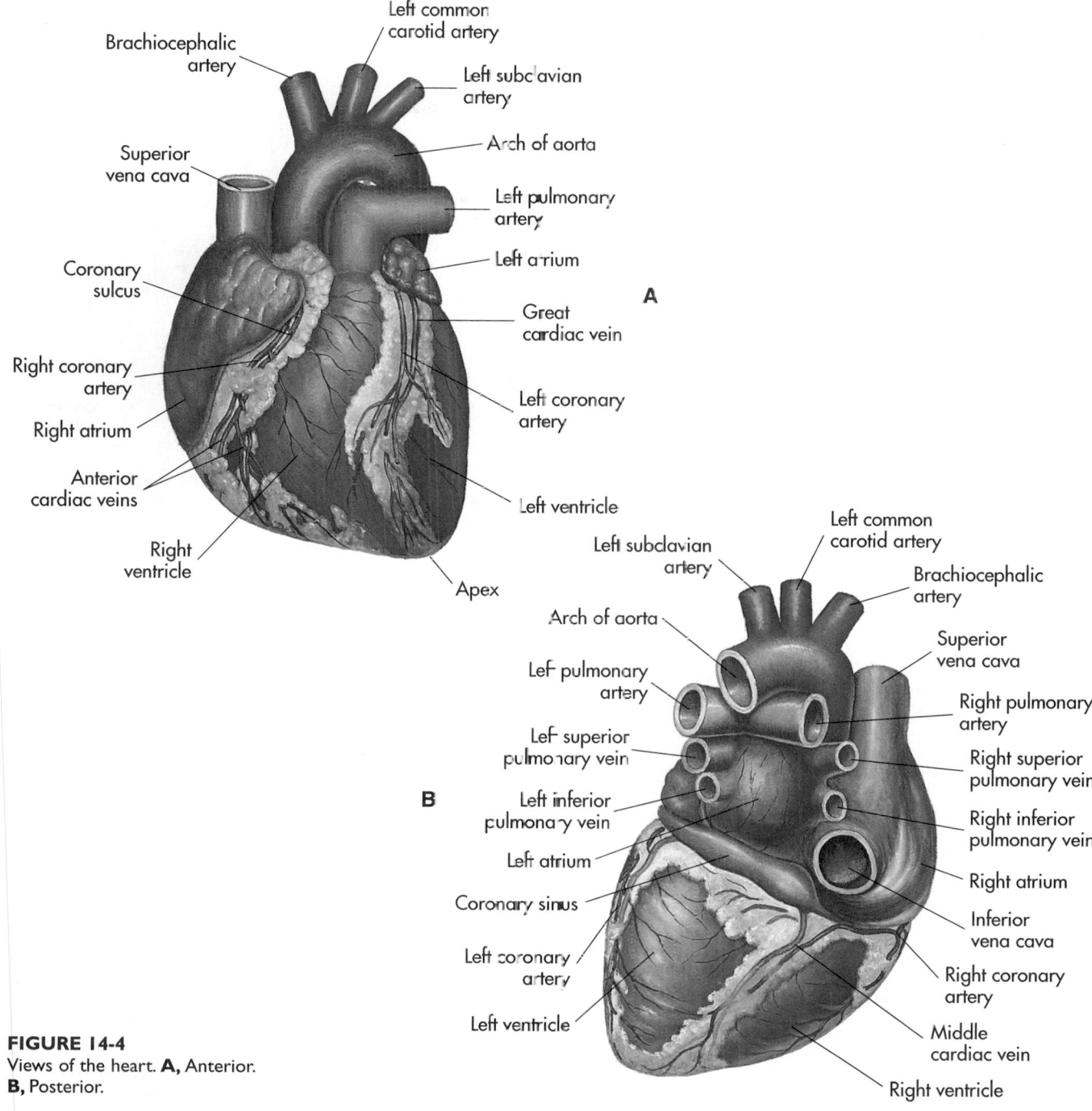

FIGURE 14-4
Views of the heart. **A,** Anterior.
B, Posterior.

CARDIAC CYCLE

The heart contracts and relaxes rhythmically to ensure proper circulation, a process that creates two phases in the cardiac cycle. During systole, the ventricles contract, ejecting blood from the left ventricle into the aorta and from the right ventricle into the pulmonary artery. During diastole, the ventricles dilate, an energy-requiring effort that draws blood into the ventricles as the atria contract, thereby moving blood from the atria to the ventricles (Fig. 14-6). The volume of blood and the pressure under which it is returned to the heart vary with the degree of body activity, both physical and metabolic (e.g., with exercise or fever). As the ventricles fill, each must respond to the force under which filling takes place.

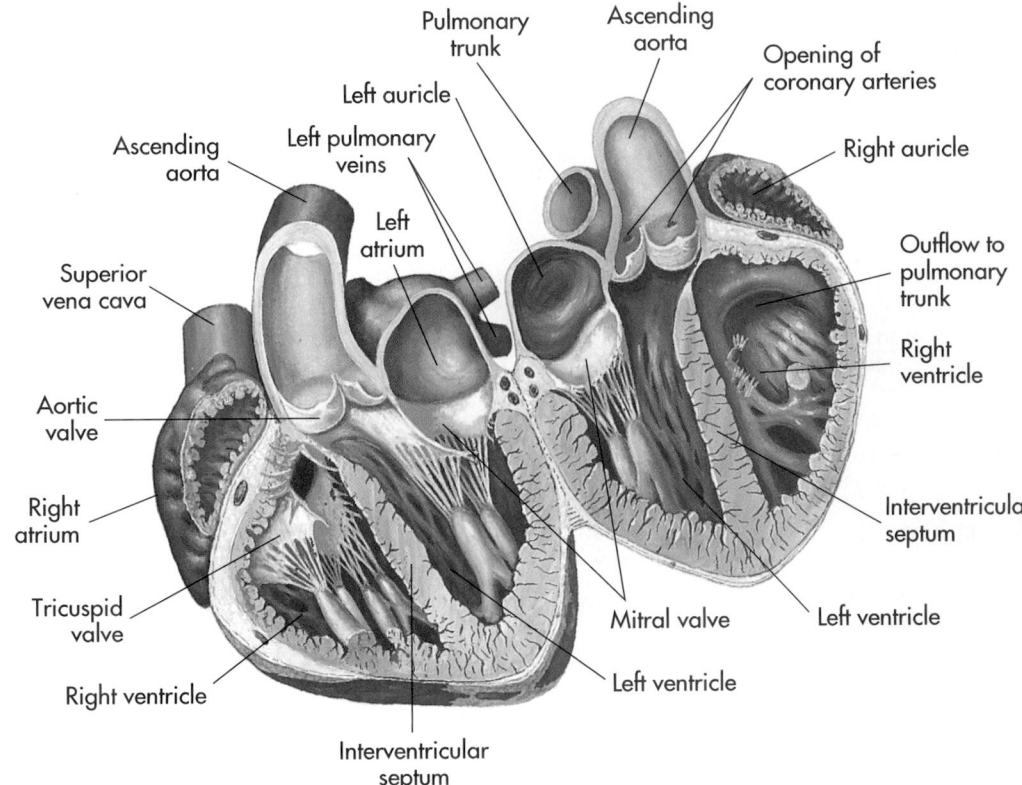

FIGURE 14-5
Anterior cross section showing the valves and chambers of the heart.

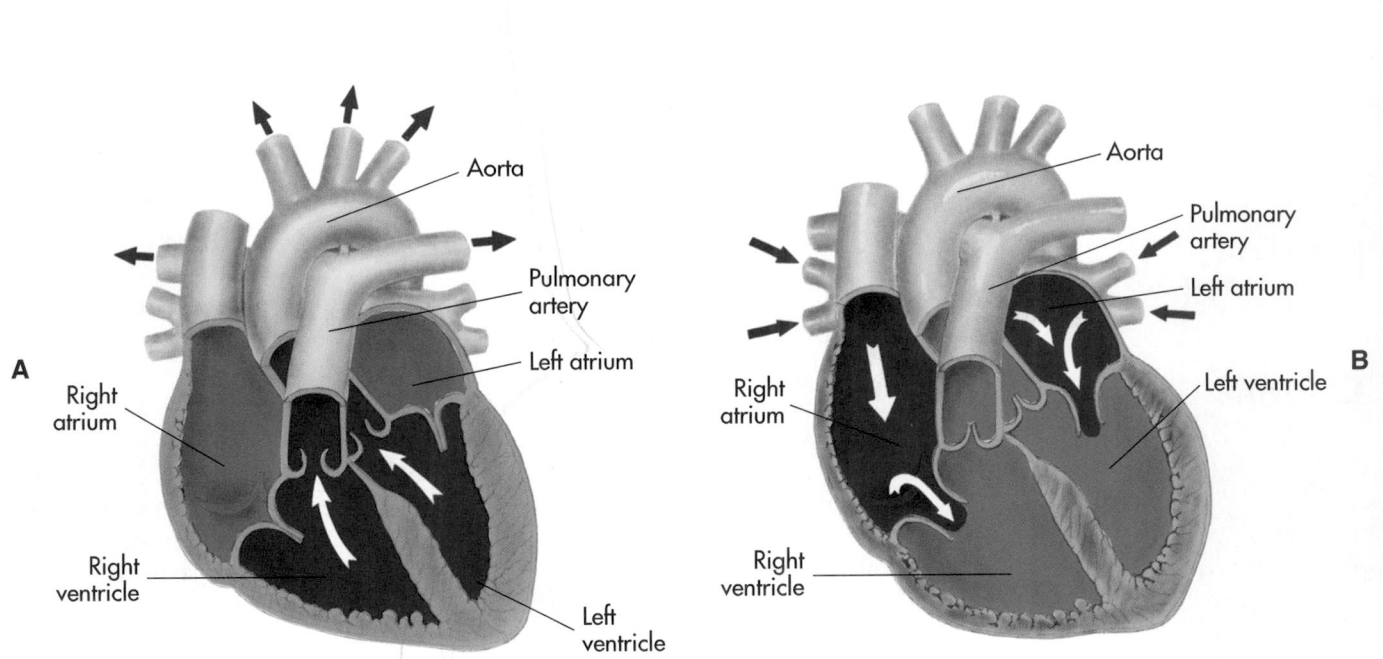

FIGURE 14-6
Blood flow through the heart. **A,** Systole. **B,** Diastole.
From Canobbio, 1990.

As systole begins, ventricular contraction raises the pressure in the ventricles and forces the mitral and tricuspid valves closed preventing backflow. This valve closure produces the first heart sound (S_1), the characteristic "lubb." The intraventricular pressure rises until it exceeds that in the aorta and pulmonary artery. Then the aortic and pulmonic valves are forced open, and ejection of blood into the arteries begins. Valve opening is usually a silent event (Fig. 14-7).

When the ventricles are almost empty, the pressure in the ventricles falls below that in the aorta and pulmonary artery, allowing the aortic and pulmonic valves to close. Closure of these valves causes the second heart sound (S_2), the "dubb." This sound has two components: A_2 is produced by aortic valve closure, and P_2 is produced by pulmonic valve closure. As ventricular pressure falls below atrial pressure, the mitral and tricuspid valves open to allow the blood collected in the atria to refill the relaxed ventricles. Diastole is a relatively passive interval until ventricular filling is almost complete. This filling sometimes produces a third heart sound (S_3). Then the atria contract to ensure the ejection of any remaining blood. This can sometimes be heard as a fourth heart sound (S_4). The cycle begins anew, with ventricular contraction and atrial refilling occurring at about the same time. The heart fulfills this impressive demand without resting and while adjusting constantly to the variable demands of work, rest, digestion, and illness.

This discussion describes the events of the cardiac cycle as virtually simultaneous on both sides of the heart. In fact, the pressures in the right ventricle, right atrium, and pulmonary artery are lower than those on the left side of the heart; and the same events occur slightly later on the right side than on the left. The effect is that heart sounds sometimes have two distinct components, the first produced by the left side and the second by the right side. For example,

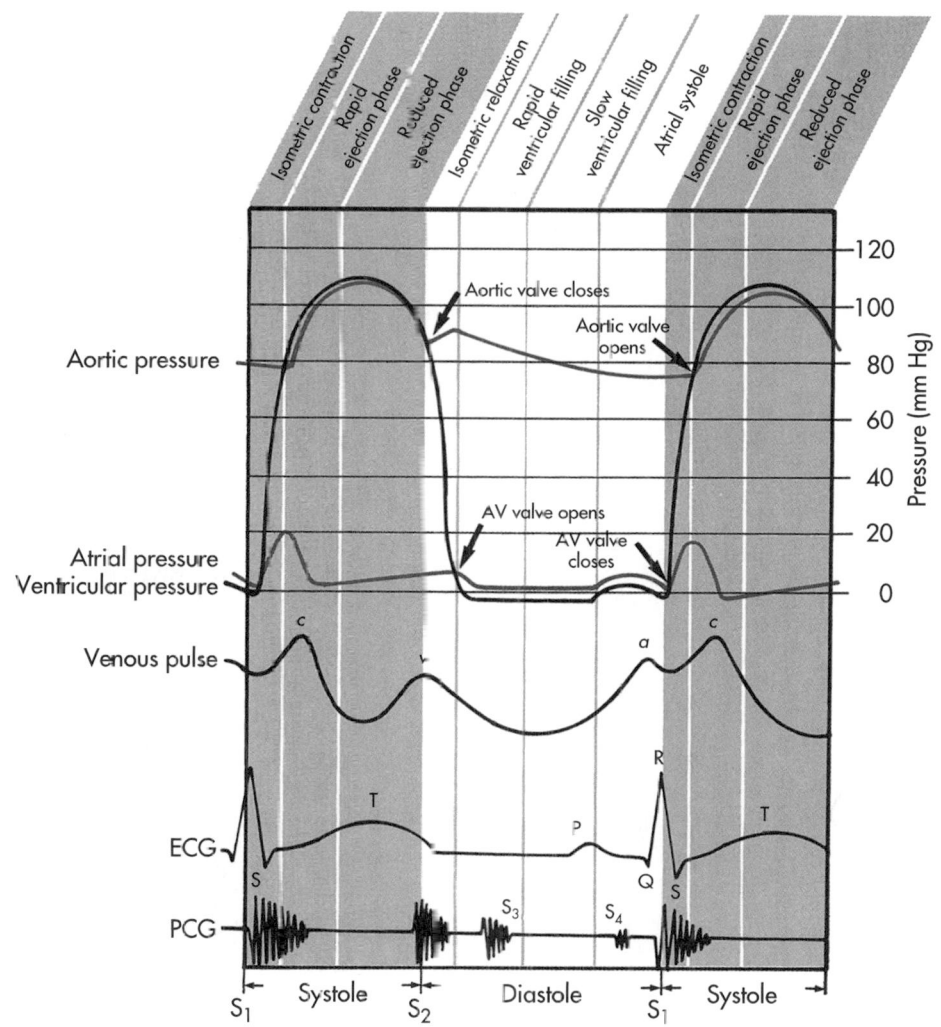

FIGURE 14-7
Events of the cardiac cycle, showing venous pressure waves, ECG, and heart sounds in systole and diastole. *PCG, Phonocardiogram.*
Modified from Guzzetta, Dossey, 1992.

the aortic valve closes slightly before the pulmonic, so that S_2 is often heard as two distinct components, referred to as "split S_2."

Closure of the heart valves during the cardiac cycle produces heart sounds in rapid succession. The simultaneous muscular tension and flow of blood give "body" to the sounds. Although the valves are anatomically close to each other, their sounds are best heard in an area away from the anatomic site (in the direction of blood flow; see Fig. 14-15).

ELECTRICAL ACTIVITY

The heart is, in a sense, autonomous: an intrinsic electrical conduction system enables it to contract within itself, free of any stimulus from elsewhere in the body. (This is not to imply that the heart rate is insensitive to other stimuli.) The electrical system coordinates the sequence of muscular contractions that take place during the cardiac cycle. An electrical current or impulse stimulates each myocardial contraction. The impulse originates in and is paced by the sinoatrial node (SA node), located in the wall of the right atrium. The impulse then travels through both atria to the atrioventricular node (AV node), located in the atrial septum. In the AV node the impulse is delayed but then passes down the bundle of His to the Purkinje fibers in the ventricular myocardium. Ventricular contraction is initiated at the apex and proceeds toward the base of the heart (Fig. 14-8).

An electrocardiogram (ECG) is a graphic recording of electrical activity during the cardiac cycle. The ECG records electrical current generated by movement of ions in and out of the myocardial cell membranes. The ECG records two basic events: depolarization, which is the spread of a stimulus through the heart muscle, and repolarization, which is the return of the stimulated heart muscle to a resting state. The ECG records electrical activity as specific waves (Fig. 14-9):

- P wave—the spread of a stimulus through the atria (atrial depolarization).
- PR interval—the time from initial stimulation of the atria to initial stimulation of the ventricles, usually 0.12 to 0.20 second.
- QRS complex—the spread of a stimulus through the ventricles (ventricular depolarization), less than 0.10 second.
- ST segment and T wave—the return of stimulated ventricular muscle to a resting state (ventricular repolarization).
- U wave—a small deflection sometimes seen just after the T wave.
- Q-T interval—the time elapsed from the onset of ventricular depolarization until the completion of ventricular repolarization. The interval varies with the cardiac rate.

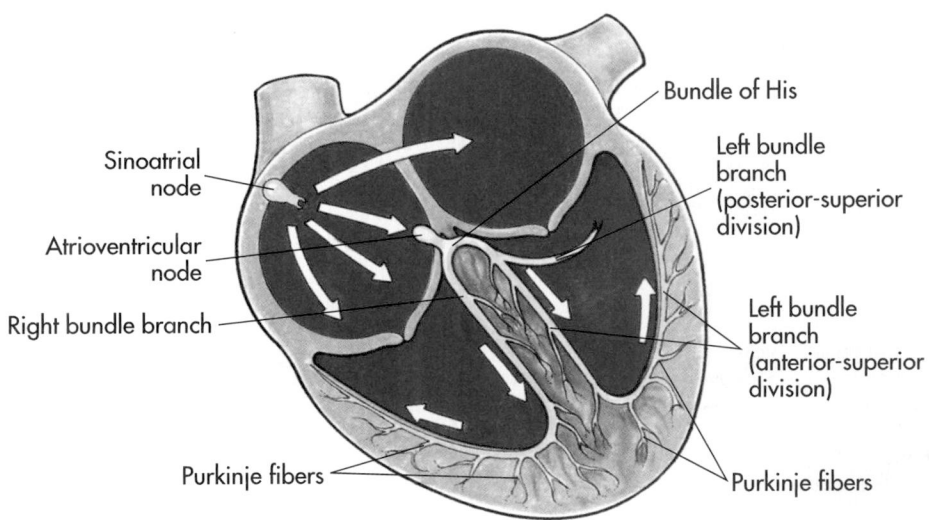

FIGURE 14-8
Cardiac conduction.
From Canobbio, 1990.

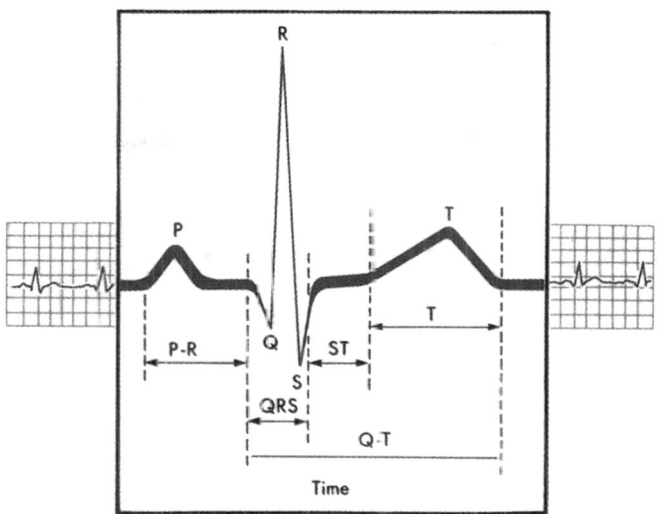

FIGURE 14-9
Usual electrocardiogram wave-
form.
From Berne, Levy, 1996.

Because the electrical stimulus starts the cycle, it must precede the mechanical response by a brief moment; the sequence of myocardial depolarization is the cause of events on the left side of the heart occurring slightly before those on the right. When the heart is beating at a rate of 68 to 72 beats per minute, ventricular systole is shorter than diastole; however, as the rate increases to about 120 because of stress or pathologic factors, the two phases of the cardiac cycle tend to approximate each other in length.

INFANTS AND CHILDREN   The heart becomes very much like the adult heart early in fetal life. The fetal circulation, including the umbilical vessels, compensates for the nonfunctional fetal lungs: the right ventricle pumps blood through the patent ductus arteriosus rather than into the lungs. The right and left ventricles are equal in weight and muscle mass because they both pump blood into the systemic circulation (Figs. 14-10 and 14-11).

The changes at birth include closure of the ductus arteriosus, usually within 24 to 48 hours; and the functional closure of the interatrial foramen ovale as pressure rises in the left atrium. The changing demand on the right ventricle as the pulmonary circulation is established, and on the left ventricle as it assumes total responsibility for the systemic circulation, result in a relative increase in the mass of the left ventricle. By 1 year of age, the relative sizes of the left and right ventricles approximate the adult ratio of 2:1.

The heart lies more horizontally in the chest in infants and young children than in the adult, and as a result the apex of the heart rides higher, sometimes well out into the fourth left intercostal space. In most cases, the adult heart position is reached by the age of 7 years.

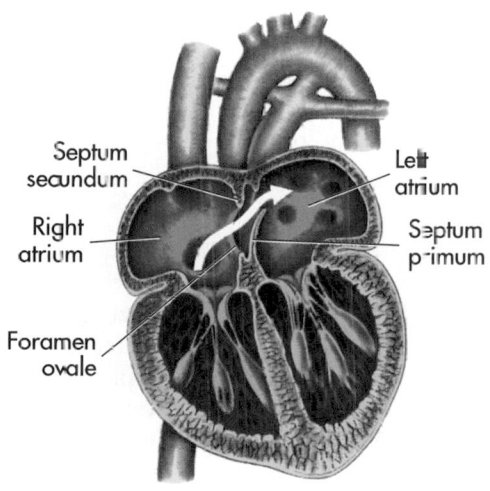

FIGURE 14-10
Anatomy of the fetal heart.
From Thompson et al, 1997.

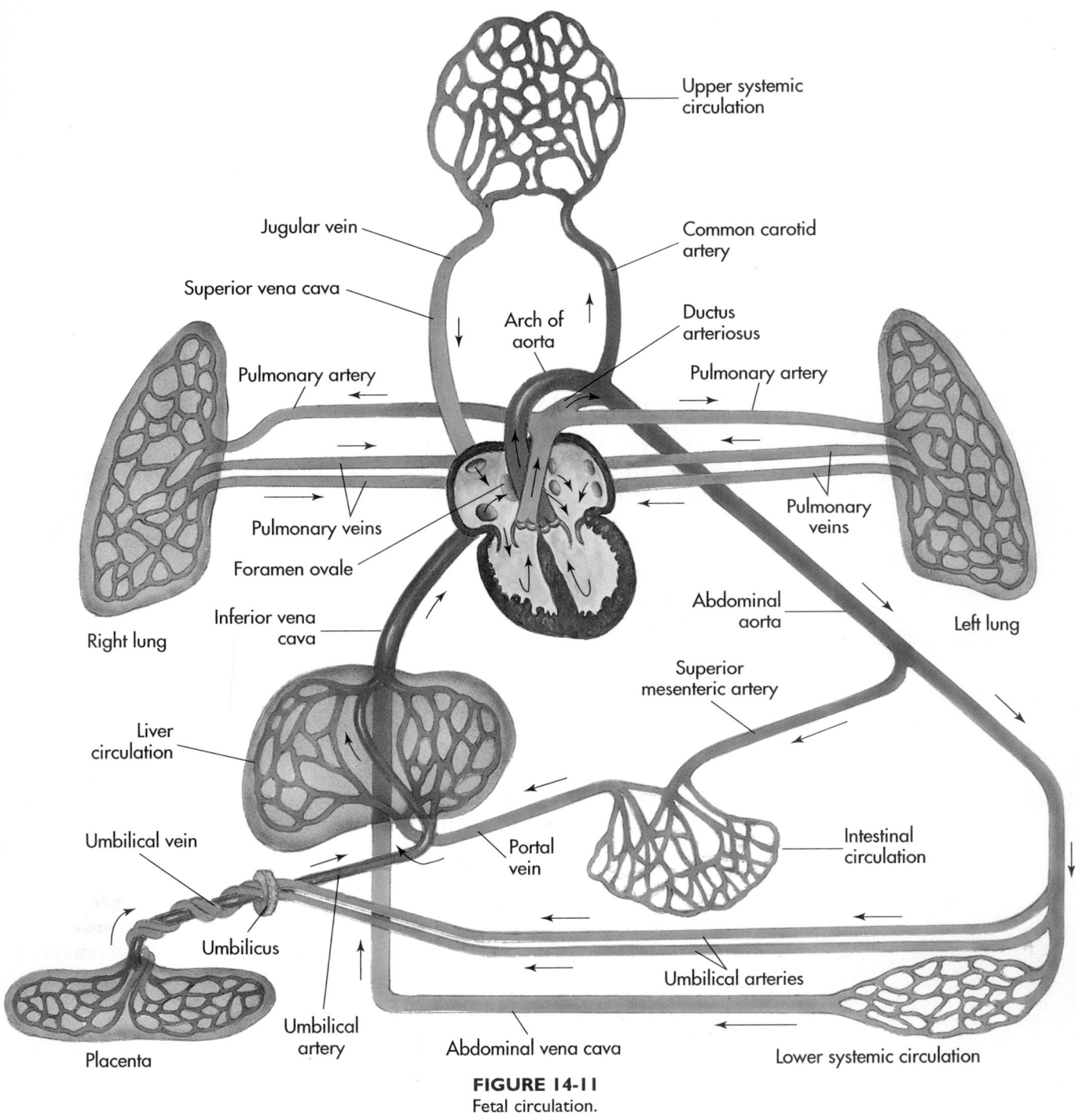

FIGURE 14-11
Fetal circulation.

PREGNANT WOMEN

The maternal blood volume increases 40% to 50% over the pre-pregnancy level. The rise is mainly due to an increase in plasma volume, which begins in the first trimester and reaches a maximum after the thirtieth week. On the average, plasma volume increases 50% with a single pregnancy and as much as 70% with a twin pregnancy. The heart works harder to accommodate the increased heart rate and stroke volume required for the expanded blood volume. The left ventricle increases in both wall thickness and mass. The blood volume returns to pre-pregnancy levels within 3 to 4 weeks after delivery (Table 14-1).

TABLE 14-1	Hemodynamic Changes During Pregnancy				
	Stage				
Hemodynamic Variable	**First Trimester**	**Second Trimester**	**Third Trimester**	**Labor and Delivery**	**Postpartum Period**
HR	Increased	Peaks at 28th week	Slightly decreased	Increased; bradycardia at delivery	Pre-pregnancy level within 2 to 6 weeks
BP	Pre-pregnancy level	Slightly decreased	Pre-pregnancy level	Pre-pregnancy level	Pre-pregnancy level
BV	Increased	Peaks at 20th week	Gradually decreased	Rises sharply	Pre-pregnancy level within 2 to 6 weeks
SV	Increased	Peaks at 28th week	Gradually decreased	Decreased	Pre-pregnancy level within 2 to 6 weeks
CO	Increased	Peaks at 20th week	Slightly decreased	Increased	Pre-pregnancy level within 2 to 6 weeks
LVEDP	Pre-pregnancy level	Pre-pregnancy level	Pre-pregnancy level	Pre-pregnancy level	Pre-pregnancy level
SVR	Decreased	Decreased	Decreased	Sharply decreased at delivery	Pre-pregnancy level within 2 to 6 weeks
PVR	Decreased	Decreased	Decreased	Decreased	Pre-pregnancy level within 2 to 6 weeks

From Walsh, 1988.
BP, Blood pressure; *BV,* blood volume; *HR,* Heart rate; *CO,* cardiac output; *LVEDP,* left ventricular end-diastolic pressure; *PVR,* pulmonary vascular resistance; *SV,* stroke volume; *SVR,* systemic vascular resistance.

The cardiac output increases approximately 30% to 40% over that of the nonpregnant state and reaches its highest level by about 25 to 32 weeks of gestation. This level is maintained until term. Cardiac output returns to pre-pregnancy levels about 2 weeks after delivery. As the uterus enlarges and the diaphragm moves upward in pregnancy, the position of the heart is shifted toward a horizontal position, and there is slight axis rotation.

OLDER ADULTS

Heart size may decrease with age unless there is enlargement associated with hypertension or heart disease. The left ventricular wall thickens and the valves tend to fibrose and calcify. The heart rate slows (although resting heart rate may not be significantly influenced by age), stroke volume decreases, and cardiac output during exercise declines by 30% to 40%. The endocardium thickens. The myocardium becomes less elastic and more rigid so that recovery of myocardial contractility is delayed. Irritability may be enhanced. Thus the response to stress and increased oxygen demand is less efficient; tachycardia is poorly tolerated; and after any type of stress, the return to an expected heart rate takes longer. Despite these age-associated changes in heart architecture and contractile properties, the aged heart continues to function reasonably well at rest; however, long-standing hypertensive disease, infarcts, and/or other insults and physical deconditioning may lead to even more severe compromise of the heart and to increasingly significant decline in cardiac output.

Cardiac function is further compromised by fibrosis and sclerosis in the region of the SA node and in the heart valves (particularly the mitral valve and aortic cusps), by increased vagal tone, and by decreased baroreceptor sensitivity.

ECG changes occur secondary to cellular alteration, to fibrosis within the conduction system, and to neurogenic changes. Common ECG changes in older patients include first-degree atrioventricular block, bundle branch blocks, ST-T wave abnormalities, premature systole (atrial and ventricular), left anterior hemiblock, left ventricular hypertrophy, and atrial fibrillation.

REVIEW OF RELATED HISTORY

For each of the conditions discussed in this section, targeted topics to include in the history of the present illness are listed. Responses to questions about these topics help fully assess the patient's condition and provide clues for focusing the physical examination.

HISTORY OF PRESENT ILLNESS

- ◆ Chest pain (Boxes 14-1 and 14-2)
  - ◆ Onset and duration: sudden, gradual, or vague onset, length of episode; cyclic nature; related to physical exertion, rest, emotional experience, eating, coughing, cold temperatures, exposure to trauma, awakens from sleep
  - ◆ Character: aching, sharp, tingling, burning, pressure, stabbing, crushing, or clenched fist sign
  - ◆ Location: radiating down arms, to neck, jaws, teeth, scapula; relief with rest or position change
  - ◆ Severity: interference with activity, need to stop all activity until subsides, disrupts sleep, how severe on a scale of 0 to 10
  - ◆ Associated symptoms: anxiety; dyspnea; diaphoresis; dizziness; nausea or vomiting; faintness; cold, clammy skin; cyanosis; pallor; swelling or edema (noted anywhere, constant or at certain times during day)

BOX 14-1

CHEST PAIN

The presence of chest pain suggests heart disease in the minds of both the clinician and the layperson. The variety of causes of chest pain, however, is great. *Angina pectoris* is traditionally described as a pressure or choking sensation substernally or into the neck. The discomfort, which can be intense, may radiate to the jaw and down the left (and sometimes the right) arm. It often begins during strenuous physical activity, eating, exposure to intense cold, windy weather, or exposure to emotional stress. Relief may occur in minutes if the activity can be stopped. There are, however, myriad variations on this theme, sometimes varying in location, intensity, and radiation, and often arising from sources other than the heart. The "precordial catch," for example, is a sudden, sharp, relatively brief pain that does not radiate, occurs most often at rest, and is unrelated to exertion and may not have a discoverable cause. It may cause concern.

Some Possible Causes of Chest Pain

Cardiac
Typical angina pectoris
Atypical angina pectoris, angina equivalent
Prinzmetal variant angina
Unstable angina
Coronary insufficiency
Myocardial infarction
Nonobstructive, nonspastic angina
Mitral valve prolapse

Aortic
Dissection of the aorta

Pleuropericardial Pain
Pericarditis
Pleurisy
Pneumothorax
Mediastinal emphysema

Gastrointestinal Disease
Hiatus hernia
Reflux esophagitis
Esophageal spasm
Cholecystitis
Peptic ulcer disease
Pancreatitis

Pulmonary Disease
Pulmonary hypertension
Pneumonia
Pulmonary embolus
Bronchial hyperreactivity

Musculoskeletal
Cervical radiculopathy
Shoulder disorder or dysfunction (e.g., arthritis, bursitis, rotator cuff injury, biceps tendonitis)
Costochondral disorder
Xiphodynia

Psychoneurotic
Illicit drug use (e.g., cocaine)

Unlike in adults, chest pain in children and adolescents is seldom due to a cardiac problem. It is often difficult to find a cause, but trauma, exercise-induced asthma and, even in a somewhat younger child, the use of cocaine should be among the considerations.

Data from Samiy, Douglas, Barondess, 1987; Harvey et al, 1988.

♦ Treatment: rest, position change, exercise, nitroglycerin, digoxin, diuretics, beta blockers, angiotensin-converting enzyme inhibitors, calcium channel blockers, nonsteroidal anti-inflammatory drugs, antihypertensives
♦ Other medications: prescription, nonprescription, alternative or complementary therapies, prophylactic penicillin

---

BOX 14-2

CHARACTERISTICS OF CHEST PAIN

Type	Characteristics
Anginal	Substernal; provoked by effort, emotion, eating; relieved by rest and/or nitroglycerin; often accompanied by diaphoresis, occasionally by nausea
Pleural	Precipitated by breathing or coughing; usually described as sharp; present during respiration; absent when breath held
Esophageal	Burning, substernal, occasional radiation to the shoulder; nocturnal occurrence, usually when lying flat; relief with food, antacids, sometimes nitroglycerin
From a peptic ulcer	Almost always infradiaphragmatic and epigastric; nocturnal occurrence and daytime attacks relieved by food; unrelated to activity
Biliary	Usually under right scapula, prolonged in duration; often occurring after eating; will trigger angina more often than mimic it
Arthritis/bursitis	Usually lasts for hours; local tenderness and/or pain with movement
Cervical	Associated with injury; provoked by activity, persists after activity; painful on palpation and/or movement
Musculoskeletal (chest)	Intensified or provoked by movement, particularly twisting or costochondral bending; long lasting; often associated with focal tenderness
Psychoneurotic	Associated with/after anxiety; poorly described; located in intramammary region

Data from Samiy, Douglas, Barondess, 1987; Harvey et al, 1988.

DIFFERENTIAL DIAGNOSIS

COMPARISON OF SOME TYPES OF CHEST PAIN

Angina Pectoris	Musculoskeletal	Gastrointestinal
Presence of cardiac risk factors	History of trauma	History of indigestion
Specifically noted time of onset	Vague onset	Vague onset
Related to physical effort or emotional or psychosocial stress	Related to physical effort	Related to food consumption
Disappears if stimulating cause can be terminated	Continues after cessation of effort	May go on for several hours; unrelated to effort
Commonly forces patients to stop effort	Patients can very often continue activity	Patients often can continue activity
Patient may awaken from sleep	Delays falling asleep	Patient may awaken from sleep, particularly during early morning
Relief at times with nitroglycerin	Relief at times with heat, nonsteroidal antiinflammatories, or rest	Relief at times with antacids
Pain often in early morning or after washing and eating	Worse in evening after a day of physical effort	No particular relationship to time of day; related to food, tension
Greater likelihood in cold weather	Greater likelihood in cold, damp weather	Anytime

Data from Samiy, Douglas, Barondess, 1987; Harvey et al, 1988.

> ### BOX 14-3
> #### EXERCISE INTENSITY
>
> **Light:** Walking 10 to 15 steps, preparing a simple meal for one, retrieving a newspaper from just outside the door, pulling down a bedspread, brushing teeth
>
> **Moderate:** Making the bed, dusting and sweeping, walking a level short block, office filing
>
> **Moderately heavy:** Climbing one or two flights of stairs, lifting full cartons, long walks, sexual intercourse
>
> **Heavy:** Jogging, vigorous athletics of any kind, cleaning the entire house in less than a day, raking a large number of leaves, mowing a large lawn, shoveling deep snow

- Fatigue
  - Unusual or persistent, inability to keep up with contemporaries, inability to maintain usual activities, bedtime earlier
  - Associated symptoms: dyspnea on exertion, chest pain, palpitations, orthopnea, paroxysmal nocturnal dyspnea, anorexia, nausea, vomiting
  - Medications: prescription, nonprescription, alternative or complementary therapies
- Cough
  - Onset and duration
  - Character: dry, wet, nighttime, aggravated by lying down
- Difficult breathing (dyspnea, orthopnea)
  - Aggravated by exertion (how much?); on level ground, climbing stairs; worsening or remaining stable (Box 14-3); lying down or eased by resting on pillows (how many?); paroxysmal nocturnal dyspnea
- Loss of consciousness (transient syncope)
  - Associated with palpitation, dysrhythmia, unusual exertion, sudden turning of neck (carotid sinus effect), looking upward (vertebral artery occlusion), change in posture

PAST MEDICAL HISTORY

- Cardiac surgery or hospitalization for cardiac evaluation or disorder
- Rhythm disorder
- Acute rheumatic fever, unexplained fever, swollen joints, inflammatory rheumatism, St. Vitus dance (Sydenham chorea)
- Chronic illness: hypertension, bleeding disorder, hyperlipidemia, diabetes, thyroid dysfunction, coronary artery disease, obesity, congenital heart defect

FAMILY HISTORY

- Diabetes
- Heart disease
- Hyperlipidemia
- Hypertension
- Obesity
- Congenital heart defects, ventricular septal defects (About 1 in 100 persons has a congenital heart problem; once it occurs in a family, the likelihood of its recurring increases to three to five times the incidence in the general population, particularly with a left-sided lesion.)
- Sudden death, particularly in young and middle-aged relatives
- Family members with risk factors, morbidity, mortality related to cardiovascular system; ages at time of illness or death

PERSONAL AND SOCIAL HISTORY

- Employment: physical demands, environmental hazards such as heat, chemicals, dust, sources of emotional stress
- Tobacco use: type (cigarettes, cigars, pipe, chewing tobacco, snuff), duration of use, amount, age started and (hopefully) stopped; pack-years (number of years smoking times number of packs per day)
- Nutritional status
  - Usual diet: proportion of fat, food preferences, history of dieting
  - Weight: loss or gain, amount and rate
  - Alcohol consumption: amount, frequency, duration of current intake
  - Known hypercholesterolemia and/or elevated triglycerides
- Personality assessment: intensity (Does the patient consider self to have a type A personality [characterized by hostile attitudes, inability to relax, and compulsive behavior] or a type D personality [characterized by negative emotions, pessimistic attitude, and failure to share emotions]?)
- Relaxation
  - Hobbies
  - Exercise: type, amount, frequency, intensity
  - Sexual activity: frequency of intercourse, sexual practices, number of partners
- Use of alcohol
- Use of illegal drugs: amyl nitrate ("poppers"), cocaine

INFANTS

- Tiring easily during feeding
- Breathing changes: more heavily or more rapidly than expected during feeding or defecation
- Cyanosis: perioral during eating, more widespread and more persistent, related to crying
- Weight gain as expected
- Knee-chest position or other position favored for rest
- Mother's health during pregnancy: rubella in first trimester, unexplained fever, drug use (prescription, nonprescription, alternative or complementary therapies, and illicit drugs)

CHILDREN

- Tiring during play: amount of time before tiring, activities that are tiring, inability to keep up with other children, reluctance to go out to play
- Naps: longer than expected, usual length
- Positions: squatting instead of sitting when at play or watching television
- Headaches
- Nosebleeds
- Unexplained joint pain
- Unexplained fever
- Expected height and weight gain (and any substantiating records)
- Expected physical and cognitive development (and any substantiating records)

PREGNANT WOMEN

- History of cardiac disease or surgery
- Dizziness or faintness on standing
- Indications of heart disease during pregnancy, including progressive or severe dyspnea, progressive orthopnea, paroxysmal nocturnal dyspnea, hemoptysis, syncope with exertion, and chest pain related to effort or emotion

RISK FACTORS
CARDIAC DISABILITY

- Gender (men more at risk than women; women's risk is increased in the postmenopausal years and with oral contraceptive use)
- Hyperlipidemia*
- Elevated homocysteine level
- Smoking*
- Family history of cardiovascular disease, diabetes, hyperlipidemia, hypertension, or sudden death in young adults
- Diabetes mellitus*
- Obesity: dietary habits including an excessively fatty diet
- Sedentary lifestyle without exercise
- Personality type: intense, compulsive behavior with feelings of hostility; negative emotions, pessimistic attitude, failure to share emotions

*If all factors marked with an asterisk are present, the risk is approximately eight times greater than if none is present.

OLDER ADULTS

- Common symptoms of cardiovascular disorders
  - Confusion, dizziness, blackouts, syncope
  - Palpitations
  - Coughs and wheezes
  - Hemoptysis
  - Shortness of breath
  - Chest pains or chest tightness
  - Impotence
  - Fatigue
  - Leg edema: pattern, frequency, time of day most pronounced
- If heart disease has been diagnosed
  - Drug reactions: potassium excess (weakness, bradycardia, hypotension, confusion); potassium depletion (weakness, fatigue, muscle cramps, dysrhythmias); digitalis toxicity (anorexia, nausea, vomiting, diarrhea, headache, confusion, dysrhythmias, halo, yellow vision)
  - Interference with activities of daily living
  - Ability of the patient and family to cope with the condition, perceived and actual
  - Orthostatic hypotension

EXAMINATION AND FINDINGS

EQUIPMENT

- Marking pencil
- Centimeter rule
- Stethoscope

The examination of the heart includes the following: inspecting, palpating, percussing the chest, and auscultating the heart.

The parts of the physical examination should be performed in a sequence that is comfortable for you. Findings from examinations of other systems besides the cardiovascular, such as signs of heart failure (crackles in the lungs, engorgement of the liver, and peripheral edema),

STAYING WELL

IMPORTANCE OF A HEALTHY LIFESTYLE

Use some of the time during your cardiac examination to remind the patient of the importance of healthy lifestyle in maintaining good cardiac health:

- Enjoy a prudent diet that is low in cholesterol. If acceptable to your patient, consider referral to a dietitian. Consider oral agents if diet alone is not sufficient to reduce cholesterol to goal.
- Exercise regularly. Even brisk walking increases and maintains cardiac health.
- Cease smoking. Various behavioral programs and newly approved medications may assist.
- Monitor blood pressure, blood glucose, inflammatory markers, and lipids annually.

have a significant impact on judgments that will be made about the cardiovascular system. Other influencing factors may include the following:

- Effect of a barrel chest or pectus deformity
- Erythema marginatum of rheumatic fever
- Osler nodes or Janeway lesions of bacterial endocarditis
- Xanthelasma
- Funduscopic changes of hypertension
- Crackles, wheezes, and rubs in and over the lungs
- Ascites
- Bruit of an aortic aneurysm

No system can be appropriately evaluated outside the context of the entire examination. Performing a successful examination requires both a mastery of the mechanics of each procedure and an ability to integrate and interpret the findings in relation to the cardiac events they reflect.

In assessing cardiac function, it is a common error to listen to the heart first. Rather, it is important to follow the proper sequence, beginning with inspection and proceeding to palpation, percussion, and then auscultation. Use a tangential light source to allow shadows to accent the surface flicker of underlying cardiac movement. The room should be quiet because subtle, low-pitched sounds are hard to hear. Stand to the patient's right, at least at the start. A thorough examination of the heart requires the patient to assume a variety of positions: sitting erect and leaning forward, lying supine, and being in the left lateral recumbent position. These necessary changes in position mandate a comfortable examining table on which movement is easy. Large breasts can make examination difficult. Either you or the patient can move the left breast up and to the left. You must also learn to appreciate the differences in findings when the chest is thin and nonmuscular (i.e., sounds are louder, closer), or muscular or obese (i.e., sounds are dimmer, more distant).

INSPECTION

In most adults, the apical impulse should be visible at about the midclavicular line in the fifth left intercostal space, but it is easily obscured by obesity, large breasts, or muscularity. In some patients it may be visible in the fourth left intercostal space. It should not be seen in more than one space if the heart is healthy. The apical impulse may become visible only when the patient sits up and the heart is brought closer to the anterior wall. This is an expected finding.

A readily visible and palpable impulse when the patient is supine suggests an intensity that may be the result of a problem. The absence of an apical impulse in addition to faint heart sounds, particularly when the patient is in the left lateral recumbent position, suggests some intervening extracardiac problem, such as pleural or pericardial fluid. In any event, findings are affected by the shape and thickness of the chest wall and the amount of tissue, air, and fluid through which the impulses are transmitted.

Inspection of other organs may reflect important information about the cardiac status. For example, inspecting the skin for cyanosis or venous distention and inspecting the nail bed for cyanosis and capillary refill time provide valuable clues to the cardiac evaluation.

PALPATION

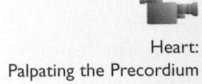

Heart:
Palpating the Precordium

Make sure that your hands are warm, and with the patient supine, feel the precordium. Use the proximal halves of the four fingers held gently together or use the whole hand. Touch gently and let the cardiac movements rise to your hand, because sensation decreases as you increase pressure.

As always, be methodical. One suggested sequence is to begin at the apex, move to the left sternal border, then move to the base, going down to the right sternal border and into the epigastrium or axillae if the circumstance dictates (Fig. 14-12).

Feel for the apical impulse and identify its location by the intercostal space and the distance from the midsternal line. Determine the width of the area in which it is felt. Usually it is palpable within a small radius—no more than 1 cm. The impulse is usually gentle and brief, not lasting as long as systole. If it is more vigorous than expected, characterize it as a *heave* or *lift*. In many adults, you may not be able to feel the apical impulse because of the thickness of the chest wall (Fig. 14-13).

An apical impulse that is more forceful and widely distributed, fills systole, or is displaced laterally and downward may indicate increased cardiac output or left ventricular hypertrophy. A lift along the left sternal border may be caused by right ventricular hypertrophy. A loss of thrust may be related to overlying fluid or air or to displacement beneath the sternum. Displacement to the right without a loss or gain in thrust suggests dextrocardia, diaphragmatic

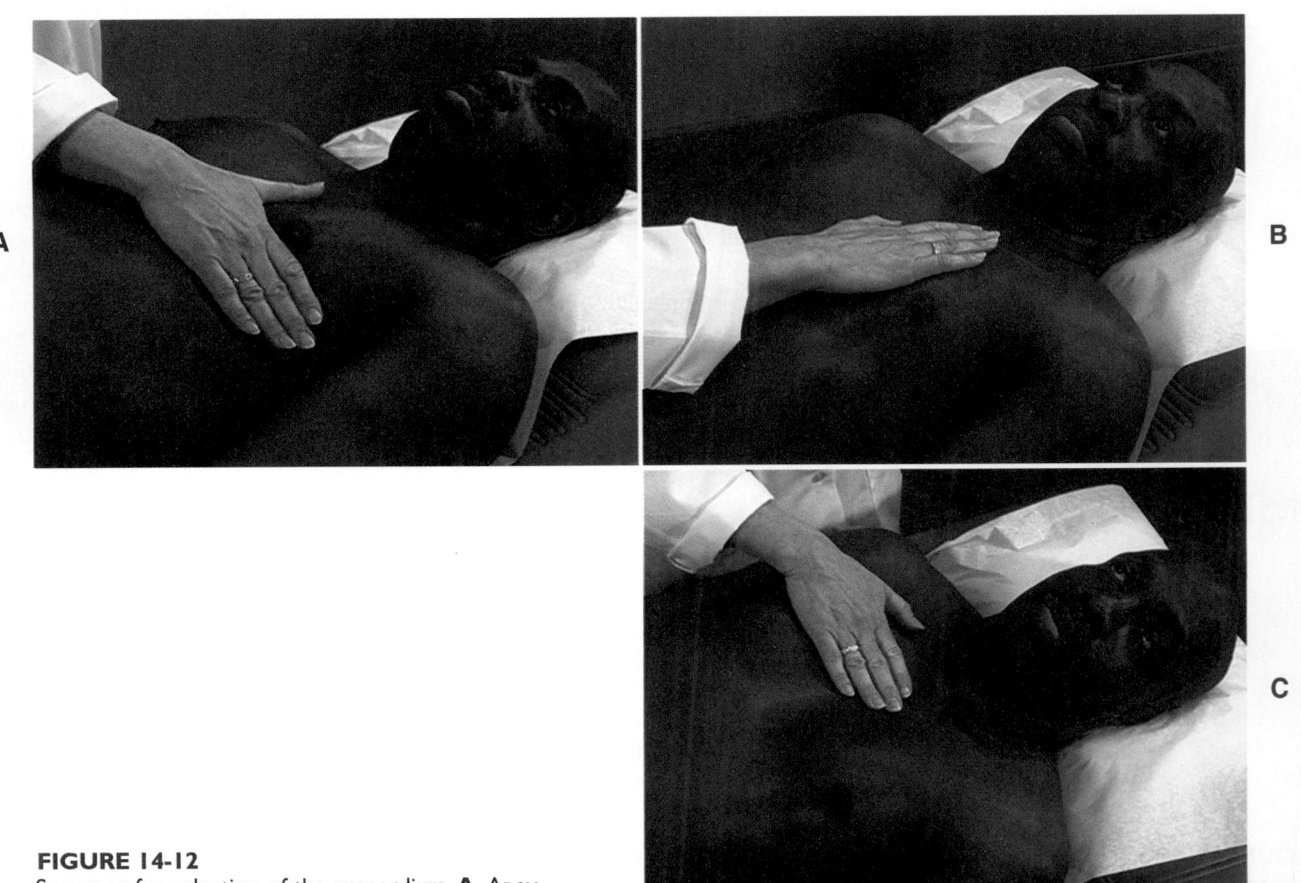

FIGURE 14-12
Sequence for palpation of the precordium. **A,** Apex.
B, Left sternal border. **C,** Base.

hernia, distended stomach, or a pulmonary abnormality. The point at which the apical impulse is most readily seen or felt should be described as the *point of maximal impulse* (PMI).

Feel for a *thrill*—a fine, palpable, rushing vibration, a palpable murmur, often, but not always, over the base of the heart in the area of the right or left second intercostal space. It generally indicates a disruption of the expected blood flow related to some defect in the closure of one of the semilunar valves (generally aortic or pulmonic stenosis), pulmonary hypertension, or atrial septal defect (Box 14-4). Locate each sensation in terms of its intercostal space and relationship to the midsternal, midclavicular, or axillary lines. Chapter 13 describes the method for counting ribs and intercostal spaces.

While palpating the precordium, use your other hand to palpate the carotid artery so that you can describe the carotid pulse in relation to the cardiac cycle. The carotid pulse and S_1 are practically synchronous. The carotid pulse is located just medial to and below the angle of the jaw (Fig. 14-14).

BOX 14-4

THE THRILL OF HEART EXAMINATION

A murmur at the grade IV level or more can be felt (see Tables 14-4 and 14-5). The sensation delivered to your probing fingers is called a *thrill*. It may be appreciated in systole or diastole. The following are among the more common:

Timing	Location	Probable Cause
Systole	Suprasternal notch and/or second and third right intercostal spaces	Aortic stenosis
	Suprasternal notch and/or second and third left intercostal spaces	Pulmonic stenosis
	Fourth left intercostal space	Ventricular septal defect
	Apex	Mitral regurgitation
	Left lower sternal border	Tetralogy of Fallot
	Left upper sternal border, often with extensive radiation	Patent ductus arteriosus
Diastole	Right sternal border	Aortic regurgitation Aneurysm of ascending aorta
	Apex	Mitral stenosis

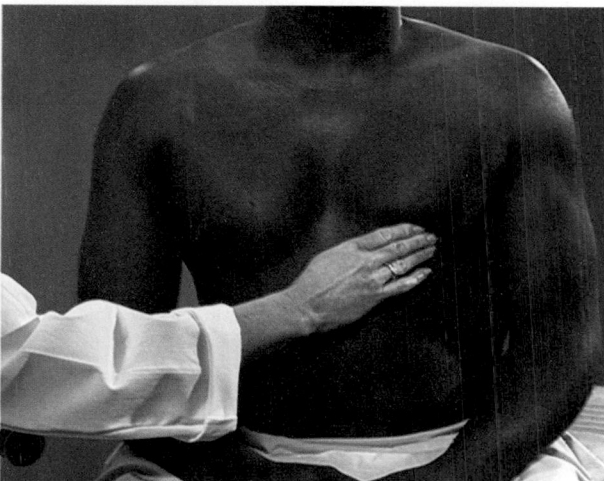

FIGURE 14-13
Palpation of the apical pulse.

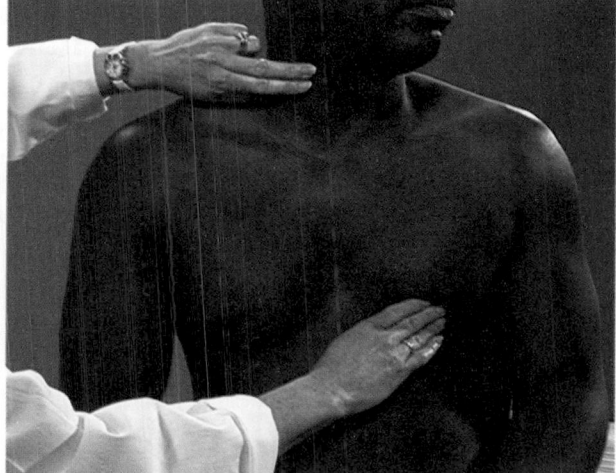

FIGURE 14-14
Palpation of the carotid artery to time events felt over the precordium.

PERCUSSION

Percussion is of limited value in defining the borders of the heart or determining its size, because the shape of the chest is relatively rigid and can make the more malleable heart conform. Left ventricular size is better judged by the location of the apical impulse. The right ventricle tends to enlarge in the anteroposterior diameter rather than laterally, thus diminishing the value of percussion of the right heart border. A chest x-ray is far more useful in defining the heart borders.

If other facilities are unavailable, you can estimate the size of the heart by percussion. Begin tapping at the anterior axillary line, moving medially along the intercostal spaces toward the sternal border. The change from a resonant to a dull note marks the cardiac border. Note these points with a marking pencil and the outline of the heart is visually defined. On the left, the loss of resonance will generally be close to the point of maximal impulse at the apex of the heart. Measure this point from the midsternal line at each intercostal space and record that distance. When percussing the right cardiac border, one does not note a change in resonance until the right sternal border is encountered. Obesity, unusual muscular development, and some pathologic conditions (such as presence of air or fluids) can easily distort the findings.

AUSCULTATION

CLINICAL PEARL

Heart Sounds
It is a common error to try to hear all of the sounds in the cardiac cycle at one time. Take the time to isolate each sound and each pause in the cardiac cycle, listening separately and selectively for as many beats as necessary to evaluate the sounds. It takes time to tune in, so you must not rush. Avoid jumping the stethoscope from one site to another; instead, inch the endpiece along the route. This maneuver helps prevent missing important sounds, particularly more widely transmitted abnormal sounds, and it allows tracking of a sound from its loudest point to its farthest reach (e.g., into the axilla or the back).

Because all heart sounds are of relatively low frequency, in a range somewhat difficult for the human ear to detect, you must be compulsive about ensuring ambient quiet. Because shivering and movement increase adventitious sound, and because comfort is important, make certain the patient is warm and relaxed before beginning. Always place a comfortably warm stethoscope on the naked chest.

Because sound is transmitted in the direction of blood flow, specific heart sounds are best heard in areas where the blood flows after it passes through a valve. Approach each of the precordial areas systematically in a sequence that is comfortable for you, working your way from base to apex or apex to base (Box 14-5). Because the site of the apex of the heart may be changed by elevation of the diaphragms because of pregnancy, ascites, or other intraabdominal conditions, many clinicians prefer to begin their examination at the base of the heart.

Auscultation should be performed in, but not be limited to, each of the five cardiac areas, using first the diaphragm and then the bell of the stethoscope. Use firm pressure with the diaphragm and light pressure with the bell.

BOX 14-5

PROCEDURE FOR AUSCULTATING THE HEART

Adopt a routine for the various positions the patient is asked to assume, although you should be prepared to alter the sequence if the patient's condition requires it. Instruct the patient when to breathe comfortably and when to hold the breath in expiration and inspiration. Listen carefully for each heart sound, isolating each component of the cardiac cycle, especially while the respirations are momentarily suspended. The following sequence is suggested:

- Patient sitting up and leaning slightly forward and, preferably, in expiration: listen in all five areas (Fig. 14-16, *A*). This is the best position to hear relatively high-pitched murmurs with the stethoscope diaphragm.
- Patient supine: listen in all five areas (Fig. 14-16, *B*).
- Patient left lateral recumbent: listen in all five areas. This is the best position to hear the low-pitched filling sounds in diastole with the stethoscope bell (Fig. 14-16, *C*).
- Other positions depend on your findings. Patient right lateral recumbent: this is best position for evaluating right rotated heart of dextrocardia. Listen in all five areas.
- Inch, don't jump, your way from area to area.

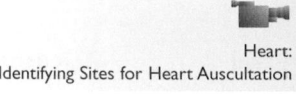

There are five traditionally designated auscultatory areas, located as follows (Fig. 14-15):
- ◆ Aortic valve area: second right intercostal space at the right sternal border
- ◆ Pulmonic valve area: second left intercostal space at the left sternal border
- ◆ Second pulmonic area: third left intercostal space at the left sternal border
- ◆ Tricuspid area: fourth left intercostal space along the lower left sternal border
- ◆ Mitral (or apical) area: at the apex of the heart in the fifth left intercostal space at the midclavicular line

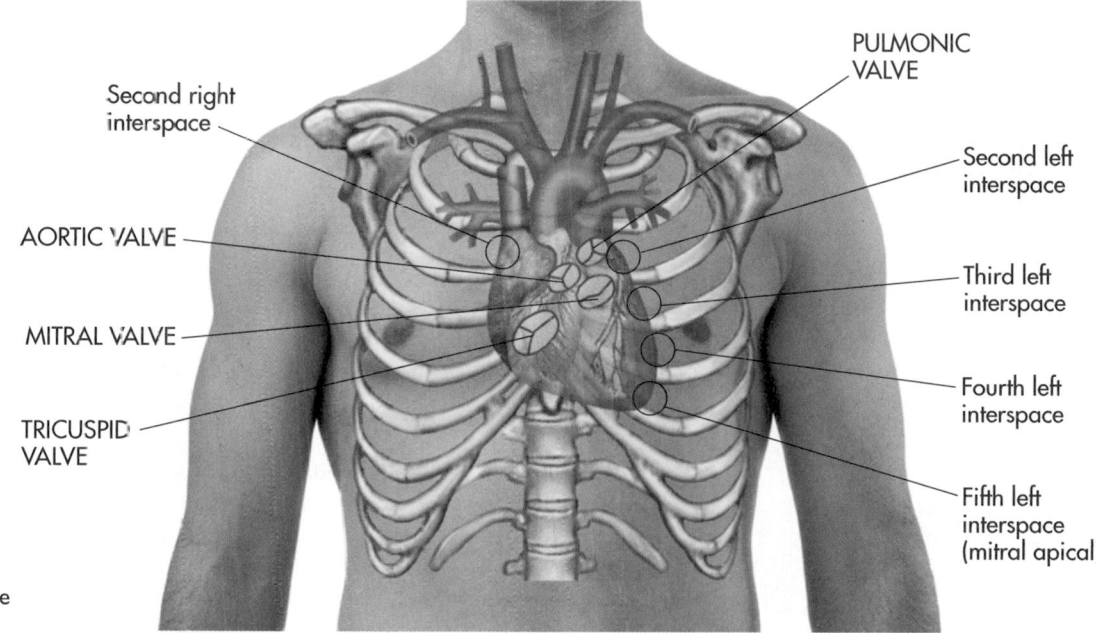

FIGURE 14-15
Areas for auscultation of the heart.

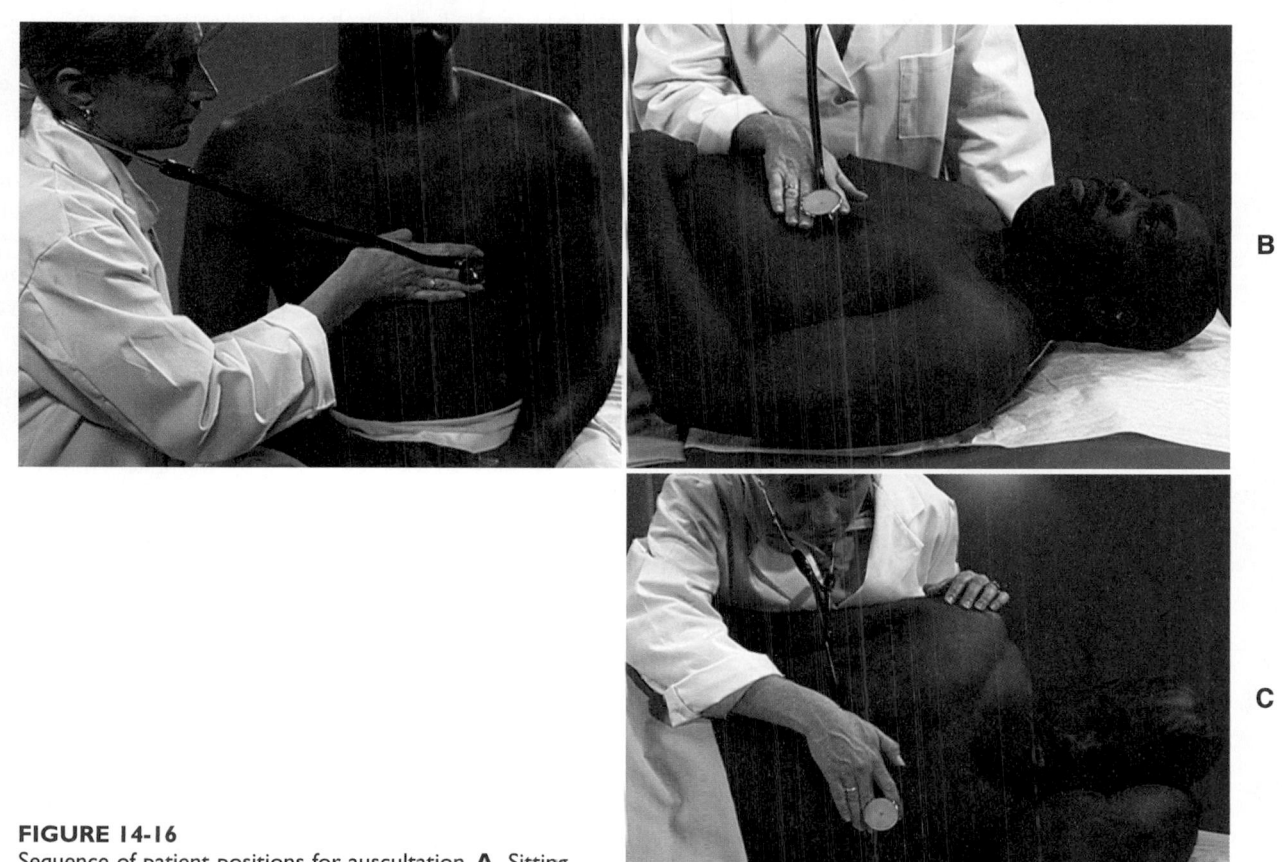

FIGURE 14-16
Sequence of patient positions for auscultation. **A,** Sitting up, leaning slightly forward. **B,** Supine. **C,** Left lateral recumbent.

TABLE 14-2	Heart Sounds According to Auscultatory Area				
	Aortic	**Pulmonic**	**Second Pulmonic**	**Mitral**	**Tricuspid**
Pitch	$S_1 < S_2$	$S_1 < S_2$	$S_1 < S_2$	$S_1 > S_2$	$S_1 = S_2$
Loudness	$S_1 < S_2$	$S_1 < S_2$	$S_1 < S_2$*	$S_1 > S_2$†	$S_1 > S_2$
Duration	$S_1 > S_2$	$S_1 > S_2$	$S_1 > S_2$	$S_1 > S_2$	$S_1 > S_2$
S_2 split	> inhale < exhale	> inhale < exhale	> inhale < exhale	> inhale‡ < exhale	> inhale < exhale
A_2	Loudest	Loud	Decreased		
P_2	Decreased	Louder	Loudest		

*S_1 is relatively louder in second pulmonic area than in aortic area.
†S_1 may be louder in mitral area than in tricuspid area.
‡S_2 split may not be audible in mitral area if P_2 is inaudible.

As you examine each of the five auscultatory areas, remember to inch along. At each site, pause and listen selectively for each component of the cardiac cycle. Let your stethoscope follow the sounds wherever they lead.

- Assess the rate and rhythm of the heart at one auscultatory site where the tones are easily heard. Note that site. If the cardiac rhythm is irregular, compare the beats per minute over the heart with the number of beats per minute at the radial pulse. Note any deficit.
- Instruct the patient to breathe normally and then hold the breath in expiration. Listen for S_1 while you palpate the carotid pulse. S_1 marks the beginning of systole. S_1 coincides with the rise (upswing) of the carotid pulse. Note the intensity, any variations, the effect of respirations, and any splitting of S_1.
- Concentrate on systole, listening for any extra sounds or murmurs.
- S_2 marks the initiation of diastole. Concentrate on diastole, which is a longer interval than systole, listening for any extra sounds or murmurs. (However, systole and diastole are equal in duration when the heart rate is rapid.)
- Instruct the patient to inhale deeply, listening closely for S_2 to become two components (split S_2) during inspiration. Split S_2 is best heard in the pulmonic auscultatory area.

Areas for inspection, palpation, and auscultation change if the heart is not located in its expected place in the left mediastinum. In situs inversus and in dextrocardia the heart is rotated to the right. In such a circumstance, adjust to the anatomic alteration by thinking of the examination sites as they would be in a mirror image of the expected.

BASIC HEART SOUNDS

Heart sounds are characterized in much the same way as respiratory and other body sounds: by pitch, intensity, duration, and timing in the cardiac cycle. Heart sounds are relatively low in pitch, except in the presence of significant pathologic events. Table 14-2 summarizes their relative differences according to auscultatory area (also see Fig. 14-19).

There are four basic heart sounds: S_1, S_2, S_3, and S_4. Of these, S_1 and S_2 are the most distinct heart sounds and should be characterized separately, because variations can offer important clues to cardiac function. S_3 and S_4 may or may not be present; their absence is not an unusual finding, but their presence does not necessarily indicate a pathologic condition. Thus S_3 and S_4 must be evaluated in relation to other sounds and events in the cardiac cycle.

S_1 and S_2. S_1, which results from closure of the AV valves, indicates the beginning of systole and is best heard toward the apex where it is usually louder than S_2 (Box 14-6). At the base, S_1 is louder on the left than on the right but softer than S_2 in both areas. It is lower in pitch and a bit longer than S_2, and it occurs immediately after diastole (Fig. 14-17).

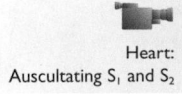

Heart:
Auscultating S_1 and S_2

BOX 14-6

S_1 INTENSITY: DIAGNOSTIC CLUES

When systole begins with the mitral valve open, the valve snaps shut more vigorously, producing a louder S_1. This occurs in the following situations:

- Blood velocity is increased, such as occurs in anemia, fever, hyperthyroidism, anxiety, and during exercise.
- The mitral valve is stenotic.

If the mitral valve is not completely open, ventricular contraction forces it shut. The loudness produced by valve closure depends on the degree of opening, so the intensity of S_1 varies in the following situations:

- Complete heart block is present.
- Gross disruption of rhythm occurs, such as during fibrillation.

The intensity of S_1 is decreased in the following situations:

- Increased overlying tissue, fat, or fluid (such as occurs in emphysema, obesity, or pericardial fluid) obscures sounds.
- Systemic or pulmonary hypertension is present, which contributes to more forceful atrial contraction. If the ventricle is noncompliant, the contraction may be delayed or diminished, especially if the valve is partially closed when contraction begins.
- Fibrosis and calcification of a diseased mitral valve can result from rheumatic heart disease. Calcification diminishes valve flexibility so that it closes with less force.

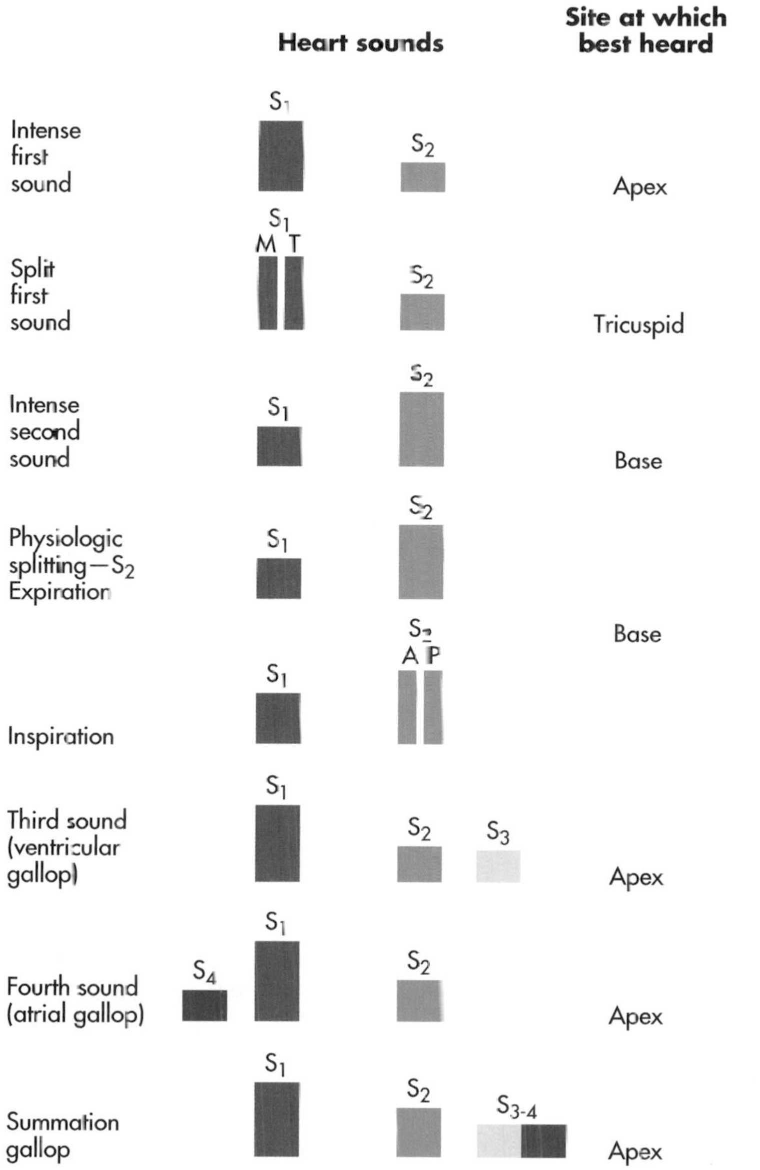

FIGURE 14-17
Heart sounds.

BOX 14-7

S₂ INTENSITY: DIAGNOSTIC CLUES

The intensity of S_2 increases in the following conditions:
- Systemic hypertension (S_2 may ring or boom), syphilis of the aortic valve, exercise, or excitement accentuates S_2.
- Pulmonary hypertension, mitral stenosis, and congestive heart failure accentuate P_2.
- The valves are diseased but still fully mobile; the component of S_2 affected depends on which valve is compromised.

The intensity of S_2 decreases in the following conditions:
- A shocklike state with arterial hypotension causes loss of valvular vigor.
- The valves are immobile, thickened, or calcified; the component of S_2 affected depends on which valve is compromised.
- Aortic stenosis affects A_2.
- Pulmonic stenosis affects P_2.
- Overlying tissue, fat, or fluid mutes S_2.

Although there is some asynchrony between closure of the mitral and tricuspid valves, S_1 is usually heard as one sound. If the asynchrony is more marked than usual, the sound may be split and is then best heard in the tricuspid area. Other variations in S_1 depend on the competency of the pulmonary and systemic circulations, the structure of the heart valves, their position when ventricular contraction begins, and the force of the contraction.

S_2, the result of closure of the semilunar valves, indicates the end of systole and is best heard in the aortic and pulmonic areas. It is of higher pitch and shorter duration than S_1. S_2 is louder than S_1 at the base of the heart; still it is usually softer than S_1 at the apex (Box 14-7).

Splitting. *Splitting* is a term used to define the failure of the mitral and tricuspid valves or the pulmonic and aortic vales to close simultaneously. Splitting of S_1 is not usually heard because the sound of the tricuspid valve closing is too faint to hear. Rarely, however, it may be audible in the tricuspid area, particularly on deep inspiration.

S_2 is actually two sounds that merge during expiration. The closure of the aortic valve (A_2) contributes most of the sound of S_2 when it is heard in the aortic or pulmonic areas. A_2 tends to mask the sound of pulmonic valve closure (P_2). During inspiration, P_2 occurs slightly later, giving S_2 two distinct components; this is a split S_2. Splitting is more often heard and easier to detect in the young; it is not well heard in older adults. This may be because of the tendency of the anteroposterior diameter of the chest to increase with age.

Splitting of S_2 is an expected event, because pressures are higher and depolarization occurs earlier on the left side of the heart. Ejection times on the right are longer, and the pulmonic valve closes a bit later than the aortic valve. If P_2 is heard outside the pulmonary area, it is most often unusually loud or delayed.

Splitting of S_2 is greatest at the peak of inspiration (see Fig. 14-17). During expiration, the disparity in ejection times tends to diminish, and the split may disappear. Ejection times tend to equalize when the breath is held in expiration, so this maneuver also tends to eliminate the split. Thus the degree of S_2 splitting is most evident during inspiration. It may vary from easily heard to nondetectable. The respiratory cycle is not always the dominant factor; the interval between the components may remain easily discernible throughout the respiratory cycle (Box 14-8).

S₃ and S₄. During diastole, the ventricles fill in two steps: an early, passive flow of blood from the atria is followed by a more vigorous atrial ejection. The passive phase occurs relatively early in diastole, distending the ventricular walls and causing vibration. The resultant sound, S_3, is quiet, low pitched, and often difficult to hear (see Fig. 14-17).

In the second phase of ventricular filling, vibration in the valves, papillae, and ventricular walls produces S_4 (see Fig. 14-17). Because it occurs so late in diastole (presystole), S_4 may be confused with a split S_1.

> **BOX 14-8**
> ### UNEXPECTED SPLITTING OF HEART SOUNDS
>
> **Wide Splitting**
> The split becomes wider when there is delayed activation of contraction or emptying of the right ventricle resulting in delay in pulmonic closure. This occurs, for example, in right bundle branch block, which splits both S_1 and S_2. Wide splitting of S_2 also occurs when stenosis delays closure of the pulmonic valve, when pulmonary hypertension delays ventricular emptying, or when mitral regurgitation induces early closure of the aortic valve. The split becomes narrower and is even eliminated or paradoxic when closure of the aortic valve is delayed, such as in left bundle branch block.
>
> **Fixed Splitting**
> Splitting is said to be fixed when it is unaffected by respiration. This occurs with delayed closure of the pulmonic valve when output of the right ventricle is greater than that of the left (such as occurs in large atrial septal defects, a ventricular septal defect with left to right shunting, or right ventricular failure).
>
> **Paradoxic (Reversed) Splitting**
> Paradoxic splitting occurs when closure of the aortic valve is delayed (such as in left bundle branch block) so that P_2 occurs first, followed by A_2. In this case, the interval between P_2 and A_1 is heard during expiration and disappears during inspiration.
>
> See Fig. 14-18 for visual depiction of variations in splitting of S_2 heart sounds.

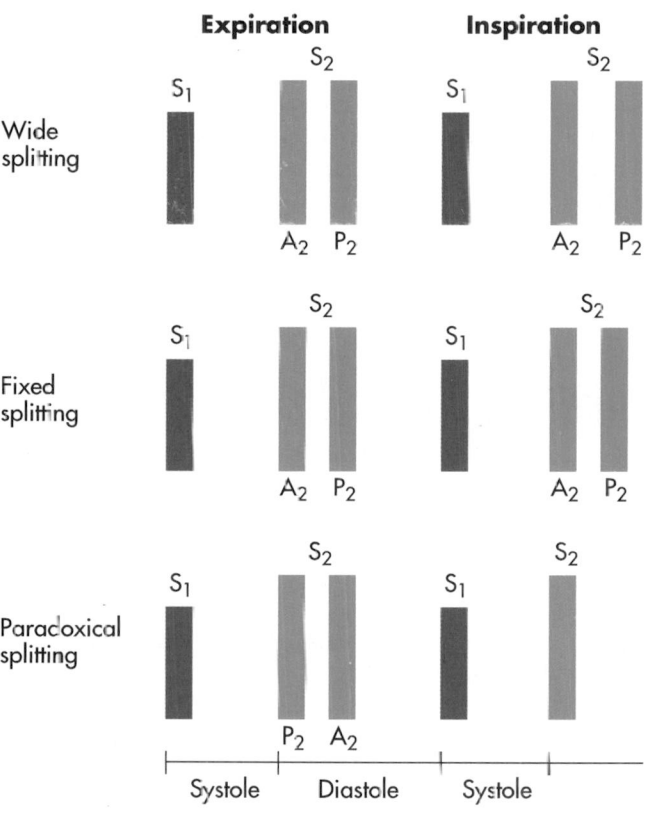

FIGURE 14-18
Variations in splitting of S_2.

S_3 and S_4 should be quiet and therefore somewhat difficult to hear. Increasing venous return (by asking the patient to raise a leg) or arterial pressure (by asking the patient to grip your hand vigorously and repeatedly) may make these sounds easier to hear. When S_3 becomes intense and easy to hear, the resultant sequence of sounds simulates a gallop; this is the proto-diastolic gallop rhythm. S_3 may be louder if filling pressure is increased or if ventricular compliance is reduced. It may be best heard when the patient is in the left lateral decubitus (recumbent) position. S_4 may also become more intense, producing a readily discernible presystolic gallop rhythm. S_4 is most commonly heard in older patients, but it may be heard at any age when there is increased resistance to filling because of loss of compliance of the ventricular walls (e.g., in hypertensive disease and coronary artery disease) or the increased stroke volume of high-output states (e.g., in profound anemia, pregnancy, and thyrotoxicosis). The rhythm of the heart sound when an S_3 is heard resembles the rhythm of pronouncing the word *Ken-TUCK-y*. When an S_4 is heard, it resembles the rhythm of pronouncing the word *TEN-nes-see*. A loud S_4 always suggests pathology and deserves additional evaluation. The cardiac valves generally open noiselessly unless thickened, roughened, or otherwise altered as a result of disease. Valvular stenosis may produce an opening snap (mitral valve), ejection clicks (semilunar valves), or mid-to-late nonejection systolic clicks (mitral prolapse). The pulmonary ejection click is best heard on expiration and is seldom heard on inspiration; aortic ejection clicks are less sharp, are less involved with S_1, and may be heard as distant as the anterior axillary line. Extra heart sounds often accompany murmurs and should always be considered indicative of a pathologic process.

EXTRA HEART SOUNDS

A pericardial friction rub can be easily mistaken for cardiac-generated sounds. Inflammation of the pericardial sac causes a roughening of the parietal and visceral surfaces, which produces a rubbing sound audible through the stethoscope. It occupies both systole and diastole and overlies the intracardiac sounds. Pericardial friction rub may have three components that are associated in sequence with the atrial component of systole, ventricular systole, and ventricular diastole. It is usually heard widely but is more distinct toward the apex. A three-component friction rub is a grating sound that may be intense enough to obscure the heart sounds. If there are only one or two components, the sound may not be intense or machine-like and may then be more difficult to distinguish from an intracardiac murmur. The detection of extra heart sounds is detailed in Table 14-3, along with associated causes (see Fig. 14-19 on pp. 440 and 441).

You should always be aware, based on the history and inspection of the chest, of a patient's having had a cardiac surgical procedure. If this involves the placement of a prosthetic mitral valve, listen for a distinct click early in diastole, loudest at the apex and transmitted precordially. A prosthetic aortic valve causes a sound in early systole. The intensity of these sounds depends on the type of material used for the prosthesis. Animal tissue is the quietest and may even be silent. Pacemakers no longer cause a sound.

TABLE 14-3	Extra Heart Sounds	
Sounds	**Detection**	**Description**
Increased S_3	Bell at apex; patient left lateral recumbent	Early diastole, low pitch
Increased S_4	Bell at apex, patient supine or in the left lateral recumbent position	Late diastole or early systole, low pitch
Gallops	Bell at apex; patient supine or left lateral recumbent position	Presystole, intense, easily heard
Mitral valve opening snap	Diaphragm medial to apex, may radiate to base; any position, second left intercostal space	Early diastole briefly, before S_3; high pitch, sharp snap or click; not affected by respiration; easily confused with S_2
Ejection clicks	Diaphragm; patient sitting or supine	
Aortic valve	Apex, base in second right intercostal space	Early systole, intense, high pitch; radiates; not affected by respirations
Pulmonary valve	Second left intercostal space at sternal border	Early systole, less intense than aortic click; intensifies on expiration, decreased on inspiration
Pericardial friction rub	Widely heard, sound clearest toward apex	May occupy all of systole and diastole; intense, grating, machine-like; may have three components and obliterate heart sounds; if only one or two components, may sound like murmur

HEART MURMURS

Heart murmurs are relatively prolonged extra sounds heard during systole or diastole; they often indicate a problem. Murmurs are caused by some disruption in the flow of blood into, through, or out of the heart. The characteristics of a murmur depend on the adequacy of valve function, the size of the opening, the rate of blood flow, the vigor of the myocardium, and the thickness and consistency of the overlying tissues through which the murmur must be heard.

Diseased valves, a common cause of murmurs, either do not open or do not close well. When the leaflets are thickened and the passage narrowed, forward blood flow is restricted (stenosis). When valve leaflets, which are intended to fit together snugly, lose competency, the slack openings allow backward flow of blood (regurgitation). Table 14-4 summarizes the characteristics of the heart murmurs. Murmurs are described in many ways (e.g., harsh, blowing, seagull). Such descriptions may or may not be consistent with the way you hear the sounds. Do not hesitate to use words that best suit your interpretation.

The discovery of a heart murmur requires careful assessment and diagnosis. Although some murmurs are benign (Box 14-9), others represent a pathologic process. Therefore solid evidence from additional testing is often mandatory before a murmur is dismissed as functional.

TABLE 14-4	Characterization of Heart Murmurs	
	Classification	**Description**
Timing and duration*	Early systolic	Begins with S_1, decrescendos, ends well before S_2
	Midsystolic (ejection)	Begins after S_1, ends before S_2; crescendo-decrescendo quality sometimes difficult to discern
	Late systolic	Begins mid to late systole, crescendos, ends at S_2; often introduced by mid to late systolic clicks
	Early diastolic	Begins with S_2
	Mid diastolic	Begins at clear interval after S_2
	Late diastolic (presystolic)	Begins immediately before S_1
	Holosystolic (pansystolic)	Begins with S_1, occupies all of systole, ends at S_2
	Holodiastolic (pandiastolic)	Begins with S_2, occupies all of diastole, ends at S_1
	Continuous	Starts in systole, continues without interruption through S_2, into all or part of diastole; does not necessarily persist throughout entire cardiac cycle
Pitch	High, medium, low	Depends on pressure and rate of blood flow; low pitch is heard best with the bell
Intensity†	Grade I	Barely audible in quiet room
	Grade II	Quiet but clearly audible
	Grade III	Moderately loud
	Grade IV	Loud, associated with thrill
	Grade V	Very loud, thrill easily palpable
	Grade VI	Very loud, audible with stethoscope not in contact with chest, thrill palpable and visible
Pattern	Crescendo	Increasing intensity caused by increased blood velocity
	Decrescendo	Decreasing intensity caused by decreased blood velocity
	Square or plateau	Constant intensity
Quality	Harsh, raspy, machine-like, vibratory, musical, blowing	Quality depends on several factors, including degree of valve compromise, force of contractions, blood volume
Location	Anatomic landmarks (e.g., second left intercostal space on sternal border)	Area of greatest intensity, usually area to which valve sounds are normally transmitted
Radiation	Anatomic landmarks (e.g., to axilla or carotid arteries)	Site farthest from location of greatest intensity at which sound is still heard; sound usually transmitted in direction of blood flow
Respiratory phase variations	Intensity, quality, and timing may vary	Venous return increases on inspiration and decreases on expiration

*Systolic murmurs are best described according to time of onset and termination; diastolic murmurs are best classified according to time of onset only.
†Discrimination among the six grades is more difficult for the diastolic murmur than for the systolic.

	First heart sound $[S_1(M_1T_1)]$	Second heart sound $[S_2(A_2P_2)]$	Third heart sound (S_3, ventricular gallop)	Fourth heart sound (S_4, atrial gallop)
Heart sounds	Systole / Diastole; S_1 S_2 S_1 S_2	S_1 S_2 S_1 S_2	S_1 S_2 S_3 S_1 S_2 S_3	$S_4$$S_1$ S_2 $S_4$$S_1$ S_2
Anatomic reference	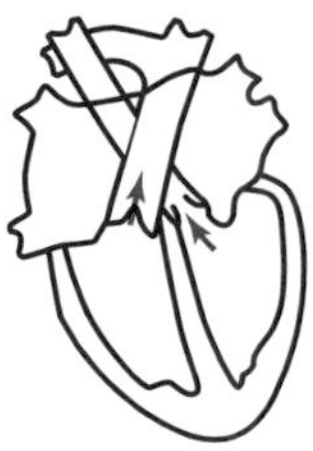	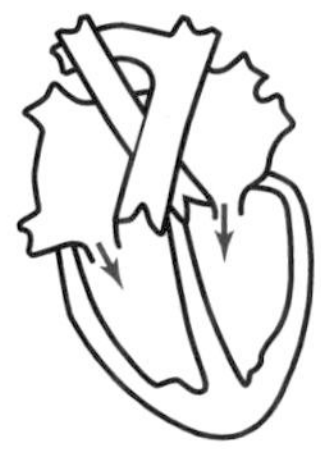	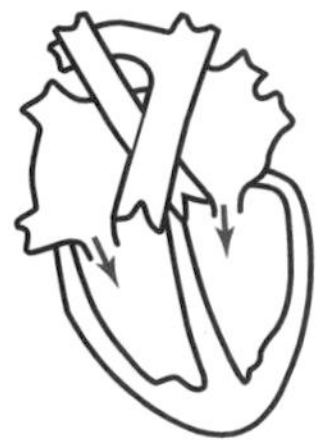	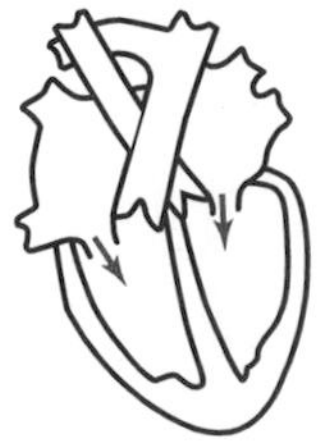
Preferable position of patient	Any position	Sitting or supine	Supine or left lateral	Supine or left semilateral
Area for auscultation	Entire precordium (apex)	A_2 at 2nd RICS P_2 at 2nd LICS	Apex	Apex
Endpiece	Diaphragm	Diaphragm	Bell	Bell
FINDINGS Pitch	High	High	Low	Low
Effects of respiration	Softer on inspiration	Fusion of A_2P_2 on expiration; physiologic split on inspiration	Increased on inspiration	Increased on inspiration
External influences	Increased with excitement, exercise, amyl nitrate, epinephrine, and atropine	Increased with thin chest walls and with exercise	Increased with exercise, fast heart rate, elevation of legs and increased venous return	Increased with exercise, fast heart rate, elevation of legs and increased venous return
Cause	Closure of tricuspid and mitral valves	Closure of pulmonic and aortic valves	Rapid ventricular filling	Forceful atrial ejection into distended ventricle

FIGURE 14-19
Assessment of heart sounds. *LICS,* Left intercostal space; *RICS,* right intercostal space.
Modified from Guzzetta, Dossey, 1992.

Quadruple rhythm	Summation gallop (triple gallop)	Ejection sounds	Systolic click	Opening snap
S_4S_1 $S_2 S_3$ $S_4 S_1 S_2$	S_{3-4} $S_1 S_2$ S_{3-4} S_1 S_2	S_1 S_2 S_1 ↑ S_2	S_1 ↑ S_2 S_1 ↑ S_2	S_1 S_2 ↑ S_1 S_2 ↑
Supine or left lateral	Supine or left lateral	Sitting or supine	Sitting or supine	Any position
Apex	Apex	2nd RICS, 2nd LICS, or apex	Apex	Apex
Bell	Bell	Diaphragm	Diaphragm	Diaphragm
Low	Low	High	High	High
Increased on inspiration	Increased on inspiration	Increased on expiration with pulmonary stenosis	Increased on inspiration	Uninfluenced by inspiration
Aortic ejection sound same as S_1 and S_2; pulmonary ejection sound increased on expiration	Aortic ejection sound same as S_1 and S_2; pulmonary ejection sound increased on expiration	Aortic ejection sound same as S_1 and S_2; pulmonary ejection sound increased on expiration	Occurs later in systole with increased venous return (e.g., with elevated legs or supine position)	May be confused with S_3
S_1, S_2, S_3, and S_4, all heard separately	S_3 and S_4 fuse with fast heart rates	Opening of deformed semi-lunar valves	Prolapse of mitral valve leaflet	Abrupt recoil of stenotic mitral or tricuspid valve

Not all murmurs, however, are the result of valvular defects. Other causes include the following:

- High output demands that increase speed of blood flow (e.g., thyrotoxicosis, anemia, pregnancy)
- Structural defects, either congenital or acquired, that allow blood to flow through inappropriate pathways (e.g., the myocardial septum)
- Diminished strength of myocardial contraction
- Altered blood flow in the major vessels near the heart
- Transmitted murmurs resulting from valvular aortic stenosis, ruptured chordae tendineae of the mitral valve, or severe aortic regurgitation
- Vigorous left ventricular ejection (more common in children than in adults)
- Obstructive disease in cervical arteries, such as atherosclerotic carotid arteries, fibromuscular hyperplasia, or arteritis

It is not always possible on physical examination to identify with consistency the cause of a systolic murmur; however, a number of maneuvers can narrow the choices before diagnostic laboratory studies are performed.

BOX 14-9
ARE SOME MURMURS INNOCENT?

Many murmurs—particularly in children, adolescents, and especially in young athletes—have no apparent cause. They are presumably a result of vigorous myocardial contraction, the consequent stronger blood flow in early systole or midsystole, and the rush of blood from the larger chamber of the heart into the smaller bore of a blood vessel. The thinner chests of the young make these sounds easier to hear, particularly with a lightly held bell. They are usually grade I or II, usually midsystolic, without radiation, or medium pitch, blowing, brief, and often accompanied by splitting of S_2. They are often located in the second left intercostal space near the left sternal border. Such murmurs heard in a recumbent position may disappear when the patient sits or stands because of the tendency of the blood to pool. Do not confuse an "innocent" murmur with one that is "benign," the result of a structural anomaly that is not severe enough to cause a clinical problem.

DIFFERENTIAL DIAGNOSIS
COMPARISON OF SYSTOLIC MURMURS

Origin	Maneuver	Effect of Intensity
Right-sided chambers	Inspiration	Increase
	Expiration	Decrease
Hypertrophic cardiomyopathy	Valsalva	Increase
	Squatting to standing (rapidly for 30 seconds)	Increase
	Standing to squatting (rapidly)	Decrease
	Passive leg elevation to 45 degrees, patient supine	Decrease
Mitral regurgitation*	Handgrip	Increase
Ventricular septal defect*	Transient arterial occlusion (sphygmomanometer placed on each of patient's upper arms and simultaneously inflated to 20 to 40 mm Hg above patient's previously recorded blood pressures; intensity noted after 20 seconds)	Increase
	Inhalation of amyl nitrate (three rapid breaths from a broken ampule) *(Not routinely recommended)*	Decrease
Aortic stenosis	No maneuver distinguishes this murmur; the diagnosis can be made by exclusion	

Modified from Lembo et al, 1988.

*The combination of handgrip, transient arterial occlusion, and inhalation of amyl nitrate will distinguish mitral regurgitation and ventricular septal defect from other causes of systolic murmurs; more than just auscultation is needed to make further distinction.

RHYTHM DISTURBANCE

Determine the steadiness of the heart rhythm, which should be regular. If it is irregular, determine whether there is a consistent pattern. A heart rate that is irregular but occurs in a repeated pattern may indicate sinus dysrhythmia, a cyclic variation of the heart rate characterized by an increasing rate on inspiration and decreasing rate on expiration. A patternless, unpredictable, irregular rhythm may indicate heart disease or conduction system impairment.

INFANTS

Examination of the newborn presents a challenge because of the immediate change from fetal to systemic and pulmonary circulation. Examine the heart within the first 24 hours of life and again at about 2 to 3 days of age.

Complete evaluation of heart function includes examination of the skin, lungs, and liver. Infants with right-sided congestive heart failure have large, firm livers with the inferior edge as much as 5 to 6 cm below the right costal margin. Unlike adults, this finding may precede that of pulmonary crackles.

Inspect the color of the skin and mucous membranes. The well newborn should be reassuringly pink. A purplish plethora is associated with polycythemia; an ashy white color indicates shock; and central cyanosis (i.e., cyanosis of the skin and mucous membranes of the face and upper body) suggests congenital heart disease. Note the distribution and intensity of discoloration, as well as the extent of change after vigorous exertion. Acrocyanosis, cyanosis of the hands and feet without central cyanosis, is of little concern; it usually disappears within a few days, or even a few hours, after birth.

Cyanosis is distinctive of the problems that lead to admixture of arterial and venous blood or that prevent the expected oxygenation of blood. Severe cyanosis evident at birth or shortly thereafter suggests transposition of the great vessels, tetralogy of Fallot, tricuspid atresia, a severe septal defect, or severe pulmonic stenosis. Cyanosis that does not appear until after the neonatal period suggests a pure pulmonic stenosis, Eisenmenger complex, tetralogy of Fallot, or large septal defects.

The apical impulse in the newborn is usually seen and felt at the fourth to fifth left intercostal space just medial to the midclavicular line. The smaller the baby or the thinner the chest, the more obvious it will be. It may be somewhat farther to the right in the first few hours of life, sometimes even substernal.

Note any enlargement of the heart. It is especially important to note the position of the heart if a baby is having trouble breathing. A pneumothorax shifts the apical impulse away from the area of the pneumothorax. A diaphragmatic hernia, more commonly found on the left, shifts the heart to the right. Dextrocardia results in an apical impulse on the right.

The right ventricle is relatively more vigorous than the left in a well, full-term newborn. If the baby is thin, you might even be able to feel the closure of the pulmonary valve in the second left intercostal space.

S_2 in infants is somewhat higher in pitch and more discrete than S_1. The vigor and quality of the heart sounds of the newborn (and throughout infancy and early childhood) are major indicators of the function of the heart. Diminished vigor may be the only apparent change when an infant is already in heart failure. Splitting of the heart sounds is common. S_2 is usually heard without a split at birth, then often splits within a few hours.

S_3 and S_4 are commonly heard in pediatric patients. Increased intensity of either sound is suspect.

Murmurs are relatively common in the newborn until about 48 hours of age. Most are innocent, caused by the transition from fetal to pulmonic circulation rather than by a significant congenital abnormality. These murmurs are usually of grade I or II intensity, systolic, and unaccompanied by other signs and symptoms; they usually disappear within 2 to 3 days. Paradoxically, a significant congenital abnormality may be unaccompanied by a murmur.

If you cannot tell a murmur from respiration, pinch the nares briefly, listen while the baby is feeding, or time the sound with the carotid pulsation. Because of the rapid heart rate in infants, the heart sounds are more difficult to evaluate. A murmur heard immediately at birth is apt to be less significant than one continuously noted after the first few hours of life. If a murmur persists beyond the second or third day of life, is intense, fills systole, occupies diastole to any extent, or radiates widely, it must be investigated. If you push up on the liver, thereby increasing right atrial pressure, the murmur of a left-to-right shunt through a septal opening or patent ductus will disappear briefly, whereas the murmur of a right-to-left shunt will intensify.

Murmurs that extend beyond S_2 and occupy diastole are said to have a machine-like quality; they may be associated with a patent ductus arteriosus. The murmur should disappear when the patent ductus closes in the first 2 or 3 days of life. Diastolic murmurs, almost always significant, may nevertheless be transient and possibly related to an early closing ductus arteriosus or a mild, brief, pulmonary insufficiency.

Infants' heart rates are more variable than those of older children. Eating, sleeping, and waking can change the rate considerably. The variation is greatest at birth or shortly after and is even more marked in premature infants. Rates close to 200 beats per minute are not uncommon, but they may also indicate paroxysmal atrial tachycardia. Ordinarily, the decrease in rate is relatively rapid, and at a few hours of age the rate may be much closer to 120. A relatively fixed tachycardia is a clue to some difficulty.

CHILDREN

The precordium of a child tends to bulge over an enlarged heart if the enlargement is of long standing. A child's thoracic cage, being more cartilaginous and yielding than that of an adult, responds more to the thrust of cardiac enlargement.

Sinus arrhythmia is a physiologic event during childhood. The heart rate varies in a cyclic pattern, usually faster on inspiration and slower on expiration. Most often, other dysrhythmias in children are ectopic in origin (e.g., supraventricular and ventricular ectopic beats). These and a variety of other seeming irregularities require extensive investigation only occasionally.

The heart rates of children are more variable than those of adults, reacting with wider swings to stress of any sort (e.g., exercise, fever, or tension). It is not uncommon to discover an increase of 10 to 20 beats in the heart rate for each degree of temperature elevation. The expected heart rates in children vary with age:

Age	Rate (Beats Per Minute)
Newborn	120-170
1 year	80-160
3 years	80-120
6 years	75-115
10 years	70-110

Most organic murmurs in infants and children are the result of congenital heart disease; however, acute rheumatic fever still accounts for most acquired murmurs, and its occurrence has been on the rise in this country in recent years.

Some murmurs are innocent. A Still murmur, so named after the physician who first described it, occurs in active, healthy children between the ages of 3 to 7 years. Caused by the vigorous expulsion of blood from the left ventricle into the aorta, it increases in intensity with activity and diminishes when the child is quiet. It is often described as musical (see Box 14-9).

When examining a child with known heart disease, take careful note of weight gain (or loss), developmental delay, cyanosis, and clubbing of fingers and toes. Cyanosis is a major clue to congenital heart defects that impede oxygenation of blood.

PREGNANT WOMEN

The heart rate gradually increases throughout pregnancy until it is 10% to 30% higher at term. There is no significant change in the ECG.

The heart position is shifted during pregnancy, but the position varies with the size and position of the uterus. The apical impulse is upward and more lateral by 1 to 1.5 cm. Some changes in auscultated heart sounds are expected because of the increased blood volume and extra effort of the heart. There is more audible splitting of S_1 and S_2, and S_3 may be readily heard after 20 weeks of gestation. A fourth heart sound is abnormal. In addition, systolic ejection murmurs may be heard over the pulmonic area in 90% of pregnant women. The murmur is intensified during inspiration or expiration but should not be louder than grade II.

The presence of cyanosis, clubbing, persistent neck vein distention, or the development of a diastolic murmur suggests an abnormality.

OLDER ADULTS

You may need to slow the pace of your examination when asking an older patient to assume positions that may be uncomfortable or perhaps too difficult. Some older patients may not be able to lie flat for an extended time, and some may not be able to control their breathing pattern at your request. Because the cardiac response to even minimal demand may be slowed or insufficient, even a moderately abrupt position change may cause a transient lightheadedness, as may the drop in arterial pressure after a moderate meal.

The heart rate may be slower because of increased vagal tone, or more rapid, with a wide range that may vary from the low 40s to more than 100 beats per minute. Occasional ectopic beats are fairly common and may or may not be significant.

The apical impulse may be harder to find in many persons because of the increased anteroposterior diameter of the chest. In obese older adults, the diaphragm is raised and the heart is more transverse.

Older adults who exercise regularly may reverse or deter some of the age-associated changes.

S_4 is more common in older adults and may indicate decreased left ventricular compliance. Early, soft physiologic murmurs may be heard, caused by aortic lengthening, tortuosity, and sclerotic changes.

SAMPLE DOCUMENTATION
HISTORY AND PHYSICAL EXAMINATION

Subjective

A 56-year-old man comes to the emergency department complaining of substernal chest pain radiating to the jaw and into the left shoulder for past hour. No relief with antacid tablets. Nauseated. Rates pain as 8 on a scale of 10. Known history of hyperlipidemia.

For additional sample documentation, see Chapter 26.

Objective

Diaphoretic, pale, and grimacing in pain. Heart rate of 124 beats per minute, S_4 noted with a regular rhythm. Blood pressure 100/66 mm Hg. Precordium with no visible pulsations and no palpable lifts, heaves, or thrills.

SUMMARY OF EXAMINATION
HEART

The following steps are performed with the patient sitting and leaning forward, supine, and in the left lateral recumbent positions; these positions are all used to compare findings or enhance the assessment.

1. Inspect the precordium for the following (p. 429):
   - Apical impulse
   - Pulsations
   - Heaves or lifts
2. Palpate the precordium to detect the following (p. 430):
   - Apical impulse
   - Thrills, heaves, or lifts
3. Percussion to estimate the heart size (optional) (p. 432)
4. Systematically auscultate in each of the five areas while the patient is breathing regularly and holding breath for the following (p. 432):
   - Rate

   - Rhythm
   - S_1
   - S_2
   - Splitting
   - S_3 and/or S_4
   - Extra heart sounds (snaps, clicks, friction rubs, or murmurs)
5. Assess the following characteristics of murmurs (p. 439):
   - Timing and duration
   - Pitch
   - Intensity
   - Pattern
   - Quality
   - Location
   - Radiation
   - Variation with respiratory phase

COMMON ABNORMALITIES

HEART MURMURS

The most common source of significant murmurs is anatomic disorder of the valves of the heart (Fig. 14-20; Table 14-5).

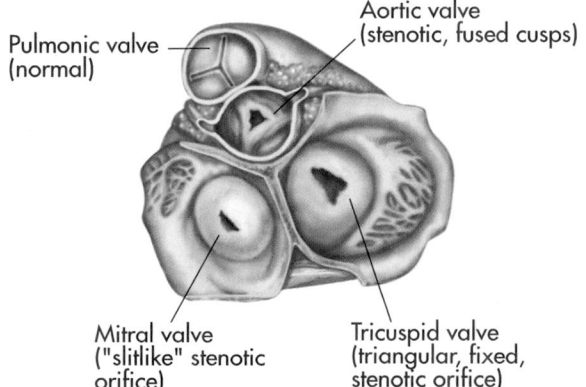

FIGURE 14-20
Valvular heart disease.
Modified from Canobbio, 1990.

TABLE 14-5	Heart Murmurs	
Type and Detection	**Findings on Examination**	**Description**
MITRAL STENOSIS Heard with bell at apex, patient in left lateral decubitus position	Low-frequency diastolic rumble, more intense in early and late diastole, does not radiate; systole usually quiet; palpable thrill at apex in late diastole common; S_1 increased and often palpable at left sternal border; S_2 split often with accented P_2; opening snap follows P_2 closely Visible lift in right parasternal area if right ventricle hypertrophied Arterial pulse amplitude decreased	Narrowed valve restricts forward flow; forceful ejection into ventricle Often occurs with mitral regurgitation Caused by rheumatic fever or cardiac infection	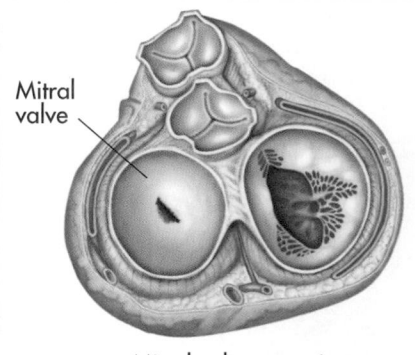 Mitral valve stenosis
AORTIC STENOSIS Heard over aortic area; ejection sound at second right intercostal border	Midsystolic (ejection) murmur, medium pitch, coarse, diamond shaped,* crescendo-decrescendo; radiates along left sternal border (sometimes to apex) and to carotid with palpable thrill; S_1 often heard best at apex, disappearing when stenosis is severe, often followed by ejection click; S_2 soft or absent and may not be split; S_4 palpable; ejection sound muted in calcified valves; the more severe the stenosis, the later the peak of the murmur in systole Apical thrust shifts down and left and is prolonged if left ventricular hypertrophy is also present	Calcification of valve cusps restricts forward flow; forceful ejection from ventricle into systemic circulation Caused by congenital bicuspid (rather than the usual tricuspid) valve, rheumatic heart disease, atherosclerosis May be the cause of sudden death, particularly in children and adolescents, either at rest or during exercise; risk apparently related to degree of stenosis	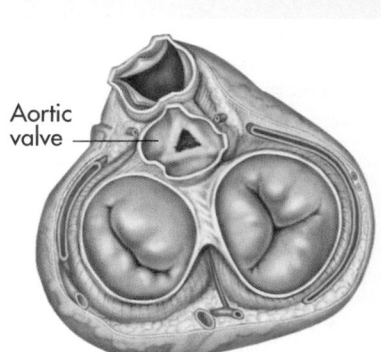 Aortic valve stenosis

*Diamond-shaped murmur is named for its recorded shape on phonocardiogram (a crescendo-decrescendo sound).

TABLE 14-5   Heart Murmurs—cont'd

Type and Detection	Findings on Examination	Description	
SUBAORTIC STENOSIS			
Heard at apex and along left sternal border	Murmur fills systole, diamond shaped, medium pitch, coarse; thrill often palpable during systole at apex and right sternal border; multiple waves in apical impulses; S_2 usually split; S_3 and S_4 often present Arterial pulse brisk, double wave in carotid common; jugular venous pulse prominent	Fibrous ring, usually 1 to 4 mm below aortic valve; most pronounced on ventricular septal side; may become progressively severe with time; difficult to distinguish from aortic stenosis on clinical grounds alone	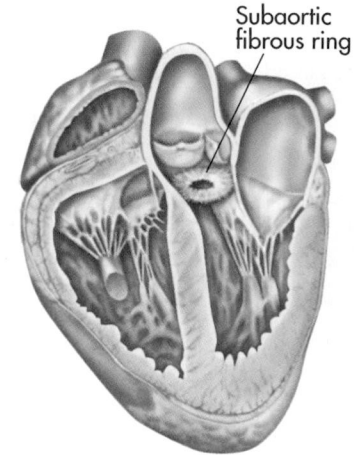 Subaortic stenosis
PULMONIC STENOSIS			
Heard over pulmonic area radiating to left and into neck; thrill in second and third left intercostals space	Systolic (ejection) murmur, diamond shaped, medium pitch, coarse; usually with thrill; S_1 often followed quickly by ejection click; S_2 often diminished, usually wide split; P_2 soft or absent; S_4 common in right ventricular hypertrophy; murmur may be prolonged and confused with that of a ventricular septal defect	Valve restricts forward flow; forceful ejection from ventricle into pulmonary circulation Cause is almost always congenital	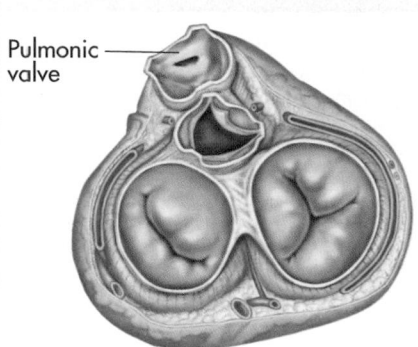 Pulmonic valve stenosis
TRICUSPID STENOSIS			
Heard with bell over tricuspid area	Diastolic rumble accentuated early and late in diastole, resembling mitral stenosis but louder on inspiration; diastolic thrill palpable over right ventricle; S_2 may be split during inspiration Arterial pulse amplitude decreased; jugular venous pulse prominent, especially a wave; slow fall of v wave (see Chapter 15)	Calcification of valve cusps restricts forward flow; forceful ejection into ventricles Usually seen with mitral stenosis, rarely occurs alone Caused by rheumatic heart disease, congenital defect, endocardial fibroelastosis, right atrial myxoma	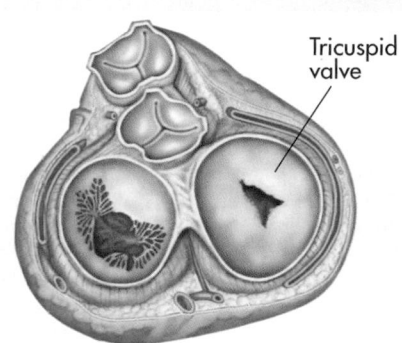 Tricuspid valve stenosis

Continued

TABLE 14-5 **Heart Murmurs—cont'd**

Type and Detection	Findings on Examination	Description	
MITRAL REGURGITATION			
Heard best at apex; loudest there, transmitted into left axilla	Holosystolic, plateau-shaped intensity, high pitch, harsh blowing quality, often quite loud and may obliterate S_2; radiates from apex to base or to left axilla; thrill may be palpable at apex during systole; S_1 intensity diminished; S_2 more intense with P_2 often accented; S_3 often present; S_3-S_4 gallop common in late disease If mild, late systolic murmur crescendos; if severe, early systolic intensity decrescendos; apical thrust more to left and down in ventricular hypertrophy	Valve incompetence allows backflow from ventricle to atrium Caused by rheumatic fever, myocardial infarction, myxoma, rupture of chordae	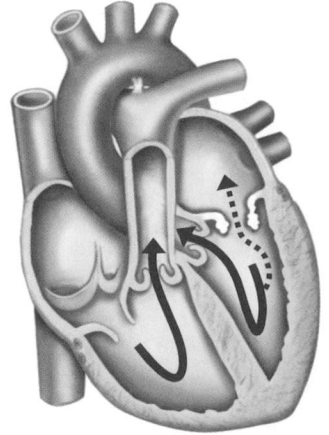Mitral regurgitation (heart in systole)
MITRAL VALVE PROLAPSE			
Heard at apex and left lower sternal border; easily missed in supine position; also listen with patient upright	Typically late systolic murmur preceded by midsystolic clicks, but both murmur and clicks highly variable in intensity and timing	Valve is competent early in systole but prolapses into atrium later in systole; may become progressively severe, resulting in a holosystolic murmur; often concurrent with pectus excavatum	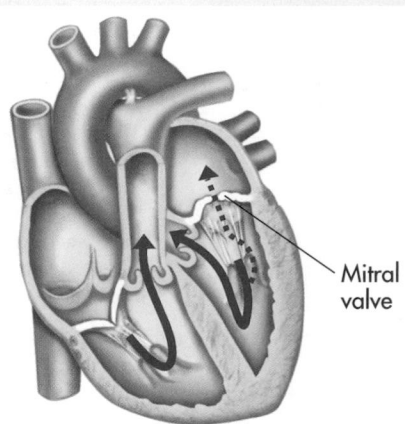Mitral valve Mitral valve prolapse (heart in systole)
AORTIC REGURGITATION			
Heard with diaphragm, patient sitting and leaning forward; Austin-Flint murmur heard with bell; ejection click heard in second intercostal space	Early diastolic, high pitch, blowing, often with diamond-shaped midsystolic murmur, sounds often not prominent; duration varies with blood pressure; low-pitched, rumbling murmur at apex common (Austin-Flint); early ejection click sometimes present; S_1 soft; S_2 split may have tambour-like quality; M_1 and A_2 often intensified, S_3-S_4 gallop common In left ventricular hypertrophy, prominent prolonged apical impulse down and to left Pulse pressure wide; water-hammer or bisferiens pulse common in carotid, brachial, and femoral arteries (Chapter 15)	Valve incompetence allows backflow from aorta to ventricle Caused by rheumatic heart disease, endocarditis, aortic diseases (Marfan syndrome, medial necrosis), syphilis, ankylosing spondylitis, dissection, cardiac trauma	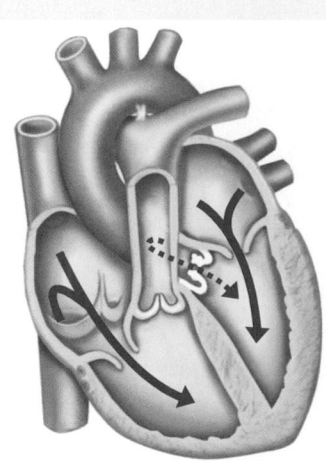Aortic regurgitation (heart in diastole)

TABLE 14-5	Heart Murmurs—cont'd	
Type and Detection	**Findings on Examination**	**Description**

PULMONIC REGURGITATION

	Difficult to distinguish from aortic regurgitation on physical examination	Valve incompetence allows backflow from pulmonary artery to ventricle Secondary to pulmonary hypertension or bacterial endocarditis

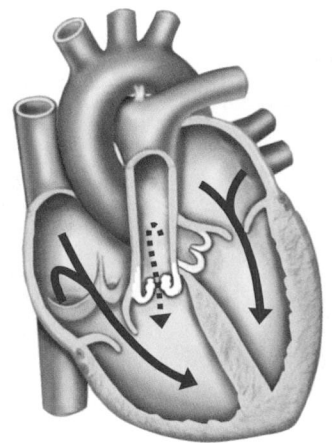

Pulmonic regurgitation
(heart in diastole)

TRICUSPID REGURGITATION

Heard at left lower sternum, occasionally radiating a few centimeters to left	Holosystolic murmur over right ventricle, blowing, increased on inspiration; S_3 and thrill over tricuspid area common In pulmonary hypertension, pulmonary artery impulse palpable over second left intercostal space and P_2 accented; in right ventricular hypertrophy, visible lift to right of sternum Jugular venous pulse has large v waves (see Chapter 15)	Valve incompetence allows backflow from ventricle to atrium Caused by congenital defects, bacterial endocarditis (especially in IV drug abusers), pulmonary hypertension, cardiac trauma

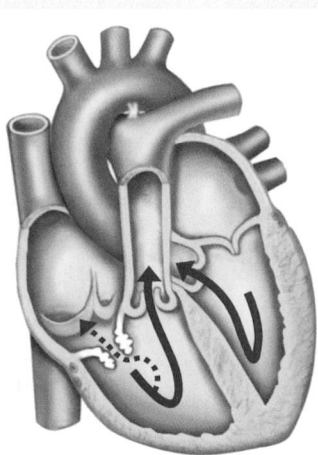

Tricuspid regurgitation
(heart in systole)

LEFT VENTRICULAR HYPERTROPHY	The left ventricle works harder and longer with each beat when it meets increased resistance to the emptying of blood into the systemic circulation (e.g., with aortic stenosis, volume overload, and systemic hypertension). As it hypertrophies because of the extra exercise, the left ventricle increases in mass and becomes displaced laterally. A vigorous sustained lift is then often palpable during ventricular systole, sometimes over a broader area than usual, as much as 2 cm or more. The displacement of the apical impulse can be most impressive, well lateral to the midclavicular line and downward.
RIGHT VENTRICULAR HYPERTROPHY	The right ventricle works harder and enlarges with defects of the pulmonary vascular bed, pulmonary hypertension, and left-to-right shunts. This condition is less common than left ventricular hypertrophy. It can cause a lift along the left sternal border in the third and fourth left intercostal spaces accompanied by occasional systolic retraction at the apex. The left ventricle is not itself particularly affected, but it is displaced and turned posteriorly by the enlarged right ventricle.

SICK SINUS SYNDROME In sick sinus syndrome, sinoatrial dysfunction occurs secondary to hypertension, arteriosclerotic heart disease, or rheumatic heart disease; it may also occur idiopathically. The condition causes dysrhythmias with subsequent fainting, transient dizzy spells, light-headedness, seizures, palpitations, and symptoms of angina or congestive heart failure.

BACTERIAL ENDOCARDITIS

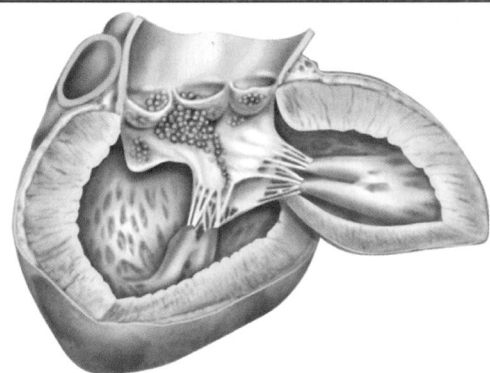

FIGURE 14-21
Bacterial endocarditis.
Modified from Canobbio, 1990.

A bacterial infection of the endothelial layer of the heart and valves should be suspected with prolonged fever, signs of neurologic dysfunctions, and sudden onset of congestive heart failure. A murmur may or may not be present. Individuals with valvular defects, congenital or acquired, and those who use intravenous drugs are particularly susceptible (Fig. 14-21). Janeway lesions and Osler nodes are characteristic. Janeway lesions are small erythematous or hemorrhagic macules appearing on the palms and soles. Osler nodes appear on the tips of fingers or toes. They are caused by septic emboli from the infected heart valve.

CONGESTIVE HEART FAILURE

Congestive heart failure (CHF) is a syndrome in which the heart fails to propel blood forward with its usual force, resulting in congestion in the pulmonary or systemic circulation. Decreased cardiac output causes decreased blood flow to the tissues. Congestive heart failure may be predominantly left or right sided. Left sided CHF is often characterized as being either systolic or diastolic. Systolic is characterized by a narrow pulse pressure while diastolic CHF has a wide pulse pressure. Systolic CHF results from reduction in myocardial tissue after myocardial infarction or as a consequence of atherosclerotic cardiovascular disease (ASCVD). The diastolic form is the result of advanced glycation products which crosslink collagen and thereby create a stiff ventricle that is unable to dilate actively. It occurs in older adults whose tissue is exposed to glucose for a longer period of time and in individuals with diabetes mellitus. Symptoms can develop gradually or suddenly with acute pulmonary edema. The prevalence of each form increases more markedly with age, particularly after 50 years, and more rapidly among women than among men.

EVIDENCE-BASED PRACTICE IN PHYSICAL EXAMINATION

CAN THE CLINICAL EXAMINATION DIAGNOSE LEFT-SIDED HEART FAILURE IN ADULTS?

Badgett and colleagues conducted an evaluation of what physical findings are most helpful in the diagnosis of left-sided congestive heart failure. The researchers found that the most helpful finding is jugular venous distention (see Chapter 15). Somewhat helpful were the following:

- Dyspnea
- Orthopnea
- Tachycardia

- Decreased systolic or pulse pressure
- Third heart sound
- Crackles on examination of the lungs
- Abdominojugular reflux

Edema was found to be helpful diagnostically only if present; the absence of edema is not helpful in ruling out the diagnosis.

Badgett, Lucey, Mulrow, 1997.

PERICARDITIS

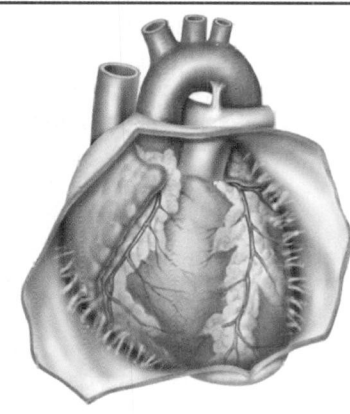

FIGURE 14-22
Pericarditis.
Modified from Canobbio, 1990.

Pericardial disease, which is relatively rare, may be confused with more common and occasionally life-threatening cardiac conditions. Chest pain is the usual initial symptom in acute pericarditis (sudden inflammation of the pericardium). The key physical finding is the triphasic friction rub, which comprises ventricular systole, early diastolic ventricular filling, and late diastolic atrial systole. It occurs in more than 90% of patients with the disease. It is best heard just to the left of the sternum in the third and fourth intercostal spaces and is characteristically scratchy, grating, and very easily heard even in the presence of considerable pericardial effusion. As an acute pericarditis persists and becomes subacute or chronic, the effusion may increase and result in cardiac tamponade (Fig. 14-22).

CARDIAC TAMPONADE

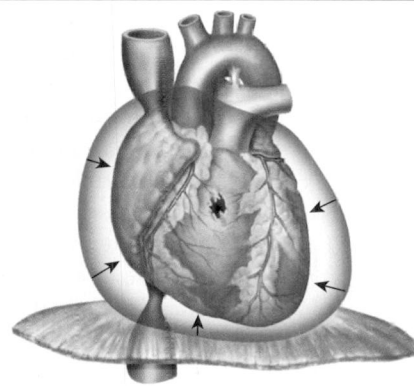

FIGURE 14-23
Hemopericardium and cardiac tamponade.
Modified from Canobbio, 1990.

An "excessive" accumulation of effused fluids or blood between the pericardium and heart results in cardiac tamponade (Fig. 14-23). *Excessive* is difficult to define because as much as 300 mL of fluid may not constrain cardiac function in the adult. In any event, a sufficient amount seriously constrains cardiac relaxation, impairing access of blood to the right heart and ultimately causing the signs and symptoms of systemic venous congestion: edema, ascites, and dyspnea. A chronically and severely involved pericardium may also scar and constrict, forming in a sense a shell around the heart that limits cardiac filling. In this circumstance, heart sounds are muffled, blood pressure drops, the pulse becomes weakened and rapid, and the paradoxic pulse (see Chapter 15) becomes exaggerated. Pericarditis, aortic dissection, and trauma are common causes of tamponade.

COR PULMONALE

Cor pulmonale is the enlargement of the right ventricle secondary to pulmonary malfunction. Usually chronic but occasionally acute, cor pulmonale results from chronic obstructive pulmonary disease. Alterations in the pulmonary circulation lead to pulmonary arterial hypertension, which imposes a mechanical load on right ventricular emptying. Signs include left parasternal systolic lift and a loud S_2 exaggerated in the pulmonic region.

HYPERLIPIDEMIA

Elevated serum cholesterol is a potent risk factor for myocardial infarction. It is also one of the most common metabolic diseases in the American population. Its frequency is great because of the increasing obesity in the population as well as evidence from clinical trials that ever lower levels of total cholesterol and low-density lipoprotein (LDL) cholesterol further reduce the risk of myocardial infarction. These studies have led the National Institutes of Health to lower the desirable level of total cholesterol to 200 mg/dL and the LDL cholesterol to 100 mg/dL. The LDL goal for individuals with a previous myocardial infarction or with diabetes mellitus is now 70 mg/dL.

MYOCARDIAL INFARCTION

Ischemic myocardial necrosis is caused by an abrupt decrease in coronary blood flow to a segment of the myocardium. It most commonly affects the left ventricle, but damage may extend into the right ventricle or atria. Symptoms commonly include deep substernal or visceral pain that often radiates to the jaw, neck, and left arm, although discomfort may be mild, especially in older adults or patients with diabetes mellitus. Dysrhythmias are common, and S_4 is usually present. Heart sounds are typically distant, with a soft, systolic, blowing apical murmur.

Pulse may be thready, and blood pressure varies, although hypertension is usual in the early phases. Atherosclerosis and thrombosis are the common underlying causes.

MYOCARDITIS

Focal or diffuse inflammation of the myocardium can result from infectious agents, toxins, or autoimmune diseases such as amyloidosis. Initial symptoms are typically vague and include fatigue, dyspnea, fever, and palpitations. As the disease process advances, cardiac enlargement, murmurs, gallop rhythms, tachycardia, dysrhythmias, and pulsus alternans develop.

ABNORMALITIES IN HEART RATE AND RHYTHM

CONDUCTION DISTURBANCES

MNEMONICS

Causes of Syncope:
CANADA

C Cardiac: valve stenosis, Stokes-Adams attacks, other conduction disturbances

A Arteriovenous: "steal" syndromes

N Nervous: psychologic, autonomic, vagal, coughing

A Anemia, altered blood (CO)

D Drugs, diabetes, alcohol, poisons

A Altitude, acute fevers

Conduction disturbances occur either proximal to the bundle of His or diffusely throughout the conduction system. They may produce symptoms of transient weakness, fainting spells, or strokelike episodes. Some patients note only a rapid or irregular heart beat. Heart block may result from a variety of disturbances: ischemic; infiltrative; or more rarely, neoplastic. Unusual dysrhythmias—whether fast or slow, with or without block—may result in fainting, particularly in older adults. Antidepressant drugs, digitalis, quinidine, and many other medications can be precipitating factors. With these attacks, cardiac syncope may occur acutely and without particular warning; sometimes a diminished sensibility, a "gray-out" instead of a "black-out," may precede the event. Heart rates are often labile and disturbances in rhythm are not unusual (Table 14-6).

TABLE 14-6	**Abnormalities in Rates and Rhythms**	
Type and Detection	**Findings on Examination**	**Description**
ATRIAL (AURICULAR) FLUTTER	Atrial rate far in excess of ventricular rate; heart sounds not necessarily weak	Regular uniform atrial contractions occur in excess of 200/min, but the ventricular response is limited as a result of physiologic heart block. The conduction system cannot respond to the rapidity of the atrial rate, causing variance from the ventricular rate. The ECG may look like a saw-tooth cog.
Atrial flutter with a constant 4:1 conduction ratio. From Guzzetta, Dossey, 1992.		
SINUS BRADYCARDIA	Slow rate, sometimes below 50 or 60/min	There is no disruption in conduction; not necessarily suggestive of a problem.
Sinus bradycardia From Guzzetta, Dossey, 1992.		

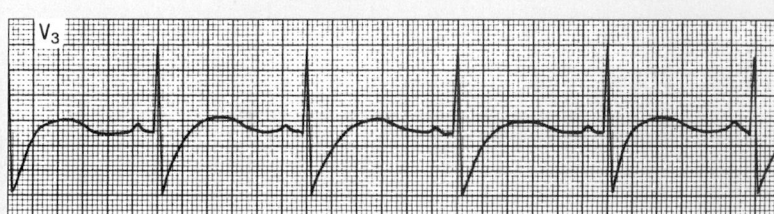

TABLE 14-6   Abnormalities in Rates and Rhythms—cont'd

Type and Detection	Findings on Examination	Description

ATRIAL FIBRILLATION

| | Dysrhythmic contraction of the atria gives way to rapid series of irregular spasms of the muscle wall; no discernible regularity in rhythm or pattern | The conduction system is malfunctioning and is in an anarchic state. Any contraction of the atria that gets through to the ventricle is irregular. The sounds are best described as irregularly irregular. |

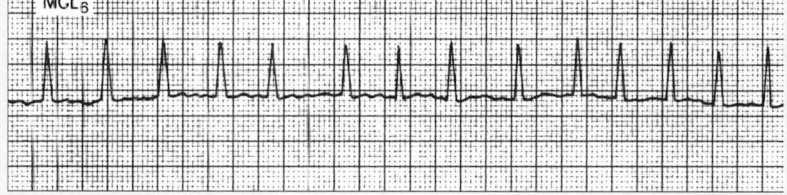

Atrial fibrillation with rapid ventricular response.

From Guzzetta, Dossey, 1992.

HEART BLOCK

| | Heart rate slower than expected, often 25-45/min at rest | Conduction from atria to ventricles partially or completely disrupted. If conduction is completely disrupted, the ventricle may be left to beat on its own and the heart rate slows considerably. ECG is necessary to determine the extent and nature of heart block in conduction. |

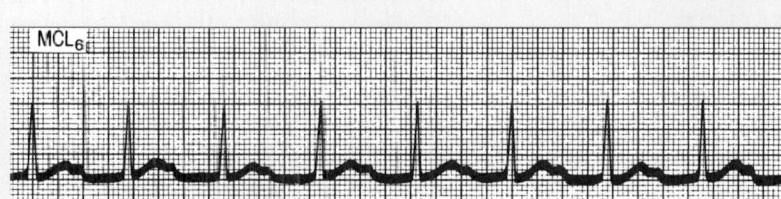

Sinus rhythm with first-degree AV block characterized by prolonged PR interval.

From Guzzetta, Dossey, 1992.

ATRIAL TACHYCARDIA

| | Rapid, regular heart rate (200/min) without disruption of the rhythm; may be heard only on occasion (in paroxysms) and without loss of vigor in heart sounds | This is the result of electrical stimulus originating in a focus in the atrium separate from the SA node. Conduction through to the ventricle is usually complete. Often there is no other evidence of disease, and the patient is usually a young adult. The rate will occasionally decrease with vagal stimulation, holding a deep breath, or gentle massage of a carotid sinus. (Massage must always be done with care.) (See Chapter 15.) |

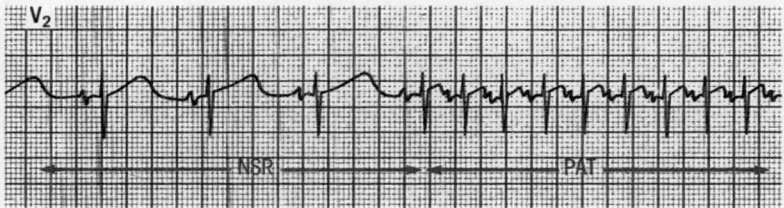

Paroxysmal atrial tachycardia (PAT).

From Guzzetta, Dossey, 1992.

VENTRICULAR TACHYCARDIA

| | Rapid, relatively regular heartbeat (often nearly 200/min) without loss in apparent strength | The electrical source of the beat is in an unusual focus somewhere in the ventricles. This usually arises in serious heart disease and is a grave prognostic sign. |

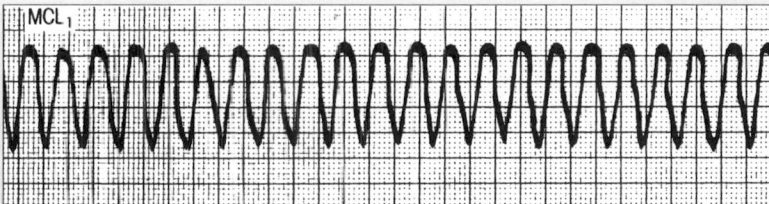

Ventricular tachycardia.

From Guzzetta, Dossey, 1992.

Continued

TABLE 14-6	Abnormalities in Rates and Rhythms—cont'd	
Type and Detection	**Findings on Examination**	**Description**
VENTRICULAR FIBRILLATION		
Ventricular fibrillation.	Complete loss of regular heart rhythm with expected conduction pattern absent; if weakened and rapid, ventricular contraction is irregular	The ventricle has lost the rhythm of its expected response, and all evidence of vigorous contraction is gone. It calls for immediate action and may immediately precede sudden death.

From Guzzetta, Dossey, 1992.

INFANTS AND CHILDREN

TETRALOGY OF FALLOT

Four cardiac defects make up the tetralogy of Fallot: ventricular septal defect, pulmonic stenosis, dextroposition of the aorta, and right ventricular hypertrophy. Infants with tetralogy of Fallot often have paroxysmal dyspnea with loss of consciousness and central cyanosis; older children develop clubbing of fingers and toes. There is a parasternal heave and precordial prominence. A systolic ejection murmur is heard over the third intercostal space, sometimes radiating to the left side of the neck. A single S_2 is heard (Fig. 14-24). Surgical correction, currently initiated after the first "spell" in infancy, may allow the tolerance of effort to approach the expected for ordinary day-to-day living.

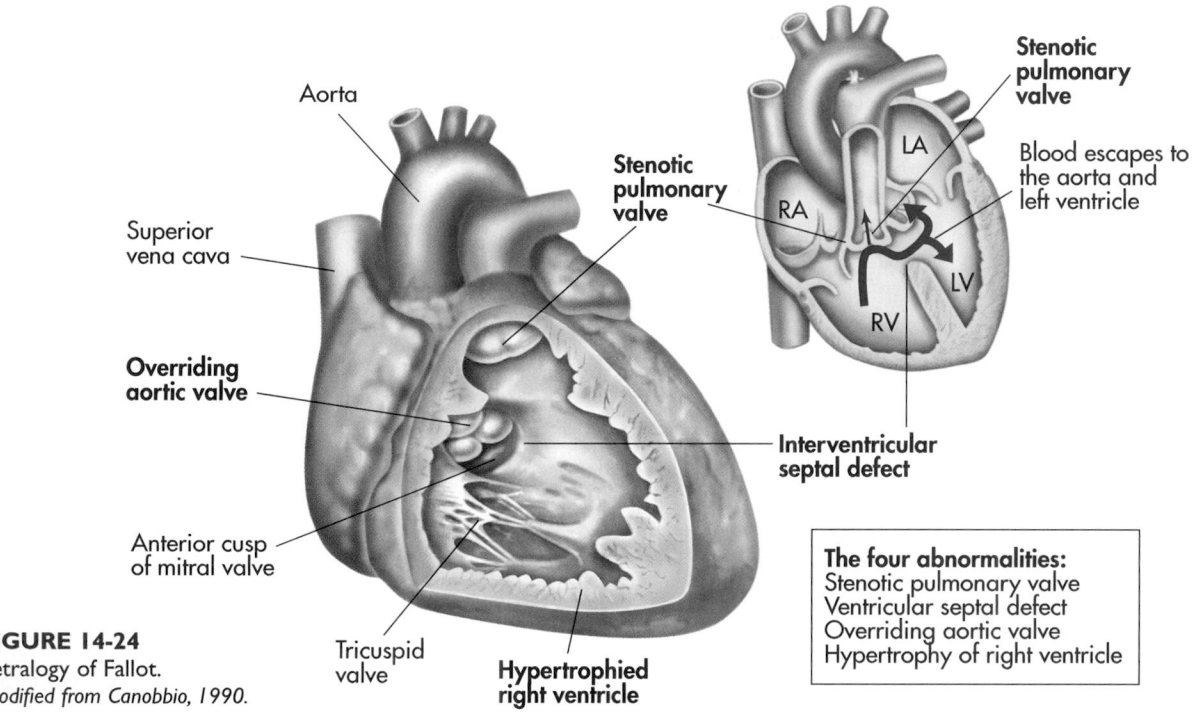

FIGURE 14-24
Tetralogy of Fallot.
Modified from Canobbio, 1990.

The four abnormalities:
Stenotic pulmonary valve
Ventricular septal defect
Overriding aortic valve
Hypertrophy of right ventricle

VENTRICULAR SEPTAL DEFECT

Ventricular septal defect is an opening between the left and right ventricles. The arterial pulse is small, and the jugular venous pulse is unaffected. Regurgitation occurs through the septal defect; as a result, the murmur tends to be holosystolic. It is often loud, coarse, high-pitched, and best heard along the left sternal border in the third to fifth intercostal spaces. A distinct lift is often discernible along the left sternal border and the apical area. A smaller defect causes a louder murmur and a more easily felt thrill than a large one (Fig. 14-25). This murmur does not radiate to the neck, whereas a similar murmur—the result of subaortic stenosis (see Table 14-5)—does.

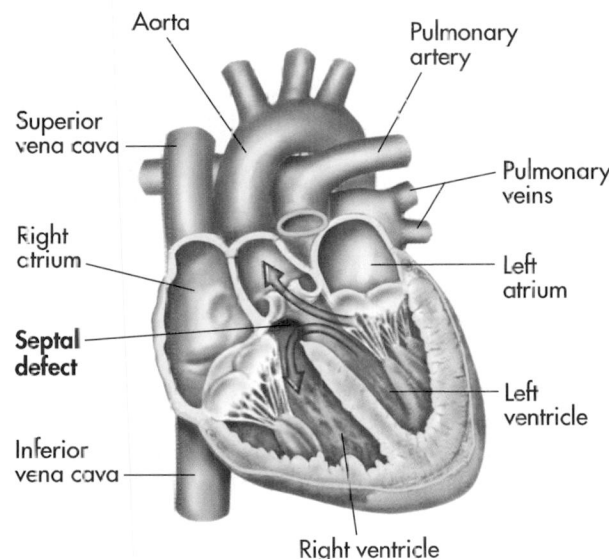

FIGURE 14-25
Ventricular septal defect.
Modified from Canobbio, 1990.

PATENT DUCTUS ARTERIOSUS

Sometimes the ductus arteriosus, which is patent in the fetal circulation, fails to close after birth. Blood flows through the ductus during systole and diastole, increasing the pressure in the pulmonary circulation and consequently the workload of the right ventricle. A small shunt can be asymptomatic; a larger one causes dyspnea on exertion. The neck vessels are dilated and pulsate, and the pulse pressure is wide. A harsh, loud, continuous murmur is often heard at the first to third intercostal spaces and the lower sternal border. It has a machine-like quality (Fig. 14-26). This murmur is usually, but not always, unaltered by postural change, quite unlike the murmur of a venous hum.

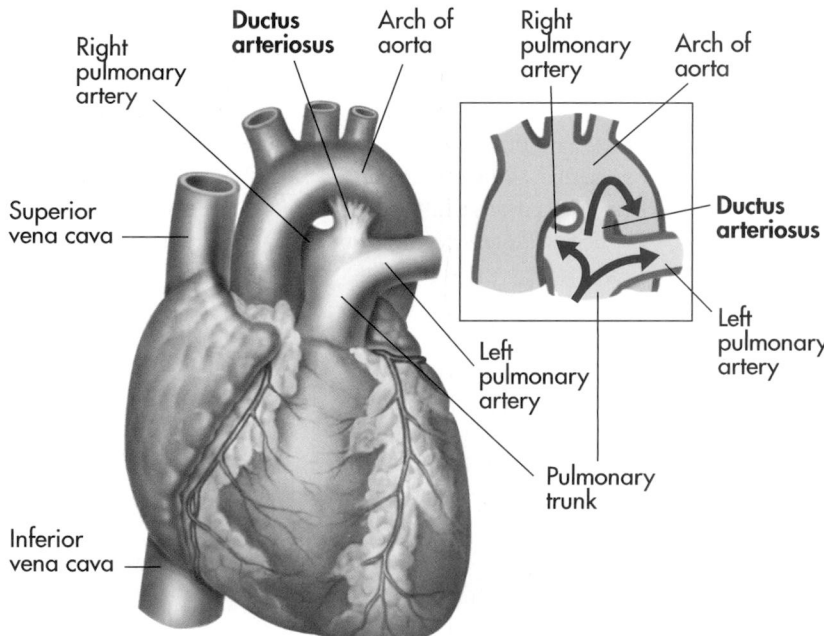

FIGURE 14-26
Patent ductus arteriosus.
Modified from Canobbio, 1990.

ATRIAL SEPTAL DEFECT

A congenital defect in the septum dividing the left and right atria causes a systolic ejection murmur that is diamond shaped, often loud, high in pitch, and harsh. It is heard best over the pulmonic area and not over the lesion, and may be accompanied by a brief, rumbling, early diastolic murmur. It does not usually radiate beyond the precordium. A systolic thrill may be felt over the area of the murmur, along with a palpable parasternal thrust. S_2 may be split fairly widely (Fig. 14-27). Sometimes this murmur may not sound particularly impressive and, especially in an overweight child, may seem of little consequence. Still, if there is a palpable thrust and radiation through to the back, it is more apt to be significant.

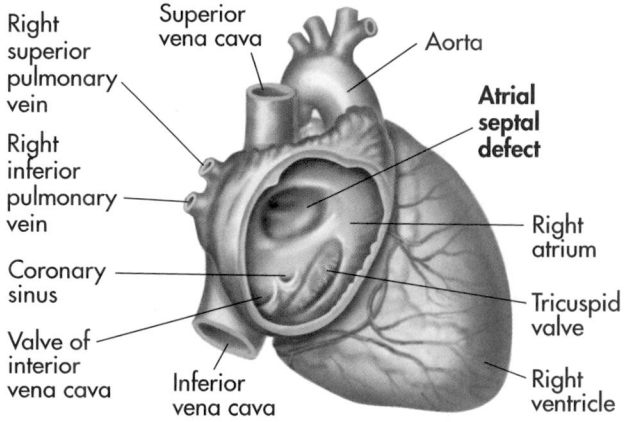

FIGURE 14-27
Atrial septal defect.
From Canobbio, 1990.

DEXTROCARDIA AND SITUS INVERSUS	Congenital abnormality of the heart in the presence of situs inversus is not very common; however, a right thoracic heart with normally placed stomach and liver should suggest congenital abnormalities such as pulmonic stenosis, ventricular or atrial septal defects, and transposition of the great vessels. As an affected infant matures, an unusually placed heart can change the clinical manifestations of disease by adulthood. For example, the substernal pressure of myocardial ischemia may be felt to the right of the precordium and may more often radiate into the right arm rather than to the left, the usual site when the heart is in its expected place.
ACUTE RHEUMATIC FEVER	Acute rheumatic fever is a systemic connective tissue disease that occurs after a streptococcal pharyngitis or skin infection; it is characterized by a variety of major and minor manifestations (Box 14-10). It may result in serious cardiac valvular involvement of the mitral or aortic valve. Often the affected valve becomes both stenotic and regurgitant. The tricuspid and pulmonic valves may be, but are not often, affected. The major physical findings may include the murmurs of mitral regurgitation and aortic insufficiency; cardiomegaly; the friction rub of pericarditis; congestive heart failure; a migratory polyarthritis (most commonly in the larger joints); chorea (at times without other manifestations); a transient erythema marginatum (pink margins with pale centers); and, rarely in recent years, firm, painless subcutaneous nodules, particularly on, but not limited to, the elbows, knees, and wrists. Although there has been a marked diminution in the incidence of rheumatic fever in the last 20 years, there is a recent worrisome resurgence. Children between 5 and 15 years of age are most commonly affected. Prevention—adequate treatment for streptococcal pharyngitis or skin infections—is the best therapy.

BOX 14-10

REVISED JONES CRITERIA FOR GUIDANCE IN THE DIAGNOSIS OF RHEUMATIC FEVER

Major Manifestations	**Minor Manifestations**
Carditis	*Clinical*
Polyarthritis	Previous rheumatic fever or rheumatic heart disease
Chorea	Arthralgia
Erythema marginatum	Fever
Subcutaneous nodules	*Laboratory*
	Acute phase reactions: erythrocyte sedimentation rate, C-reactive protein, leukocytosis
	Prolonged P-R interval on ECG

Supporting Evidence of Streptococcal Infection
- Increased titer of antistreptolysin antibodies (antistreptolysin O in particular)
- Positive throat culture for group A streptococci
- Recent scarlet fever

   The presence of two major or one major and two minor manifestations suggests a high probability of acute rheumatic fever, if supported by evidence of a preceding group A streptococcal infection. You should never make the diagnosis on the basis of laboratory findings and two minor manifestations alone.

From the American Heart Association, 1984.

Older Adults

ATHEROSCLEROTIC HEART DISEASE	Atherosclerotic heart disease, a condition caused by deposition of cholesterol, other lipids, and by a complex inflammatory process, leads to vascular wall thickening and ultimate narrowing of the vascular lumen. It may cause myocardial insufficiency, angina pectoris, dysrhythmias, and congestive heart failure.
MITRAL INSUFFICIENCY	Mitral insufficiency is usually silent and painless until it produces sudden heart failure, stroke, or dysrhythmias. It also occurs after infarction involving the mitral chordae, along with tachycardia, pallor, a variety of alterations in the heart sounds, occasional pericardial friction rub, various murmurs, and dysrhythmias.
ANGINA	The definition of angina is pain. With reference to the heart, it indicates a substernal pain or intense pressure radiating at times to the neck; jaws; and the arms, particularly the left. It is often accompanied by shortness of breath, fatigue, diaphoresis, faintness, and syncope. Although angina is listed as a common abnormality in the older adult, it can occur, of course, in much younger men and women.
SENILE CARDIAC AMYLOIDOSIS	Amyloid deposits in the heart cause heart failure. Amyloid is itself a fibrillary protein produced by chronic inflammation or neoplastic disease. Electrocardiography or echocardiography shows a small, thickened left ventricle, and the right ventricle may also be thickened. The contractility of the heart may at times be reduced.
AORTIC SCLEROSIS	Older adults, and even some persons of middle age, may develop thickening and calcification of the aortic valves. The result need not be a significant obstruction to left ventricular outflow, but regardless of severity, there may be a midsystolic (ejection) murmur.

ELECTRONIC RESOURCES

For Weblinks and additional resources, go to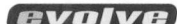

http://evolve.elsevier.com/Seidel

or to the Companion CD-ROM.

Additional information related to the content in Chapter 14 can be found on the companion website at evolve.elsevier.com/Seidel/ or on the interactive companion CD-ROM. Resources and activities for Chapter 14 include:

- Sound and Vision Theater
- Printouts for Your Practice
- Interactive Challenge
- Spanish Assessment Terms with Pronunciation Guide
- Instant Calculator

BLOOD VESSELS

ANATOMY AND PHYSIOLOGY

The great vessels, the arteries leading from and the veins leading to the heart, are located in a cluster at the base of the heart. They include the aorta, superior and inferior vena cavae, pulmonary arteries, and pulmonary veins (Fig. 15-1). The aorta carries oxygenated blood out of the left ventricle to the body. The pulmonary artery, which leaves the right ventricle and divides almost immediately into right and left branches, carries blood to the lungs. The superior and inferior vena cavae carry blood from the upper and lower body, respectively, to the right atrium. The pulmonary veins return oxygenated blood from the lungs to the left atrium.

BLOOD CIRCULATION

Once it leaves the heart, blood flows through two circulatory systems: the pulmonary and the systemic. The heart and these two systems create a closed system that distributes oxygen and nutrients to all parts of the body (Fig. 15-2).

The pulmonary circulation routes blood through the lungs, where it is reoxygenated before moving on to the rest of the body. Venous blood arrives at the right atrium via the superior and inferior vena cavae and moves through the tricuspid valve to the right ventricle. During systole, unoxygenated blood is ejected through the pulmonic valve into the pulmonary artery; it travels through increasingly smaller and more numerous arteries, arterioles, and capillaries of the lungs until it reaches the alveoli, where gas exchange occurs.

Oxygenated blood returns to the heart through the pulmonary veins into the left atrium, then through the mitral valve into the left ventricle. The left ventricle contracts, forcing a volume of blood with each beat (stroke volume) through the aortic valve into the aorta, and then through the arterial system and capillaries. In the capillary bed, oxygen is provided to the tissues of the body; the deoxygenated blood, now carbon dioxide rich, then passes into the venous system and returns to the heart (Fig. 15-3). The stroke volume (SV) multiplied by the heart rate per minute (R) gives the cardiac output (CO), a measure of the heart's ability to adapt to the changing demands of the body.

The structure of the arteries and veins reflects their function. The arteries are tougher, more tensile, and less distensible. They are subjected to much more pressure than are the veins. The veins are less sturdy and more passive than the arteries (Fig. 15-4). Because venous return is less forceful than blood flow through the arteries, veins contain valves to keep blood

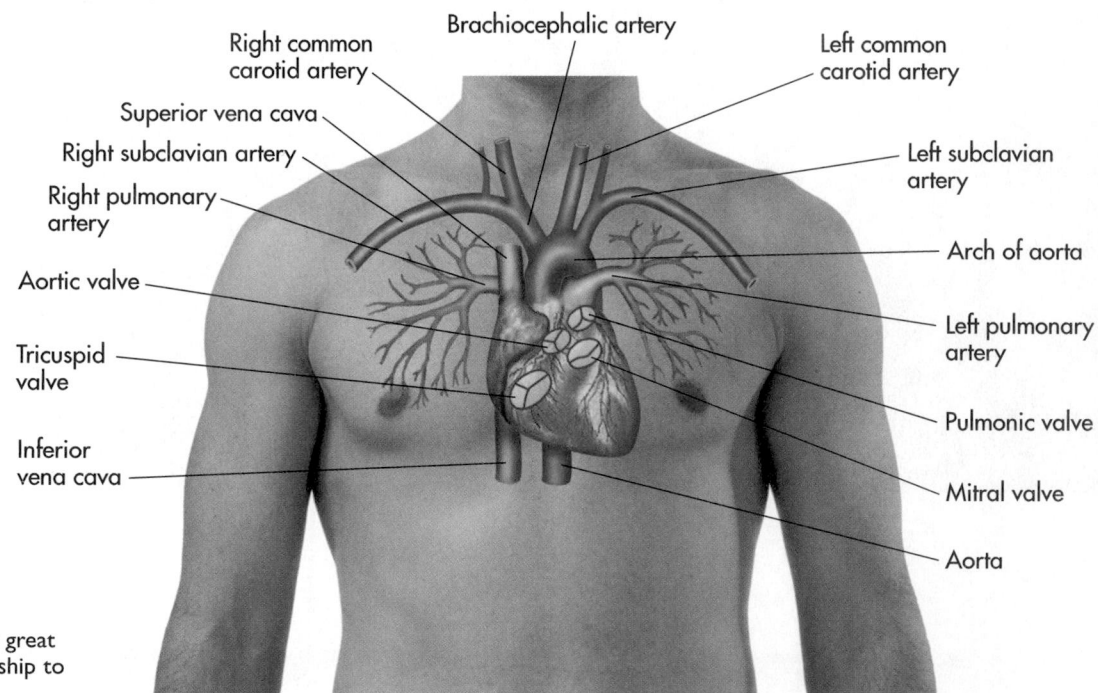

FIGURE 15-1
Anatomic location of the great vessels and their relationship to the heart valves.

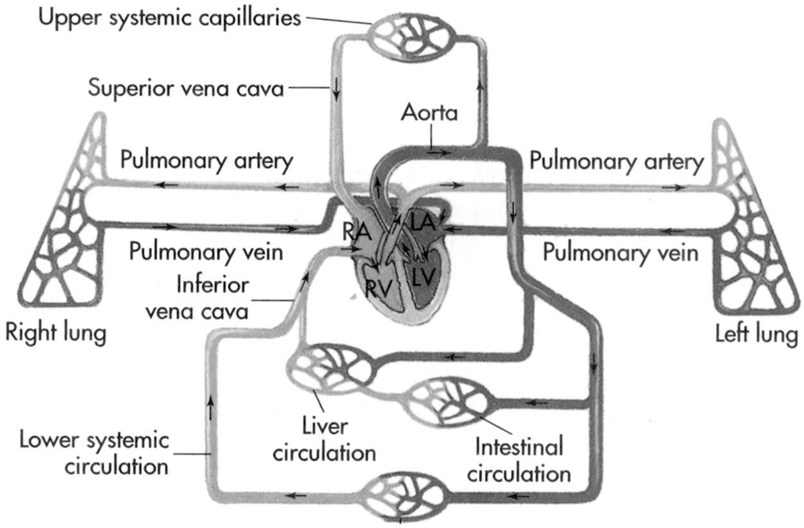

FIGURE 15-2
Circulatory system.
From Canobbio, 1990.

flowing in one direction. If blood volume increases significantly, the veins can expand and act as a repository for extra blood. This compensatory mechanism helps diminish stress on the heart.

ARTERIAL PULSE AND PRESSURE

The palpable and sometimes visible arterial pulses are the result of ventricular systole, which produces a pressure wave throughout the arterial system (arterial pulse). It takes barely 0.2 second for the impact of this wave to be felt in the dorsalis pedis artery, and considerably more than 2 seconds for a red blood cell to travel the same distance. The arterial blood pressure is the force exerted by the blood against the wall of an artery as the ventricles of the heart contract and relax.

The pulse usually is felt as a forceful wave that is smooth and more rapid on the ascending part of the wave; it becomes domed, less steep, and slower on the descending part. Because the carotid arteries are the most accessible of the arteries closest to the heart, they have the most definitive pulse for evaluation of cardiac function (Fig. 15-5).

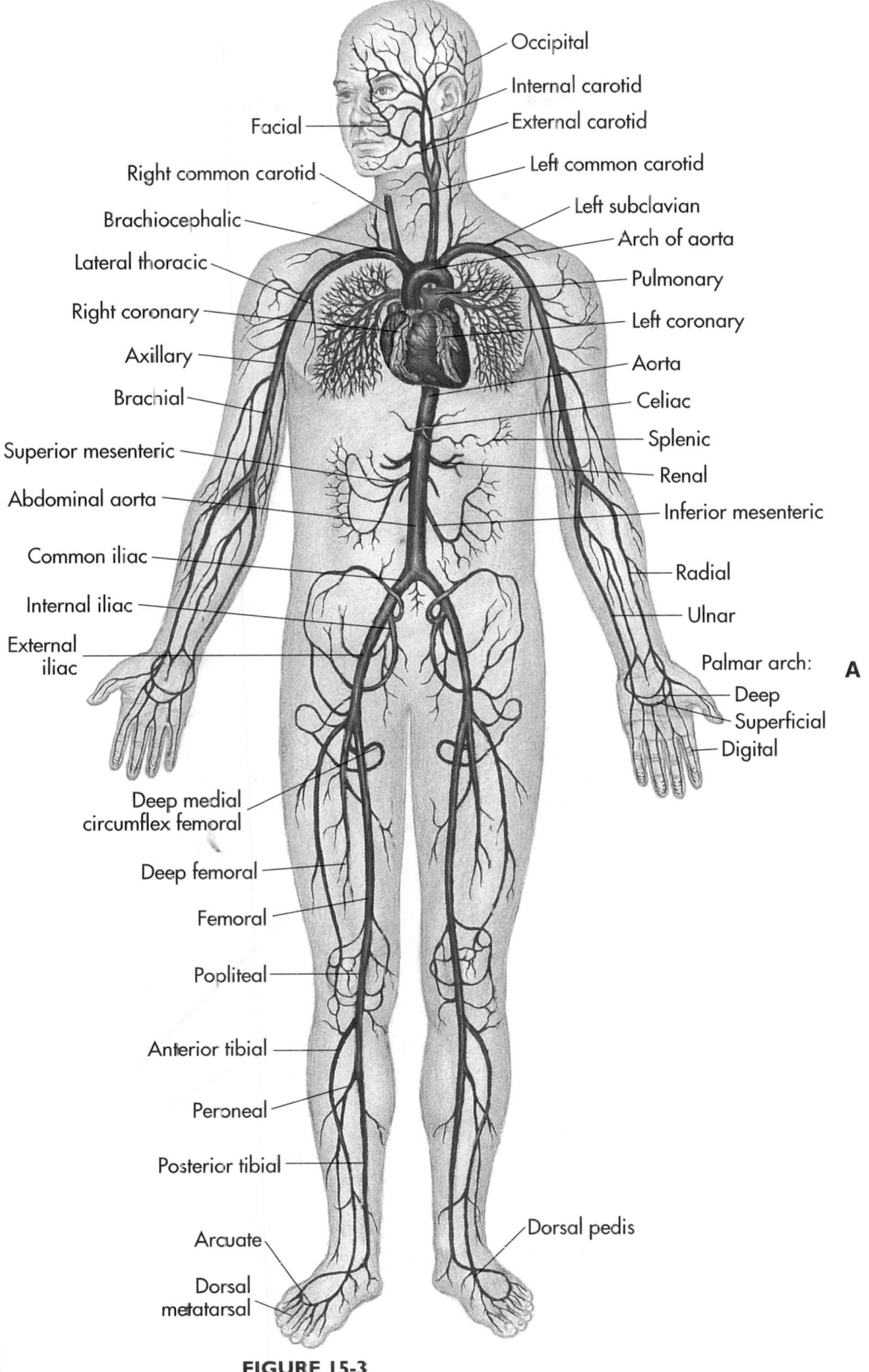

FIGURE 15-3
Systemic circulation. **A,** Arteries.

Continued

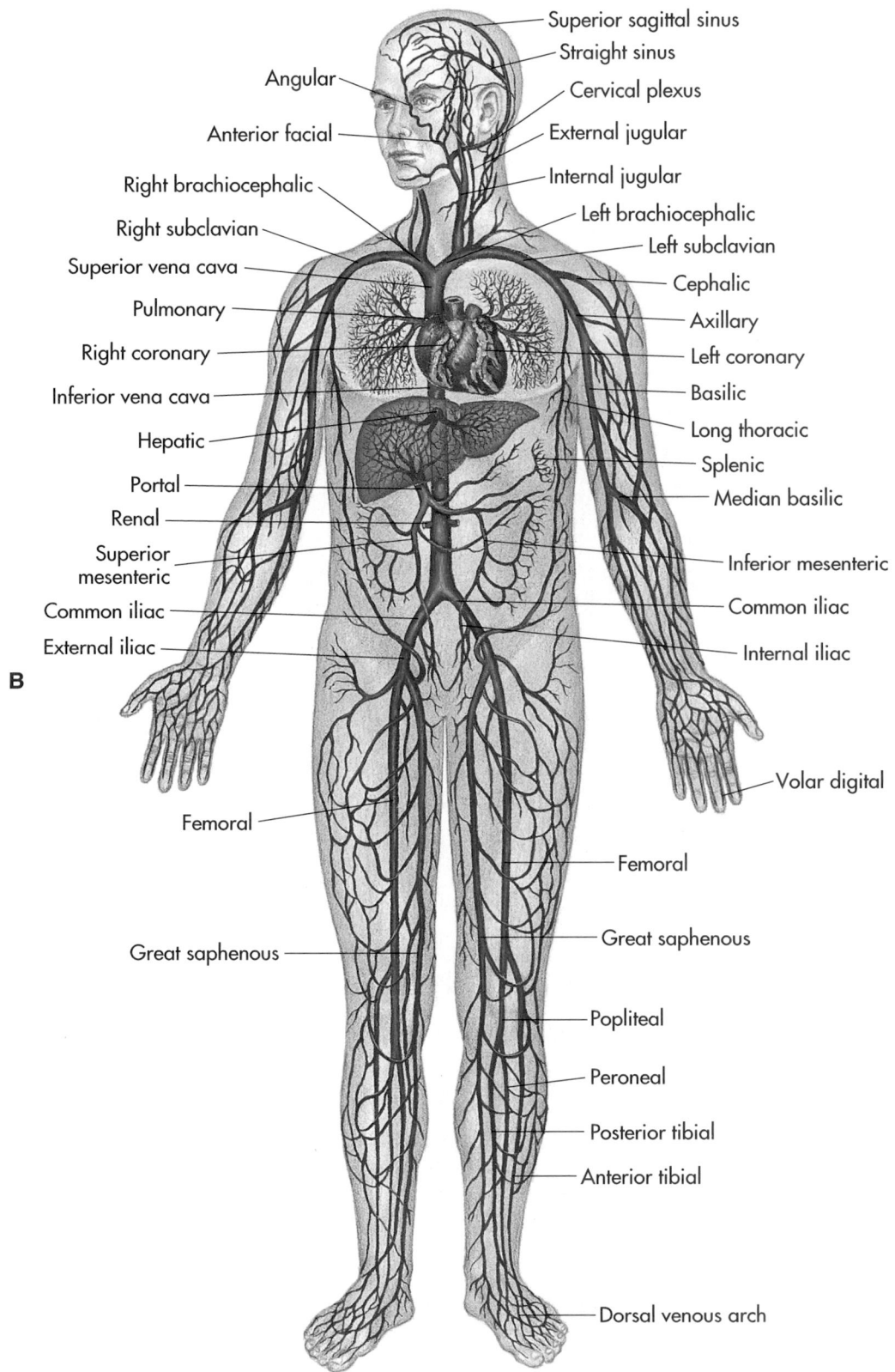

Superior sagittal sinus
Straight sinus
Cervical plexus
External jugular
Internal jugular
Left brachiocephalic
Left subclavian
Cephalic
Axillary
Left coronary
Basilic
Long thoracic
Splenic
Median basilic
Inferior mesenteric
Common iliac
Internal iliac
Volar digital

Angular
Anterior facial
Right brachiocephalic
Right subclavian
Superior vena cava
Pulmonary
Right coronary
Inferior vena cava
Hepatic
Portal
Renal
Superior mesenteric
Common iliac
External iliac

B

Femoral
Femoral
Great saphenous
Great saphenous
Popliteal
Peroneal
Posterior tibial
Anterior tibial
Dorsal venous arch

FIGURE 15-3, cont'd
Systemic circulation. **B,** Veins.

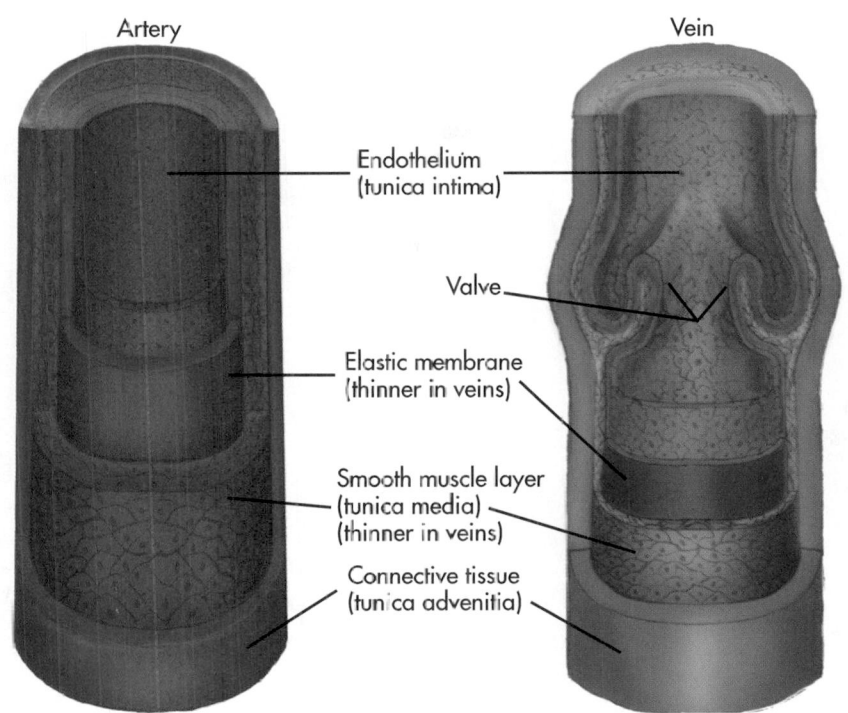

FIGURE 15-4
Structure of arteries and veins. Note the relative thickness of the arterial wall.

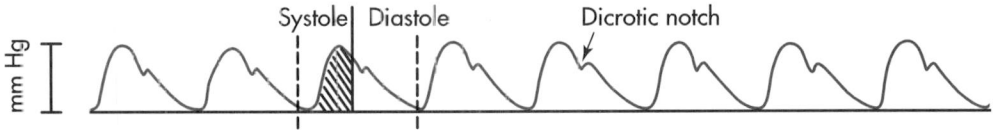

FIGURE 15-5
Diagram of usual pulse.
From Barkauskas et al, 1998.

Arterial blood pressure has both systolic and diastolic components. Systolic pressure is the force exerted against the wall of the artery when the ventricles contract; it is largely the result of cardiac output, blood volume, and compliance of the arterial tree. Blood pressure is its highest during systole. Diastolic pressure is the force exerted against the wall of the artery when the heart is in the filling or relaxed state and is primarily the function of peripheral vascular resistance. During diastole, pressure falls to its lowest point. Pulse pressure is the difference between systolic and diastolic pressures. The following variables contribute to the characteristics of the pulses:

- Volume of blood ejected (stroke volume)
- Distensibility of the aorta and large arteries
- Viscosity of the blood
- Peripheral arteriolar resistance

JUGULAR VENOUS PULSE AND PRESSURE

The jugular veins, which empty directly into the superior vena cava, reflect the activity of the right side of the heart and offer clues to its competency. The level at which the jugular venous pulse is visible gives an indication of right atrial pressure.

The external jugular veins are more superficial and are more visible bilaterally above the clavicle, close to the insertion of the sternocleidomastoid muscles. The larger internal jugular veins run deep to the sternocleidomastoids, near the carotid arteries, and are less accessible to inspection (Fig. 15-6).

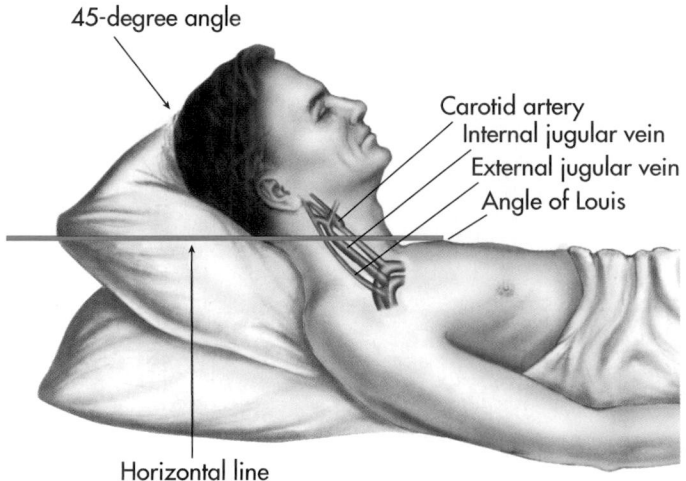

FIGURE 15-6
Inspection of jugular venous pressure.
From Thompson et al, 1997.

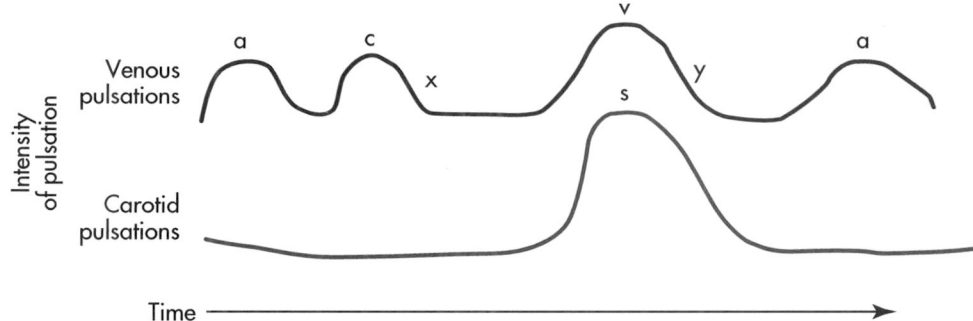

FIGURE 15-7
Expected venous pulsations.

The activity of the right side of the heart is transmitted back through the jugular veins as a pulse* that has five identifiable components—three peaks and two descending slopes (Fig. 15-7):

a wave	The a wave, the first and most prominent component, is the result of a brief backflow of blood to the vena cava during right atrial contraction.
c wave	The c wave is a transmitted impulse from the vigorous backward push produced by closure of the tricuspid valve during ventricular systole.
v wave	The v wave is caused by the increasing volume and concomitant increasing pressure in the right atrium. It occurs a split moment after the c wave, late in ventricular systole.
x slope	The downward x slope is caused by passive atrial filling.
y slope	The y slope following the v wave reflects the open tricuspid valve and the rapid filling of the ventricle.

INFANTS AND CHILDREN

At birth the cutting of the umbilical cord, through which oxygen has been provided in utero, necessitates that the lungs begin their work and that the infant begins to breathe. The onset of respiration expands the lungs and carries air to the alveoli. Pulmonary vascular resistance drops and systemic vascular resistance increases. Blood, therefore, flows more freely to the lungs and less freely systemically. The ductus arteriosus closes, usually within the first 12 to 14 hours of life. Once pulmonary vascular resistance is lower than systemic, blood is shunted from the aorta to the pulmonary arteries so that the interatrial foramen ovale is functionally closed by the shifting pressures.

PREGNANT WOMEN

Systemically, vascular resistance decreases and peripheral vasodilation occurs, often resulting in palmar erythema and spider telangiectases. The systolic blood pressure decreases slightly. There is a greater decrease in the diastolic pressure. The lowest levels occur in the second trimester and then rise but still remain below pre-pregnancy levels. Blood pressure determinations can be affected by maternal position. Hypotension is more often noted when the patient is supine during the third trimester. The hypotension is secondary to venous occlusion

---

*Although often referred to as a pulse, this is not the same as an arterial pulse because it is reflected back from the right heart rather than pushed forward by the left heart. Unlike arterial pulses, it cannot be palpated, only visualized.

of the vena cava and impaired venous return. Blood in the lower extremities tends to stagnate in later pregnancy—except when the woman is in the lateral recumbent position—as a result of occlusion of the pelvic veins and inferior vena cava from pressure created by the enlarged uterus. The occlusion results in an increase in dependent edema, varicosities of the legs and vulva, and hemorrhoids.

Older Adults

Calcification and other changes noted histologically in the walls of the arteries, at first proximally and then throughout, cause dilation and tortuosity of the aorta, aortic branches, and the carotid arteries. The superficial vessels of the forehead, neck, and extremities also become tortuous and more prominent. The arterial walls lose elasticity and vasomotor tone, thus diminishing the ability of the artery to comply with changing body needs. Increased peripheral vascular resistance usually elevates blood pressure. Increased vasopressor lability tends to increase both systolic and diastolic pressures progressively.

REVIEW OF RELATED HISTORY

For each of the conditions discussed in this section, targeted topics to include in the history of the present illness are listed. Responses to questions about these topics help fully assess the patient's condition and provide clues for focusing the physical examination.

HISTORY OF PRESENT ILLNESS

- Leg pain or cramps
  - Onset and duration: with activity or rest, with elevation of legs, recent injury or immobilization
  - Character
    Continuous burning in toes, pain when pointing toes, pain in thighs or buttocks, "charley horses," aching, pain over specific location, induced by activity, amount of activity
    Skin changes: Cold skin, pallor, hair loss, sores, redness or warmth over vein, visible veins, region of skin darkening, becoming black, development of odor
  - Increased tendency to bruise easily or bleed excessively
- Dizziness (see Chapter 12)
  - Fatigue or limping: Occurs with walking, improves with walking
  - Wake up at night
- Severe headaches
  - Onset and duration: upon first awakening, diminishing as day progresses, disappearing in the afternoon
  - Location: over the occiput, in the frontal area
  - Character: throbbing, dull, stabbing
  - Known history of hypertension
- Swollen ankles
  - Onset and duration: present in the morning, appearing as the day progresses, sudden onset, insidious onset
  - Related circumstances: recent and long airplane travel, recent travel to high elevations
  - Associated symptoms: onset of nocturia, increased frequency of urination, increasing shortness of breath
- Treatment attempted
  - Rest
  - Massage
  - Heat

Clinical Pearl
Antihypertensives and Bone Loss
Some antihypertensive medications, particularly thiazide-type diuretics and beta blockers, protect against bone loss and the possibility of fractures, an added benefit, particularly in older adults.

- Elevation
- Medication: heparin, warfarin, diuretics, antihypertensive medications, nonprescription medications (including nonsteroidal antiinflammatory drugs), complementary or alternative therapies

PAST MEDICAL HISTORY

- Cardiac surgery or hospitalization for cardiac evaluation or disorder, congenital heart defect, procedures to correct vascular disease
- Acute rheumatic fever, unexplained fever, swollen joints, inflammatory rheumatism, St. Vitus dance (Sydenham chorea)
- Chronic illness: hypertension and studies to define its cause, bleeding disorder, hyperlipidemia, diabetes, thyroid dysfunction, coronary artery disease, atrial fibrillation or other type of dysrhythmia, thrombophlebitis

FAMILY HISTORY

- Diabetes
- Heart disease
- Hyperlipidemia
- Hypertension
- Family members with risk factors, morbidity, mortality related to cardiovascular system; hypertension, peripheral vascular disease, ages at time of illness or death

PERSONAL AND SOCIAL HISTORY

- Employment: physical demands; environmental hazards such as heat, chemicals, dust; sources of emotional stress
- Tobacco: type (cigarettes, cigars, pipe, chewing tobacco, snuff), duration of use, amount, age started and, perhaps, stopped; pack-years (number of years smoking times number of packs per day)
- Nutritional status
  - Usual diet: proportion of fat, food preferences, history of dieting
  - Weight: loss or gain, amount and rate
  - Known hypercholesterolemia and/or hypertriglyceridemia
- Personality assessment: intensity, hostile attitudes, inability to relax, compulsive behavior
- Relaxation
  - Hobbies
  - Exercise: type, amount, frequency, intensity (see Box 14-3)
  - Sexual activity: frequency of intercourse, sexual practices, number of partners

STAYING WELL
COMPONENTS OF A HEALTHY DIET

Those whose nutritional lives center on a diet common to the region around the Mediterranean Sea have taught us that we should use olive oil consistently in our diets. This, in addition to a disciplined, *moderate* intake of wine, is helpful in the effort to decrease the risk of hypertension and associated cardiac problems. An undisciplined, immoderate habit of alcohol consumption negates any advantage. The message then: olive oil in abundance, wine in moderation. More than two glasses of wine a day becomes inappropriate and an additional bottle of beer is too much.

- Use of alcohol: amount consumed, frequency, duration of current intake
- Use of illegal drugs: amyl nitrate ("poppers"), cocaine
- Use of nonprescription drugs, complementary or other alternative therapies

INFANTS AND CHILDREN
- Hemophilia
- Renal disease
- Coarctation of the aorta
- Leg pains during exercise

PREGNANT WOMEN
- Blood pressure: pre-pregnancy levels, elevation during pregnancy; associated symptoms and signs, such as headaches, visual changes, nausea and vomiting, epigastric pain, right upper quadrant pain, oliguria, rapid onset of edema (facial, abdominal, or peripheral), hyperreflexia, proteinuria, unusual bruising or bleeding
- Legs: edema, varicosities, pain or discomfort
- Use of nonprescription drugs, complementary or alternative therapies. Ask specifically about calcium supplementation, particularly during the second trimester. (It is now known that calcium intake can reduce the risk of hypertension in pregnancy; it may also reduce the risk of hypertension in the offspring.)

OLDER ADULTS
- Leg edema: pattern, frequency, time of day most pronounced
- Interference with activities of daily living
- Ability of the patient and family to cope with the condition, perceived and actual
- Claudication: area involved, unilateral or bilateral, distance one can walk before its onset, characteristic sensation, length of time required for relief
- Medications used for relief; efficacy of drugs

RISK FACTORS
PREECLAMPSIA

- Older than 40 years of age
- First pregnancy
- Black
- Preexisting chronic hypertension
- Renal disease or diabetes mellitus
- Multifetal gestation
- Family history of preeclampsia or gestational hypertension
- Previous preeclampsia or gestational hypertension
- Obesity

RISK FACTORS
VARICOSE VEINS

- Gender: women four times more often than men (during pregnancy in particular, increased hormonal levels weaken the walls of the vein and result in failure of the valves)
- Genetic predisposition (persons of Irish or German descent, daughters of women with varicosities, and genetically predisposed women taking birth control pills)
- Sedentary lifestyle (habitual inactivity allows blood to pool in the veins, resulting in edema; thus the valves are compromised)
- Age (the veins of older adults are less elastic and, as a result, more apt to succumb to varicosity)
- Race (blacks have a lower incidence of varicosities than whites, probably because they have more venous valves in the lower legs than whites)

EXAMINATION AND FINDINGS

EQUIPMENT

- Marking pencil
- Centimeter rule, both tape and folding rulers at least 15 cm long
- Stethoscope with bell and diaphragm
- Sphygmomanometer with appropriately sized cuff (see Fig. 3-2)

The examination of the vascular system includes the following: (1) observing and palpating the pulses, comparing each with the contralateral pulse and comparing pulses of the upper extremity with those of the lower; (2) inspecting the veins, particularly the jugular veins; (3) measuring blood pressure in both upper extremities with the patient sitting, standing, and supine, when there is clinical indication; and measuring the blood pressure in both lower extremities when there is a clinical indication.

The parts of the physical examination should be performed in a sequence that is comfortable for you. Findings from examinations of other systems besides the vascular (e.g., the funduscopic changes of hypertension) are exceedingly valuable. As already noted, no system can be appropriately evaluated outside the context of the entire examination, and performing a successful examination requires a mastery of the mechanics of each procedure.

PERIPHERAL ARTERIES

PALPATION

Blood Vessels:
Palpating the Carotid Arteries

CLINICAL PEARL

Carotid Palpation
When palpating the carotid arteries, never palpate both sides simultaneously. Excessive carotid sinus massage can cause slowing of the pulse, a drop in blood pressure, and compromise of blood flow to the brain. The resultant effect could be possible circulatory embarrassment, particularly in older adults who may already have compromised cardiovascular function. If you have difficulty feeling the pulse, rotate the patient's head to the side being examined to relax the sternocleidomastoid muscle.

The pulses are best palpated over arteries that are close to the surface of the body and that lie over bones. These include the carotid, brachial, radial, femoral, popliteal, dorsalis pedis, and posterior tibial (Table 15-1; Fig. 15-8).

An arterial pulsation is essentially a bounding wave of blood with varying vigor that diminishes with increasing distance from the heart. Of all the arterial pulses, the carotids are most easily accessible and closest to the cardiac source and thus most useful in evaluating heart activity. The arterial pulses in the extremities are examined to determine the sufficiency of the entire arterial circulation. Palpate at least one pulse point in each extremity, usually at the most distal point.

Examine the arterial pulses with the digital pads of the second and third fingers. Despite traditional advice to the contrary, the thumb may also be used; if vessels have a tendency to move when probed by fingers, the thumb is particularly useful in "fixing" the brachial and even the femoral pulses. Palpate firmly but not so hard as to occlude the artery.

TABLE 15-1	Locations of Palpable Pulses
Pulse	**Location**
Carotid	In the neck, just medial to and below angle of the jaw (do not palpate both sides simultaneously)
Brachial	Just medial to biceps tendon
Radial	Medial and ventral side of wrist (gentle pressure)
Femoral	Below the inguinal ligament midway between the symphysis pubis and the anterior superior iliac spine
Popliteal	Popliteal fossa (press firmly); the patient should be prone with the knee flexed
Dorsalis pedis	Medial side of dorsum of foot with foot slightly dorsiflexed (pulse may be hard to feel and may not be palpable in some well persons)
Posterior tibial	Behind and slightly inferior to medial malleolus of ankle (pulse may be hard to feel and may not be palpable in some well persons)

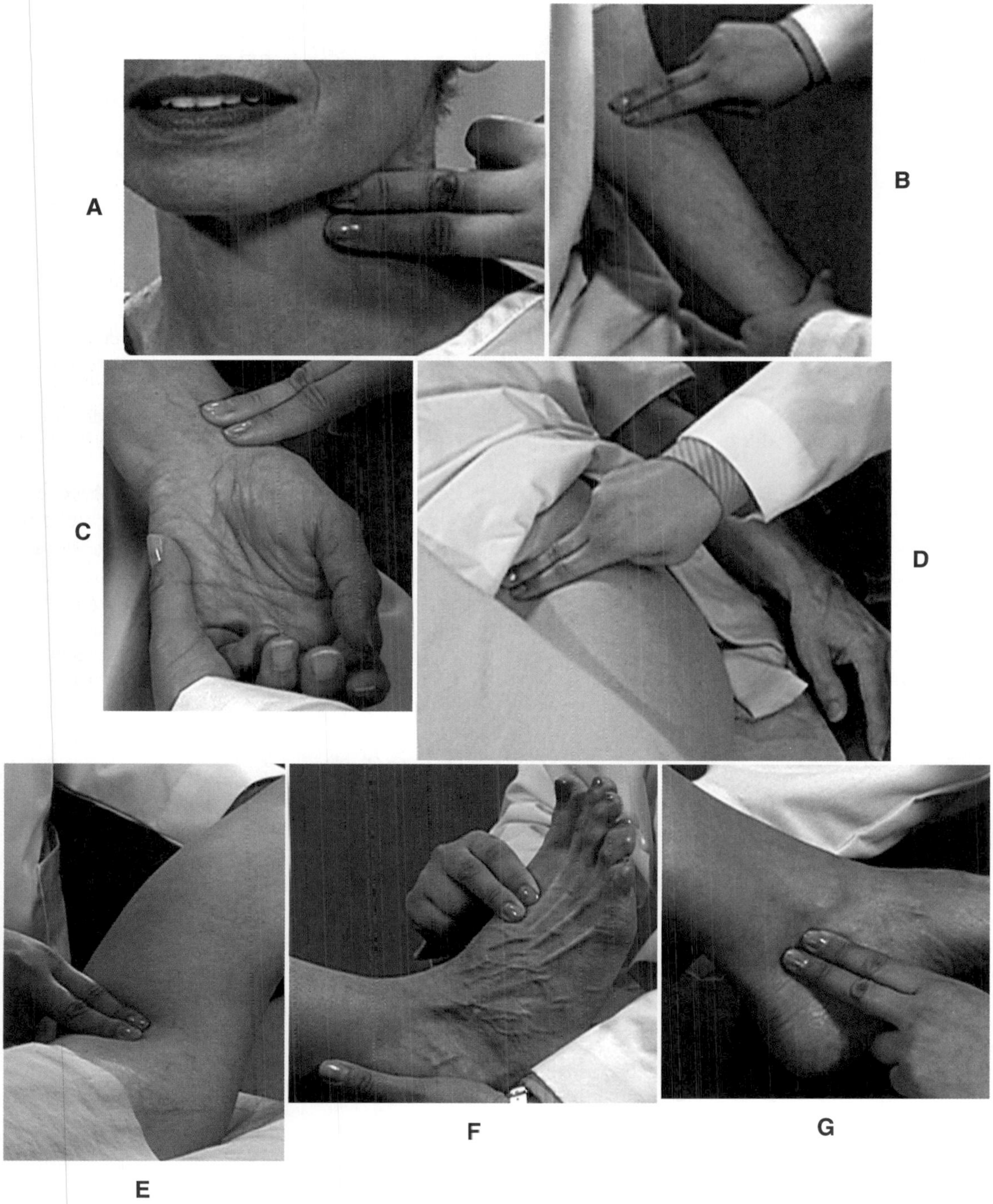

A

B

C

D

E

F

G

FIGURE 15-8
Palpation of arterial pulses. **A,** Carotid. **B,** Brachial. **C,** Radial. **D,** Femoral. **E,** Popliteal. **F,** Dorsalis pedis. **G,** Posterior tibial.

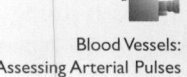

Blood Vessels:
Assessing Arterial Pulses

If you have difficulty finding a pulse, try varying your pressure, feeling carefully throughout the area. Make sure when you locate the pulse that you are not feeling your own pulse. A pulse is most readily felt over a bony prominence; therefore in some areas (particularly the feet), fat or edema may make it difficult to feel the pulse.

Palpate the arterial pulses (most often the radial) to assess the heart rate and rhythm; pulse contour (waveform); amplitude (force); symmetry; and, sometimes, obstructions to blood flow. Variations from the expected findings are described in Table 15-2 and Fig. 15-9.

TABLE 15-2	Arterial Pulse Abnormalities	
Type	**Description**	**Associated Conditions**
Alternating pulse (pulsus alternans)	Regular rate; amplitude varies from beat to beat with weak and strong beats	Left ventricular failure (see Fig. 15-9, A)
Pulsus bisferiens	Two strong systolic peaks separated by a midsystolic dip	Aortic regurgitation alone or with stenosis (see Fig. 15-9, B)
Bigeminal pulse (pulsus bigeminus)	Two beats in rapid succession followed by longer interval; easily confused with alternating pulse	Regularly occurring ventricular premature beats (see Fig. 15-9, C)
Bounding pulse	Increased pulse pressure; contour may have rapid rise, brief peak, rapid fall	Atherosclerosis, aortic rigidity, patent ductus arteriosus, fever, anemia, hyperthyroidism, anxiety, exercise (see Fig. 15-9, D)
Bradycardia	Rate less than 60	Hypothermia, hypothyroidism, drug intoxication, impaired cardiac conduction, excellent physical conditioning
Labile pulse	Pulse amplitude increased when patient is sitting or standing when compared with amplitude while supine	Not necessarily associated with disease; not a specific indicator of a problem
Paradoxic pulse (pulsus paradoxus)	Amplitude decreases on inspiration	Chronic obstructive pulmonary disease, constrictive pericarditis, pericardial effusion (see Fig. 15-9, E)
Pulsus differens	Unequal pulses between left and right extremities	Impaired circulation, usually from unilateral local obstruction
Tachycardia	Rate over 100	Fever, hyperthyroidism, anemia, shock, heart disease, anxiety, exercise
Trigeminal pulse (pulsus trigeminus)	Three beats followed by a pause	Often benign, such as after exercise, but may occur with cardiomyopathy, severe ventricular hypertrophy, severe aortic stenosis, dysfunctional right ventricle
Water-hammer pulse (Corrigan pulse)	Jerky pulse with full expansion followed by sudden collapse	Aortic regurgitation, patent ductus arteriosus (see Fig. 15-9, F)

The contour of the pulse wave is pliable: Healthy arteries have a smooth, rounded, or domed shape. Attention should be paid to the ascending portion, the peak, and the descending portion. Each wave crest should be compared with the next to detect cyclic differences.

The amplitude of the pulse is described on a scale of 0 to 4:

4	Bounding
3	Full, increased
2	Expected
1	Diminished, barely palpable
0	Absent, not palpable

The pulse rate (heart rate) is determined by counting the pulsations for 60 seconds (or by counting for 30 seconds and doubling the count). The duration of counting really depends on both the heart rate and the regularity. An irregular rhythm requires a longer period of counting. The resting pulse rate should range between 60 and 90 beats per minute.

Determine the steadiness of the heart rhythm; it should be regular. If it is irregular, determine whether there is a consistent pattern. A heart rate that is irregular but that occurs in a repeated pattern may indicate sinus arrhythmia, a cyclic variation of the heart rate characterized by an increasing rate on inspiration and decreasing rate on expiration. A patternless, unpredictable, irregular rate may indicate heart disease or conduction system impairment. If an irregularity in rate is noted, record the beats per minute and compare it with the rate heard when examining the heart (see Chapter 14). Record any deficit in the transmitted pulse.

Lack of symmetry (in contour or amplitude) between the left and right extremities suggests impaired circulation. Compare the amplitude of the upper extremity pulses with those of the lower extremities and the left with the right. Ordinarily, the femoral is as strong as or stronger than the radial pulse. If this is reversed or if the femoral pulsation is absent, coarctation of the aorta must be suspected.

PULSE   **POSSIBLE CAUSE**

Alternating pulse (pulsus alternans)

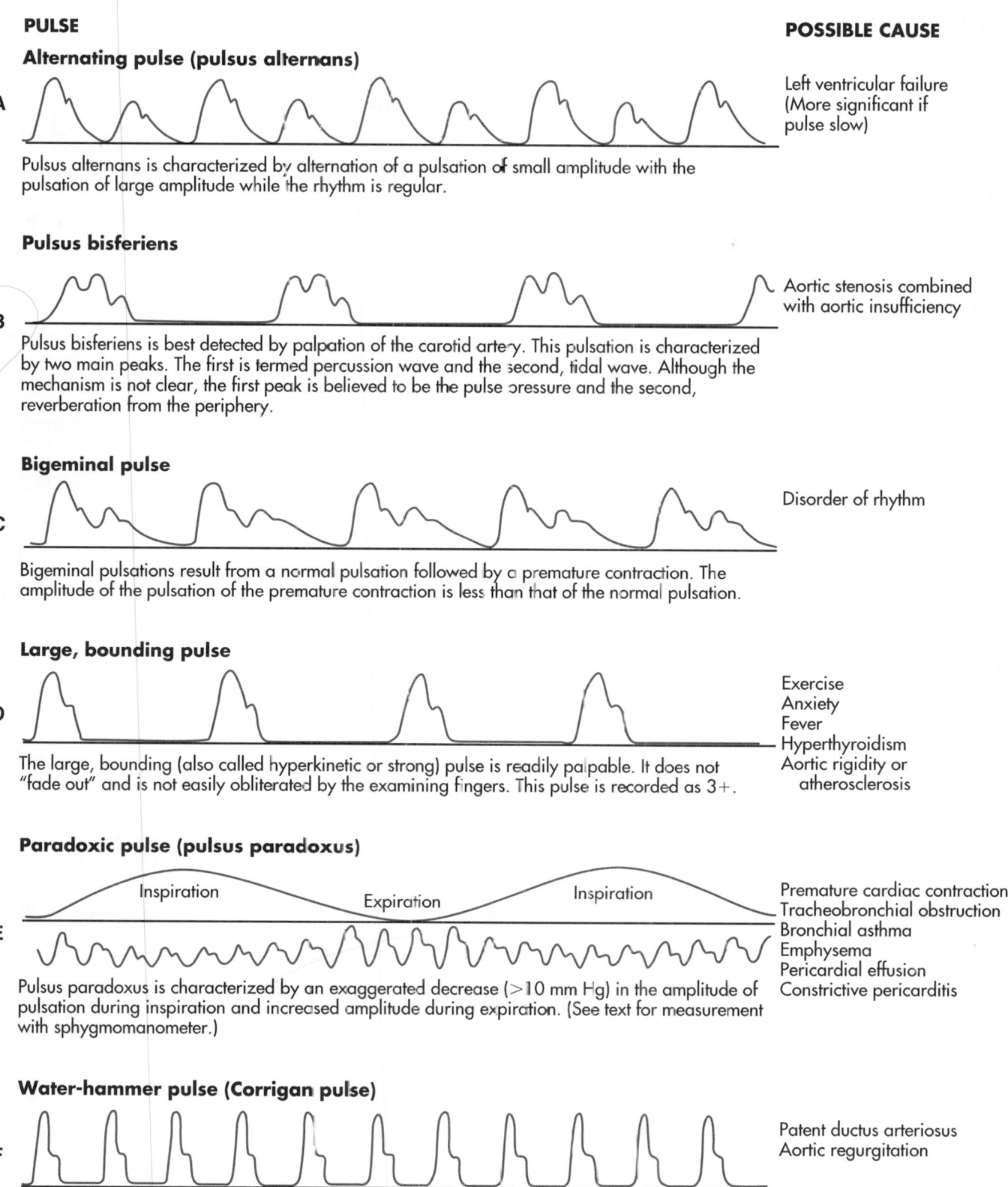

A

Pulsus alternans is characterized by alternation of a pulsation of small amplitude with the
pulsation of large amplitude while the rhythm is regular.

Left ventricular failure
(More significant if
pulse slow)

Pulsus bisferiens

B

Pulsus bisferiens is best detected by palpation of the carotid artery. This pulsation is characterized
by two main peaks. The first is termed percussion wave and the second, tidal wave. Although the
mechanism is not clear, the first peak is believed to be the pulse pressure and the second,
reverberation from the periphery.

Aortic stenosis combined
with aortic insufficiency

Bigeminal pulse

C

Bigeminal pulsations result from a normal pulsation followed by a premature contraction. The
amplitude of the pulsation of the premature contraction is less than that of the normal pulsation.

Disorder of rhythm

Large, bounding pulse

D

The large, bounding (also called hyperkinetic or strong) pulse is readily palpable. It does not
"fade out" and is not easily obliterated by the examining fingers. This pulse is recorded as 3+.

Exercise
Anxiety
Fever
Hyperthyroidism
Aortic rigidity or
    atherosclerosis

Paradoxic pulse (pulsus paradoxus)

E

Inspiration   Expiration   Inspiration

Pulsus paradoxus is characterized by an exaggerated decrease (>10 mm Hg) in the amplitude of
pulsation during inspiration and increased amplitude during expiration. (See text for measurement
with sphygmomanometer.)

Premature cardiac contraction
Tracheobronchial obstruction
Bronchial asthma
Emphysema
Pericardial effusion
Constrictive pericarditis

Water-hammer pulse (Corrigan pulse)

F

Patent ductus arteriosus
Aortic regurgitation

The water-hammer pulse (also known as collapsing) has a greater amplitude than expected, a
rapid rise to a narrow summit, and a sudden descent.

FIGURE 15-9
Pulse abnormalities.
Modified from Barkauskas, 1998.

AUSCULTATION

Auscultate over an artery for a bruit (i.e., a murmur or unexpected sound) if you are following the radiation of murmurs first noted during the cardiac examination or looking for evidence of local obstruction. These sounds are usually low pitched and relatively hard to hear. Place the bell of the stethoscope directly over the artery. Sites to auscultate for a bruit are over the temporal, carotid, subclavian, abdominal aorta, renal, iliac, and femoral arteries. When listening over the carotid vessels, ask the patient to hold a breath for a few heartbeats so that respiratory sounds will not interfere with auscultation (Fig. 15-10).

Carotid artery bruits are best heard at the anterior margin of the sternocleidomastoid muscle. These may include the following types:

- Transmitted murmurs resulting from valvular aortic stenosis, ruptured chordae tendineae of the mitral valve, or severe aortic regurgitation
- Vigorous left ventricular ejection (more common in children than in adults) (Box 15-1)
- Obstructive disease in carotid arteries (e.g., atherosclerotic carotid arteries, fibromuscular hyperplasia, or arteritis)

BOX 15-1

LISTENING TO THE NECK

Venous Hum
- Heard at medial end of clavicle and anterior border of sternocleidomastoid muscle
- Usually of no clinical significance
- Confused with carotid bruit, patent ductus arteriosus, and aortic regurgitation
- In adults, usually occurs with anemia, pregnancy, thyrotoxicosis, and intracranial arteriovenous malformation

Carotid Artery Bruits
- Heard at medial end of clavicle and anterior margin of sternocleidomastoid muscle
- Transmitted murmurs: valvular aortic stenosis, ruptured chordae tendineae of mitral valve, and severe aortic regurgitation
- Can be heard with vigorous left ventricular ejection (more commonly in children than in adults)
- Occur with obstructive disease in cervical arteries (e.g., atherosclerotic carotid arteries, fibromuscular hyperplasia, and arteritis)

Mild obstruction produces a short, not particularly intense, localized bruit; greater obstruction lengthens the duration and increases the pitch. Virtual or complete obstruction will eliminate the bruit.

A 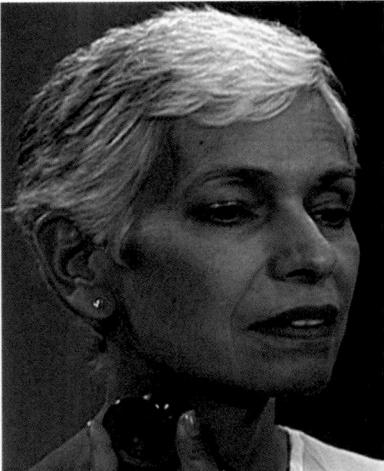 B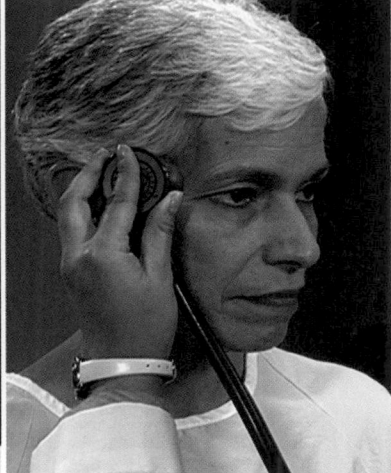

FIGURE 15-10
Auscultation for bruits.
A, Carotid artery. **B,** Temporal artery.

ASSESSMENT FOR ARTERIAL OCCLUSION AND INSUFFICIENCY

Arteries in any location can become occluded or traumatized in some manner, making them insufficient to their task. The resultant diminution in circulation to the tissues will lead to signs and symptoms that are related to the following:

- Site
- Degree of occlusion
- Ability of collateral channels to compensate
- Rapidity with which the problem develops

The first symptom is pain that results from muscle ischemia, referred to as claudication (Box 15-2). This pain can be characterized as a dull ache with accompanying muscle fatigue and, often, with crampiness. It usually appears during sustained exercise, such as walking a distance or climbing several flights of stairs. Just a few minutes of rest will ordinarily relieve it. It recurs again with the same amount of activity. Continued activity causes worsening pain.

The site of pain is distal to the occlusion. After determining the distinguishing characteristics of the pain, you should note the following:

- Pulses (weak and thready, or possibly absent)
- Possible systolic bruits over the arteries that may extend through diastole
- Loss of expected body warmth in the affected area
- Localized pallor and cyanosis
- Collapsed superficial veins, with delay in venous filling
- Thin, atrophied skin; muscle atrophy; or loss of hair (particularly in the case of long-term insufficiency)
- Long-term insufficiency also accentuates skin mottling and increases the likelihood of ulceration, localized anesthesia, and tenderness

To judge the degree of occlusion and the potential severity of the arterial occlusion, perform the following steps:

- Have the patient lie supine.
- Elevate the extremity.
- Note the degree of blanching.
- Have the patient sit on the edge of the bed or examining table in order to lower the extremity.
- Note the time for maximal return of color after the extremity is elevated. Slight pallor on elevation and a return to full color as soon as the leg becomes dependent is the expected finding. If there is a delay of many seconds or even minutes before the extremity regains full color, arterial occlusion is present. When return to full color takes as long as 2 minutes, the problem is severe.

A measurement of the *capillary refill time* provides another method of assessing severity (Box 15-3).

MNEMONICS

Arterial Occlusion: The Ps
Pallor
Pain
Pulselessness
Paresthesias (if a major artery is occluded)
Paralysis (rarely)

The presence of all Ps comprises the *compartment syndrome.*

BOX 15-2

COMPARISON OF PAIN FROM VASCULAR INSUFFICIENCIES AND MUSCULOSKELETAL DISORDERS

Arterial
- Comes on during exercise
- Quickly relieved by rest
- Intensity increases with the intensity and duration of exercise

Venous and Musculoskeletal
- Comes on during or often several hours after exercise
- Relieved by rest but sometimes only after several hours or even days; pain tends to be constant
- Greater variability than arterial pain in response to intensity and duration of exercise

---

BOX 15-3

CAPILLARY REFILL TIME

The capillary bed joins the arterial and venous systems. It is the bodywide structure that allows fluid exchange between the vascular and interstitial spaces, as a result of the competitive and complementary interaction of the hydrostatic pressures of the blood and interstitial tissues and the colloid osmotic pressures of plasma and interstitial fluids. This interplay in the healthy person allows dominance of hydrostatic pressure at the arterial end of the capillary bed (pushing fluid out) and of the colloid osmotic pressure at the venous end (pulling fluid in), thereby maintaining the balance of fluids in the intravascular and extravascular spaces.

The time it takes the capillary bed to fill after it is occluded by pressure gives some indication of the health of the system. This is referred to as the capillary refill time. To gauge the *capillary refill time,* perform the following:

- Blanch the nail bed with a sustained pressure of several seconds on a fingernail or toenail.
- Release the pressure.
- Observe the time elapsed before the nail regains its full color.

If the system is intact, this should occur almost instantly—in less than 2 seconds. If, however, the system is compromised (e.g., during arterial occlusion, hypovolemic shock, or hypothermia), the refill time will be *more than 2 seconds,* and much longer if circulatory compromise is severe.

CAUTION: Environmental influences, such as even moderately decreased ambient temperature, may influence capillary time by prolonging it, thus suggesting a problem that may not exist. In addition, there is variability among examiners in defining the time. Therefore the capillary refill time should not be considered an observation with exquisite sensitivity and specificity and should be used more to confirm a clinical judgment.

The following list provides a general guideline for assessment of possible causes of pain:

Location	Probable Obstructed Artery
Calf muscles	Superficial femoral artery
Thigh	Common femoral artery or external iliac artery
Buttock	Common iliac artery or distal aorta (impotence may accompany occlusion of distal aorta)

If the pain is constant, the occlusion is probably acute; if it is excruciating, a major artery has probably been severely compromised.

BLOOD PRESSURE

Blood pressure is usually measured in the patient's arm, and should be measured in both arms at least once annually and during a hospitalization (Box 15-4). The patient's arm should be slightly flexed and comfortably supported on a table, pillow, or your hand. Be sure that the arm is free of clothing. Apply an appropriately sized cuff (see Chapter 3) snugly and securely because a loose cuff will give an inaccurate diastolic measurement. Center the deflated bladder over the brachial artery, just medial to the biceps tendon, with the lower edge 2 to 3 cm above the antecubital crease.

Checking the palpable systolic blood pressure first will help you avoid being misled by an auscultatory gap when you listen with the stethoscope. Place the fingers of one hand over the brachial or radial artery. Rapidly inflate the cuff with the handbulb 20 to 30 mm Hg above the point at which you no longer feel the peripheral pulse. Deflate the cuff slowly at a rate of 2 to 3 mm Hg per second until you again feel at least two beats of the pulse. This point is the palpable systolic blood pressure. Immediately deflate the cuff completely (Fig. 15-11, *A*).

Now place the bell of the stethoscope over the brachial artery and, pausing for 30 seconds, again inflate the cuff until it is 20 to 30 mm Hg above the palpable systolic blood pressure (Fig. 15-11, *B*). The bell of the stethoscope is more effective than the diaphragm in transmitting the

BOX 15-4

GUIDES TO A PROPER APPROACH TO MEASURING BLOOD PRESSURE

- In general, it is better to use a bigger cuff than a smaller cuff, provided it fits comfortably on the arm. The size of the cuff is measured by the width of bladder and not the width of the cloth.
- Hypertension is a diagnosis to be made over time. A few readings on any given day may not be conclusive. This, of course, does not hold when the patient has a malignant hypertension requiring immediate care.
- The mercury column is the most reliable of the available mechanisms for measuring blood pressure. The use of a mercury column risks exposure of the patient to this dangerous element and is no longer permitted in many public sites including hospitals and nursing homes. Remember that the aneroid sphygmomanometer tends to lose its accuracy with age and use.
- Pressures taken when the patient is supine tend to be lower than those taken when the patient is sitting. The preferred position for monitoring blood pressure is with the patient seated and the cuff at the level of the heart. When documenting a patient's blood pressure measurements over time, use the same position. The standards currently used in the health care field have been set for patients (except infants) in the seated position. For them, the standards have been adjusted by the addition of 7 to 8 mm Hg. It is acceptable to add this amount in the very young, if the blood pressure is taken while the child is supine.
- Blood pressure generally increases with age (see Tables 15-3, 15-5, and 15-6).
- The taller and heavier the individual (whether he or she is an adult or a child), the more likely the blood pressure will be higher than in a shorter or leaner person of the same age. A blood pressure measurement in the very high (yet not unusual) range for age can often be attributed to greater height or excess weight.

Modified from Dillon, 1987

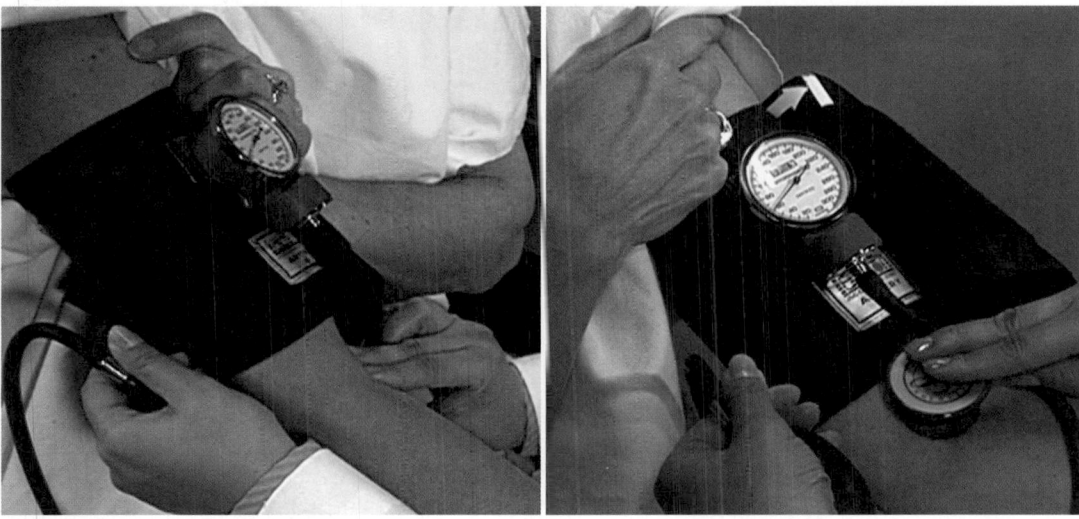

FIGURE 15-11
Blood pressure measurement. **A,** Checking palpable systolic pressure. **B,** Using bell of stethoscope.

low-pitched sound produced by the turbulence of blood flow in the artery (Korotkoff sounds). Deflate the cuff slowly as previously described, listening for the following sounds (Fig. 15-12):

- Two consecutive beats indicate the systolic pressure as well as the beginning of phase 1 of the Korotkoff sounds.
- Occasionally, the Korotkoff sounds will be heard, will disappear, and will reappear 10 to 15 mm Hg lower (phase 2). The period of silence is the auscultatory gap. You should be

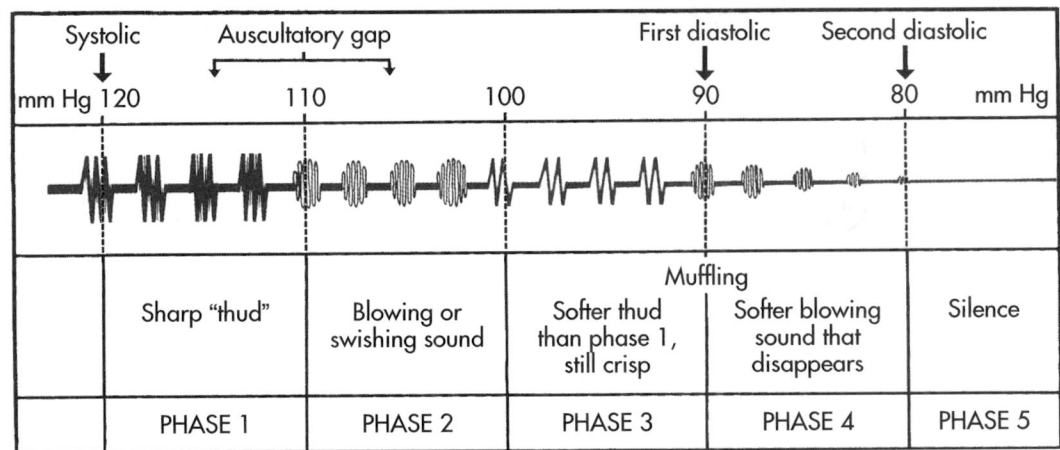

FIGURE 15-12
Phases of Korotkoff sounds, including an example of auscultatory gap.

aware of the possibility of this gap or you may underestimate the systolic pressure or overestimate the diastolic pressure. The auscultatory gap widens in the instance of systolic hypertension in older persons (with loss of arterial pliability) or with a drop in diastolic pressure (with chronic severe aortic regurgitation). It narrows in the event of pulsus paradoxus with cardiac tamponade or other constrictive cardiac events.

♦ Note the point at which the sounds that are first crisp (phase 3) become muffled (phase 4). This is the first diastolic sound, which is considered to be the closest approximation of direct diastolic arterial pressure. It signals imminent disappearance of the Korotkoff sounds.

♦ Note the point at which the sounds disappear (phase 5). This is the second diastolic sound. Now deflate the cuff completely.

Repeat the process in the other arm. Readings between the arms may vary by as much as 10 mm Hg and tend to be higher in the right arm; the higher reading should be accepted as closest to the patient's blood pressure. Record both sets of measurements.

The American Heart Association recommends recording three values for the blood pressure: the systolic and both diastolic measures (e.g., 110/76/68). If only two values are recorded, they are the systolic and the second diastolic pressures (e.g., 110/68). The difference between the systolic and diastolic pressures is the pulse pressure. The expected range is approximately 100 to 140 mm Hg for the systolic pressure and 60 to 90 mm Hg for the (second) diastolic sound. The pulse pressure should range from 30 to 40 mm Hg, even to as much as 50 mm Hg.

Electronic sphygmomanometers with a Doppler or other oscillometric technique work by sensing vibrations, converting them to electrical impulses, and transmitting them to a device that produces a digital readout. They are relatively sensitive and are increasingly popular and available. They can also simultaneously measure the pulse rate. If the readout and clinical impression are not consistent, you may validate the readout by taking the pressure with a manual cuff. Doppler devices, however, are more sensitive than stethoscopes to the first Korotkoff sound.

Because the systolic pressure is more labile and more readily responsive to a wide range of physical, emotional, and pharmacologic (caffeine) stimuli, hypertension is usually defined on the basis of several measurements taken over time. The Joint National Committee on prevention, detection, evaluation, and treatment of high blood pressure has classified blood pressure for adults (Table 15-3). Some studies suggest that the pulse pressure may be a more important predictor of heart disease than either the systolic or diastolic pressure alone. Most cases of hypertension in adults have no discoverable cause and are referred to as essential hypertension. Because the elevation of blood pressure may, for a time, be the only significant clinical finding, persons with hypertension are often asymptomatic. Individuals who complain of frequent epistaxis or recurrent morning headaches that disappear as the day progresses certainly deserve careful monitoring of their blood pressure.

If the diastolic pressure in the arms is above 90 mm Hg, or if you suspect coarctation of the aorta, measure the blood pressure in the legs. The patient should be prone, if possible; if

PHYSICAL VARIATIONS

Blood Pressure

Blood pressure differs by race in many comparative studies, with blacks having higher blood pressure than whites. This observed difference is partly due to environment—blacks from higher socioeconomic levels generally have lower blood pressure than do blacks at lower socioeconomic levels. But there is also a genetic component to the increase in blood pressure—blacks show differences related to renin activity, and blacks retain salt better under heat stress than whites do, which may affect their blood pressure levels.

TABLE 15-3	Classification of Blood Pressure for Adults Age 18 and Older*		
Category	**Systolic (mm Hg)**		**Diastolic (mm Hg)**
Optimal†	<120	and	<80
Prehypertension	120-139	or	80-89
Hypertension‡			
Stage 1	140-159	or	90-99
Stage 2	160-179	or	100-109
Stage 3	≥180	or	≥110

*Not taking antihypertensive drugs and not acutely ill. When systolic and diastolic blood pressures fall into different categories, the higher category should be selected to classify the individual's blood pressure status (e.g., 160/93 mm Hg should be classified as stage 2 hypertension, and 174/120 mm Hg should be classified as stage 3 hypertension). Isolated systolic hypertension is defined as systolic blood pressure of 140 mm Hg or greater and diastolic blood pressure below 90 mm Hg and staged appropriately (e.g., 170/82 mm Hg is defined as stage 2 isolated systolic hypertension). In addition to classifying stages of hypertension on the basis of average blood pressure levels, clinicians should specify presence or absence of target organ disease and additional risk factors. This specificity is important for risk classification and treatment.
†Optimal blood pressure with respect to cardiovascular risk is below 120/80 mm Hg; however, unusually low readings should be evaluated for clinical significance. Prehypertension should be treated with lifestyle modifications to prevent the progressive rise in blood pressure and cardiovascular disease. The diagnosis of hypertension is based on the average of two or more readings taken at each of two or more visits after an initial screening.
‡From NIH Publication No. 04-5230, June 2003.

supine, the leg should be flexed as little as possible. Center the thigh cuff bladder over the posterior surface and wrap the cuff securely on the distal third of the femur. Measure the pressure over the popliteal artery using the same procedure as for the brachial artery. A Doppler measurement may be helpful in this regard. Leg pressures, which are usually higher than arm pressures, will be lower with coarctation of the aorta or aortic stenosis.

If the patient is taking antihypertensive medications, has a depleted blood volume, or complains of fainting or postural lightheadedness, blood pressure in the arm should also be measured with the patient standing. Ordinarily, as a patient changes position from supine to standing, there is a slight or no drop in systolic pressure and a slight rise in diastolic pressure. However, if postural hypotension is present, expect to see a significant drop in systolic pressure (greater than 15 mm Hg) and a drop in diastolic pressure. Even a mild blood loss (such as from blood donation), drugs, autonomic nervous system disease, or prolonged time in a recumbent position can contribute to postural hypotension. Indeed, patients who have active gastrointestinal bleeding will often have dramatic changes in blood pressure with postural change. Patients at risk in this regard should have the blood pressure taken at first when supine, then standing.

With even impeccable technique, the accuracy of the blood pressure reading may be undermined by some conditions:

- Cardiac dysrhythmias: An infrequent odd beat may be ignored, but if the irregularity is sustained, it is a good idea to take the average of several pressures and to write a note about the uncertainty.
- Aortic regurgitation: The sounds of aortic regurgitation may not disappear, thus obscuring the diastolic pressure.
- Venous congestion: Sluggish venous flow from a pathologic event can cause the systolic pressure to be heard lower than it actually is and the diastolic pressure higher. Repeated, slow inflations of the cuff can also cause venous congestion.
- Valve replacement: The sounds may be heard all the way down to a zero gauge reading; listen carefully for the first muffling of the sound (Korotkoff phase 4) to determine the diastolic pressure. More modern valves do not cause this discrepancy.

In addition, measurement of blood pressure during the respiratory phase may suggest constrictive disease involving the heart or pulmonary disease (Box 15-5).

BOX 15-5

DETERMINATION OF A PARADOXIC PULSE* BY SPHYGMOMANOMETER

Determination of a paradoxic pulse may be an important diagnostic finding. The difference in systolic pressure between expiration and inspiration should be 5 mm Hg. If it is greater than 10 mm Hg, the paradoxic pulse is *exaggerated*. This may be associated with a serious constraint on the heart's action caused by cardiac tamponade or constrictive pericarditis or by great respiratory effort as occurs with emphysema. Associated findings include low blood pressure and a weak and rapid pulse.

- Ask the patient to breathe as easily and comfortably as possible; this can be a difficult assignment for the patient while being observed.
- Apply the sphygmomanometer and inflate it until no sounds are audible.
- Deflate the cuff *gradually* until sounds are audible only during expiration.
- Note the pressure.
- Deflate the cuff further until sounds are also audible during inspiration.
- Note the pressure.

*Paradoxic pulse is the exaggerated fall in systolic pressure during inspiration.

PERIPHERAL VEINS

JUGULAR VENOUS PRESSURE

Careful measurement of the jugular venous pressure (JVP) is an important and, in some instances, critical portion of the physical examination. Several techniques may be used. The simplest, most reproducible and reliable method requires a ruler at least 15 cm long. Folding rulers with guides for ECG analysis are widely available and useful for this purpose. In the most convenient mode of examination, a bed or examining table is used with an angle of back support that can be adjusted. Use a light to supply tangential illumination across the neck to accentuate the appearance of the jugular venous pulsations (see Fig. 15-13).

Blood Vessels:
Assessing the Jugular Veins

The patient initially is placed in the supine position. This position results in engorgement of the jugular veins. The head of the bed is raised gradually until the jugular venous pulsations become evident between the angle of the jaw and the clavicle (see Fig. 15-6). Palpating the contralateral carotid pulse helps identify the venous pulsations and distinguish them from the carotid pulsations. Table 15-4 provides instructions on differentiating between jugular and carotid pulses. The jugular pulse can only be visualized; it cannot be palpated.

Several conditions may make the examination more difficult: (1) Severe right heart failure, tricuspid insufficiency, constrictive pericarditis, and cardiac tamponade may each cause ex-

---

TABLE 15-4	**Comparison of the Jugular and Carotid Pulse Waves**	
	Jugular	**Carotid**
Quality and Character	Three positive waves in normal sinus rhythm	One wave
Palpate the carotid artery on one side of the neck and look at the jugular vein on the other to tell the difference	More undulating	More brisk
Effect of Respiration	Level of pulse wave decreased on inspiration and increased on expiration	No effect
Venous Compression Apply gentle pressure over vein at base of neck above clavicle	Easily eliminates pulse wave	No effect
Abdominal Pressure Place the palm moderately firmly over the right upper quadrant of the abdomen for half a minute	May cause some increased prominence even in well persons; with right-sided heart failure, jugular vein may be more visible	No effect

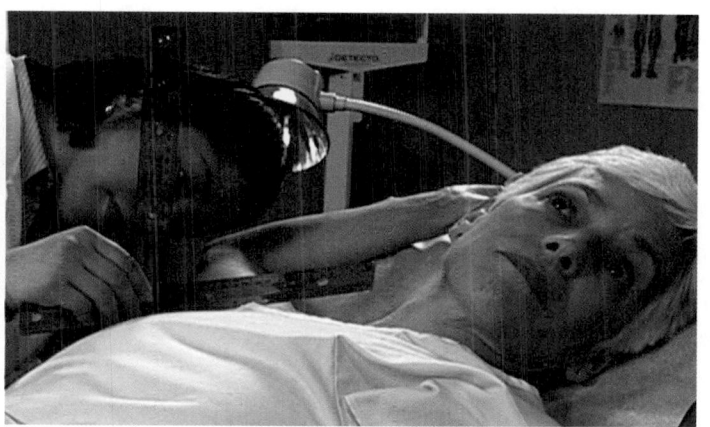

FIGURE 15-13
Measuring jugular venous pressure.

treme elevation of the JVP so that it is not apparent until the patient is sitting upright; (2) severe volume depletion makes it difficult to detect the JVP even when the patient is supine; and (3) in extreme obesity, overlying adipose tissue obscures the jugular venous pulsations.

A ruler is placed with its tip at the midaxillary line (the position of the heart within the chest) at the level of the nipple and extended vertically. Another ruler, placed at the level of the meniscus of the JVP, is extended horizontally to where it intersects the vertical ruler, and the vertical distance above the level of the heart is noted as the mean JVP in centimeters of water (Fig. 15-13). A value of less than 9 cm H_2O is the expected value. The number can be divided by 1.3 to calculate its value in millimeters of mercury.

Maneuvers useful for confirming the JVP measurement include hepatojugular reflux and evaluation of the venous engorgement of the hands at various levels of elevation above the heart.

HEPATOJUGULAR REFLUX

Some have erroneously suggested that the hepatojugular reflux is a sign of right heart failure. All patients will have elevation of the JVP with this maneuver, depending on the elevation of their head with respect to the heart and their underlying venous pressure. Still, the hepatojugular reflux is exaggerated when right heart failure is present and its measurement is used to evaluate that condition.

To assess the hepatojugular reflux maneuver, use your hand to apply firm and sustained pressure to the abdomen in the midepigastric region while the patient is instructed to breathe regularly. Observe the neck for an elevation in JVP followed by an abrupt fall in JVP as the hand pressure is released. The JVP quickly equilibrates to its true level between the positions it achieved with and immediately after removal of the abdominal hand pressure.

This maneuver is analogous to focusing a camera by turning the focus ring one way and then the other until the picture is the sharpest. If the JVP is not obvious with this maneuver, the pressure is either much higher or much lower than the patient's current neck position with relation to the heart. The maneuver should then be repeated with the patient more supine, if you suspect the pressure to be lower; or with the patient more upright, if you suspect the JVP to be higher.

EVALUATION OF HAND VEINS

The veins of the hand can be used as an "auxiliary manometer" of the right heart pressure in the absence of thrombosis in the hand or subclavian vein, the absence of an A-V fistula in that arm, and in the absence of the superior vena cava syndrome. With the patient semirecumbent, place the hand on the examination table or mattress. Palpate the hand veins, which should be engorged, to make sure they are compressible and not thrombosed. Slowly raise the hand until the hand veins collapse (Fig. 15-14). Use a ruler to note the vertical distance between the midaxillary line at the nipple level (level of the heart) and the level of collapse of the hand veins. Confirm this level by lowering the hand slowly until the veins distend again and raise it back until they once again collapse. This distance should be identical to the mean JVP.

The hand vein measurement is particularly helpful at the extremes of JVP: severe right heart failure where the pressure may be 20 to 30 cm H_2O (i.e., not evident with the patient sitting upright) or volume depletion (i.e., not visible with the patient supine).

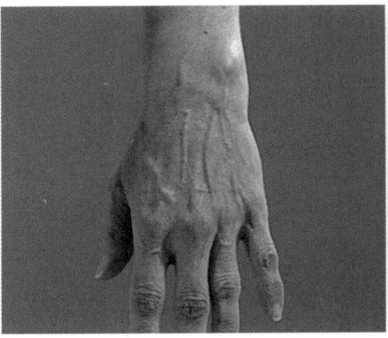
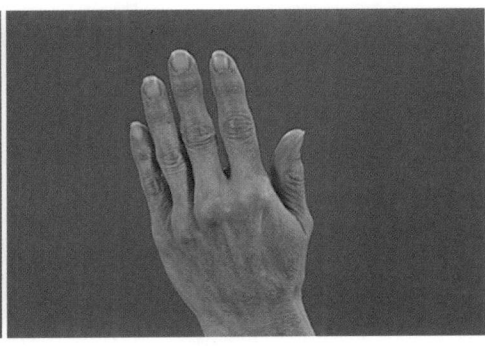

A

B

FIGURE 15-14
Evaluation of hand veins. **A,** Engorged veins in dependent hand. **B,** Collapsed veins in elevated hand.

ASSESSMENT FOR VENOUS OBSTRUCTION AND INSUFFICIENCY

Obstruction of the venous system and a consequent insufficiency results in signs and symptoms that vary depending on the rapidity with which the occlusion develops and on the degree of localization. An acute process may result from injury, external compression, or thrombophlebitis. A constant pain is one of the first symptoms (see Box 15-2). In the affected area, pain occurs simultaneously with the following:

- Swelling and tenderness over the muscles
- Engorgement of superficial veins
- Erythema and/or cyanosis

Inspect the extremities for signs of venous insufficiency (e.g., thrombosis, varicose veins, or edema). Examine the patient in both the standing and supine positions, particularly in the case of a suspected chronic venous occlusion.

Thrombosis. Note any redness, thickening, and tenderness along a superficial vein; together, these findings suggest thrombophlebitis of a superficial vein. Suspect a deep vein thrombosis if swelling, pain, and tenderness occur over a vein. It cannot be confirmed on physical examination alone. (An occluded artery does not result in swelling.)

Homans Sign. Flex the patient's knee slightly with one hand and, with the other, dorsiflex the foot. The complaint of calf pain with this procedure is a positive sign and often indicates venous thrombosis. Absence of Homans sign does not preclude venous thrombosis.

Edema. Inspect the extremities for edema, manifested as a change in the usual contour of the leg. Press your index finger over the bony prominence of the tibia or medial malleolus for several seconds. A depression that does not rapidly refill and resume its original contour indicates orthostatic (pitting) edema. This finding is not usually accompanied by thickening or pigmentation of the overlying skin. Right-sided heart failure leads to an increased fluid volume, which in turn elevates the hydrostatic pressure in the vascular space, causing edema in dependent parts of the body.

Edema accompanied by some thickening and ulceration of the skin is associated with deep venous obstruction or venous valvular incompetence. Edema related to valvular incompetence or an obstruction of a deep vein (usually in the legs) is caused by the mechanical pressure of increased blood volume in the area served by the affected vein. Circulatory disorders that cause edema so tense that it does not pit must be distinguished from lymphedema (see Chapter 9).

The severity of edema may be characterized by grading 1+ through 4+ (Fig. 15-15). Any concomitant pitting can be mild or severe, as evidenced by the following:

1+ Slight pitting, no visible distortion, disappears rapidly
2+ A somewhat deeper pit than in 1+, but again no readily detectable distortion, and it disappears in 10 to 15 seconds
3+ Noticeably deep pit that may last more than a minute; the dependent extremity looks fuller and swollen
4+ Very deep pit that lasts as long as 2 to 5 minutes, and the dependent extremity is grossly distorted

Varicose Veins. Varicose veins are dilated and swollen, with a diminished rate of blood flow and an increased intravenous pressure. These characteristics result from incompetence of the vessel wall or venous valves, or an obstruction in a more proximal vein.

CLINICAL PEARL

Calf Pain

Be certain that you do not confuse calf pain with Achilles tendon pain, a common finding in athletes who frequently stress the Achilles tendon and in women who wear high-heeled shoes. Avoid this confusion by keeping the knee slightly flexed when you dorsiflex the foot.

CLINICAL PEARL

Edema

If edema is unilateral, suspect the occlusion of a major vein. If edema is bilateral, consider congestive heart failure. If edema occurs without pitting, suspect arterial disease and occlusion or lymphedema.

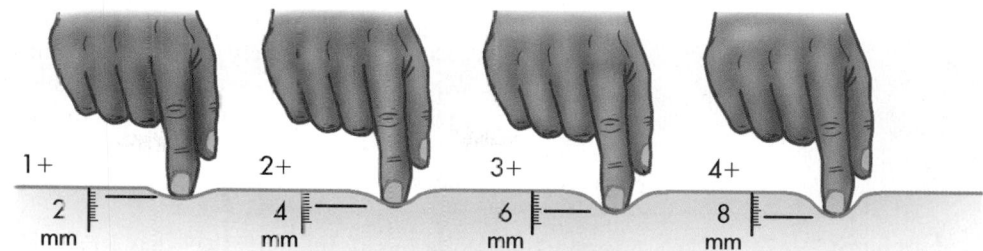

FIGURE 15-15
Assessing for pitting edema.
Modified from Canobbio, 1990.

Superficial varicosities are easy to detect on inspection, particularly when the patient is standing. The veins appear dilated and often tortuous when the extremities are dependent. If varicose veins are suspected, have the patient stand on the toes 10 times in succession. This will build a palpable pressure in the veins. If the venous system is competent, the pressure in the veins will disappear in just a few seconds. If not, the feeling of pressure in the veins will be sustained for a longer time, and the return to the pretest state will be sluggish.

When varicosities are present, use the Trendelenburg test to evaluate venous incompetence. With the patient supine, lift the leg above the level of the heart until the veins empty. Then lower the leg quickly. An incompetent system allows rapid filling of the veins.

The Perthes test is used to evaluate the patency of deep veins. With the patient supine and the extremity elevated, occlude the subcutaneous veins with a tourniquet just above the knee to prevent filling of superficial varicosities from above. As the patient walks, muscular tension will act on the deep veins and empty the dilated superficial varicosities. When these superficial veins fail to empty, suspect that the deep veins are also incompetent.

To evaluate the direction of blood flow and the competency of the valves in the venous system, distend visible veins by putting the limb in a dependent position. Compress the vein with the finger or thumb of one hand and strip the vein of blood by compressing it with fingers of the second hand. If the compressed vessel fills before either compressing finger is released, there is collateral circulation. If the compressing finger nearest the heart is released, the vessel should fill backward to the first valve only. If the entire venous column fills, the valves in that vessel are incompetent.

INFANTS

The brachial, radial, and femoral pulses of the newborn are easily palpable. When the pulse is weaker or thinner than expected, the cardiac output may be diminished, or peripheral vasoconstriction may be present. A bounding pulse is associated with a large left-to-right shunt produced by a patent ductus arteriosus. A difference in pulse amplitude between the upper extremities or between the femoral and radial pulses suggests a coarctation of the aorta, as does absence of the femoral pulses.

The usual blood pressure measurement techniques may be difficult to implement in infants and very young children. A small arm and the problem of obtaining cooperation suggest the alternative of the "flush technique":

1. Place the cuff on the upper arm (or thigh).
2. Elevate and wrap the arm firmly with an elastic bandage from fingers to the antecubital space, thus emptying the veins and capillaries.
3. Inflate the cuff to a pressure above the systolic reading you expect.
4. Lower the arm and remove the bandage. (The arm will be pale.)
5. Diminish the pressure gradually until you see a sudden flush and a return to usual color in the forearm and hand, a quite definitive endpoint.

The resultant value is generally both lower than the systolic pressure and higher than the diastolic pressure obtained through auscultation and palpation.

Electronic sphygmomanometers with a Doppler or other oscillometric technique are available for infants and for children and are now widely available in the hospital setting. The usual newborn blood pressure ranges from 60 to 96 mm Hg systolic and 30 to 62 mm Hg diastolic. A sustained increase in blood pressure is almost always significant.

CLINICAL PEARL

Blood Pressure in Infants
A very sick infant has a "good" blood pressure. Do not be comfortable about a possibly lesser potential for shock or even cardiac arrest. A very ill baby with a "good" pressure can crash. Check the capillary refill (see p. 474). It can be as long as 6 to 7 seconds with the pressure seemingly OK. The lesson: Get both measurements to evaluate well.

Hypertension in the newborn may be the result of thrombosis after the use of an umbilical catheter, stenosis of the renal artery, coarctation of the aorta, cystic disease of the kidney, neuroblastoma, Wilms tumor, hydronephrosis, adrenal hyperplasia, or central nervous system disease. Capillary refill times in infants and children younger than 2 years of age are rapid, less than 1 second. A prolonged capillary refill time, longer than 2 seconds, indicates dehydration or hypovolemic shock.

CHILDREN

A venous hum, common in children, usually has no pathologic significance (see Box 15-1). It is caused by the turbulence of blood flow in the internal jugular veins. To detect a venous hum, ask the child to sit with the head turned to the left and tilted slightly upward (to the right if you are listening on the left). Auscultate over the right supraclavicular space at the medial end of the clavicle and along the anterior border of the sternocleidomastoid muscle (Fig. 15-16). The intensity of the hum is increased when the patient is sitting with the head turned away from the area of auscultation, and it is diminished with a Valsalva maneuver. When present, the hum is a continuous low-pitched sound that is louder during diastole. It may be interrupted by gentle pressure over the vein in the space between the trachea and the sternocleidomastoid muscle at about the level of the thyroid cartilage. The venous hum can be confused with patent ductus arteriosus, aortic regurgitation, and the murmur of valvular aortic stenosis transmitted into the carotid arteries.

Blood pressure is easy to measure in children older than 2 or 3 years of age. The correct cuff size is mandatory (see Fig. 3-2). Korotkoff phase 4 sound should be considered the appropriate diastolic reading until adolescence, when Korotkoff phase 5 is used. Children like to explore the sphygmomanometer, and full explanation of the process and a moment for playing with the instrument can facilitate examination. If your ability to hear is compromised by the child's crying or a deeply placed brachial artery, palpate the radial artery if a digital sphygmomanometer is not available. Its use will yield a systolic pressure about 10 mm Hg less than that at the brachial artery.

Do not make the diagnosis of hypertension on the basis of one reading. Many readings should be taken over time. If the systolic pressure is elevated and the diastolic is not, anxiety may be responsible. Take time to reassure the child to alleviate the anxiety. Studies suggest that in children the blood pressure varies with gender and height at any age. Values for normal (less than 90th percentile), prehypertensive (90th to 95th percentile) and hypertensive (more than 95th percentile) blood pressure have been compiled by the Task Force on High Blood Pressure in Children (Tables 15-5 and 15-6).

To use the tables, measure and record the child's systolic and diastolic blood pressures. Determine the child's height percentile using the standard length or height growth curve (Appendix C). Find the child's age on the left side of the table and follow the age row horizontally across the table to the intersection of the line for the child's height percentile. In that column find the blood pressure closest to the child's. Then determine whether the child's systolic and

CLINICAL PEARL

Facial Palsy

Severe hypertension in children may be accompanied by a facial palsy that disappears when the hypertension is treated. When there is such a palsy, always be sure to check the blood pressure.

Siegler, 1991.

CLINICAL PEARL

Obesity in Adolescents

There has been an increase in the number of adolescents who are obese. There has also been an increase in hypertension unrelated to secondary factors such as renal artery abnormalities. About 50% of the time, hypertension is now primary in adolescents; however, hypertension in children younger than 10 years of age is almost certainly secondary.

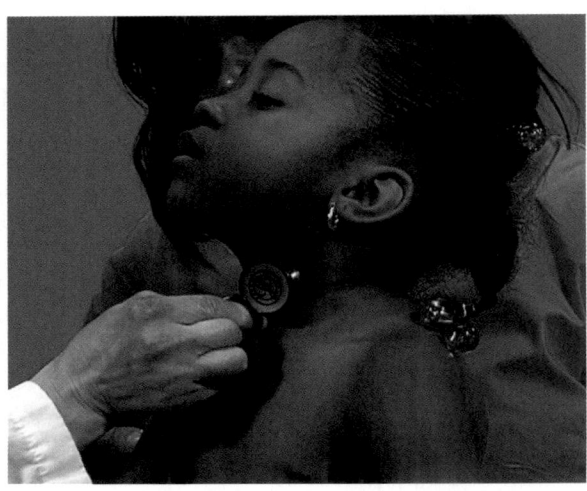

FIGURE 15-16
Auscultation for venous hum.

TABLE 15-5	Blood Pressure Levels for the 90th and 95th Percentiles of Blood Pressure for Boys 1 to 17 Years of Age by Percentiles of Height

		Systolic Blood Pressure by Percentile of Height (mm Hg†)							Diastolic Blood Pressure by Percentile of Height (mm Hg†)						
Age (yr)	Blood Pressure Percentile*	5%	10%	25%	50%	75%	90%	95%	5%	10%	25%	50%	75%	90%	95%
1	90th	94	95	97	99	100	102	103	49	50	51	52	53	53	54
	95th	98	99	101	103	104	106	106	54	54	55	56	57	58	58
2	90th	97	99	100	102	104	105	106	54	55	56	57	58	58	59
	95th	101	102	104	106	108	109	110	59	59	60	61	62	63	63
3	90th	100	101	103	105	107	108	109	59	59	60	61	62	63	63
	95th	104	105	107	109	110	112	113	63	63	64	65	66	67	67
4	90th	102	103	105	107	109	110	111	62	63	64	65	66	66	67
	95th	106	107	109	111	112	114	115	66	67	68	69	70	71	71
5	90th	104	105	106	108	110	111	112	65	66	67	68	69	69	70
	95th	108	109	110	112	114	115	116	69	70	71	72	73	74	74
6	90th	105	106	108	110	111	113	113	68	68	69	70	71	72	72
	95th	109	110	112	114	115	117	117	72	72	73	74	75	76	76
7	90th	106	107	109	111	113	114	115	70	70	71	72	73	74	74
	95th	110	111	113	115	117	118	119	74	74	75	76	77	78	78
8	90th	107	109	110	112	114	115	116	71	72	72	73	74	75	76
	95th	111	112	114	116	118	119	120	75	76	77	78	79	79	80
9	90th	109	110	112	114	115	117	118	72	73	74	75	76	76	77
	95th	113	114	116	118	119	121	121	76	77	78	79	80	81	81
10	90th	111	112	114	115	117	119	119	73	73	74	75	76	77	78
	95th	115	116	117	119	121	122	123	77	78	79	80	81	81	82
11	90th	113	114	115	117	119	120	121	74	74	75	76	77	78	78
	95th	117	118	119	121	123	124	125	78	78	79	80	81	82	82
12	90th	115	116	118	120	121	123	123	74	75	75	76	77	78	79
	95th	119	120	122	123	125	127	127	78	79	80	81	82	82	83
13	90th	117	118	120	122	124	125	126	75	75	76	77	78	79	79
	95th	121	122	124	126	128	129	130	79	79	80	81	82	83	83
14	90th	120	121	123	125	126	128	128	75	76	77	78	79	79	80
	95th	124	125	127	128	130	132	132	80	80	81	82	83	84	84
15	90th	122	124	125	127	129	130	131	76	77	78	79	80	80	81
	95th	126	127	129	131	133	134	135	81	81	82	83	84	85	85
16	90th	125	126	128	130	131	133	134	78	78	79	80	81	82	82
	95th	129	130	132	134	135	137	137	82	83	83	84	85	86	87
17	90th	127	128	130	132	134	135	136	80	80	81	82	83	84	84
	95th	131	132	134	136	138	139	140	84	85	86	87	87	88	89

From National High Blood Pressure Education Program Working Group on High Blood Pressure in Children and Adolescents, 2004.
*Blood pressure percentile was determined by a single measurement.
†Height percentile was determined by standard growth curves.

diastolic blood pressures are below, at, or above the 90th or 95th percentile values. The child's systolic and diastolic blood pressure values should be below the 90th percentile for age and height percentile.

If the blood pressure is in the 90th to 95th percentile range, it should be taken twice on the same visit and the systolic and diastolic pressures averaged. If the pressure is more than the 95th percentile, it should be carefully studied and followed. Primary (essential) hypertension in children is becoming more common because of the increasing prevalence of overweight children. Still, most often hypertension in children is caused by kidney disease, renal arterial disease, coarctation of the aorta, or pheochromocytoma.

Venous thrombosis occurs less commonly in children than in adults and is most often associated with placement of venous access devices. They can occur in any peripheral vessel and cause swollen, painful extremities.

TABLE 15-6 | Blood Pressure Levels for the 90th and 95th Percentiles of Blood Pressure for Girls 1 to 17 Years of Age by Percentiles of Height

Age (yr)	Blood Pressure Percentile*	Systolic Blood Pressure by Percentile of Height (mm Hg†)							Diastolic Blood Pressure by Percentile of Height (mm Hg†)						
		5%	10%	25%	50%	75%	90%	95%	5%	10%	25%	50%	75%	90%	95%
1	90th	97	97	98	100	101	102	103	52	53	53	54	55	55	56
	95th	100	101	102	104	105	106	107	56	57	57	58	59	59	60
2	90th	98	99	100	101	103	104	105	57	58	58	59	60	61	61
	95th	102	103	104	105	107	108	109	61	62	62	63	64	65	65
3	90th	100	100	102	103	104	106	106	61	62	62	63	64	64	65
	95th	104	104	105	107	108	109	110	65	66	66	67	68	68	69
4	90th	101	102	103	104	106	107	108	64	64	65	66	67	67	68
	95th	105	106	107	108	110	111	112	68	68	69	70	71	71	72
5	90th	103	103	105	106	107	109	109	66	67	67	68	69	69	70
	95th	107	107	108	110	111	112	113	70	71	71	72	73	73	74
6	90th	104	105	106	108	109	110	111	68	68	69	70	70	71	72
	95th	108	109	110	111	113	114	115	72	72	73	74	74	75	76
7	90th	106	107	108	109	111	112	113	69	70	70	71	72	72	73
	95th	110	111	112	113	115	116	116	73	74	74	75	76	76	77
8	90th	108	109	110	111	113	114	114	71	71	71	72	73	74	74
	95th	112	112	114	115	116	118	118	75	75	75	76	77	78	78
9	90th	110	110	112	113	114	116	116	72	72	72	73	74	75	75
	95th	114	114	115	117	118	119	120	76	76	76	77	78	79	79
10	90th	112	112	114	115	116	118	118	73	73	73	74	75	76	76
	95th	116	116	117	119	120	121	122	77	77	77	78	79	80	80
11	90th	114	114	116	117	118	119	120	74	74	74	75	76	77	77
	95th	118	118	119	121	122	123	124	78	78	78	79	80	81	81
12	90th	116	116	117	119	120	121	122	75	75	75	76	77	78	78
	95th	119	120	121	123	124	125	126	79	79	79	80	81	82	82
13	90th	117	118	119	121	122	123	124	76	76	76	77	78	79	79
	95th	121	122	123	124	126	127	128	80	80	80	81	82	83	83
14	90th	119	120	121	122	124	125	125	77	77	77	78	79	80	80
	95th	123	123	125	126	127	129	129	81	81	81	82	83	84	84
15	90th	120	121	122	123	125	126	127	78	78	78	79	80	81	81
	95th	124	125	126	127	129	130	131	82	82	82	83	84	85	85
16	90th	121	122	123	124	126	127	128	78	78	79	80	81	81	82
	95th	125	126	127	128	130	131	132	82	82	83	84	85	85	86
17	90th	122	122	123	125	126	127	128	78	79	79	80	81	81	82
	95th	125	126	127	129	130	131	132	82	83	83	84	85	85	86

From National High Blood Pressure Education Program Working Group on High Blood Pressure in Children and Adolescents, 2004.
*Blood pressure percentile was determined by a single reading.
†Height percentile was determined by standard growth curves.

PREGNANT WOMEN

Blood pressure readings gradually fall until they reach a nadir at 16 to 20 weeks of gestation, and then gradually rise to pre-pregnant levels at term. Blood pressures that would typically be considered usual in a nonpregnant woman may indicate impending problems in a pregnant one. In the second trimester, a systolic blood pressure greater than or equal to 125 mm Hg or a diastolic blood pressure greater than or equal to 75 mm Hg indicates a problem. In the third trimester, systolic blood pressure greater than 130 mm Hg or diastolic of 85 mm Hg or more is a concern. A rise in systolic pressure of more than 30 mm Hg or diastolic of 15 mm Hg over the first trimester baseline should be monitored closely. A sustained systolic blood pressure of 140 mm Hg or greater or a diastolic pressure of 90 mm Hg or greater should alert you to the probability of a blood pressure disorder in pregnancy.

OLDER ADULTS

The dorsalis pedis and posterior tibial pulses may be more difficult to find, and the superficial vessels are more apt to appear tortuous and distended.

Because of loss of elasticity of the vessels in the process of aging, the systolic blood pressure may increase. Hypertension in older adults is defined as a pressure greater than 140/90. The suggestion that the systolic blood pressure should be less than 120 plus the patient's age is no longer acceptable. Many practitioners do consider other factors, in addition to the blood pressure itself, when deciding to undertake therapy. Recent studies suggest that individuals who are normotensive at 55 years of age will have a 90% lifetime risk of developing hypertension.

SAMPLE DOCUMENTATION

HISTORY AND PHYSICAL EXAMINATION

Subjective

A 67-year-old man with a history of carcinoma of the breast noted the onset of pain in his right leg 1 day ago, accompanied by erythema. Pain is severe when he tries to stand upright and is reduced when supine. On a scale of 0 to 10, the patient judges his pain to be a 6.

For additional sample documentation, see Chapter 26.

Objective

Circumference of the leg 7 cm above the medial malleolus is 23 cm on the left and 27 cm on the right. Fifteen cm below the patellar tip, the circumference is 37 cm on the left and 40 cm on the right. The lower extremity is diffusely erythematous. The Homans sign is positive on the right.

SUMMARY OF EXAMINATION

BLOOD VESSELS

1. Palpate the arterial pulses in distal extremities, comparing characteristics bilaterally for the following (p. 468):
   - Rate
   - Rhythm
   - Contour
   - Amplitude
2. Auscultate the carotid, temporal, abdominal aorta, renal, iliac, and femoral arteries for bruits (p. 472).
3. Measure the blood pressure in both arms, first seated and then, in patients at risk for orthostatic hypotension, standing (p. 474).
4. With the patient reclining at a 45-degree angle elevation, inspect for jugular venous pulsations and distention; differentiate jugular and carotid pulse waves, and measure jugular venous pressure (p. 478).

5. Inspect the extremities for sufficiency of arteries and veins through the following (p. 480):
   - Color, skin texture, and nail changes
   - Presence of hair
   - Muscular atrophy
   - Edema or swelling
   - Varicose veins
6. Palpate the extremities for the following (p. 480):
   - Warmth
   - Pulse quality
   - Tenderness along any superficial vein
   - Pitting edema

COMMON ABNORMALITIES

VESSEL DISORDERS

CRANIAL ARTERITIS (GIANT CELL ARTERITIS)	Chronic generalized inflammatory disease of the branches of the aortic arch principally affects arteries of the carotid system and the temporal and occipital arteries. Temporal arteritis usually affects persons older than 50 years of age. Flu-like symptoms (e.g., low-grade fever, malaise, anorexia) are accompanied by polymyalgia involving the trunk and proximal muscles. Headache may be severe; there is throbbing in the temporal region on one or both sides; and the area over the temporal artery becomes red, swollen, tender, and nodular. The temporal pulse may be variously strong, weak, or absent. Ocular symptoms, including loss of vision, are common.
ARTERIAL ANEURYSM	An aneurysm is a localized dilation of an artery caused by a weakness in the arterial wall (Fig. 15-17). It is noticed as a pulsatile swelling along the course of an artery. Aneurysms occur most commonly in the aorta, although renal, femoral, and popliteal arteries are also common sites. A thrill or bruit may be evident over the aneurysm. An aortic aneurysm is usually the result of atherosclerosis. Abdominal aneurysms are four times more common in men than in women.

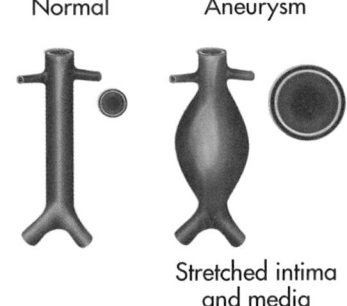

Normal   Aneurysm

Stretched intima
and media

FIGURE 15-17
Type I aortic dissection.

ARTERIOVENOUS FISTULA	An arteriovenous fistula is a pathologic communication between an artery and a vein. It may result in an aneurysmal dilation. A continuous bruit or thrill over the area of the fistula suggests its presence. Fistulas may be found in a variety of locations such as intracranially with a potential of intracranial hemorrhage (not uncommon), in the gastrointestinal tract (a not unusual source of gastrointestinal bleeding), and in the lungs (rare). Damage to vessels caused by ever more common catheterization procedures may also occasionally lead to A-V fistula formation.
PERIPHERAL ATHEROSCLEROTIC DISEASE (ARTERIOSCLEROSIS OBLITERANS)	Occlusion of the blood supply to the extremities by atherosclerotic plaques causes symptoms that vary in severity. Intermittent claudication produces pain, ache, or cramp in the exercised muscle that is receiving an inadequate blood supply. The amount of exercise necessary to cause the discomfort is predictable (e.g., occurring each time the same distance is walked). A brief rest relieves the pain. After resting the patient can walk the same distance as before and then again experiences the same symptoms. The limb appears healthy, but pulses are weak or absent. Progressive occlusion results in severe ischemia, in which the foot or leg is painful at rest, is cold and numb, and has skin changes (e.g., dry and scaling, with poor hair and nail growth). Edema seldom accompanies this disorder, but ulceration is common in severe disease, and the muscles may atrophy.
RAYNAUD PHENOMENON AND DISEASE	Idiopathic, intermittent spasm of the arterioles in the digits (occasionally in the nose and tongue) causes skin pallor. The vasospasm may last from minutes to hours. It can occur bilaterally, and the skin over the digits eventually appears smooth, shiny, and tight from loss of subcutaneous tissue. Ulcers may appear on tips of the digits. Raynaud disease occurs most

commonly in young, otherwise healthy women in whom episodes recur for at least 2 years with no evidence of underlying cause. Raynaud phenomenon is secondary to connective tissue diseases, neurogenic lesions, drug intoxication, primary pulmonary hypertension, and trauma. It is rare in childhood, and although it has been associated with immunologic abnormalities in this age-group, there is no evidence of serious prognostic significance (Fig. 15-18).

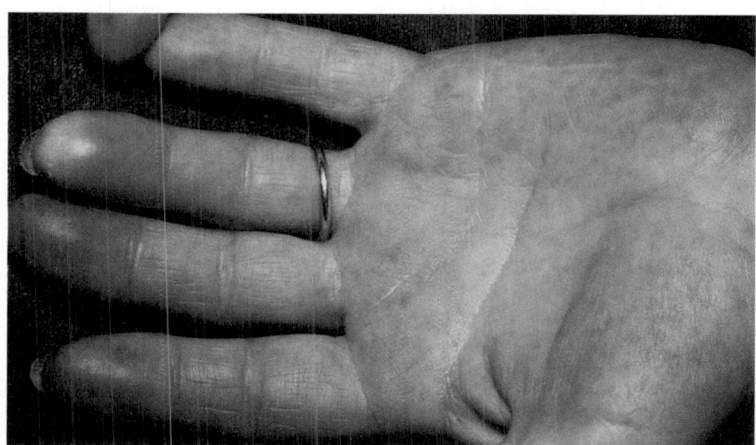

FIGURE 15-18
Raynaud phenomenon.
From Zitelli, Davis, 2002.

ARTERIAL EMBOLIC DISEASE

Dilation of the left atrium because of mitral regurgitation can lead to atrial fibrillation and clot formation within the atrium. If the clot is unstable, emboli may be disbursed throughout the arterial system, giving rise to occlusion of small arteries and necrosis of the tissue supplied by that vessel (Fig. 15-19).

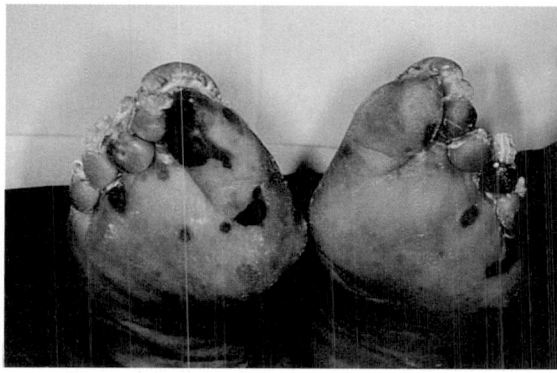

FIGURE 15-19
Embolic phenomenon.
Courtesy Charles W. Bradley, DPM, MPA; and Caroline Harvey, DPM, California College of Podiatric Medicine, San Bruno, CA.

VENOUS THROMBOSIS

Thrombosis can occur suddenly or gradually and with varying severity of symptoms. It can be the result of trauma or prolonged immobilization. Clinical findings of thrombosis in a superficial vein include redness, thickening, and tenderness along the involved segment. Deep vein thrombosis in the femoral and pelvic circulations may be asymptomatic; and pulmonary embolism, sometimes fatal, may occur without warning. Signs and symptoms suggestive of deep vein thrombosis include tenderness along the iliac vessels and the femoral canal, in the popliteal space, and over the deep calf veins; slight swelling that may be distinguished only by measuring and comparing the upper and lower legs bilaterally; minimal ankle edema; low-grade fever; and tachycardia. Homans' sign can be helpful but is not absolutely reliable in suggesting deep vein thrombosis. Doppler flow studies are diagnostic.

EVIDENCE-BASED PRACTICE IN PHYSICAL EXAMINATION
DOES A PATIENT HAVE DEEP VEIN THROMBOSIS?

Evaluation of what historical and physical examination clues are valuable in making the diagnosis of deep vein thrombosis suggest a scoring system (Anand et al, 1998). One point is given for each of the following risk factors:

- Active cancer
- Paralysis, paresis, or recent cast immobilization of a lower extremity
- Having been recently bedridden for more than 3 days after major surgery within the last 4 weeks
- Localized tenderness along the distribution of a deep venous system

- Swelling of an entire leg
- Calf swelling of more than 3 cm when compared to the asymptomatic leg
- Pitting edema greater in the symptomatic leg
- Presence of collateral superficial veins

Two points are subtracted if an alternative diagnosis is as likely as, or more likely than, that of deep vein thrombosis.

A score of 3 or more suggests a high probability of deep vein thrombosis; 1 to 2 suggests a moderate probability; 0 or less suggests a low probability. Definitive diagnosis requires additional laboratory testing including ultrasound studies.

HYPERTENSION

Hypertension is one of the most common diseases in the world. It is often responsible for cerebrovascular accidents (CVAs), renal failure, and certainly contributes to congestive heart failure. Hypertension continues to be defined as a blood pressure consistently at 140/90 mm Hg or higher. The Joint National Committee on Prevention, Detection, Evaluation, and Treatment of High Blood Pressure (JNC7) has suggested a new classification of *prehypertension*. This state is defined by a systolic blood pressure between 120 and 139 mm Hg or a diastolic pressure between 80 and 89 mm Hg. Prehypertension does not require pharmacologic intervention but should be treated by reducing fats and salt in the diet, succeeding in weight reduction, and enjoying increased physical activity. Hypertension itself will require medication for its control (see Table 15-3). Perhaps because of the increasing obesity in the American population, the JNC7 predicts that the great majority of individuals now 55 years of age will develop hypertension in their lifetime.

JUGULAR VENOUS PRESSURE DISORDERS

TRICUSPID REGURGITATION

With severe tricuspid regurgitation, the v wave is much more prominent and occurs earlier, often merging with the c wave (Fig. 15-20; see also Fig. 15-7). Physical findings might include a holosystolic murmur in the tricuspid region, a pulsatile liver, and peripheral edema (see Table 14-5).

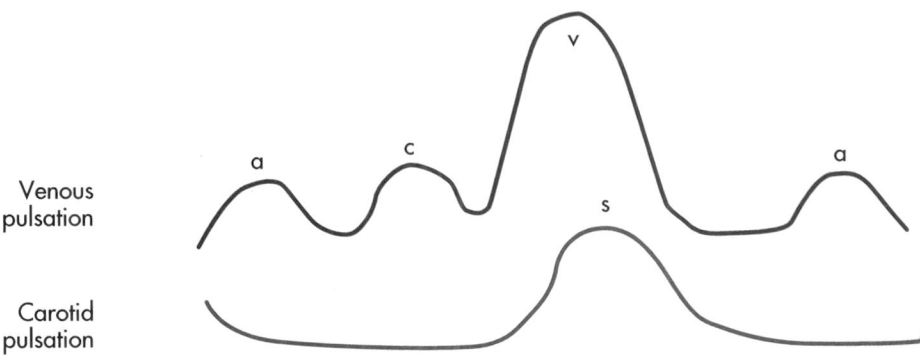

Venous pulsation

Carotid pulsation

FIGURE 15-20
Diagram of pulsation in tricuspid regurgitation.

ATRIAL FIBRILLATION

With atrial fibrillation, the a wave is absent and the pulse is typically irregular. Therefore there are only two venous pulsations for each arterial pulsation, and the time interval between v waves is variable.

CARDIAC TAMPONADE The JVP is particularly helpful for evaluating patients with pericardial disease. With cardiac tamponade, the Y-descent is abolished and the JVP is markedly elevated (15 to 25 cm H_2O). Additionally, the JVP fails to fall with inspiration as it usually does and may actually increase (Kussmaul sign). Other physical findings may include tachycardia and pulsus paradoxus (decrease in systolic blood pressure greater than 15 mm Hg with inspiration) (see Box 15-5; see Fig. 14-23).

CONSTRICTIVE PERICARDITIS In constrictive pericarditis, the JVP is elevated, just as with cardiac tamponade, but there is a prominent Y-descent. Additional physical findings in constrictive pericarditis may include signs of severe right heart failure such as ascites and severe peripheral edema (Fig. 15-21).

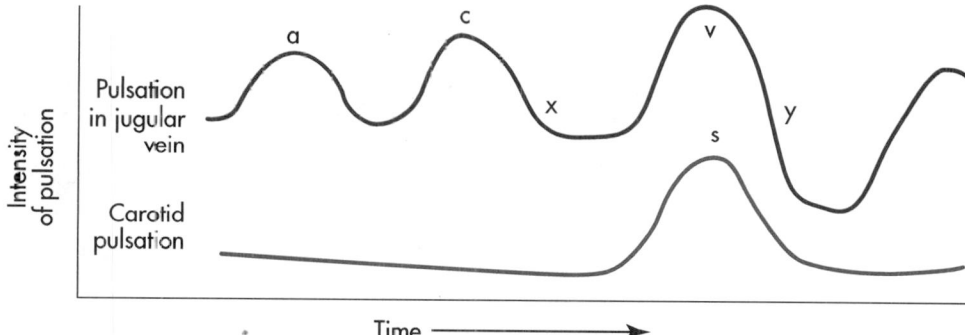

FIGURE 15-21
Diagram of pulsation in constrictive pericarditis.

CHILDREN

COARCTATION OF THE AORTA

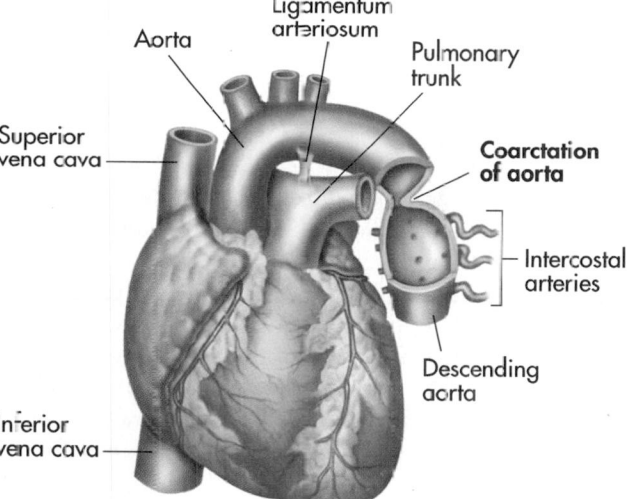

FIGURE 15-22
Coarctation of the aorta.
Modified from Canobbio, 1990.

Coarctation of the aorta is a congenital stenosis or narrowing seen most commonly in the descending aortic arch near the origin of the left subclavian artery and ligamentum arteriosum (Fig. 15-22). If present, it will be detected most often during infancy and should be routinely sought. When the radial and femoral pulses are palpated simultaneously, they will ordinarily be perceived to peak at the same time, the femoral slightly earlier than the radial. If there is a delay and/or a palpable diminution of amplitude (not necessarily an absence) of the femoral pulse, coarctation must be suspected. The findings will be the same on both sides of the body. Differences in blood pressure readings taken in the arms and legs should confirm the suspicion. They will be distinctly, even severely, higher in the arms than in the legs. (Blood pressure in the legs will ordinarily be the same or even slightly higher than that in the arms.) A systolic murmur will be audible over the precordium and, at times, radiate over the back relative to the area of the coarctation. In older children and adults, x-ray film may show notching of the ribs and a figure three sign in the contour of the left upper border of the heart, caused by dilation of the aorta distal to the area of the coarctation, which is then adjacent to the shadow of the descending thoracic aorta. If coarctation remains undetected, the aorta may dissect or rupture. Endocarditis and congestive heart failure are also possible. The results of surgery are usually excellent; rarely, the coarctation may recur.

KAWASAKI DISEASE

Kawasaki disease is an acute illness of uncertain cause affecting the young, and affecting males more often than females. The manifestations are diffuse and are typified by fever lasting a few days to 3 weeks and by the effects of a systemic vasculitis with conjunctival injection, strawberry tongue, edema of the hands and feet, some lymphadenopathy, and polymorphous non-vesicular rashes, among a variety of other findings (Fig. 15-23). The critical concern, however, is cardiac involvement. As the disease progresses and as the vasculitis takes hold, aneurysms of a coronary artery may develop, sometimes very early, sometimes later. Other arteries may be involved, and early death may be the result of myocardial infarction, rupture of an aneurysm, or generalized vasculitis of the smaller vessels of the heart. An aneurysm may rupture even years later. Effective therapy requires early diagnosis and treatment in the first few days of the illness with high-dose intravenous immunoglobulins. Corticosteroids are not given because they may exaggerate the risk of aneurysmal dilations.

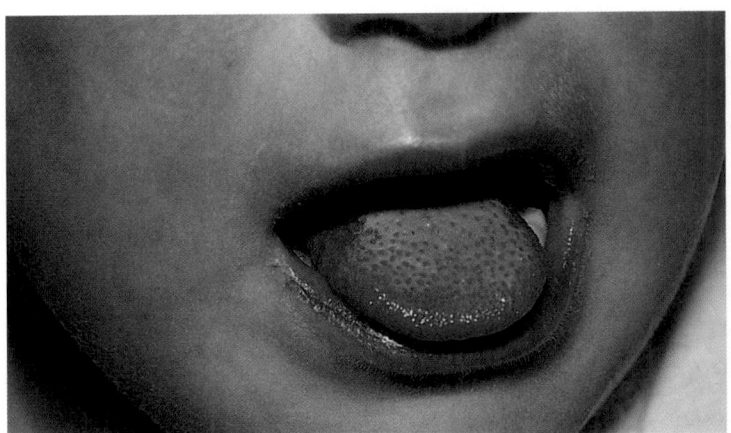

FIGURE 15-23
Strawberry tongue.
From Zitelli, Davis, 2002.

PREGNANT WOMEN

CHRONIC HYPERTENSION

Chronic hypertension is hypertension that was present before conception or detected before the 20th week of gestation and does not resolve in the early postpartum period. This includes women whose systolic blood pressure is 140 mm Hg or higher or diastolic blood pressure is 90 mm Hg or higher.

PREECLAMPSIA-ECLAMPSIA

Preeclampsia-eclampsia defines a syndrome specific to pregnancy. It is determined by hypertension that occurs after the 20th week of pregnancy and the presence of proteinuria. It may be diagnosed *without* proteinuria if other systemic symptoms are present (e.g., visual changes, headache, abdominal pain, or abnormal laboratory values). Eclampsia is preeclampsia with seizures when no other cause for the seizures can be found.

PREECLAMPSIA SUPERIMPOSED ON CHRONIC HYPERTENSION

Preeclampsia superimposed on chronic hypertension has the worst prognosis and is associated with severe maternal and fetal complications. It is suspected in women with hypertension before 20 weeks of gestation with a new onset of proteinuria, in women with hypertension and proteinuria both before 20 weeks of gestation, in women with previously controlled hypertension whose blood pressure suddenly increases, and in women with thrombocytopenia and elevated liver enzymes.

GESTATIONAL HYPERTENSION

Gestational hypertension may be transient or chronic in nature and the specific diagnosis may not be made until the postpartum period. Transient hypertension occurs, without proteinuria or symptoms, late in pregnancy and blood pressure returns to normal by 12 weeks postpartum. Chronic gestational hypertension describes a woman whose blood pressure remains elevated beyond 12 weeks postpartum.

OLDER ADULTS

ARTERIOSCLEROSIS OBLITERANS OF THE EXTREMITIES

This is an age-related progressive arterial disease paralleling the development of atherosclerosis elsewhere. The particular and sole specific symptom is intermittent claudication, pain, spasm, or weakness in a muscle at work, especially during walking, that is almost immediately relieved by rest. It is severe enough to force the patient to stop and to sit because it is too painful to continue or the muscle gives way and the patient falls.

VENOUS ULCERS

These ulcers are generally found on the medial or lateral aspects of the lower limbs, most often in older adults (Fig. 15-24). Induration, edema, and hyperpigmentation are common associated findings. Heart failure, hypoalbuminemia, and nutritional deficiency may be factors adding to the result of the aging of the veins. Peripheral neuropathy and diabetes mellitus, as well as arterial disease, may be causal.

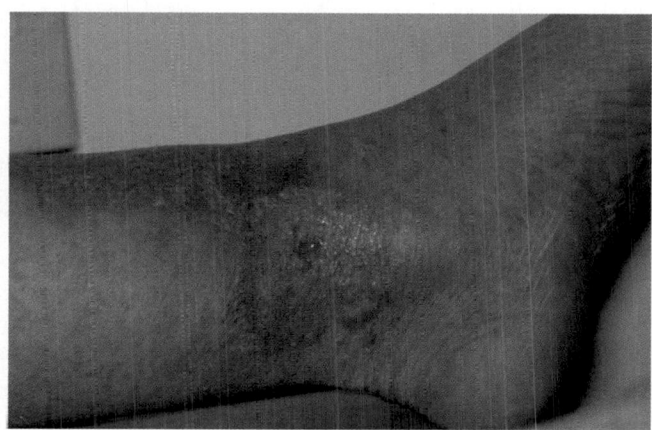

FIGURE 15-24
Venous stasis ulcer.
From Lemmi, Lemmi, 2000.

ELECTRONIC RESOURCES

For Weblinks and additional resources, go to **evolve**

http://evolve.elsevier.com/Seidel

or to the Companion CD-ROM.

Additional information related to the content in Chapter 15 can be found on the companion website at evolve.elsevier.com/Seidel/ or on the interactive companion CD-ROM. Resources and activities for Chapter 15 include:
- Sound and Vision Theater
- Printouts for Your Practice
- Interactive Challenge
- Spanish Assessment Terms with Pronunciation Guide
- Instant Calculator

BREASTS AND AXILLAE

ANATOMY AND PHYSIOLOGY

The breasts are paired mammary glands located on the anterior chest wall, superficial to the pectoralis major and serratus anterior muscles (Fig. 16-1). In women, the breast extends from the second or third rib to the sixth or seventh rib, and from the sternal margin to the midaxillary line. The nipple is located centrally, surrounded by the areola. The male breast consists of a small nipple and areola overlying a thin layer of breast tissue that is indistinguishable by palpation from surrounding tissue.

The female breast is composed of glandular and fibrous tissue and subcutaneous and retromammary fat. The glandular tissue is arranged into 15 to 20 lobes per breast that radiate about the nipple. Each lobe is composed of 20 to 40 lobules; each lobule consists of milk-producing acini cells that empty into lactiferous ducts. These cells are small and inconspicuous in nonpregnant, nonlactating women. A lactiferous duct drains milk from each lobe onto the surface of the nipple.

The layer of subcutaneous fibrous tissue provides support for the breast. Suspensory ligaments (Cooper ligaments) extend from the connective tissue layer through the breast and attach to the underlying muscle fascia, providing further support. The muscles forming the floor of the breast are the pectoralis major, pectoralis minor, serratus anterior, latissimus dorsi, subscapularis, external oblique, and rectus abdominis.

Vascular supply to the breast is primarily through branches of the internal mammary artery and the lateral thoracic artery. This network provides most of the blood supply to the deeper tissues of the breast and to the nipple. The intercostal arteries assist in supplying the more superficial tissues.

The subcutaneous and retromammary fat that surrounds the glandular tissue constitutes most of the bulk of the breast. The proportions of each of the component tissues vary with age, nutritional status, pregnancy, lactation, and genetic predisposition.

For the purposes of examination the breast is divided into five segments: four quadrants and a tail (Fig. 16-2). The greatest amount of glandular tissue lies in the upper outer quadrant. Breast tissue extends from this quadrant into the axilla, forming the tail of Spence. In the axillae the mammary tissue is in direct contact with the axillary lymph nodes.

The nipple, onto which the lactiferous ducts empty, is located centrally on the breast and is surrounded by the pigmented areola. The nipple is composed of epithelium that is infiltrated with circular and longitudinal smooth muscle fibers. Contraction of the smooth muscle, induced by tactile, sensory, or autonomic stimuli, produces erection of the nipple and causes the

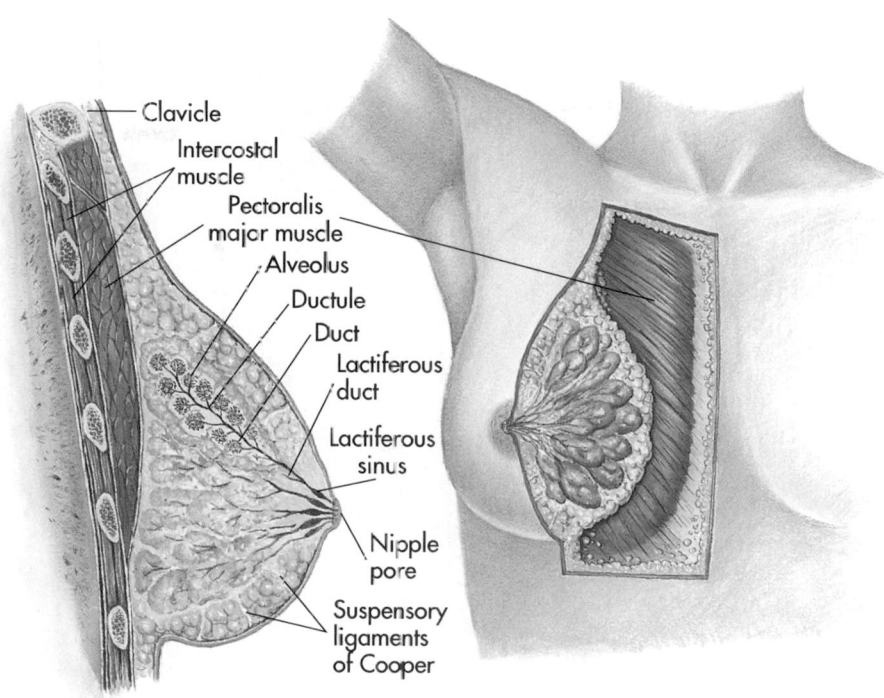

FIGURE 16-1
Anatomy of the breast showing position and major structures.

Clavicle
Intercostal muscle
Pectoralis major muscle
Alveolus
Ductule
Duct
Lactiferous duct
Lactiferous sinus
Nipple pore
Suspensory ligaments of Cooper

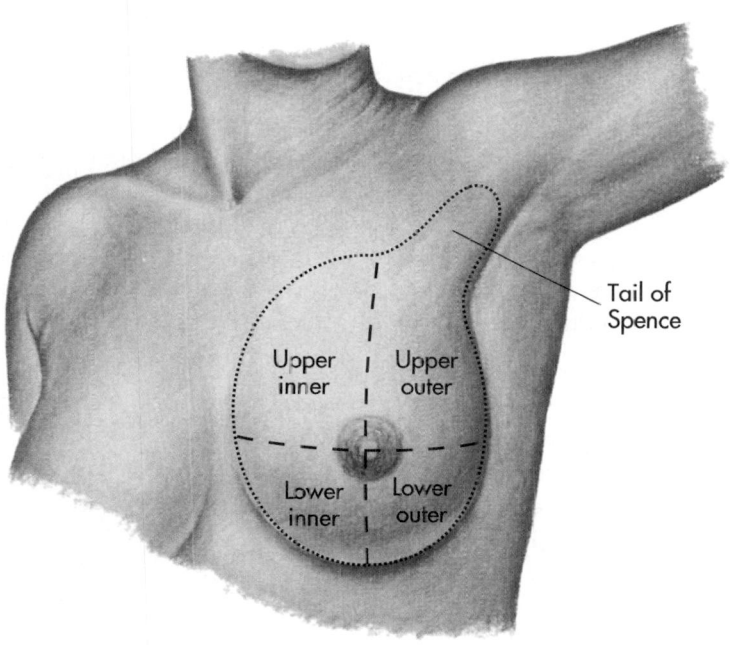

FIGURE 16-2
Quadrants of the left breast and axillary tail of Spence.

Tail of Spence
Upper inner
Upper outer
Lower inner
Lower outer

lactiferous ducts to empty. The process of erection is supported by venous stasis in the erectile vascular tissue. Tiny sebaceous glands may be apparent on the areola surface (Montgomery tubercles or follicles). Some hair follicles may be found about the circumference of the areola. Supernumerary nipples or breast tissue is sometimes present along the mammary ridge that extends from the axilla during embryonic development (see Fig. 16-10).

Each breast contains a lymphatic network that drains the breast radially and deeply to underlying lymphatics. Superficial lymphatics drain the skin, and deep lymphatics drain the mammary lobules. Table 16-1 summarizes the patterns of lymph drainage.

The complex of lymph nodes, their locations, and direction of drainage are illustrated in Fig. 16-3. The axillary nodes are more superficial and are therefore more accessible and rela-

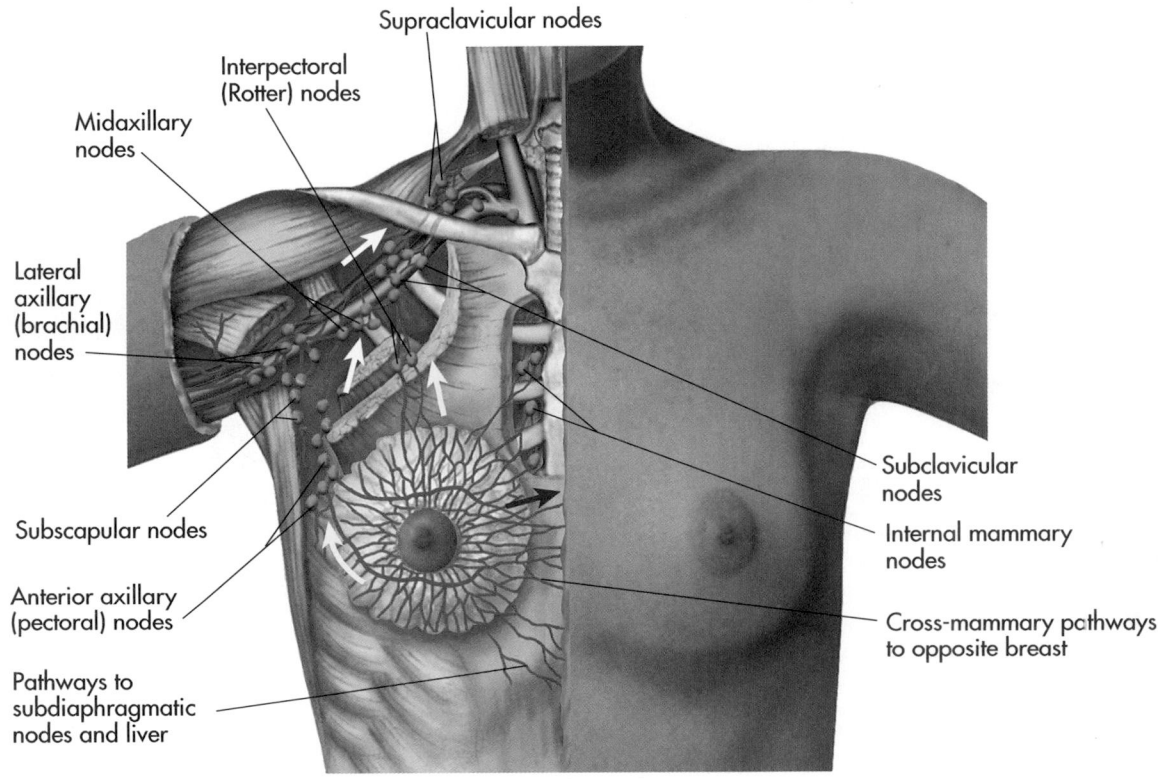

FIGURE 16-3
Lymphatic drainage of the breast.

PHYSICAL VARIATIONS

Breast Size
As adolescents develop, they may wonder about their breast size. Asian women generally have smaller breasts than white women, but data are lacking regarding breast size in other groups.

Data from Alagaratnam, Wong, 1985.

TABLE 16-1	Patterns of Lymph Drainage
Area of Breast	**Drainage**
SUPERFICIAL	
Upper outer quadrant	Scapular, brachial, intermediate nodes toward axillary nodes
Medial portion	Internal mammary chain toward opposite breast and abdomen
DEEP	
Posterior chest wall and portion	Posterior axillary nodes (subscapular) of the arm
Anterior chest wall	Anterior axillary nodes (pectoral)
Upper arm	Lateral axillary nodes (brachial)
Retroareolar area	Interpectoral (Rotter) nodes into the axillary chain
AREOLA AND NIPPLE	Midaxillary, subclavicular, and supraclavicular nodes

tively easy to palpate when enlarged. The anterior axillary (pectoral) nodes are located along the lower border of the pectoralis major inside the lateral axillary fold. The midaxillary (central) nodes are high in the axilla close to the ribs. The posterior axillary (subscapular) nodes lie along the lateral border of the scapula and deep in the posterior axillary fold, whereas the lateral axillary (brachial) nodes can be felt along the upper humerus.

CHILDREN AND ADOLESCENTS

The breast evolves in structure and function throughout life. Childhood and preadolescence represent a latent phase of breast development during which only minimal branching of primary ducts occurs. Thelarche (breast development) represents an early sign of puberty in adolescent girls. The developmental process has been classified and described in a number of ways. Tanner's five stages of developing sexual maturity, discussed in Chapter 5, is the classification most commonly used.

In using the Tanner charts to stage breast development, it is important to note certain temporal relationships. It is unusual for the onset of menses to occur before stage 3. About 25% of females begin menstruation at stage 3. Approximately 75% are menstruating at stage 4 and are beginning a reasonably regular menstrual cycle. Some 10% of young women do not begin to menstruate until stage 5. The average interval from the appearance of the breast bud (stage 2) to menarche is 2 years. Stage 4 may not occur in as many as 25% of all adolescents and may be only minimal in another 25%. Breasts develop at different rates in the individual, which can result in asymmetry.

PREGNANT WOMEN

Striking changes occur in the breasts during pregnancy. In response to luteal and placental hormones, the lactiferous ducts proliferate and the alveoli increase extensively in size and number, which may cause the breasts to enlarge two to three times their pre-pregnancy size. The increase in glandular tissue displaces connective tissue and, as a result, the tissue becomes softer and looser. Toward the end of pregnancy, as epithelial secretory activity increases, colostrum is produced and accumulates in the acinus cells (alveoli).

The areolae become more deeply pigmented and their diameter increases. The nipples become more prominent, darker, and more erectile. Montgomery tubercles often develop as sebaceous glands hypertrophy.

Mammary vascularization increases, causing veins to engorge and become visible as a blue network beneath the surface of the skin.

LACTATING WOMEN

In the first few days after delivery, small amounts of colostrum are secreted from the breasts. Colostrum contains more protein and minerals than does mature milk. Colostrum also contains antibodies and other host resistance factors. Milk production to replace colostrum begins 2 to 4 days after delivery in response to surging prolactin levels, declining estrogen levels, and the stimulation of sucking. As the alveoli and lactiferous ducts fill, the breasts may become full and tense. This, combined with tissue edema and a delay in effective ejection reflexes, produces breast engorgement.

At the termination of lactation, involution occurs over a period of about 3 months. Breast size decreases without loss of lobular and alveolar components; the breasts rarely return to their prelactation size.

OLDER ADULTS

Before menopause there is a moderate decrease in glandular tissue and some decomposition of alveolar and lobular tissue. After menopause, glandular tissue continues to atrophy gradually and is replaced by fat deposited in the breasts. The inframammary ridge at the lower edge of the breast thickens. The breasts tend to hang more loosely from the chest wall because of these tissue changes and the relaxation of the suspensory ligaments. The nipples become smaller, flatter, and lose some erectile ability.

The skin may take on a relatively dry, thin texture. Loss of axillary hair may also occur.

REVIEW OF RELATED HISTORY

For each of the conditions discussed in this section, targeted topics to include in the history of the present illness are listed. Responses to questions about these topics help fully assess the patient's condition and provide clues for focusing the physical examination.

HISTORY OF PRESENT ILLNESS

- Breast discomfort/pain
  - Temporal sequence: onset gradual or sudden; length of time symptom has been present; does symptom come and go or is it always present

- ◆ Relationship to menses: timing, severity
- ◆ Character: stinging, pulling, burning, drawing, stabbing, aching, throbbing; unilateral or bilateral; localization; radiation
- ◆ Associated symptoms: lump or mass, discharge from nipple
- ◆ Contributory factors: skin irritation under breasts from tissue-to-tissue contact or from rubbing of brassiere; strenuous activity; recent injury to breast
- ◆ Medications: nonprescription or prescription
- ◆ Breast mass or lump
  - ◆ Temporal sequence: length of time since lump first noted; does lump come and go or is it always present; relationship to menses
  - ◆ Symptoms: tenderness or pain (characterize as described previously), dimpling or change in contour
  - ◆ Changes in lump: size, character, relationship to menses (timing or severity)
  - ◆ Associated symptoms: nipple discharge or retraction, tender lymph nodes
  - ◆ Medications: nonprescription or prescription
- ◆ Nipple discharge
  - ◆ Character: spontaneous or provoked; unilateral or bilateral, onset gradual or sudden, duration, color, consistency, odor, amount
  - ◆ Associated symptoms: nipple retraction; breast lump or discomfort
  - ◆ Associated factors: relationship to menses or other activity; recent injury to breast
  - ◆ Medications: nonprescription or prescription; contraceptives; phenothiazines, digitalis, diuretics, steroids

PAST MEDICAL HISTORY

- ◆ Previous breast disease: cancer, fibroadenomas, fibrocystic changes
- ◆ Known BRCA1 or BRCA2 mutation; other known hereditary cancer syndrome (hereditary nonpolyposis colorectal cancer [HNPCC], Li-Fraumeni syndrome, or Cowden syndrome)
- ◆ Previous other related cancers: ovarian, colorectal, endometrial
- ◆ Surgeries: breast biopsies, aspirations, implants, reductions, plasties; oophorectomy
- ◆ Any changes in breast characteristics: pain, tenderness, lumps, discharge, skin changes, size or shape changes
- ◆ Changes in the breast that occur with the menstrual cycle: tenderness, swelling, pain, enlarged nodes
- ◆ Risk factors for breast cancer (see the Risk Factors box on p. 497)
- ◆ Mammography history: how frequently, date of last mammogram, results
- ◆ Menstrual history: first day of last menstrual period; age at menarche or menopause; cycle length, duration and amount of flow, regularity; associated breast symptoms (nipple discharge; pain or discomfort)
- ◆ Pregnancy: age at each pregnancy, length of each pregnancy, date of delivery or termination
- ◆ Lactation: number of children breast-fed; duration of time for breast-feeding; date of termination of last breast-feeding; medications used to suppress lactation
- ◆ Menopause: onset, course, associated problems, residual problems
- ◆ Use of hormonal medications: name and dosage, reason for use (contraception, menstrual control, menopausal symptom relief), length of time on hormones, date of termination
- ◆ Other medications: nonprescription or prescription; tamoxifen, raloxifene

FAMILY HISTORY

- ◆ Breast cancer: primary relatives, secondary relatives; type of cancer; age at time of occurrence; treatment and results; known BRCA1 or BRCA2 mutation
- ◆ Other cancers: ovarian, colorectal; known hereditary cancer syndromes (hereditary nonpolyposis colorectal cancer [HNPCC], Li-Fraumeni syndrome, or Cowden syndrome)
- ◆ Other breast disease in female and male relatives: type of disease; age at time of occurrence; treatment and results

RISK FACTORS
BREAST CANCER

Nonmodifiable Factors

Age: Risk increases with aging. About 18% of breast cancer diagnoses are in women in their 40s; about 77% of breast cancer diagnoses are in women older than 50 years of age. Only about 5% of breast cancer occurs in women younger than 40 years of age.

Gender: Female. More women than men develop breast cancer. The incidence of male breast cancer is less than 1% of that of female breast cancer.

Genetic risk factors: About 5% to 10% of breast cancer cases are hereditary as a result of gene mutations, most commonly those of the BRCA1 and BRCA2 genes. Women with an inherited BRCA1 or BRCA2 mutation have a 35% to 85% chance of developing breast cancer during their lifetime. Women with these inherited mutations also have an increased risk for developing ovarian cancer.

Personal history of breast cancer: A woman with cancer in one breast has a threefold to fourfold increased risk of developing a new cancer in the other breast or in another part of the same breast. This is different from a recurrence of the first cancer.

Family history of breast cancer: Having one first-degree relative (mother, sister, or daughter) with breast cancer approximately doubles a woman's risk, and having two first-degree relatives increases her risk fivefold

The risk of developing breast cancer is increased with:
- Two or more relatives with breast or ovarian cancer
- Breast cancer that occurs before age 50 years in a relative (mother, sister, grandmother, or aunt) on either side of the family; the risk is higher if the mother or sister has a history of breast cancer
- Relatives with both breast and ovarian cancer
- One or more relatives with two cancers (breast and ovarian, or two different breast cancers)
- A male relative (or relatives) with breast cancer
- A family history of breast or ovarian cancer and Ashkenazi Jewish heritage
- A family history that includes a history of diseases associated with hereditary breast cancer such as hereditary nonpolyposis colorectal cancer, Li-Fraumeni syndrome, or Cowden syndrome

Previous breast biopsies: Proliferative breast disease without atypia or unusual hyperplasia slightly increases the risk

of breast cancer (1.5 to 2 times greater risk). Atypical hyperplasia increases a woman's breast cancer risk by 4 to 5 times. Fibrocystic changes without proliferative breast disease does not affect breast cancer risk.

Race: White women are slightly more likely to develop breast cancer than are black women, but black women are more likely to die of this cancer.

Previous breast radiation: Women and men who as children or young adults had radiation therapy to the chest area as treatment for another cancer (such as Hodgkin disease or non-Hodgkin lymphoma) have a significantly increased risk for breast cancer.

Menstrual periods: Women who started menstruating at an early age (before age 12) or who went through menopause at a late age (after age 55) have a slightly higher risk of breast cancer.

Diethylstilbestrol (DES) therapy: Women who received diethylstilbestrol in the 1940s through the 1960s during their pregnancies have a slightly increased risk of developing breast cancer.

Modifiable/Lifestyle Factors

Childbirth: Nulliparity or late age at birth of first child (after age 30) is associated with an increased risk of breast cancer.

Hormone therapy: Use of combined estrogen and progesterone hormone replacement therapy (HRT) after menopause (greater than 4 years of use) increases the risk of breast cancer by 26% compared to the risk in women who have not used HRT.

Alcohol: Use of alcohol is clearly linked to a slightly increased risk of developing breast cancer. Compared with nondrinkers, women who consume one alcoholic drink a day have a very small increase in risk, and those who have two to five drinks daily have about $1\frac{1}{2}$ times the risk of women who drink no alcohol.

Obesity and high-fat diets: Obesity is associated with an increased risk of developing breast cancer, especially for women after menopause. Having more fat tissue can increase estrogen levels and increase the likelihood of developing breast cancer. Overweight women are 60% more likely to die of breast cancer as compared to normal weight women.

PERSONAL AND SOCIAL HISTORY

- Age
- Breast support used with strenuous exercise or sports activities
- Amount of caffeine intake
- Breast self-examination: frequency; at what time in the menstrual cycle; see the Staying Well box on Breast Awareness and Self-Examination on p. 498
- Use of alcohol; daily amounts

STAYING WELL

BREAST AWARENESS AND SELF-EXAMINATION

Breast self-examination (BSE) remains an important tool in the detection of breast cancer. Women should be told about benefits and limitations of BSE. Women can notice changes by being aware of how their breasts normally feel and feeling their breasts for changes (breast awareness) or by choosing to use a step-by-step approach and using a specific schedule to examine her breasts. The lesson learned from a recent randomized clinical trial is that intensive teaching of BSE does not improve its effectiveness (Thomas, et al 2002). Every woman should be familiar with her own breasts and should report any breast change promptly to her health care provider. The American Cancer Society recommends BSE as an option for women starting in their 20s. The technique for BSE is shown in Box 16-1. As you discuss BSE it would be an appropriate time to review the accepted recommendations for early breast cancer detection (Box 16-2) and to discuss the issues related to breast cancer screening.

BOX 16-1

BREAST SELF-EXAMINATION

Breast self-examination (BSE) should be done once a month so that you become familiar with the usual appearance and feel of your breasts. Familiarity makes it easier to notice any changes in the breast from one month to another. Early discovery of a change from what is baseline is the main idea behind BSE.

If you menstruate, the best time to do BSE is 2 or 3 days after your period ends, when your breasts are least likely to be tender or swollen. If you no longer menstruate, pick a day, such as the first day of the month, to remind yourself it is time to do BSE.

Here is how to do BSE:
1. Stand before a mirror. Inspect both breasts for anything unusual, such as any discharge from the nipples, puckering, dimpling, or scaling of the skin.

The next two steps are designed to emphasize any change in the shape or contour of your breasts. As you do them, you should be able to feel your chest muscles tighten.
2. Watching closely in the mirror, clasp hands behind your head and swing elbows forward.
3. Next, press hands firmly on hips and bow slightly toward your mirror as you pull your shoulders and elbows forward.

Some women do the next part of the examination in the shower. Fingers glide over soapy skin, making it easy to appreciate the texture underneath.

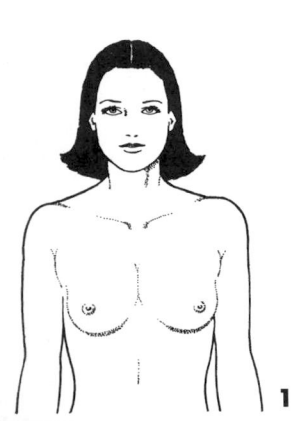

1

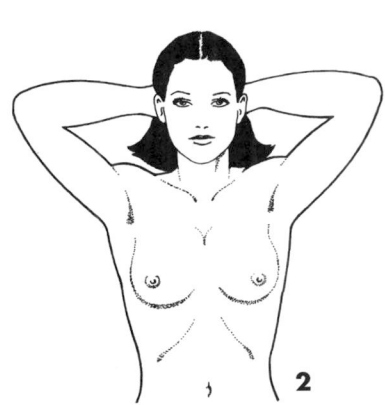

2

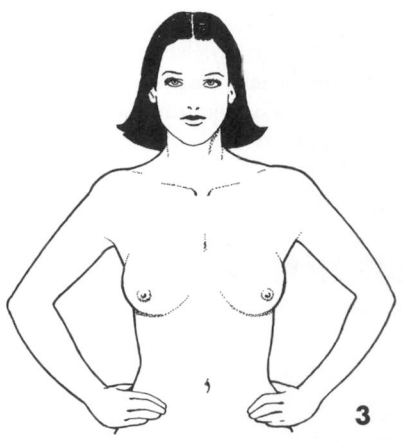

3

EVIDENCE-BASED PRACTICE IN PHYSICAL EXAMINATION

BREAST CANCER SCREENING

Are breast self-examination (BSE), clinical breast examination (CBE), and mammography effective in screening for breast cancer? A clear distinction must be made between screening asymptomatic women and the clinical assessment of women who have breast symptoms. The evidence from recent studies is controversial and mixed.

BSE

In a randomized controlled trial of BSE instruction, breast cancer incidence and mortality were similar in women instructed in BSE and in those who received no instruction. However women in both groups performed BSE and both groups detected breast lumps. Women in the instruction group detected more benign lesions. There is no study of BSE effectiveness, i.e., doing BSE vs. not doing BSE.

CBE

The sensitivity of CBE in detecting breast cancer ranges from 40% to 69% and the specificity from 88% to 99%. No trial has compared CBE alone with no screening. In a trial that compared annual CBE and mammography to mammography alone,

the relative risk for death suggested that mammography added little benefit to a careful and detailed CBE. The mortality reductions in trials of CBE with mammography are similar to those in trials including mammography only.

Mammography

Estimates of the sensitivity and specificity of mammography in detecting breast cancer vary. Sensitivity is lower among women who are younger than 50 years of age, have denser breasts, or are taking hormone replacement therapy. Specificity is increased with a shorter screening interval and the availability of prior mammograms. In a review of randomized clinical trials, for a 1-year screening interval, the sensitivity of first mammography ranged from 71% to 96%. Sensitivity was substantially lower for women in their 40s than for older women. The specificity of a single mammogram was 94% to 97%.

Until the evidence is clear, we must educate patients about the likelihood and significance of both false-positive and false-negative test results and address the associated issues of uncertainty, anxiety, and cost.

Data from Humphrey et al, 2002.

BOX 16-1

BREAST SELF-EXAMINATION—cont'd

4. Raise your left arm. Use three or four fingers of your right hand to explore your left breast firmly, carefully, and thoroughly. Beginning at the outer edge, press the flat part of your fingers in small circles, moving the circles slowly around the breast. Gradually work toward the nipple. Be sure to cover the entire breast. Pay special attention to the area between the breast and the armpit, including the armpit itself. Feel for any unusual lump or mass under the skin.

5. Step 4 should be repeated lying down. Lie flat on your back, left arm over your head and a pillow or folded towel under your left shoulder. This position flattens the breast and makes it easier to examine. Use the same circular motion described earlier.

6. Repeat on your right breast.

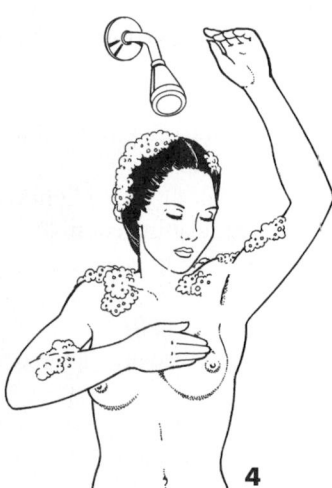

4

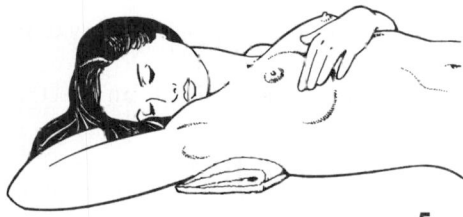

5

BOX 16-2

SCREENING FOR BREAST CANCER

Breast cancer is the most common type of cancer among women in the United States and is the second leading cause of cancer death in women. Early detection through screening is important for timely treatment and prevention of death. Authorities do not completely agree on the need for, frequency of, and timing of screening (see the Evidence-Based Practice box on p. 499). Clinical breast examination (CBE), mammography, and breast self-examination (BSE), are the currently available mechanisms for screening asymptomatic women.

The following is a summary of the various recommendations:

CBE	Older than 40 years of age: annually
	Younger than 40 years of age: every 1 to 3 years
Mammogram	Women at average risk: yearly starting at 40 years of age and continuing for as long as a woman is in good health
	Women at increased risk (e.g., family history, genetic tendency, past breast cancer): consider more frequent CBE, earlier mammographic screening, additional tests (e.g., breast ultrasound or magnetic resonance imaging)
BSE	Optional. Monthly starting during age 20s. Women should be familiar with their breasts and report any changes to their health care provider.

PREGNANT WOMEN

- Sensations: fullness, tingling, tenderness
- Presence of colostrum and knowledge about how to care for breasts and nipples during pregnancy
- Use of supportive brassiere
- Knowledge and information about breast-feeding
- Plans to breast-feed, experience, expectations (all women should be encouraged to consider breast-feeding because of the positive health benefits for the newborn)

LACTATING WOMEN

- Cleaning procedures for breasts: use of soap products that can remove natural lubricants, frequency of use; nipple preparations
- Use of nursing brassiere
- Nipples: tenderness, pain, cracking, bleeding; retracted; related problems with feeding; exposure to air
- Associated problems: engorgement, leaking breasts, plugged duct (localized tenderness and lump), fever, infection; treatment and results; infant with oral candidal infection
- Nursing routine: length of feeding, frequency, rotation of breasts, positions used
- Breast milk pumping devices used, frequency of use
- Cultural beliefs about nursing
- Food and environmental agents that can affect breast milk (e.g., chocolate, photography chemicals)
- Medications that can cross the milk-blood barrier (e.g., cimetidine, clemastine, thiouracil); all medications—prescription and nonprescription—should be evaluated for potential side effects in the newborn

OLDER ADULTS

- Skin irritation under pendulous breasts from tissue-to-tissue contact or from rubbing of brassiere; treatment
- Hormone therapy during or since menopause: name and dosage of medication; duration of therapy

EXAMINATION AND FINDINGS

EQUIPMENT

- ◆ Flashlight with transilluminator
- ◆ Ruler
- ◆ Small pillow or folded towel
- ◆ Glass slide and cytologic fixative, if nipple discharge is present

Adequate lighting is essential for revealing shadows and subtle variations in skin color and texture. Adequate exposure is also essential, requiring that the patient be disrobed to the waist. Simultaneous observation of both breasts is necessary to detect minor differences between them that may be significant. Modesty is a concern, however, and you or the patient may be uncomfortable at first. A matter-of-fact and composed approach with attention to the patient as a person will go a long way in reassuring the patient of your regard and sensitivity.

INSPECTION

BREASTS

With the patient in a sitting position with arms hanging loosely at the sides, inspect each breast and compare it with the other for size, symmetry, contour, skin color and texture, venous patterns, and lesions. Perform this portion of the examination for both women and men. With female patients, lift the breasts with your fingertips, inspecting the lower and lateral aspects to determine whether there are any changes in the color or texture of the skin.

Women's breasts vary somewhat in shape, from convex to pendulous or conical, and often one breast is somewhat smaller than the other (Fig. 16-4). Men's breasts are generally even

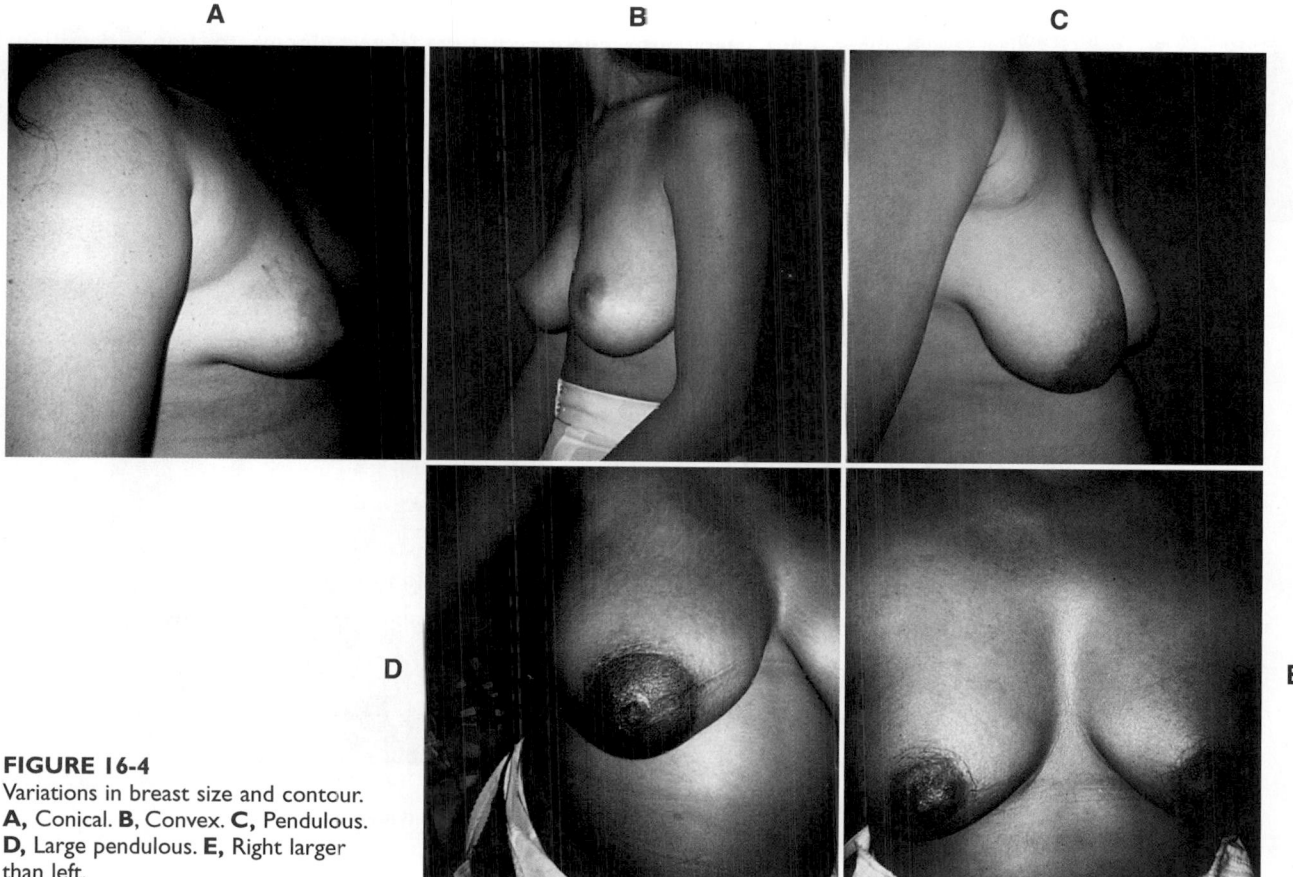

A   **B**   **C**   **D**   **E**

FIGURE 16-4
Variations in breast size and contour.
A, Conical. **B,** Convex. **C,** Pendulous.
D, Large pendulous. **E,** Right larger than left.

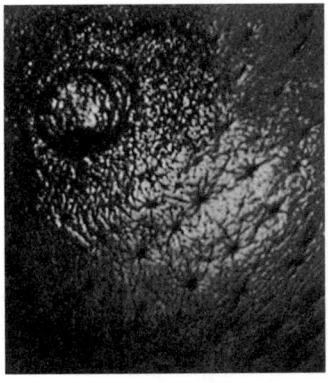

FIGURE 16-5
Peau d'orange appearance from edema.
From Gallager, 1978.

with the chest wall, although some men, particularly those who are overweight, have breasts with a convex shape.

The skin texture should appear smooth and the contour should be uninterrupted. Retractions and dimpling signify the contraction of fibrotic tissue that occurs with carcinoma. Alterations in contour are best seen on bilateral comparison of one breast with the other. A *peau d'orange* appearance of the skin indicates edema of the breast caused by blocked lymph drainage in advanced or inflammatory carcinoma (Fig. 16-5). The skin appears thickened with enlarged pores and accentuated skin markings. Healthy skin may look similar if the pores of the skin are large.

Venous patterns should be bilaterally similar. Venous networks may be visible, although these are usually pronounced only in the breasts of pregnant or obese women. If these are bilateral, there is no cause for concern; however, unilateral venous patterns can be produced by dilated superficial veins from increased blood flow to a malignancy. This finding should alert you to the need for further investigation.

Other markings and nevi that are long-standing, unchanging, or nontender are of little concern. Changes in or the recent appearance of any lesions always signals the need for closer investigation: a mammogram, ultrasound, or biopsy is indicated.

NIPPLE AND AREOLA

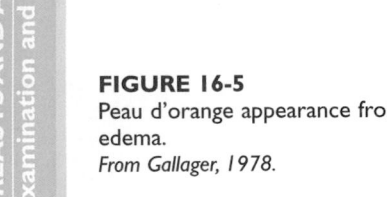

MNEMONICS

Five Ds Related to Nipples

D Discharge
D Depression or inversion
D Discoloration: pregnancy
D Dermatologic changes: Paget disease
D Deviation: compare opposite side

Inspect the areolae and nipples of both men and women. The areola should be round or oval and bilaterally equal or nearly so. The color ranges from pink to black. In light-skinned women the areola usually turns brown with the first pregnancy and remains dark. In women with dark skin, the areola is brown before pregnancy. A peppering of nontender, nonsuppurative Montgomery tubercles is a common expected finding (Fig. 16-6). The surface should be otherwise smooth. The peau d'orange skin associated with carcinoma is often seen first in the areola.

Most nipples are everted, but one or both nipples may be inverted (Fig. 16-7). In these instances, ask whether there is a lifetime history of inversion. Recent unilateral inversion or retraction of a previously everted nipple suggests malignancy.

Simultaneous bilateral inspection is necessary to detect nipple retraction or deviation. Retraction is seen as a flattening, withdrawal, or inversion of the nipple and indicates inward pulling by inflammatory or malignant tissue (Fig. 16-8). The fibrotic tissue of carcinoma can also change the axis of the nipple, causing it to point in a direction different from that of the other nipple.

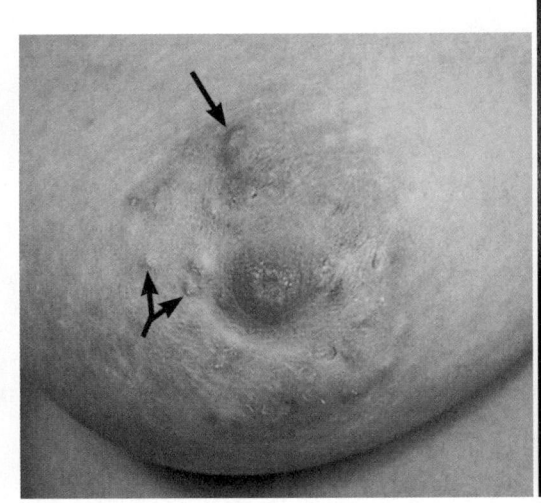
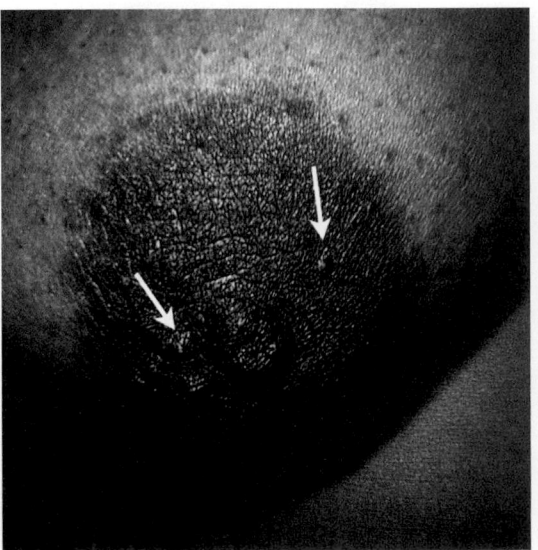

FIGURE 16-6
Montgomery tubercles. **A,** Light-skinned woman. **B,** Dark-skinned woman.
A from Mansel, Bundred, 1995.

The nipples should be a homogenous color and match that of the areolae. Their surface may be either smooth or wrinkled, but should be free of crusting, cracking, or discharge. Areola color varies from light pink to very dark brown or black (Fig. 16-9).

Supernumerary nipples, which are more common in black women than in white women, appear as one or more extra nipples located along the embryonic mammary ridge (the "milk line") (Fig. 16-10). These nipples and areolae may be pink or brown, are usually small, and are commonly mistaken for moles (Fig. 16-11). Infrequently, some glandular tissue may accom-

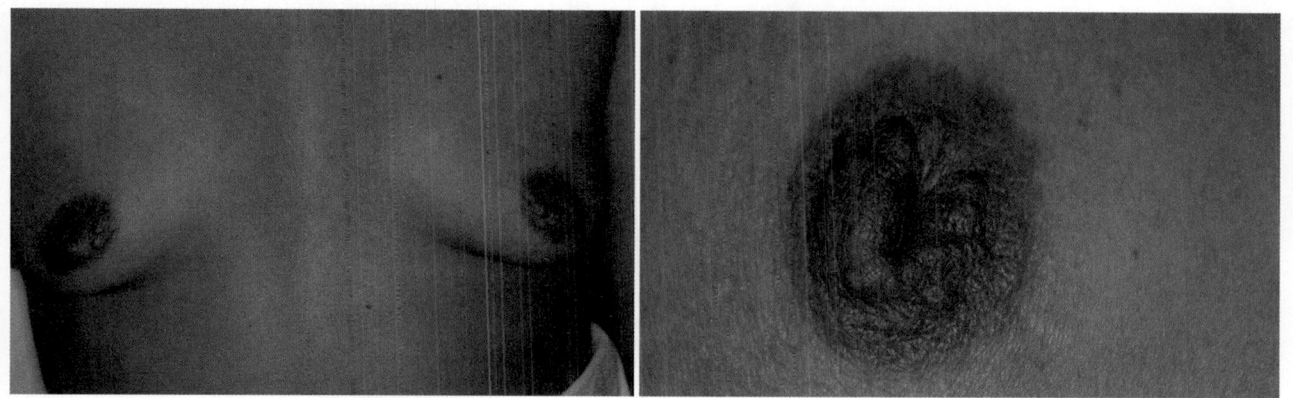

FIGURE 16-7
A, Left nipple inverted; right nipple everted. **B,** Close-up of nipple inversion.
From Lemmi, Lemmi, 2000.

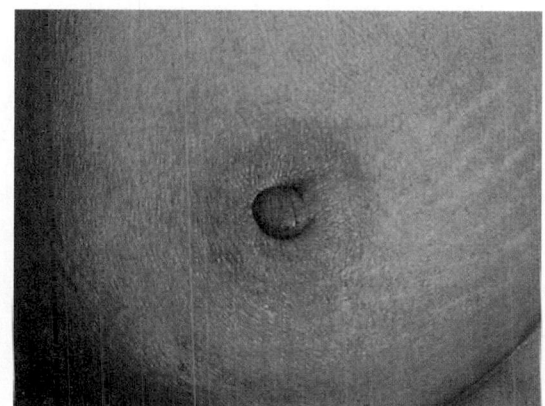

FIGURE 16-8
Nipple retraction laterally and swelling behind right nipple in Asian woman with breast cancer.
From Mansel, Bundred, 1995.

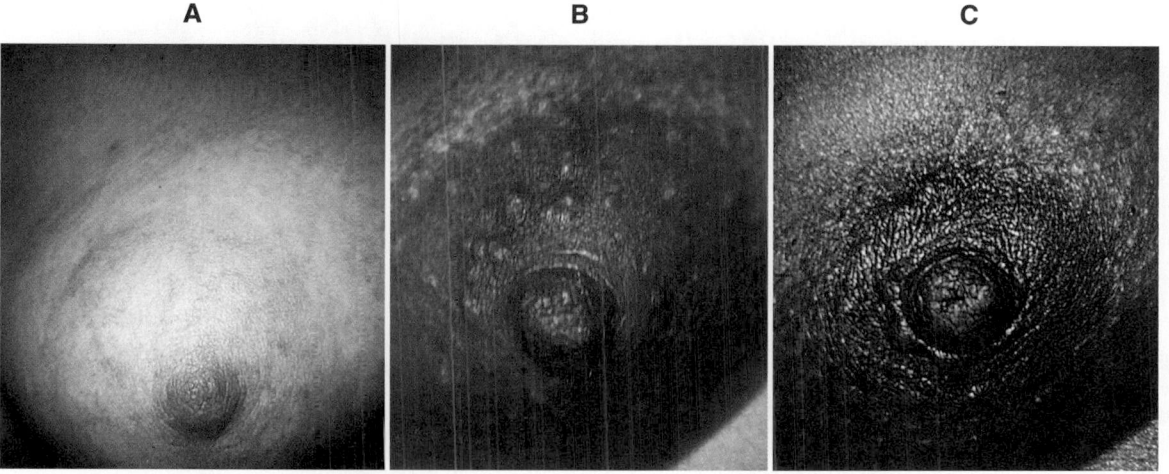

FIGURE 16-9
Variations in color of areola. **A,** Pink. **B,** Brown. **C,** Black.

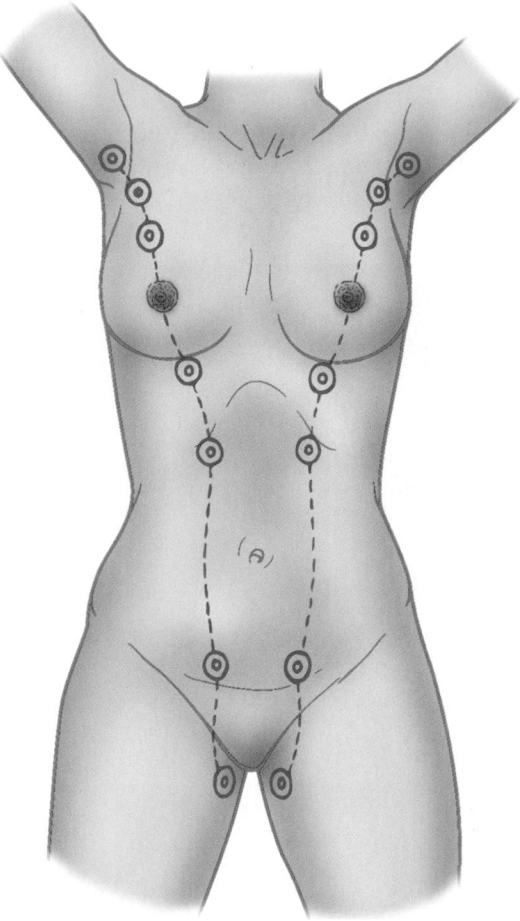

FIGURE 16-10
Supernumerary nipples and tissue may arise along the "milk line," an embryonic ridge.
From Thompson et al, 1997.

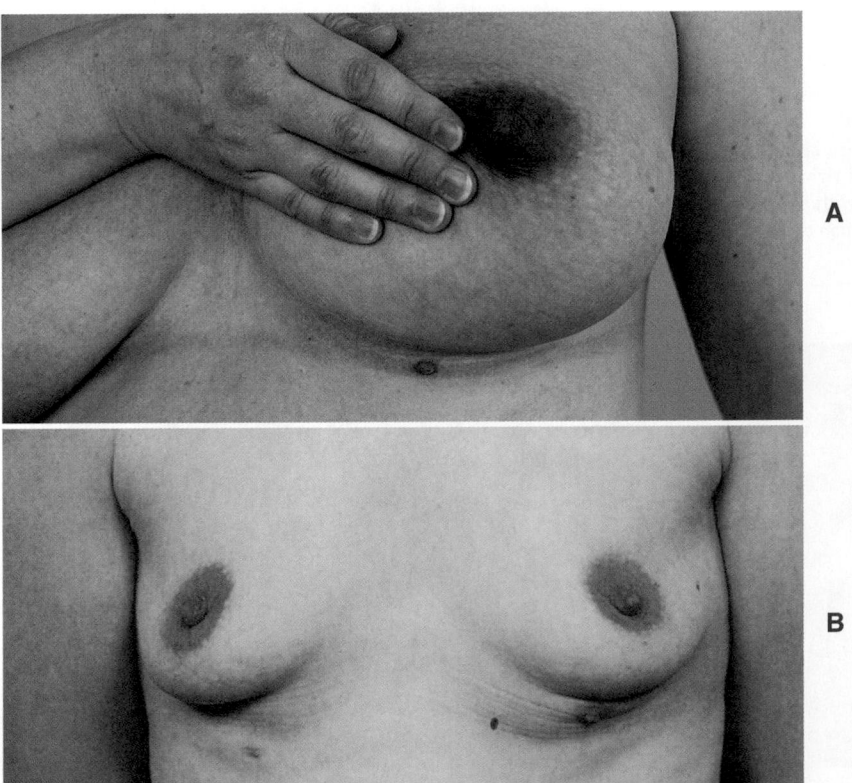

A

B

FIGURE 16-11
A, Supernumerary nipple without glandular tissue. **B,** Supernumerary breast and nipple on left side and supernumerary nipple alone on right side.
From Mansel, Bundred, 1995.

pany these nipples. In some cases, supernumerary nipples may be associated with congenital renal or cardiac anomalies, particularly in whites.

REINSPECTION IN VARIED POSITIONS

Breasts and Axillae: Inspecting the Breasts in Different Positions

Reinspect the woman's breasts with the patient in the following positions:

- Seated with arms over the head or flexed behind the neck: This adds tension to the suspensory ligaments, accentuates dimpling, and may reveal variations in contour and symmetry (Fig. 16-12, *A*).
- Seated with hands pressed against hips with shoulders rolled forward (or alternatively have the patient push her palms together): This contracts the pectoral muscles, which can reveal deviations in contour and symmetry (Fig. 16-12, *B* and *C*).
- Seated and leaning forward from the waist: This also causes tension in the suspensory ligaments. The breasts should hang equally. This maneuver can be particularly helpful in assessing the contour and symmetry of large breasts, because the breasts fall away from the chest wall and hang freely. As the patient leans forward, support her by the hands (Fig. 16-12, *D*).

For all patient positions, the breasts should appear bilaterally equal, with an even contour and absence of dimpling, retraction, or deviation.

PALPATION

After a thorough inspection, systematically palpate the breasts, axillae, and supraclavicular and infraclavicular regions. Palpation of male breasts can be brief but should not be omitted.

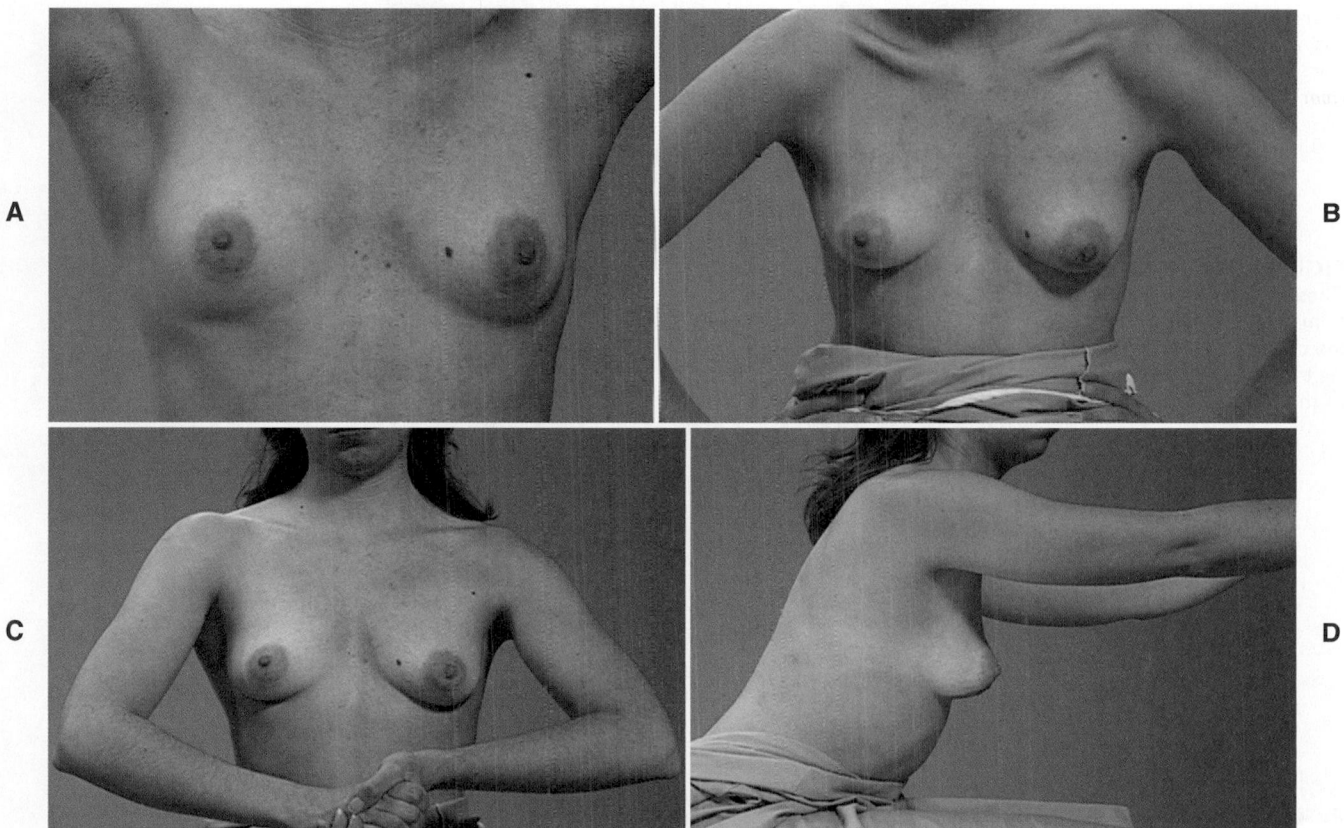

FIGURE 16-12
Inspect the breasts in the following positions. **A,** Arms extended overhead. **B,** Hands pressed against hips. **C,** Pressing hands together (an alternative way to flex the pectoral muscles). **D,** Leaning forward from the waist.

PATIENT IN SEATED POSITION

Breasts and Axillae:
Palpating Lymph Nodes Near the Breasts

Chest Wall Sweep. Have the patient sit with arms hanging freely at the sides. Place the palm of your right hand at the patient's right clavicle at the sternum. Sweep downward from the clavicle to the nipple feeling for superficial lumps. Repeat the sweep until you have covered the entire right chest wall. Repeat the procedure using your left hand for the left chest wall (Fig. 16-13).

Bimanual Digital Palpation. Place one hand, palmar surface facing up, under the patient's right breast. Position your hand so that it acts as a flat surface against which to compress the breast tissue. With the fingers of the other hand walk across the breast tissue, feeling for lumps as you compress the tissue between your fingers and your flat hand. Repeat the procedure for the other breast (Fig. 16-14).

Lymph Node Palpation. Palpate for lymph nodes in both male and female patients. To palpate the axillae, have the patient seated with arms flexed at the elbow. Support the patient's left lower arm with your left hand while examining the left axilla with your right hand, as shown in Fig. 16-15. With the palmar surface of your fingers, reach deeply into the axillary hollow, pushing firmly but not too aggressively upward. Use the first rib as your landmark. Then bring your fingers downward so that you gently roll the soft tissue against the chest wall and muscles of the axilla. Be sure to explore all sections of the axilla. From the apex palpate downward to the bra line, and also along the inner aspect of the upper arm down to the elbow. Reposition your fingers to palpate the medial aspect along the rib cage and into the anterior wall along the pectoral muscles. Reposition again to palpate the posterior wall along the border of the scapula. Repeat the mirror image of this maneuver for the right axilla.

The supraclavicular and infraclavicular areas also should be palpated for the presence of enlarged nodes. Hook your fingers over the clavicle and rotate them over the entire supra-

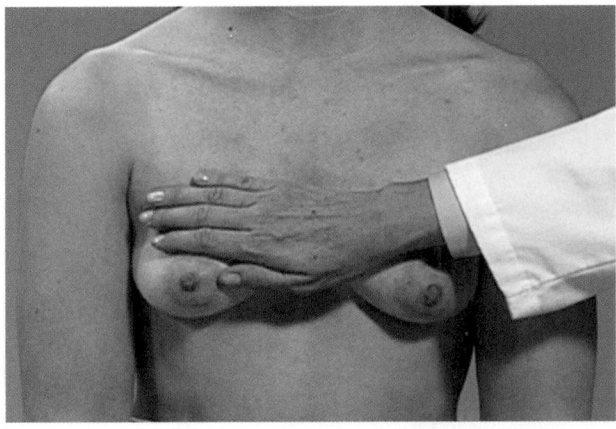

FIGURE 16-13
Chest wall sweep. With the palm of your hand sweep from the clavicle to the nipple, covering the area from the sternum to the midaxillary line.

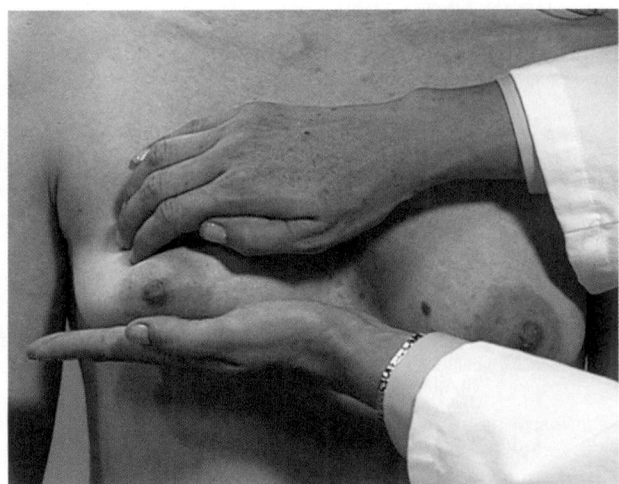

FIGURE 16-14
Bimanual digital palpation. Walk your fingers across the breast tissue, compressing it between your fingers and the palmar surface of your other hand.

clavicular fossa. Have the patient turn his or her head toward the side being palpated and raise the same shoulder, allowing your fingers to reach more deeply into the fossa. Have the patient bend the head forward to relax the sternocleidomastoid muscle. These nodes are considered to be sentinel nodes (Virchow nodes), so any enlargement is highly significant. Virchow nodes are the first sign of invasion of the lymphatics by abdominal or thoracic carcinoma. Move your fingers to the infraclavicular area and palpate along the clavicle using a rotary motion with your fingers.

Nodes are not usually palpable in the adult. Palpable nodes may be the result of an inflammatory or malignant process. Nodes that are detected should be described according to location, size, shape, consistency, tenderness, fixation, and delineation of borders (see Chapter 9).

PATIENT IN SUPINE POSITION

Have the patient raise one arm behind her head; then place a small pillow or folded towel under that shoulder to spread the breast tissue more evenly over the chest wall (Fig. 16-16). The ideal position for examination is to have the nipple pointing toward the ceiling. Women with large breasts may need to roll slightly to achieve this position. Palpate each breast separately.

Palpate all areas of breast tissue, feeling for lumps or nodules (Box 16-3). Remember that the breast tissue extends from the second or third rib to the sixth or seventh rib, and from the sternal margin to the midaxillary line. It is essential to include the tail of Spence in palpation. Recall that the greatest amount of glandular tissue lies in the upper outer quadrant of the breast with tissue extending from this quadrant into the axilla to form the tail of Spence (Fig. 16-17).

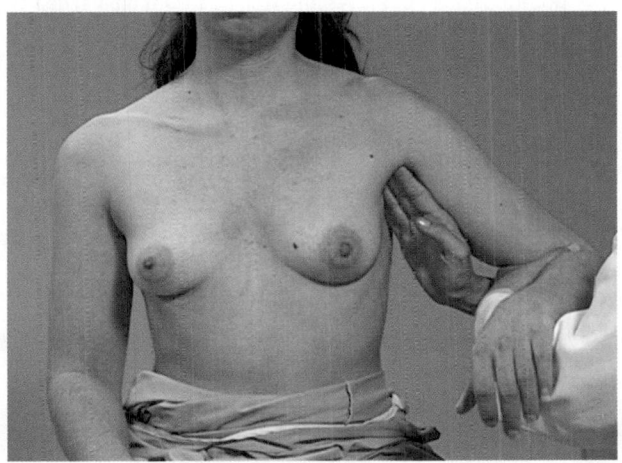

FIGURE 16-15
Palpation of the axilla for lymph nodes.

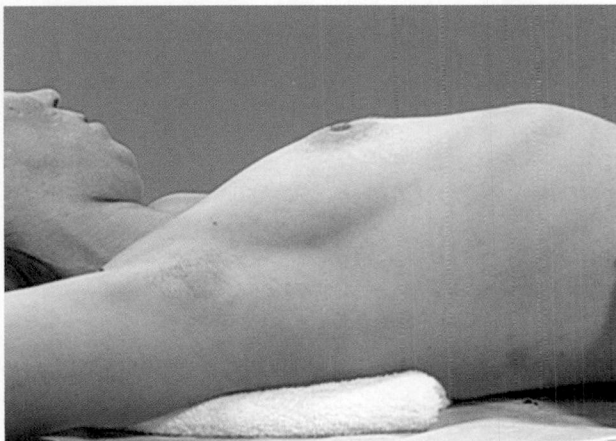

FIGURE 16-16
Supine position for palpation.

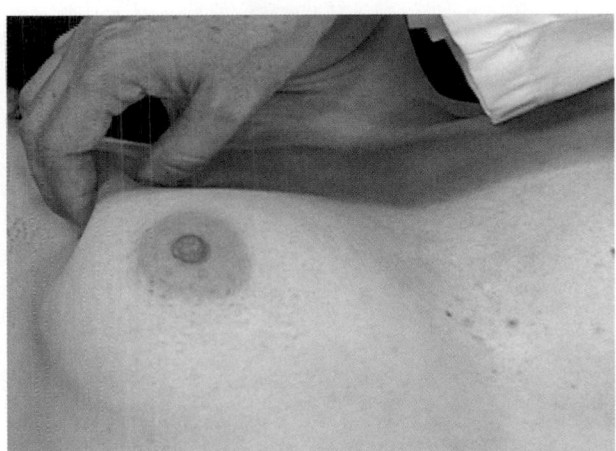

FIGURE 16-17
Palpation of the tail of Spence.

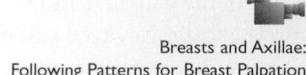

Breasts and Axillae:
Following Patterns for Breast Palpation

Palpate using your finger pads because they are more sensitive than your fingertips. Palpate systematically, pushing gently but firmly, toward the chest with your fingers rotating in a clockwise or counterclockwise pattern. Fig. 16-18 illustrates three methods that are commonly used for ensuring palpation of the entire breast. Many methods are used; any are acceptable, as long as every part of the breast is palpated. In the vertical strip technique, begin at the top of the breast and palpate, first downward, then upward, working your way down over the entire breast. In the concentric circle technique, begin at the outermost edge of the breast tissue and spiral your way inward toward the nipple. To use the wedge method, palpate from the center of the breast in radial fashion, returning to the areola to begin each spoke. Regardless of the method, glide your fingers from one point to the next. Avoid lifting your fingers off the breast tissue because doing so makes it easy to miss tissue. At each point, press inward, using three depths of palpation: light, then medium, and finally deep.

BOX 16-3

DOCUMENTING BREAST MASSES

If a breast mass is felt, characterize it by its location, size, shape, consistency, tenderness, mobility, delineation of borders, and retraction (see Figs. 16-21 and 16-22). Transillumination can be used to confirm the presence of fluid in certain masses. These characteristics are not diagnostic by themselves; but, in conjunction with a thorough history, they provide a great deal of clinical information for correlation with findings from diagnostic testing.

Any and all breast masses or lumps that you encounter should be described by the following characteristics:

- Location: clock positions and distance from nipple; depict in an illustration in the medical record
- Size: in centimeters: length, width, thickness
- Shape: round, discoid, lobular, stellate regular or irregular
- Consistency: firm, soft, hard
- Tenderness: to what degree
- Mobility: movable (in what directions) or fixed to overlying skin or subadjacent fascia
- Borders: discrete or poorly defined
- Retraction: presence or absence of dimpling; altered contour

All new solitary or dominant masses must be investigated with further diagnostic testing.

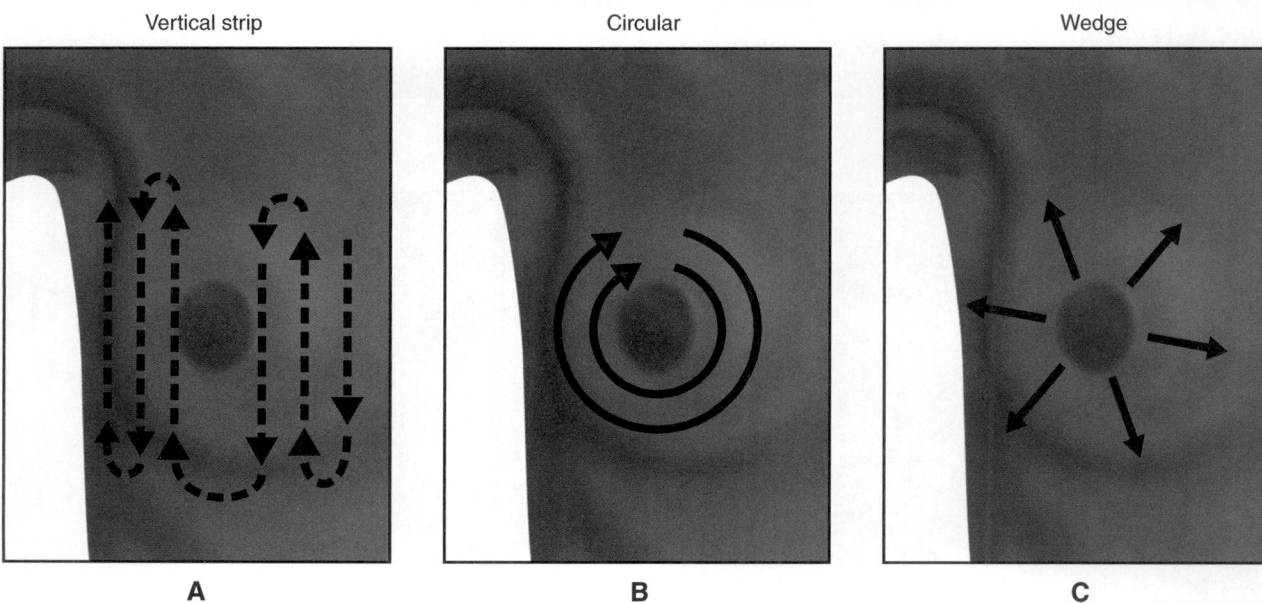

Vertical strip	Circular	Wedge
A	**B**	**C**

FIGURE 16-18
Various methods for palpation of the breast. **A,** Palpate from top to bottom in vertical strips. **B,** Palpate in concentric circles. **C,** Palpate out from the center in wedge sections.

At the completion of the examination, return to the nipple and with two fingers gently depress the tissue inward into the well behind the areola. Your fingers and tissue should move easily inward (Fig. 16-19).

Nipple compression should be performed only if the patient reports spontaneous nipple discharge. Determine whether the discharge is bilateral or unilateral. Use a magnifying glass to look closely at the nipple to determine whether the discharge is from a single duct or multiple ducts. Characteristics of concern include spontaneous discharge that is unilateral and from a single duct. Fig. 16-20 shows various types of nipple discharge.

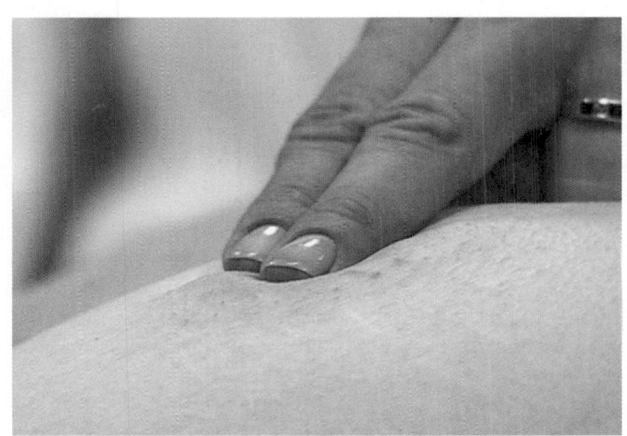

FIGURE 16-19
Depressing nipple inward into well behind the areola.

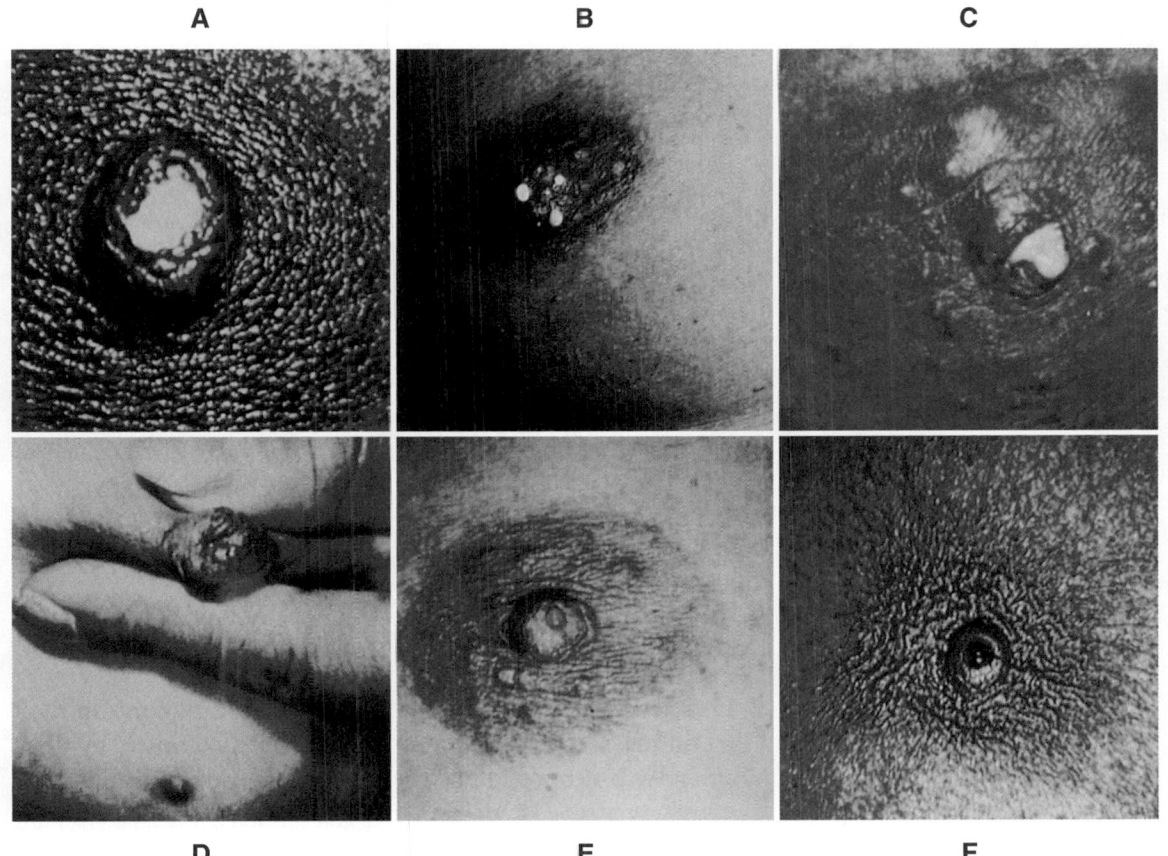

FIGURE 16-20
Types of nipple discharge. **A,** Milky discharge. **B,** Multicolored sticky discharge. **C,** Purulent discharge. **D,** Watery discharge. **E,** Serous discharge. **F,** Serosanguineous discharge.
From Gallager, 1978.

Early lesions can be tiny and may be detected only through meticulous technique. The exact sequence you select for palpation is not critical, but it is essential to develop a systematic approach that always begins and ends at a fixed point. This will help ensure that all portions of the breast are examined. If a breast mass is felt, note its characteristics and palpate its dimensions, consistency, and mobility (Figs. 16-21 and 16-22; see also Box 16-3). See the Staying Well box below.

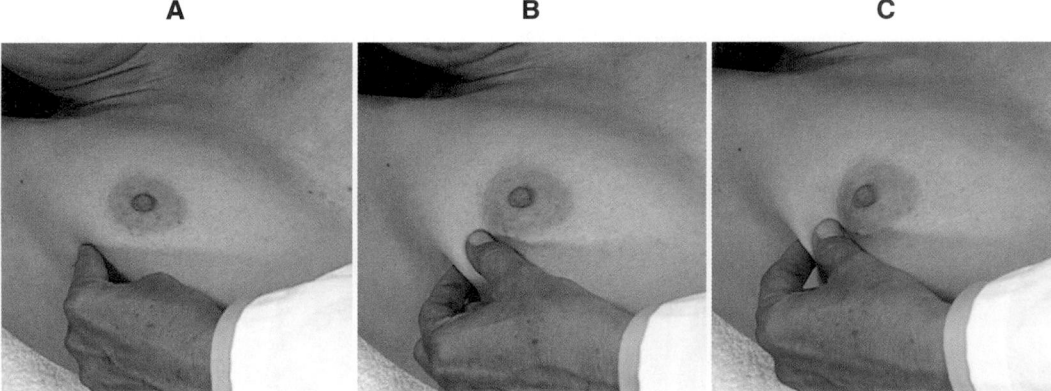

FIGURE 16-21
A, Palpating for consistency of a breast lesion. **B,** Palpating for delineation of borders of breast mass. **C,** Palpating for mobility of breast mass.

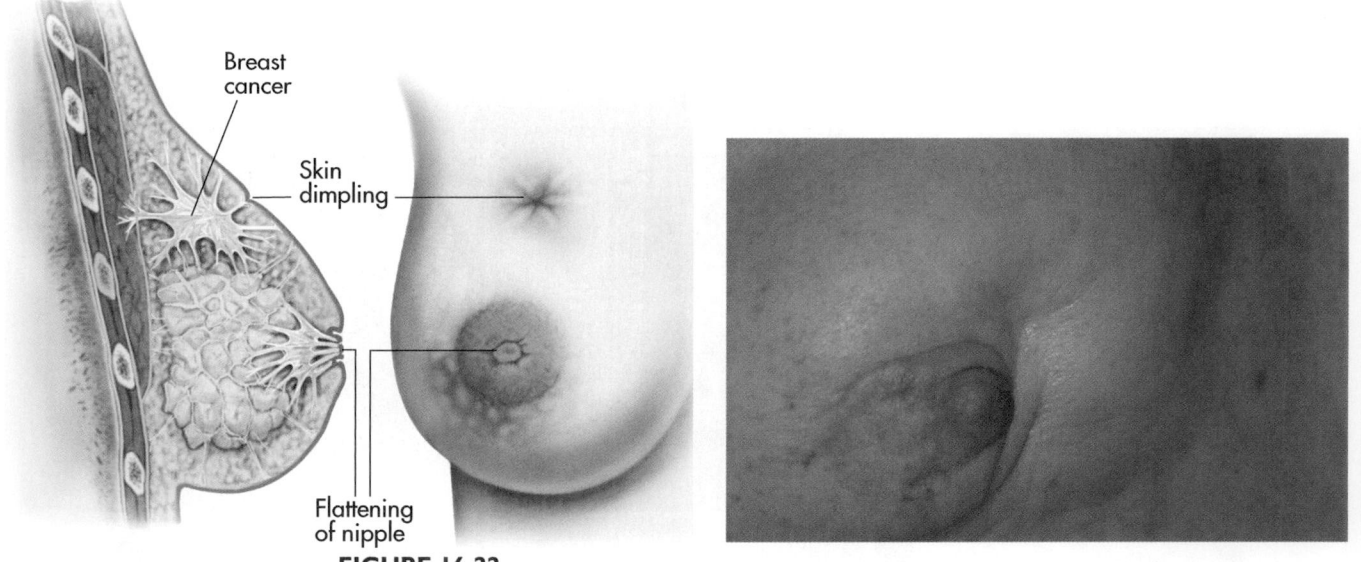

FIGURE 16-22
A, Clinical signs of cancer. **B,** Nipple retraction and dimpling of skin.
B from Lemmi, Lemmi, 2000.

STAYING WELL

BREAST HEALTH: CAN BREAST CANCER BE PREVENTED?

At this time there is no guaranteed way to prevent breast cancer. The best preventive health strategy is to reduce known risk factors whenever possible. Maintaining a healthy weight, engaging in regular physical activity, reducing alcohol intake to no more than one drink a day for women, and avoiding the use of postmenopausal combination hormone therapy are lifestyle changes that can decrease the risk of breast cancer.

Women who are at increased risk of breast cancer may consider chemoprevention. Tamoxifen has been shown to reduce the risk by almost 50% in women who are at high risk (Fisher et al, 1998). Women at very high risk may elect prophylactic mastectomy, which has been shown to reduce the risk of developing breast cancer by about 90% (Hartmann et al, 2001).

Females. The breast tissue of adult women will feel dense, firm, and elastic. Expected variations include the lobular feel of glandular tissue (this feels like tiny granular bumps widely dispersed throughout the breast tissue) and the fine, granular feel of breast tissue in older women. A firm transverse ridge of compressed tissue (the inframammary ridge) may be felt along the lower edge of the breast. It is easy to mistake this for a breast mass. A cyclical pattern of breast enlargement, increased nodularity, and tenderness is a common response to hormonal changes during the menstrual cycle. Be aware of where the woman is in her cycle because these changes are most likely to occur premenstrually and during menses. They are least noticeable during the week after menstrual flow.

The patient who has had a mastectomy has special examination needs. The procedure for examining the patient who has had a mastectomy is described in Box 16-4.

Males. In most men, expect to feel a thin layer of fatty tissue overlying muscle. Obese men may have a somewhat thicker fatty layer, giving the appearance of breast enlargement. A firm disk of glandular tissue can be felt in some men.

BOX 16-4

EXAMINING THE PATIENT WHO HAS HAD A MASTECTOMY

The patient who has had a mastectomy has special examination needs. In addition to examining the unaffected breast in the usual manner, you must examine the mastectomy site, with particular attention to the scar. If malignancy recurs, it may be at the scar site. Be aware that a woman who has had a mastectomy may feel uncomfortable removing her brassiere and prosthesis if she wears one.

Inspect the mastectomy site and axilla for any visible signs of swelling, lumps, thickening, redness, color change, rash, or irritation to the scar. Note muscle loss or lymphedema that may be present, depending on the type and extent of the surgical procedure.

Palpate the surgical scar with two fingers, using small, circular motions to assess for swelling, lumps, thickening, or tenderness. Then palpate the chest wall using three or four fingers in a sweeping motion across the area, being sure not to miss any spots. Intercostal residual breast tissue may exist. Position your fingers on either side of each rib and run your fingers along the anterior ribs, using a stripping motion. Remember to use your finger pads and not your fingertips. If the patient has had breast reconstruction, augmentation, or a lumpectomy, perform breast examination in the usual manner, with particular attention to any scars and new tissue.

Finally, palpate for lymph nodes in the axillary and supraclavicular areas.

Have this patient demonstrate her breast self-examination procedures. Regular monthly breast self-examination is an essential component of continuing health care for these women.

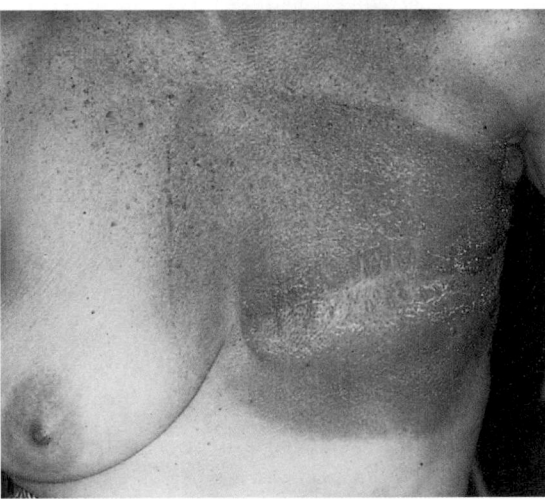

From Skarin, 1996.

INFANTS

The breasts of many well infants, male and female, are enlarged for a relatively brief time during the newborn period. The enlargement may be noted at birth and is the result of passively transferred maternal estrogen. If you squeeze the breast bud gently, a small amount of clear or milky white fluid, commonly called "witch's milk," is sometimes expressed. The enlargement is rarely more than 1 to 1.5 cm in diameter and can be easily palpated behind the nipple. It usually disappears within 2 weeks, and rarely lasts beyond 3 months of age.

ADOLESCENTS

The right and left breasts of the adolescent female may not develop at the same rate. Reassure the girl that this asymmetry is common and that her breasts are developing appropriately. Chapter 5 describes the stages of breast development. Breast tissue of the adolescent female feels homogenous, dense, firm, and elastic. Although malignancy in this age-group is rare, routine examination provides an excellent opportunity for reassurance and education. Starting breast self-examination early can also help establish a healthful habit for life.

Many males at puberty have transient unilateral or bilateral subareolar masses. These are firm, sometimes tender, and are often a source of great concern to the patient and his parents. Reassure them that these breast buds will most likely disappear, usually within a year. They seldom enlarge to a point of cosmetic difficulty.

Occasionally, however, pubescent males experience gynecomastia, an unusual and unexpected enlargement that is readily noticeable. Fortunately, it is usually temporary and benign and resolves spontaneously. If the enlargement is extreme, it can be corrected surgically for psychologic or cosmetic reasons. In rare instances, biopsy is required to rule out the presence of cancer. Gynecomastia can be associated with the use of either illicit or prescription drugs. Symptoms resolve after the drugs are discontinued.

PREGNANT WOMEN

Many changes in the breasts occur during pregnancy. Most become obvious during the first trimester. The woman may experience a sensation of fullness with tingling, tenderness, and a bilateral increase in size. It is important to ascertain that the woman is providing adequate support for her breasts with a properly fitting brassiere. As her breasts continue to enlarge, she may need to alter the size and style of the brassiere.

Generally, the nipples enlarge and are more erectile. As the pregnancy progresses, the nipples sometimes become flattened or inverted. A crust caused by dried colostrum can be evident on the nipple. The areola begins to broaden and darken, and Montgomery tubercles may appear (Fig. 16-23).

Palpation reveals a generalized coarse nodularity, and the breasts feel lobular because of hypertrophy of the mammary alveoli. Dilated subcutaneous veins may create a network of blue tracing across the breasts.

During the second trimester, vascular spiders may develop on the upper chest, arms, neck, and face as a result of elevated levels of circulating estrogen. The spiders are bluish in color and do not blanch with pressure. Striae may be evident as a result of stretching as the breasts increase in size.

LACTATING WOMEN

During lactation, it is important to assess whether the breasts are adequately supported with a properly fitting brassiere. Palpate the breasts to determine the degree of softness. Full breasts, which are firm, dense, and slightly enlarged, may become engorged. Engorged breasts feel hard and warm and are enlarged, shiny, and painful. Engorgement is not an unusual condition in the first 24 to 48 hours after the breasts fill with milk; however, its later development may signal the onset of mastitis.

Clogged milk ducts are a relatively common occurrence in lactating women. A clogged duct may result from either inadequate emptying of the breast or a brassiere that is too tight. The clogged duct will create a tender spot on the breast that may feel lumpy and hot. Frequent nursing and/or expression of the milk, along with local application of heat, will help open the duct. A clogged duct left unattended will probably result in the development of mastitis.

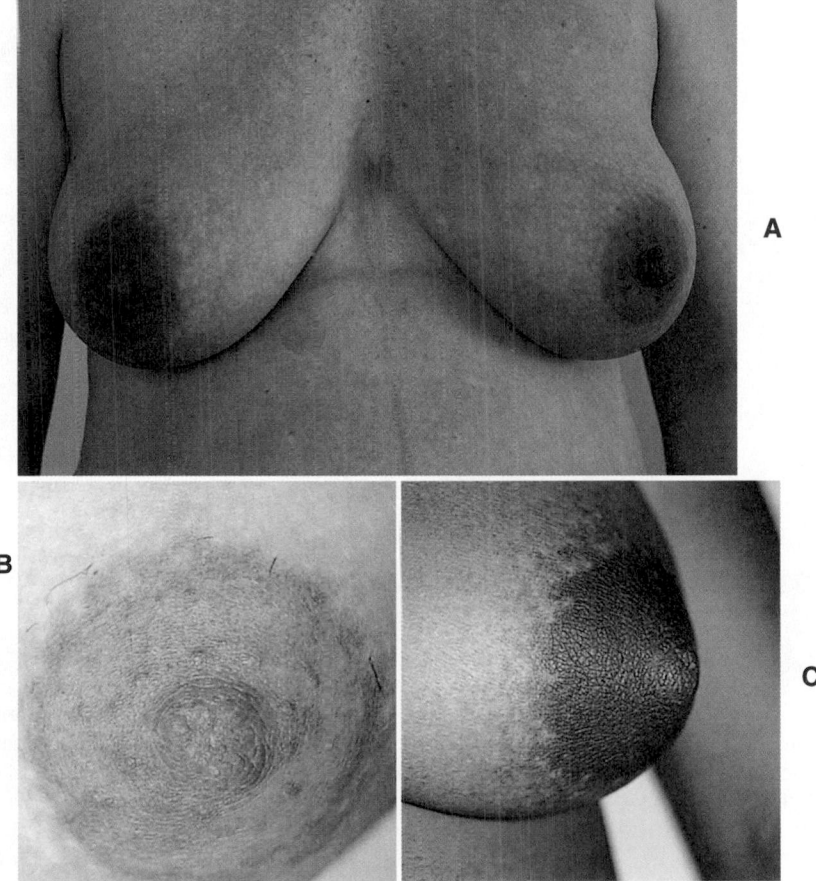

FIGURE 16-23
Breast changes in pregnancy.
A, Note venous network, darkened areolae and nipples, and vascular spider. **B,** Increased pigmentation and the development of raised sebaceous glands known as Montgomery tubercles. **C,** Marked pigmentation in woman with dark skin.
B, C from Symonds, Macpherson, 1994.

Examine the nipples for signs of irritation (redness and tenderness) and for blisters or petechiae, which are precursors of overt cracking. If the nipples are already cracked, they will be sore and may be bleeding. There is no correlation between color of the nipple and nipple damage from breast-feeding, which has to do with placement of the nipple in the infant's mouth. Lighter-colored nipples are no more prone to damage than are darker nipples.

After pregnancy and lactation, there is regression of most of these changes. The areolae and nipples tend to retain their darker color, and the breasts become less firm than in their pre-pregnant state.

OLDER ADULTS

The breasts in postmenopausal women may appear flattened, elongated, and suspended more loosely from the chest wall as the result of glandular tissue atrophy and relaxation of the suspensory ligaments. A finer, granular feel on palpation replaces the lobular feel of glandular tissue. The inframammary ridge thickens and can be felt more easily. The nipples become smaller and flatter.

Postmenopausal women should be encouraged to continue monthly breast self-examination as an option. Because the breasts are no longer subject to hormonal changes of menstruation, these women should choose a convenient date and regularly examine their breasts on this date. Hormone replacement therapy can result in fluid-filled breast cysts, which can be painful.

SAMPLE DOCUMENTATION

HISTORY AND PHYSICAL EXAMINATION

Subjective

A 42-year-old woman noticed a knot in her right lower breast last week. Denies nipple discharge or skin changes. Reports normal mammogram 2 years ago. Has never had a breast lump before. Currently on last day of menses. Has breast tenderness just before menses but denies breast pain today. No family history of breast cancer.

For additional sample documentation, see Chapter 26.

Objective

Breasts: moderate size, conical shape, left slightly larger than right. No skin lesions; contour smooth without dimpling or retraction; venous patterns symmetric. Nipples symmetric without discharge; Montgomery tubercles bilaterally. Tissue dense, particularly in upper quadrants; 3 cm × 3 cm × 2 cm soft mass in LLQ of right breast, 5 cm from nipple. Mobile, nontender, borders smooth. No supraclavicular, infraclavicular, or axillary lymphadenopathy.

SUMMARY OF EXAMINATION

BREASTS AND AXILLAE

Females

1. Inspect with patient seated and arms hanging loosely at the sides. Inspect both breasts and compare them for the following (p. 501):
   - Size
   - Symmetry
   - Contour
   - Retractions or dimpling
   - Skin color and texture
   - Venous patterns
   - Lesions
   - Supernumerary nipples
2. Inspect both areolae and nipples and compare them for the following (p. 502):
   - Shape
   - Symmetry
   - Color
   - Smoothness
   - Size
   - Nipple inversion, eversion, or retraction
3. Reinspect breasts with the patient in the following positions (p. 505):
   - Arms extended over head or flexed behind the neck
   - Hands pressed on hips with shoulder rolled forward
   - Seated and leaning over
   - In recumbent position
4. With patient seated, perform a chest wall sweep (p. 506)
5. With patient seated, perform bimanual digital palpation (p. 506)

6. With patient seated, palpate for lymph nodes in the apex, medial and lateral aspects, anterior and posterior walls of the axilla and down the arm to the elbow. Palpate the supraclavicular and infraclavicular areas (p. 506).
7. Continue palpation of breast tissue with patient supine, one arm behind head and towel under shoulder (p. 507). Palpate breasts systematically in all four quadrants and the tail of Spence using light, medium, and deep pressure, feeling for lumps or nodules.
8. Depress the nipple into the well behind the areola (p. 509)

Males

1. Inspect breasts for the following (p. 501):
   - Symmetry
   - Enlargement
   - Surface characteristics
2. Inspect both areolae and nipples and compare them for the following (p. 502):
   - Shape
   - Symmetry
   - Color
   - Smoothness
   - Size
   - Nipple inversion, eversion, or retraction
3. Palpate breasts and over areolae for lumps or nodules (p. 505).
4. With patient seated, palpate for lymph nodes in the apex, medial and lateral aspects, anterior and posterior walls of the axilla and down the arm to the elbow. Palpate the supraclavicular and infraclavicular areas (p. 506).

COMMON ABNORMALITIES

FIBROCYSTIC CHANGES

Benign cyst formation caused by ductal enlargement is associated with a long follicular or luteal phase of the menstrual cycle. The lesions are filled with fluid and are usually bilateral and multiple. Characteristically the cysts are tender and painful with an increase in these symptoms premenstrually. Fibrocystic disease occurs most commonly in women between 30 and 55 years of age. The Differential Diagnosis box below details the differences between fibrocystic changes, fibroadenoma, and breast cancer.

DIFFERENTIAL DIAGNOSIS

DIFFERENTIATING SIGNS AND SYMPTOMS OF BREAST MASSES

	Fibrocystic Changes	Fibroadenoma	Cancer
Age range (yr)	20 to 49	15 to 55	30 to 80
Occurrence	Usually bilateral	Usually bilateral	Usually unilateral
Number	Multiple or single	Single; may be multiple	Single
Shape	Round	Round or discoid	Irregular or stellate
Consistency	Soft to firm; tense	Firm, rubbery	Hard, stonelike
Mobility	Mobile	Mobile	Fixed
Retraction signs	Absent	Absent	Often present
Tenderness	Usually tender	Usually nontender	Usually nontender
Borders	Well delineated	Well delineated	Poorly delineated; irregular
Variation with menses	Yes	No	No

FIBROADENOMA

Fibroadenomas are benign tumors composed of stromal and epithelial elements that represent a hyperplastic or proliferative process in a single terminal ductal unit. Fibroadenomas may occur in girls and women of any age during their reproductive years and account for the majority of breast tumors in young women. Fibroadenomas are generally asymptomatic and do not change with the menstrual cycle. Biopsy is often performed to rule out carcinoma. After menopause, the tumors often regress. Fibroadenomas rarely appear in older women; therefore any new solid lesion in an older woman should be considered malignant until proven otherwise. While fibroadenomas are not considered to have malignant potential because they contain epithelium, a risk of neoplasia exists.

MALIGNANT BREAST TUMORS

Peak incidence of malignancy is between ages 40 and 75 years, with the majority of malignant breast tumors occurring in women older than 50 years of age. About 80% of patients with breast cancer have a painless lump in the breast as the initial symptom. Metastases occur through the lymph and vascular systems. The following findings are associated with breast cancer: mass or thickening in the breast; marked asymmetry of breasts; prominent unilateral veins; discolorations (erythema or ecchymosis); peau d'orange; ulcerations; dimpling, puckering, or retraction of skin or areola; fixed inversion or deviation in position of the nipple; crusting or erosion of the nipple or areola; or change in surface characteristics (e.g., moles or scars) (Fig. 16-24).

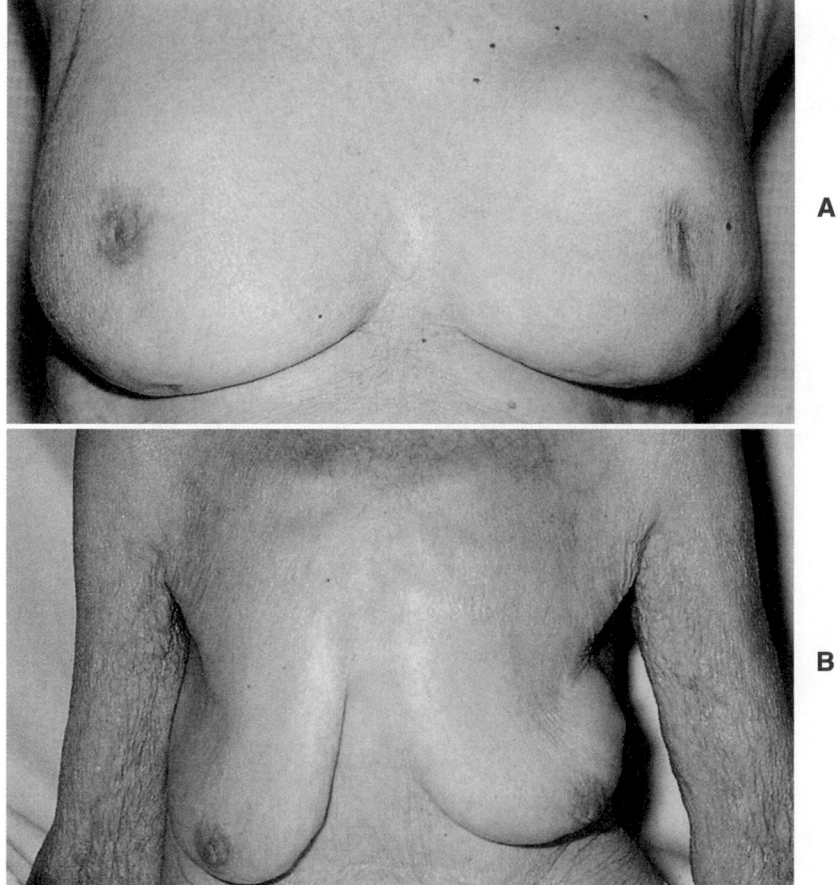

A

B

FIGURE 16-24
A, Patient with lump and nipple retraction in left breast. **B,** Patient with altered nipple height resulting from breast cancer in left breast.
From Mansel, Bundred, 1995.

FAT NECROSIS

Fat necrosis is a response to local injury. It is felt as a firm, irregular mass, often appearing as an area of discoloration (Fig. 16-25).

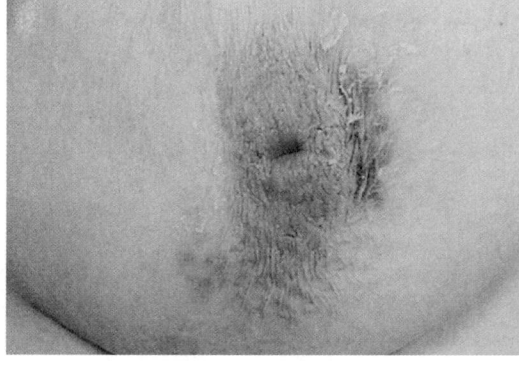

FIGURE 16-25
Fat necrosis presenting as a hard mass in the breast following an episode of trauma sufficient to cause bruising.
From Mansel, Bundred, 1995.

INTRADUCTAL PAPILLOMAS AND PAPILLOMATOSIS

These benign 2- to 3-cm tumors of the subareolar ducts may occur singly or in multiples. Papillomas are a common cause of serous or bloody nipple discharge. They need to be excised and examined to rule out malignancy.

PAGET DISEASE

Paget disease of the breast is a surface manifestation of underlying ductal carcinoma. A red, scaling, crusty patch forms on the nipple, areola, and surrounding skin. The lesion appears eczematous but, unlike eczema, may occur unilaterally, and does not respond to steroids (Fig. 16-26).

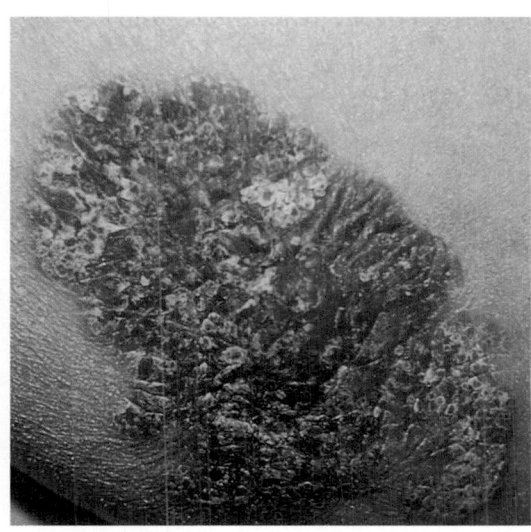

FIGURE 16-26
Paget disease.
From Habif, 2004.

ADULT GYNECOMASTIA

Gynecomastia is a smooth, firm, mobile, tender disk of breast tissue located behind the areola in males. It may be unilateral or bilateral. In adult men it can be caused by hormone imbalance; by testicular, pituitary, or hormone-secreting tumors; by liver failure; or by antihypertensive medications or those containing estrogens or steroids (Fig. 16-27).

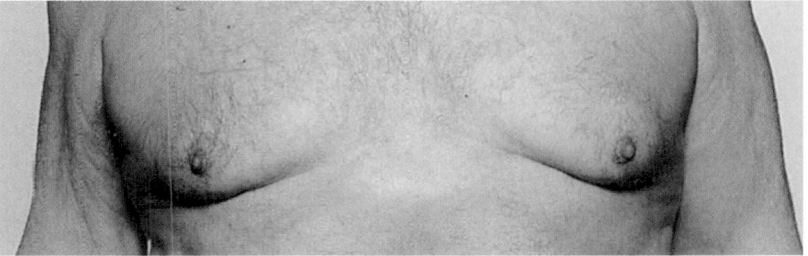

FIGURE 16-27
Adult gynecomastia.
From Mansel, Bundred, 1995.

RETENTION CYSTS

Inflammation of the sebaceous glands in the areola results in retention cysts. They may become tender and suppurative.

GALACTORRHEA

Lactation not associated with childbearing is most commonly caused by drugs, especially phenothiazines, tricyclic antidepressants, some antihypertensive agents, and estrogens. Intrinsic causes of galactorrhea include prolactin-secreting tumors, pituitary tumors (Fig. 16-28), hypothyroidism, Cushing syndrome, and hypoglycemia.

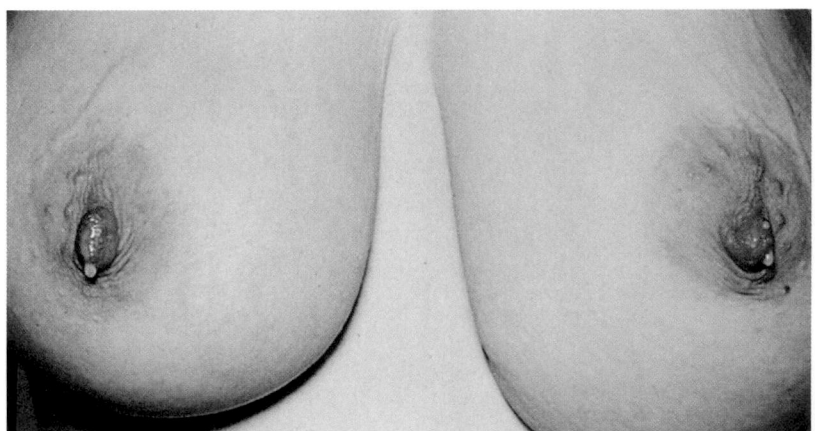

FIGURE 16-28
Galactorrhea produced by a prolactin-secreting pituitary tumor.
From Mansel, Bundred, 1995.

CHILDREN

GYNECOMASTIA

Enlargement of breast tissue in boys is caused by puberty, hormonal imbalance, testicular or pituitary tumors, and medications containing estrogens or steroids (Fig. 16-29).

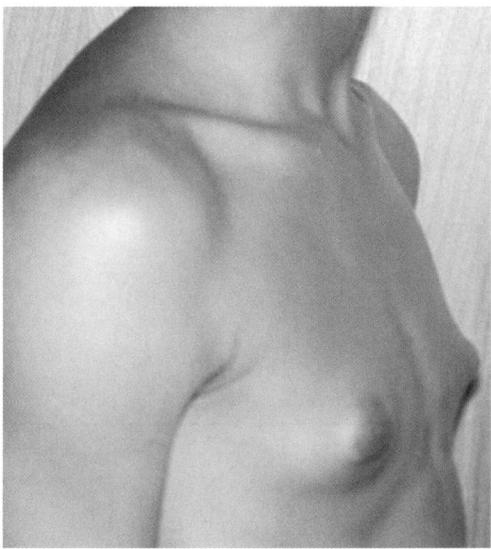

FIGURE 16-29
Prepubertal gynecomastia, small and subareolar.
Courtesy Wellington Hung, MD, Children's National Medical Center, Washington, DC.

PREMATURE THELARCHE

Prepubertal breast enlargement of unknown cause in girls can occur in the absence of other signs of sexual maturation. The degree of enlargement varies from very slight to fully developed breasts. It usually occurs bilaterally, with the breasts continuing to enlarge slowly throughout childhood until full development is reached during adolescence (Fig. 16-30).

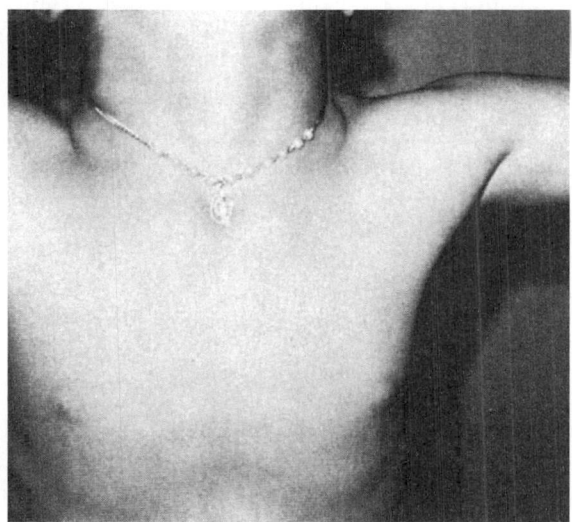

FIGURE 16-30
Premature thelarche.
Courtesy Wellington Hung, MD, Children's National Medical Center, Washington, DC.

LACTATING WOMEN

MASTITIS

Mastitis is inflammation and infection of the breast tissue characterized by sudden onset of swelling, tenderness, erythema, and heat; it is usually accompanied by chills, fever, and increased pulse rate. Most infections are staphylococcal, often *Staphylococcus aureus*. Mastitis is most common in lactating women after milk is established, usually the second to third week after delivery; however, it may occur at any time. Mastitis is not an indication to discontinue breast-feeding. Abscess formation can result, which presents as discharge of pus (suppuration) and a large, hardened mass with an area of fluctuation, erythema, and heat. The underlying pus-filled abscess may impart a bluish tinge to the skin (Fig. 16-31).

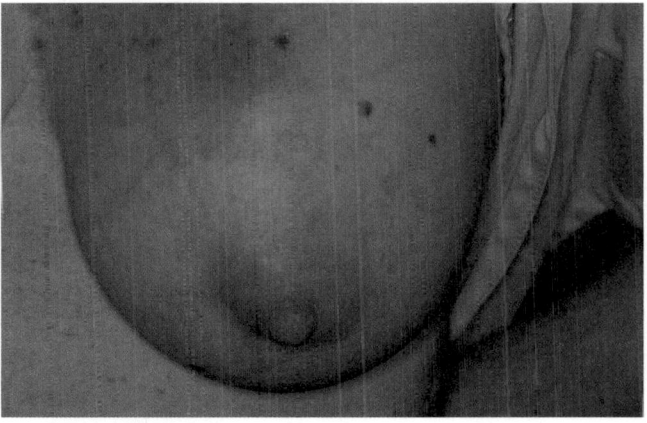

FIGURE 16-31
Mastitis.
From Lemmi, Lemmi, 2000.

OLDER ADULTS

MAMMARY DUCT ECTASIA

Mammary duct ectasia occurs most commonly in menopausal women. The subareolar ducts become blocked with desquamating secretory epithelium, necrotic debris, and chronic inflammatory cells. This condition is often bilateral and is characterized by pain, tenderness, periods of inflammation, and a nipple discharge that is spontaneous, sticky, multicolored, and from multiple ducts. Nipple retraction may occur. There is no known association with malignancy.

ELECTRONIC RESOURCES

For Weblinks and additional resources, go to

http://evolve.elsevier.com/Seidel

or to the Companion CD-ROM.

Additional information related to the content in Chapter 16 can be found on the companion website at http://evolve.elsevier.com/Seidel/ or on the interactive companion CD-ROM. Resources and activities for Chapter 16 include:
- Sound and Vision Theater
- Printouts for Your Practice
- Interactive Challenge
- Spanish Assessment Terms with Pronunciation Guide
- Instant Calculator

ABDOMEN

ANATOMY AND PHYSIOLOGY

The abdominal cavity contains several of the body's vital organs (Fig. 17-1). The peritoneum, a serous membrane, lines the cavity and forms a protective cover for many of the abdominal structures. Double folds of the peritoneum around the stomach constitute the greater and lesser omentum. The mesentery, a fan-shaped fold of the peritoneum, covers most of the small intestine and anchors it to the posterior abdominal wall.

ALIMENTARY TRACT

The alimentary tract is a tube approximately 27 feet long that runs from the mouth to the anus and includes the esophagus, stomach, small intestine, and large intestine. It functions to ingest and digest food; absorb nutrients, electrolytes, and water; and excrete waste products. Food and the products of digestion are moved along the length of the digestive tract by peristalsis, which is under autonomic nervous system control.

The esophagus is a collapsible tube about 10 inches long, connecting the pharynx to the stomach. Passing just posterior to the trachea, the esophagus descends through the mediastinal cavity, travels through the diaphragm, and enters the stomach at the cardiac orifice.

The flask-shaped stomach lies transversely in the upper abdominal cavity, just below the diaphragm. It consists of three sections: the fundus, which lies above and to the left of the cardiac orifice; the middle two thirds, or body; and the pylorus, the most distal portion that narrows and terminates in the pyloric orifice. The stomach secretes hydrochloric acid and digestive enzymes that break down fats and proteins. Pepsin acts to digest proteins, whereas gastric lipase acts on emulsified fats. Very little absorption takes place in the stomach.

The small intestine, about 21 feet long, begins at the pyloric orifice. Coiled in the abdominal cavity, it joins the large intestine at the ileocecal valve. The first 12 inches of the small intestine, the duodenum, forms a C-shaped curve around the head of the pancreas. The common bile duct and pancreatic duct open into the duodenum at the duodenal papilla, about 3 inches below the pylorus of the stomach. The next 8 feet of intestine, the jejunum, gradually becomes larger and thicker. The ileum makes up the remaining 12 feet of the small intestine. The ileocecal valve between the ileum and large intestine prevents backward flow of fecal material.

The small intestine completes digestion through the action of pancreatic enzymes, bile, and several enzymes. Nutrients are absorbed through the walls of the small intestine, whose functional surface area is enormously increased by its circular folds and villi.

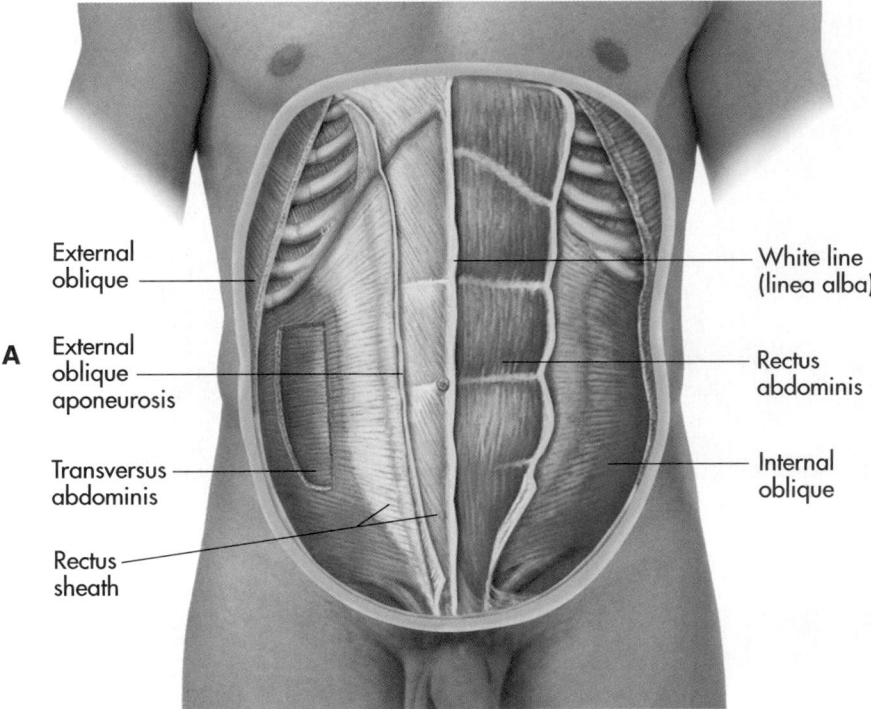

A

External
oblique

External
oblique
aponeurosis

Transversus
abdominis

Rectus
sheath

White line
(linea alba)

Rectus
abdominis

Internal
oblique

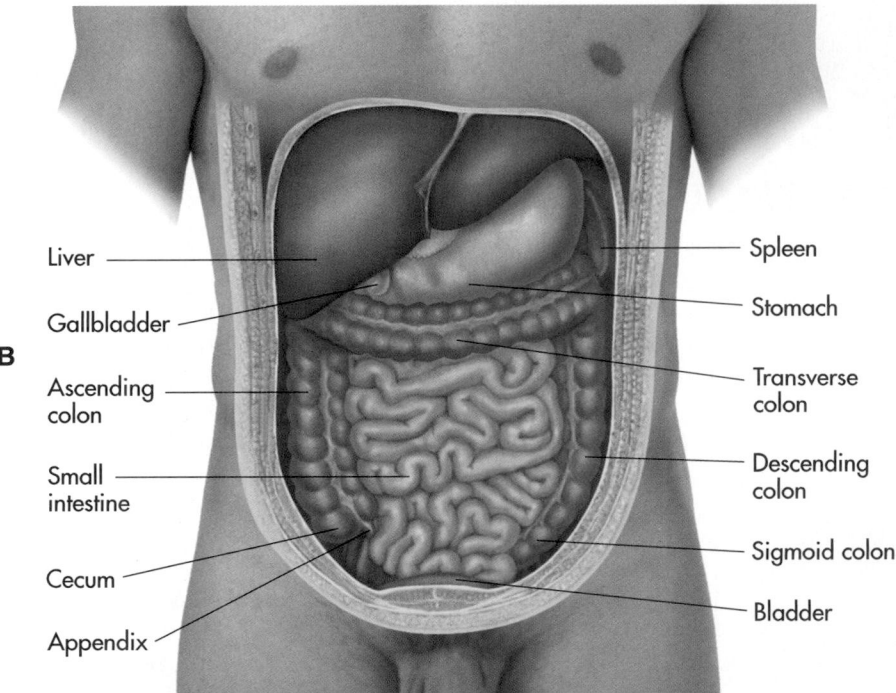

B

Liver

Gallbladder

Ascending
colon

Small
intestine

Cecum

Appendix

Spleen

Stomach

Transverse
colon

Descending
colon

Sigmoid colon

Bladder

FIGURE 17-1
Anatomic structures of the abdominal cavity.

The large intestine begins at the cecum, a blind pouch about 2 to 3 inches long. The ileal contents empty into the cecum through the ileocecal valve, and the vermiform appendix extends from the base of the cecum. The ascending colon rises from the cecum along the right posterior abdominal wall to the undersurface of the liver, where it turns toward the midline (the hepatic flexure), becoming the transverse colon. The transverse colon crosses the abdominal cavity toward the spleen, turning downward at the splenic flexure. The descending colon continues along the left abdominal wall to the rim of the pelvis, where it turns medially and in-

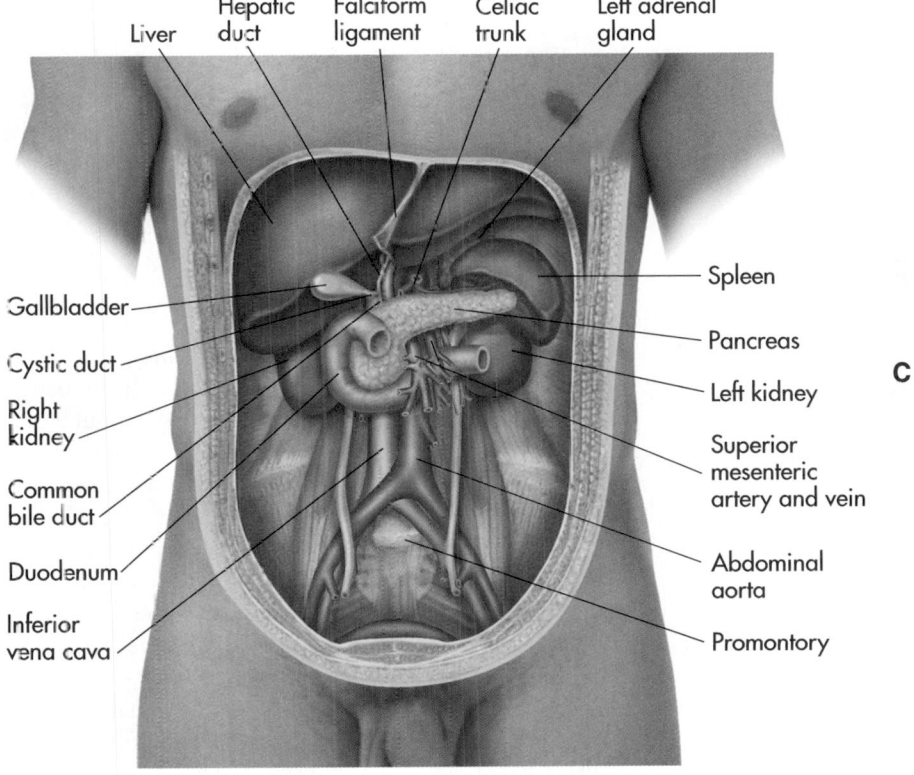

C

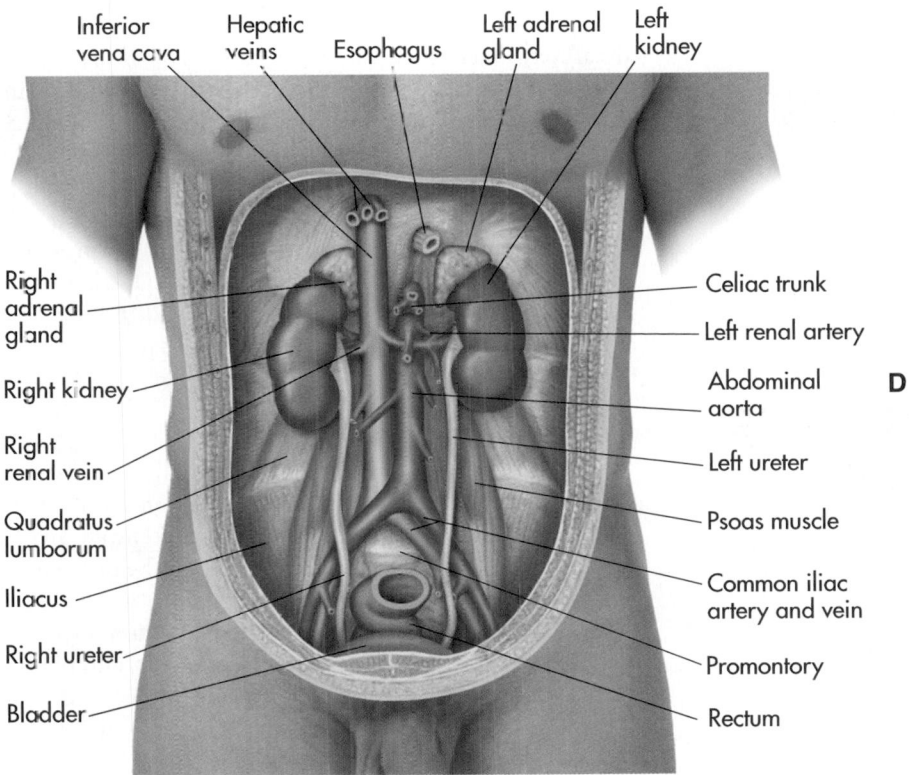

D

FIGURE 17-1, cont'd
Anatomic structures of the abdominal cavity.

feriorly to form the S-shaped sigmoid colon. The rectum extends from the sigmoid colon to the muscles of the pelvic floor, where it continues as the anal canal and terminates at the anus.

The large intestine is about $4\frac{1}{2}$ to 5 feet long, with a diameter of $2\frac{1}{2}$ inches. Water absorption takes place here. Mucous glands secrete large quantities of alkaline mucus that lubricate the intestinal contents and neutralize acids formed by intestinal bacteria. Live bacteria decompose undigested food residue, unabsorbed amino acids, cell debris, and dead bacteria through a process of putrefaction.

LIVER

The liver lies in the right upper quadrant of the abdomen, just below the diaphragm. Its inferior surface almost embraces the gallbladder, stomach, duodenum, and hepatic flexure of the colon. The heaviest organ in the body, the liver weighs about 3 pounds in the adult. It is composed of four lobes containing lobules, the functional units. Each lobule is made up of liver cells radiating around a central vein. Branches of the portal vein, hepatic artery, and bile duct embrace the periphery of the lobules. Bile secreted by the liver cells drains from the bile ducts into the hepatic duct, which joins the cystic duct from the gallbladder to form the common bile duct.

The hepatic artery transports blood to the liver directly from the aorta, and the portal vein carries blood from the digestive tract and spleen to the liver. Repeated branching of both vessels makes the liver a highly vascular organ. Three hepatic veins carry blood from the liver and empty into the inferior vena cava.

The liver plays an important role in the metabolism of carbohydrates, fats, and proteins. Glucose is converted and stored as glycogen until, in response to varying levels of insulin and regulator hormones, it is reconverted and released again as glucose. The liver also has the capacity to convert amino acids to glucose (gluconeogenesis). Fats, arriving at the liver in the form of fatty acids, are oxidized to two-carbon components in preparation for entry into the tricarboxylic acid cycle. Cholesterol is used by the liver to form bile salts. Synthesis of fats from carbohydrates and proteins also occurs in the liver. Proteins are broken down to amino acids through hydrolysis, and their waste products are converted to urea for excretion.

Other functions of the liver include storage of several vitamins and iron; detoxification of potentially harmful substances; production of antibodies; conjugation and excretion of steroid hormones; and the production of prothrombin, fibrinogen, and other substances for blood coagulation. The liver is responsible for the production of the majority of proteins circulating in the plasma. It serves a vital role as an excretory organ through the synthesis of bile, the secretion of organic wastes into bile, and the conversion of fat-soluble wastes to water-soluble material for renal excretion.

GALLBLADDER

The gallbladder is a saclike, pear-shaped organ about 4 inches long, lying recessed in the inferior surface of the liver. Its function is to concentrate and store bile from the liver. In response to cholecystokinin, a hormone produced in the duodenum, the gallbladder releases bile into the cystic duct which, along with the hepatic duct, forms the common bile duct. Contraction of the gallbladder propels bile along the common duct and into the duodenum at the duodenal papilla. Composed of cholesterol, bile salts, and pigments, bile serves to maintain the alkaline pH of the small intestine to permit emulsification of fats so that absorption can be accomplished.

PANCREAS

The pancreas lies behind and beneath the stomach, with its head resting in the curve of the duodenum and its tip extending across the abdominal cavity to almost touch the spleen. As part of the pancreas' function as an exocrine gland, the acinar cells of the pancreas produce digestive juices containing inactive enzymes for the breakdown of proteins, fats, and carbohydrates. Collecting ducts empty the juice into the pancreatic duct (duct of Wirsung), which runs the length of the organ. The pancreatic duct empties into the duodenum at the duodenal papilla, alongside the common bile duct. Once introduced into the duodenum, the digestive enzymes are activated. As an endocrine gland, islet cells scattered throughout the pancreas produce the hormones insulin and glucagon. These are secreted directly into the blood to regulate the body's level of glucose. Insulin, a major anabolic hormone of the body, also serves several other vital functions.

SPLEEN

The spleen is in the left upper quadrant, lying above the left kidney and just below the diaphragm. White pulp (lymphoid tissue) constitutes most of the organ and functions as part of the reticuloendothelial system to filter blood and to manufacture lymphocytes and monocytes. The red pulp of the spleen contains a capillary network and venous sinus system that allow for the storage and release of blood, permitting the spleen to accommodate up to several hundred milliliters at once.

KIDNEYS, URETERS, AND BLADDER

The two kidneys, the excretory organs responsible for the removal of water-soluble waste, are located in the retroperitoneal space of the upper abdomen. Each extends from about the vertebral level of T12 to L3. The right kidney is usually slightly lower than the left, presumably because of the large, heavy liver just above it. Both kidneys are imbedded in fat and fascia, which anchor and protect these organs. Each contains more than 1 million nephrons, the structural and functional units of the kidneys. The nephrons are composed of a tuft of capillaries, the glomerulus, a proximal convoluted tubule, the loop of Henle, and a distal convoluted tubule. The distal tube empties into a collecting tubule.

Each kidney receives about one eighth of the cardiac output through its renal artery. The glomeruli filters blood at a rate of about 125 mL/min in the adult male and about 110 mL/min in the adult female. Most of the filtered material, including electrolytes, glucose, water, and small proteins, is actively resorbed in the proximal tubule. Some organic acids are also actively secreted in the distal tubule. Urinary volume is carefully controlled by antidiuretic hormone (ADH) to maintain a constant total body fluid volume. Urine passes into the renal pelvis via the collecting tubules and then into the ureter. Peristaltic waves move it on to a reservoir, the urinary bladder, which has a capacity of about 400 to 500 mL in the adult.

The kidney also serves as an endocrine gland responsible for the production of renin, which is important for the ultimate control of aldosterone secretion. It is the primary source of erythropoietin production in adults, thus influencing the body's red cell mass. In addition to synthesizing several prostaglandins, the kidney produces the biologically active form of vitamin D.

MUSCULATURE AND CONNECTIVE TISSUES

The rectus abdominis muscles anteriorly and the internal and external oblique muscles laterally form and protect the abdominal cavity The linea alba, a tendinous band, is located in the midline of the abdomen between the rectus abdominis muscles. It extends from the xiphoid process to the symphysis pubis and contains the umbilicus. The inguinal ligament (Poupart ligament) extends from the anterior superior spine of the ilium on each side to the pubis.

VASCULATURE

The abdominal portion of the descending aorta travels from the diaphragm through the abdominal cavity, just to the left of midline. At about the level of the umbilicus the aorta branches into the two common iliac arteries. The splenic and renal arteries, which supply their respective organs, also branch off within the abdomen.

INFANTS

The pancreatic buds, liver, and gallbladder all begin to form during week 4 of gestation, by which time the intestine already exists as a single tube. The motility of the gastrointestinal tract develops in a cephalocaudal direction, permitting amniotic fluid to be swallowed by 17 weeks of gestation. Production of meconium, an end product of fetal metabolism, begins shortly thereafter. By 36 to 38 weeks of gestation, the gastrointestinal tract is capable of adapting to extrauterine life; however, its elasticity, musculature, and control mechanisms continue to develop, reaching adult levels of function at 2 to 3 years of age.

During gestation, the liver begins to form blood cells at about week 6, to synthesize glycogen by week 9, and to produce bile by week 12. The liver's role as a metabolic and glycogen storage organ accounts for its large size at birth. Its growth during infancy is not as rapid as skeletal growth, but it remains the heaviest organ in the body.

Pancreatic islet cells are developed by 12 weeks of gestation and begin producing insulin. The spleen is active in blood formation during fetal development and the first year of life. After that time, the spleen aids in the destruction of blood cells and in the formation of hemoglobin.

Nephrogenesis begins during the second embryologic month. By 12 weeks the kidney is able to produce urine, and the bladder expands as a sac. Development of new nephrons ceases by 36 weeks of gestation. After birth the kidney increases in size incrementally because of enlargement of the more than 1 million existing nephrons and adjoining tubules—a process that parallels body growth. The glomerular filtration rate is approximately 0.5 mL/min before 34 weeks of gestation and gradually increases in a linear fashion to 125 mL/min.

PREGNANT WOMEN

As the uterus enlarges, the muscles of the abdominal wall stretch and ultimately lose some tone (Fig. 17-2). During the third trimester the rectus abdominis muscles may separate, allowing abdominal contents to protrude at the midline.

The umbilicus flattens or protrudes. The abdominal contour changes when lightening occurs (about 2 weeks before term in a nullipara), and the fetal presenting part descends into the true pelvis. Striae may form as the skin is stretched. A line of pigmentation at the midline (linea nigra) often develops (Fig. 17-3). Abdominal muscles have less tone and are less active. After pregnancy, the muscles gradually regain tone, although separation of the rectus abdominis muscles (diastasis recti) may persist.

During the second trimester there is decreased pressure of the lower esophageal sphincter. Peristaltic wave velocity in the distal esophagus also decreases. Gastric emptying appears to be normal; however, gastrointestinal transit time is prolonged in the second and third trimesters. Incompetence of the pyloric sphincter may result in alkaline reflux of duodenal contents into the stomach. Heartburn is a common complaint.

The gallbladder may become distended, accompanied by decreased emptying time and change in tone. The combination of gallbladder stasis and secretion of lithogenic bile increases

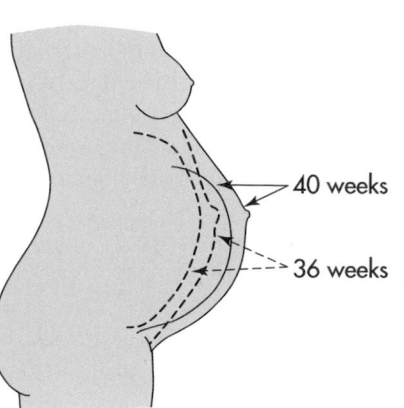

FIGURE 17-2
Contour changes in the abdomen during pregnancy.
From Lowdermilk, Perry, Bobak, 1997.

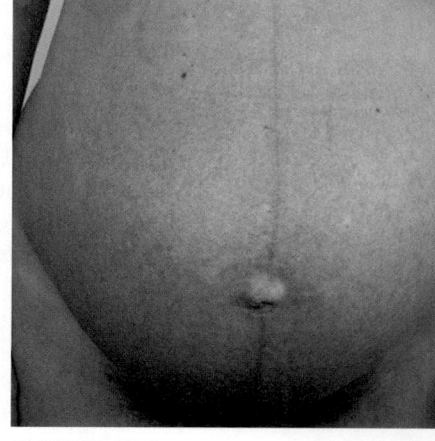

FIGURE 17-3
Linea nigra in the third trimester of pregnancy.

formation of cholesterol crystals in the development of gallstones. Gallstones are more common in the second and third trimesters.

The kidneys enlarge slightly (by about 1 cm in length) during pregnancy. The renal pelvis and ureters dilate from the effects of hormones and pressure from the enlarging uterus. Dilation of the ureter is greater on the right side than on the left, probably because it is affected by displacement of the uterus to the right by an enlarged right ovarian vein. The ureters also elongate and form single and double curves of varying sizes and angulation. These changes lead to urinary stasis and pyelonephritis in gravid women with asymptomatic bacteriuria. Renal function is most efficient if the woman lies in the lateral recumbent position, which helps prevent compression of the vena cava and aorta. These changes can last up to 3 or 4 months after delivery.

The bladder has increased sensitivity and compression during pregnancy, which may lead to frequency and urgency of urination during the first and third trimesters. After the fourth month the increase in uterine size, hyperemia, and hyperplasia of muscle and connective tissue cause elevation of the bladder trigone and thickening of the posterior margin, which produce a marked deepening and widening of the trigone by the end of the pregnancy and an increased incidence of microhematuria. During the third trimester, compression may also result from the descent of the fetus into the pelvis; this, in turn, causes a sense of urgency and/or incontinence, even if there is only a small amount of urine in the bladder.

The colon is displaced laterally upward and posteriorly, peristaltic activity may decrease, and water absorption is increased. As a result, bowel sounds are diminished, and constipation and flatus are more common. The appendix is displaced upward and laterally so that it is high and to the right, away from the McBurney point. Blood flow to the pelvis increases, as does venous pressure, contributing to hemorrhoid formation.

In the postpartum period the uterus involutes rapidly. Immediately after delivery the uterus is approximately the size of a 20-week pregnancy (at the level of the umbilicus). By the end of the first week, it is about the size of a 12-week pregnancy, palpable at the symphysis pubis. The muscles of the pelvic floor and the pelvic supports gradually regain their tone during the postpartum period and may require 6 to 7 weeks to recover. Stretching of the abdominal wall during pregnancy may result in persistent striae and diastasis of the rectus muscles.

OLDER ADULTS

The process of aging brings about changes in the functional abilities of the gastrointestinal tract. Motility of the intestine is the most severely affected; secretion and absorption are affected to a lesser degree. Altered motility may be caused in part by age-related changes in neurons of the central nervous system and by changes in collagen properties that increase the resistance of the intestinal wall to stretching. Reduced circulation to the intestine often follows other system changes associated with hypoxia and hypovolemia. Thus functional abilities of the intestine can decrease secondary to adverse changes occurring elsewhere in the older adult.

As a result of epithelial atrophy, the secretion of both digestive enzymes and protective mucus in the intestinal tract is decreased. Particular elements of the mucosal cells show a lesser degree of differentiation and are associated with reduction in secretory ability. These cells are also more susceptible to both physical and chemical agents, including ingested carcinogens. Bacterial flora of the intestine can undergo both qualitative and quantitative changes and become less biologically active. These changes may impair digestive ability and thereby cause food intolerances in the older adult.

Liver size decreases after 50 years of age, which parallels the decrease in lean body mass. Hepatic blood flow decreases as a result of the decline in cardiac output associated with aging. The liver loses some ability to metabolize certain drugs. Increasing obesity and the development of type 2 diabetes mellitus also put the liver at risk of the appearance of nonalcoholic steatohepatitis.

The size of the pancreas is unaffected by aging, although the main pancreatic duct and its branches widen. With aging there is an increase in fibrous tissue and fatty deposition with acinar cell atrophy; however, the large reserve of the organ results in no significant physiologic changes. The functional reserve of the pancreas may be reduced, although this can occur as a result of delayed gastric emptying rather than pancreatic changes.

There may be an increase of biliary lipids, specifically the phospholipids and cholesterol. This can result in the formation of gallstones.

REVIEW OF RELATED HISTORY

For each of the conditions discussed in this section, targeted topics to include in the history of the present illness are listed. Responses to questions about these topics help fully assess the patient's condition and provide clues for focusing the physical examination.

HISTORY OF PRESENT ILLNESS

- Abdominal pain
  - Onset and duration: when it began; sudden or gradual; persistent, recurrent, intermittent
  - Character: dull, sharp, burning, gnawing, stabbing, cramping, aching, colicky
  - Location: of onset, change in location over time, radiating to another area, superficial or deep
  - Associated symptoms: vomiting, diarrhea, constipation, passage of flatus, belching, jaundice, change in abdominal girth
  - Relationship to: menstrual cycle, abnormal menses, urination, defecation, inspiration, change in body position, food or alcohol intake, stress, time of day, trauma
  - Recent stool characteristics: color, consistency, odor, frequency
  - Urinary characteristics: frequency, color, volume congruent with fluid intake, force of stream, ease of starting stream, ability to empty bladder
  - Medications: prescription or nonprescription; high doses of aspirin, acetaminophen; steroids; nonsteroidal antiinflammatory drugs (NSAIDs)
  - Use of complementary/alternative therapies to treat
- Indigestion
  - Character: feeling of fullness, heartburn, discomfort, excessive belching, flatulence, loss of appetite, severe pain
  - Location: localized or general, radiates to arms or shoulders
  - Association with: food intake, timing of food intake, amount, type; date of last menstrual period
  - Onset of symptoms: time of day or night, sudden or gradual
  - Symptom relieved by antacids, rest, activity
  - Medications: prescription or nonprescription; antacids
  - Use of complementary/alternative therapies to treat
- Nausea: associated with vomiting; particular stimuli (odors, activities, time of day, food intake); date of last menstrual period
  - Medications: prescription or nonprescription; antiemetics
  - Use of complementary/alternative therapies to treat
- Vomiting
  - Character: nature (color, fresh blood or coffee grounds, undigested food particles), quantity, duration, frequency, ability to keep any liquids or food in stomach
  - Relationship to: previous meal, change in appetite, diarrhea or constipation, fever, weight loss, abdominal pain, medications, headache, nausea, date of last menstrual period
  - Medications: prescription or nonprescription; antiemetics
  - Use of complementary/alternative therapies to treat
- Diarrhea
  - Character: watery, copious, explosive; color; presence of blood, mucus, undigested food, oil, or fat; odor; number of times per day, duration; change in pattern
  - Associated symptoms: chills, fever, thirst, weight loss, abdominal pain or cramping, fecal incontinence
  - Relationship to: timing and nature of food intake, stress
  - Travel history
  - Medications: prescription or nonprescription; laxatives or stool softeners; antidiarrheals
  - Use of complementary/alternative therapies to treat

- Constipation
  - Character: presence of bright blood, black or tarry appearance of stool; diarrhea alternating with constipation; accompanied by abdominal pain or discomfort
  - Pattern: last bowel movement, pain with passage of stool, change in pattern or size of stool
  - Diet: recent change in diet, inclusion of high-fiber foods
  - Medications: prescription or nonprescription; laxatives, stool softeners, diuretics; iron
  - Use of complementary/alternative therapies to treat
- Fecal incontinence
  - Character: stool characteristics, timing in relation to meals, number of episodes per day; occurring with or without warning sensation
  - Associated with: use of laxatives, presence of underlying disease (cancer, inflammatory bowel disease, diverticulitis, colitis, proctitis, diabetic neuropathy)
  - Relationship to: fluid and dietary intake, immobilization
  - Medications: prescription or nonprescription; laxatives, stool softeners, iron, diuretics
  - Use of complementary/alternative therapies to treat
- Jaundice
  - Onset and duration
  - Color of stools or urine
  - Associated with abdominal pain, chills, fever
  - Exposure to hepatitis
  - Medications: prescription or nonprescription; high doses of acetaminophen
  - Use of club/recreational drugs
  - Use of complementary/alternative therapies to treat
- Dysuria
  - Character: location (suprapubic, distal urethra), pain or burning, frequency or volume changes
  - Exposure to: tuberculosis, fungal or viral infection, parasitic infection, bacterial infection
  - Increased frequency of sexual intercourse
  - Amount of daily fluid intake
  - Use of complementary/alternative therapies to treat

RISK FACTORS

PERSONS AT RISK FOR VIRAL HEPATITIS

Hepatitis A	Hepatitis B	Hepatitis C
Household/sexual contacts of infected persons	Persons with multiple sex partners or diagnosis of a sexually transmitted infection	Drug users who inject
Unimmunized travelers to countries where hepatitis A is common	Men who have sex with men	Recipients of clotting factors made before 1987
Person living in areas with increased rates of hepatitis A	Drug users who inject	Hemodialysis patients
Men who have sex with men	Sexual/household contacts of infected persons	Recipients of blood and/or solid organs before 1992
Injecting and noninjecting drug users	Infants born to infected mothers	People with undiagnosed liver problems
	Infants/children of immigrants from areas with high rates of hepatitis B infection	Infants born to infected mothers
	Health care and public safety workers	Health care/public safety workers
	Hemodialysis patients	People having sex with multiple partners
		People having sex with an infected steady partner

Modified from CDC, 2004.

- Urinary frequency
  - Change in usual pattern and/or volume
  - Associated with dysuria or other urinary characteristics: urgency, hematuria, incontinence, nocturia
  - Change in urinary stream; dribbling
  - Medications: prescription or nonprescription; diuretics
  - Use of complementary/alternative therapies to treat
- Urinary incontinence
  - Character: amount and frequency, constant or intermittent, dribbling versus frank incontinence
  - Associated with: urgency, previous surgery, coughing, sneezing, walking up stairs, nocturia, menopause
  - Medications: prescription or nonprescription; diuretics
  - Use of complementary/alternative therapies to treat
- Hematuria
  - Character: color (bright red, rusty brown, cola-colored); present at beginning, end, or throughout voiding
  - Associated symptoms: flank or costovertebral pain, passage of wormlike clots, pain on voiding
  - Alternate possibilities: ingestion of foods containing red vegetable dyes (may cause red urinary pigment); ingestion of laxatives containing phenolphthalein
  - Medications: prescription or nonprescription; aspirin, NSAIDs, anticoagulants, diuretics, antibiotics
  - Use of complementary/alternative therapies to treat
- Chyluria (milky urine)
  - Exposure to parasitic infections through travel
  - Exposure to tuberculosis
  - Medications: prescription or nonprescription
  - Use of complementary/alternative therapies to treat

PAST MEDICAL HISTORY

- Gastrointestinal disorder: peptic ulcer, polyps, inflammatory bowel disease, intestinal obstruction, pancreatitis, history of hyperlipidemia
- Hepatitis or cirrhosis of the liver
- Abdominal or urinary tract surgery or injury
- Urinary tract infection: number, treatment
- Major illness: cancer, arthritis (steroids or aspirin use), kidney disease, cardiac disease
- Blood transfusions
- Hepatitis vaccines
- Colorectal cancer or related cancers—breast, ovarian, endometrial

FAMILY HISTORY

- Familial Mediterranean fever (periodic peritonitis)
- Gallbladder disease
- Kidney disease: renal stone, polycystic disease, renal tubular acidosis, renal or bladder carcinoma
- Malabsorption syndrome: cystic fibrosis, celiac disease
- Hirschsprung disease, aganglionic megacolon
- Familial colorectal cancer syndromes—Familial adenomatous polyposis, hereditary nonpolyposis colorectal cancer
- Colorectal cancer

PERSONAL AND SOCIAL HISTORY

- Nutrition: 24-hour recall intake, food preferences and dislikes, ethnic foods frequently eaten, religious food restrictions, food intolerances, lifestyle effects on food intake, weight gain or loss
- First day of last menstrual period
- Alcohol intake: frequency and usual amounts
- Recent stressful life events: physical and psychologic changes
- Exposure to infectious diseases: hepatitis, flu; travel history
- Trauma: through type of work, physical activity, abuse
- Use of street/club/recreational/intravenous drugs
- Tobacco use—smoking: frequency, amount, duration, pack-years

INFANTS

- Birth weight (less than 1500 g at higher risk for necrotizing enterocolitis)
- Passage of first meconium stool within 24 hours
- Jaundice: in newborn period, exchange transfusions, phototherapy, breast-fed infant, appearance later in first month of life
- Vomiting: increasing in amount or frequency, forceful or projectile, failure to gain weight, insatiable appetite, blood in emesis (pyloric stenosis or gastroesophageal reflux)
- Diarrhea, colic, failure to gain weight, weight loss, steatorrhea (malabsorption syndrome)
- Apparent enlargement of abdomen (with or without pain), constipation, or diarrhea

CHILDREN

- Constipation: toilet training methods; diet; soiling; diarrhea; abdominal distention; pica; size, shape, consistency, and time of last stool; rectal bleeding; painful passage of stool
- Abdominal pain: splinting of abdominal movement, resists movement, keeps knees flexed

PREGNANT WOMEN

- Urinary symptoms: frequency, urgency, nocturia (common in early and late pregnancy); burning, dysuria, odor (signs of infection)
- Abdominal pain: weeks of gestation (pregnancy can alter the usual location of pain)
- Fetal movement
- Contractions: onset, frequency, duration, intensity; accompanying symptoms; lower back pain; leakage of fluid, vaginal bleeding

OLDER ADULTS

- Urinary symptoms: nocturia, change in stream, dribbling, frank incontinence
- Change in bowel patterns, constipation, diarrhea, incontinence
- Dietary habits: inclusion of fiber in diet, change in ability to tolerate certain foods, change in appetite, daily fluid intake

RISK FACTORS

COLORECTAL CANCER

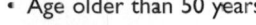

- Age older than 50 years
- Family history of colon cancer, familial adenomatous polyposis (FAP), familial hereditary nonpolyposis colorectal cancer (HNPCC), Gardner syndrome
- Personal history of colorectal cancer, intestinal polyps, chronic inflammatory bowel disease (Crohn disease, ulcerative colitis), Gardner syndrome
- Personal history of ovarian, endometrial or breast cancer
- Ethnic background: Ashkenazi Jewish descent
- Diet high in beef and animal fats, low in fiber
- Obesity
- Smoking
- Physical inactivity (regular physical activity reduces risk)
- Alcohol intake: risk increases with increased amounts

EXAMINATION AND FINDINGS

EQUIPMENT

- ◆ Stethoscope
- ◆ Centimeter ruler and nonstretchable measuring tape
- ◆ Marking pen

PREPARATION

To perform the abdominal examination satisfactorily, you will need a good source of light; full exposure of the abdomen; warm hands with short fingernails; and a comfortable, relaxed patient. Have the patient empty his or her bladder before the examination begins; a full bladder interferes with accurate examination of nearby organs and makes the examination uncomfortable for the patient. Place the patient in a supine position with arms at the sides. Approach the patient from the right side. The patient's abdominal musculature should be as relaxed as possible to allow access to the underlying structures. It may be helpful to place a small pillow under the patient's head and another small pillow under slightly flexed knees. Drape a towel or sheet over the patient's chest for warmth and privacy. Ask the patient to breathe slowly through the mouth. Make your approach slow and gentle, avoiding sudden movements. Ask the patient to point to any tender areas, and examine those last.

For the purposes of examination, the abdomen can be divided into either four quadrants or nine regions. To divide the abdomen into quadrants, draw an imaginary line from the sternum to the pubis through the umbilicus. Draw a second imaginary line perpendicular to the first, horizontally across the abdomen through the umbilicus (Fig. 17-4). The nine regions are created by the following imaginary lines: two horizontal lines, one across the lowest edge of the costal margin and the other across the edge of the iliac crest; and two vertical lines running bilaterally from the midclavicular line to the middle of the Poupart ligament, approximating the lateral borders of the rectus abdominis muscles (Fig. 17-5). Choose one of these mapping methods and use it consistently. The quadrant method is the more common of the

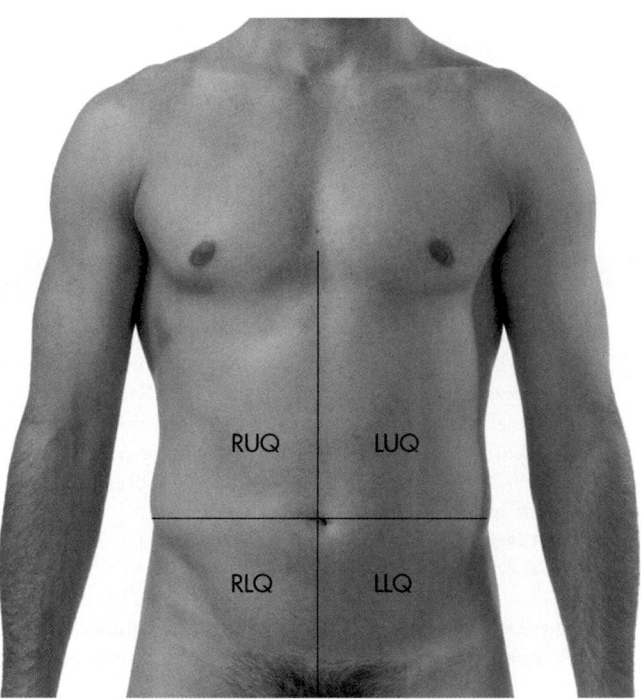

FIGURE 17-4
Four quadrants of the abdomen.
From Wilson, Giddens, 2005.

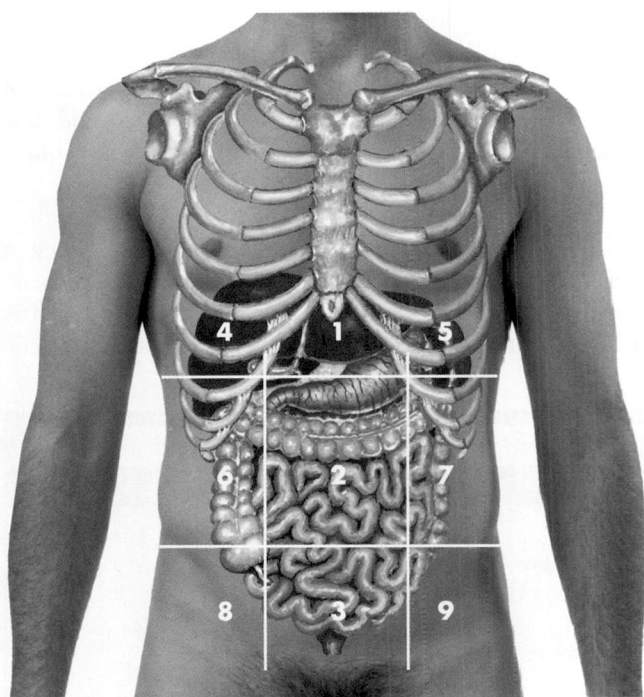

FIGURE 17-5
Nine regions of the abdomen: 1, Epigastric; 2, umbilical; 3, hypogastric (pubic); 4 and 5, right and left hypochondriac; 6 and 7, right and left lumbar; 8 and 9, right and left inguinal.
From Wilson, Giddens, 2005.

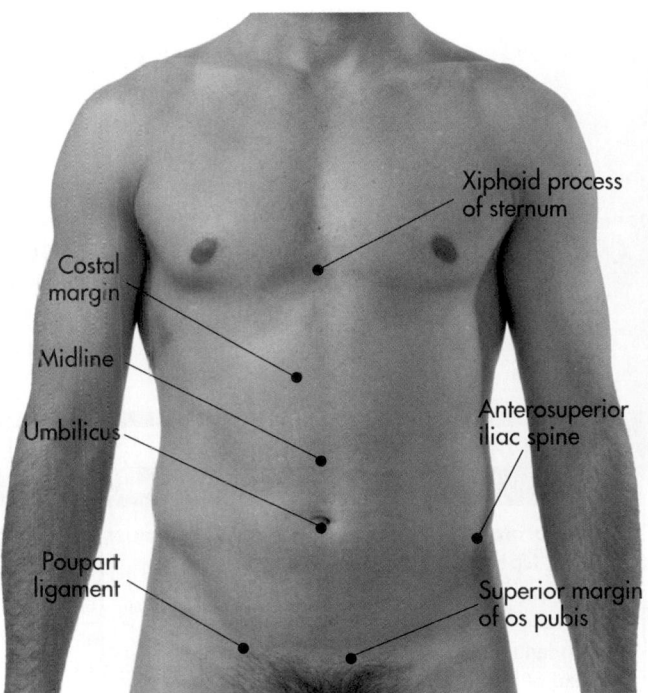

FIGURE 17-6
Landmarks of the abdomen.
From Wilson, Giddens, 2005.

two. Box 17-1 lists the contents of the abdomen in each of the quadrants and regions. Become accustomed to mentally visualizing the underlying organs and structures in each of the zones as you proceed with the examination.

Certain other anatomic landmarks are useful in describing the location of pain, tenderness, and other findings. These landmarks are illustrated in Fig. 17-6.

INSPECTION

SURFACE CHARACTERISTICS

Begin by inspecting the abdomen from a seated position at the patient's right side. This position allows a tangential view that enhances shadows and contouring. Observe the skin color and surface characteristics. The skin of the abdomen is subject to the same expected variations in color and surface characteristics as the rest of the body. The skin may be somewhat paler if it has not been exposed to the sun. Tanning lines are often visible on light-colored skin. A fine venous network is often visible. Above the umbilicus, venous return should be toward the head; below the umbilicus it should be toward the feet (Fig. 17-7, *A*). To determine the direction of venous return, use the following procedure. Place the index fingers of both hands side by side over a vein. Press laterally, separating the fingers and milking empty a section of vein. Release one finger and time the refill. Release the other finger and time the refill. The flow of venous blood is in the direction of the faster filling. Flow patterns are altered in some disease states (Fig. 17-7, *B* and *C*).

Unexpected findings include generalized color changes such as jaundice or cyanosis. A glistening, taut appearance suggests ascites. Inspect for bruises and localized discoloration. Areas of redness may indicate inflammation. A bluish periumbilical discoloration (Cullen sign) suggests intraabdominal bleeding. Striae often result from pregnancy or weight gain. Striae of recent origin are pink or blue in color but turn silvery white over time. Abdominal tumor or ascites that stretches the skin also produces striae. The striae of Cushing disease remain purplish.

Inspect for any lesions, particularly nodules. Lesions are of particular importance because gastrointestinal diseases often produce secondary skin changes. A pearl-like, enlarged umbilical node may signal intraabdominal lymphoma. Skin and gastrointestinal lesions may arise from the same cause or may occur without relationship to one another.

Note any scars and draw their location, configuration, and relative size on an illustration of the abdomen. If the cause of a scar was not explained during the history, now is a good time to pursue that information. The presence of scarring should alert you to the possibility of internal adhesions.

CONTOUR

Inspect the abdomen for contour, symmetry, and surface motion, using tangential lighting to illuminate contour and visible peristalsis. Contour is the abdominal profile from the rib margin to the pubis, viewed on the horizontal plane. The expected contours can be described as flat, rounded, or scaphoid (Fig. 17-8). A flat contour is common in well-muscled, athletic

---

BOX 17-1

LANDMARKS FOR ABDOMINAL EXAMINATION

Anatomic Correlates of the Four Quadrants of the Abdomen

Right Upper Quadrant (RUQ)	*Left Upper Quadrant (LUQ)*
Liver and gallbladder	Left lobe of liver
Pylorus	Spleen
Duodenum	Stomach
Head of pancreas	Body of pancreas
Right adrenal gland	Left adrenal gland
Portion of right kidney	Portion of left kidney
Hepatic flexure of colon	Splenic flexure of colon
Portions of ascending and transverse colon	Portions of transverse and descending colon

Right Lower Quadrant (RLQ)	*Left Lower Quadrant (LLQ)*
Lower pole of right kidney	Lower pole of left kidney
Cecum and appendix	Sigmoid colon
Portion of ascending colon	Portion of descending colon
Bladder (if distended)	Bladder (if distended)
Ovary and salpinx	Ovary and salpinx
Uterus (if enlarged)	Uterus (if enlarged)
Right spermatic cord	Left spermatic cord
Right ureter	Left ureter

Anatomic Correlates of the Nine Regions of the Abdomen

4 Right Hypochondriac	*1 Epigastric*	*5 Left Hypochondriac*
Right lobe of liver	Pyloric end of stomach	Stomach
Gallbladder	Duodenum	Spleen
Portion of duodenum	Pancreas	Tail of pancreas
Hepatic flexure of colon	Portion of liver	Splenic flexure of colon
Portion of right kidney		Upper pole of left kidney
Suprarenal gland	*2 Umbilical*	Suprarenal gland
	Omentum	
6 Right Lumbar	Mesentery	*7 Left Lumbar*
Ascending colon	Lower part of duodenum	Descending colon
Lower half of right kidney	Jejunum and ileum	Lower half of left kidney
Portion of duodenum and jejunum		Portions of jejunum and ileum
	3 Hypogastric (Pubic)	
8 Right Inguinal	Ileum	*9 Left Inguinal*
Cecum	Bladder	Sigmoid colon
Appendix	Uterus (in pregnancy)	Left ureter
Lower end of ileum		Left spermatic cord
Right ureter		Left ovary
Right spermatic cord		
Right ovary		

From Barkauskas et al, 1998.

adults. The rounded or convex contour is characteristic of young children, but in adults it is the result of subcutaneous fat or poor muscle tone from inadequate exercise. The abdomen should be evenly rounded with the maximum height of convexity at the umbilicus. The scaphoid or concave contour is seen in thin adults.

Note the location and contour of the umbilicus. It should be centrally located without displacement upward, downward, or laterally. The umbilicus may be inverted or protrude slightly, but it should be free of inflammation, swelling, or bulges that may indicate a hernia.

Inspect for symmetry from a seated position at the patient's side, then move to a standing position behind the patient's head. Contralateral areas of the abdomen should be symmetric in appearance and contour. Look for any distention or bulges.

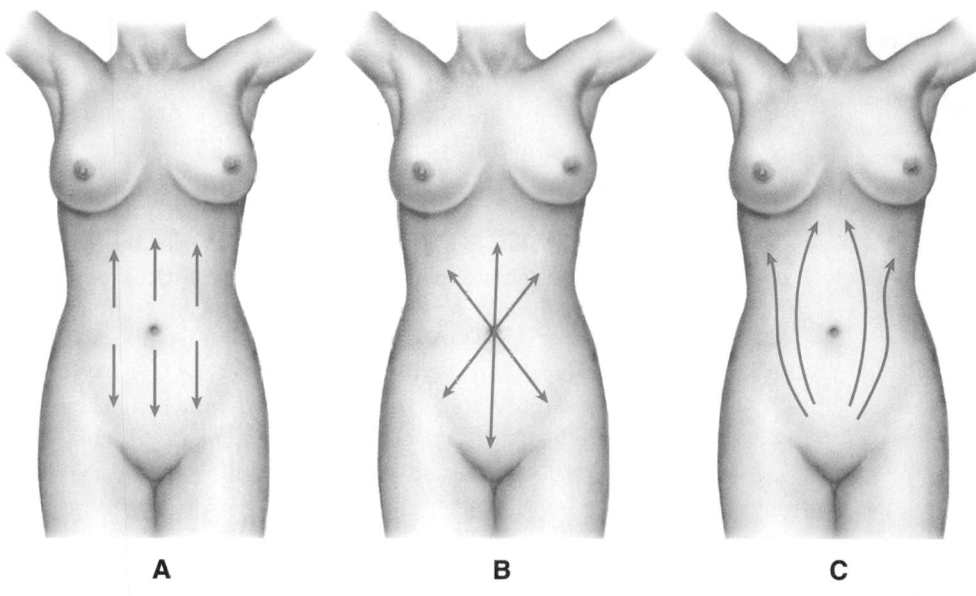

FIGURE 17-7
Abdominal venous patterns.
A, Expected. **B,** Portal hypertension. **C,** Inferior vena cava obstruction.

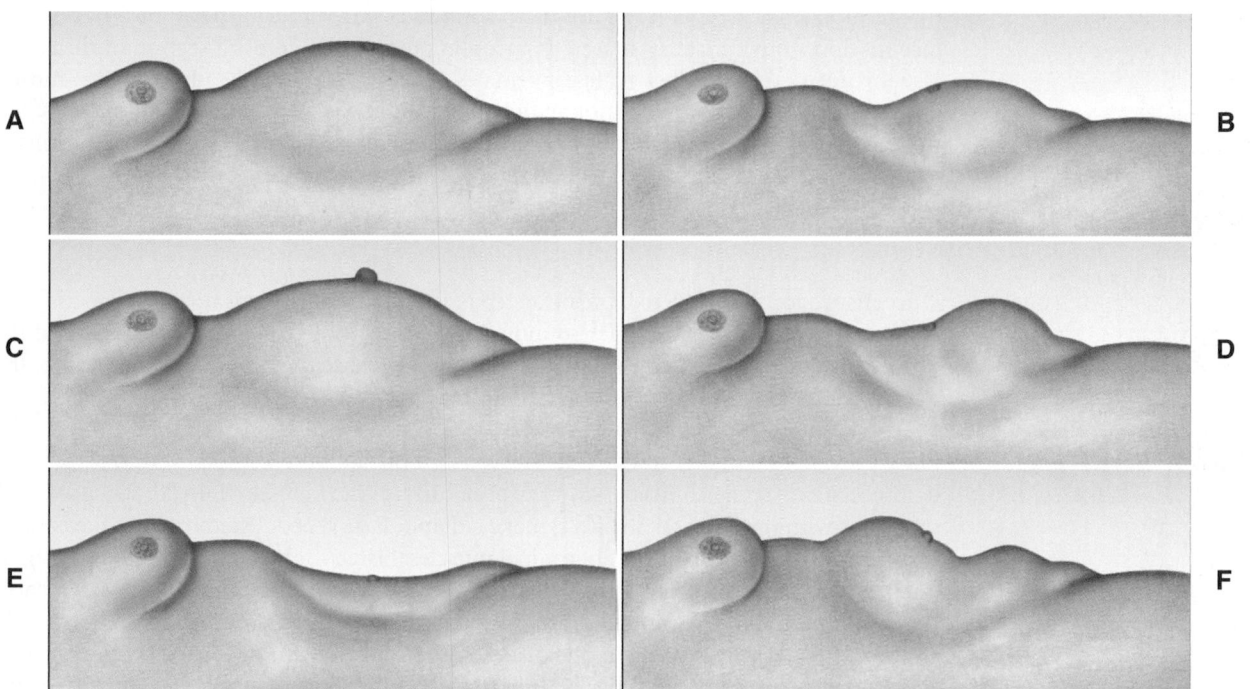

FIGURE 17-8
Abdominal profiles. **A,** Fully rounded or distended, umbilicus inverted. **B,** Distended lower half.
C, Fully rounded or distended, umbilicus everted. **D,** Distended lower third. **E,** Scaphoid. **F,** Distended upper half.

CLINICAL PEARL

Abdominal Distention

You are with a patient whose abdomen is significantly distended and whose bowel sounds are hypoactive or even absent. There is no particular pain and you feel no masses. The reflexes are hypoactive. You know that the patient is on diuretics for treatment of hypertension. Think hypokalemia. Diuretics/distention/deficiency of K$^+$. Steroids can do the same thing.

Generalized symmetric distention may occur as a result of obesity, enlarged organs, and fluid or gas. Distention from the umbilicus to the symphysis can be caused by an ovarian tumor, pregnancy, uterine fibroids, or a distended bladder. Distention of the upper half, above the umbilicus, can mean carcinoma, pancreatic cyst, or gastric dilation. Asymmetric distention or protrusion may indicate hernia, tumor, cysts, bowel obstruction, or enlargement of abdominal organs.

Ask the patient to take a deep breath and hold it. The contour should remain smooth and symmetric. This maneuver lowers the diaphragm and compresses the organs of the abdominal cavity, which may cause previously unseen bulges or masses to appear. Next ask the patient to raise his or her head from the table. This contracts the rectus abdominis muscles, which produces muscle prominence in thin or athletic adults. Superficial abdominal wall masses may become visible. If a hernia is present, the increased abdominal pressure may cause it to protrude.

An incisional hernia is caused by a defect in the abdominal musculature that develops after a surgical incision. The hernia will protrude in the area of the surgical scar. Protrusion of the navel indicates an umbilical hernia. The adult type develops during pregnancy, in longstanding ascites, or when intrathoracic pressure is repeatedly increased, as occurs in chronic respiratory disease. Hernias may also occur in the midline of the epigastrium (i.e., hernia of the linea alba). This type of hernia contains a bit of fat and is felt as a small, tender nodule. Most hernias are reducible, meaning that the contents of the hernial sac are easily replaced. If not, the hernia is nonreducible or incarcerated. A nonreducible hernia in which the blood supply to the protruded contents is obstructed is strangulated and requires immediate surgical intervention.

In addition to hernias, separation of the rectus abdominis muscles may become apparent when the patient raises his or her head from the table. Diastasis recti is often caused by pregnancy or obesity. The condition is of little clinical significance.

MOVEMENT

With the patient's head again resting on the table, inspect the abdomen for movement. Smooth, even movement should occur with respiration. Males exhibit primarily abdominal movement with respiration, whereas females show mostly costal movement. Limited abdominal motion associated with respiration in adult males may indicate peritonitis or disease. Surface motion from peristalsis is seen as a rippling movement across a section of the abdomen. Usually not visible in either males or females, it indicates a definite abnormality, most often an intestinal obstruction. Pulsation in the upper midline is often visible in thin adults. Marked pulsation may occur as the result of increased pulse pressure or abdominal aortic aneurysm.

AUSCULTATION

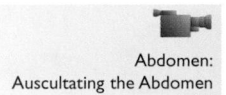
Abdomen:
Auscultating the Abdomen

Once inspection is completed, the next step is auscultation. Use this technique to assess bowel motility and to discover vascular sounds. Unlike the usual sequence, auscultation of the abdomen always precedes percussion and palpation, because these maneuvers may alter the frequency and intensity of bowel sounds.

BOWEL SOUNDS

Place the diaphragm of a warmed stethoscope on the abdomen and hold it in place with very light pressure. (Some clinicians say they prefer to use the bell; in reality, they tend to pull the skin tight with the bell and, in effect, make a diaphragm.) A cold stethoscope, like cold hands, may initiate contraction of the abdominal muscles. Listen for bowel sounds and note their frequency and character. They are usually heard as clicks and gurgles that occur irregularly and range from 5 to 35 per minute. Bowel sounds are generalized so they most often can be assessed adequately by listening in one place. Loud prolonged gurgles called borborygmi (stomach growling) are sometimes heard. Increased bowel sounds may occur with gastroenteritis, early intestinal obstruction, or hunger. High-pitched tinkling sounds suggest intestinal fluid and air under pressure, as in early obstruction. Decreased bowel sounds occur with peritonitis and paralytic ileus. Auscultate in all four quadrants if you have a concern. The absence of bowel sounds is established only after 5 minutes of continuous listening.

VASCULAR SOUNDS

Listen with the bell of the stethoscope in the epigastric region and for bruits in the aortic, renal, iliac, and femoral arteries. Vascular sounds are usually well localized. Keep their specific locations in mind as you listen at those sites (Fig. 17-9). Listen with the diaphragm for friction rubs over the liver and spleen. Friction rubs are high pitched and are heard in association with respiration. Although friction rubs in the abdomen are rare, they indicate inflammation of the peritoneal surface of the organ from tumor, infection, or infarct.

Auscultate with the bell of the stethoscope in the epigastric region and around the umbilicus for a venous hum, which is soft, low pitched, and continuous. A venous hum occurs with increased collateral circulation between portal and systemic venous systems.

PERCUSSION

Percussion (generally indirect) is used to assess the size and density of the organs in the abdomen and to detect the presence of fluid (as with ascites), air (as with gastric distention), and fluid-filled or solid masses. Percussion is used either independently or concurrently with palpation while specific organs are evaluated, and it can validate palpatory findings. For simplicity, percussion and palpation are discussed separately; however, either approach is acceptable.

First percuss all quadrants or regions of the abdomen for a sense of overall tympany and dullness (Table 17-1). Tympany is the predominant sound because air is present in the stomach and intestines. Dullness is heard over organs and solid masses. A distended bladder produces dullness in the suprapubic area. Develop a systematic route for percussion, as shown in Fig. 17-10.

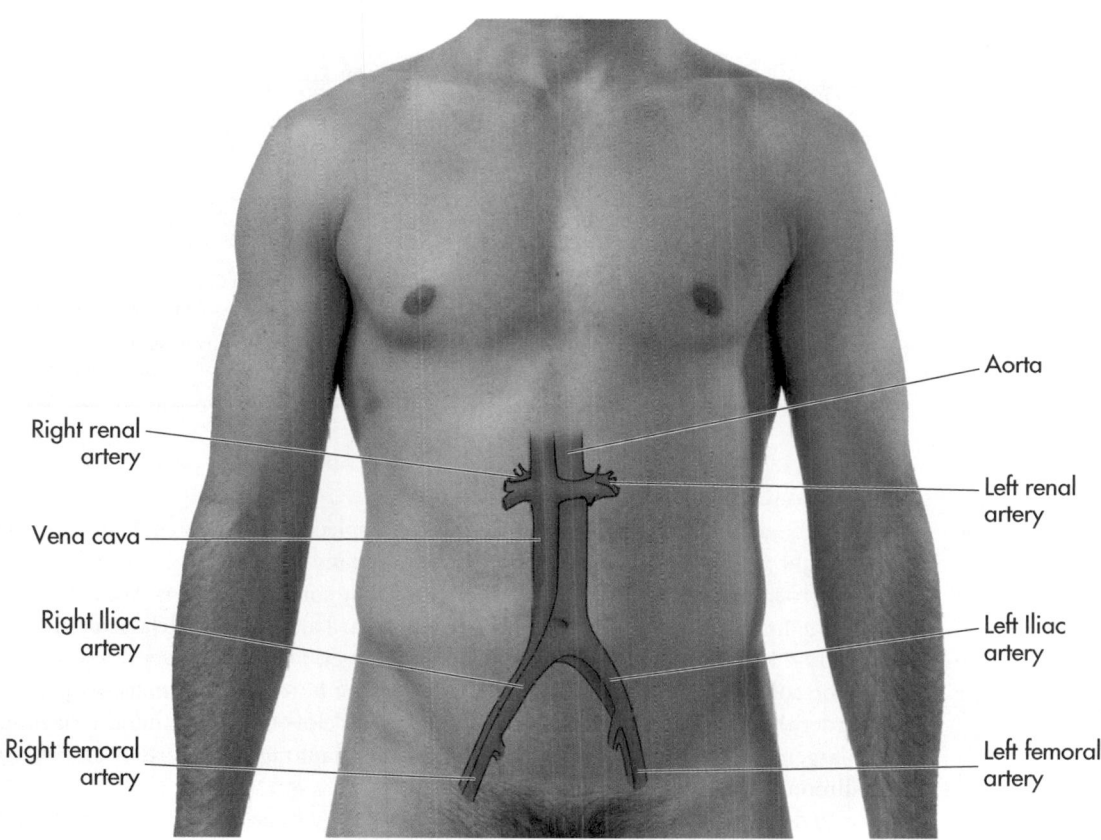

Right renal artery

Vena cava

Right Iliac artery

Right femoral artery

Aorta

Left renal artery

Left Iliac artery

Left femoral artery

FIGURE 17-9
Sites to auscultate for bruits: renal arteries, iliac arteries, aorta, and femoral arteries.
Modified from Wilson, Giddens, 2005.

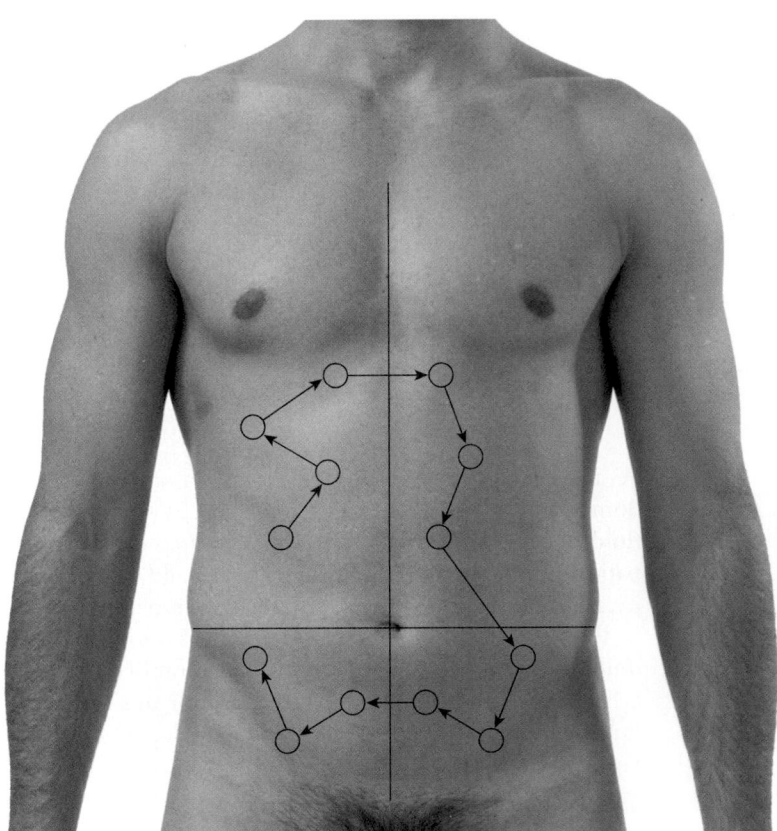

FIGURE 17-10
Systematic route for abdominal percussion.
From Wilson, Giddens, 2005.

TABLE 17-1	**Percussion Notes of the Abdomen**	
Note	**Description**	**Location**
Tympany	Musical note of higher pitch than resonance	Over air-filled viscera
Hyperresonance	Pitch lies between tympany and resonance	Base of left lung
Resonance	Sustained note of moderate pitch	Over lung tissue and some times over the abdomen
Dullness	Short, high-pitched note with little resonance	Over solid organs adjacent to air-filled structures

LIVER SPAN

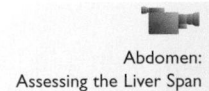

Abdomen:
Assessing the Liver Span

Now go back and percuss individually the liver, spleen, and stomach. Begin liver percussion at the right midclavicular line over an area of tympany. (Always begin with an area of tympany and proceed to an area of dullness, because that sound change is easier to detect than the change from dullness to tympany.) Percuss upward along the midclavicular line, as shown in Fig. 17-11, to determine the lower border of the liver. The area of liver dullness is usually heard at the costal margin or slightly below it. Mark the border with a marking pen. A lower liver border that is more than 2 to 3 cm (¾ to 1 inch) below the costal margin may indicate organ enlargement or downward displacement of the diaphragm because of emphysema or other pulmonary disease.

To determine the upper border of the liver, begin percussion on the right midclavicular line at an area of lung resonance. Continue downward until the percussion tone changes to one of dullness; this marks the upper border of the liver. Mark the location with the pen. The upper border usually begins at the fifth to seventh intercostal space. An upper border below this may

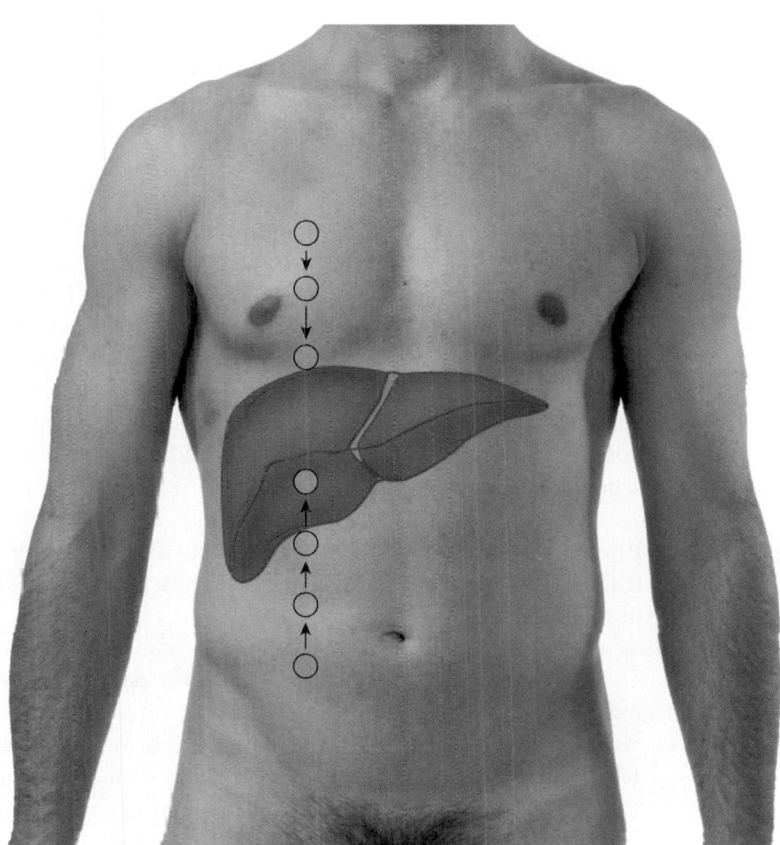

FIGURE 17-11
Liver percussion routes along midclavicular and midsternal lines.
Modified from Wilson, Giddens, 2005.

indicate downward displacement or liver atrophy. Dullness extending above the fifth intercostal space suggests upward displacement from abdominal fluid or masses.

Measure the distance between the marks to estimate the vertical span of the liver. The usual span is approximately 6 to 12 cm (2½ to 4½ inches). A span greater than this may indicate liver enlargement, whereas a lesser span suggests atrophy. Age and gender influence liver size. Obviously, the liver will be larger in adults than in children. Liver span is usually greater in males and in tall individuals than in females and short people. Interestingly, in the early years of life, the liver tends to be somewhat larger in the female; but usually by about 2 years of age, the liver of the male will be larger. Of course, individuals at any age vary, and the generalization will not hold true in all cases.

Although percussion provides the most accurate clinical measure of liver size, the measure remains only a gross estimate. Errors in estimating liver span can occur when the dullness of pleural effusion or lung consolidation obscures the upper liver border, leading to overestimation of size. Similarly, gas in the colon may produce tympany in the right upper quadrant and obscure the dullness of the lower liver border, leading to underestimation of liver size.

LIVER DESCENT

To assess the descent of the liver, ask the patient to take a deep breath and hold it while you percuss upward again from the abdomen at the right midclavicular line. The area of lower border dullness should move downward 2 to 3 cm. This maneuver will guide subsequent palpation of the organ.

ADDITIONAL LIVER ASSESSMENT

If liver enlargement is suspected, additional percussion maneuvers can provide further information. Percuss upward and then downward over the right midaxillary line. Liver dullness is usually detected in the fifth to seventh intercostal space. Dullness beyond those limits suggests a problem. You can also percuss along the midsternal line to estimate the midsternal liver span. Percuss upward from the abdomen and downward from the lungs, marking the upper and lower borders of dullness. The usual span at the midsternal line is 4 to 8 cm (1½ to 3 inches). Spans exceeding 8 cm suggest liver enlargement.

It is best to report the size of the liver in two ways: liver span as determined from percussing the upper and lower borders; and the extent of liver projection below the costal margin. When the size of a patient's liver is important in assessing the clinical condition, projection below the costal margin alone will not provide enough comparative information.

SPLEEN

Percuss the spleen just posterior to the midaxillary line on the left side. Percuss in several directions as shown in Fig. 17-12, beginning at areas of lung resonance. You may hear a small area of splenic dullness from the sixth to the tenth rib. A large area of dullness suggests spleen enlargement; however, a full stomach or feces-filled intestine may mimic the dullness of splenic enlargement. Percuss the lowest intercostal space in the left anterior axillary line before and after the patient takes a deep breath. The area should remain tympanic. With splenic enlargement, tympany changes to dullness as the spleen is brought forward and downward with inspiration. Remember that it is not possible to distinguish between the dullness of the posterior flank and that of the spleen. In addition, the dullness of a healthy spleen is often obscured by the tympany of colonic air.

GASTRIC BUBBLE

Percuss for the gastric air bubble in the area of the left lower anterior rib cage and left epigastric region. The tympany produced by the gastric bubble is lower in pitch than the tympany of the intestine.

KIDNEYS

To assess each kidney for tenderness, ask the patient to assume a sitting position. Place the palm of your hand over the right costovertebral angle and strike your hand with the ulnar surface of the fist of your other hand. Repeat the maneuver over the left costovertebral angle (Fig. 17-13, *A*). Direct percussion with the fist over each costovertebral angle may also be used (Fig. 17-13, *B*). The patient should perceive the blow as a thud, but it should not cause tenderness or pain. For efficiency of time and motion, assessment for kidney tenderness is usually performed while examining the back rather than the abdomen.

PALPATION

Use palpation to assess the organs of the abdominal cavity and to detect muscle spasm, masses, fluid, and areas of tenderness. Evaluate the abdominal organs for size, shape, mobility, consistency, and tension. Stand at the patient's side (usually the right) with the patient in the supine position. Make certain that the patient is comfortable and that the abdomen is as relaxed as possible; bending the patient's knees may help relax the muscles. Your hands should be warm to avoid producing muscle contraction, which will hinder further examination. Ticklishness may also create a problem (Box 17-2).

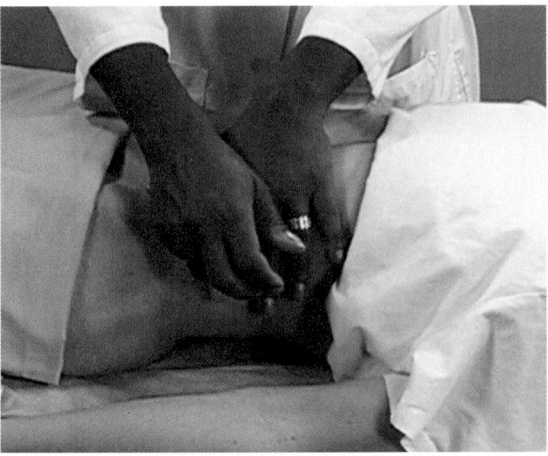

FIGURE 17-12
Percussion of the spleen.

LIGHT PALPATION

Begin with a light, systematic palpation of all four quadrants, initially avoiding any areas that have already been identified as problem spots. Lay the palm of your hand lightly on the abdomen, with the fingers extended and approximated (Fig. 17-14). With the palmar surface of your fingers, depress the abdominal wall no more than 1 cm, using a light and even pressing motion. Avoid short, quick jabs. The abdomen should feel smooth, with a consistent softness. The patient's abdomen may tense if you press too deeply, if your hands are cold, if the patient

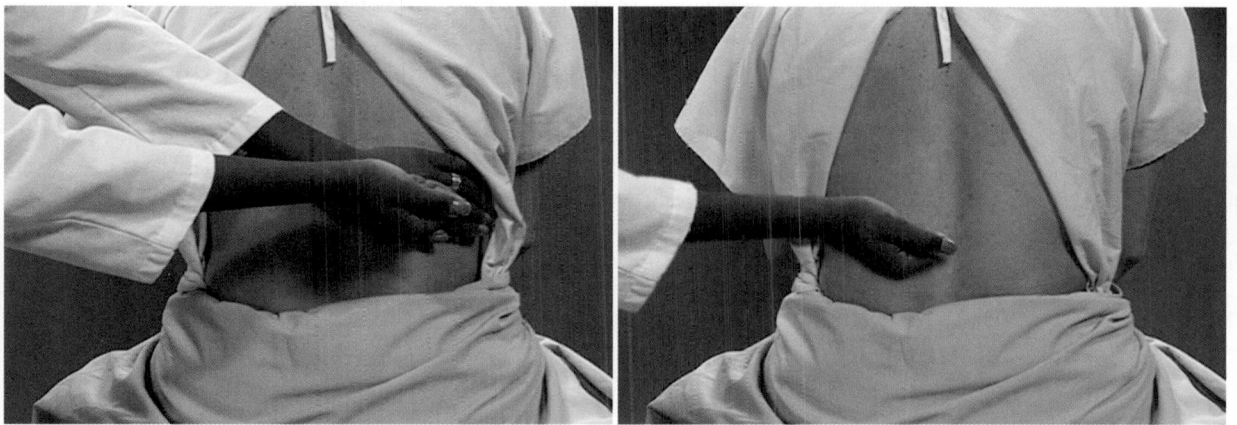

A   **B**

FIGURE 17-13
Fist percussion of the costovertebral angle for kidney tenderness. **A,** Indirect percussion. **B,** Direct percussion.

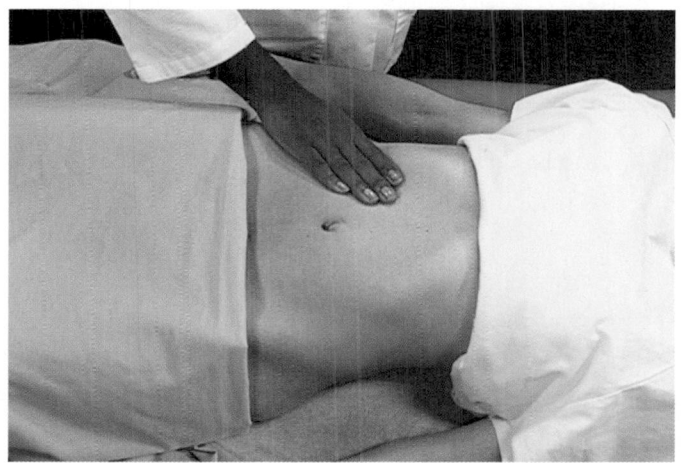

FIGURE 17-14
Light palpation of the abdomen. With fingers extended and approximated, press in no more than 1 cm.

BOX 17-2

EXAMINING THE ABDOMEN IN A TICKLISH PATIENT

The ticklishness of a patient can sometimes make it difficult for you to palpate the abdomen satisfactorily; however, there are ways to overcome this problem. Ask the patient to perform self-palpation, and place your hands over the patient's fingers, not quite touching the abdomen itself. After a time, let your fingers drift slowly onto the abdomen while still resting primarily on the patient's fingers. You can still learn a good deal, and ticklishness might not be so much of a problem. You might also use the diaphragm of the stethoscope (making sure it is warm enough) as a palpating instrument. This serves as a starting point, and again your fingers can drift over the edge of the diaphragm and palpate without eliciting an excessively ticklish response. Applying a stimulus to another, less sensitive part of the body with your nonpalpating hand can also decrease a ticklish response. In some instances a patient's ticklishness cannot be overcome, and you just have to palpate as best you can.

is ticklish, or if inflammation is present. Guarding should alert you to move cautiously through the remainder of the examination.

Light palpation is particularly useful in identifying muscular resistance and areas of tenderness. A large mass or distended structure may be appreciated on light palpation as a sense of resistance. If resistance is present, try to determine whether it is voluntary or involuntary in the following way: Place a pillow under the patient's knees and ask the patient to breathe slowly through the mouth as you feel for relaxation of the rectus abdominis muscles on expiration. If the tenseness remains, it is probably an involuntary response to localized or generalized rigidity. Rigidity is a boardlike hardness of the abdominal wall overlying areas of peritoneal irritation.

Specific zones of peritoneal irritation may be identified through cutaneous hypersensitivity (Fig. 17-15). To evaluate hypersensitivity, gently lift a fold of skin away from the underlying muscle or stimulate the skin with a pin or other object and have the patient describe the local sensation (Fig. 17-16). In the event of hypersensitivity, the patient will perceive pain or an exaggerated sensation in response to this maneuver.

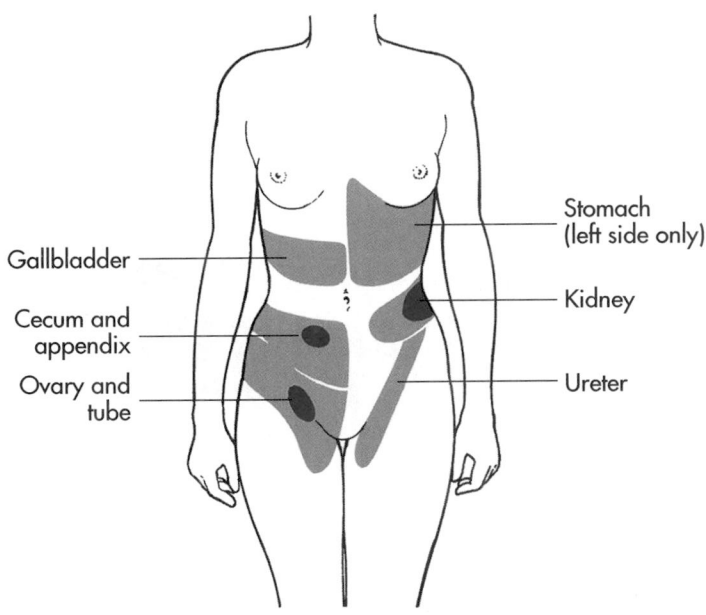

FIGURE 17-15
Areas of cutaneous hypersensitivity.

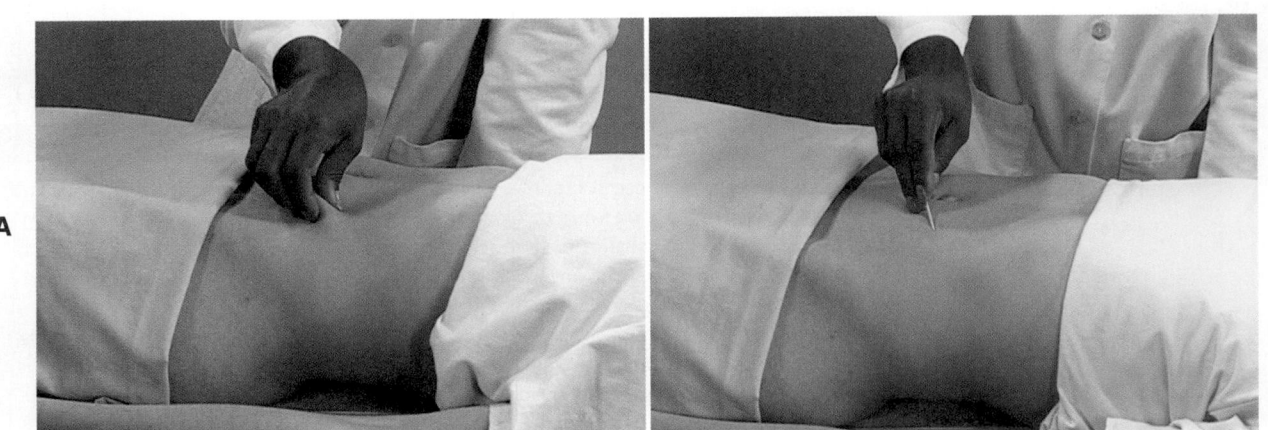

FIGURE 17-16
Testing for cutaneous hypersensitivity. **A,** Lift a fold of skin away from underlying muscle or, **B,** stimulate the skin with a sharp point or a broken tongue blade.

MODERATE PALPATION

Continue palpation of all four quadrants with the same hand position as for light palpation, exerting moderate pressure as an intermediate step to gradually approach deep palpation. Tenderness not elicited on gentle palpation may become evident with deeper pressure. An additional maneuver of moderate palpation is performed with the side of your hand (Fig. 17-17). This maneuver is useful in assessing organs that move with respiration, specifically the liver and spleen. Palpate during the entire respiratory cycle; as the patient inspires, the organ is displaced downward, and you may be able to feel it as it bumps gently against your hand.

DEEP PALPATION

Deep palpation is necessary to thoroughly delineate abdominal organs and to detect less obvious masses. Use the palmar surface of your extended fingers, pressing deeply and evenly into the abdominal wall (Fig. 17-18). Palpate all four quadrants, moving the fingers back and forth over the abdominal contents. (The abdominal wall may also slide back and forth as you do this.) Often you are able to feel the borders of the rectus abdominis muscles, the aorta, and portions of the colon. Tenderness not elicited with light or moderate palpation may become evident. Deep pressure may also evoke tenderness in the healthy person over the cecum, sigmoid colon, aorta, and in the midline near the xiphoid process.

MASSES

Identify any masses and note the following characteristics: location, size, shape, consistency, tenderness, pulsation, mobility, and movement with respiration. To determine whether a mass is superficial (i.e., located in the abdominal wall) or intraabdominal, have the patient lift his or her head from the examining table, thus contracting the abdominal muscles. Masses in the abdominal wall will continue to be palpable, whereas those located in the abdominal cavity will be more difficult to feel because they are obscured by abdominal musculature. The presence of feces in the colon, often mistaken for an abdominal mass, can be felt as a soft, rounded, boggy mass in the cecum and in the ascending, descending, or sigmoid colons. Other structures that are sometimes mistaken for masses are the lateral borders of the rectus abdominis muscles, the uterus, aorta, sacral promontory, and common iliac artery (Fig. 17-19). If you can mentally visualize the placement of the abdominal structures, it will be easier to distinguish between what you know ought to be there and an unexpected finding.

UMBILICAL RING

Palpate the umbilical ring and around the umbilicus. The area should be free of bulges, nodules, and granulation. The umbilical ring should be round and free of irregularities. Note whether it is incomplete or soft in the center, which suggests the potential for herniation. The umbilicus may be either slightly inverted or everted, but it should not protrude.

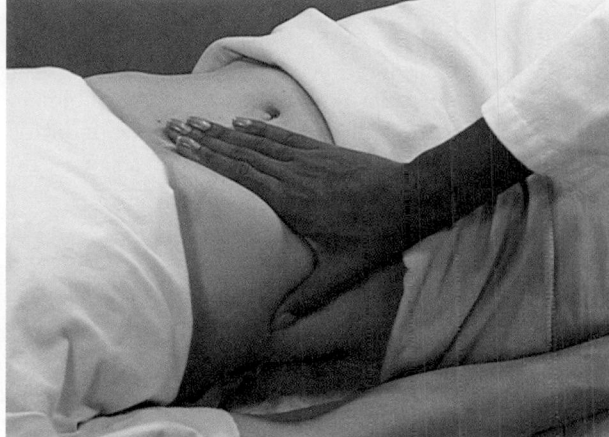

FIGURE 17-17
Moderate palpation using the side of the hand.

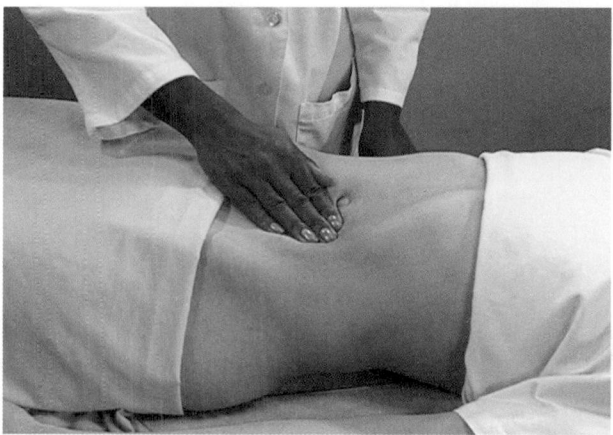

FIGURE 17-18
Deep palpation of the abdomen. Press deeply and evenly with the palmar surface of extended fingers.

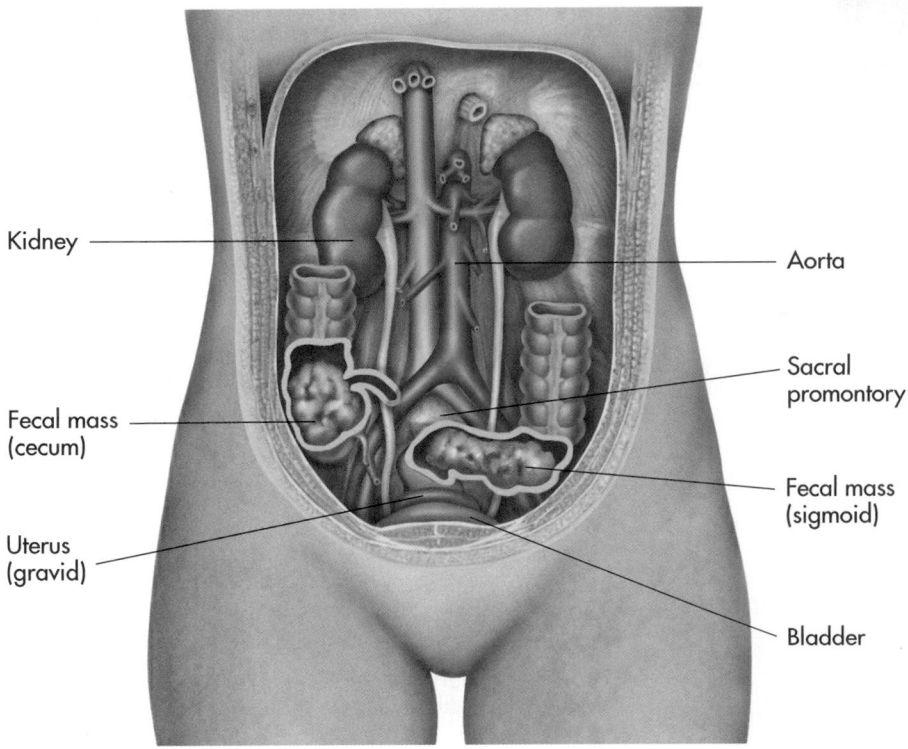

Kidney

Aorta

Sacral
promontory

Fecal mass
(cecum)

Fecal mass
(sigmoid)

Uterus
(gravid)

Bladder

FIGURE 17-19
Abdominal structures commonly
felt as masses.

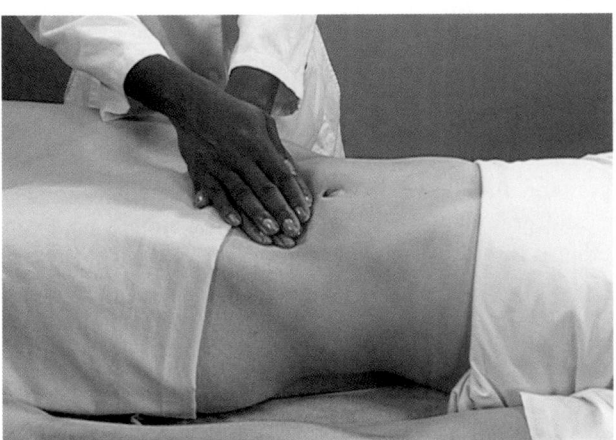

FIGURE 17-20
Deep bimanual palpation.

BIMANUAL TECHNIQUE	If deep palpation is difficult because of obesity or muscular resistance, you can use a bimanual technique with one hand atop the other as shown in Fig. 17-20. Exert pressure with the top hand while concentrating on sensation with the other hand. Some examiners prefer to use the bimanual technique for all patients.
PALPATION OF SPECIFIC STRUCTURES	**Liver.** Place your left hand under the patient at the eleventh and twelfth ribs, pressing upward to elevate the liver toward the abdominal wall. Place your right hand on the abdomen, fingers pointing toward the head and extended so the tips rest on the right midclavicular line below the level of liver dullness, as shown in Fig. 17-21, *A*. As an alternative, you can place your right hand parallel to the right costal margin, as shown in Fig. 17-21, *B*. In either case, press your right hand gently but deeply in and up. Have the patient breathe regularly a few times and then take a deep breath. Try to feel the liver edge as the diaphragm pushes it down to meet your fingertips. Ordinarily, the liver is not palpable, although it may be felt in some thin persons even when no pathologic condition exists. If the liver edge is felt, it should be firm,

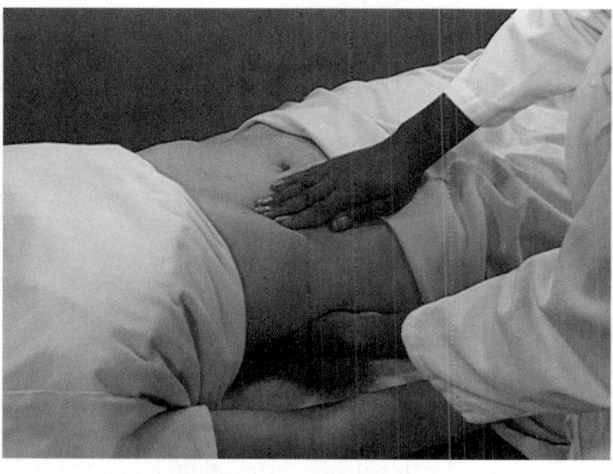 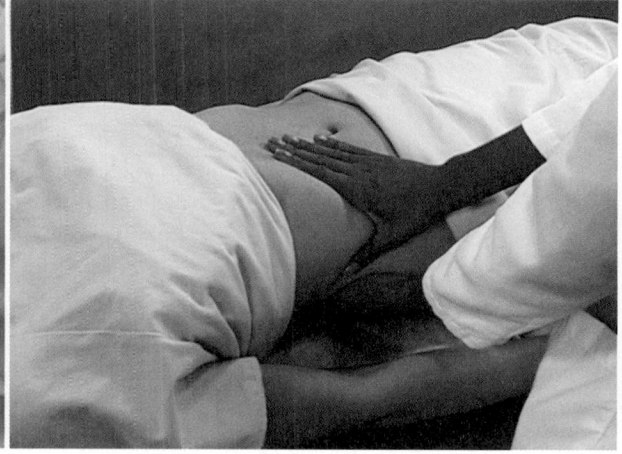

A

B

FIGURE 17-21
Palpating the liver. **A,** Fingers are extended, with tips on right midclavicular line below the level of liver tenderness and pointing toward the head. **B,** Alternative method for liver palpation with fingers parallel to the costal margin.

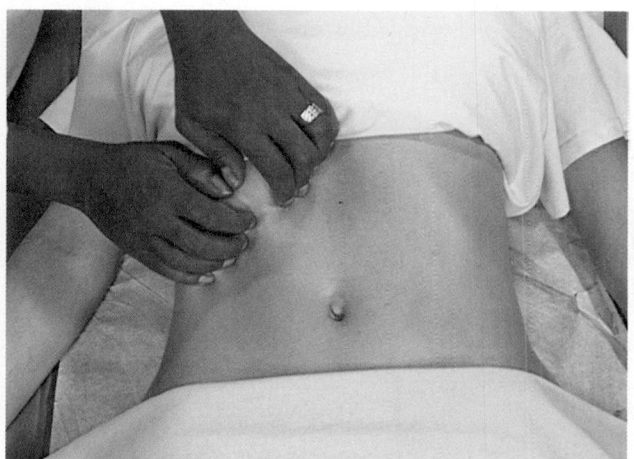

FIGURE 17-22
Palpating the liver with fingers hooked over the costal margin.

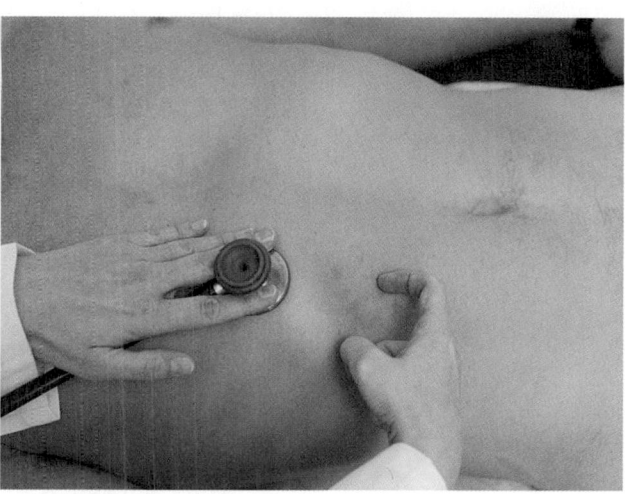

FIGURE 17-23
Scratch technique for auscultating the liver. With stethoscope over the liver, lightly scratch the abdominal surface, moving toward the liver. The sound will be intensified over the liver.

smooth, even, and nontender. Feel for nodules, tenderness, and irregularity. If the liver is palpable, repeat the maneuver medially and laterally to the costal margin to assess the contour and surface of the liver.

Liver: Alternative Techniques. An alternative technique is to hook your fingers over the right costal margin below the border of liver dullness, as shown in Fig. 17-22. Stand on the patient's right side facing his or her feet. Press in and up toward the costal margin with your fingers and ask the patient to take a deep breath. Try to feel the liver edge as it descends to meet your fingers.

If the abdomen is distended or the abdominal muscles tense, the usual techniques for determining the lower liver border may be unproductive. At such a point, the scratch test may be useful (Fig. 17-23). This technique uses auscultation to detect the differences in sound transmission over solid and hollow organs. Place the stethoscope over the liver and with the finger of your other hand scratch the abdominal surface lightly, moving toward the liver border. When you encounter the liver, the sound you hear in the stethoscope will be intensified.

To check for liver tenderness when the liver is not palpable, use indirect fist percussion. Place the palmar surface of one hand over the lower right rib cage, and then strike your hand with the ulnar surface of the fist of your other hand as shown in Fig. 17-24. The healthy liver is not tender to percussion.

Gallbladder. Palpate below the liver margin at the lateral border of the rectus abdominis muscle for the gallbladder. A healthy gallbladder will not be palpable. A palpable, tender gallbladder indicates cholecystitis, whereas nontender enlargement suggests common bile duct obstruction. If you suspect cholecystitis, have the patient take a deep breath during deep palpation. As the inflamed gallbladder comes in contact with the examining fingers, the patient will experience pain and abruptly halt inspiration (Murphy sign).

Spleen. While still standing on the patient's right side, reach across with your left hand and place it beneath the patient over the left costovertebral angle. Press upward with that hand to lift the spleen anteriorly toward the abdominal wall. Place the palmar surface of your right hand with fingers extended on the patient's abdomen below the left costal margin (Fig. 17-25, *A*). Use findings from percussion as a guide. Press your fingertips inward toward the spleen as you ask the patient to take a deep breath. Try to feel the edge of the spleen as it moves downward toward your fingers. The spleen is not usually palpable in an adult; if you can feel it, it is probably enlarged (Box 17-3). Be sure to palpate with your fingers below the costal margin so that you will not miss the lower edge of an enlarged spleen. Be gentle in palpation to avoid rupturing an enlarged spleen.

Repeat the palpation while the patient is lying on the right side with hips and knees flexed (see Fig. 17-25, *B*). Still standing on the right side, press inward with your left hand to assist

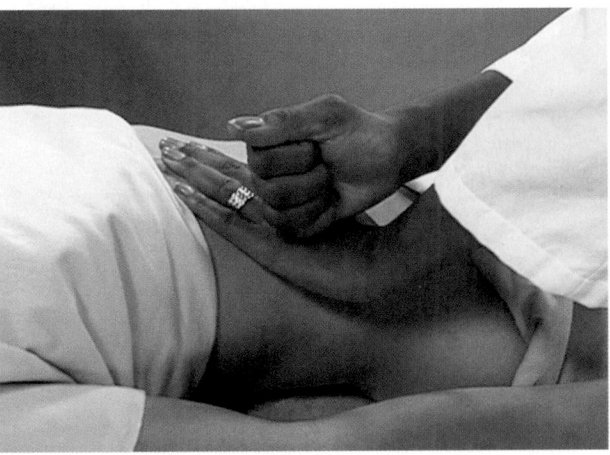

FIGURE 17-24
Fist percussion of the liver.

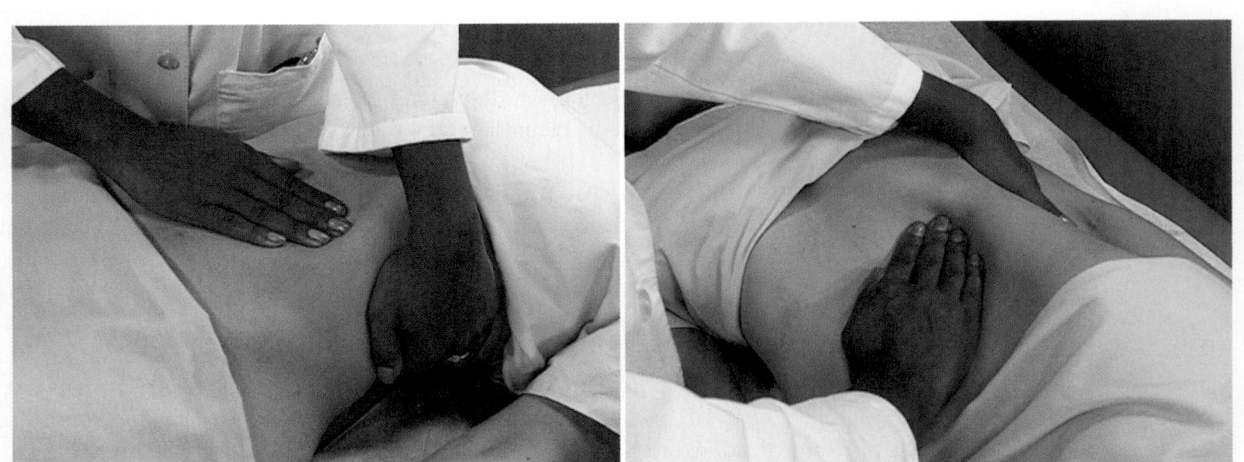

FIGURE 17-25
Palpating the spleen. **A,** Press upward with the left hand at the patient's left costovertebral angle. Feel for the spleen with the right hand below the left costal margin. **B,** Palpating the spleen with the patient lying on the side. Press inward with left hand and tips of the right fingers.

BOX 17-3

AN ENLARGED SPLEEN OR AN ENLARGED LEFT KIDNEY?

When an organ is palpable below the left costal margin, it may be difficult to differentiate an enlarged spleen from an enlarged left kidney. Percussion should help distinguish between the organs. The percussion note over an enlarged spleen is dull because the spleen displaces bowel. The usual area of splenic dullness will be increased downward and toward the midline. The percussion note over an enlarged kidney is resonant because the kidney is deeply situated behind the bowel. In addition, the edge of the spleen is sharper than that of the kidney. A palpable notch along the medial border suggests an enlarged spleen rather than an enlarged kidney.

gravity in bringing the spleen forward and to the right. Press inward with the fingertips of your right hand and feel for the edge of the spleen. Again, you will not usually feel it; if you can, it is probably enlarged.

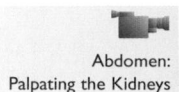

Abdomen:
Palpating the Kidneys

Left Kidney. Ask the patient to lie supine. Standing on the patient's right side, reach across with your left hand as you did in spleen palpation and place the hand over the left flank. Place your right hand at the patient's left costal margin. Have the patient take a deep breath and then elevate the left flank with your left hand and palpate deeply (because of the retroperitoneal position of the kidney) with your right hand (Fig. 17-26). Try to feel the lower pole of the kidney with your fingertips as the patient inhales. The left kidney is ordinarily not palpable.

Another approach is to capture the kidney. Move to the patient's left side and position your hands as before, with the left hand over the patient's left flank and the right hand at the left costal margin. Ask the patient to take a deep breath. At the height of inspiration, press the fingers of your two hands together to capture the kidney between the fingers. Ask the patient to breathe out and hold the exhalation while you slowly release your fingers. If you have captured the kidney you may feel it slip beneath your fingers as it moves back into place. Although the patient may feel the capture and release, the maneuver should not be painful. Again, a left kidney is seldom palpable.

Right Kidney. Stand on the patient's right side, placing one hand under the patient's right flank and the other hand at the right costal margin. Perform the same maneuvers as you did for the left kidney (Fig. 17-27). Because of the anatomic position of the right kidney, it is more commonly palpable than the left kidney. If it is palpable, it should be smooth, firm, and nontender. It may be difficult to distinguish the kidney from the liver edge. The liver edge tends to be sharp, whereas the kidney is more rounded. The liver also extends more medially and laterally and cannot be captured.

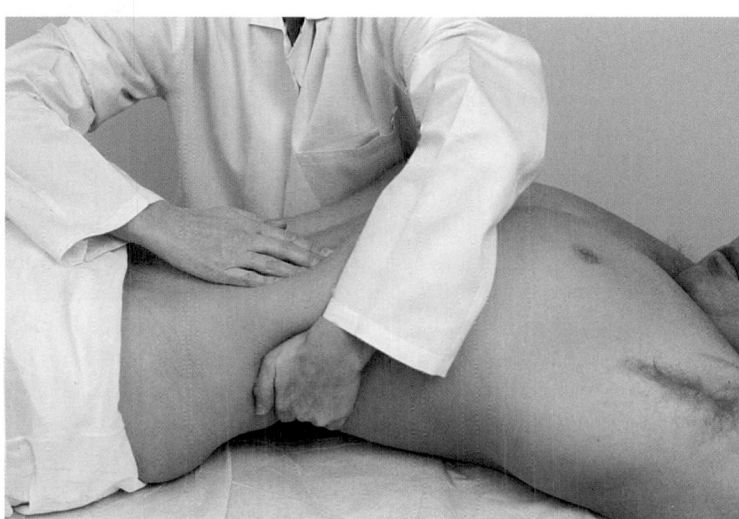

FIGURE 17-26
Palpating the left kidney. Elevate the left flank with the left hand. Palpate deeply with the right hand.

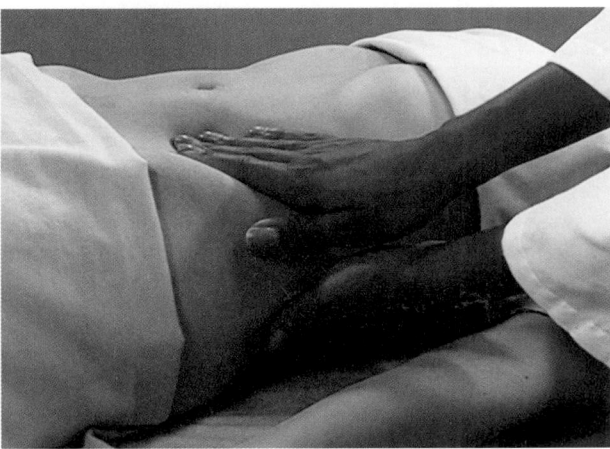

FIGURE 17-27
Capture technique for palpating the kidney (left kidney palpation shown). As the patient takes a deep breath, press the fingers of both hands together. As the patient exhales, slowly release the pressure and feel for the kidney to slip between the fingers.

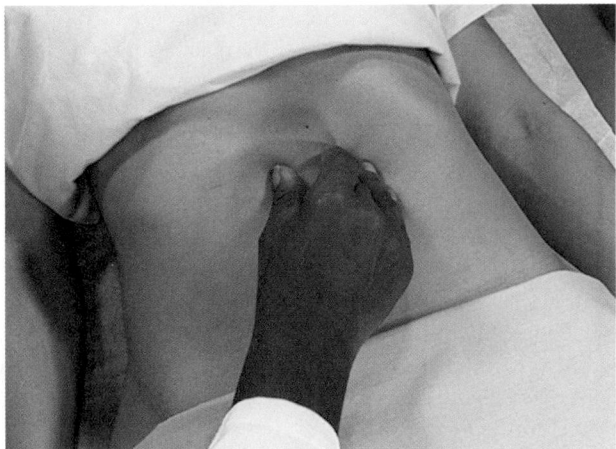

FIGURE 17-28
Palpating the aorta. Place the thumb on one side of the aorta and the fingers on the other side.

Aorta. With the patient in the supine position, palpate deeply slightly to the left of the midline and feel for the aortic pulsation. If the pulsation is prominent, try to determine the direction of pulsation. A prominent lateral pulsation suggests an aortic aneurysm. Although the aortic pulse may be felt, particularly in thin adults, the pulse should be in an anterior direction.

If you are unable to feel the pulse on deep palpation, an alternate technique may help. Place the palmar surface of your hands with fingers extended on the midline. Press the fingers deeply inward on each side of the aorta and feel for the pulsation. In thin individuals, you can use one hand, placing the thumb on one side of the aorta and the fingers on the other side (Fig. 17-28).

Urinary Bladder. The urinary bladder is not palpable in a healthy patient unless the bladder is distended with urine. When the bladder is distended, you can feel it as a smooth, round, tense mass. You can determine the distended bladder outline with percussion; a distended bladder will elicit a lower percussion note than the surrounding air-filled intestines.

Abdominal Reflexes. With the patient supine, stroke each quadrant of the abdomen with the end of a reflex hammer or edge of a tongue blade. The upper abdominal reflexes are elicited by stroking upward and away from the umbilicus; lower abdominal reflexes are elicited by stroking downward and away from the umbilicus (Fig. 17-29). With each stroke, expect to see contraction of the rectus abdominis muscles and pulling of the umbilicus toward the stroked side. A diminished reflex may be present in patients who are obese or whose abdominal muscles have been stretched during pregnancy. Absence of the reflex may indicate a pyramidal tract lesion.

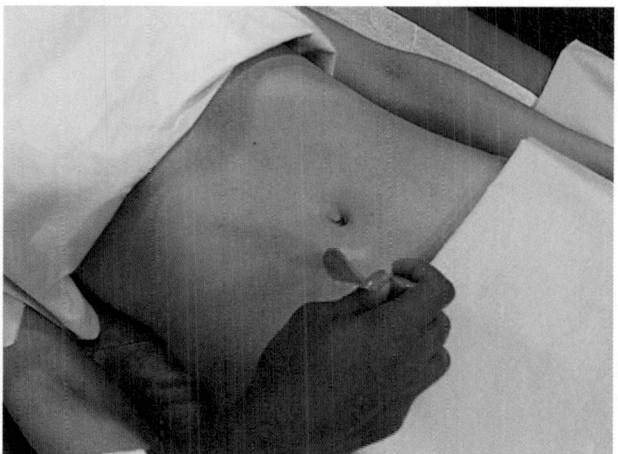

FIGURE 17-29
Examination of the superficial abdominal reflexes. One of several approaches is illustrated. Stroke the upper abdominal area upward, away from the umbilicus, and the lower abdominal area downward, away from the umbilicus.

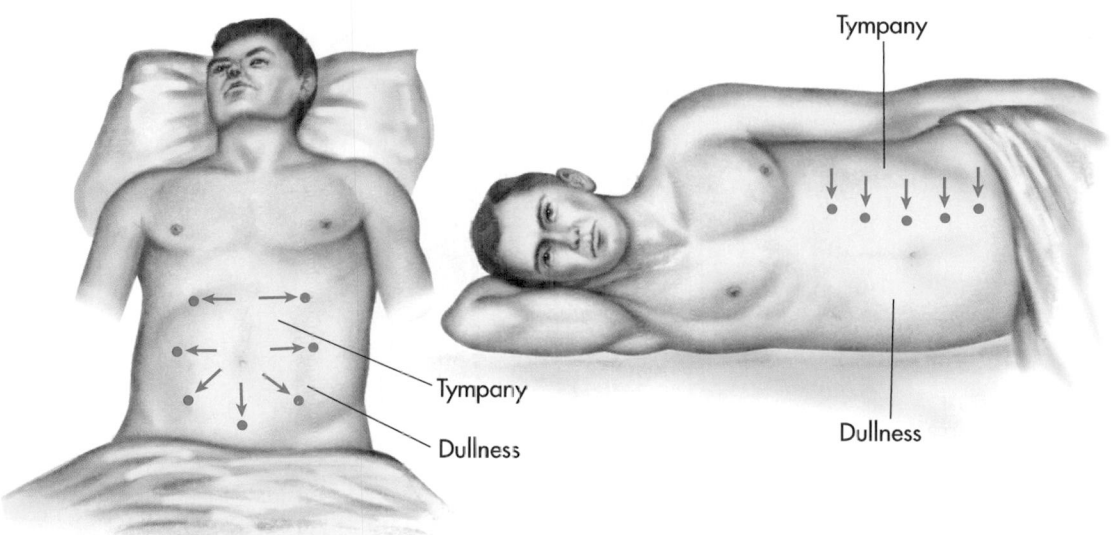

FIGURE 17-30
Testing for shifting dullness. Dullness shifts to the dependent side.

ADDITIONAL PROCEDURES

ASCITES ASSESSMENT

Ascites may be suspected in patients who have protuberant abdomens or flanks that bulge in the supine position. Percuss for areas of dullness and resonance with the patient supine. Because ascites fluid settles with gravity, expect to hear dullness in the dependent parts of the abdomen and tympany in the upper parts where the relatively lighter bowel has risen. Mark the borders between tympany and dullness.

Shifting Dullness. Test for shifting dullness to help ascertain the presence of fluid. Have the patient lie on one side and again percuss for tympany and dullness and mark the borders. In the patient without ascites, the borders will remain relatively constant. In ascites, the border of dullness shifts to the dependent side (approaches the midline) as the fluid resettles with gravity (Fig. 17-30).

Fluid Wave. Another maneuver is to test for a fluid wave. This procedure requires three hands, so you will need assistance from the patient or another examiner (Fig. 17-31). With the patient supine, ask him or her or another person to press the edge of the hand and forearm firmly along the vertical midline of the abdomen. This positioning helps stop the transmission of a wave through adipose tissue. Place your hands on each side of the abdomen and strike one side sharply with your fingertips. Feel for the impulse of a fluid wave with the fingertips of your other hand. An easily detected fluid wave suggests ascites, but be cautioned that the

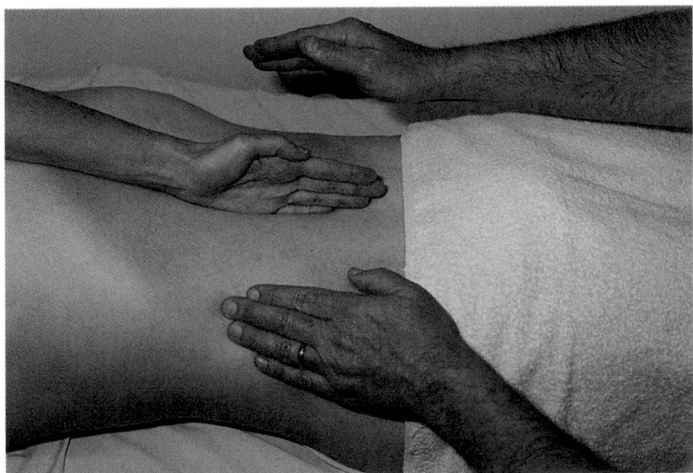

FIGURE 17-31
Testing for fluid wave. Strike one side of the abdomen sharply with the fingertips. Feel for the impulse of a fluid wave with the other hand.

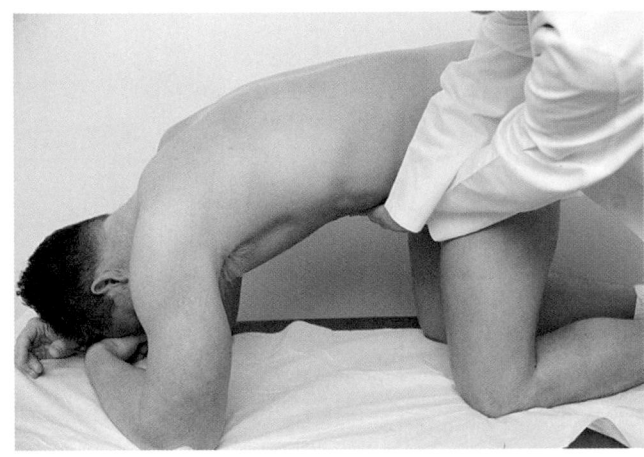

FIGURE 17-32
Testing for pooling abdominal fluid. Percuss the umbilical area for dullness.

findings of this maneuver are not conclusive. A fluid wave can sometimes be felt in people without ascites and, conversely, may not occur in people with early ascites.

Auscultatory Percussion. Auscultatory percussion has been suggested as an additional maneuver for detecting ascites. Have the patient void and then stand for 3 minutes to allow fluid to gravitate to the pelvis. Hold the diaphragm of the stethoscope immediately above the symphysis pubis in the midline with one hand. With the other hand, apply finger-flicking percussion to three or more sites from the costal margin perpendicularly downward toward the pelvis. In the healthy person the percussion note is first dull and then changes sharply to a loud note at the pelvic border. In patients with ascites the percussion note changes above the pelvic border at the fluid level.

Puddle Sign. Another maneuver allows you to test for fluid pooling (puddle sign). Ask the patient to assume the knee-chest position and maintain that position for several minutes to allow any fluid to pool by gravity. Percuss the umbilical area for dullness to determine the presence of fluid (Fig. 17-32). The area will remain tympanic if no fluid is present.

None of these previously discussed maneuvers is specific or reliable, and generally all have been replaced by sonographic examination of the abdomen. Their importance is now largely historical.

PAIN ASSESSMENT

Abdominal pain is a common complaint, but one that is often difficult to evaluate. How bad is the pain? Is there an underlying physical cause? Has there been recent trauma? Pain that is severe enough to make the patient unwilling to move, that is accompanied by nausea and vomiting, and that is marked by areas of localized tenderness generally has an underlying physical cause. While examining the abdomen, keep your eyes on the patient's face. The facial response is as important in your evaluation as the patient's verbal response to questions about

CLINICAL PEARL

Continuous Pain

The sudden onset of severe epigastric pain is, of course, unsettling. If that pain is continuous, unrelieved, and radiating (often) to the groin and back, think acute pancreatitis.

CLINICAL PEARL

Smell the Vomitus

A variety of odors from vomitus are possible:
- Fetid (gastrointestinal obstruction)
- Kerosene (hydrocarbon ingestion)
- Violets (sometimes from turpentine)
- Garlic (arsenic)

MNEMONICS

Features of Peritonitis: PERITONITIS

P Pain: front, back, sides, shoulders

E Electrolytes fall, shock ensues

R Rigidity or rebound of anterior abdominal wall

I Immobile abdomen and patient

T Tenderness (rebound)

O Obstruction

N Nausea and vomiting

I Increasing pulse, decreasing blood pressure

T Temperature falls then rises

I Increasing girth of abdomen

S Silent abdomen (no bowel sounds)

From Shipman, 1984.

BOX 17-4

CLUES IN DIAGNOSING ABDOMINAL PAIN

There are all types of rules for telling whether pain in the abdomen has significance. The following are a few of them:

- Patients may give a "touch-me-not" warning—that is, to not touch in a particular area; however, these patients may not actually have pain if their faces seem relaxed and unconcerned, even smiling. When you touch they might recoil, but the unconcerned face persists. (This sign is helpful in other areas of the body, as well as the abdomen.)
- Patients with an organic cause for abdominal pain are generally not hungry. A negative response to the "Do you want something to eat?" question is probable, particularly with appendicitis or intraabdominal infection.
- Ask the patient to point a finger to the location of the pain. If it is not directed to the navel but goes immediately to a fixed point, there is a great likelihood that this has significant physical importance. The farther from the navel the pain, the more likely it will be organic in origin (Apley rule). If the finger goes to the navel and the patient seems otherwise well to you, you should include psychogenic causes in the list of differential diagnoses.
- Patients with nonspecific abdominal pain may keep their eyes closed during abdominal palpation, whereas patients with organic disease usually keep their eyes open.

BOX 17-5

SOME CAUSES OF PAIN PERCEIVED IN ANATOMIC REGIONS

Right Upper Quadrant
Duodenal ulcer
Hepatitis
Hepatomegaly
Pneumonia
Cholecystitis

Right Lower Quadrant
Appendicitis
Salpingitis
Ovarian cyst
Ruptured ectopic pregnancy
Renal/ureteral stone
Strangulated hernia
Meckel diverticulitis
Regional ileitis
Perforated cecum

Periumbilical
Intestinal obstruction
Acute pancreatitis
Early appendicitis
Mesenteric thrombosis
Aortic aneurysm
Diverticulitis

Left Upper Quadrant
Ruptured spleen
Gastric ulcer
Aortic aneurysm
Perforated colon
Pneumonia

Left Lower Quadrant
Sigmoid diverticulitis
Salpingitis
Ovarian cyst
Ruptured ectopic pregnancy
Renal/ureteral stone
Strangulated hernia
Perforated colon
Regional ileitis
Ulcerative colitis

Modified from Judge, Zuidema, Fitzgerald, 1988.

---

the quality and degree of pain. Ask the patient to cough or take a deep breath. Assess the patient's willingness to jump or to walk. Is the pain exacerbated? A time-honored test is to ask the patient, "Do you want something to eat?" It is unlikely that hunger will persist in the face of acute intraabdominal infection (Box 17-4).

Common causes of abdominal pain are described in Tables 17-2 and 17-3. Careful assessment of the quality (Table 17-4) and location of pain (Box 17-5) can usually narrow the possible causes, allowing you to select additional diagnostic studies with greater efficiency. Findings associated with peritoneal irritation are summarized in Box 17-6. Table 17-5 delineates symptoms found in other body systems that help direct the abdominal examination. The Evidence-Based Practice box on p. 554 describes the use of history and physical examination in diagnosing appendicitis.

TABLE 17-2	Common Conditions Producing Acute Abdominal Pain	
Condition	**Usual Pain Characteristics**	**Possible Associated Findings**
Appendicitis	Initially periumbilical or epigastric; colicky; later becomes localized to RLQ, often at McBurney point	Guarding, tenderness; + iliopsoas and + obturator signs, RLQ skin hyperesthesia; anorexia, nausea, or vomiting after onset of pain; low-grade fever; + Aaron, Rovsing, Markle, and McBurney signs*
Peritonitis	Onset sudden or gradual; pain generalized or localized, dull or severe and unrelenting; guarding; pain on deep inspiration	Shallow respiration; + Blumberg, Markle, and Ballance signs; reduced or absent bowel sounds, nausea and vomiting; + obturator and iliopsoas tests
Cholecystitis	Severe, unrelenting RUQ or epigastric pain; may be referred to right subscapular area	RUQ tenderness and rigidity, + Murphy sign, palpable gallbladder, anorexia, vomiting, fever, possible jaundice
Pancreatitis	Dramatic, sudden, excruciating LUQ, epigastric, or umbilical pain; may be present in one or both flanks; may be referred to left shoulder	Epigastric tenderness, vomiting, fever, shock; + Grey Turner sign; + Cullen sign: both signs occur 2 to 3 days after onset
Salpingitis	Lower quadrant, worse on left	Nausea, vomiting, fever, suprapubic tenderness, rigid abdomen, pain on pelvic examination
Pelvic inflammatory disease	Lower quadrant, increases with activity	Tender adnexa and cervix, cervical discharge, dyspareunia
Diverticulitis	Epigastric, radiating down left side of abdomen especially after eating; may be referred to back	Flatulence, borborygmus, diarrhea, dysuria, tenderness on palpation
Perforated gastric or duodenal ulcer	Abrupt RUQ; may be referred to shoulders	Abdominal free air and distention with increased resonance over liver; tenderness in epigastrium or RUQ; rigid abdominal wall, rebound tenderness
Intestinal obstruction	Abrupt, severe, spasmodic; referred to epigastrium, umbilicus	Distention, minimal rebound tenderness, vomiting, localized tenderness, visible peristalsis; bowel sounds absent (with paralytic obstruction) or hyperactive high pitched (with mechanical obstruction)
Volvulus	Referred to hypogastrium and umbilicus	Distention, nausea, vomiting, guarding; sigmoid loop volvulus may be palpable
Leaking abdominal aneurysm	Steady throbbing midline over aneurysm; may radiate to back, flank	Nausea, vomiting, abdominal mass, bruit
Biliary stones, colic	Episodic, severe, RUQ, or epigastrium lasting 15 min to several hours; may be referred to subscapular area, especially right	RUQ tenderness, soft abdominal wall, anorexia, vomiting, jaundice, subnormal temperature
Renal calculi	Intense; flank, extending to groin and genitals; may be episodic	Fever, hematuria; + Kehr sign
Ectopic pregnancy	Lower quadrant; referred to shoulder; with rupture is agonizing	Hypogastric tenderness, symptoms of pregnancy, spotting, irregular menses, soft abdominal wall, mass on bimanual pelvic examination; ruptured: shock, rigid abdominal wall, distention; + Kehr, Cullen signs
Ruptured ovarian cyst	Lower quadrant, steady, increases with cough or motion	Vomiting, low-grade fever, anorexia, tenderness on pelvic examination
Splenic rupture	Intense; LUQ, radiating to left shoulder; may worsen with foot of bed elevated	Shock, pallor, lowered temperature

LUQ, Left upper quadrant; *RLQ,* right lower quadrant; *RUQ,* right upper quadrant.
*See Table 17-6 for explanation of signs.

TABLE 17-3	Common Conditions Producing Chronic Abdominal Pain	
Condition	**Usual Pain Characteristics**	**Possible Associated Findings**
Irritable bowel syndrome	Hypogastric pain; crampy, variable, infrequent; associated with bowel function	Negative physical examination Pain associated with gas, bloating, distention; relief with passage of flatus, feces
Lactose intolerance	Crampy pain after eating milk or milk products	Associated diarrhea; negative physical examination
Diverticular disease	Localized pain	Abdominal tenderness, fever
Constipation	Colicky or dull and steady pain that does not progress and worsen	Fecal mass palpable, stool in rectum
Uterine fibroids	Pain related to menses, intercourse	Palpable myoma(s)
Hernia	Localized pain that increase with exertion or lifting	Hernia on physical examination
Esophagitis/gastro-esophageal reflux disease	Burning gnawing pain in mid-epigastrium, worsens with recumbency	Negative physical examination
Peptic ulcer	Burning or gnawing pain	May have epigastric tenderness on palpation
Gastritis	Constant burning pain in epigastrium	May be accompanied by nausea, vomiting, diarrhea, or fever Physical examination negative

Modified from Dains, Baumann, Scheibel, 2003.

CLINICAL PEARL

Ectopic Pregnancy

Unhappily, ectopic pregnancy is often not diagnosed before rupture because symptoms are mild. Big clue: a sudden, dramatic change from mild, even vague abdominal pain that is there but not particularly distressing to a sudden onset of severe abdominal tenderness in the hypogastric area, particularly on the involved side. Rigidity and rebound may come on early or late. The main point: If a woman presents with vague abdominal complaints, check out the sexual contact and menstrual history, do a pelvic examination, and do not disregard the mild tenderness that might be evoked. Try, at least, to anticipate the emergency of a rupture.

TABLE 17-4	Quality and Onset of Abdominal Pain
Characteristic	**Possible Related Condition**
Burning	Peptic ulcer
Cramping	Biliary colic, gastroenteritis
Colic	Appendicitis with impacted feces; renal stone
Aching	Appendiceal irritation
Knifelike	Pancreatitis
Ripping, tearing	Aortic dissection
Gradual onset	Infection
Sudden onset	Duodenal ulcer, acute pancreatitis, obstruction, perforation

BOX 17-6

FINDINGS IN PERITONEAL IRRITATION

- Involuntary rigidity of abdominal muscles
- Tenderness and guarding
- Absent bowel sounds
- Positive obturator test (p. 555)
- Positive iliopsoas test (p. 555)
- Rebound tenderness (Blumberg sign and McBurney sign; see Table 17-6)
- Abdominal pain on walking
- Positive heel jar test (Markle sign, see Table 17-6)
- Right lower quadrant pain intensified by left lower quadrant abdominal palpation (positive Rovsing sign, see Table 17-6)

TABLE 17-5	Symptoms or Signs Elicited in Other Systems That May Relate to the Abdominal Examination		
Symptom or Sign	**Possible Pathologic Condition**	**Symptom or Sign**	**Possible Pathologic Condition**
Shock	Acute pancreatitis, ruptured tubal pregnancy	Flank tenderness	Renal inflammation, pyelonephritis Renal stone Renal infarct Renal vein thrombosis
Mental status deficit	Hemorrhage—duodenal ulcer Abdominal epilepsy	Leg edema	Iliac obstruction, pelvic mass Renal disease
Hypertension	Aortic dissection Abdominal aortic aneurysm Renal infarction Glomerulonephritis Vasculitis	Lymphadenopathy	Renal vein thrombosis Hepatitis Lymphoma
Orthostatic hypotension	Hypovolemia—blood loss, fluid	Jaundice	Mononucleosis Liver-biliary disease
Pulse deficit/asymmetric pulses	Aortic dissection Aortic aneurysm or thrombosis	Dark yellow to brown urine	Excessive hemolysis Liver-biliary disease Blood resulting from kidney stone, infarct, glomerulonephritis, or pyelonephritis
Bruits	Aortic dissection Aortic aneurysm Dissection or aneurysm of arteries—splenic, renal, or iliac		
Low-output cardiac symptoms—atrial fibrillation	Ischemia of mesentery	Fever (39.4° C [103° F]) and chills	Peritonitis Pelvic infection Cholangitis
Valvular disease, congestive heart failure	Embolus	White blood cell count >10,000 mm^3 or shift to left (more than 80% polymorphonuclear cells) >20,000 mm^3	Pyelonephritis Appendicitis (95%) Acute cholecystitis (90%) Localized peritonitis Bowel strangulation Bowel infarction
Pleural effusion	Esophageal rupture Pancreatitis Ovarian tumor		

Modified from Barkauskas et al, 2002.

EVIDENCE-BASED PRACTICE IN PHYSICAL EXAMINATION

DIAGNOSING APPENDICITIS

Appendicitis is a common cause of acute abdominal pain. Until recently, history and physical examination were at least as accurate as other modalities in diagnosing or excluding appendicitis. Historical symptoms that increase the likelihood of appendicitis are RLQ pain, initial periumbilical pain with migration to the RLQ, and the presence of pain before vomiting. The presence of rigidity, a positive psoas sign, fever, or rebound tenderness are physical examination findings that increase the likelihood of appendicitis. Conversely, the absence of RLQ pain, the absence of the migration of the pain, and the presence of similar pain previously are historical findings that make appendicitis less likely. On physical examination, the lack of RLQ pain,

rigidity, or guarding makes appendicitis less likely. Clinicians rarely rely on a single symptom or sign to make a diagnosis; however, the precision and accuracy of combinations of these findings have not been reported. No finding effectively rules out appendicitis (Wagner, McKinney, Carpenter, 1996).

Although no systematic review has been done to date, individual studies indicate that computed tomography has had equivocal success in improving diagnostic accuracy (Brandt & Wahl, 2003; Herskho et al, 2002; Patrtrick et al, 2003; Perez et al, 2003). Newer biotechnology using radioactively labeled antibodies for scintigraphic imaging should enable quicker and more accurate diagnosis (FDA, 2004; Kipper et al, 2000).

REBOUND TENDERNESS

The following maneuver is considered crude and unnecessary by many examiners, because light percussion produces a mild localized response in the presence of peritoneal inflammation. If the patient is experiencing abdominal pain, this maneuver can be used to determine peritoneal irritation (see Box 17-6). Place the patient in the supine position. Hold your hand at a 90-degree angle to the abdomen with the fingers extended, then press gently and deeply into a region remote from the area of discomfort. Rapidly withdraw your hand and fingers

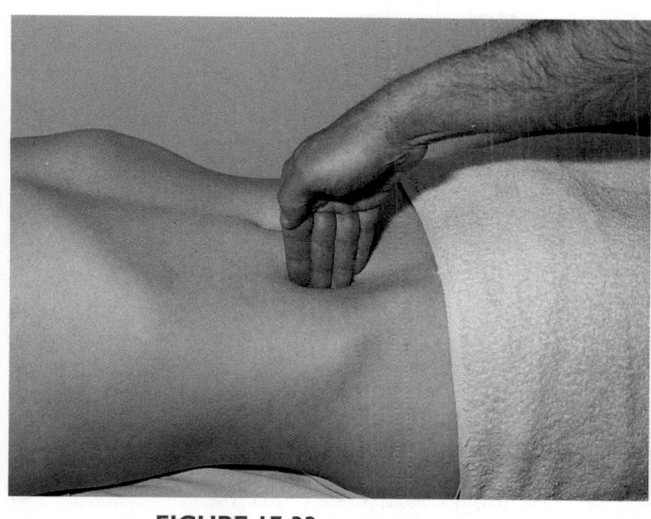 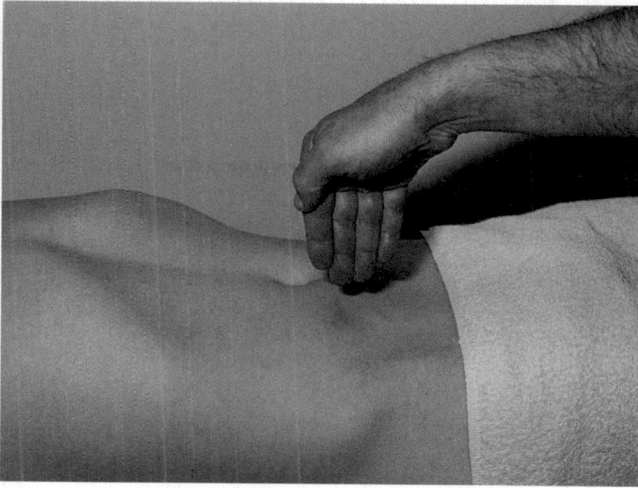

FIGURE 17-33
Testing for rebound tenderness. **A,** Press deeply and gently into the abdomen. **B,** Then rapidly withdraw the hands and fingers.

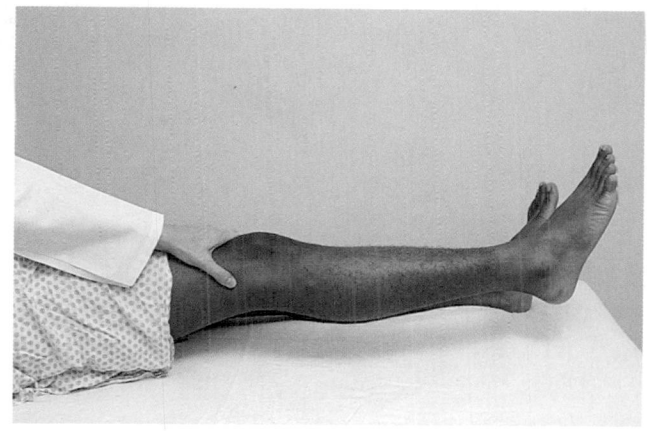

FIGURE 17-34
Iliopsoas muscle test. The patient raises the leg from the hip while the examiner pushes downward against it.

(Fig. 17-33). The return to position (rebound) of the structures that were compressed by your fingers causes a sharp stabbing pain at the site of peritoneal inflammation (positive Blumberg sign). Rebound tenderness over the McBurney point in the lower right quadrant suggests appendicitis (positive McBurney sign). The maneuver for rebound tenderness should be performed at the end of the examination because a positive response produces pain and muscle spasm that can interfere with any subsequent examination.

ILIOPSOAS MUSCLE TEST

A patient with a positive iliopsoas sign will experience lower quadrant pain. Perform this test when you suspect appendicitis, because an inflamed appendix may cause irritation of the lateral iliopsoas muscle. Ask the patient to lie supine and then place your hand over the lower thigh. Ask the patient to raise the leg, flexing at the hip, while you push downward against the leg (Fig. 17-34). An alternative technique is to position the patient on the left side and ask that the right leg be raised from the hip while you press downward against it. A third technique is to hyperextend the leg by drawing it backward while the patient is lying on the right side.

OBTURATOR MUSCLE TEST

Perform this test when you suspect a ruptured appendix or a pelvic abscess, because these conditions can cause irritation of the obturator muscle. Pain in the hypogastric region is a positive sign, indicating irritation of the obturator muscle. The patient should be supine for this test. Ask the patient to flex the right leg at the hip and knee to 90 degrees. Hold the leg just above the knee, grasp the ankle, and rotate the leg laterally and medially (Fig. 17-35).

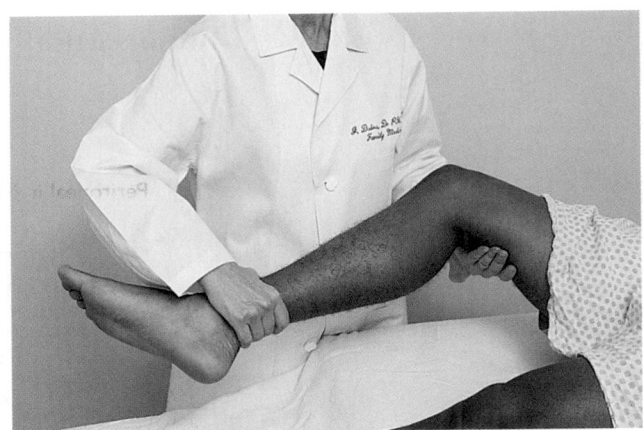

FIGURE 17-35
Obturator muscle test. With the right leg flexed at the hip and knee, rotate the leg laterally and medially.

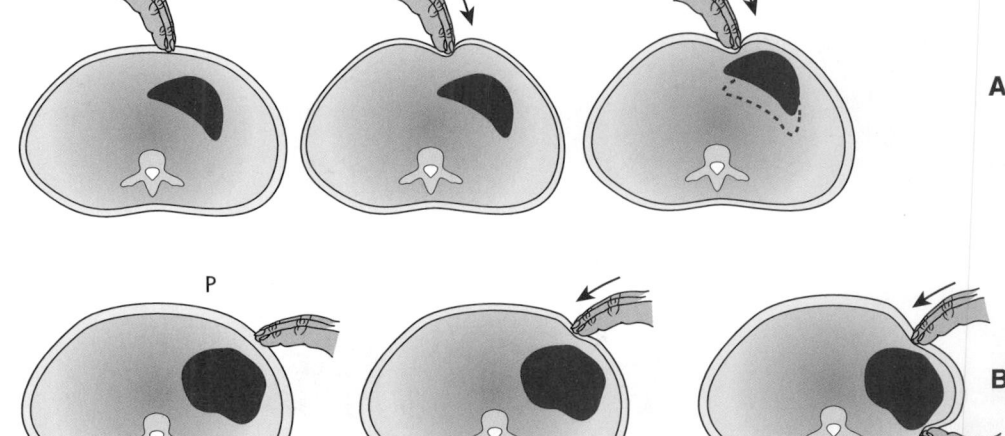

FIGURE 17-36
Ballottement technique.
A, Single-handed ballottement. Push inward at a 90-degree angle. If the object is freely movable, it will float upward to touch the fingertips. **B,** Bimanual ballottement; *P,* pushing; *R,* receiving hand.

BALLOTTEMENT

Ballottement is a palpation technique used to assess a floating mass, such as the head of a fetus. To perform abdominal ballottement with one hand, place your extended fingers, hand, and forearm at a 90-degree angle to the abdomen. Push in toward the mass with the fingertips (Fig. 17-36, *A*). If the mass is freely movable, it will float upward and touch the fingertips as fluid and other structures are displaced by the maneuver.

To perform bimanual ballottement, place one hand on the anterior abdominal wall and one hand against the flank. Push inward on the abdominal wall while palpating with the flank hand to determine the presence and size of the mass (Fig. 17-36, *B*).

ABDOMINAL SIGNS

"Classic" abdominal pain signs have often been given the name of the person who first described them. Some of the most common are included in Table 17-6.

INFANTS AND CHILDREN

If possible, the infant's abdomen should be examined during a time of relaxation and quiet. It is often best to do this at the start of the overall examination, especially before initiating any procedure that might cause distress (Fig. 17-37). Sucking a bottle or pacifier may help relax the infant. The parent's lap makes the best examining surface, much better than having the child lie fixed and supine on a table. Sit facing the parent, knees touching, and conduct the abdominal examination entirely on the parent's lap. This works well during the first several months, and often the first 2 to 3 years, of life. The infant will be most secure.

TABLE 17-6	Abdominal Signs Associated with Common Abnormalities	
Sign	**Description**	**Associated Conditions**
Aaron	Pain or distress occurs in the area of the patient's heart or stomach on palpation of McBurney point	Appendicitis
Ballance	Fixed dullness to percussion in left flank, and dullness in right flank that disappears on change of position	Peritoneal irritation
Blumberg	Rebound tenderness	Peritoneal irritation; appendicitis
Cullen	Ecchymosis around umbilicus	Hemoperitoneum; pancreatitis; ectopic pregnancy
Dance	Absence of bowel sounds in right lower quadrant	Intussusception
Grey Turner	Ecchymosis of flanks	Hemoperitoneum; pancreatitis
Kehr	Abdominal pain radiating to left shoulder	Spleen rupture; renal calculi; ectopic pregnancy
Markle (heel jar)	Patient stands with straightened knees, then raises up on toes, relaxes, and allows heels to hit floor, thus jarring body. Action will cause abdominal pain if positive	Peritoneal irritation; appendicitis
McBurney	Rebound tenderness and sharp pain when McBurney point is palpated	Appendicitis
Murphy	Abrupt cessation of inspiration on palpation of gallbladder	Cholecystitis
Romberg-Howship	Pain down the medial aspect of the thigh to the knees	Strangulated obturator hernia
Rovsing	Right lower quadrant pain intensified by left lower quadrant abdominal palpation	Peritoneal irritation; appendicitis

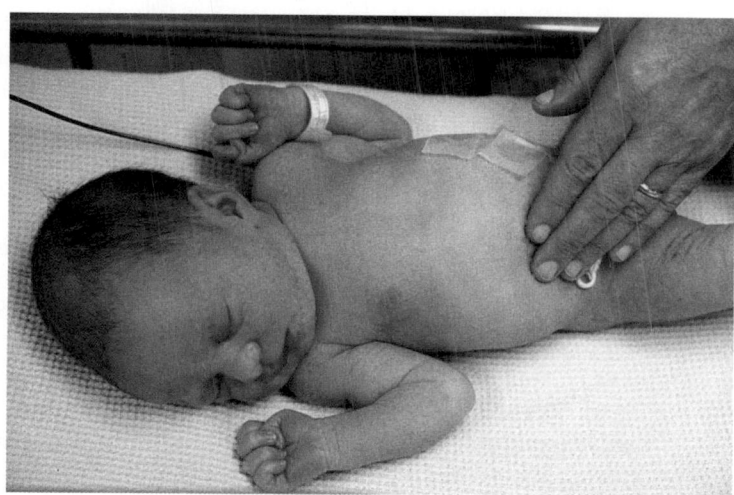

FIGURE 17-37
Positioning to examine the infant's abdomen.

INSPECTION

Inspect the abdomen, noting its shape, contour, and movement with respiration. It should be rounded and dome-shaped because the abdominal musculature has not fully developed. Note any localized fullness. Abdominal and chest movements should be synchronous, with a slight bulge of the abdomen at the beginning of respiration. Note whether the abdomen protrudes above the level of the chest or is scaphoid. A distended or protruding abdomen can result from feces, a mass, or organ enlargement. A scaphoid abdomen suggests that the abdominal contents are displaced into the thorax.

Note any pulsations over the abdomen. Pulsations in the epigastric area are common in newborns and infants. Superficial veins are usually visible in the thin infant; however, distended veins across the abdomen are an unexpected finding suggestive of vascular obstruction or abdominal distention or obstruction. If any distended veins are present, identify the direction of blood flow. Spider nevi may indicate liver disease.

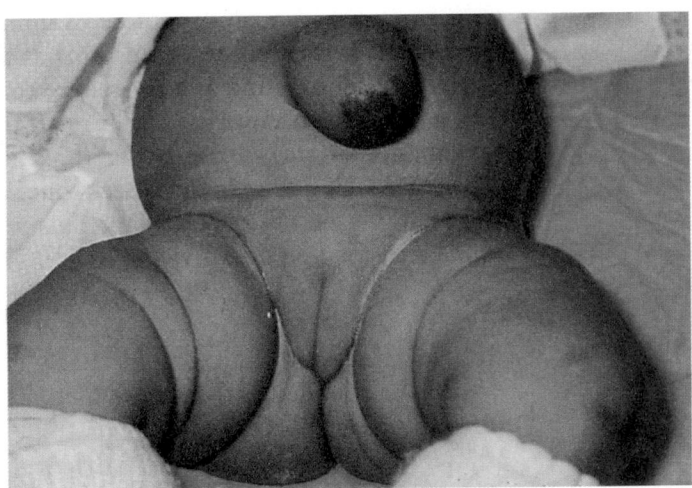

FIGURE 17-38
Umbilical hernia in an infant.

> **CLINICAL PEARL**
> ***Umbilical Cord***
> A thick umbilical cord suggests a well-nourished fetus; a thin cord suggests otherwise.

Inspect the umbilical cord of the newborn, counting the number of vessels. Two arteries and one vein should be present. A single umbilical artery should alert you to the possibility of congenital anomalies. Any intestinal structure present in the umbilical cord or protruding into the umbilical area and visible through a thick transparent membrane suggests an omphalocele.

The umbilical stump area should be dry and odorless. Inspect it for discharge, redness, induration, and skin warmth. Once the stump has separated, serous or serosanguineous discharge may indicate a granuloma when no other signs of infection are present. Inspect all folds of skin in the umbilicus for a nodule of granulomatous tissue.

Note any protrusion through the umbilicus or rectus abdominis muscles when the infant strains. The umbilicus is usually inverted. An umbilical hernia (i.e., the protrusion of omentum and intestine through the umbilical opening, forming a visible and palpable bulge) is a common finding in infants (Fig. 17-38).

The umbilicus often everts with increased abdominal pressure (e.g., with coughing or sneezing). Umbilical hernias can be very large and impressive. It is ordinarily easy to reduce them temporarily by pushing the contents back into a more appropriate intraabdominal position. Usually, however, they pop right out again. The apparent size is not cause for alarm, and generally it pays to temporize. Measure the diameter of the umbilical opening rather than the protruding contents to determine the size. The maximum size is generally reached by 1 month of age, and the hernia will generally close spontaneously by 1 to 2 years of age. Diastasis rectus abdominis, a separation 1 to 4 cm wide in the midline usually between the xiphoid and the umbilicus, is a common finding when the rectus abdominis muscles do not approximate each other. Ordinarily, there is no need to repair this. Herniation through the rectus abdominis muscles, however, is a problem.

If the infant is vomiting frequently, use tangential lighting and observe the abdomen at eye level for peristaltic waves. Peristalsis is not usually visible. Peristaltic waves may sometimes be seen in thin, malnourished infants, but their presence usually suggests an intestinal obstruction such as pyloric stenosis.

AUSCULTATION AND PERCUSSION

The procedures of auscultation and percussion of the abdomen do not differ from those used for adults. Peristalsis is detected when metallic tinkling is heard every 10 to 30 seconds, and bowel sounds should be present within 1 to 2 hours after birth. Because a scaphoid abdomen suggests a diaphragmatic hernia in the newborn, auscultate the chest for bowel sounds. No bruits or venous hums should be detected on abdominal auscultation.

Renal bruits are associated with renal artery stenosis and rarely with renal arteriovenous fistula. The bruit of stenosis has a high frequency and is soft; the bruit of arteriovenous fistula is continuous. Both are hard to hear. Try first with the patient held upright or sitting, listening at the posterior flank; then try with the patient supine, listening over the abdomen.

> **BOX 17-7**
>
> **PALPATING AN INFANT'S ABDOMEN**
>
> The abdomen of an infant can seem very tiny in relation to the size of your hand. One technique for palpating a very small abdomen is as follows: Place your right hand gently on the abdomen with the thumb at the right upper quadrant and the index finger at the left upper quadrant. Press very gently at first, only gradually increasing pressure (never too vigorously) as you palpate over the entire abdomen.

CLINICAL PEARL
Enlarged Liver
An infant of a mother with poorly controlled diabetes may more often than not have an enlarged liver, a finding that, by itself, presents no problem.

The abdomen may produce more tympany on percussion than is found in adults, because infants swallow air when feeding or crying. As with adults, tympany in a distended abdomen is usually the result of gas, whereas dullness may indicate fluid or a solid mass. The upper edge of the liver should be detected within 1 cm of the fifth intercostal space at the right midclavicular line. Before 2 years of age, females have a slightly larger liver span than males. The mean range of liver spans in infants and children is as follows:

Age	Liver Span (cm)	Age	Liver Span (cm)
6 months	2.4 to 2.8	5 years	4.5 to 4.8
12 months	2.8 to 3.1	6 years	4.8 to 5.1
24 months	3.5 to 3.6	8 years	5.1 to 5.6
3 years	4.0	10 years	5.5 to 6.1
4 years	4.3 to 4.4		

PALPATION

Palpate the abdomen with the infant's feet slightly elevated and knees flexed to promote relaxation of the abdominal musculature (Box 17-7). Begin with superficial palpation to detect the spleen, liver, and masses close to the surface. The spleen is usually palpable 1 to 2 cm below the left costal margin during the first few weeks after birth. A detectable spleen tip at the left costal margin is a common finding in well infants and young children. Any increase in spleen size may indicate blood dyscrasias or septicemia.

LIVER PALPATION

To assess the liver, superficially palpate at the right midclavicular line 3 to 4 cm below the costal margin. As the infant inspires, wait to feel a narrow mass tap your finger. Gradually move your fingers up the midclavicular line until the sensation is felt. The liver edge is usually palpable just below the right costal margin in the newborn. The liver edge may be palpable at 1 to 3 cm below the right costal margin in infants and toddlers. Estimation of true liver size can be accomplished only by percussing the upper border, as well as palpating the lower edge. Together the techniques provide an estimate of liver span, rather than just a projection of size below the costal margin. Hepatomegaly is present when the liver is more than 3 cm below the right costal margin, suggesting infection, cardiac failure, or liver disease.

DEEP PALPATION

CLINICAL PEARL
Palpate with Caution!
Once a mass is felt near the kidney, do not repeatedly or aggressively palpate the mass. Such palpation could cause the release of cells that have metastatic potential.

Following light palpation, perform deep palpation in all quadrants. Note the location, size, shape, tenderness, and consistency of any masses. Use transillumination to distinguish cystic masses from solid masses. Fluid-filled masses will transilluminate, whereas solid masses will not. When pulsations are seen, palpate the aorta for any sign of enlargement. Fixed masses that are laterally mobile, pulsatile, or located along the vertebral column should be investigated further with special studies. If any suspicion of neoplasm exists, limit palpation of the mass because manipulation may cause injury or spread of malignancy.

A sausage-shaped mass in the left lower quadrant may indicate feces in the sigmoid colon associated with constipation. A midline suprapubic mass suggests Hirschsprung disease, in which feces fill the rectosigmoid colon. A sausage-shaped mass in the left or right upper quadrant may indicate intussusception. The almond-shaped mass of pyloric stenosis can often be detected with deep palpation in the right upper quadrant immediately after the infant vom-

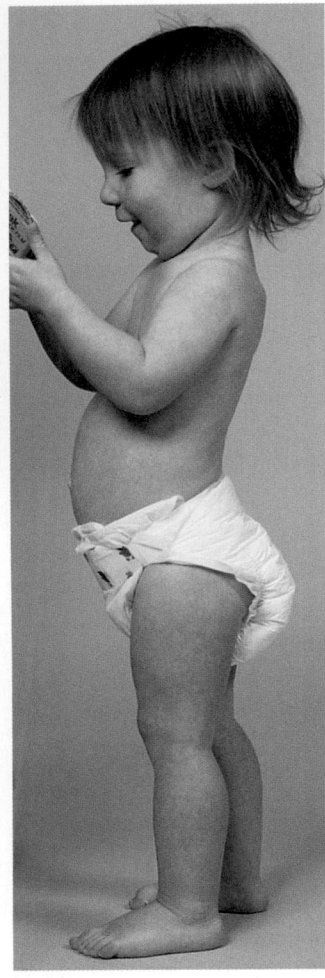

FIGURE 17-39
Potbellied stance of a toddler.

its. It may be helpful to sit the infant in your lap, folding the upper body gently against your palpating hand, bringing the pyloric mass into opposition with your hand. Almost all other palpable masses in the abdomen of the newborn are renal in origin.

In the infant and toddler, the bladder can usually be palpated and percussed in the suprapubic area. Determine the size of the bladder to detect any sign of distention. A distended bladder, felt as a firm, central dome-shaped structure in the lower abdomen, may indicate urethral obstruction or central nervous system defects.

Palpate the femoral arteries as described in Chapter 15.

Tenderness or pain on palpation may be difficult to detect in the infant; however, pain and tenderness are assessed by such behaviors as change in the pitch of crying, facial grimacing, rejection of the opportunity to suck, and drawing the knees to the abdomen with palpation. When an infant will not stop crying, seize the quiet moment in the respiratory cycle to palpate in order to distinguish between a hard and soft abdomen. The abdomen should be soft during inspiration. If the abdomen remains hard with a noticeable rigidity or resistance to pressure during both respiratory phases, peritoneal irritation may be present. It is often necessary to delay examination of a distressed infant for a little while, waiting for a quieter moment, unless there is reason for urgency.

> **MNEMONICS**
>
> **Intussusception in Infants: ABCDEF**
> **A** Abdominal or anal "sausage"
> **B** Blood from the rectum (red currant jelly)
> **C** Colic: babies draw up their legs
> **D** Distention, dehydration, and shock
> **E** Emesis
> **F** Face pale
>
> From Shipman, 1984.

The abdomen of the young child protrudes slightly, giving a potbellied appearance when the child is standing, sitting, and supine (Fig. 17-39). After age 5 years, the contour of the child's abdomen, when supine, may become convex and will not extend above an imaginary line drawn from the xiphoid process to the symphysis pubis. Respirations will continue to be abdominal until the child is 6 to 7 years old. Abdominal respiration beyond this age suggests thoracic problems. Restricted abdominal respiration in young children can be caused by peritoneal irritation or an acute abdomen. Diastasis rectus abdominis ordinarily resolves by 6 years of age.

The upper edge of the liver should be detected by percussion at the sixth intercostal space. The lower edge of the liver may be palpated either at, or 1 to 2 cm below, the right costal margin.

Palpate the abdomen of a child who is ticklish with a firm rather than feathery touch. If this is unsuccessful, place the child's hand under the palm of your examining hand, leaving your fingers free to palpate. Localization of abdominal tenderness or pain may be difficult in the young child who cannot verbalize about the site or character of pain. Distract the child with a toy, or question the child about a favorite activity as you begin palpating in the abdominal region believed most distant from the area of pain. Observe for changes in facial expression and for constriction of the pupils during palpation to identify the location of greatest pain. Check for rebound tenderness and make the same observations of the child's facial expression and pupils. As with adults, check rebound tenderness cautiously. Too vigorous an approach may be cruel and inhumane. Once a child has experienced palpation that is too intense, a subsequent examiner has little chance for easy access to the abdomen.

ADOLESCENTS

The techniques of abdominal examination of the adolescent are the same as those used for adults. Do not overlook the possibility of pregnancy as a cause of a mass in the lower abdomen, even in young adolescent females.

PREGNANT WOMEN

Uterine changes that can be detected on pelvic examination are discussed in Chapter 18. Bowel sounds will be diminished as a result of decreased peristaltic activity. Striae and a midline band of pigmentation (linea nigra) may be present. Gastrointestinal complaints of nausea and vomiting are common in the first trimester. Constipation is a common occurrence, and hemorrhoids often develop later in pregnancy.

Assessment of the abdomen of pregnant women includes uterine size estimation for gestational age, fetal growth, position of the fetus, monitoring of fetal well-being, and the presence of uterine contractions. Evaluation techniques for fetal well-being, such as ultrasound examination and electronic fetal monitoring, are not reviewed in this text.

GESTATIONAL AGE

Before assessment of the abdomen, calculation is performed to determine the estimated date of delivery or confinement (EDC). One of the most common methods is to use the Naegele rule: Add 7 days to the first day of the last normal menstrual period and count back 3 months.

The average duration of pregnancy is considered to be 280 days, or 40 weeks. The pregnancy is then divided into trimesters, each of which is slightly more than 13 weeks, or 3 calendar months. The clinically appropriate unit of measure, however, is weeks of gestation completed. Weeks of gestation completed can be easily calculated by using an obstetric wheel or a web-based electronic pregnancy calculator. Assessment of the abdomen of pregnant women includes measurement of fundal height. This technique provides an estimate for the length of the pregnancy and growth of the fetus. To measure fundal height, perform the following steps:

1. Have the patient empty her bladder before the procedure.
2. Ask the patient to lie supine.
3. With a nonstretchable tape measure, measure from the upper part of the pubis symphysis to the superior fundus uterus over the middle portion of the fundus (Fig. 17-40). The measurement is recorded in centimeters.

The same person should perform the measurement each time to decrease chances of individual variations.

This measurement is most accurate between 20 and 30 weeks of gestation when the fundal height in centimeters may be equal to the gestational age in weeks. A 1-cm increase per week in fundal height is an expected pattern. Twin pregnancy or other conditions that enlarge the uterus should be suspected if during the second trimester the uterine size is larger than usually occurs during the expected week of gestation. A variation of more than 2 cm may indicate a need for further evaluation. If the uterine size is smaller than is expected, the possibility of intrauterine growth retardation should be considered. The accuracy of fundal height as a screening tool for intrauterine growth retardation is poor, but can provide clinical suspicion for sonography. Customized charts based on maternal height, weight, parity, and ethnicity are more accurate.

During the second and third trimesters, the McDonald rule can also be used to estimate the duration of the pregnancy from fundal height measurement. Using the McDonald rule, divide the height of the fundus (in centimeters) by 3.5; the resultant figure is said to equal the duration of pregnancy in lunar months.

Factors that can affect the accuracy of the fundal height measurement are obesity, amount of amniotic fluid, myomata, multiple gestation, fetal size and attitude, and position of the uterus.

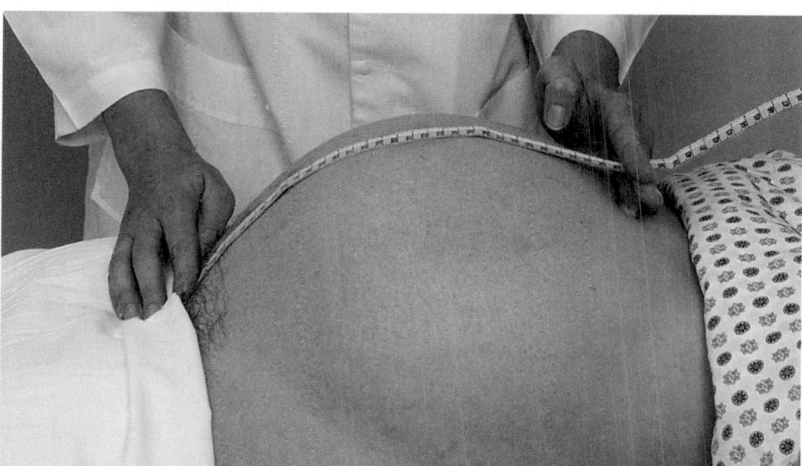

FIGURE 17-40
Measurement of fundal height from the symphysis to the superior fundus uterus.

FETAL WELL-BEING

Assessment of fetal well-being includes, but is not limited to, measurement of fetal heart rate (FHR) and fetal movements. To determine the fetal heart rate, count the FHR or impulse for 1 minute (using a Doppler or fetoscope), and compare it with the mother's pulse during that time. Also note the quality and rhythm of the fetal heart rate. Charting of the results is usually done using a two-line figure in which the point of intersection is the umbilicus and the four quadrants are the maternal abdomen. Use an X or the FHR obtained to identify the point on the maternal abdomen in which the maximal impulse was heard (see example).

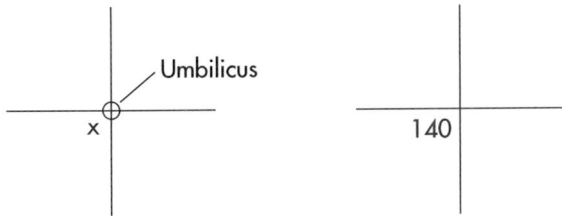

Kick counts can be used as an indicator of fetal well-being. Instruct the woman to note the pattern of movement over a given time. If the pattern shows a decrease, or if movement ceases, the woman should notify her health care professional. Different techniques exist for monitoring fetal movement (FM). A simple technique is to count 10 movements and note the length of time for them to occur. The woman should be in the left lateral position. There are no universally accepted FM count criteria. The standard ranges from 10 times in 1 hour to 10 times in 12 hours. Begin FM recording based on the woman's situation. If there are no identifiable risks of uteroplacental insufficiency, start recording between 34 and 36 weeks of gestation. If there are risk factors, monitoring should start as early as 28 weeks. Individual assessment of circumstances is necessary. If no monitoring technique is used, the occurrence of three or fewer FMs in 2 hours for 2 consecutive days while the woman is at rest in left lateral position signals the need for further evaluation of fetal well-being.

FETAL POSITION

Assessment of fetal position can be performed using the four steps of the Leopold maneuvers (Fig. 17-41). After positioning the woman supine with her head slightly elevated and knees slightly flexed, place a small towel under her right hip. If you are right-handed, stand at the woman's right side facing her and perform the first three steps, then turn and face her feet for the last step; if you are left-handed, stand on the woman's left for the first three steps, then turn and face her feet for the last step. The maneuvers are performed as follows:

1. Place hands over the fundus and identify the fetal part (Fig. 17-41, *A*). The head feels round, firm, and freely movable, and is detectable by ballottement. The buttocks feel softer and less mobile and regular.
2. With the palmar surface of your hand, locate the back of the fetus by applying gentle but deep pressure (Fig. 17-41, *B*). The back feels smooth and convex, whereas the small parts (the feet, hands, knees, and elbows) will feel more irregular.
3. With the right hand (if you are right-handed) or with the left (if you are left-handed), using the thumb and third finger, gently grasp the presenting part over the symphysis pubis (Fig. 17-41, *C*). The head will feel firm and, if not engaged, will be movable from side to side and easily displaced upward. If the buttocks are presenting, they will feel softer and irregular. If the presenting part is not engaged, the fourth step is used.
4. Turn and face the woman's feet and use two hands to outline the fetal head (Fig. 17-41, *D*). If the head is presenting and is deep into the pelvis, only a small portion may be felt. Palpation of the cephalic prominence (the part of the fetus that prevents descent of the examiner's hand) on the same side as the small parts suggests that the head is flexed and

Back of fetus

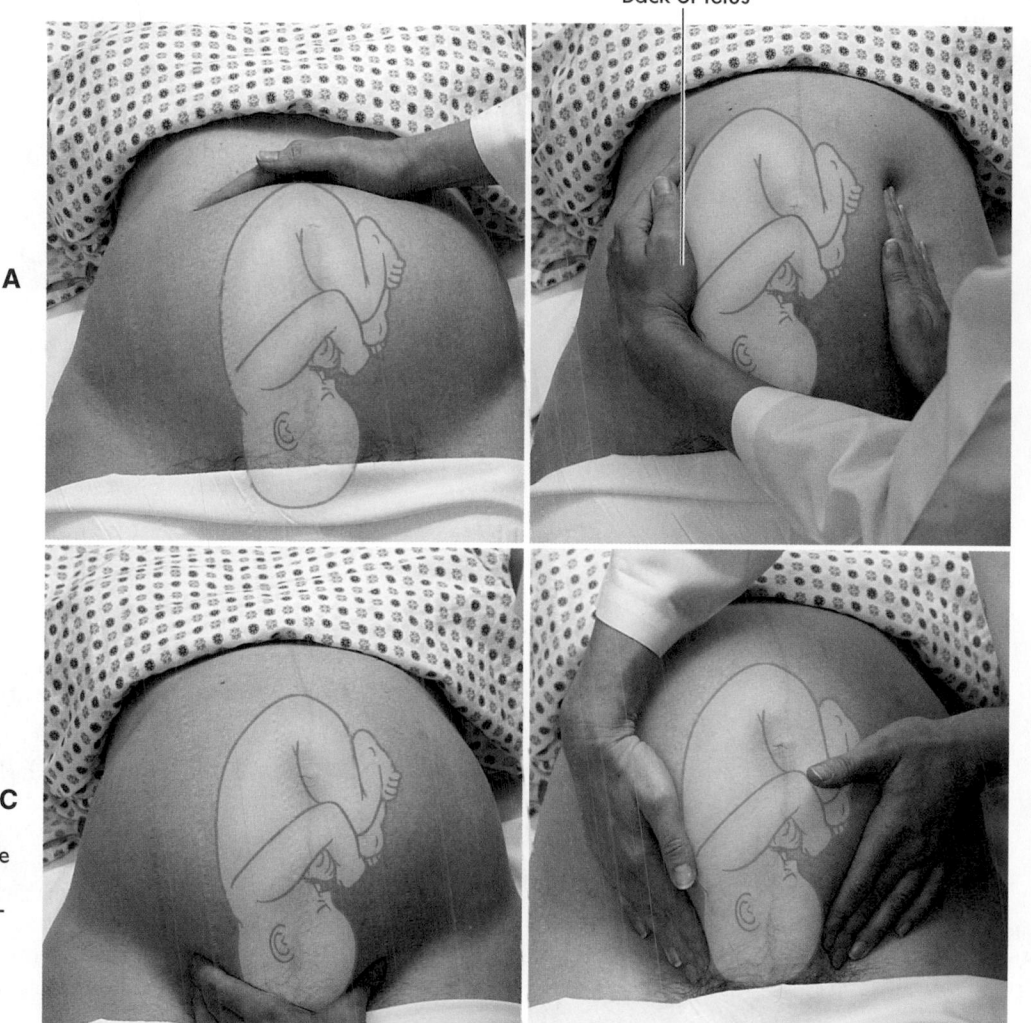

FIGURE 17-41
Leopold maneuvers. **A,** First maneuver. Place hand(s) over fundus and identify the fetal part. **B,** Second maneuver. Use the palmar surface of one hand to locate the back of the fetus. Use the other hand to feel the irregularities, such as hands and feet. **C,** Third maneuver. Use thumb and third finger to grasp presenting part over the symphysis pubis. **D,** Fourth maneuver. Use both hands to outline the fetal head. With a head presenting deep in the pelvis, only a small portion may be felt.

the vertex presenting. This is the optimal position. Palpation of the cephalic prominence on the same side as the back suggests that the presenting part is extended.

When recording the information obtained from the abdominal palpation, include the presenting part (i.e., vertex if the head, or breech if the buttocks), the lie (the relationship of the long axis of the fetus to the long axis of the mother) as either longitudinal or vertical, and the attitude of the fetal head if it is the presenting part (flexed or extended). With experience you will also be able to estimate the weight of the fetus. A bedside ultrasound can confirm the position.

Twins are a variation, often suspected when there is the presence of two fetal heart tones or on abdominal palpation when a second set of fetal parts is detected. Diagnosis is made by ultrasound examination. The technique for abdominal palpation in twin pregnancy is depicted in Fig. 17-42.

The FHR can also be used to estimate position of the fetus. The areas of maximal intensity of the FHR and the position of the fetus are depicted in Fig. 17-43.

CONTRACTIONS

Uterine contractions begin as early as the third month of gestation. These contractions are a natural condition of pregnancy and are called Braxton Hicks contractions. They may go unnoticed by the woman but may become painful at times, especially as the pregnancy progresses and with increased gravidity. The regular occurrence of more than 4 to 6 uterine contractions per hour before 37 weeks of gestation requires evaluation.

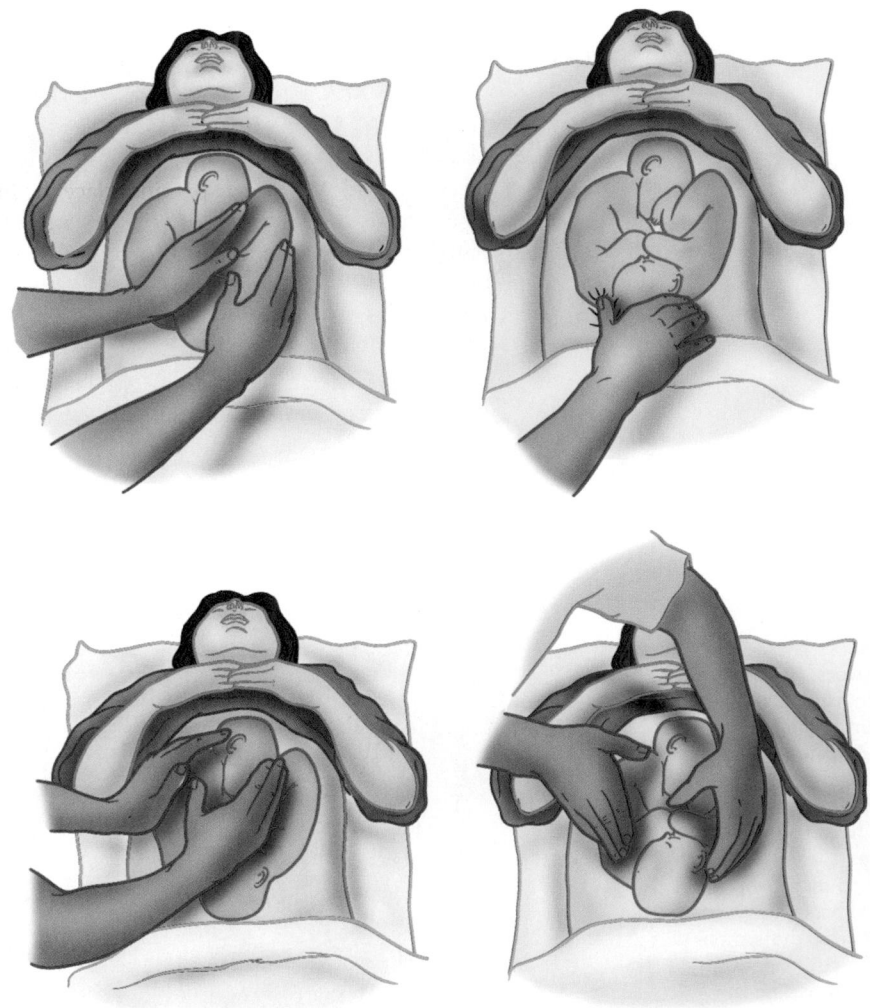

FIGURE 17-42
Abdominal palpation of twin pregnancy.

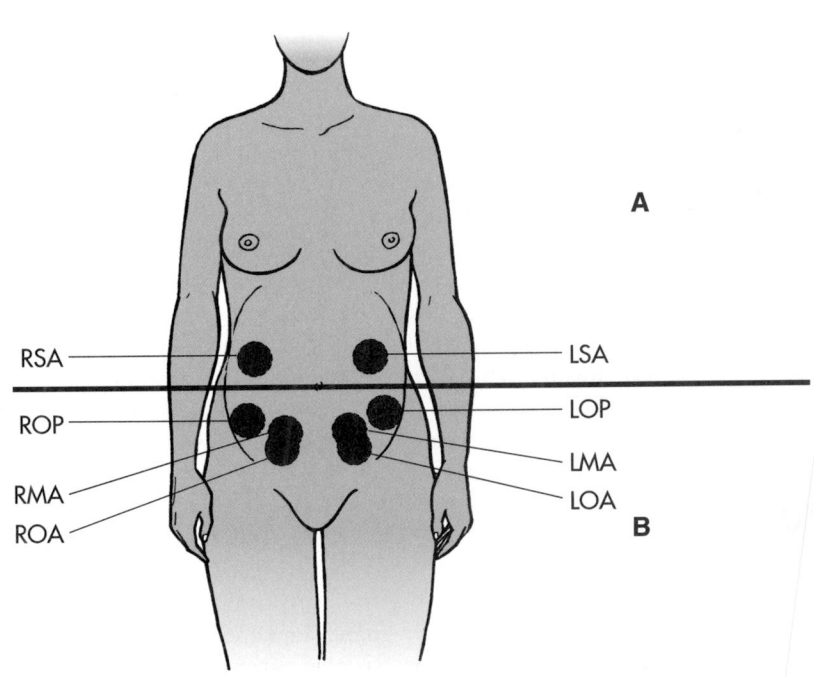

FIGURE 17-43
Areas of maximal intensity of fetal heart rate for differing positions: RSA, right sacrum anterior; ROP, right occipitoposterior; RMA, right mentum anterior; ROA, right occipitoanterior; LSA, left sacrum anterior; LOP, left occipitoposterior; LMA, left mentum anterior; and LOA, left occipitoanterior. **A,** Presentation is breech if FHR is heard above umbilicus. **B,** Presentation is vertex if FHR is heard below umbilicus.
From Lowdermilk, Perry, Bobak, 1997.

Uterine contractions can be assessed with abdominal palpation, but more accuracy is obtained through use of electronic monitoring equipment, either indirectly through the abdominal wall or directly with the placement of an intrauterine pressure catheter. Assessment through abdominal palpation is helpful when equipment is not available to determine the onset or course of labor, either preterm or term. Practice is needed to determine the difference between mild, moderate, and strong contractions. Place the fingertips on the abdomen so that you are able to detect the contraction and relaxation of the uterus, and keep them there throughout the entire contraction, including the period of relaxation.

The strength of the contraction is classified as follows:

- Mild: slightly tense fundus that is easy to indent with the fingertips
- Moderate: firm fundus that is difficult to indent with the fingertips
- Strong: rigid or hard, boardlike fundus or one that does not indent with fingertips

The duration of the contraction is measured in seconds from the beginning until relaxation occurs. The frequency of contractions is measured from the beginning of one contraction to the beginning of the next. The frequency of contractions is assessed for regularity (at regular intervals, such as every 5 minutes; or at irregular or sporadic intervals). Each woman's experience of the discomfort created by the contracting uterus varies because of physiologic makeup, past experiences, cultural influences, expectations, prenatal education, support, and other factors. Her sense of the event should not be discounted based on physiologic and subjective measures.

OLDER ADULTS

The techniques of examination are the same as those used for younger adults. The abdominal wall of the older adult becomes thinner and less firm as a result of the loss of connective tissue and muscle mass that accompanies aging. Palpation therefore may be relatively easier and yield more accurate findings. A pulsating abdominal aortic aneurysm may be more readily palpable than in younger patients. Deposition of fat over the abdominal area is common despite concurrent loss of fatty tissue over the extremities. The abdominal contour is often rounded as a result of loss of muscle tone.

The only modifications in examination techniques require some common sense. Use judgment in determining whether a patient is able to assume a particular position, such as the kneeling position to test for fluid pooling in assessing ascites. Similarly, remember that rotation of joints, such as with the obturator muscle test, may cause discomfort in patients who have decreased muscle flexibility or increased joint tenderness.

Be aware that respiratory changes can produce corresponding findings in the abdominal examination. The liver of the patients with hyperexpanded lungs and depressed diaphragm may be displaced downward. In this case, both the upper and lower borders of the liver may be detected 1 to 2 cm below the usual markers, but the liver span should still be between 6 and 12 cm. On the other hand, with the decrease in liver size after 50 years of age, you may find that the midclavicular liver span is somewhat less.

With decreased intestinal motility associated with aging, intestinal disorders are common in older adults, so be particularly sensitive to patient complaints and related findings in this regard. Constipation is a common complaint, and you are more likely to feel stool in the sigmoid colon. Accompanying complaints of gas and a sensation of bloatedness may be reflected in increased tympany on percussion. Fecal impaction is a common finding in older adults with severe or chronic constipation.

Obstruction may be a problem with older adults, occurring as a result of hypokalemia, myocardial infarction, and infections such as pneumonia, septicemia, peritonitis, and pancreatitis. Vomiting, distention, diarrhea, and constipation can signal obstruction.

The incidence of gastrointestinal cancer increases with age; its various symptoms depend on the site of the tumor. Symptoms can range from dysphagia to nausea, vomiting, anorexia, and hematemesis; and can include changes in stool frequency, size, consistency, or color. See Chapter 20 for a discussion of rectal digital examination, an important step in the detection of colon cancer.

Pain perception may be altered as part of the aging process, and older patients may exhibit atypical pain symptoms. These can include less severe or totally absent pain with disease states that characteristically produce pain in younger adults. Therefore evaluation of pain in the older adult must take into account concurrent symptoms and accompanying findings.

MNEMONICS

Causes of Constipation: CONSTIPATED

C Congenital: Hirschsprung disease
O Obstruction
N Neoplasms
S Stricture of colon
T Topical: painful hemorrhoids or fissure
I Impacted feces
P Prolapse of the rectum
A Anorexia and depression
T Temperature high, dehydration results
E Endocrine: hypothyroidism
D Diet, diverticulitis, and drugs

From Shipman, 1984.

SAMPLE DOCUMENTATION
HISTORY AND PHYSICAL EXAMINATION

Subjective

A 44-year-old woman complains of burning sensation in epigastric area and chest. Occurs after eating, especially spicy foods. Lasts 1 to 2 hours. Is worse when lying down. Sometimes causes bitter taste in mouth. Also feels bloated. Antacids do not relieve the symptoms. Denies nausea/vomiting/diarrhea. No cough or shortness of breath.

For additional sample documentation, see Chapter 26.

Objective

Abdomen rounded and symmetric with white striae adjacent to umbilicus in all quadrants. A well-healed, 5-cm white surgical scar evident in right lower quadrant. No areas of visible pulsations or peristalsis. Active bowel sounds audible in all four quadrants. Percussion tones tympanic over epigastrium and resonant over remainder of abdomen. Liver span 8 cm at right midclavicular line. On inspiration, liver edge firm, smooth, and nontender. No splenomegaly. Musculature soft and relaxed to light palpation. No masses or areas of tenderness to deep palpation. Superficial reflexes intact. No costovertebral angle tenderness.

SUMMARY OF EXAMINATION
ABDOMEN

1. Inspect the abdomen for the following (p. 533):
   - Skin characteristics
   - Venous return patterns
   - Symmetry
   - Surface motion
2. Inspect abdominal muscles as patient raises head to detect presence of the following (p. 536):
   - Masses
   - Hernia
   - Separation of muscles
3. Auscultate with stethoscope diaphragm for the following (p. 536):
   - Bowel sounds
   - Friction rubs over liver and spleen
4. Auscultate with bell of stethoscope for the following (p. 537):
   - Venous hums in epigastric area and around umbilicus
   - Bruits over aorta and renal and femoral arteries
5. Percuss the abdomen for the following (p. 537):
   - Tone in all four quadrants
   - Liver borders to estimate span

   - Splenic dullness in left midaxillary line
   - Gastric air bubble
6. Lightly palpate in all quadrants for the following (p. 541):
   - Muscular resistance
   - Tenderness
   - Masses
7. Deeply palpate all quadrants for the following (p. 543):
   - Bulges and masses around the umbilicus and umbilical ring
   - Liver border in right costal margin
   - Gallbladder below liver margin at lateral border of the rectus muscle
   - Spleen in left costal margin
   - Right and left kidneys
   - Aortic pulsation in midline
   - Other masses
8. Elicit the abdominal reflexes (p. 548).
9. With patient sitting, percuss the left and right costovertebral angles for kidney tenderness (p. 540).

COMMON ABNORMALITIES

ALIMENTARY TRACT

ACUTE DIARRHEA	An acute onset of diarrhea in a previously healthy patient without signs or symptoms or other organ involvement suggests an infectious cause. Acute diarrhea in adults usually has an abrupt onset and lasts less than 2 weeks. Most of the disorders cause some combination of abdominal pain, diarrhea, nausea, vomiting, fever, and tenesmus. Acute diarrhea in adults is commonly viral in origin. The viral illnesses are self-limited. Travel outside of the United States carries the potential to acquire foodborne infection (such as enterotoxigenic *Escherichia coli*, *Salmonella*, *Shigella*, or *Entamoeba histolytica*). Camping exposes individuals to *Giardia* and *Campylobacter* through untreated water. Outbreaks of diarrhea caused by *Cryptosporidium* have been linked to contaminated water in urban areas of the United States. Undercooked poultry is a potential cause of *Salmonella* or *Campylobacter jejuni* diarrhea. Undercooked beef or unpasteurized milk are food sources that contain *E. coli* 0157:H7. Raw shellfish is a potential for source of Norwalk virus. Food poisoning should be considered if diarrhea develops in two or more persons following ingestion of the same food.
GASTROESOPHAGEAL REFLUX DISEASE	Relaxation or incompetence of the lower esophagus produces gastroesophageal reflux. Gastroesophageal reflux refers to the backward flow of acid from the stomach up into the esophagus. Patients experience heartburn, also known as acid indigestion, when excessive amounts of acid reflux into the esophagus. Symptoms of acid indigestion are more common among older adults and in women during pregnancy. Symptoms in infants and children include regurgitation and vomiting, which can be severe enough to cause weight loss and failure to thrive. Patients describe heartburn as a feeling of burning chest pain, localized behind the breastbone that moves up toward the neck and throat. Some experience the bitter or sour taste of the acid in the back of the throat. Others complain of hoarseness. The condition can cause respiratory problems from aspiration, and bleeding from esophagitis.
IRRITABLE BOWEL SYNDROME	Irritable bowel syndrome (IBS) is a functional disorder of the intestine that produces a cluster of symptoms, consisting most commonly of abdominal pain, bloating, constipation, and diarrhea. Some IBS patients experience alternating diarrhea and constipation. Mucus may be present around or within the stool. There is no sign of the disease that can be seen or measured, but the intestine is not functioning normally. It is common, occurring in about one in

STAYING WELL

AVOIDING FOODBORNE INFECTION

Adults and children are susceptible to foodborne infection, both at home and while traveling. Prevention measures that you can recommend:

- Cook all ground beef and poultry thoroughly. Send restaurant food back if it is not cooked well. Eat only food that has been cooked thoroughly and is still hot.
- Don't drink unpasteurized juices or milk.
- Refrigerate ground beef and perishable food right away after shopping.
- Wash hands and food utensils with hot, soapy water after handling meat and poultry.
- Avoid cooked food that has been kept at room temperature for several hours.

Travelers can minimize their risk for "traveler's diarrhea" by practicing the following effective preventive measures:

- Avoid eating foods or drinking beverages purchased from street vendors or other establishments where unhygienic conditions are present.
- Avoid eating raw or undercooked meat and seafood.
- Avoid eating raw fruits (e.g., oranges, bananas, avocados) and vegetables unless the traveler peels them.
- Avoid ice unless it has been made from safe water.
- Avoid dishes containing raw or undercooked eggs.

five Americans, more commonly in women, and more often at times of emotional stress. It usually begins in late adolescence or early adult life and rarely appears for the first time after the age of 50 years.

HIATAL HERNIA WITH ESOPHAGITIS	A hiatal hernia occurs when a part of the stomach has passed through the esophageal hiatus in the diaphragm into the chest cavity. The condition is very common and occurs most often in women and older adults. It is associated with obesity, pregnancy, ascites, and the use of tight-fitting belts and clothes; muscle weakness is a primary factor in developing this condition. A hiatal hernia is clinically significant when accompanied by acid reflux, producing esophagitis. Patients complain of epigastric pain and/or heartburn that worsens with lying down and is relieved by sitting up or with antacids, of water brash (the mouth fills with fluid from the esophagus), and of dysphagia. Incarceration of the hernia can occur, requiring surgical intervention. Symptoms of incarceration include sudden onset of vomiting, pain, and complete dysphagia.
DUODENAL ULCER (DUODENAL PEPTIC ULCER DISEASE)	The most common form of peptic ulcer disease, duodenal ulcer, is a chronic circumscribed break in the duodenal mucosa that scars with healing (Fig. 17-44). The ulcers may occur as a result of infection with *Helicobacter pylori* and cause increased gastric acid secretion. The condition occurs approximately twice as often in men as in women. Duodenal ulcers occur on both the anterior and posterior walls; anterior wall ulcers may produce tenderness on palpation of the abdomen. Patients generally complain of localized epigastric pain that occurs when the stomach is empty and that is relieved by food or antacids. Upper gastrointestinal bleeding can occur as a result of ulceration, producing symptoms that include hematemesis, melena, dizziness or syncope, decreased blood pressure, increased pulse rate, and decreased hematocrit level. Perforation of the duodenum is a life-threatening event that requires immediate surgical intervention. The patient exhibits signs of an acute abdomen. Anterior ulcers are more likely to perforate, whereas posterior ulcers are more likely to bleed.

FIGURE 17-44
Peptic ulcer. **A** and **B,** Two endoscopic views of the duodenum demonstrate the grayish-white base of an ulcer crater. **B** also demonstrates slightly erythematous, boggy tissue at the margin of the ulcer.
From Zitelli, Davis, 1997.

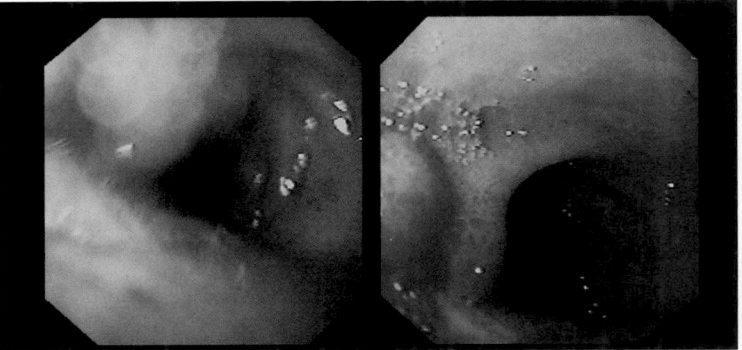

A   B

CROHN DISEASE

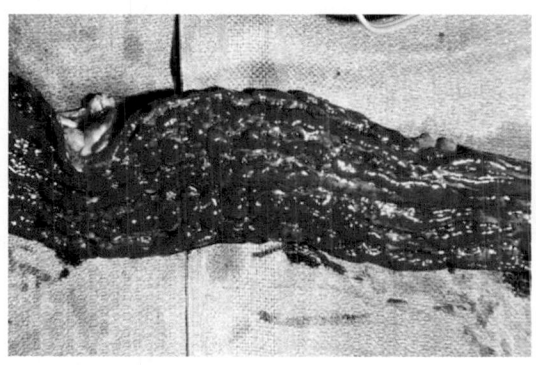

> ### CLINICAL PEARL
> #### Crohn Disease
> A reminder: Crohn disease does not always reveal itself dramatically at the start with bowel signs and symptoms. Something else may bring the patient in first (e.g., cheilitis, gingival redness and swelling, or mouth sores). Obviously, these conditions occur far more often than Crohn disease; but remember, although perhaps not always pathologically appropriate, that the connection is constant from entry to exit.

Crohn disease is a chronic inflammatory disorder of the gastrointestinal tract that produces ulceration, fibrosis, and malabsorption. Inflammation may occur anywhere along the gastrointestinal tract; the terminal ileum and colon are the most common sites. The cause of Crohn disease is unknown. On colonoscopy the mucosa has a characteristic cobblestone appearance (Fig. 17-45). Fissure and fistula formation, sometimes extending to the skin, is common (Fig. 17-46). Patients exhibit chronic diarrhea, compromised nutritional status, and often other systemic manifestations such as arthritis, iritis, and erythema nodosum.

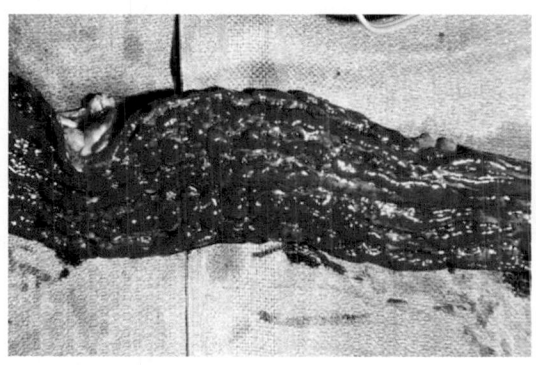

FIGURE 17-45
Crohn disease showing deep ulcers and fissures, creating "cobblestone" effect.
From Doughty, Jackson, 1993.

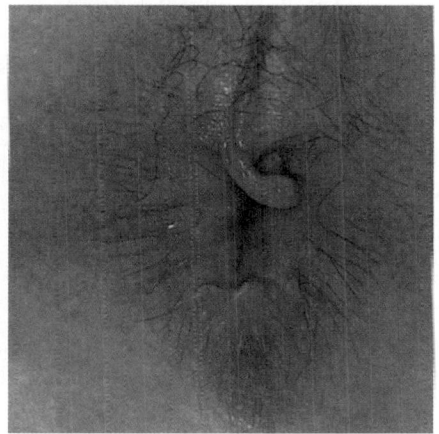

FIGURE 17-46
Crohn disease. Note a scar from previous incision and drainage. Perianal skin tags are common in Crohn disease and a good clue to diagnosis.
From Zitelli, Davis, 1997.

DIFFERENTIAL DIAGNOSIS

COMPARISON OF CROHN DISEASE AND ULCERATIVE COLITIS

Disease	Pathologic Conditions	Characteristics
Crohn disease	Inflammation, transmural bowel wall thickens, lumen narrows; mucosa ulcerated, cobblestone appearance (see Fig. 17-45); mesenteric fibrosis	Cramping diarrhea, mild bleeding, occurs anywhere in gastrointestinal tract; fissure, fistula, abscess formation; periumbilical colic; malabsorption; folate deficiency
Ulcerative colitis	Inflammation confined to mucosa; starts in rectum, progresses through colon; vascular engorgement of submucosa; mucosa ulcerated and denuded with granulation tissue (see Fig. 17-47); minimal fibrosis	Mild to severe symptoms; bloody, watery diarrhea; no localized peritoneal signs; weight loss, fatigue, general debility; may progress to carcinoma of colon

ULCERATIVE COLITIS

Ulcerative colitis is a chronic inflammatory disorder of the colon and rectum that produces mucosal friability and areas of ulceration; fibrosis is minimal. The etiologic factor is unknown, but immunologic and genetic factors have been implicated. The condition is not caused by psychosomatic mechanisms. Ulcerative colitis is characterized by bloody, frequent, watery diarrhea, with patients reporting as many as 20 to 30 diarrheal stools per day. Patients may also exhibit weight loss, fatigue, and general debilitation. Ulcerative colitis may range from mild to severe, depending on the degree of involvement of the colon (Fig. 17-47). The condition may remain in remission for years after an acute phase of the illness. Active chronic ulcerative colitis predisposes an individual to carcinoma of the colon.

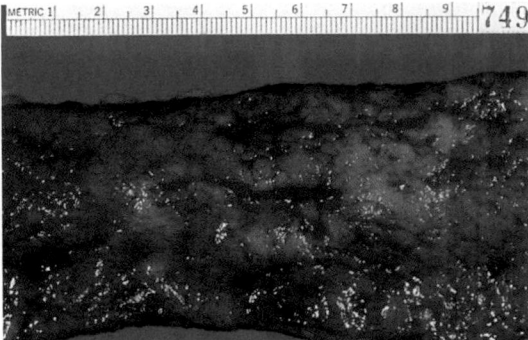

FIGURE 17-47
Ulcerative colitis showing severe mucosal edema and inflammation with ulcerations and bleeding.
From Doughty, Jackson, 1993.

STOMACH CANCER

Gastric carcinomas are most commonly found in the lower half of the stomach. These neoplasms arise from epithelial cells of the mucous membrane. In early stages, the growth is confined to the mucosa and submucosa; but as the disease progresses, the muscular layer of the stomach will also be involved. Metastases, local and distant, are common. Symptoms may be vague and nonspecific, and include loss of appetite, feeling of fullness, weight loss, dysphagia, and persistent epigastric pain. Physical examination may reveal tenderness in the midepigastrium, an enlarged liver, positive supraclavicular nodes, and ascites. An epigastric mass is not palpable until late stages of the disease.

DIVERTICULOSIS

Inflammation of existing diverticula produces left lower quadrant pain, anorexia, nausea, vomiting, and altered bowel habits, usually constipation. The pain usually becomes localized at the site of the inflammatory process (Fig. 17-48). The abdomen may be distended and tympanic with decreased bowel sounds and localized tenderness.

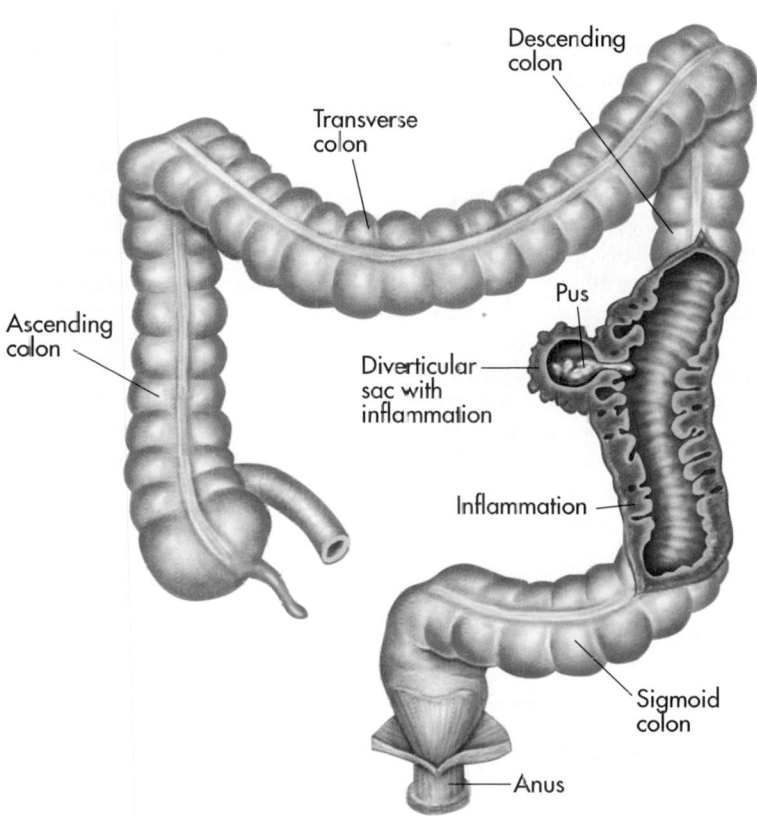

FIGURE 17-48
Diverticulosis (diverticulitis).
From Doughty, Jackson, 1993.

COLON CANCER (COLORECTAL CANCER)

Carcinoma of the colon usually occurs in the rectum, sigmoid, and lower descending colon, but it may also appear in the proximal colon. The earliest sign is often occult blood in the stool detectable by fecal occult blood testing. The patient often gives a history of changes in the frequency or character of stools. There are few early physical findings unless a lesion is felt on rectal examination (see Chapter 20). A tumor may be palpable in the right or left lower quadrant. The Evidence-Based Practice box on p. 572 highlights some of the colon cancer screening test concerns and recommendations.

EVIDENCE-BASED PRACTICE IN PHYSICAL EXAMINATION

SCREENING FOR COLON CANCER

The third leading cause of cancer deaths in the United States is colorectal cancer. Most of these deaths are preventable through appropriate screening. Persons are defined as being at average risk for colorectal cancer if they are 50 years or older and have no risk factors for colorectal cancer other than age.

Options for average-risk screening for colon cancer include the following:

- Annual fecal occult blood test (FOBT)
- Flexible sigmoidoscopy every 5 years
- Annual FOBT plus flexible sigmoidoscopy every 5 years
- Double-contrast barium enema every 5 to 10 years
- Screening colonoscopy every 10 years

Which to recommend? Each has costs and benefits that need to be considered.

The U.S. Preventive Services Task Force (USPSTF) found good evidence that periodic fecal occult blood testing reduces mortality from colorectal cancer and fair evidence that sigmoidoscopy alone or in combination with fecal occult blood testing (FOBT) reduces mortality. The USPSTF did not find direct evidence that screening colonoscopy or double-contrast barium enema is effective in reducing colorectal cancer *mortality. The USPSTF found insufficient evidence that newer screening technologies (for example, computed tomography colonography) are effective in improving health outcomes* (USPSTF, 2002).

The Agency for Healthcare Research and Quality recommends sigmoidoscopy every 5 years and annual fecal blood testing as the two most cost-effective strategies (Khandker et al, 2000). The preferred screening strategy, according to the American College of Gastroenterology, is colonoscopy every 10 years in the average-risk patient (Rex et al, 2000; American College of Gastroenterology, 2004). The American Association of Gastroenterology recommends presenting multiple options to patients since no single test is of unequivocal superiority, with the rationale that giving patients a choice allows them to apply personal preferences and may increase the likelihood that screening will occur (Winawer, 2003).

HEPATOBILIARY SYSTEM

HEPATITIS	Hepatitis is an inflammatory process of the liver characterized by diffuse or patchy hepatocellular necrosis. The condition is most commonly caused by viral infection, alcohol, drugs, or toxins. Symptoms include jaundice, hepatomegaly, anorexia, abdominal and gastric discomfort, clay-colored stools, and tea-colored urine. Liver function tests are abnormal. Systemic infection may produce small focal areas of hepatic necrosis and inflammation (reactive hepatitis). Reactive hepatitis causes minor liver function abnormalities and is usually asymptomatic. Acute viral hepatitis is caused by at least five distinct agents (see the Differential Diagnosis box on p. 573). Hepatitis D occurs only in persons infected with hepatitis B, either as a co-infection in acute hepatitis B, or as a superinfection in chronic hepatitis B. Hepatitis E (epidemic) is a self-limited type of hepatitis that may occur after natural disasters because of fecal-contaminated water or food.
CIRRHOSIS	Cirrhosis is characterized by destruction of the liver parenchyma. Often the liver is initially enlarged with a firm, nontender border on palpation; but as scarring progresses, the liver mass is reduced, and it generally cannot be palpated. Associated symptoms include ascites, jaundice, prominent abdominal vasculature, cutaneous spider angiomas, dark urine, light-colored stools, and spleen enlargement. The patient often complains of fatigue, and in late stages muscle wasting may be evident.
LIVER CARCINOMA	Invasion of the liver by malignant cells produces liver enlargement and a hard, irregular border on palpation. Nodules may be present and palpable, and the liver may be either tender or nontender. Associated symptoms can include ascites, jaundice, anorexia, fatigue, dark urine, and light-colored stools.
CHOLELITHIASIS	Stone formation in the gallbladder is responsible for most gallbladder diseases. Many patients are asymptomatic; however, symptoms of indigestion, colic, and mild transient jaundice are not unusual. The condition commonly produces episodes of acute cholecystitis and pancreatitis.

DIFFERENTIAL DIAGNOSIS

COMPARISON OF VIRAL HEPATITIS INFECTIONS

Type	Mode of Transmission	Statistics	Clinical Sequelae	Prevention
Hepatitis A virus (HAV)	Fecal-oral, food/waterborne outbreaks, blood-borne (rare)	33% of Americans have evidence of past infection (immunity) Occurs in epidemics both nationwide and in communities	No chronic infection Prolonged or relapsing hepatitis over 6- to 9-month period in about 15% of infected persons	Vaccine; immune globulin before and after exposure; good hygiene and sanitation
Hepatitis B virus (HBV)	Blood and body fluids; sexual; perinatal	New infections have declined since 1980s especially in children and adolescents due to routine vaccination Highest rate in 20- to 49-year-olds 1 to 1.25 million Americans chronically infected	Chronic infection in 90% of infants infected at birth, 30% of children infected at ages 1 to 5 years, 6% of persons infected after age 5 years Death from chronic liver disease in 15% to 25% of chronically infected persons	Vaccine; screen pregnant women and treat infected infants; screen blood/organ/tissue donors; avoid needle sharing (injectable drug users); avoid tattoos and body piercings
Hepatitis C virus (HCV)	Blood and body fluid; sexual; perinatal	New infections have declined since 1980s 3.9 million Americans have been infected with 2.7 million chronically infected Most infections due to illegal drug use	Chronic infection in 75% to 85%; chronic liver disease in 70% of chronically infected 1%-5% with chronic liver disease die	No vaccine; screen blood/organ/tissue donors
Hepatitis D virus (HDV)	Blood and body fluids, sexual, perinatal (rare) HDV infection can be acquired either as a co-infection with HBV or as a superinfection of persons with chronic HBV infection	The global pattern of HDV infection corresponds to the prevalence of chronic HBV infection In the United States and in other countries with a low prevalence of chronic HBV infection, HDV prevalence is generally low; HDV infection in these countries occurs most commonly among injecting drug users and persons with hemophilia In countries with moderate and high levels of chronic HBV prevalence, the prevalence of HDV infection is highly variable	Chronic HBV carriers who acquire HDV superinfection usually develop chronic HDV infection, with evidence of chronic liver diseases with cirrhosis (70% to 80%)	No vaccine; co-infection can be prevented with either preexposure or postexposure prophylaxis for HBV; however, no products exist to prevent HDV superinfection of persons with chronic HBV infection. Prevention of HDV superinfection depends primarily on education to reduce risk behaviors
Hepatitis E virus (HEV)	Fecal-oral route and fecally contaminated drinking water; nosocomial transmission, presumably by person-to-person contact, has been reported	Accounts for 50% of acute sporadic hepatitis in both children and adults in some high endemic areas; U.S. cases are in travelers returning from high HEV-endemic areas	No evidence of chronic infection has been detected	No vaccine; clean water supply; hygienic practices for travelers to endemic countries: avoid drinking water (and beverages with ice) of unknown purity, uncooked shellfish, and uncooked fruits or vegetables that are not peeled or prepared by the traveler

GALLBLADDER CANCER	Invasion of the gallbladder by malignant cells results in abdominal pain, jaundice, and weight loss. A mass may be palpable in the upper abdomen.
CHOLECYSTITIS	Cholecystitis is an inflammatory process of the gallbladder that may be either acute or chronic. Acute cholecystitis has associated stone formation (cholelithiasis) in 90% of all cases, causing obstruction and inflammation. Acute cholecystitis without stones results from any condition that affects the regular emptying and filling of the gallbladder, such as immobilization or sudden starvation. The primary symptom of acute cholecystitis is pain in the right upper quadrant with radiation around the midtorso to the right scapular region. The pain is abrupt and severe, and lasts for 2 to 4 hours. Chronic cholecystitis refers to repeated attacks of acute cholecystitis in a gallbladder that is scarred and contracted. These patients will exhibit fat intolerance, flatulence, nausea, anorexia, and nonspecific abdominal pain and tenderness of the right hypochondriac region.

PHYSICAL VARIATIONS
Gallbladder Disease
Native Americans/American Indians have a much higher incidence of gallbladder disease than do individuals of other groups.

PANCREAS

CHRONIC PANCREATITIS	Chronic inflammation of the pancreas produces constant, unremitting abdominal pain; epigastric tenderness; weight loss; steatorrhea; and glucose intolerance.
PANCREATIC CANCER	Malignant degeneration results in abdominal pain that radiates from the epigastrium to the upper quadrants or back, weight loss, anorexia, and jaundice.

SPLEEN

SPLEEN LACERATION/ RUPTURE	The spleen is the organ most commonly injured in abdominal trauma because of its anatomic location. The mechanism of injury can be either blunt or penetrating, but is more often blunt (e.g., from motor vehicle accidents). The symptoms of splenic rupture are pain in the left upper quadrant with radiation to the left shoulder (positive Kehr sign), hypovolemia, and peritoneal irritation. Diagnosis is made by paracentesis or computed tomography. Surgical intervention may be required.

KIDNEYS

GLOMERULO-NEPHRITIS	Inflammation of the capillary loops of the renal glomeruli usually produces nonspecific symptoms. The patient complains of nausea, malaise, and arthralgias. Hematuria may occur. Pulmonary infiltrates may be present.
HYDRONEPHROSIS	Hydronephrosis is the dilation of the renal pelvis from back pressure of urine that cannot flow past an obstruction in the ureter. If secondary infection is present the patient experiences hematuria, pyuria, and fever.
PYELONEPHRITIS	Infection of the kidney and renal pelvis is characterized by flank pain, bacteriuria, pyuria, dysuria, nocturia, and frequency. Costovertebral angle tenderness may be evident.
RENAL ABSCESS	Renal abscess is a localized infection within the cortex of the kidney. The patient may complain of chills, fever, and aching flanks. Fist percussion produces costovertebral angle tenderness.
RENAL CALCULI	Renal calculi are stones formed in the pelvis of the kidney from a physiochemical process; calculus formation is associated with obstruction and infections in the urinary tract. Renal calculi are composed of calcium salts, uric acid, cystine, and struvite. Any situation leading to an alkaline urine is conducive to stone formation because uric acid, calcium, and phosphate are all more soluble in a low pH. Urine temperature, ionic strength, and concentration also affect

stone formation. The condition is much more prevalent in men than in women. Symptoms include fever, hematuria, and flank pain that may extend to the groin and genitals.

ACUTE RENAL FAILURE	This is the sudden, severe impairment of renal function causing an acute uremic episode. The impairment may be prerenal, renal, or postrenal. Urine output may be normal, decreased, or absent. The patient may show signs of either fluid overload or deficit.
CHRONIC RENAL FAILURE	Chronic renal failure is a slow, insidious, and irreversible impairment of renal function. Uremia usually develops gradually. The patient may experience oliguria or anuria and have signs of fluid overload.
RENAL ARTERY EMBOLI	Numerous small or a few major emboli can occlude the renal artery, causing either acute or chronic renal failure. The condition may be a silent event or a full-blown syndrome of flank pain and tenderness, hematuria, hypertension, fever, and decreased renal function.
MALODOROUS URINE	Many (but not all) diseases or disorders signaled by malodorous urine are inborn errors of metabolism (Box 17-8).

BOX 17-8

DISEASES AND CONDITIONS SIGNALED BY MALODOROUS URINE

Odor	Disease/Condition
Maple syrup	Maple syrup urine disease
Mousy, musty	Phenylketonuria
Dead fish	Fish odor syndrome (trimethylaminuria)
Cat's urine	Cat syndrome (similar to Werdnig-Hoffman disease)
Yeastlike, celery	Oasthouse urine disease (methionine)
Fishy, musty	Tyrosinemia/tyrosinosis
Rancid butter	Rancid butter syndrome (hypermethioninemia)
Ammonia	Urea-splitting bacteria (especially *Proteus*)
Rotting fish	Uremia (di-, trimethylamines)
Stale water	Acute tubular necrosis
Violets	Turpentine ingestion
Medicinal	Antibiotics: penicillin, cephalosporins

Modified from Wilson, 1997; and Mace et al, 1976.

INFANTS

INTUSSUSCEPTION	The prolapse of one segment of the intestine into another causes intestinal obstruction. Intussusception commonly occurs in infants between 3 and 12 months old. The cause is unknown. Symptoms include acute intermittent abdominal pain, abdominal distention, vomiting, and passage at first of normal brown stool. Subsequent stools may be mixed with blood and mucus with a red currant jelly appearance. A sausage-shaped mass may be palpated in the right or left upper quadrant, whereas the lower quadrant feels empty (positive Dance sign). Intussusception in an infant can be dramatic in onset. The apparently well child starts crying suddenly, in severe pain, sometimes awakening from sleep. The child is inconsolable, sometimes doubling up with pain. The episode can cease abruptly, but the symptoms will most likely recur.
PYLORIC STENOSIS	Hypertrophy of the circular muscle of the pylorus leads to obstruction of the pyloric sphincter during the first month after birth. Symptoms include regurgitation progressing to projectile vomiting (i.e., vigorous, shoots out of the mouth, and carries a short distance); feeding eagerly (even after a vomiting episode); failure to gain weight; and signs of dehydration. A small,

rounded mass is often palpable in the right upper quadrant, particularly after the infant vomits.

MECONIUM ILEUS	Meconium ileus is a lower intestinal obstruction caused by thickening and hardening of meconium in the lower intestine. Identified by the failure to pass meconium in the first 24 hours after birth and by abdominal distention, it is often the first manifestation of cystic fibrosis.
BILIARY ATRESIA	Biliary atresia is a congenital obstruction or absence of some or all of the bile duct system. Symptoms include jaundice that usually becomes apparent at 2 to 3 weeks of age, hepatomegaly, abdominal distention, poor weight gain, and pruritus. Stools become lighter in color and urine darkens.
MECKEL DIVERTICULUM	An outpouching of the ileum varies in size from a small appendiceal process to a segment of bowel several inches long, often in the proximity of the ileocecal valve. It is the most common congenital anomaly of the gastrointestinal tract. The symptoms, if any, are those of intestinal obstruction or diverticulitis. In many cases, there is bright or dark red rectal bleeding with little abdominal pain, although symptoms like those of acute appendicitis are not uncommon.
NECROTIZING ENTEROCOLITIS	An inflammatory disease of the gastrointestinal mucosa, necrotizing enterocolitis is associated with prematurity and immaturity of the gastrointestinal tract. Signs include abdominal distention, occult blood in stool, and respiratory distress. The condition is often fatal, complicated by perforation and septicemia.

CHILDREN

NEUROBLASTOMA	A common solid malignancy in early childhood, neuroblastoma often appears as a mass in the adrenal medulla of the young child, but a mass may occur anywhere along the craniospinal axis. A firm, fixed, nontender, irregular and nodular abdominal mass that crosses the midline is often found. Symptoms include malaise, loss of appetite, weight loss, and protrusion of one or both eyes. Other symptoms arise from compression of the mass or metastasis to adjacent organs.
WILMS TUMOR (NEPHROBLASTOMA)	Nephroblastoma, the most common intraabdominal tumor of childhood, usually appears at 2 to 3 years of age. It is a firm, nontender mass deep within the flank, only slightly movable and not usually crossing the midline. It is sometimes bilateral. Painless enlargement of the abdomen is the usual sign; however, a low-grade fever and hypertension may be present.
HIRSCHSPRUNG DISEASE (CONGENITAL AGANGLIONIC MEGACOLON)	The primary absence of parasympathetic ganglion cells in a segment of the colon interrupts the motility of the intestine. The absence of peristalsis causes feces to accumulate proximal to the defect, leading to an intestinal obstruction. Symptoms include failure to thrive, constipation, abdominal distention, and episodes of vomiting and diarrhea. The newborn may fail to pass meconium in the first 24 to 48 hours after birth. Symptoms in older infants and young children are generally intestinal obstruction or severe constipation.
HEMOLYTIC UREMIC SYNDROME (HUS)	HUS is one of the most common causes of acute renal failure in children. Diarrhea and upper respiratory infection are the most common precipitating factors. The child typically presents with decreased or absent urine output, fever and irritability, with a history of bloody diarrhea. Gastrointestinal involvement may lead to symptoms of an acute abdomen, with occasional perforation. The number one bacterial cause of HUS in the United States is *E. coli* 0157:H7.

Pregnant Women

HYDRAMNIOS (POLYHYDRAMNIOS)	Hydramnios is an excessive quantity of amniotic fluid, an amniotic fluid index greater than the 95th percentile, which can range from 2000 mL of fluid to as much as 15 L. Hydramnios is associated with maternal diabetes; with an increased incidence of fetal malformations, especially of the central nervous system and gastrointestinal tract; and with other conditions including fetal polyuria, fetal cardiac failure, and congenital infections although the majority of cases are idiopathic. There is usually difficulty in palpating fetal small parts and in hearing fetal heart tones. A large uterus and tense uterine wall may also be present. Symptoms are primarily due to pressure on the surrounding organs from the distended uterus and include dyspnea, edema, and pain. Hydramnios may lead to perinatal mortality from premature labor and fetal abnormalities.
OLIGOHYDRAMNIOS	Oligohydramnios is a reduced amount of amniotic fluid identified on ultrasound. An amniotic fluid index (AFI) of less than the fifth percentile for gestational age is associated with premature rupture of membranes, intrauterine growth restriction, post maturity, and fetal anomalies of renal origin. On examination, the uterine size may be small for gestational age, with the fetal parts easily palpated. Fetal mortality is increased due to underlying etiology and increased risk for cesarean delivery.

Older Adults

FECAL INCONTINENCE	Fecal incontinence in older adults is associated with three major causes: fecal impaction, underlying disease, and neurogenic disorders. The most common cause, fecal impaction, is associated with immobilization and poor fluid and dietary intake. Typically these patients will have an "overflow incontinence" or a soft stool that oozes around the impaction. Underlying diseases such as cancer, inflammatory bowel disease, diverticulitis, colitis, proctitis, or diabetic neuropathy may all have fecal incontinence as a presenting symptom. Overuse of laxatives may also be a cause of incontinence. Neurogenic disorders take two forms: local or cognitive. Local refers to any process that causes degeneration of the mesenteric plexus and lower bowel, resulting in a lax sphincter muscle, diminished sacral reflex, and decreased puborectal muscle tone. Cognitive neurogenic disorders usually result from stroke or dementia. These patients are unable to recognize rectal fullness and have an inability to inhibit intrinsic rectal contraction. Their stools are normally formed and occur in a set pattern, usually after a meal. Incontinence in the older patient is diagnosed through digital rectal examination, abdominal films, history, and assessment of cognitive abilities.

Clinical Pearl

Constipation with Diarrhea

Be aware: People with apparent diarrhea may still be seriously constipated. Some may have loose stools around a major impaction of feces. Message: A person can be constipated and still have diarrhea.

URINARY INCONTINENCE	The most common types of urinary incontinence in older adults are stress, urge, overflow, and functional (see the Differential Diagnosis box on p. 578). Stress incontinence is a leakage of urine due to increased intraabdominal pressure that can occur from coughing, laughing, exercise, or lifting heavy things. Causes of stress incontinence include weakness of bladder neck supports and anatomic damage to the urethral sphincter, both often associated with childbirth. Urge incontinence is the inability to hold urine once the urge to void occurs. Causes of this abnormality can be local genitourinary conditions, such as infection or tumor; or central nervous system disorders, such as stroke. Reflex incontinence, a type of urge incontinence, is caused by uninhibited bladder contractions and no urge to void. Overflow incontinence is a mechanical dysfunction resulting from an overdistended bladder. This type of incontinence has many causes: anatomic obstruction by prostatic hypertrophy and strictures; neurologic abnormalities that impair detrusor contractility, such as multiple sclerosis; or spinal lesions. With functional incontinence there is an intact urinary tract, but other factors such as cognitive abilities, immobility, or musculoskeletal impairments lead to incontinence. Assessment of the incontinent patient can often be accomplished by a thorough history, physical examination, and urinary analysis. Note that many older patients will have more than one type of incontinence at any given time.

Mnemonics

Reversible Causes of Urinary Incontinence: DRIP

D Delirium, dehydration

R Retention, restricted mobility

I Impaction, infection

P Polyuria, pharmaceuticals, psychologic

From Penninger, 1993.

DIFFERENTIAL DIAGNOSIS

URINARY INCONTINENCE

Condition	History	Physical Findings
Stress incontinence	Small volume incontinence with cough, sneezing, laughing, running; history of prior pelvic surgery	Pelvic floor relaxation; cystocele, rectocele; lax urethral sphincter; loss of urine with provocative testing; atrophic vaginitis; postvoid residual less than 100 mL
Urge incontinence	Uncontrolled urge to void; large volume incontinence; history of central nervous system disorders such as stroke, multiple sclerosis, parkinsonism	Unexpected findings only as related to central nervous system disorder; postvoid residual less than 100 mL
Overflow incontinence	Small volume incontinence, dribbling, hesitancy; in men, symptoms of enlarged prostate; nocturia, dribbling, hesitance, deceased force and caliber of stream In neurogenic bladder: history of bowel problems, spinal cord injury, or multiple sclerosis	Distended bladder; prostate hypertrophy; stool in rectum, fecal impaction; postvoid residual greater than 100 mL Evidence of spinal cord disease or diabetic neuropathy; lax sphincter; gait disturbance
Functional incontinence	Change in mental status; impaired mobility; new environment Medications: hypnotics, diuretics, anticholinergic agents, alpha-adrenergic agents, calcium-channel blockers	Impaired mental status; impaired mobility Impaired mental status or unexpected findings only as related to other physical conditions

ELECTRONIC RESOURCES

For Weblinks and additional resources, go to

http://evolve.elsevier.com/Seidel

or to the Companion CD-ROM.

Additional information related to the content in Chapter 17 can be found on the companion website at http://evolve.elsevier.com/Seidel/ or on the interactive companion CD-ROM. Resources and activities for Chapter 17 include:

- Sound and Vision Theater
- Printouts for Your Practice
- Interactive Challenge
- Spanish Assessment Terms with Pronunciation Guide
- Instant Calculator

FEMALE GENITALIA

ANATOMY AND PHYSIOLOGY

EXTERNAL GENITALIA

The vulva, or external female genital organs, include the mons pubis, labia majora, labia minora, clitoris, vestibular glands, vaginal vestibule, vaginal orifice, and urethral opening (Fig. 18-1). The symphysis pubis is covered by a pad of adipose tissue called the mons pubis or mons veneris, which in the postpubertal female is covered with coarse terminal hair. Extending downward and backward from the mons pubis are the labia majora, two folds of adipose tissue covered by skin. The labia majora vary in appearance depending on the amount of adipose tissue present. The outer surfaces of the labia majora are also covered with hair in the postpubertal female.

Lying inside and usually hidden by the labia majora are the labia minora, two hairless, flat, reddish folds. The labia minora meet at the anterior of the vulva, where each labium divides into two lamellae, the lower pair fusing to form the frenulum of the clitoris and the upper pair forming the prepuce. Tucked between the frenulum and the prepuce is the clitoris, a small bud of erectile tissue, the homolog of the penis and a primary center of sexual excitement. Posteriorly, the labia minora meet as two ridges that fuse to form the fourchette.

The labia minora enclose the area designated as the vestibule, which contains six openings: the urethra, the vagina, two ducts of Bartholin glands, and two ducts of Skene glands. The lower two thirds of the urethra lies immediately above the anterior vaginal wall and terminates in the urethral meatus at the midline of the vestibule just above the vaginal opening and below the clitoris. Skene ducts drain a group of urethral glands and open onto the vestibule on each side of the urethra. The ductal openings may be visible.

The vaginal opening occupies the posterior portion of the vestibule and varies in size and shape. Surrounding the vaginal opening is the hymen, a connective tissue membrane that may be circular, crescentic, or fimbriated. After the hymen tears and becomes permanently divided, the edges either disappear or cicatrize, leaving hymenal tags. Bartholin glands, located posteriorly on each side of the vaginal orifice, open onto the sides of the vestibule in the groove between the labia minora and the hymen. The ductal openings are not usually visible. During sexual excitement, Bartholin glands secrete mucus into the introitus for lubrication.

The pelvic floor consists of a group of muscles that form a supportive sling for the pelvic contents. The muscle fibers insert at various points on the bony pelvis and form functional sphincters for the vagina, rectum, and urethra (Fig. 18-2).

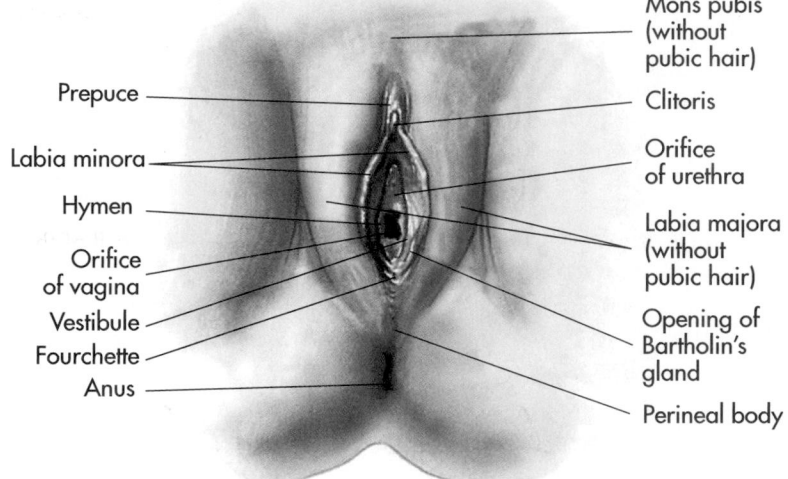

FIGURE 18-1
External female genitalia.
From Lowdermilk, Perry, 2004.

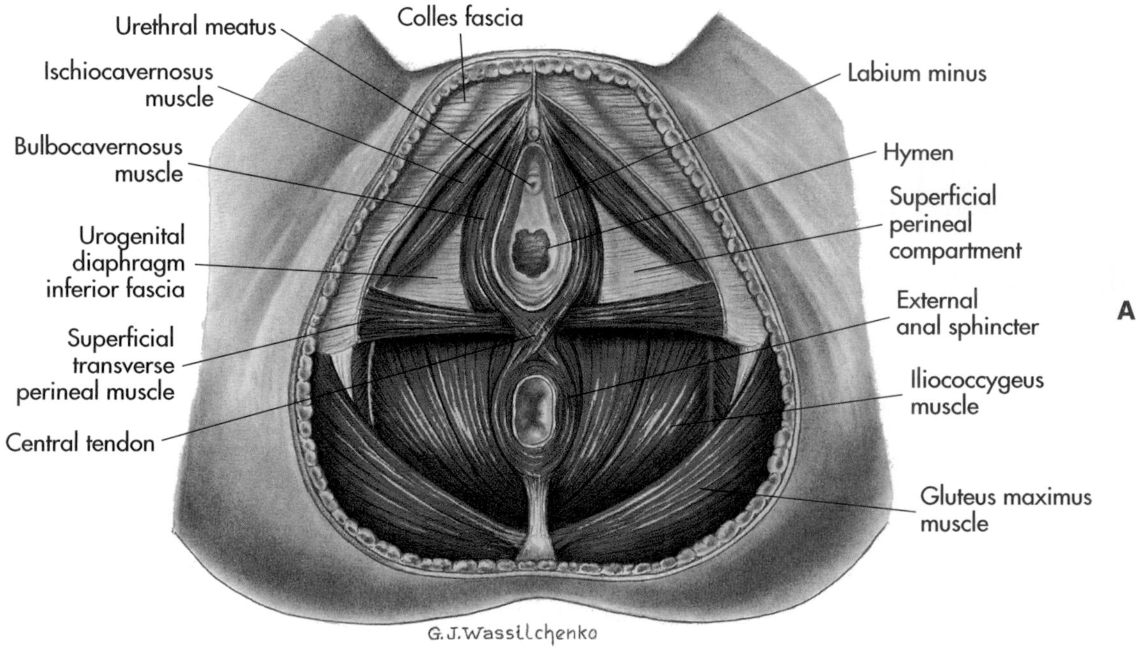

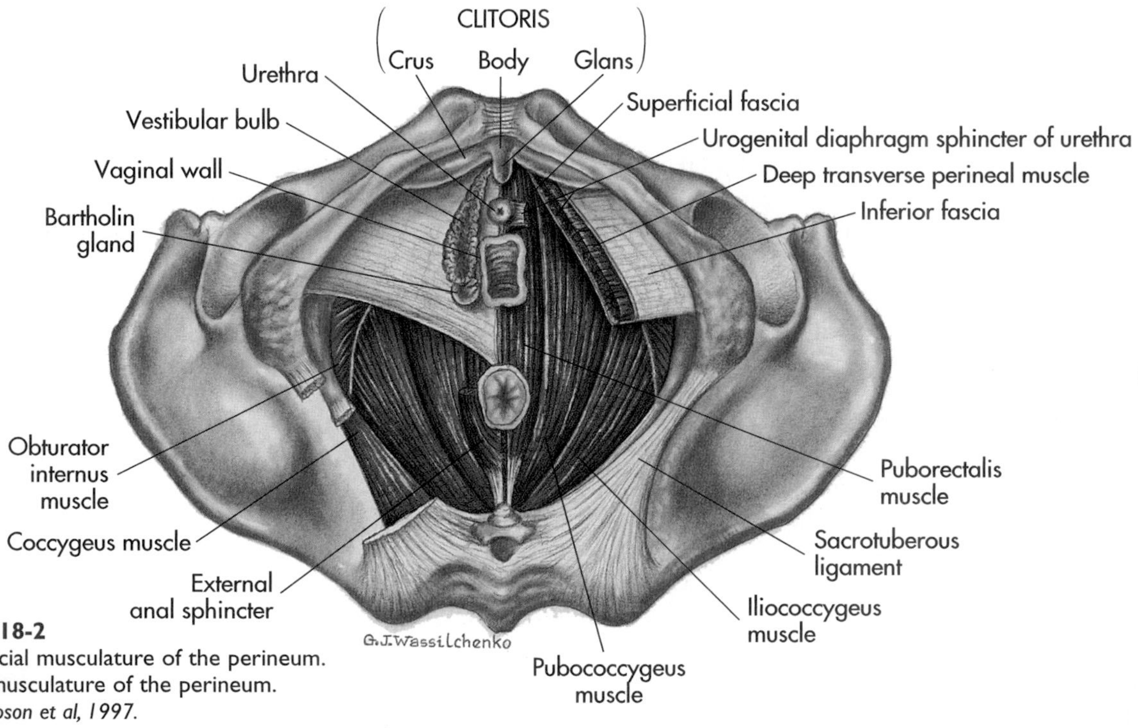

Prepuce

Labia minora

Hymen

Orifice of vagina

Vestibule

Fourchette

Anus

Mons pubis (without pubic hair)

Clitoris

Orifice of urethra

Labia majora (without pubic hair)

Opening of Bartholin's gland

Perineal body

Urethral meatus

Ischiocavernosus muscle

Bulbocavernosus muscle

Urogenital diaphragm inferior fascia

Superficial transverse perineal muscle

Central tendon

Colles fascia

Labium minus

Hymen

Superficial perineal compartment

External anal sphincter

Iliococcygeus muscle

Gluteus maximus muscle

A

G.J.Wassilchenko

CLITORIS

Crus   Body   Glans

Urethra

Vestibular bulb

Vaginal wall

Bartholin gland

Superficial fascia

Urogenital diaphragm sphincter of urethra

Deep transverse perineal muscle

Inferior fascia

Obturator internus muscle

Coccygeus muscle

External anal sphincter

Puborectalis muscle

Sacrotuberous ligament

Iliococcygeus muscle

Pubococcygeus muscle

B

G.J.Wassilchenko

FIGURE 18-2
A, Superficial musculature of the perineum.
B, Deep musculature of the perineum.
From Thompson et al, 1997.

INTERNAL GENITALIA

The vagina is a musculomembranous tube that is transversely rugated during the reproductive phase of life. It inclines posteriorly at an angle of approximately 45 degrees with the vertical plane of the body (Fig. 18-3). The anterior wall of the vagina is separated from the bladder and urethra by connective tissue called the vesicovaginal septum. The posterior vaginal wall is separated from the rectum by the rectovaginal septum. Usually the anterior and posterior walls of the vagina lie in close proximity, with only a small space between them. The upper end of the vagina is a blind vault into which the uterine cervix projects. The pocket formed around the cervix is divided into the anterior, posterior, and lateral fornices. These are of clinical importance because the internal pelvic organs can be palpated through their thin walls. The vagina carries menstrual flow from the uterus, serves as the terminal portion of the birth canal, and is the receptive organ for the penis during sexual intercourse.

The uterus sits in the pelvic cavity between the bladder and the rectum. It is an inverted pear-shaped, muscular organ that is relatively mobile (Fig. 18-4). The uterus is covered by the peritoneum and lined by the endometrium, which is shed during menstruation. The rectouterine cul-de-sac (pouch of Douglas) is a deep recess formed by the peritoneum as it covers the lower posterior wall of the uterus and upper portion of the vagina, separating it from the rectum. The uterus is flattened anteroposteriorly and usually inclines forward at a 45-degree angle, although it may be anteverted, anteflexed, retroverted, or retroflexed. In nulliparous women the size is approximately 5.5 to 8 cm long, 3.5 to 4 cm wide, and 2 to 2.5 cm thick. The uterus of a parous woman may be larger by 2 to 3 cm in any of the dimensions. The nonpregnant uterus weighs approximately 60 to 90 g (Fig. 18-5).

The uterus is divided anatomically into the corpus and cervix. The corpus consists of the fundus, which is the convex upper portion between the points of insertion of the fallopian tubes; the main portion or body; and the isthmus, which is the constricted lower portion adjacent to the cervix. The cervix extends from the isthmus into the vagina. The uterus opens into the vagina via the external cervical os.

The adnexa of the uterus comprise the fallopian tubes and ovaries. The fallopian tubes insert into the upper portion of the uterus and extend laterally to the ovaries. Each tube ranges from 8 to 14 cm long and is supported by a fold of the broad ligament called the *mesosalpinx*. The isthmus end of the fallopian tube opens into the uterine cavity. The fimbriated end opens into the pelvic cavity, with a projection that extends to the ovary and captures the ovum. Rhythmic contractions of the tubal musculature transport the ovum to the uterus.

The ovaries are a pair of oval organs resting in a slight depression on the lateral pelvic wall at the level of the anterosuperior iliac spine. The ovaries are approximately 3 cm long, 2 cm wide, and 1 cm thick in the adult woman during the reproductive years. Ovaries secrete estrogen and progesterone, hormones that have several functions, including controlling the menstrual cycle (Fig. 18-6 and Table 18-1) and supporting pregnancy.

The internal genitalia are supported by four pairs of ligaments: the cardinal, uterosacral, round, and broad ligaments.

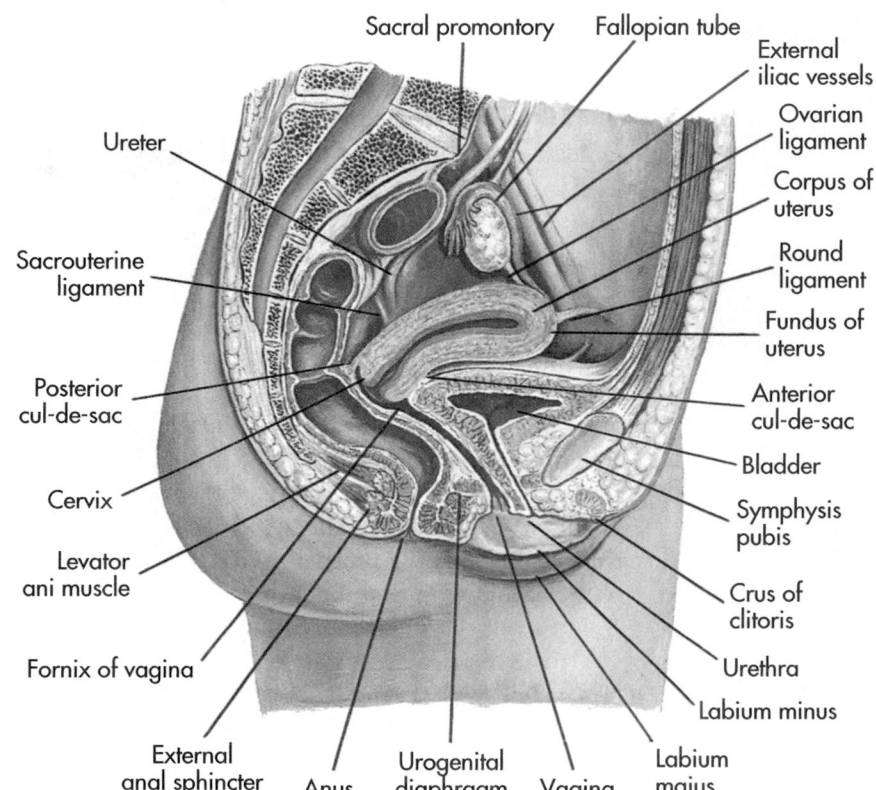

FIGURE 18-3
Midsagittal view of the female pelvic organs.

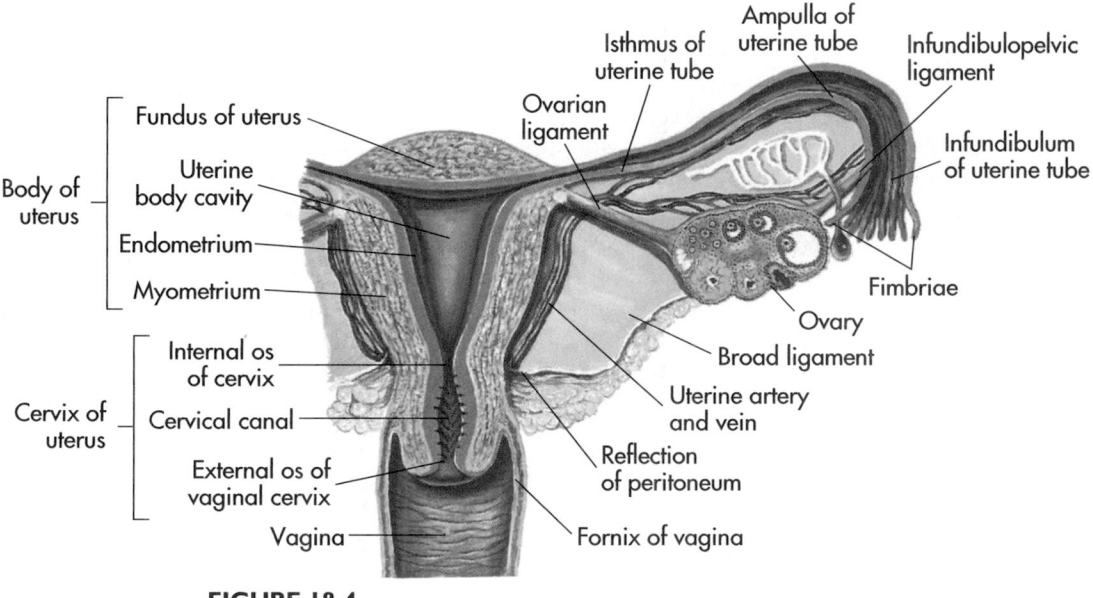

FIGURE 18-4
Cross-sectional view of internal female genitalia and pelvic contents.

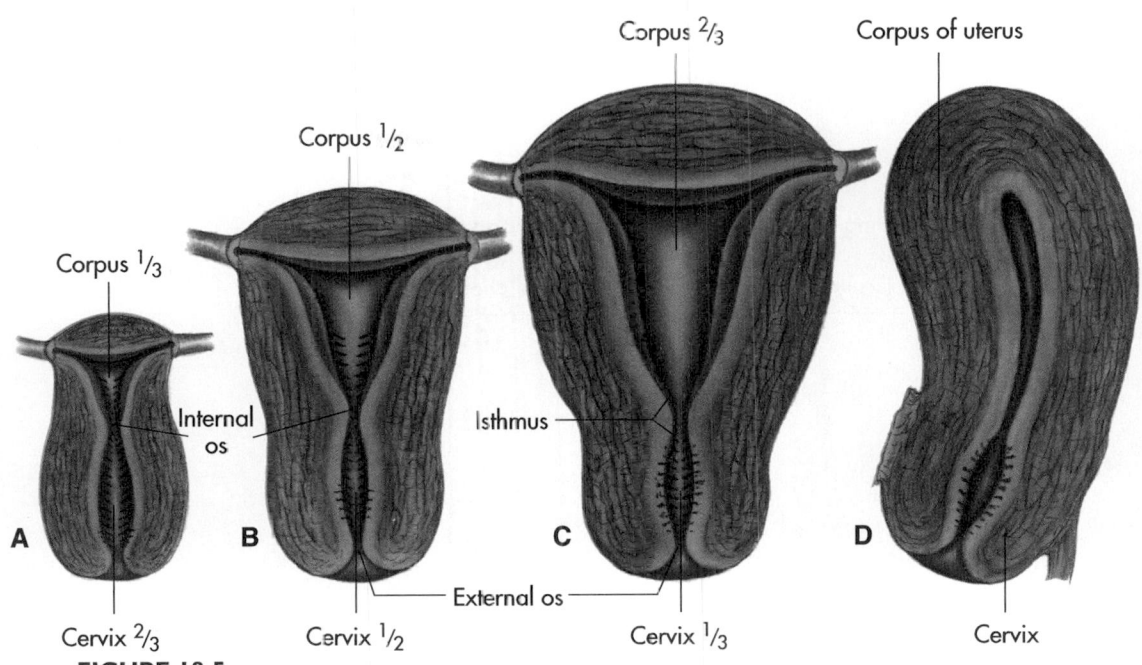

FIGURE 18-5
Comparative sizes of uteri at various stages of development. **A,** Prepubertal. **B,** Adult nulliparous.
C, Adult multiparous. **D,** Lateral view, adult multiparous. The fractions give the relative proportion of
the size of the corpus and the cervix.

BONY PELVIS

The pelvis is formed from four bones: two innominate (each consisting of ilium, ischium, and pubis), the sacrum, and the coccyx (Fig. 18-7). The bony pelvis is important in accommodating a growing fetus during pregnancy and in the birth process. The four pelvic joints—the symphysis pubis, the sacrococcygeal, and the two sacroiliac joints—usually have little movement. During pregnancy, increased levels of the circulating hormones estrogen and relaxin contribute to the strengthening and elasticity of pelvic ligaments and softening of the cartilage. As a result, the pelvic joints separate slightly, allowing some mobility. Later in pregnancy, the symphysis pubis separates appreciably, which may cause discomfort when walking. Protrusion of the abdomen as the uterus grows causes the pelvis to tilt forward, placing additional strain on the back and sacroiliac joints.

The pelvis is divided into two parts. The shallow upper section is considered the false pelvis, which consists mainly of the flared-out iliac bones. The true pelvis is the lower curved bony canal, including the inlet, cavity, and outlet; through these the fetus must pass during birth. The upper border of the outlet is at the level of the ischial spines, which project into the pelvic cavity and serve as important landmarks during labor. The lower border of the outlet is bounded by the pubic arch and the ischial tuberosities (Fig. 18-8).

INFANTS AND CHILDREN The vagina of the female infant is a small narrow tube with fewer epithelial layers than that of the adult. The uterus is approximately 35 mm long, with the cervix constituting about two thirds of the entire length of the organ. The ovaries are tiny and functionally immature. The labia minora are relatively avascular, thin, and pale. The labia majora are hairless and nonprominent. The hymen is a thin diaphragm just inside the introitus, usually with a crescent-shaped opening in the midline. The clitoris is small.

During childhood, the genitalia, except for the clitoris, grow incrementally at varying rates. Anatomic and functional development accelerates with the onset of puberty and the accompanying hormonal changes.

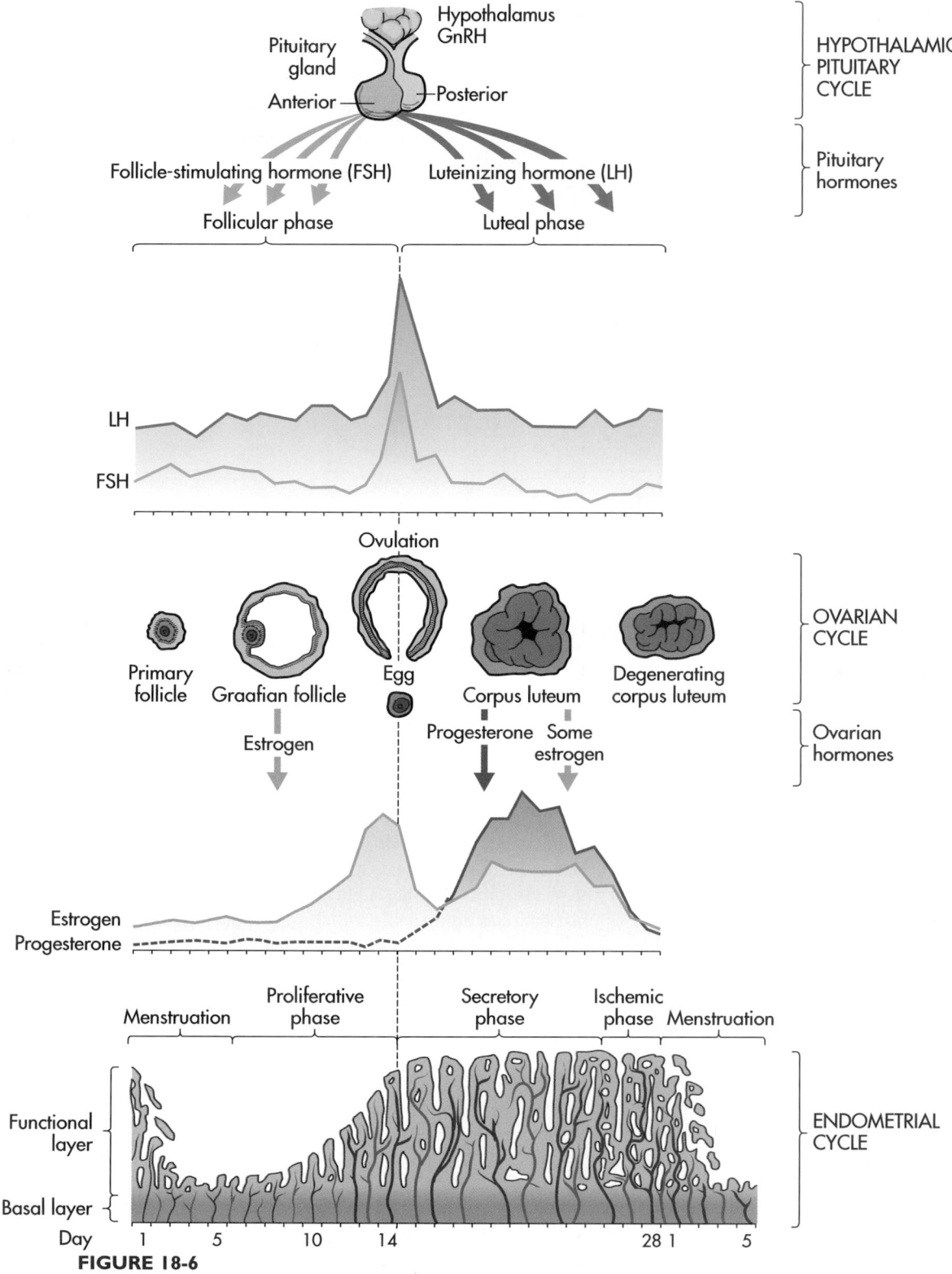

FIGURE 18-6

Female menstrual cycle. Diagram shows the interrelationship of the cerebral, hypothalamic, pituitary, and uterine functions throughout a standard 28-day menstrual cycle.
From Lowdermilk, Perry, 2004.

TABLE 18-1	The Menstrual Cycle	
Phase		**Process Description**

MENSTRUAL PHASE: DAYS 1 TO 4

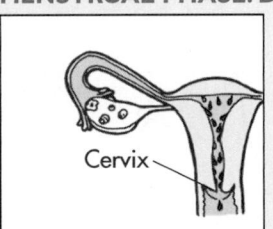

	Ovary	Estrogen levels begin to rise, preparing follicle and egg for next cycle
	Uterus	Progesterone stimulates endometrial prostaglandins that cause vasoconstriction; upper layers of endometrium shed
	Breast	Cellular activity in the alveoli decreases; breast ducts shrink
	Central nervous system (CNS) hormones	Follicle-stimulating hormone (FSH) and luteinizing hormone (LH) levels decrease
	Symptoms	Menstrual bleeding may vary, depending on hormones and prostaglandins

POSTMENSTRUAL, PREOVULATORY PHASE: DAYS 5 TO 12

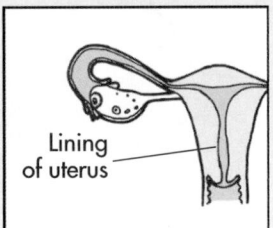

	Ovary	Ovary and maturing follicle produce estrogen; *follicular phase*—egg develops within follicle
	Uterus	*Proliferative phase*—uterine lining thickens
	Breast	Parenchymal and proliferation (increased cellular activity) of breast ducts occurs
	CNS hormones	FSH stimulates ovarian follicular growth

OVULATION: DAY 13 OR 14

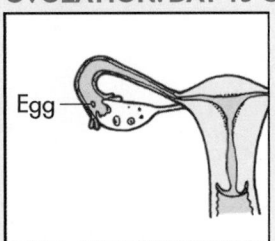

	Ovary	Egg is expelled from follicle into abdominal cavity and drawn into the uterine (fallopian) tube by fimbriae and cilia; follicle closes and begins to form corpus luteum; fertilization of egg may occur in outer one third of tube if sperm are unimpeded
	Uterus	End of proliferative phase; progesterone causes further thickening of the uterine wall
	CNS hormones	LH and estrogen levels increase rapidly; LH surge stimulates release of egg
	Symptoms	Mittelschmerz may occur with ovulation; cervical mucus is increased and is stringy and elastic (spinnbarkeit)

SECRETORY PHASE: DAYS 15 TO 20

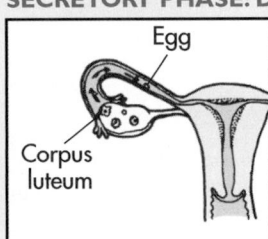

	Ovary	Egg (ovum) is moved by cilia into the uterus
	Uterus	After the egg is released, the follicle becomes a corpus luteum; secretion of progesterone increases and precominates
	CNS hormones	LH and FSH decrease

PREMENSTRUAL, LUTEAL PHASE: DAYS 21 TO 28

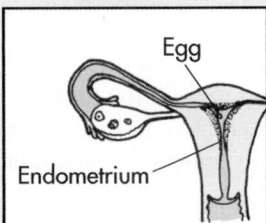

	Ovary	If implantation does not occur, the corpus luteum degenerates; progesterone production decreases, and estrogen production drops and then begins to rise as a new follicle develops
	Uterus	Menstruation starts around day 28, which begins day 1 of the menstrual cycle
	Breast	Alveolar breast cells differentiate into secretory cells
	CNS hormones	Increased levels of gonadotropin-releasing hormone (GnRH) cause increased secretion of FSH
	Symptoms	Vascular engorgement and water retention may occur

Modified from Edge, Miller, 1994.

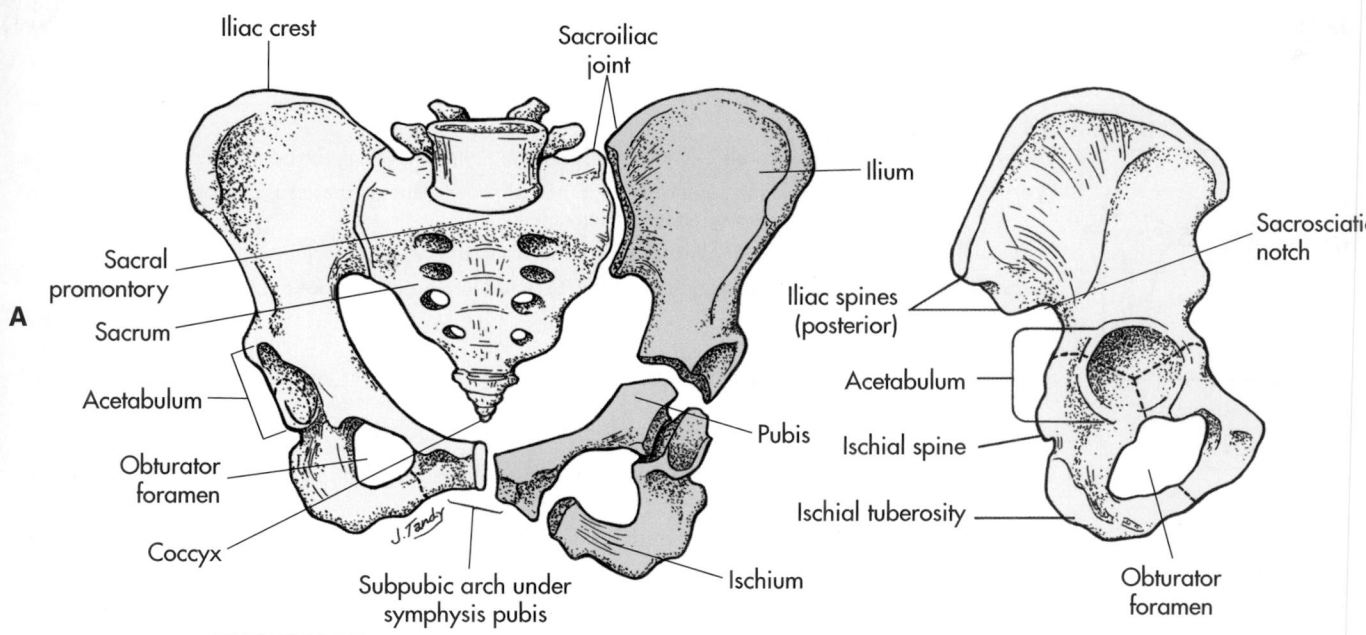

FIGURE 18-7
Adult female pelvis. **A,** Anterior view. The three embryonic parts of the left innominate bone are lightly shaded. **B,** External view of right innominate bone (fused).
From Lowdermilk, Perry, 2004.

FIGURE 18-8
Female pelvis. **A,** Cavity of the false pelvis is a shallow basin above the inlet; the true pelvis is a deeper cavity below the inlet. **B,** Cavity of the true pelvis is an irregularly curved canal *(arrows).*
From Lowdermilk, Perry, 2004.

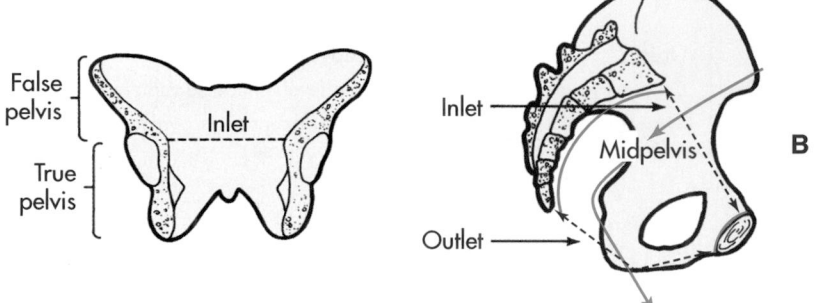

ADOLESCENTS

During puberty, the external genitalia increase in size and begin to assume adult proportions. The clitoris becomes more erectile and the labia minora more vascular. The labia majora and mons pubis become more prominent and begin to develop hair, often occurring simultaneously with breast development. Growth changes and secondary sex characteristic developments that occur during puberty are discussed in Chapter 5.

If the hymen is intact, the vaginal opening is about 1 cm. The vagina lengthens, and the epithelial layers thicken. The vaginal secretions become acidic.

The uterus, ovaries, and fallopian tubes increase in size and weight. The uterine musculature and vascular supply increase. The endometrial lining thickens in preparation for the onset of menstruation (menarche), which on the average, occurs between 11 and 14 years of age in the United States. Just before menarche, vaginal secretions increase. Functional maturation of the reproductive organs is reached during puberty.

PREGNANT WOMEN

The high levels of estrogen and progesterone that are necessary to support pregnancy are responsible for uterine enlargement during the first trimester. After the third month, uterine enlargement is primarily the result of mechanical pressure of the growing fetus. As the uterus enlarges, the muscular walls strengthen and become more elastic. As the uterus becomes larger and more ovoid, it rises out of the pelvis; by 12 weeks of gestation it reaches into the abdom-

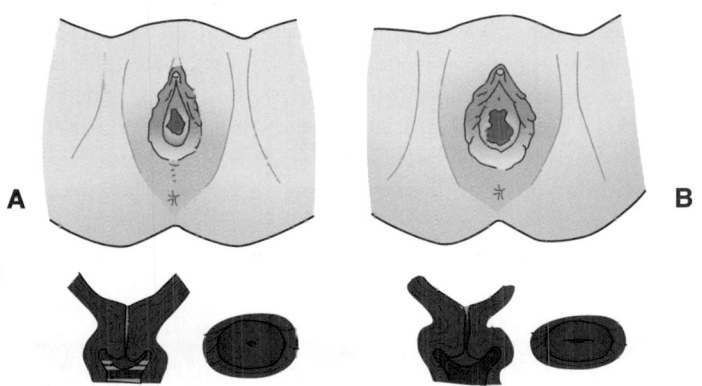

FIGURE 18-9
Comparison of vulva and cervix in a nullipara **(A)** and a multipara **(B)** woman at the same stage of pregnancy.
From Lowdermilk, Perry, 2004.

inal cavity. During the first months the walls become thicker, but then gradually thin to about 1.5 cm or less at term. Uterine weight at term, excluding the fetus and placenta, will usually have increased more than 10-fold, to a weight of about 100 g and the capacity increases 500 to 1000 times that of the nonpregnant uterus.

Hormonal activity (relaxin and progesterone) is responsible for the softening of the pelvic cartilage and strengthening of the pelvic ligaments. As a consequence, the pelvic joints separate slightly, allowing some mobility; this results in the characteristic "waddle" gait. The symphysis pubis relaxes and increases in width, and there is marked mobility of the pelvis at term with resolution of changes occurring within 3 to 5 months postpartum.

During pregnancy, an increase in uterine blood flow and lymph causes pelvic congestion and edema. As a result the uterus, cervix, and isthmus soften, and the cervix takes on a bluish color. The cervical canal is obstructed by thick mucus soon after conception. The glands near the external os proliferate with eversion of the columnar endocervical glands, which tend to be friable. The softness and compressibility of the isthmus result in exaggerated uterine anteflexion during the first 3 months of pregnancy, causing the fundus to press on the urinary bladder.

The vaginal changes are similar to the cervical changes and result in the characteristic violet color. Both the mucosa of the vaginal walls and the connective tissue thicken, and smooth muscle cells hypertrophy. These changes result in an increased length of the vaginal walls, so that at times they can be seen protruding from the vulvar opening. The papillae of the mucosa have a hobnailed appearance. The vaginal secretions increase and have an acidic pH due to an increase in lactic acid production by the vaginal epithelium. Fig. 18-9 compares the changes that occur in a woman experiencing her first pregnancy with those in a woman who has experienced more than one pregnancy.

OLDER ADULTS

Concurrent with endocrine changes, ovarian function diminishes during a woman's 40s, and menstrual periods begin to cease between 40 and 55 years of age, although fertility may continue. Menopause is conventionally defined as 1 year with no menses. Just as menarche in the adolescent is one aspect of puberty, so menopause is only one aspect of this transitional phase of the life cycle. During this time, estrogen levels decrease, causing the labia and clitoris to become smaller. The labia majora also become flatter as body fat is lost. Pubic hair turns gray and is usually sparser. Other hormone levels change as well. Both adrenal androgens and ovarian testosterone levels markedly decrease after menopause, which may account in part for decreases in libido and in muscle mass and strength.

The vaginal introitus gradually constricts. The vagina narrows, shortens, and loses its rugation; and the mucosa becomes thin, pale, and dry, which may result in dyspareunia. The cervix becomes smaller and paler. The uterus decreases in size, and the endometrium thins.

The ovaries also decrease to approximately 1 to 2 cm. Follicles gradually disappear, and the surface of the ovary convolutes. Ovulation usually ceases about 1 to 2 years before menopause.

The ligaments and connective tissue of the pelvis sometimes lose their elasticity and tone, thus weakening the supportive sling for the pelvic contents. The vaginal walls may lose some of their structural integrity.

Menopause has systemic effects, which include an increase in body fat and intraabdominal deposition of body fat (tendency toward male pattern of body fat distribution). Levels of total and low-density lipoprotein cholesterol increase. Thermoregulation is altered, which produces the hot flushes associated with menopause. After menopause, women experience an increased risk of cardiovascular disease. Postmenopausal hormone replacement (estrogen with or without progestin) is prescribed to reduce the impact of menopausal symptoms and sequelae.

REVIEW OF RELATED HISTORY

For each of the conditions discussed in this section, targeted topics to include in the history of the present illness are listed. Responses to questions about these topics help fully assess the patient's condition and provide clues for focusing the physical examination.

HISTORY OF PRESENT ILLNESS

- Abnormal bleeding
  - Character: shortened interval between periods (less than 19 to 21 days), lengthened interval between periods (more than 37 days), amenorrhea, prolonged menses (more than 7 days), bleeding between periods; postmenopausal bleeding
  - Change in flow: nature of change, number of pads or tampons used in 24 hours (tampons/pads soaked?), presence of clots
  - Temporal sequence: onset, duration, precipitating factors, course since onset
  - Associated symptoms: pain, cramping, abdominal distention, pelvic fullness, change in bowel habits, weight loss or gain
  - Medications: prescription or nonprescription; oral contraceptives; hormones; Tamoxifen
- Pain
  - Temporal sequence: date and time of onset, sudden versus gradual onset, course since onset, duration, recurrence
  - Character: specific location, type, and intensity of pain
  - Associated symptoms: vaginal discharge or bleeding, gastrointestinal symptoms, abdominal distention or tenderness, pelvic fullness
  - Association with menstrual cycle: timing, location, duration, changes
  - Relationship to body functions and activities: voiding, eating, defecation, flatus, exercise, walking up stairs, bending, stretching, sexual activity
  - Aggravating or relieving factors
  - Previous medical care for this problem
  - Efforts to treat
  - Medications: prescription or nonprescription
- Vaginal discharge
  - Character: amount, color, odor, consistency, changes in characteristics
  - Occurrence: acute or chronic
  - Douching habits
  - Clothing habits: use of cotton or ventilated underwear and pantyhose, tight pants or jeans
  - Sexual history—see in personal and social history
  - Presence of discharge or symptoms in sexual partner
  - Use of condoms
  - Associated symptoms: itching; tender, inflamed, or bleeding external tissues; dyspareunia; dysuria or burning on urination; abdominal pain or cramping; pelvic fullness
  - Efforts to treat: antifungal vaginal cream
  - Medications: prescription or nonprescription; oral contraceptives, antibiotics

- Premenstrual symptoms complaint
  - Symptoms: headaches, weight gain, edema, breast tenderness, irritability or mood changes
  - Frequency: every period?
  - Interference with activities of daily living
  - Relief measures
  - Aggravating factors
  - Medications: prescription or nonprescription
- Menopausal symptoms complaint
  - Age at menopause or currently experiencing
  - Symptoms: menstrual changes, mood changes, tension, hot flashes
  - Postmenopausal bleeding
  - General feelings about menopause: self-image, effect on intimate relationships
  - Mother's experience with menopause
  - Birth control measures during menopause
  - Medications: hormone therapy, dose and duration, related side effects: breast tenderness, bloating, vaginal bleeding; serum estrogen receptor modulators, related side effects: hot flashes, breast tenderness; other medications prescription or nonprescription
  - Use of complementary/alternative therapies, soy, other natural estrogen products
- Infertility
  - Length of time attempting pregnancy, sexual activity pattern, knowledge of fertile period in menstrual cycle, length of cycle
  - Abnormalities of vagina, cervix, uterus, fallopian tubes, ovaries
  - Contributing factors: stress, nutrition, chemical substances
  - Partner factors (see Chapter 19)
  - Diagnostic evaluation to date
- Urinary symptoms: dysuria, burning on urination, frequency, urgency
  - Character: acute or chronic; frequency of occurrence; last episode; onset; course since onset; feel like bladder is empty or not after voiding; pain at start, throughout, or at cessation of urination
  - Description of urine: color, presence of blood or particles, clear or cloudy
  - Associated symptoms: vaginal discharge or bleeding, abdominal pain or cramping, abdominal distention, pelvic fullness, flank pain
  - Medications: prescription or nonprescription

PAST MEDICAL HISTORY

- Menstrual history
  - Age of menarche
  - Date of last normal menstrual period: first day of last cycle
  - Number of days in cycle and regularity of cycle
  - Character of flow: amount (number of pads or tampons used in 24 hours on heaviest days), duration, presence and size of clots
  - Dysmenorrhea: characteristics, duration, frequency (occurs with each cycle?), relief measures
  - Intermenstrual bleeding or spotting: amount, duration, frequency, timing in relation to phase of cycle
  - Intermenstrual pain: severity, duration, timing; association with ovulation
  - Premenstrual symptoms: headaches, weight gain, edema, breast tenderness, irritability or mood changes, frequency (occur with every period?), interference with activities of daily living, relief measures
- Obstetric history
  - G: Gravity: total number of pregnancies
  - T: number of term pregnancies
  - P: number of preterm pregnancies

- ◆ A: number of abortions, spontaneous or induced
- ◆ L: number of living children
- ◆ Complications of pregnancy, delivery, abortion, or with fetus or neonate
- ◆ Menopausal history
  - ◆ Age of menopause or currently experiencing
  - ◆ Associated symptoms: menstrual changes, mood changes, tension, hot flashes
  - ◆ Postmenopausal bleeding
  - ◆ Birth control measures during menopause
  - ◆ General feelings about menopause: self-image, effect on intimate relationships
  - ◆ Mother's experience with menopause
  - ◆ Medications: hormone therapy; dose and duration, related side effects: breast tenderness, bloating, vaginal bleeding; serum estrogen receptor modulators, related side effects: hot flashes, breast tenderness; other medications, prescription or nonprescription
  - ◆ Use of complementary/alternative therapies

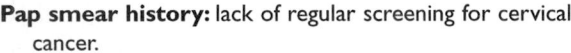

RISK FACTORS
CERVICAL CANCER

Pap smear history: lack of regular screening for cervical cancer.

HPV infection: human papillomavirus (HPV) infection is common and only a small percentage of women infected with untreated HPV will develop cervical cancer. The "high-risk" types include HPV 16, HPV 18, HPV 31, HPV 33, and HPV 45, as well as some others.

Sexual history: sexual intercourse before 16 years of age; multiple sexual partners (increases risk of HPV infection).

Cigarette smoking: doubles the risk; tobacco by-products have been found in the cervical mucus of women who smoke.

HIV infection: increased susceptibility to HPV infections.

Diet: diets low in fruits and vegetables may increase risk for cervical cancer; overweight women are more likely to develop this cancer.

Race: invasive cancer rates are higher in blacks, Hispanics, and Native Americans/American Indians.

DES exposure: women whose mothers took diethylstilbestrol (DES) during pregnancy (prescribed to women at high risk of miscarriages between 1940 and 1971).

Oral contraceptives: data are inconsistent and it is difficult to separate the risk of using oral contraceptives from other risk factors such as early age at first sexual intercourse and a history of multiple sexual partners. Some evidence indicates that long-term use (more than 5 years) may slightly increase the risk of cervical cancer.

Low socioeconomic status: likely related to access to health care services, including Pap tests and treatment of precancerous cervical disease.

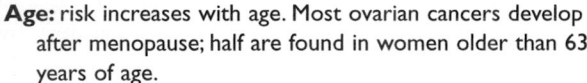

RISK FACTORS
OVARIAN CANCER

Age: risk increases with age. Most ovarian cancers develop after menopause; half are found in women older than 63 years of age.

Reproductive history: early menarche (before age 12), infertility, nulliparity, or first child after age 30, menopause after age 50. Relationship between the number of menstrual cycles in a woman's lifetime and her risk of developing ovarian cancer.

Use of fertility drugs: increased risk in some studies, especially if pregnancy is not achieved.

Family history: one or more first-degree relatives (mother, sister, daughter) with ovarian and/or breast cancer; strong family history of colon cancers; Ashkenazi Jewish descent and a family history of breast and/or ovarian cancer.

Personal history: breast, endometrial, and/or colon cancers.

Inherited genetic mutation: known inherited mutation of the BRCA1 or BRCA2 gene.

Race: occurs 50% more frequently in white women than black women.

Hormone replacement therapy: in postmenopausal women, very slightly increases the risk for ovarian cancer.

Diet: high-fat diet associated with higher rates of ovarian cancer in industrialized nations, but the link remains unproven.

Talcum powder: use of cosmetic talc in feminine hygiene sprays or in sanitary napkins has been suggested as a risk factor, although this is not a consistent finding. No evidence at present links cornstarch powders with any female cancers.

- Gynecologic history
  - Prior Papanicolaou (Pap) smears and results
  - Prior abnormal Pap smears, when, how treated, follow-up
  - Recent gynecologic procedures
  - Past gynecologic procedures or surgery (tubal ligation, hysterectomy, oophorectomy, laparoscopy, cryosurgery, conization)
  - Sexually transmitted infections
  - Pelvic inflammatory disease
  - Vaginal infections
  - Diabetes
  - Cancer of reproductive organs or related cancers (breast, colorectal)

FAMILY HISTORY

- Diabetes
- Cancer of reproductive organs
- Mother received diethylstilbestrol (DES) while pregnant with patient
- Multiple pregnancies
- Congenital anomalies

PERSONAL AND SOCIAL HISTORY

- Cleansing routines: use of sprays, powders, perfume, antiseptic soap, deodorants, or ointments
- Contraceptive history
  - Current method: length of time used, effectiveness, consistency of use, side effects, satisfaction with method
  - Previous methods: duration of use for each, side effects, and reasons for discontinuing each

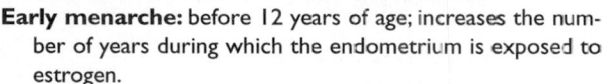
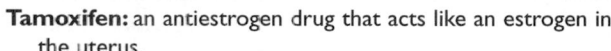

RISK FACTORS

ENDOMETRIAL CANCER

Early menarche: before 12 years of age; increases the number of years during which the endometrium is exposed to estrogen.

Late menopause: after 50 years of age; increases the number of years during which the endometrium is exposed to estrogen. Women with increased bleeding during perimenopause have an increased risk (4 times greater) of endometrial cancer.

Total length of menstruation span: may be a more important factor than age at menarche or menopause. For example, early menarche is less a risk factor for women who also have early menopause. Likewise early menarche *and* late menopause would be higher risk.

Infertility or nulliparity: during pregnancy, the hormonal balance shifts toward more progesterone. Therefore, having many pregnancies reduces endometrial cancer risk, and women who have not been pregnant have a higher risk.

Obesity: having more fat tissue can increase a woman's estrogen levels and therefore increase her endometrial cancer risk. Obesity increases a woman's risk of endometrial cancer by 2 to 5 times.

Tamoxifen: an antiestrogen drug that acts like an estrogen in the uterus.

Estrogen replacement therapy (ERT): estrogen alone (without progestins) in women with a uterus.

Ovarian diseases: polycystic ovaries and some ovarian tumors such as granulosa-theca cell tumors cause an increase in estrogen relative to progestin.

Diet: diet high in animal fat

Diabetes: endometrial cancer more common in women with both type I and type II diabetes.

Age: risk increases with age; 95% of endometrial cancers occur in women 40 years of age or older. The average age at diagnosis is 60.

Family history: of endometrial breast, ovarian or colorectal cancers.

Personal history: breast, ovarian, or colorectal cancer; known genetic mutation in BRCA1 or BRCA2.

Prior pelvic radiation therapy: radiation used to treat some other cancers can damage the DNA of cells, sometimes increasing the risk of developing a second type of cancer such as endometrial cancer.

Staying Well

Genital Self-Examination for Women

Genital self-examination (GSE) is now recommended for anyone who is at risk for contracting a sexually transmitted infection (STI). This includes sexually active persons who have had more than one sexual partner or whose partner has had other partners. The purpose of GSE is to detect any signs or symptoms that might indicate the presence of an STI. Many people who have an STI do not know that they have one, and some STIs can remain undetected for years. GSE should become a regular part of routine self-health care practices.

You should explain and demonstrate the following procedure to your patients and give them the opportunity to perform a GSE under your guidance. Emphasize hand-washing before and afterward.

Instruct the patient to start by examining the area that the pubic hair covers. Patients may want to use a mirror and position it so that they can see their entire genital area. The pubic hair should then be spread apart with the fingers, and the woman should carefully look for any bumps, sores, or blisters on the skin. Bumps and blisters may be red or light-colored or resemble pimples. Also instruct the patient to look for warts, which may look similar to warts on other parts of the body. At first they may be small, bumpy spots; left untreated, however, they could develop a fleshy, cauliflower-like appearance (see Fig. 18-44).

Next, instruct the patient to spread the outer vaginal lips and look closely at the hood of the clitoris. She should gently pull the hood up to see the clitoris and again look for any bumps, blisters, sores, or warts. Then both sides of the inner vaginal lips should be examined for the same signs.

Have the patient move on to examine the area around the urinary and vaginal openings, looking for any bumps, blisters, sores, or warts (see Figs. 18-44 through 18-48). Some signs of STIs may be out of view—in the vagina or near the cervix; therefore, if patients believe that they have come in contact with an STI, they should see their health care provider even if no signs or symptoms are discovered during self-examination.

Also educate patients about other symptoms associated with STIs: specifically, pain or burning on urination, pain in the pelvic area, bleeding between menstrual periods, or an itchy rash around the vagina. Some STIs may cause a vaginal discharge. Because most women have a vaginal discharge from time to time, they should try to be aware of what their normal discharge looks like. Discharge caused by an STI will be different from the usual; it may be yellow and thicker and have an odor.

Instruct patients to see a health care provider if they have any of the above signs or symptoms.

- Douching history
  - Frequency: length of time since last douche; number of years douching
  - Method
  - Solution used
  - Reason for douching
- Sexual history
  - Current sexual activity: number of current and previous partners; number of their partners; gender of partner(s), sexual preference
  - Method(s) of contraception: current and past; satisfaction with
  - Use of barrier protection for sexually transmitted infections (STIs)
  - Prior STIs
  - Satisfaction with relationship(s), sexual pleasure achieved, frequency
  - Problems: pain on penetration (entry or deep); decreased lubrication, lack of orgasm
- Performance of genital self-examination (see the Staying Well box above)
- Date of last pelvic examination
- Date of last Pap smear and results
- Use of club/street/recreational drugs

Infants and Children

Usually no special questions are required unless there is a specific complaint from the parent or child.

- Bleeding
  - Character: onset, duration, precipitating factor if known, course since onset
  - Age of mother at menarche
  - Associated symptoms: pain, change in crying of infant, child fearful of parent or other adults
  - Parental suspicion about insertion of foreign objects by child
  - Parental suspicion about possible sexual abuse

BOX 18-1

EVALUATION OF MASTURBATION IN CHILDREN

Masturbation is a common, healthy, self-discovery activity in children. Parents sometimes express concern about their child's masturbation activity. The following guidelines can help you determine when such activity might be a cause for concern.

Healthy Activity	**Needs Further Assessment**
Occasional	Frequent, compulsive
Discreet, private	No regard for privacy
Not preferred over other activity or play	Often preferred over other activity or play
No physical signs or symptoms	Produces genital discomfort, irritation, or physical signs
External stimulation of genitalia only	Involves penetration of the genital orifices; includes bizarre practices or rituals

From Haka-Ikse, Mian, 1993.

---

* Pain
    * Character: type of pain, onset, course since onset, duration
    * Specific location
    * Associated symptoms: vaginal discharge or bleeding, urinary symptoms, gastrointestinal symptoms, child fearful of parent or other adults
    * Contributory problems: use of bubble bath, irritating soaps, or detergents; parental suspicion about insertion of foreign objects by child or about possible sexual abuse
* Vaginal discharge
    * Relationship to diapers: use of powder or lotions, how frequently diapers are changed
    * Associated symptoms: pain, bleeding
    * Contributory problems: parental suspicion about insertion of foreign objects by child or about possible sexual abuse
* Urinary symptoms in infants and young children
* Diarrhea
* Excessive crying that cannot be resolved by typical measures (e.g., feeding, holding)
* Loss of appetite
* Fever
* Nausea and vomiting
* Masturbation (Box 18-1)

ADOLESCENTS

As the older child matures, you should ask her the same questions that you ask adult women. You should not assume that youthful age precludes sexual activity or any of the related concerns. While taking the history, it is necessary at some point to talk with the child alone while the parent is out of the room. Your questions should be posed in a gentle, matter-of-fact, and nonjudgmental manner.

PREGNANT WOMEN

* Expected date of delivery (EDC) or weeks of gestation
* Previous obstetric history: GPTAL, prenatal complications, infertility treatment
* Previous birth history: length of gestation at birth, birth weight, fetal outcome, length of labor, fetal presentation, type of delivery, use of forceps, lacerations and/or episiotomy, complications (natal and postnatal)
* Previous menstrual history (see menstrual history under Past Medical History)
* Surgical history: prior uterine surgery and type of scar
* Family history: diabetes mellitus, multiple births, preeclampsia, genetic disorder
* Involuntary passage of fluid, which may result from rupture of membranes (ROM); determine onset, duration, color, odor, amount, and if still leaking

- Bleeding
  - Character: onset, duration, precipitating factor if known (e.g., intercourse, trauma), course since onset, amount
  - Associated symptoms
  - Pain: type (e.g., sharp or dull, intermittent or continuous), onset, location, duration
- Gastrointestinal symptoms: nausea, vomiting, heartburn

OLDER ADULTS

- See Past Medical History: Menopausal history
- Symptoms associated with age-related physiologic changes: itching, urinary symptoms, dyspareunia
- Changes in sexual desire or behavior in self or partner(s)

EXAMINATION AND FINDINGS

EQUIPMENT

- Drapes
- Speculum
- Gloves
- Water-soluble lubricant
- Specimen collection equipment:
  - Sterile cotton swabs
  - Glass slides
  - Wooden or plastic spatula
  - Cervical brush or broom devices
  - Cytologic fixative
  - Culture plates or media
- DNA probe kits for chlamydia and gonorrhea, if needed
- Lamp or light source

PREPARATION

The pelvic examination may be accompanied by some anxiety on the part of both the patient and a novice examiner. Although most women express lack of enthusiasm in anticipation of a pelvic examination, most do not experience anxiety. Marked anxiety before an examination may be a sign that something is not quite right. Before beginning you should find out the source of the anxiety. It could be a bad experience either in a patient's personal life (e.g., child abuse, sexual assault) or during a previous pelvic examination. It could be the lack of familiarly with what she can expect during the examination; it could be worry about possible findings or their meaning. Do not assume you know—use your skills and ask. It is your job to minimize the patient's apprehension and discomfort. Explain in general terms what you are going to do. Maintain eye contact with the patient, both before and, as much as possible, during the examination. Women from some various cultural or ethnic groups may not return eye contact as a show of respect. Be sensitive to cultural variations in behavior. If the patient has not seen the equipment before, show it to her, and explain its use.

Assure the patient that you will explain to her what you are doing as the examination proceeds. Let her know that you will be as gentle as possible, and to let you know if she feels any discomfort.

Make sure that the room temperature is comfortable and that privacy is ensured. The door should be securely closed and should be opened only with permission of both the patient and examiner. The examination table should be positioned so that the patient faces away from it during the examination. A crawn curtain can ensure that any door opening will not expose the patient. Ideally, examiners of either gender will be accompanied by a female assistant. An assistant or chaperone is often required by policy and protects both the examiner and patient. Some patients may be reluctant to reveal confidential and sensitive material in the presence of an observer.

Have the patient empty her bladder before the examination. Bimanual examination is extremely uncomfortable for the woman if her bladder is full. A full bladder also makes it difficult to palpate the pelvic organs.

POSITIONING

Assist the patient into the lithotomy position on the examining table. (If a table with stirrups is not available or if the woman is unable to assume the lithotomy position, the examination can be performed in other positions (see pp. 620 and 621). Help the woman stabilize her feet in the stirrups and slide her buttocks down to the edge of the examining table. Place your hand at the edge of the table and instruct her to move down until she touches your hand. If the patient is not positioned correctly, you will have difficulty with the speculum examination.

DRAPING AND GLOVING

CLINICAL PEARL

Gloving

Once you have touched any of the patient's genital skin, assume that your glove is "contaminated." Do not touch any surfaces or instruments that will not be discarded or immediately disinfected until you remove or change your gloves. This includes lights, drawers, door handles, counter surfaces, examining table surfaces, fixative and specimen bottles and jars, and patient records. Change gloves as often as you need to. Some clinicians prefer to double or triple glove at the beginning of an examination and then remove a glove when a clean hand is needed.

The patient can be draped in such a way that allows minimal exposure. A good method is to cover her knees and symphysis, depressing the drape between her knees. This allows you to see the woman's face (and she, yours) throughout the examination (Fig. 18-10).

Once the patient is positioned and draped, make sure that any equipment is nearby and in easy reach. Arrange the examining lamp so that the external genitalia are clearly visible. Wash your hands and put gloves on both hands.

Ask the woman to separate or drop open her knees. Never try to spread her legs forcibly or even gently. The pelvic examination is an intrusive procedure, and you may need to wait a moment until the woman is ready. Tell her that you are going to begin, then start with a neutral touch on her lower thigh, moving your examining hand along the thigh without breaking contact, to the external genitalia.

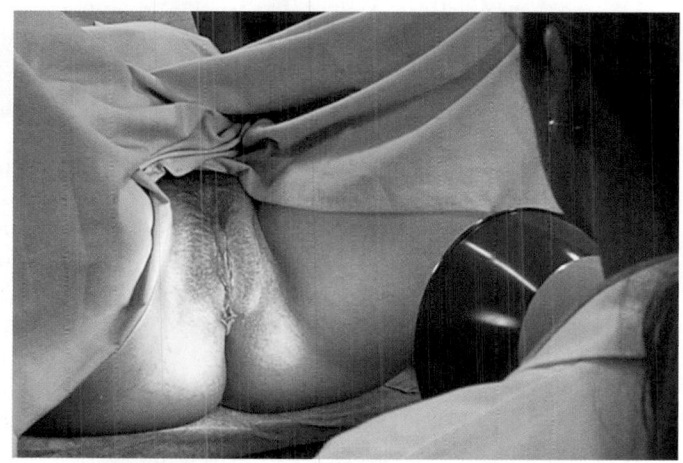

FIGURE 18-10
Draped patient in dorsal lithotomy position.

EXTERNAL EXAMINATION

INSPECTION AND PALPATION

Sit at the end of the examining table and inspect and palpate the external genitalia. Look at the hair distribution and notice the surface characteristics of the mons pubis and labia majora. The skin should be smooth and clean, the hair free of nits or lice.

LABIA MAJORA

The labia majora may be gaping or closed and may appear dry or moist. They are usually symmetric and may be either shriveled or full. The tissue should feel soft and homogeneous. Labial swelling, redness, or tenderness, particularly if unilateral, may be indicative of a Bartholin gland abscess. Look for excoriation, rashes, or lesions, which suggest an infectious or inflammatory process. If any of these signs are present, ask the woman if she has been scratching. Observe for discoloration, varicosities, obvious stretching, or signs of trauma or scarring.

LABIA MINORA

Separate the labia majora with the fingers of one hand and inspect the labia minora. Use your other hand to palpate the labia minora between your thumb and second finger; then separate the labia minora and inspect and palpate the inside of the labia minora, clitoris, urethral orifice, vaginal introitus, and perineum (Fig. 18-11).

The labia minora may appear symmetric or asymmetric, and the inner surface should be moist and dark pink. The tissue should feel soft, homogeneous, and without tenderness (Fig. 18-12). Look for inflammation, irritation, excoriation, or caking of discharge in the tissue folds, which suggests vaginal infection or poor hygiene. Discoloration or tenderness may be the result of traumatic bruising. Ulcers or vesicles may be signs of a sexually transmitted infection. Feel for irregularities or nodules.

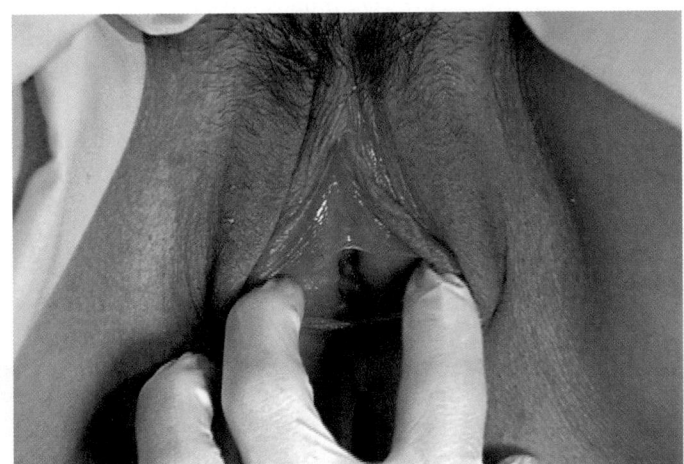

FIGURE 18-11
Separation of the labia.

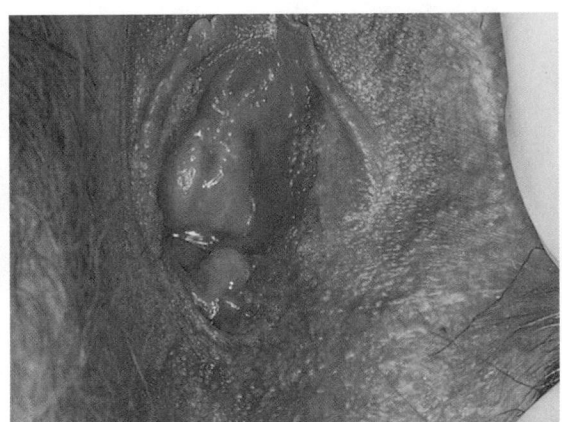

FIGURE 18-12
Normal vulva with finely textured papular sebaceous glands on the inner labia majora and labia minora.
From Morse et al, 2003.

CLITORIS

Inspect the clitoris for size. Generally the clitoris is about 2 cm or less in length and 0.5 cm in diameter. Enlargement may be a sign of a masculinizing condition. Observe also for atrophy, inflammation, or adhesions.

URETHRAL ORIFICE

The urethral orifice appears as an irregular opening or slit. It may be close to or slightly within the vaginal introitus and is usually in the midline. Inspect for discharge, polyps, caruncles, and fistulas. Signs of irritation, inflammation, or dilation suggest repeated urinary tract infections or insertion of foreign objects. Ask questions about any findings at a later time—not during the pelvic examination when the woman feels most vulnerable.

VAGINAL INTROITUS

The vaginal introitus can be a thin vertical slit or a large orifice with irregular edges from hymenal remnants (myrtiform caruncles). The tissue should be moist. Look for swelling, discoloration, discharge, lesions, fistulas, or fissures.

SKENE AND BARTHOLIN GLANDS

With the labia still separated, examine the Skene and Bartholin glands. Tell the woman you are going to insert one finger in her vagina and that she will feel you pressing forward with it. With your palm facing upward, insert the index finger of the examining hand into the vagina as far as the second joint of the finger. Exerting upward pressure, milk the Skene glands by moving the finger outward. Do this on both sides of the urethra, and then directly on the urethra (Fig. 18-13). Look for discharge and note any tenderness. If a discharge occurs, note its color, consistency, and odor, and obtain a culture. Discharge from the Skene glands or urethra usually indicates an infection, most commonly, but not necessarily, gonococcal.

With your finger still in place, you can then locate the cervix and note the direction in which it points. This may help you locate the cervix when you insert the speculum.

Maintaining labial separation and with your finger still in the vaginal opening, tell the patient that she will feel you pressing around the entrance to the vagina. Palpate the lateral tissue between your index finger and thumb. Palpate the entire area, paying particular attention to the posterolateral portion of the labia majora where the Bartholin glands are located. Note any swelling, tenderness, masses, heat, or fluctuation. Observe for discharge from the opening of the Bartholin gland duct. Palpate and observe bilaterally, because each gland is separate (Fig. 18-14). Note the color, consistency, and odor of any discharge, and obtain a specimen for culture. Swelling that is painful, hot to the touch, and fluctuant is indicative of an abscess of the Bartholin gland. The abscess is usually gonococcal or staphylococcal in origin and is pus filled. A nontender mass is indicative of a Bartholin cyst, which is the result of chronic inflammation of the gland.

MUSCLE TONE

Test muscle tone if the woman has borne children or has told you about signs of weak muscle tone (e.g., urinary incontinence or the sensation of something "falling out"). To test, ask the patient to squeeze the vaginal opening around your finger, explaining that you are testing

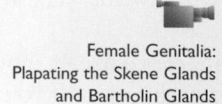

Female Genitalia: Plapating the Skene Glands and Bartholin Glands

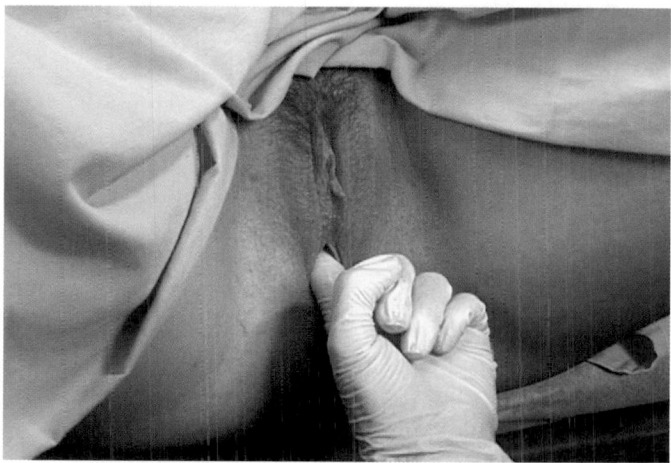

FIGURE 18-13
Palpation of Skene glands.

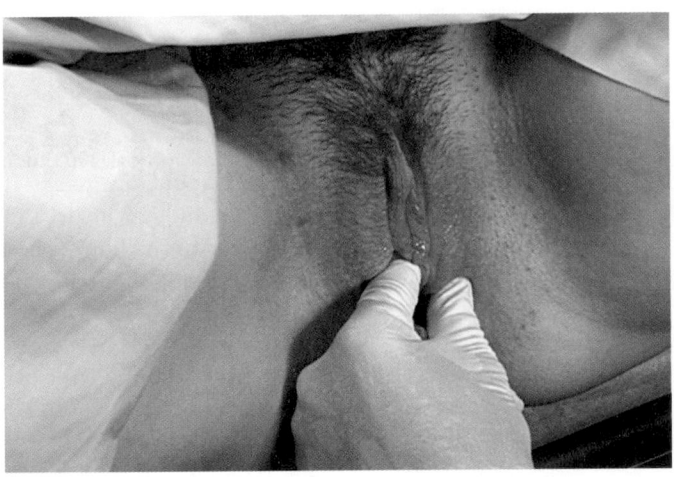

FIGURE 18-14
Palpation of Bartholin glands.

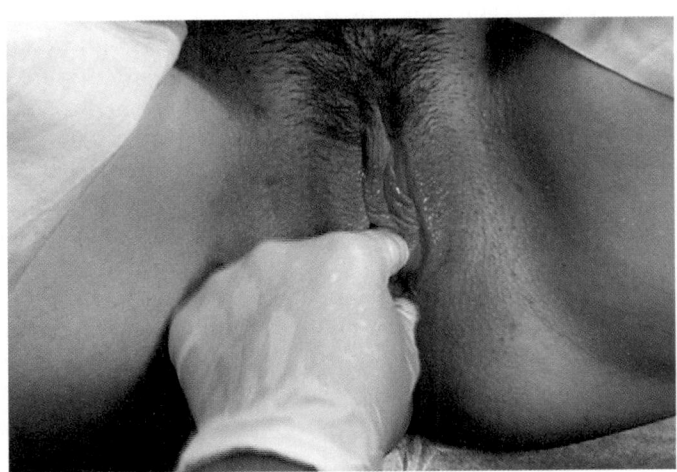

FIGURE 18-15
Palpating the perineum.

muscle tone. Then ask the patient to bear down as you watch for bulging and urinary incontinence. Bulging of the anterior wall and urinary incontinence indicate the presence of a cystocele. Bulging of the posterior wall indicates a rectocele. Uterine prolapse is marked by protrusion of the cervix or uterus on straining.

PERINEUM

Inspect and palpate the perineum. The perineal surface should be smooth; episiotomy scarring may be evident in women who have borne children. The tissue will feel thick and smooth in the nulliparous woman. It will be thinner and rigid in multiparous women. In either case, it should not be tender. Look for inflammation, fistulas, lesions, or growths (Fig. 18-15).

ANUS

The anal surface is more darkly pigmented, and the skin may appear coarse. It should be free of scarring, lesions, inflammation, fissures, lumps, skin tags, or excoriation. If you touch the anus or perianal skin, be sure to change your gloves so that you do not introduce bacteria into the vagina during the internal examination.

INTERNAL EXAMINATION

PREPARATION

It is essential that you become familiar with how the speculum operates before you begin the examination, so that you do not inadvertently hurt the woman through mishandling of the instrument. Chapter 3 describes the proper use of the speculum. Become familiar with both the reusable stainless steel and the disposable plastic specula, because their mechanisms of action are somewhat different.

EVIDENCE-BASED PRACTICE IN PHYSICAL EXAMINATION

LUBRICATING THE SPECULUM

The conventional wisdom has been that gel lubricants should not be used when collecting a pap smear specimen because the gel could obscure cellular elements and interfere with specimen analysis and interpretation. Two recent studies (Amies et al, 2002; Harer et al, 2002) and an earlier report (Cassleman et al, 1997) question this premise and show evidence that using a water-soluble gel lubricant does not adversely affect cellular analysis with conventional Pap smears. However, a recent report (Zardawi et al, 2003) documents contamination by excess gel in some instances with both conventional and liquid-based pap smears. Our advice: Until further studies conclusively determine that gel lubricant does not adversely interfere with specimen analysis, we continue to recommend lubrication with water. However, if gel lubricant is used, a thin layer on the external surface of the blades only will help avoid contamination of the specimen.

Lubricate the speculum (and the gloved fingers) with water or a water-soluble lubricant. Most clinicians routinely lubricate with water only. An added advantage of using water as a lubricant is that a cold speculum can be warmed by rinsing in warm (but not hot) water. A speculum can also be warmed by holding it in your hand (if it is warm) or under the lamp for a few minutes.

Select the appropriate size speculum (see Chapter 3) and hold it in your hand with the index finger over the top of the proximal end of the anterior blade and the other fingers around the handle. This position controls the blades as the speculum is inserted into the vagina.

INSERTION OF SPECULUM

Tell the patient that she is going to feel you touching her again, and gently insert a finger of your other hand just inside the vaginal introitus and apply pressure downward. Ask the woman to breathe slowly and to try to consciously relax her muscles or the muscles of her buttocks. Wait until you feel the relaxation (Fig. 18-16, *A*). Use the fingers of that hand to separate the labia minora very widely so that the hymenal opening becomes clearly visible. Then slowly insert the speculum along the path of least resistance, often slightly downward, avoiding trauma to the urethra and vaginal walls. Some clinicians insert the speculum blades at an oblique angle; others prefer to keep the blades horizontal. In either case, avoid touching the clitoris, catching pubic hair, or pinching labial skin (Fig. 18-16, *B* and *C*).

Insert the speculum the length of the vaginal canal. While maintaining gentle downward pressure with the speculum, open it by pressing on the thumb piece. Sweep the speculum slowly upward until the cervix comes into view. Gently reposition the speculum, if necessary, to locate the cervix. Adjust the light source.

Once the cervix is visualized, manipulate the speculum so that the cervix is well exposed between the anterior and posterior blades. Lock the speculum blades into place to stabilize the distal spread of the blades, and adjust the proximal spread as needed (Fig. 18-16, *D*).

CERVIX

Inspect the cervix for color, position, size, surface characteristics, discharge, and size and shape of the os.

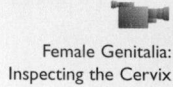

Female Genitalia:
Inspecting the Cervix

Color. The cervix should be pink, with the color evenly distributed. A bluish color indicates increased vascularity, which may be a sign of pregnancy. Symmetric, circumscribed erythema around the os is an expected finding that indicates exposed columnar epithelium from the cervical canal. However, beginning practitioners should consider any reddened areas as an unexpected finding, especially if patchy or if the borders are irregular. A pale cervix is associated with anemia.

Position. The position of the cervix correlates with the position of the uterus. A cervix that is pointing anteriorly indicates a retroverted uterus; one pointing posteriorly indicates an anteverted uterus. A cervix in the horizontal position indicates a uterus in midposition. The cervix should be located in the midline. Deviation to the right or left may indicate a pelvic mass, uterine adhesions, or pregnancy. The cervix may protrude 1 to 3 cm into the vagina. Projection greater than 3 cm may indicate a pelvic or uterine mass. The cervix of a woman of childbearing age is usually 2 to 3 cm in diameter. An enlarged cervix is generally indicative of a cervical infection.

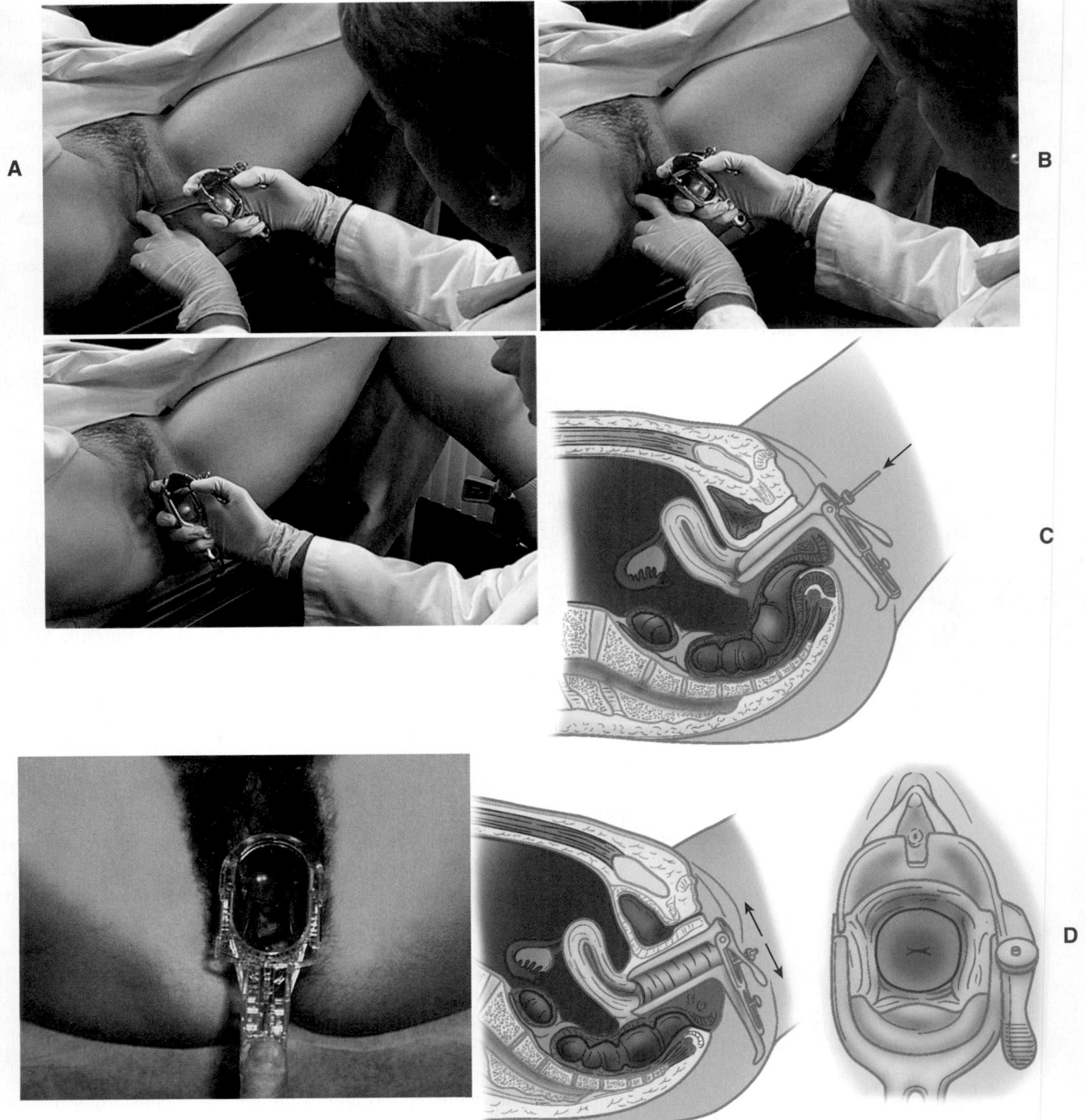

FIGURE 18-16
Examination of the internal genitalia with a speculum. Begin by inserting a finger and applying downward pressure to relax the vaginal muscles. **A,** Gently insert the closed speculum blades into the vagina. **B,** Direct the speculum along the path of least resistance. **C,** Insert the speculum the length of the vaginal canal. **D,** Speculum is in place, locked, and stabilized. Note cervix in full view.
D (photo) from Edge, Miller, 1994.

Surface Characteristics. The surface of the cervix should be smooth. Some squamocolumnar epithelium of the cervical canal may be visible as a symmetric reddened circle around the os (Fig. 18-17). Nabothian cysts may be observed as small, white or yellow, raised, round areas on the cervix. These are retention cysts of the endocervical glands and are considered an expected finding. An infected nabothian cyst becomes swollen with fluid and distorts the shape of the cervix, giving it an irregular appearance. Look for friable tissue, red patchy areas, granular areas, and white patches that could indicate cervicitis, infection, or carcinoma.

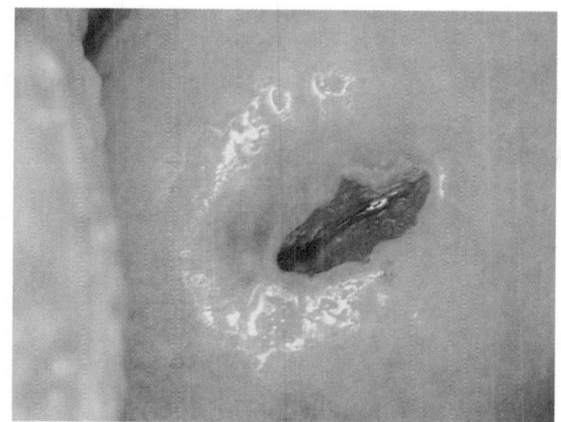

FIGURE 18-17
Normal cervix. The squamo-columnar junction and lower part of the endocervical canal are seen.
From Morse et al, 2003.

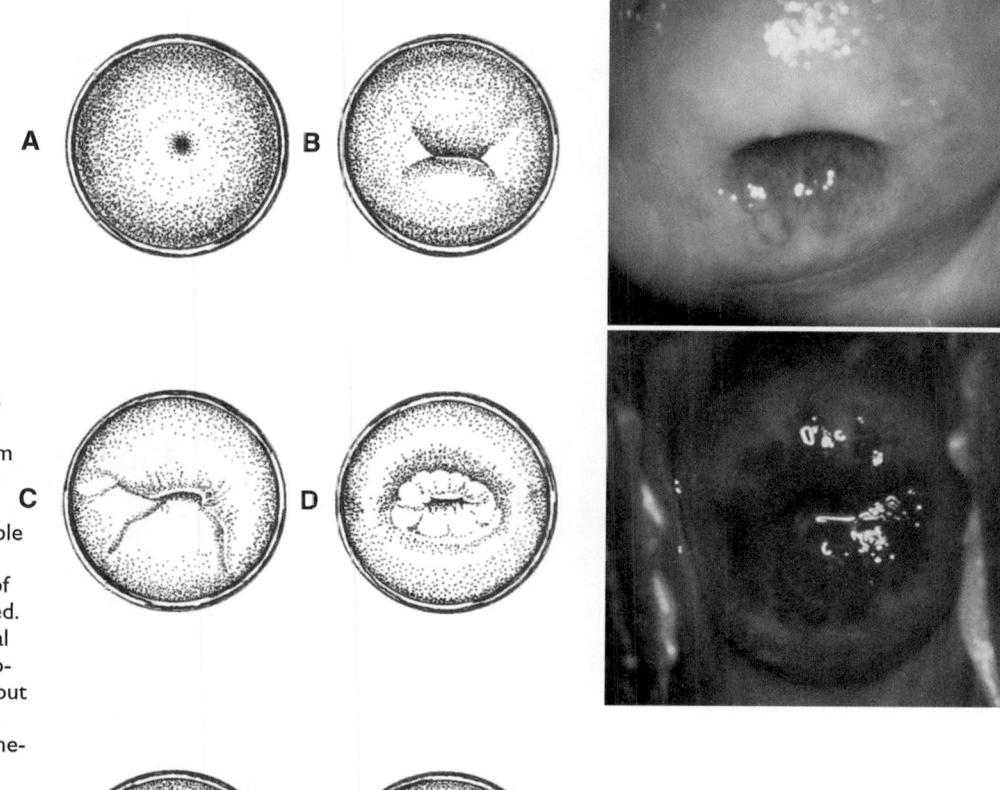

FIGURE 18-18
Common appearances of the cervix. **A,** Normal nulliparous cervix. The surface is covered with pink squamous epithelium that is uniform in consistency. The os is small and round. A small area of ectropion is visible inferior to the os. **B,** Parous cervix. Note slit appearance of os. **C,** Multigravidous, lacerated. **D,** Everted. Columnar mucosal cells usually found in the endocervical canal have extended out into the surface of the cervix, creating a circular raised erythematous appearance. Note the normal nonpurulent cervical mucus. This normal variant is not to be confused with cervicitis. **E,** Eroded. **F,** Nabothian cysts.
Photos from Zitelli, Davis, 1997; A courtesy C. Stevens; D courtesy E. Jerome, MD.

Discharge. Note any discharge. Determine whether the discharge comes from the cervix itself, or whether it is vaginal in origin and has only been deposited on the cervix. Usual discharge is odorless; may be creamy or clear; may be thick, thin, or stringy; and is often heavier at midcycle or immediately before menstruation. The discharge of a bacterial or fungal infection will more likely have an odor and will vary in color from white to yellow, green, or gray.
Size and Shape. The os of the nulliparous woman is small and round or oval. The os of a multiparous woman is usually a horizontal slit or may be irregular and stellate. Trauma from induced abortion or difficult removal of an intrauterine device may change the shape of the os to a slit (Fig. 18-18). Obtain specimens for Pap smear, culture, or other laboratory analysis as indicated in Box 18-2.

BOX 18-2

OBTAINING VAGINAL SMEARS AND CULTURES

Very often during the speculum examination, you will be obtaining vaginal specimens for smears and cultures. Vaginal specimens are obtained while the speculum is in place in the vagina, but after the cervix and its surrounding tissue have been inspected. Collect specimens as indicated for Pap smear, sexually transmitted infection screening, and wet mount. Label the specimen with the patient's name and a description of the specimen (e.g., cervical smear, vaginal smear, and culture). Be sure to follow Standard Precautions for the safe collection of human secretions.

Papanicolaou Smear

Brushes and brooms are now being used in conjunction with, or instead of, the conventional spatula to improve the quality of cells obtained. The cylindric-type brush collects endocervical cells only. First, collect a sample from the ectocervix with

a spatula (Figs. 18-19 and 18-20, A). Insert the longer projection of the spatula into the cervical os; rotate it 360 degrees, keeping it flush against the cervical tissue. Withdraw the spatula, and spread the specimen on a glass slide. A single light stroke with each side of the spatula is sufficient to thin the specimen out over the slide. Immediately spray with cytologic fixative and label the slide as the ectocervical specimen. Then introduce the brush device into the vagina and insert it into the cervical os until only the bristles closest to the handle are exposed (Fig. 18-20, B,C). Slowly rotate one half turn. Remove and prepare the endocervical smear by rolling and twisting the brush with moderate pressure across a glass slide. Fix the specimen with spray and label as the endocervical specimen.

The broom-type device is used for collecting both ectocervical and endocervical cells at the same time (see Fig. 18-20, D). This broom utilizes flexible plastic bristles, which are reported to cause less blood spotting after the examination. Introduce the brush into the vagina and insert the central long bristles into the cervical os until the lateral bristles

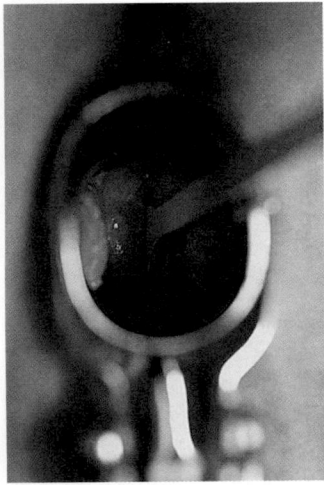

FIGURE 18-19
Scrape the cervix with the bifid end of the spatula for obtaining Pap smear.
From Symonds, Macpherson, 1994.

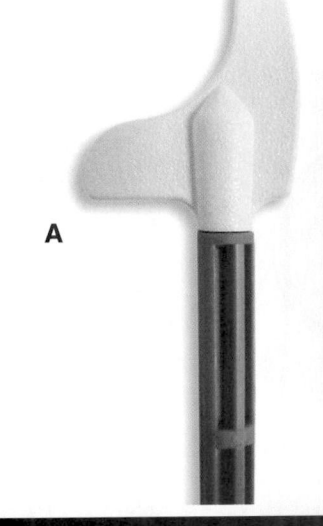

A

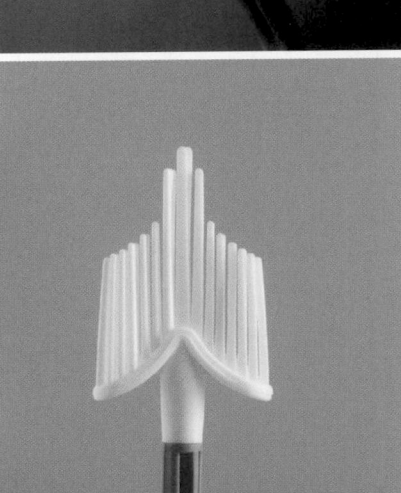

B

D

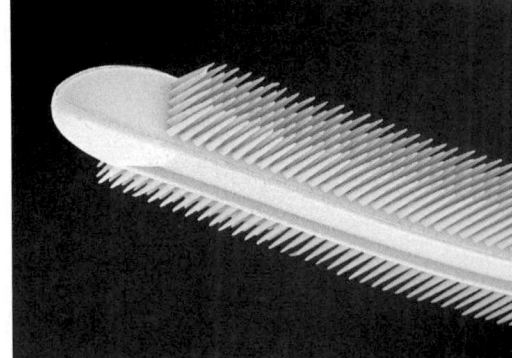

C

FIGURE 18-20
Implements used to obtain a Pap smear. **A,** Close-up of spatula. **B,** Brush device. **C,** Close-up of brush. **D,** Broom device.
Courtesy Therapak Corporation, Irwindale, CA.

BOX 18-2

OBTAINING VAGINAL SMEARS AND CULTURES—cont'd

bend fully against the ectocervix. Maintain gentle pressure and rotate the brush by rolling the handle between the thumb and forefinger three to five times to the left and right. Withdraw the brush, and transfer the sample to a glass slide with two single paint strokes: Apply first one side of the bristle, turn the brush over, and paint the slide again in exactly the same area. Apply fixative and label as the ectocervical and endocervical specimen.

For the thin prep technology procedure using the broom type device, insert the central bristles of the broom into the endocervical canal deep enough to allow the shorter bristles to fully contact the ectocervix. Push gently, and rotate the broom in a clockwise direction five times. Rinse the broom into the solution vial by pushing the broom into the bottom of the vial 10 times, forcing the bristles apart. As a final step, swirl the broom vigorously to further release material. Discard the collection device. Alternatively, deposit the broom end of the device directly into the collection vial. With any collection device, be sure to follow the manufacturer's and laboratory instructions to collect and preserve the specimen appropriately. Close the thin prep vial tightly to prevent leakage and loss of the sample during transport.

Gonococcal Culture Specimen

Immediately after the Pap smear is obtained, introduce a sterile cotton swab into the vagina and insert it into the cervical os (Fig. 18-21); hold it in place for 10 to 30 seconds. With-

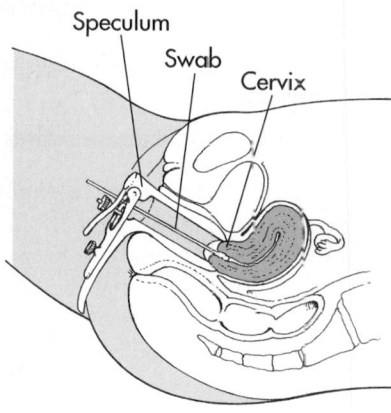

FIGURE 18-21
Obtaining a cervical specimen by inserting a swab into the cervical os.
From Grimes, 1991.

draw the swab and spread the specimen in a large Z pattern over the culture medium, rotating the swab at the same time. Label the tube or plate, and follow agency routine for transporting and warming the specimen. If indicated, an anal culture can be obtained after the vaginal speculum has been removed. Insert a fresh, sterile cotton swab about 2.5 cm into the rectum and rotate it full circle; hold it in place for 10 to 30 seconds. Withdraw the swab and prepare the specimen as described for the vaginal culture. Gonococcal cultures are now used less commonly than the combined DNA probe for chlamydia and gonorrhea.

DNA Probe for Chlamydia and Gonorrhea

This test involves the construction of nucleic acid sequence (called a probe) that will match to a sequence in the DNA or RNA of the target tissue. The results are rapid and sensitive. Use a Dacron swab (with plastic or wire shaft) when collecting your specimen, because wooden cotton-tipped applicators may interfere with the test results. Also be sure to check the expiration date so as not to use out-of-date materials. Insert the swab into the cervical os and rotate the swab in the endocervical canal for 30 seconds to ensure adequate sampling and absorption by the swab. Avoid contact with the vaginal mucous membranes, which would contaminate the specimen. Remove the swab and place it in the tube containing the specimen reagent.

Wet Mount and Potassium Hydroxide (KOH) Procedures

In a woman with vaginal discharge, these microscope examinations can demonstrate the presence of *Trichomonas vaginalis*, bacterial vaginosis, or candidiasis. For the wet mount, obtain a specimen of vaginal discharge using a swab. Smear the sample on a glass slide and add a drop of normal saline. Place a coverslip on the slide, and view under the microscope. The presence of trichomonads indicates *T. vaginalis*. The presence of bacteria-filled epithelial cells (clue cells) indicates bacterial vaginosis. On a separate glass slide, place a specimen of vaginal discharge, apply a drop of aqueous 10% KOH, and put a coverslip in place. The presence of fishy odor (the "whiff test") suggests bacterial vaginosis. The KOH dissolves epithelial cells and debris and facilitates visualization of the mycelia of a fungus. View under the microscope for the presence of mycelial fragments, hyphae, and budding yeast cells, which indicate candidiasis.

WITHDRAWAL OF SPECULUM

Unlock the speculum and remove it slowly and carefully so that you can inspect the vaginal walls. Note color, surface characteristics, and secretions. The color should be about the same color pink as the cervix, or a little lighter. Reddened patches, lesions, or pallor indicates a local or systemic pathologic condition. The surface should be moist, smooth or rugated, and homogeneous. Look for cracks, lesions, bleeding, nodules, and swelling. Secretions that may be expected are usually thin, clear or cloudy, and odorless. Secretions indicative of infection are often profuse; may be thick, curdy, or frothy; appear gray, green, or yellow; and may have a foul odor.

Evidence-Based Practice in Physical Examination

Pap Smear After Hysterectomy?

Most experts agree that women who have had a hysterectomy for noncancer reasons, with the cervix removed, no evidence of malignancy, and no history of abnormal cancerous cell growth, can discontinue Pap smears screening for cervical can-cer. The yield of cytologic screening is very low in women after hysterectomy and there is no evidence that continuing screening improves health outcomes. Annual pelvic examination should be continued.

American Cancer Society, 2002. National Cancer Institute, 2003, U.S. Preventive Services Task Force 2003.

BOX 18-3

Examining the Woman Who Has Had a Hysterectomy

Examination of a woman who has had a hysterectomy is essentially no different from the usual procedure. The same examination steps and sequence are followed, with minor variation in what you are assessing. Getting an accurate history before the examination will assist you in knowing what to look for. Determine whether the surgical approach was vaginal or abdominal, whether the woman had a total or partial hysterectomy (i.e., whether she still has fallopian tubes and ovaries), the reason for the hysterectomy, bladder or bowel changes since the surgery, and the presence of menopausal symptoms.

Examine the external genitalia for atrophy, skin changes, decreased resilience, and discharge. In these patients, specimens for gonococci or chlamydia are often taken at the vestibule rather than internally. On speculum examination, the cervix will be absent. In the woman who has had a vaginal hysterectomy, the surgical scar (vaginal cuff) will be visible at the end of the vaginal canal and will be an identifiable white or pink suture line in the posterior fornix. If indicated, a Pap smear should be taken from this suture line with the blunt end of the spatula. Be sure to label the specimen as vaginal cells; otherwise the report may be sent back as incomplete or unsatisfactory because of a lack of endocervical cell sample. Assess the walls, mucosa, and secretions as you ordinarily would. The vaginal canal of a woman who has had a total hysterectomy might show the same changes as those that occur with menopause (e.g., a decrease in rugae and secretions), especially if the woman is not receiving hormone replacement therapy. Examine for a cystocele or rectocele. Stress incontinence may be a problem, so observe for this when having the patient bear down.

On bimanual examination the uterus will obviously not be present; further findings will depend on whether the hysterectomy was total or partial. If partial, proceed with the examination as usual, assessing the ovaries and surrounding area. If the hysterectomy was total, assess the adnexal area for masses, adhesions, or tenderness. The bladder and bowel may feel more prominent than usual.

As you withdraw the speculum, the blades will tend to close themselves. Avoid pinching the cervix and vaginal walls. Maintain downward pressure of the speculum to avoid trauma to the urethra. Hook your index finger over the anterior blade as it is removed. Keep one thumb on the handle lever and control closing of the speculum. Make sure that the speculum is fully closed when the blades pass through the hymenal ring. Note the odor of any vaginal discharge that has pooled in the posterior blade and obtain a specimen, if you have not already done so. Deposit the speculum in the proper container.

BIMANUAL EXAMINATION

Inform the woman that you are going to examine her internally with your fingers. Change your gloves or remove the outer glove and lubricate the index and middle fingers of your examining hand. Insert the tips of the gloved index and middle fingers into the vaginal opening and press downward, again waiting for the muscles to relax. Gradually and gently insert your fingers their full length into the vagina. Palpate the vaginal wall as you insert your fingers. It should be smooth, homogeneous, and nontender. Feel for cysts, nodules, masses, or growths.

Be careful where you place your thumb during the bimanual examination. You can tuck it into the palm of your hand, but that will cut down on the distance you can insert your fingers. Be aware of where the thumb is and keep it from touching the clitoris, which can produce discomfort (Fig. 18-22).

Box 18-3 describes the examination of a woman who has had a hysterectomy.

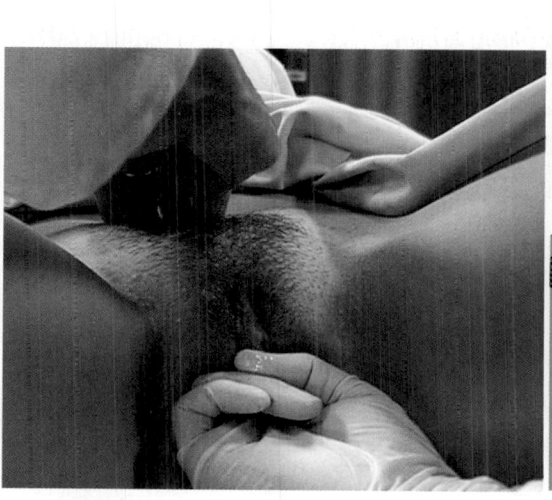 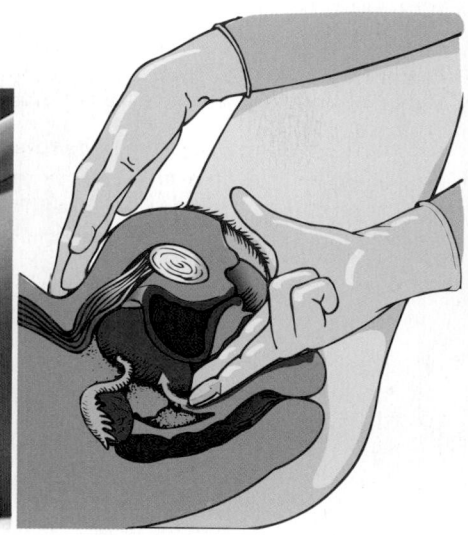

FIGURE 18-22
Bimanual palpation of the uterus.

CERVIX

Locate the cervix with the palmar surface of your fingers, feel its end, and run your fingers around its circumference to feel the fornices. Feel the size, length, and shape, which should correspond with your observations from the speculum examination. The consistency of the cervix in a nonpregnant woman will be firm, like the tip of the nose; during pregnancy the cervix is softer. Feel for nodules, hardness, and roughness. Note the position of the cervix as discussed in the speculum examination. The cervix should be in the midline and may be pointing anteriorly or posteriorly.

Grasp the cervix gently between your fingers and move it from side to side. Observe the patient for any expression of pain or discomfort with movement (cervical motion tenderness). The cervix should move 1 to 2 cm in each direction with minimal or no discomfort. Painful cervical movement suggests a pelvic inflammatory process such as acute pelvic inflammatory disease or a ruptured tubal pregnancy.

UTERUS

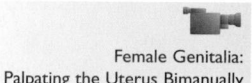

Female Genitalia:
Palpating the Uterus Bimanually

Position. Palpate the uterus. Place the palmar surface of your other hand on the abdominal midline, midway between the umbilicus and the symphysis pubis. Place the intravaginal fingers in the anterior fornix. Slowly slide the abdominal hand toward the pubis, pressing downward and forward with the flat surface of your fingers. At the same time, push inward and upward with the fingertips of the intravaginal hand while you push downward on the cervix with the backs of your fingers. Think of it as trying to bring your two hands together as you press down on the cervix. If the uterus is anteverted or anteflexed (the position of most uteri), you will feel the fundus between the fingers of your two hands at the level of the pubis (Fig. 18-23, *A* and *B*).

If you do not feel the uterus with the previous maneuver, place the intravaginal fingers together in the posterior fornix, with the abdominal hand immediately above the symphysis pubis. Press firmly downward with the abdominal hand while you press against the cervix inward with the other hand. A retroverted or retroflexed uterus should be felt with this maneuver (Fig. 18-23, *C* and D).

If you still cannot feel the uterus, move the intravaginal fingers to each side of the cervix. Keeping contact with the cervix, press inward and feel as far as you can. Then slide your fingers so that one is on top of the cervix and one is underneath. Continue pressing inward while moving your fingers to feel as much of the uterus as you can. When the uterus is in the midposition, you will not be able to feel the fundus with the abdominal hand (Fig. 18-23, *E*).

Confirm the location and position of the uterus by comparing your inspection findings with your palpation findings. The uterus should be located in the midline regardless of its position. Deviation to the right or left is indicative of possible adhesions, pelvic masses, or preg-

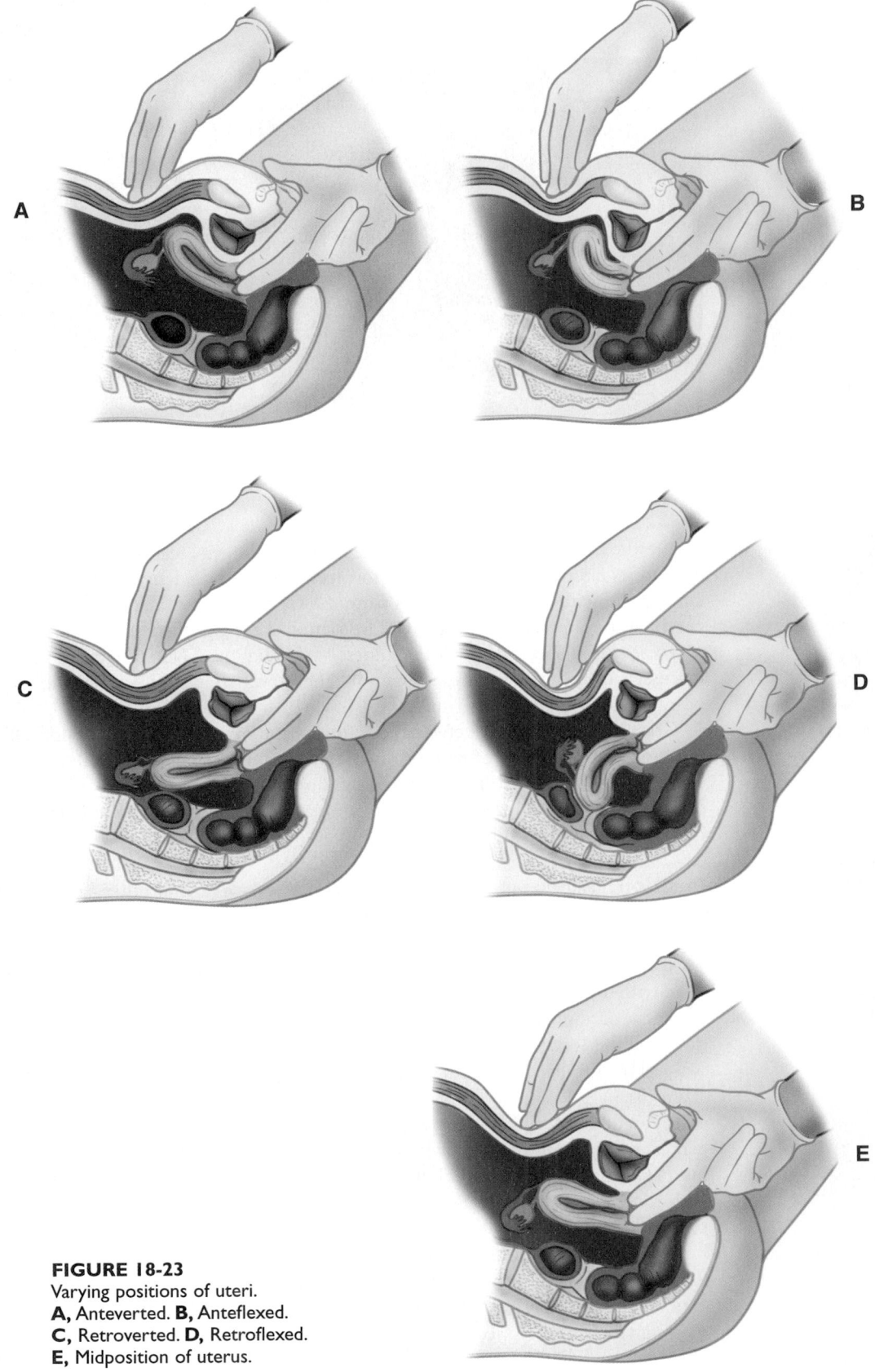

FIGURE 18-23
Varying positions of uteri.
A, Anteverted. **B,** Anteflexed.
C, Retroverted. **D,** Retroflexed.
E, Midposition of uterus.

> ● **CLINICAL PEARL**
> *Mittelschmerz*
> Mittelschmerz, lower abdominal pain associated with ovulation, may be accompanied by a degree of tenderness on the side in which ovulation took place that month and even by similarly unilateral and usually quite mild adnexal tenderness. The timing is, of course, essential in the history. The onset is usually sudden, and remission is spontaneous. If a pelvic examination is done, you may discover a bit of adnexal tenderness but it will otherwise be reassuringly negative.

nancy. Knowing the position of the uterus is essential before performing any intrauterine procedure, including insertion of an intrauterine contraceptive device.

Size, Shape, and Contour. Palpate the uterus for size, shape, and contour. It should be pear shaped and 5.5 to 8 cm long, although it is larger in all dimensions in multiparous women. A uterus larger than expected in a woman of childbearing age is indicative of pregnancy or tumor. The contour should be rounded, and walls should feel firm and smooth in the nonpregnant woman. The contour smoothness will be interrupted by pregnancy or tumor.

Mobility. Gently move the uterus between the intravaginal hand and abdominal hand to assess for mobility and tenderness. The uterus should be mobile in the anteroposterior plane. A fixed uterus indicates adhesions. Tenderness on movement suggests a pelvic inflammatory process or ruptured tubal pregnancy.

ADNEXA AND OVARIES

Palpate the adnexal areas and ovaries. Place the fingers of your abdominal hand on the right lower quadrant. With the intravaginal hand facing upward, place both fingers in the right lateral fornix. Press the intravaginal fingers deeply inward and upward toward the abdominal hand, while sweeping the flat surface of the fingers of the abdominal hand deeply inward and obliquely downward toward the symphysis pubis. Palpate the entire area by firmly pressing the abdominal hand and intravaginal fingers together. Repeat the maneuver on the left side (Fig. 18-24).

The ovaries, if palpable, should feel firm, smooth, ovoid, and approximately 3 by 2 by 1 cm in size. The healthy ovary is slightly to moderately tender on palpation. Marked tenderness, enlargement, and nodularity are unexpected. Usually no other structures are palpable except for round ligaments. Fallopian tubes are usually not palpable, so a problem may exist if they are felt. You are also palpating for adnexal masses, and if any are found they should be characterized by size, shape, location, consistency, and tenderness.

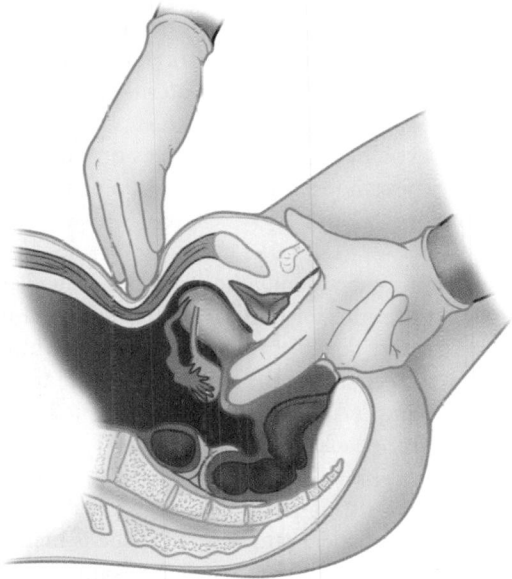

FIGURE 18-24
Bimanual palpation of adnexa. Sweep abdominal fingers downward to capture ovary.

The adnexa are often difficult to palpate because of their location and position and the presence of excess adipose tissue in some women. If you are unable to feel anything in the adnexal areas with thorough palpation, you can assume that no abnormality is present, provided no clinical symptoms exist.

RECTOVAGINAL EXAMINATION

PREPARATION

The rectovaginal exploration is an important part of the total pelvic examination. It allows you to reach almost 2.5 cm (1 inch) higher into the pelvis, which enables you to better evaluate the pelvic organs and structures. It is an uncomfortable examination for the patient, however, and she may ask you to omit it. Nevertheless, it is important to perform, and you should explain to the woman why it is necessary.

As you complete the bimanual examination, withdraw your examining fingers, change gloves, and lubricate fingers. Tell the patient that she may feel the urgency of a bowel movement. Assure her that she will not have one, and ask her to breathe slowly and consciously try to relax her sphincter, rectum, and buttocks, because tightening the muscles makes the examination more uncomfortable for her.

ANAL SPHINCTER

Place your index finger in the vagina, then press your middle finger against the anus and ask the patient to bear down. As she does, slip the tip of the finger into the rectum just past the sphincter. Palpate the area of the anorectal junction and just above it. Ask the woman to tighten and relax her anal sphincter. Observe sphincter tone. An extremely tight sphincter may be the result of anxiety about the examination; may be caused by scarring; or may indicate spasticity caused by fissures, lesions, or inflammation. A lax sphincter suggests neurologic deficit, whereas an absent sphincter may result from improper repair of third-degree perineal laceration after childbirth or trauma.

RECTAL WALLS AND RECTO-VAGINAL SEPTUM

Slide both your vaginal and rectal fingers in as far as they will go, then ask the woman to bear down. This will bring an additional centimeter within reach of your fingers. Rotate the rectal finger to explore the anterior rectal wall for masses, polyps, nodules, strictures, irregularities, and tenderness. The wall should feel smooth and uninterrupted. Palpate the rectovaginal septum along the anterior wall for thickness, tone, and nodules. You may feel the uterine body and occasionally the uterine fundus in a retroflexed uterus.

UTERUS

Press firmly and deeply downward with the abdominal hand just above the symphysis pubis while you position the vaginal finger in the posterior vaginal fornix, and press strongly upward against the posterior side of the cervix. Palpate as much of the posterior side of the uterus as possible, confirming your findings from the vaginal examination regarding location, position, size, shape, contour, consistency, and tenderness of the uterus. This maneuver is particularly useful in evaluating a retroverted uterus (Fig. 18-25).

ADNEXA

If you were unable to palpate the adnexal areas on bimanual examination or if the findings were questionable, repeat the adnexal examination using the same maneuvers described in the bimanual examination.

STOOL

As you withdraw your fingers, rotate the rectal finger to evaluate the posterior rectal wall just as you did earlier for the anterior wall. Gently remove your examining fingers and observe for secretions and stool. Note the color and presence of any blood. Prepare a specimen for occult blood testing, if indicated. Unless the woman is unable to, let her wipe off the lubricating gel herself. She can do a more thorough and comfortable job. Be sure to provide tissues and an appropriate disposal receptacle.

COMPLETION

Assist the woman into a sitting position and give her the opportunity to regain her equilibrium and composure. Provide a sanitary pad if she is menstruating. Share with her the findings and ask her to voice her feelings about the examination. This conversation may be brief,

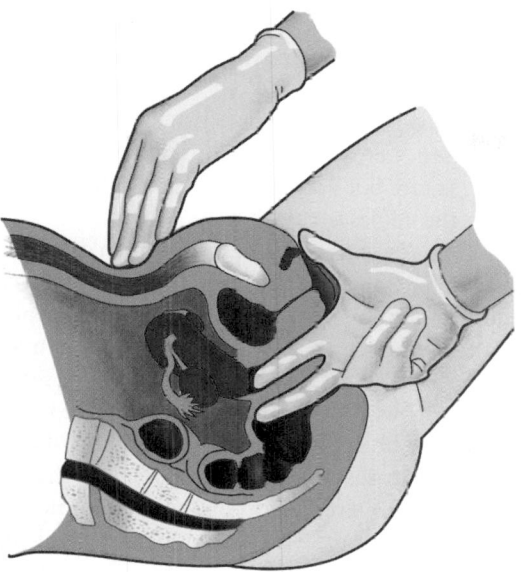

FIGURE 18-25
Rectovaginal palpation.
From Lowdermilk, Perry, 2004.

but it should never be avoided. Some clinicians prefer to leave the room and give the woman the opportunity to dress before discussing findings.

INFANTS

The appearance of the external genitalia can help in the assessment of gestational age in the newborn. Examination is conducted with the infant's legs held in a frog position. The labia majora appear widely separated, and the clitoris is prominent up to 36 weeks of gestation; but by full term the labia majora completely cover the labia minora and clitoris.

The newborn's genitalia reflect the influence of maternal hormones. The labia majora and minora may be swollen, with the labia minora often more prominent. The hymen is often protruding, thick, and vascular, and it may simulate an extruding mass. These are all transient phenomena and will disappear in a few weeks (Fig. 18-26).

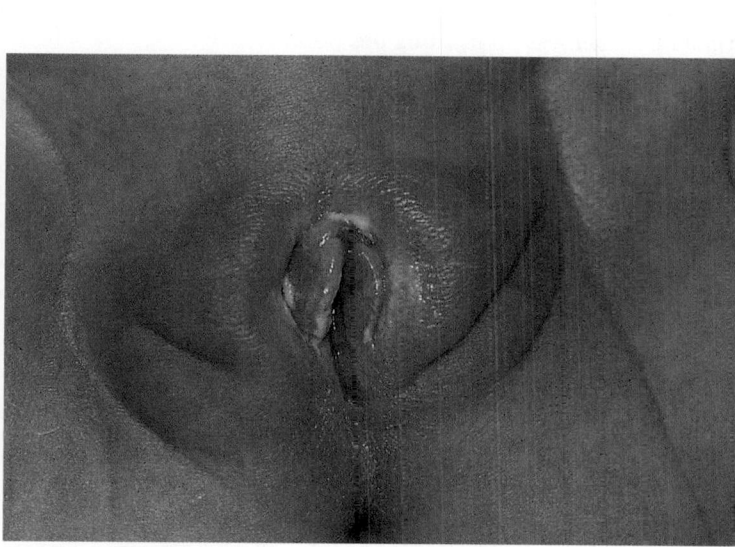

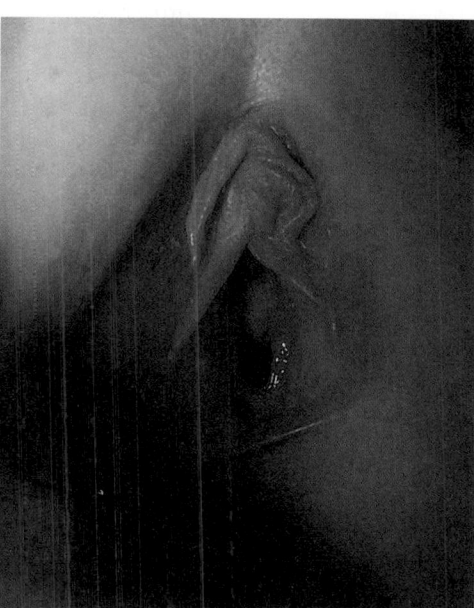

A

B

FIGURE 18-26
Normal appearance of the female genitalia. **A,** Genitalia of a newborn girl. The labia majora are full, and the thickened labia minora protrude between them. **B,** Genitalia of a 2-year-old girl. The labia majora are flattened, and the labia minora and hymen are thin and flat.
From Zitelli, Davis, 1997; A courtesy Ian Holzman, MD, NY.

The clitoris may appear relatively large; this usually has no significance. True hypertrophy is not common; however, an enlarged clitoris must always suggest adrenal hyperplasia when seen in the newborn.

The central opening of the hymen is usually about 0.5 cm in diameter. It is important to determine the presence of an opening; however, make no effort to stretch the hymen. An imperforate hymen is rare but can cause difficulty later, including hydrocolpos in the child and hematocolpos in the adolescent.

Malformations in the external genitalia are often difficult to define. If the baby was a breech delivery, her genitalia may be swollen and bruised for many days after delivery. Any ambiguous appearance or unusual orifice in the vulvar vault or perineum must be expeditiously explored before the infant is inappropriately assigned a gender.

A mucoid, whitish vaginal discharge is commonly seen during the newborn period and sometimes as late as 4 weeks after birth. The discharge is occasionally mixed with blood. This is the result of passive hormonal transfer from the mother and is an expected finding.

Thin but difficult-to-separate adhesions between the labia minora are often seen during the first few months or even years of life. Sometimes they completely cover the vulvar vestibule. There may be just the smallest of openings through which urine can escape. These may require separation, using the gentlest of teasing or the application of estrogen creams.

Vaginal discharges in infants and young children may occur as the result of irritation from the diaper or powder. These discharges are usually mucoid.

CHILDREN

INDICATIONS FOR EXAMINATION

The extent of the gynecologic examination depends on the child's age and complaints. For the well child, the examination includes only inspection and palpation of the external genitalia. The internal vaginal examination is performed on a young child only when there is a specific problem such as bleeding, discharge, trauma, or suspected sexual abuse. Bubble bath vaginitis is common in young girls and does not require an internal examination. Speculum examination on a young child requires special equipment and an experienced and knowledgeable gynecologist or pediatrician.

The young child usually cooperates with examination of the external genitalia if your approach is very matter of fact. The very young child might prefer to lie in the parent's lap, with legs held in a frog position by the parent. The preschool child can be placed on the examining table, lying back against the head of the table, which should be raised about 30 degrees. The parent can help the child hold her legs up in a frog position.

A school-age child may not like the examination, but is likely to cooperate if you take the time to reassure her that you will only look at and touch the outside. However, you must realize that a child in this circumstance, lying down, underpants off, will most often feel quite vulnerable. You might help her by having her lie on her parent's lap if her size permits and you might even leave her underpants on, simply pushing the area of the crotch aside as you do the examination. You might also have the child help by taking her hand and first having her touch herself and even retracting the labia majora herself to help you. She should be positioned on the table on her back with her knees flexed and drawn up. The examination should be approached with the same degree of respect, explanation, and caution as with the adult woman.

It is necessary to have another person chaperone during examination of the genitalia; however, the older child should be consulted about this arrangement.

INSPECTION AND PALPATION

Inspect the perineum, all the structures of the vulvar vestibule, and the urethral and vaginal orifices by separating the labia with the thumb and forefinger of one hand.

Adequate visualization of the interior of the vagina and the hymenal opening can be difficult in prepubertal girls. A technique that can be helpful is that of anterior labial traction. Firmly grasp both labia majora (not the minora) with the thumb and index finger of each hand, then gently but firmly pull the labia forward and slightly to the side. Gentle but firm traction will not cause discomfort. A previously obscured hymenal opening almost always becomes visible with this technique, as does the interior of the vagina, nearly to the cervix. Most

CLINICAL PEARL

Smell the Discharge
If sexual abuse is suspected, it is helpful to be aware of the characteristic odor of semen.

foreign bodies are visible with this method. With the help of an assistant, a swab is easily inserted through the hymenal opening to obtain cultures if needed.

Bartholin and Skene glands are usually not palpable; if they are, enlargement exists. This indicates infection, which is most often (but not always) gonococcal. Ask the girl to cough and as she does so, observe the hymen. An imperforate hymen will bulge, whereas one with an opening will not.

DISCHARGE

A vaginal discharge often irritates the perineal tissues, causing redness and perhaps excoriation. Other sources of perineal irritation are bubble baths, soaps, detergents, and urinary tract infections. Carefully question the parent for a history of hematuria, dysuria, or other symptoms that would indicate urinary tract infection. A foul odor is more likely indicative of a foreign body (particularly in preschool children), especially if a secondary infection is present. Vaginal discharge may also result from trichomonal, gonococcal, or monilial infection.

INJURIES

Swelling of vulvar tissues, particularly if accompanied by bruising or foul-smelling discharge, should alert you to the possibility of sexual abuse (Box 18-4). It must always be suspected if a young child has a sexually transmitted infection or if there is injury to the external genitalia. Injuries to the softer structure of the external genitalia are not caused by bicycle seats. A straddle injury from a bicycle seat is generally evident over the symphysis pubis where the structures are more fixed. The injuries resulting from sexual molestation are generally more posterior and may involve the perineum grossly.

BOX 18-4

RED FLAGS FOR SEXUAL ABUSE

The following signs and symptoms in children or adolescents should raise your suspicion for sexual abuse. Remember, however, that any sign or symptom by itself is of limited significance; it may be related to sexual abuse, or it may be from another cause altogether. This is an area in which good clinical judgment is imperative. Each sign or symptom must be considered in context with the particular child's health status, stage of growth and development, and entire history.
Medical complaints and findings:
- Evidence of general physical abuse or neglect
- Evidence of trauma and/or scarring in genital, anal, and perianal areas
- Unusual changes in skin color or pigmentation in genital or anal area
- Presence of sexually transmitted infection (oral, anal, genital)
- Anorectal problems such as itching, bleeding, pain, fecal incontinence, poor anal sphincter tone, bowel habit dysfunction
- Genitourinary problems such as rash or sores in genital area, vaginal odor, pain (including abdominal pain), itching,

bleeding, discharge, dysuria, hematuria, urinary tract infections, enuresis
Examples of nonspecific behavioral manifestations:
- Problems with school
- Dramatic weight changes or eating disturbances
- Depression
- Sleep problems or nightmares
- Sudden change in personality or behavior
- Aggression or destructiveness
- Sudden avoidance of certain people or places
Examples of sexual behaviors that are concerning:
- Use of sexually provocative mannerisms
- Excessive masturbation or sexual behavior that cannot be redirected
- Age-inappropriate sexual knowledge or experience
- Repeated object insertion into vagina and/or anus
- Child asking to be touched/kissed in genital area
- Sex play between children with 4 years or more age difference
- Sex play that involves the use of force, threats, or bribes

Modified from Koop, 1988; McClain et al, 2000; Hornor, 2004.

Such findings cannot be ignored, and careful questioning of the parent or custodian is mandatory.

BLEEDING

Vaginal bleeding in children is often the result of injury, manipulation with foreign bodies, or sexual abuse. Occasionally there may be an ovarian tumor or carcinoma of the cervix. Remember, too, that some girls begin menstruation well before the expected time (Box 18-5).

RECTAL EXAMINATION

On occasion a rectal examination may be indicated to determine the presence or absence of the uterus or the presence of foreign bodies in the vagina. The rectal examination is performed with the patient lying on her back, feet held together, knees bent up on the abdomen. Place one hand on the child's knees to steady her, slipping the gloved examining finger into the rectum. Most examiners prefer the index finger, but this is not mandatory. Once your finger is introduced, you may release the legs and use your free hand to simultaneously palpate the abdomen. If the child is old enough to cooperate, have her pant like a puppy to relax the muscles. Foreign bodies will be palpable, as will the cervix. The ovaries are not usually felt. There may be bleeding and even a transient mild rectal prolapse after the examination, so be sure to warn the parent of this.

ADOLESCENTS

All sexually active teenagers should have an annual pelvic examination, Pap smear, and sexually transmitted infection evaluation. Young women who are not sexually active should have their first examination by age 21 years. The adolescent requires the same examination and positioning as the adult. Ask whether this is the young woman's first gynecologic examination. The first examination is perhaps the most important, because it will set the stage for how she views future examinations. Take time to explain to her what you will be doing. Use models or illustrations to show her what will happen and what you will look for. Techniques such as deep breathing throughout the procedure, alternating tightening and relaxation of the perineal muscles, or progressive muscle relaxation may help the adolescent stay relaxed during the examination. An adolescent should be allowed the privacy, if she desires, of having the examination without her parent present. This can also provide an opportunity to talk with her in private. An interview without the parent may be necessary to obtain an accurate sexual history, including sexual abuse, and to discuss sexual play (Box 18-6). There is evidence that most sexually active adolescents prefer to be screened for sexually transmitted infection (e.g., *Chlamydia trachomatis, Neisseria gonorrhoeae,* and *Trichomonas vaginalis*) by using first-void urine specimens and self-collected vaginal swab specimens rather than pelvic examination (Serlin et al, 2002). The pelvic examination, however, is in our view central to the best care.

Choose the appropriate size speculum. A pediatric speculum with blades that are 1 to 1.5 cm wide can be used and should cause minimal discomfort. If the adolescent is sexually active, a small adult speculum may be used.

BOX 18-5

CAUSES OF GENITAL BLEEDING IN CHILDREN

Vaginal bleeding during childhood is always clinically important and requires further evaluation. Common causes in children include the following:
- Genital lesions
- Vaginitis
- Foreign body
- Trauma
- Tumors
- Endocrine changes
- Estrogen ingestion
- Precocious puberty
- Hormone-producing ovarian tumor

BOX 18-6

EVALUATION OF SEXUAL PLAY IN ADOLESCENTS

Adolescents need strong support and guidance as they experiment with independence, the search for identity, and a healthy gender role. In adolescence, sexual play and exploration may encompass the full range of sexual behavior. The critical factors in determining the significance of any sexual activity to the healthy development of sexuality are whether it fits the religious and moral codes of the youth and family and whether there is a power imbalance in the relationship. The following guidelines can help you determine whether activity is part of healthy development or requires further assessment.

Healthy Activity	Needs Further Assessment
Discreet, private	No regard for privacy
Mutual consent	One adolescent does not freely consent
No power imbalance	Power imbalance
No threats or violence	Actual or implied threats of violence
Infrequent	Frequent, compulsive
Age-appropriate language and sexual knowledge	Language beyond age-appropriate level of sexual knowledge
Does not result in injury	Causes injury
Basic, rudimentary sexual activity	Explicit, graphic, and detailed sexual activity
	Attempted or actual penetration of genital orifices

From Haka-Ikse, Mian, 1993.

As the girl goes through puberty, you will see the maturational changes of sexual development (see Fig. 5-21). Just before menarche there is a physiologic increase in vaginal secretions. The hymen may or may not be stretched across the vaginal opening. By menarche, the opening should be at least 1 cm wide. As the adolescent matures, the findings are the same as those for the adult.

PREGNANT WOMEN

The gynecologic examination for the pregnant woman follows the same procedure as that for the nonpregnant adult woman. In early pregnancy you can feel a softening of the isthmus, whereas the cervix is still firm. In the second month of pregnancy the cervix, vagina, and vulva acquire their bluish color from increased vascularity. The cervix itself softens and will feel more like lips rather than like the firmness of the nose tip. The fundus flexes easily on the cervix. There is slight fullness and softening of the fundus near the site of implantation or a lateral bulge or soft prominence with cornual implantation. These findings are summarized in Box 18-7. You will notice increased vaginal secretions as a result of increased vascularity. None of these findings is perfectly sensitive or specific for detecting pregnancy, and they should not replace human chorionic gonadotropin testing and/or ultrasound.

PELVIC SIZE

The size of the bony pelvis is estimated during one of the prenatal visits, in addition to the routine vaginal, bimanual, and rectovaginal examinations. It is usually performed during the third trimester to increase the accuracy of measurement and the comfort of the woman.

Because the bones are covered with varying amounts of soft tissue and are not directly accessible, the measurements are only approximations. Firm pressure is needed to obtain the most accurate measurements. More direct ways to measure the pelvis are through computed tomography, ultrasound, or x-ray examination; however, the last is rarely used in pregnancy.

Four pelvic types are found in women: gynecoid, android, anthropoid, and platypelloid (Table 18-2). Pelvic measurements vary depending on the type of pelvis the woman has and, to some degree, on muscle and tissue strength. The select clinical measurements that are described in Table 18-3 may help guide the practitioner in safe labor management but should not be used to predict labor outcome.

PHYSICAL VARIATIONS

Pelvic Types

Black and white women differ in their percentage of pelvic types. Both have a similar percentage of the gynecoid type, but white women more often have the android type, and black women more often have the anthropoid type.

BOX 18-7

EARLY SIGNS OF PREGNANCY

The following are physical signs that occur early in pregnancy. These signs, along with internal ballottement, palpation of fetal parts, and positive test results for urine or serum human chorionic gonadotropin, are probable indicators of pregnancy. They are considered probable because clinical conditions other than pregnancy can cause any one of them. Their occurrence together, however, creates a strong case for the presence of a pregnancy.

Sign	Finding	Approximate Weeks of Gestation
Goodell	Softening of the cervix	4 to 6
Hegar	Softening of the uterine isthmus	6 to 8
McDonald	Fundus flexes easily on the cervix	7 to 8
Braun von Fernwald	Fullness and softening of the fundus near the site of implantation	7 to 8
Piskacek	Palpable lateral bulge or soft prominence of one uterine cornu	7 to 8
Chadwick	Bluish color of the cervix, vagina, and vulva	8 to 12

From Haka-Ikse, Mian, 1993.

TABLE 18-2   Comparison of Pelvic Types

	Gynecoid (50% of Women)	Android (23% of Women)	Anthropoid (24% of Women)	Platypelloid (3% of Women)
Brim	Slightly ovoid or transversely rounded ◯ Round	Heart shaped, angulated ♡ Heart	Oval, wider anteroposteriorly ◯ Oval	Flattened anteroposteriorly, wide transversely ◯ Flat
Depth	Moderate	Deep	Deep	Shallow
Side walls	Straight	Convergent	Straight	Straight
Ischial spines	Blunt, somewhat widely separated	Prominent, narrow interspinous diameter	Prominent, often with narrow interspinous diameter	Blunted, widely separated
Sacrum	Deep, curved	Slightly curved, terminal portion often beaked	Slightly curved	Slightly curved
Subpubic arch	Wide	Narrow	Narrow	Wide
Usual mode of delivery	Vaginal Spontaneous Occiput anterior position	Cesarean Vaginal Difficult with forceps	Vaginal Forceps/spontaneous Occiput posterior or occiput anterior position	Vaginal Spontaneous

From Lowdermilk, Perry, 2004.

TABLE 18-3	Obstetric Measurements for Estimating Pelvic Size		
Name of Measurement		**Expected Measurement**	**Distance Measured**

PELVIC INLET
If the pelvis is abnormal, the AP diameter is often shortened

Diagonal conjugate: the most important clinical measurement for estimating the AP diameter of the pelvic inlet (Fig. 18-27)		12.5 to 13 cm	From the symphysis pubis (inferior border) to the sacral promontory
Obstetric conjugate: the AP diameter of the pelvic inlet obtained only by x-ray techniques or estimated from the diagonal conjugate (there may be a discrepancy) (Fig. 18-28)		Diagonal conjugate minus 1.5 to 2 cm, depending on the pubic arch; about 11 cm radiographically	From the symphysis pubis (posterior border) to the sacral promontory

MIDPLANE
Direct measurement is not possible; if the ischial spines are prominent, the side walls converge, or the concavity of the sacrum is shallow, contraction is suspected

Transverse diameter or interspinous diameter: can only be estimated (Fig. 18-29)		10.5 cm	The narrowest transverse diameter in the midplane between the interspinous processes

OUTLET
Accessible for measurement

Biischial diameter, intertuberous diameter, or transverse diameter of the outlet: provides information on the adequacy of the pelvic outlet; two techniques can be used (Figs. 18-30 and 18-31)		>8 cm	From the interior border of one ischial tuberosity to the other

AP, Anteroposterior.

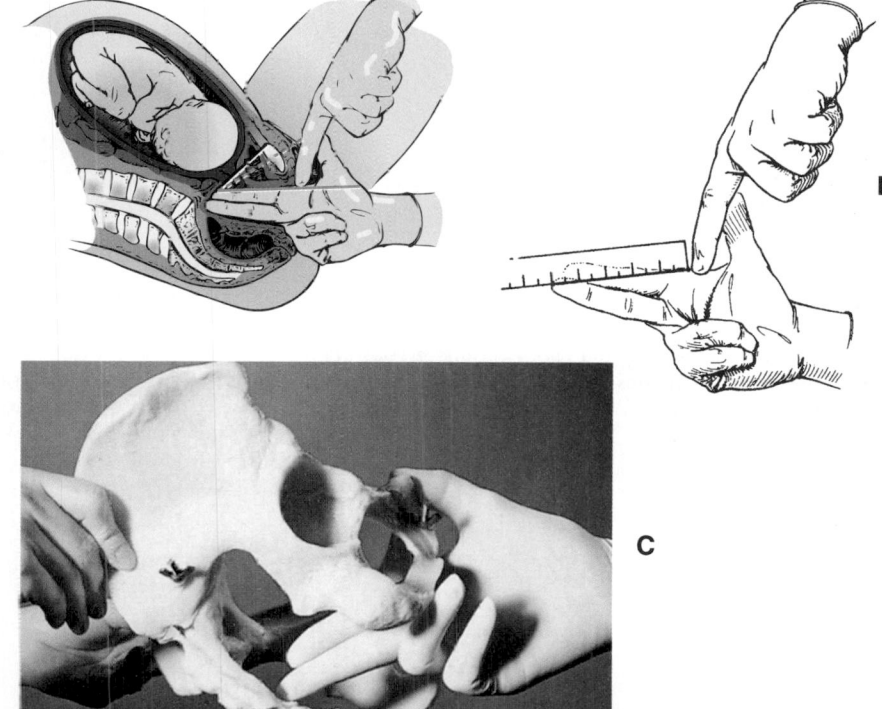

FIGURE 18-27
Measuring the diagonal conjugate. **A,** Insert the fingers until the tips reach the sacral promontory. With a finger of the other hand against the inferior border of the symphysis, mark where the symphysis pubis meets the hand. **B,** Compare the hand distance with a ruler to determine the diameter of the diagonal conjugate. **C,** Correct hand position shown with an anatomic model.
From Lowdermilk, Perry, 2004. Photo from Symonds, Macpherson, 1994.

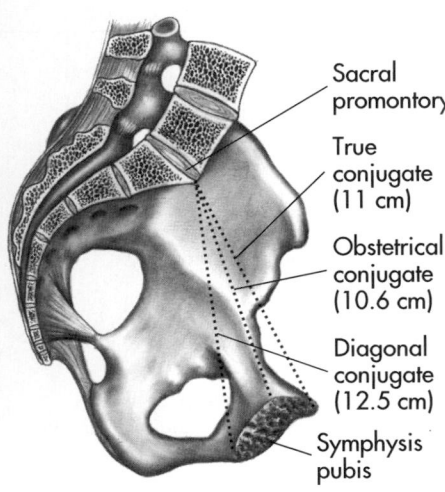

Sacral
promontory

True
conjugate
(11 cm)

Obstetrical
conjugate
(10.6 cm)

Diagonal
conjugate
(12.5 cm)

Symphysis
pubis

FIGURE 18-28
Estimate the obstetric conjugate using the diagonal conjugate. The diagonal conjugate varies in length depending on the height and inclination of the symphysis pubis.

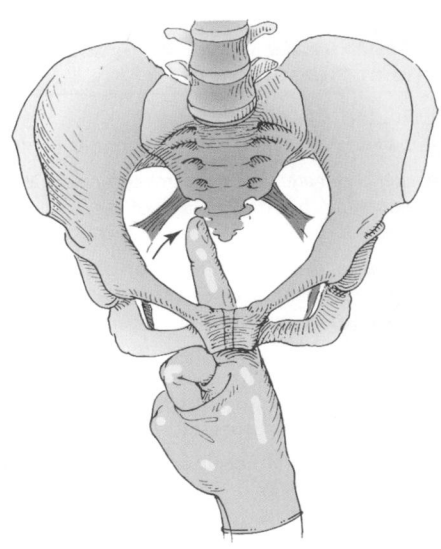

FIGURE 18-29
Estimating the transverse (interspinous) diameter. Insert the two examining fingers into the vagina and locate the ischial spines. If the spines are prominent, they may project into the pelvis similar to spikes. If they are flush with the pelvic walls, you might locate them by identifying the sacrospinous ligament and following it anteriorly to the spines. Estimate the distance between the ischial spines by moving your fingers from side to side.
From Lowdermilk, Perry, 2004.

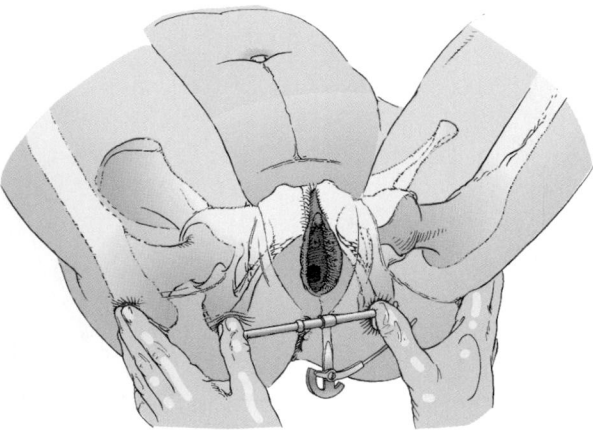

FIGURE 18-30
Determining the biischial diameter. Measure the distance between the tuberosities using the Thom pelvimeter; position it centrally and extend the tips of the crossbar until they touch the ischial tuberosities.
From Lowdermilk, Perry, 2004.

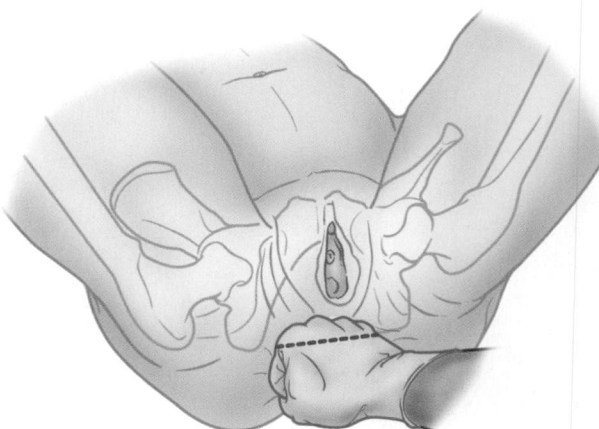

FIGURE 18-31
Alternative technique for determining the biischial diameter. First, measure your closed fist to determine its width; then place your fist against the perineum between the ischial tuberosities. Determine the distance between the tuberosities compared with your fist.

TABLE 18-4	Estimates of Uterine Size in Early Pregnancy	
Weeks of Gestation	**Uterine Length (cm)**	**Uterine Width (cm)**
6	7.3 to 9.1	3.9
8	8.8 to 10.8	5.0
10	10.2 to 12.5	6.1
12	11.7 to 14.2	7.1
14	13.2 to 15.9	8.2

From Fox, 1985.

FIGURE 18-32
Changes in fundal height with pregnancy. Weeks 10 to 12: Uterus within pelvis; fetal heartbeat can be detected with Doppler. Week 12: Uterus palpable just above symphysis pubis. Week 16: Uterus palpable halfway between symphysis and umbilicus; ballottement of fetus is possible by abdominal and vaginal examination. Week 20: Uterine fundus at lower border of umbilicus; fetal heartbeat can be auscultated with fetoscope. Weeks 24 to 26: Uterus changes from globular to avoid shape; fetus palpable. Week 28: Uterus approximately halfway between umbilicus and xiphoid; fetus easily palpable. Week 34: Uterine fundus just below xiphoid. Week 40: Fundal height drops as fetus begins to engage in pelvis.

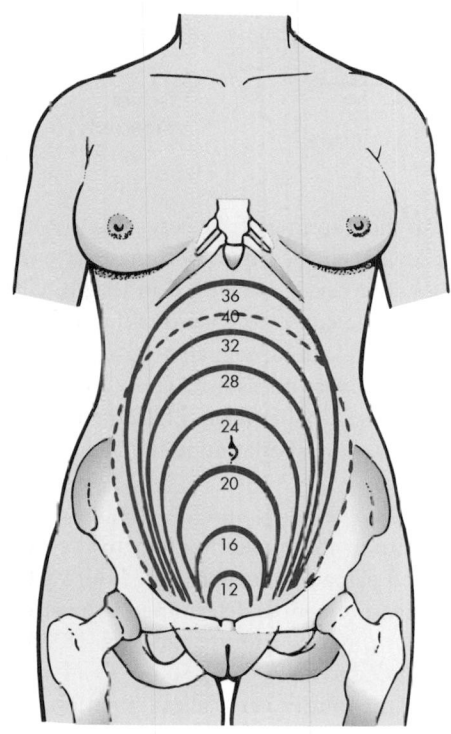

UTERUS SIZE

Early uterine enlargement may not be symmetric. Determination of the size of the uterus can be used to estimate gestational age. There is a lack of consensus about the accuracy of estimates of the size of the uterus at the various weeks; however, some estimate should be made. The size of various fruits is a common, though not reliable, means for describing the size of the uterus in early pregnancy. Centimeters are more accurate units of measurement and should be used as soon as possible. Table 18-4 provides estimates of uterine size.

Changes in fundal height at the various weeks of gestation are shown in Fig. 18-32, along with some changes that are detectable on examination. Abdominal measurements are discussed in Chapter 17, and breast and skin changes in pregnancy are discussed in Chapter 16.

CERVICAL DILATION AND LENGTH

Other pregnancy conditions that are assessed during the pelvic examination include cervical dilation and effacement. Dilation involves the opening of the cervical canal to allow for the passage of the fetus. The process is measured in centimeters and progresses from a closed os (internal) to 10 cm, which is full or complete dilation. The time may vary among women between centimeters of dilation, depending on the parity of the woman, weeks of gestation (some dilation may be present late in pregnancy), and progress of labor.

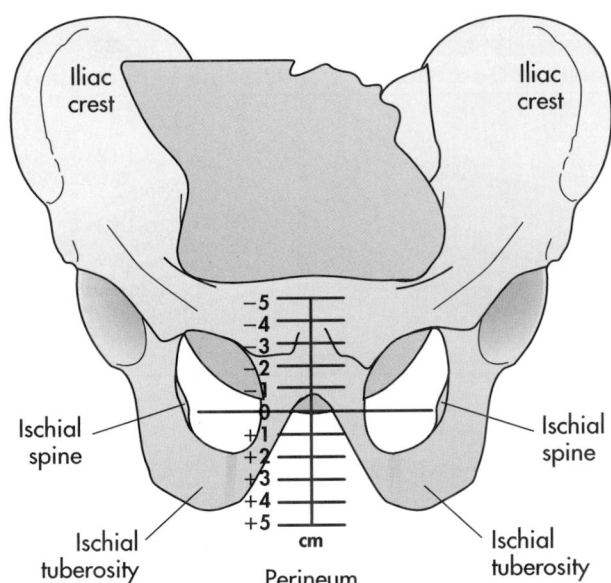

FIGURE 18-33
Stations of presenting part (degree of descent). Silhouette shows head of infant at station 0.
Courtesy Ross Products Division, Abbott Laboratories Inc., Columbus, OH. From Lowdermilk, Perry, 2004.

Effacement refers to the thinning of the cervix that results when myometrial activity pulls the cervix upward, allowing the cervix to become part of the lower uterine segment during prelabor or early labor. The cervix is reduced in length. Ultrasonographic methods estimate its length at 3 to 4 cm at the end of the third trimester. Shortening of the cervix (<29 mm) noted on vaginal ultrasound in midpregnancy indicates risk for preterm delivery. Digital examinations are not as accurate as ultrasound and may miss the problem. The cervix gradually thins to only a few millimeters (paper thin). Effacement should be recorded in centimeters. Effacement usually precedes cervical dilation in the primipara and often occurs with dilation in the multipara.

STATION

Station is the relationship of the presenting part to the ischial spines of the mother's pelvis. Vaginal examination and palpation are performed during labor to estimate the descent of the presenting part. The measurement is determined by centimeters above and below the ischial spines and is recorded by plus and minus signs (Fig. 18-33). For example, the station at 1 cm below the spines is recorded as a +1, at the spines as a 0, and at 1 cm above the spines as −1. Record (in centimeters) the routine cervical examination findings for dilation, cervical length, and station, in that order.

FETAL HEAD POSITION

The position of the fetal head can be determined by vaginal examination once dilation has begun. Insert your fingers anteriorly into the posterior aspect of the vagina and then move your fingers upward over the fetal head as you turn them, locating the sagittal suture with the posterior and anterior fontanels at either end (Fig. 18-34, *A*). The position of the fontanels is determined by examining the anterior aspect of the sagittal suture and then using a circular motion to pass alongside the head until the other fontanel is felt and differentiated (Fig. 18-34, *B*). The position of the face and breech are easier to determine because the various parts are more distinguishable.

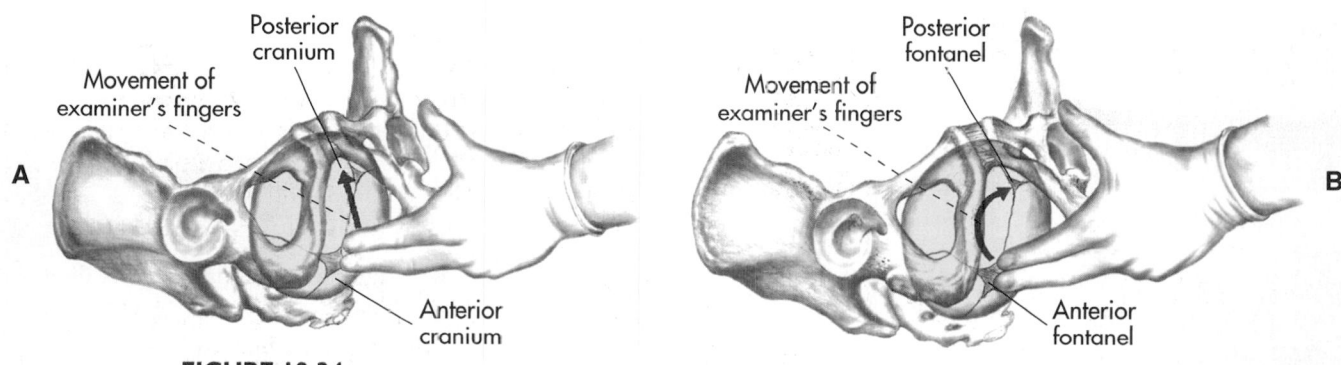

FIGURE 18-34
A, Locating the sagittal suture on vaginal examination. **B,** Differentiating the fontanels on vaginal examination.

OTHER PREGNANCY-ASSOCIATED CHANGES

The uterus may become more anteflexed during the first 3 months from softening of the isthmus. As a result, the fundus may press on the urinary bladder, causing the woman to experience urinary frequency.

Early uterine enlargement may not be symmetric, and you may feel deviation of the uterus to one side and an irregularity in its contour at the site of implantation. This uterine irregularity occurs around week 8 to 10 (Piskacek sign).

Changes in fundal height at the various weeks of gestation are shown in Fig. 18-32, along with some changes that are detectable on examination. Breast and skin changes that occur with pregnancy are discussed in Chapter 16.

OLDER ADULTS

The temptation with older women is to defer the examination because of their age. This is often not appropriate. The examination procedure for the older adult is the same as that for the adult of childbearing age, with a few modifications for comfort. The older woman may require more time and assistance to assume the lithotomy position. She may need assistance from another individual to help hold her legs, because they may tire easily when the hip joints remain in abduction for an extended period. Patients with orthopnea will need to have their head and chest elevated during examination. You may need to use a smaller speculum, depending on the degree of introital constriction that occurs with aging.

Note that the labia appear flatter and smaller, corresponding with the degree of loss of subcutaneous fat elsewhere on the body. The skin is drier and shinier than that of a younger adult, and the pubic hair is gray and may be sparse. The clitoris is smaller than that of a younger adult.

The urinary meatus may appear as an irregular opening or slit. It may be located more posteriorly, very near or within the vaginal introitus, as a result of relaxed perineal musculature.

The vaginal introitus may be constricted and may admit only one finger. In some multiparous older women, the introitus may gape, with the vaginal walls rolling toward the opening.

The vagina is narrower and shorter, and you will see and feel the absence of rugation. The cervix is smaller and paler than in younger women, and the surrounding fornices may be smaller or absent. The cervix may seem less mobile if it protrudes less far into the vaginal canal. The os may be smaller but should still be palpable.

The uterus diminishes in size and may not be palpable, and the ovaries are rarely palpable because of atrophy. Ovaries that are palpable should be considered suspicious for tumor, and additional workup, such as ultrasonography, to exclude cancer is required.

The rectovaginal septum will feel thin, smooth, and pliable. Anal sphincter tone may be somewhat diminished. Since the pelvic musculature relaxes, look particularly for stress incontinence and prolapse of the vaginal walls or uterus.

As with younger women, as you inspect and palpate you are evaluating for signs of inflammation (older women are particularly susceptible to atrophic vaginitis), infection, trauma, tenderness, growths, masses, nodules, enlargement, irregularity, and changes in consistency.

WOMEN WITH DISABILITIES

PREPARATION

The clinician and/or disabled woman can do a number of things to promote a comfortable pelvic examination experience. See Chapter 3 for a discussion of common approaches to patients who have disabilities.

ALTERNATIVE POSITIONS FOR THE PELVIC EXAMINATION

A number of alternatives in positioning for the pelvic examination are possible. A disabled woman is the best judge of which position will work for her and how to use assistants most effectively. These decisions should be made by the patient and the clinician together.

An assistant will help the disabled woman and the clinician facilitate a comfortable, thorough pelvic examination. For example, the assistant may help the woman position herself on the examination table. At least one assistant should be available throughout the examination in addition to the clinician. The assistant might be a staff member or an attendant or friend of the disabled patient.

Many disabled women cannot comfortably assume the traditional (lithotomy) pelvic examination position, which requires a woman to be on her back with knees bent, legs spread apart, and feet placed in metal stirrups at the foot of the examination table. As a result of a disability, a woman may experience one or more conditions such a joint stiffness, pain, paralysis or lack of muscle control that will require the use of an alternative position.

Some nondisabled women may experience one or more of these conditions, resulting in a need for an alternative position, just as some disabled women may wish to use the traditional pelvic examination position.

Knee-Chest Position. In the knee-chest position, the woman lies on her side with both knees bent, with her top leg brought closer to her chest (Fig. 18-35). A variation of this position would allow the woman to lie with her bottom leg straightened while the top leg is still bent close to her chest. The speculum can be inserted with the handle pointed in the direction of the woman's abdomen or back. Because the woman is lying on her side, the clinician should be sure to angle the speculum toward the small of the patient's back and not straight up toward her head. Once the speculum has been removed, the woman will need to roll onto her back.

The assistant may provide support for the patient while she is on the examination table, help the woman straighten her bottom leg if she prefers the variation of this position, or support the patient in rolling onto her back for the bimanual examination. If the patient cannot spread her legs, the assistant may help her elevate one leg.

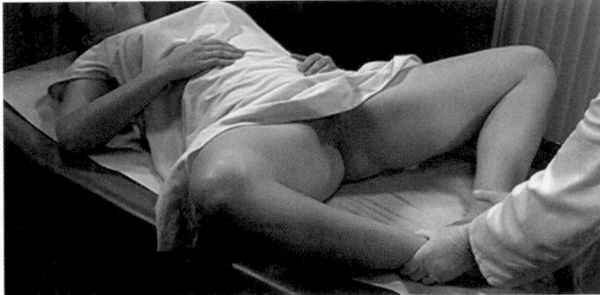

FIGURE 18-36
The diamond-shaped position.

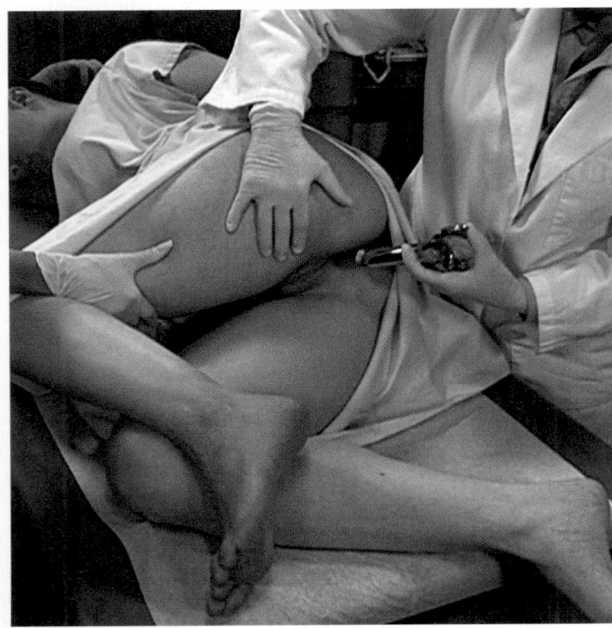

FIGURE 18-35
The knee-chest position.

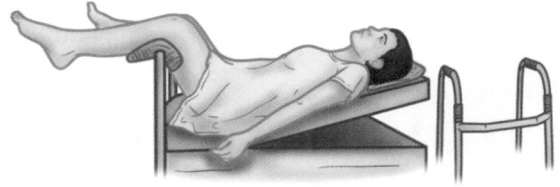

FIGURE 18-37
The obstetric stirrups position.

The knee-chest position does not require the use of stirrups. It is particularly good for a woman who feels most comfortable and balanced lying on her side.

Diamond-Shaped Position. In the diamond-shaped position the woman lies on her back with her knees bent so that both legs are spread flat and her heels meet at the foot of the table (Fig. 18-36). The speculum must be inserted with the handle up. The bimanual examination can be easily performed from the side or foot of the table.

The assistant may help the patient support herself on the table and hold her feet together in alignment with her spine to maintain this position. A woman may be more comfortable using pillows or an assistant to elevate her thighs and/or using a pillow under the small of the back.

The diamond-shaped position does not require the use of stirrups. A woman must be able to lie flat on her back to use this position. The diamond-shaped position can also be used with children.

Obstetric Stirrups Position. In the obstetric stirrups position the woman lies on her back near the foot of the table with her legs supported under the knee by obstetric stirrups (Fig. 18-37). The speculum can be inserted with the handle down. The bimanual examination can be performed from the foot of the table.

The patient may want assistance in putting her legs into the stirrups. The stirrups can be padded to increase comfort and reduce irritation. A strap can be attached to each stirrup to hold a woman's legs securely in place if the woman prefers this increased support.

Obstetric stirrups provide much more support than the traditionally used foot stirrups. This position allows a woman who has difficulty using the foot stirrups to assume the traditional pelvic examination position.

M-Shaped Position. In the M-shaped position the woman lies on her back, knees bent and apart, feet resting on the examination table close to her buttocks (Fig. 18-38). The speculum must be inserted with the handle up. The bimanual examination can be performed from the foot of the table.

If the woman feels her legs are not completely stable on the examination table, an assistant may support her feet or knees. If a woman has bilateral leg amputations, assistants may elevate her stumps to simulate this position.

The M-shaped position does not require the use of stirrups. This position allows the patient to lie with her entire body supported by the table.

V-Shaped Position. In the V-shaped position the woman lies on her back with her straightened legs spread out wide to either side of the table (Fig. 18-39). If a woman is able to put one foot in the stirrup, a variation of this position would allow the woman to hold one leg out straight and keep one foot in a stirrup. The speculum must be inserted with the handle up, and the bimanual examination can be performed from the side or foot of the table.

At least one and possibly two assistants are needed to enable the woman to maintain this position. The assistants should support each straightened leg at the knee and ankle. The patient may be more comfortable if her legs are slightly elevated or if a pillow is used under the small of her back or tailbone.

The V-shaped position may or may not require stirrups. The patient must be able to lie comfortably on her back to use this position.

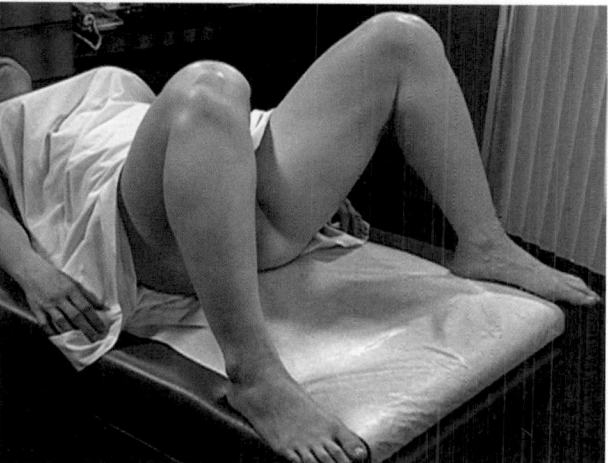

FIGURE 18-38
The M-shaped position.

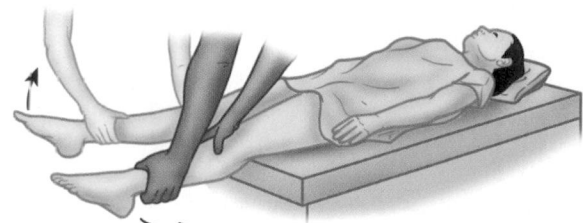

FIGURE 18-39
The V-shaped position.

WOMEN WITH SENSORY IMPAIRMENT

A woman with visual or hearing impairment will probably want to assume a foot-stirrup position for the pelvic examination (Figs. 18-40 and 18-41). Before the examination, you can ask the patient if she would like to examine the speculum, swab, or other instruments that will be used during the examination. If three-dimensional genital models are available, they can be used to familiarize the woman with the examination process. You may elevate the head of the table for a woman with a hearing impairment so that she can see the clinician and/or interpreter. The drape that is used to cover the woman's body below her waist should be eliminated or kept low between her legs.

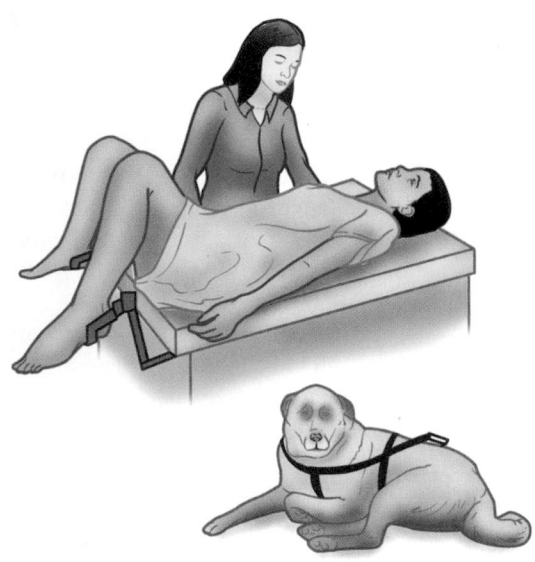

FIGURE 18-40
Positioning the visually impaired woman.

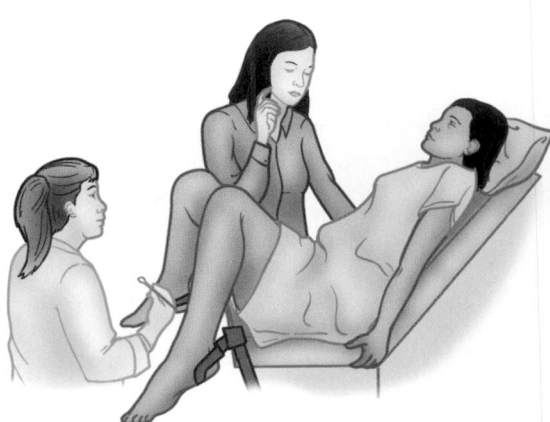

FIGURE 18-41
Positioning the hearing-impaired woman.

SAMPLE DOCUMENTATION

HISTORY AND PHYSICAL EXAMINATION

Subjective
A 45-year-old female with vaginal discharge and itching for past week. Has had yeast infections before. Completed course of antibiotics for sinusitis 2 days ago. LMP 2 weeks ago. Sexually active, one partner, mutually monogamous. No unusual vaginal bleeding. Does not douche.

Objective
External: Female hair distribution; no masses, lesions, or swelling. Urethral meatus intact without erythema or discharge. Perineum intact with a healed episiotomy scar present. No lesions.
Internal: Vaginal mucosa pink and moist with rugae present. No unusual odors. Profuse thick, white, curdy discharge. Cervix pink with horizontal slit, midline; no lesions or discharge.
Bimanual: Cervix smooth, firm, mobile. No cervical motion tenderness. Uterus midline, anteverted, firm, smooth, and nontender; not enlarged. Ovaries not palpable. No adnexal tenderness.
Rectovaginal: Septum intact. Sphincter tone intact; anal ring smooth and intact. No masses or tenderness.

For additional sample documentation, see Chapter 26.

SUMMARY OF EXAMINATION

The patient is in the lithotomy position for the following:

External Genitalia

1. Inspect the pubic hair characteristics and distribution (p. 596).
2. Inspect and palpate the labia for the following (p. 596):
   - Symmetry of color
   - Caking of discharge
   - Inflammation
   - Irritation or excoriation
   - Swelling
3. Inspect the urethral meatus and vaginal opening for the following (p. 597):
   - Discharge
   - Lesions or caruncles
   - Polyps
   - Fistulas
4. Milk the Skene glands (p. 597).
5. Palpate the Bartholin glands (p. 597).
6. Inspect and palpate the perineum for the following (p. 598):
   - Smoothness
   - Tenderness, inflammation
   - Fistulas
   - Lesions or growths
7. Inspect for bulging and urinary incontinence as the patient bears down (p. 598).
8. Inspect the perineal area and anus for the following (p. 598):
   - Skin characteristics
   - Lesions
   - Fissures or excoriation
   - Inflammation

Internal Genitalia Speculum Examination

1. Insert the speculum along the path of least resistance (p. 599).
2. Inspect the cervix for the following (p. 599):
   - Color
   - Position
   - Size
   - Surface characteristics
   - Discharge
   - Size and shape of os
3. Collect necessary specimens for culture and Pap smear (p. 602).

4. Inspect vaginal walls for the following (p. 603):
   - Color
   - Surface characteristics
   - Secretions

Bimanual Examination

1. Insert the index and middle fingers of one hand into the vagina and place the other hand on the abdominal midline (p. 604).
2. Palpate the vaginal walls for the following (p. 604):
   - Smoothness
   - Tenderness
   - Lesions (cysts, nodules, or masses)
3. Palpate the cervix for the following (p. 605):
   - Size, shape, and length
   - Position
   - Mobility
4. Palpate the uterus for the following (pp. 605 and 606):
   - Location
   - Position
   - Size, shape, and contour
   - Mobility
   - Tenderness
5. Palpate the ovaries for the following (p. 607):
   - Size
   - Shape
   - Consistency
   - Tenderness
6. Palpate adnexal areas for masses and tenderness (p. 607).

Rectovaginal Examination

1. Insert the index finger into the vagina and the middle finger into the anus (p. 608).
2. Assess sphincter tone (p. 608).
3. Palpate the rectovaginal septum for the following (p. 608):
   - Thickness
   - Tone
   - Nodules
4. Palpate the posterior aspect of the uterus (p. 608).
5. Palpate the anterior and posterior rectal wall for the following (p. 608):
   - Masses, polyps, or nodules
   - Strictures, other irregularities, tenderness
6. Note characteristics of feces when the gloved finger is removed (p. 608).

COMMON ABNORMALITIES

PREMENSTRUAL SYNDROME	Premenstrual syndrome (PMS) usually begins in a woman's late 20s and increases in incidence and severity as menopause approaches. It is characterized by edema, headache, weight gain, and behavioral disturbances such as irritability, nervousness, dysphoria, and lack of coordination. Symptoms occur 5 to 7 days before menses and subside with onset of menses.
INFERTILITY	The inability to conceive over a period of 1 year of unprotected regular intercourse has many causes, including both male and female conditions. Contributing factors in the woman include abnormalities of the vagina, cervix, uterus, fallopian tubes, and ovaries. Male infertility can be caused by insufficient, nonmotile, or immature sperm, ductal obstruction of sperm, and transport-related factors. Factors influencing both women and men include stress, nutrition, chemical substances, chromosomal abnormalities, certain disease processes, sexual and relationship problems, and immunologic response.
ENDOMETRIOSIS	The presence and growth of endometrial tissue outside the uterus causes pelvic pain, dysmenorrhea, and heavy or prolonged menstrual flow. On bimanual examination, tender nodules may be palpable along the uterosacral ligaments. Diagnosis is confirmed by laparoscopy (Figs. 18-42 and 18-43).

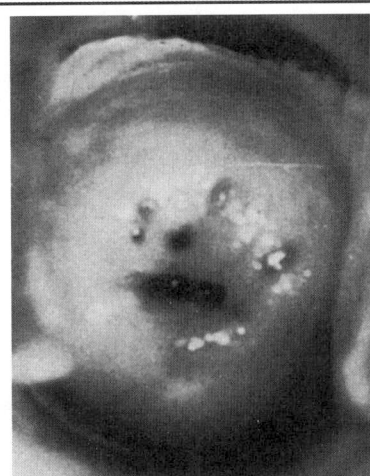

FIGURE 18-42
Superficial endometriosis of the ectocervix, resembling hemorrhagic nabothian cysts.
From Gardner, 1962.

CLINICAL PEARL

Endometriosis
Adolescents and older women can be plagued with a common problem: endometriosis. There is a possible difference in presentation. Adolescents may have pelvic pain that is cyclic and noncyclic. The pain in older women is most often cyclic. Don't let noncyclic pelvic pain in an adolescent rule out the possibility of endometriosis.

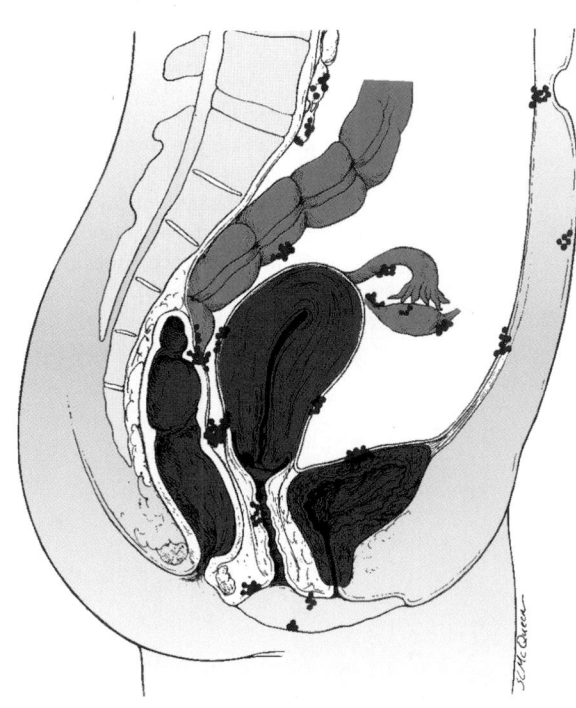

FIGURE 18-43
Common sites of endometriosis.
From Stenchever et al, 2001.

LESIONS FROM SEXUALLY TRANSMITTED INFECTIONS

CONDYLOMA ACUMINATUM (GENITAL WARTS)

Warty lesions on the labia, within the vestibule, or in the perianal region are the result of human papillomavirus (HPV) infection. Venereal warts are sexually transmitted (Fig. 18-44). They are generally flesh-colored, whitish pink to reddish brown, discrete, soft growths. They may occur singly or in clusters and may enlarge to form cauliflower-like masses.

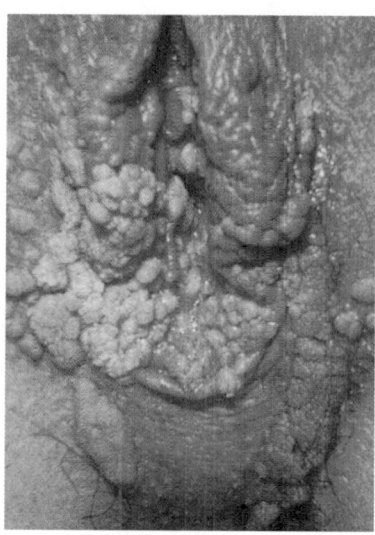

FIGURE 18-44
Condyloma acuminatum.
From Morse et al, 2003.

MOLLUSCUM CONTAGIOSUM

Caused by a poxvirus, this usually benign skin infection may be transmitted by sexual contact. The incubation period is from 2 to 7 weeks. The lesions are white or flesh-colored, dome-shaped papules that are round or oval (Fig. 18-45). The surface has a characteristic central umbilication from which a thick creamy core can be expressed. The lesions may last from several months to several years. Diagnosis is usually based on the clinical appearance of the lesions. Direct microscopic examination of stained material from the core will reveal typical molluscum bodies within the epithelial cell.

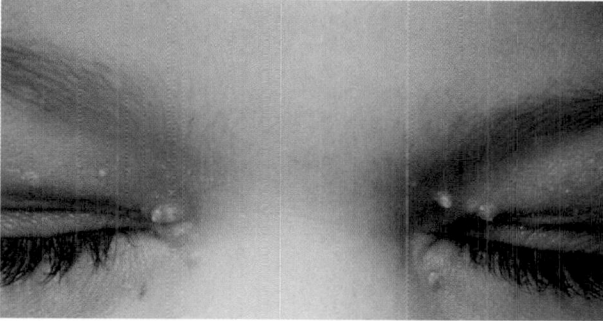

FIGURE 18-45
Molluscum contagiosum. Note that these have occurred around the eyes.
Courtesy Walter Tunnesen, MD, Chapel Hill, NC.

CONDYLOMA LATUM   Lesions of secondary syphilis appear about 6 to 12 weeks after infection. They are flat, round, or oval papules covered by a gray exudate (Fig. 18-46).

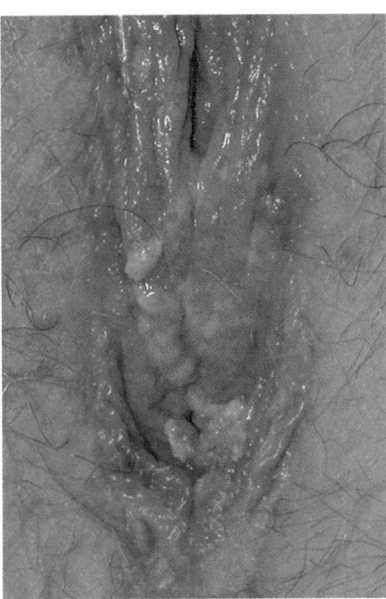

FIGURE 18-46
Condyloma latum.
From Lemmi, Lemmi, 2000.

SYPHILITIC CHANCRE (PRIMARY SYPHILIS)   A syphilitic chancre is a firm, painless ulcer. Most chancres in women develop internally and often go undetected (Fig. 18-47).

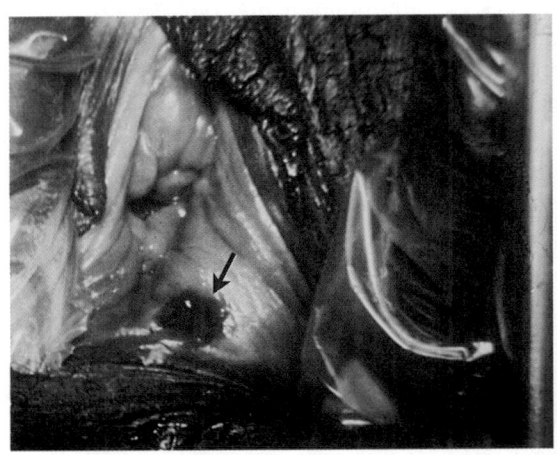

FIGURE 18-47
Primary syphilitic chancre in vagina.
From Habif, 2004.

HERPES LESIONS

Genital herpes is a sexually transmitted infection that produces small red vesicles. The lesions may itch and are usually painful. Initial infection is often extensive, whereas recurrent infection is usually confined to a small localized patch on the vulva, perineum, vagina, or cervix (Figs. 18-48 and 18-49).

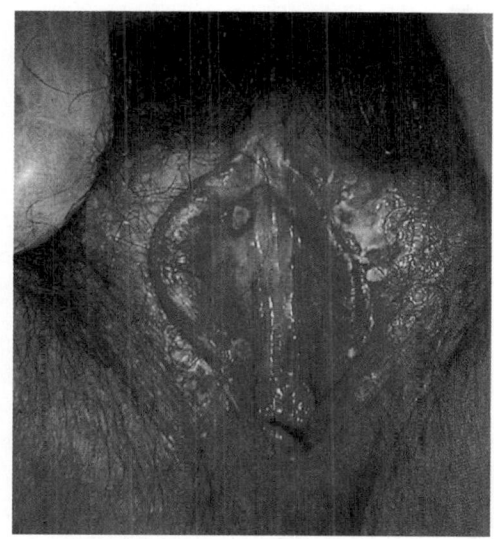

FIGURE 18-48
Herpes lesions. Scattered erosions covered with exudate.
From Habif, 2004.

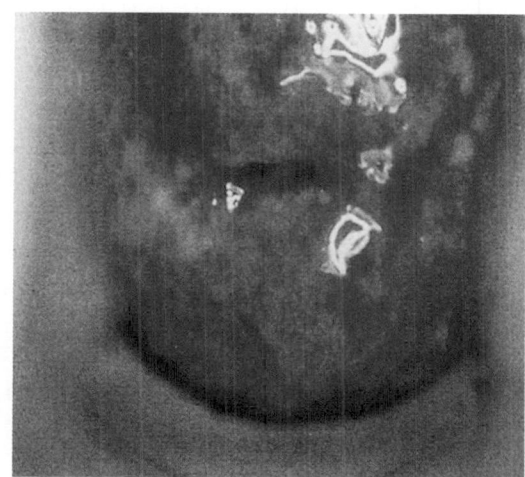

FIGURE 18-49
Herpetic cervicitis. Erythema, purulent exudate, and erosions are present on the cervix.
From Morse et al, 2003.

VULVA AND VAGINA

INFLAMMATION OF BARTHOLIN GLAND

Inflamed Bartholin glands are commonly, but not always, caused by gonococcal infection. It may be acute or chronic. Acute inflammation produces a hot, red, tender, fluctuant swelling that may drain pus. Chronic inflammation results in a nontender cyst on the labium (Fig. 18-50).

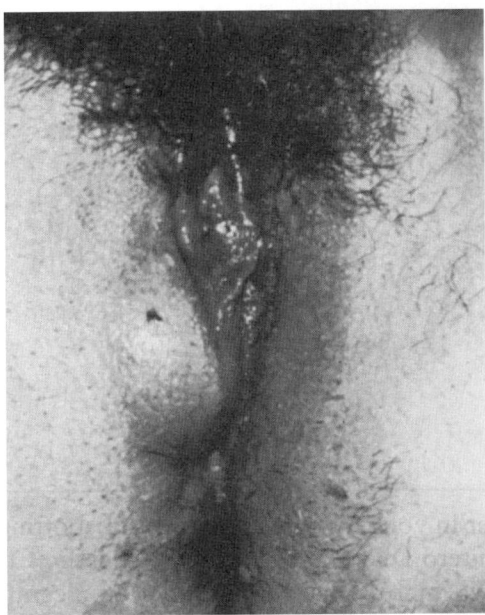

FIGURE 18-50
Inflammation of Bartholin gland.
From Kaufman, Faro, 1994.

CYSTOCELE

A cystocele is a hernial protrusion of the urinary bladder through the anterior wall of the vagina, sometimes even exiting the introitus. The bulging can be seen and felt as the woman bears down. More severe degrees of cystocele are accompanied by urinary stress incontinence (Fig. 18-51).

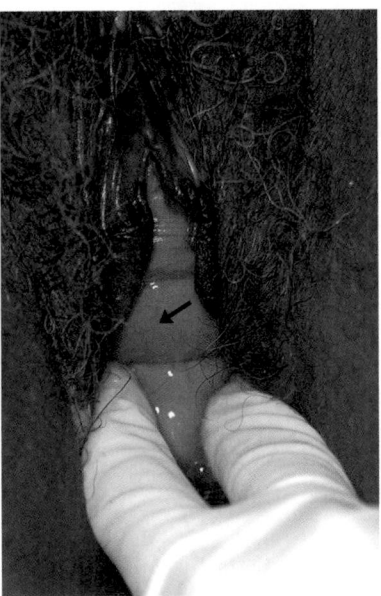

FIGURE 18-51
Cystocele.

RECTOCELE

Hernial protrusion of part of the rectum through the posterior wall of the vagina is called rectocele or proctocele. Bulging can be observed and felt as the woman bears down (Fig. 18-52).

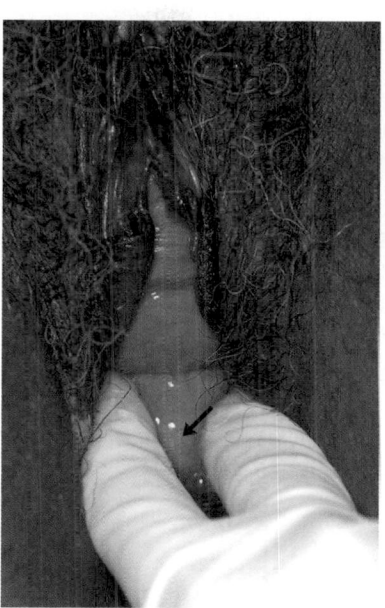

FIGURE 18-52
Rectocele.

CARCINOMA

Vaginal cancer in young women may be related to in utero DES exposure. Findings include vaginal discharge, lesions, and masses; and there may be a history of spotting, pain, and change in urinary habits. Cancer of the vulva appears as an ulcerated or raised red lesion on the vulva (Fig. 18-53).

A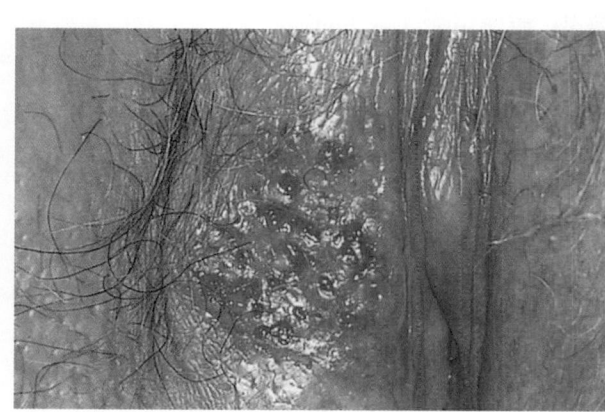

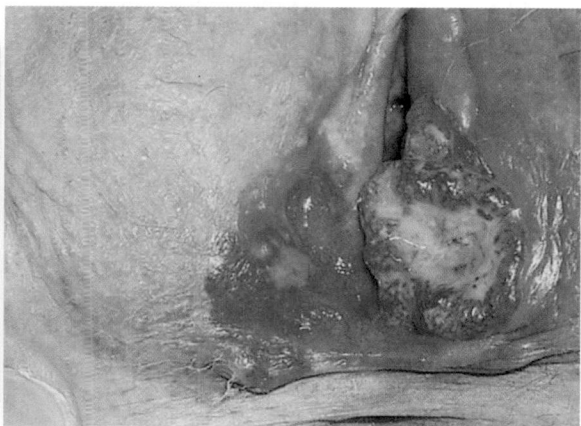 B

FIGURE 18-53
A, Basal cell carcinoma of the vulva. **B,** Ulcerative squamous cell carcinoma of the vulva.
From Symonds, Macpherson, 1994.

URETHRAL CARUNCLE A bright red polypoid growth that protrudes from the urethral meatus, most urethral caruncles cause no symptoms (Fig. 18-54).

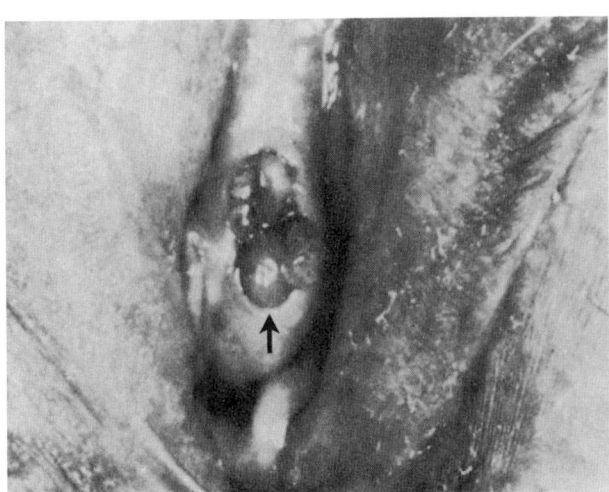

FIGURE 18-54
Urethral caruncle, a red fleshy lesion at the urethral meatus.
From Kaufman, Faro, 1994.

VAGINAL INFECTIONS Vaginal infections often produce a vaginal discharge and may be accompanied by urinary and other symptoms; however, symptoms may be entirely absent. Vaginal infections can be sexually transmitted, although candidal infections can result from antibiotics, oral contraceptives, or systemic disease (Figs. 18-55 and 18-56).

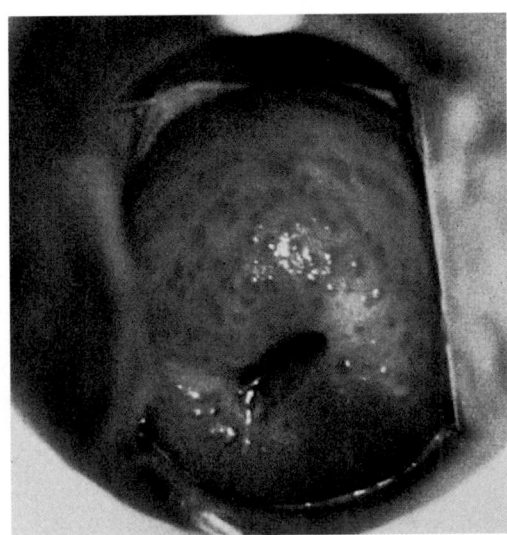

FIGURE 18-55
Trichomoniasis. The vaginal mucosa is inflamed and often speckled with petechial lesions. In adolescents, petechial hemorrhages may also be found on the cervix, resulting in the so-called strawberry cervix.
From Zitelli, Davis, 1997.

A　　　　　**B**　　　　　**C**

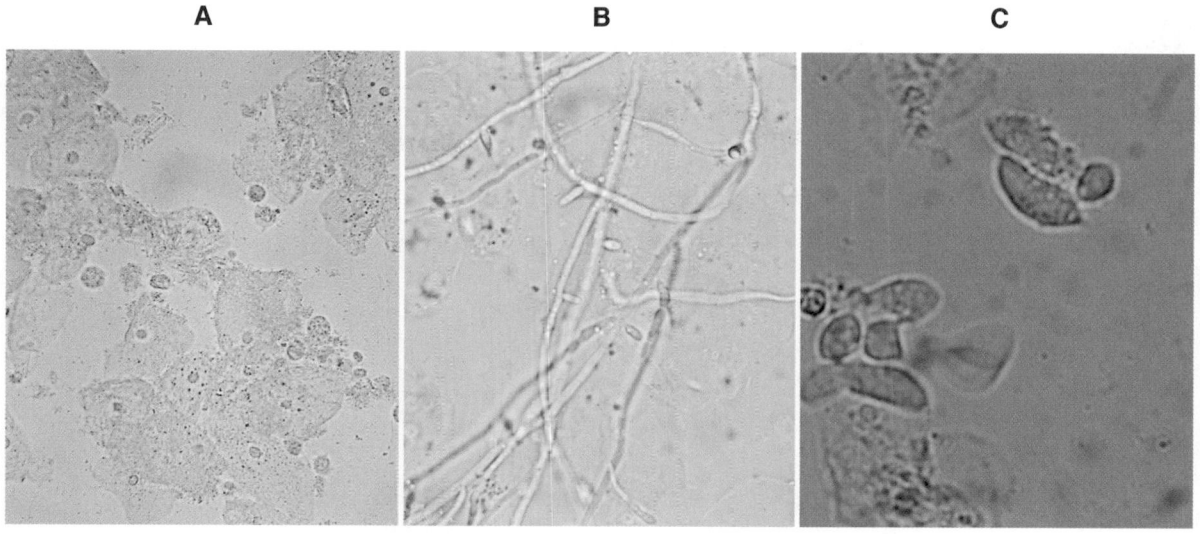

FIGURE 18-56
Microscopic differentiation of vaginal infections. **A,** Bacterial vaginosis: "clue cells." **B,** Candida vulvovaginitis: "budding, branching hyphae." **C,** Trichomoniasis: motile trichomonads.
From Zitelli, Davis, 1997.

DIFFERENTIAL DIAGNOSIS

VAGINAL DISCHARGES AND INFECTIONS

Condition	History	Physical Findings	Diagnostic Tests
Physiologic vaginitis	Increase in discharge	Clear or mucoid discharge; pH < 4.5	Wet mount: up to 3 to 5 WBCs; epithelial cells
Bacterial vaginosis (*Gardnerella vaginalis*)	No foul odor, itching or edema Foul-smelling discharge; complains of "fishy odor"	Homogenous thin, white or gray discharge; pH < 4.5	+KOH "whiff" test; wet mount: + clue cells (see Fig. 18-56, *A*)
Candida vulvovaginitis (*Candida albicans*)	Pruritic discharge; itching of labia; itching may extend to thighs	White, curdy discharge; pH 4.0 to 5.0; cervix may be red; may have erythema of perineum and thighs	KOH prep: mycelia, budding, branching yeast, pseudohypha (see Fig. 18-56, *B*)
Trichomoniasis (*Trichomonas vaginalis*)	Watery discharge; foul odor; dysuria and dyspareunia with severe infection	Profuse, frothy, greenish discharge; pH 5.0 to 6.6; red friable cervix with petechiae ("strawberry" cervix) (see Fig. 18-54)	Wet mount: round or pear-shaped protozoa; motile "gyrating" flagella (see Fig. 18-56, *C*)
Gonorrhea (*Neisseria gonorrhoeae*)	Partner with STI; often asymptomatic or may have symptoms of PID	Purulent discharge from cervix; Skene/Bartholin inflammation; cervix and vulva may be inflamed	Gram stain Culture DNA probe
Chlamydia (*Chlamydia trachomatis*)	Partner with nongonococcal urethritis; often asymptomatic; may complain of spotting after intercourse or urethritis	± purulent discharge; cervix may or may not be red or friable	DNA probe
Atrophic vaginitis	Dyspareunia; vaginal dryness; perimenopausal or postmenopausal	Pale, thin vaginal mucosa; pH < 4.5	Wet mount: folded, clumped epithelial cells
Allergic vaginitis	New bubble bath, soap, douche, or other hygiene products	Foul smell; erythema; pH <4.5	Wet mount: WBCs
Foreign body	Red and swollen vulva; vaginal discharge; history of use of tampon, condom, or diaphragm	Bloody or foul-smelling discharge	Wet mount: WBCs

KOH, Potassium hydroxide; *PID,* pelvic inflammatory disease; *STI,* sexually transmitted infection; *WBC,* white blood cell.

CERVIX

LACERATIONS

Cervical lacerations are caused by trauma, most often childbirth. Lacerations can produce lateral transverse, bilateral transverse, or stellate scarring (Fig. 18-57).

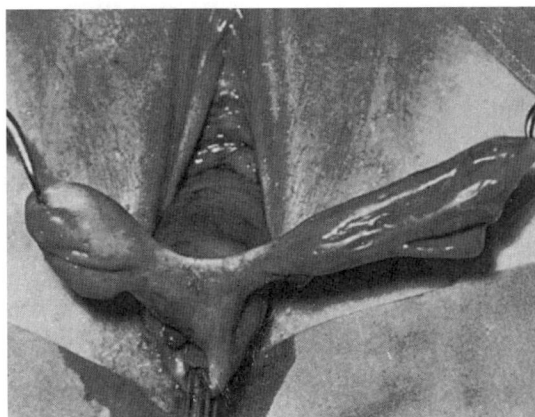

FIGURE 18-57
Severely lacerated cervix with hypertrophy and prolapse.
From Willson, Carrington, Ledger, 1987.

INFECTED NABOTHIAN CYSTS

Enlarged fluid-filled retention cysts often distort the shape of the cervix. Infected nabothian cysts vary in size and may occur singly or in multiples.

CERVICAL POLYPS

Cervical polyps are bright red, soft, and fragile. They usually arise from the endocervical canal (Fig. 18-58).

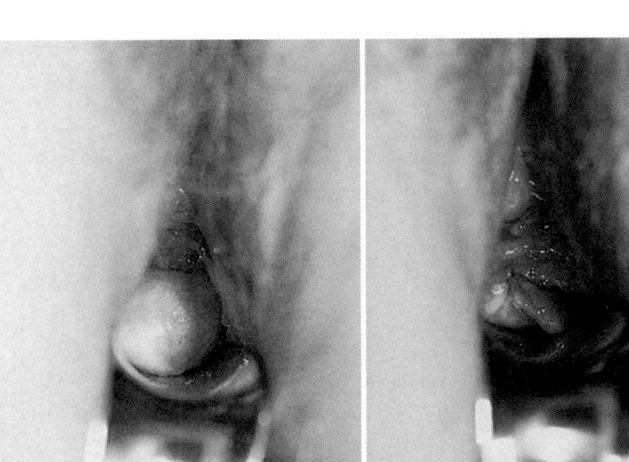

A

B

FIGURE 18-58
A, Fibroid polyp protruding through the external cervical os.
B, Small endocervical polyp.
From Symonds, Macpherson, 1994.

CERVICAL CARCINOMA Cervical cancer produces a hard granular surface at or near the cervical os. The lesion can evolve to form an extensive irregular cauliflower growth that bleeds easily. Early lesions are indistinguishable from ectropion (Fig. 18-59). Precancerous and early cancer changes are detected by Pap smear, not by physical examination.

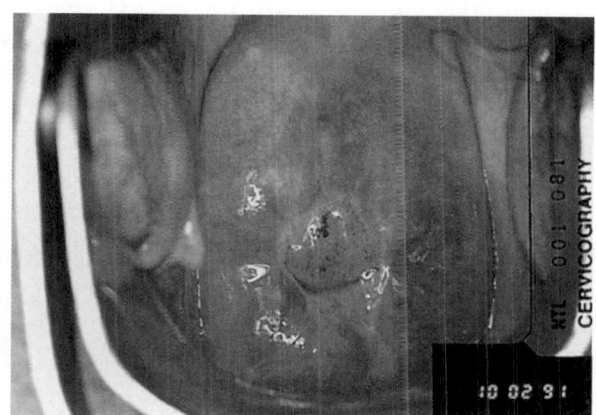

FIGURE 18-59
The cervical cancer lesion is predominantly around the external os.
From Symonds, Macpherson, 1994.

ECTROPION   Columnar epithelium from the cervical canal appears as shiny red tissue around the os that may bleed easily. Ectropion is not an abnormality, but because it is indistinguishable from early cervical carcinoma, further diagnostic studies (e.g., Pap smear, biopsy) must be performed for differential diagnosis.

UTERUS

UTERINE PROLAPSE

The uterus prolapses as the result of weakening of the supporting structures of the pelvic floor, often occurring concurrently with a cystocele and rectocele. The uterus becomes progressively retroverted and descends into the vaginal canal (Fig. 18-60). In first-degree prolapse, the cervix remains within the vagina; in second-degree prolapse, the cervix is at the introitus; in third-degree prolapse, the cervix and vagina drop outside the introitus (Fig. 18-61).

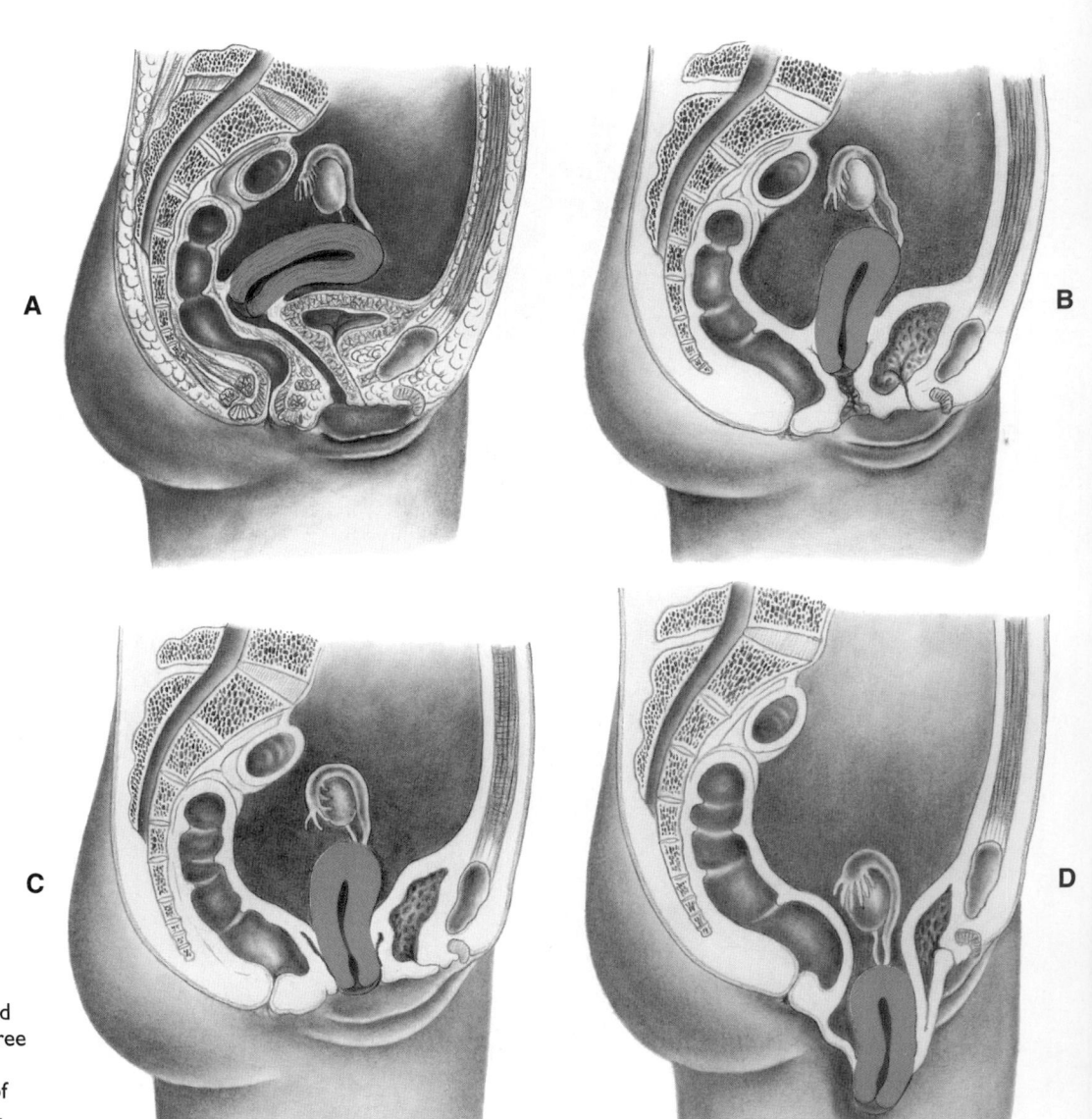

FIGURE 18-60
Uterine prolapse. **A,** Expected uterine position. **B,** First-degree prolapse of the uterus. **C,** Second-degree prolapse of the uterus. **D,** Complete prolapse of the uterus.

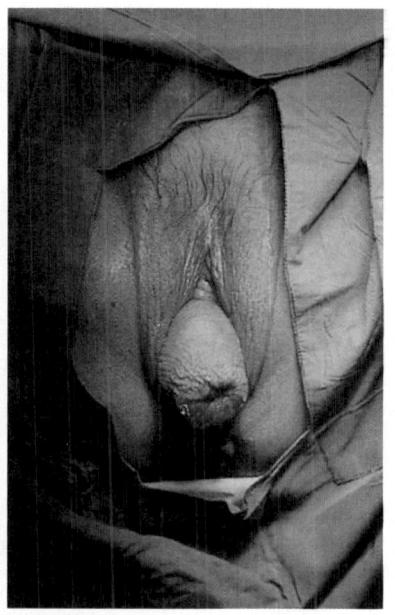

FIGURE 18-61
A third-degree prolapse of the uterus and vaginal walls.
From Symonds, Macpherson, 1994.

UTERINE BLEEDING

Abnormality in menstrual bleeding and inappropriate uterine bleeding are common gynecologic problems (Table 18-5). The following terms associated with menstrual bleeding can be found in the Glossary: *amenorrhea, dysfunctional uterine bleeding, hypermenorrhea, hypomenorrhea, menorrhagia, metrorrhagia, oligomenorrhea, postmenopausal bleeding, polymenorrhea,* and *spotting.*

TABLE 18-5	Types of Uterine Bleeding and Associated Causes
Type	**Common Causes**
Midcycle spotting	Midcycle estradiol fluctuation associated with ovulation
Delayed menstruation	Anovulation or threatened abortion with excessive bleeding
Frequent bleeding	Chronic PID, endometriosis, DUB, anovulation
Profuse menstrual	Endometrial polyps, DUB, adenomyosis, submucous bleeding leiomyomas, IUD
Intermenstrual or irregular bleeding	Endometrial polyps, DUB, uterine or cervical cancer, oral contraceptives
Postmenopausal bleeding	Endometrial hyperplasia, estrogen therapy, endometrial cancer

Modified from Thompson et al, 1997.
DUB, Dysfunctional uterine bleeding; *IUD,* intrauterine device; *PID,* pelvic inflammatory disease.

MYOMAS (LEIOMYOMAS, FIBROIDS)

Myomas are common, benign, uterine tumors that appear as firm, irregular nodules in the contour of the uterus. They may occur singly or in multiples and vary greatly in size. The uterus may become enlarged (Fig. 18-62).

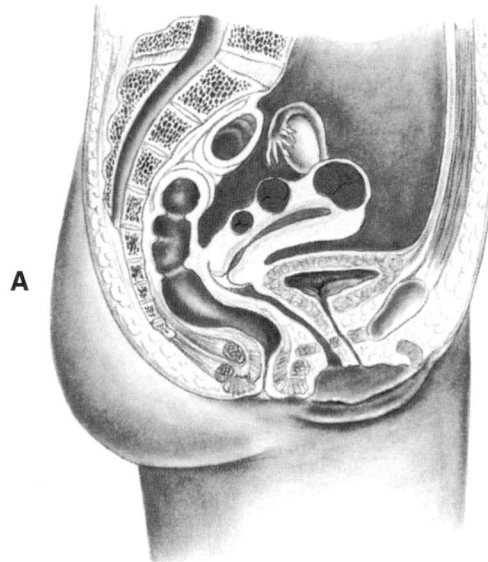
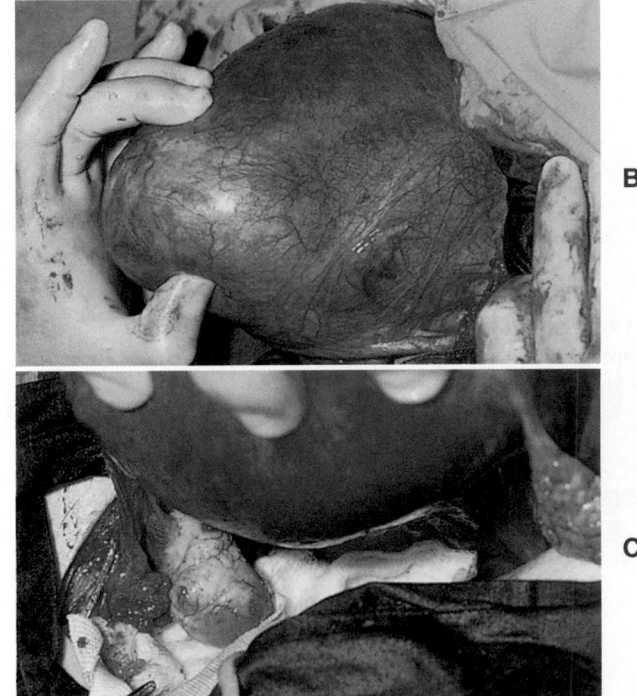

FIGURE 18-62
Myomas of the uterus (fibroids). **A,** Common location of myomas. **B,** Multiple uterine fibroids.
C, Multiple uterine fibroids with enlarged ovaries resulting from multiple small cysts.
B, C from Symonds, Macpherson, 1994.

ENDOMETRIAL CARCINOMA

Endometrial cancer occurs most often in postmenopausal women. Nearly all endometrial cancers are cancers of the glandular cells found in the lining of the uterus. Most known risk factors for endometrial cancer are linked to the balance between estrogen and progesterone in the body. Women taking Tamoxifen are at increased risk. Postmenopausal vaginal bleeding is a red flag for endometrial cancer.

ADNEXA

OVARIAN CYSTS AND TUMORS

Ovarian growths can occur unilaterally or bilaterally. Cysts tend to be smooth and sometimes compressible, whereas tumors feel more solid and nodular; neither is usually tender. A ruptured ovarian cyst will produce symptoms similar to those of ruptured tubal pregnancy (Fig. 18-63).

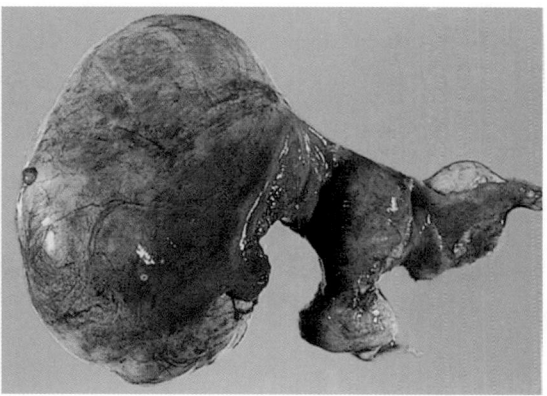

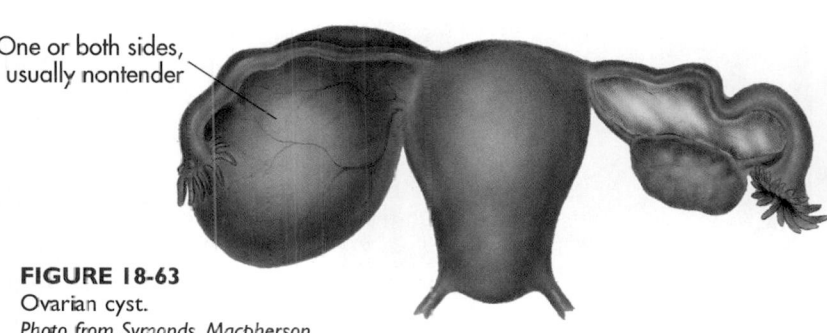

One or both sides, usually nontender

FIGURE 18-63
Ovarian cyst.
Photo from Symonds, Macpherson, 1994.

OVARIAN CARCINOMA

Ovarian cancer is difficult to detect and is often asymptomatic at first. An ovary that is enlarged should be considered suspicious for cancer, and further diagnostic tests are required. Suspect ovarian cancer in a woman older than 40 years of age with persistent and unexplained vague gastrointestinal symptoms such as generalized abdominal discomfort and/or pain, gas, indigestion, pressure, swelling, bloating, cramps or feeling of fullness even after a light meal.

RUPTURED TUBAL PREGNANCY

A ruptured tubal pregnancy causes marked pelvic tenderness, with tenderness and rigidity of the lower abdomen. Motion of the cervix produces pain. A tender, unilateral adnexal mass may indicate the site of the pregnancy. Tachycardia and shock reflect the hemorrhage into the peritoneal cavity and cardiovascular collapse. This is a surgical emergency (Fig. 18-64).

CLINICAL PEARL

Ectopic Pregnancy
Unhappily, ectopic pregnancy is often not diagnosed before rupture because symptoms are mild. Big clue: A sudden, dramatic change from mild, even vague abdominal pain that is there but not particularly distressing to a sudden onset of severe abdominal tenderness in the hypogastric area, particularly on the involved side. Rigidity and rebound may come on early or late. The main point: If a woman presents with vague abdominal complaints, check out the sexual contact and menstrual history, do a pelvic examination, and do not disregard the mild tenderness that might be evoked. Try, at least, to anticipate the emergency of a rupture.

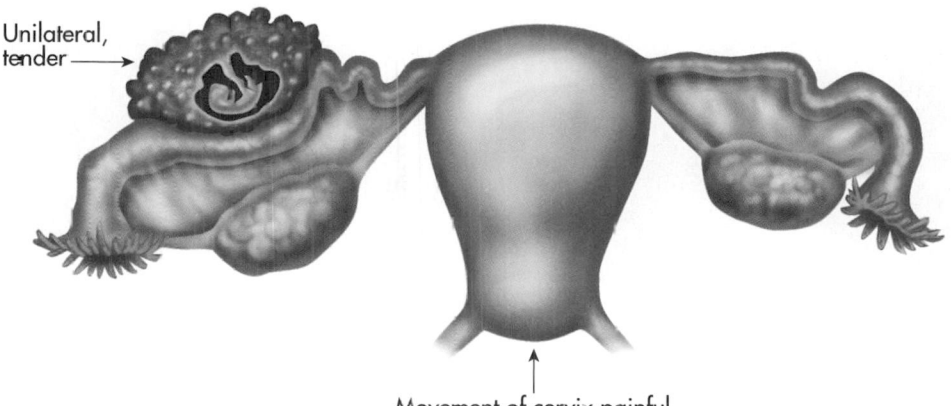

Unilateral, tender →

Movement of cervix painful

FIGURE 18-64
Ruptured tubal pregnancy.

PELVIC INFLAMMATORY DISEASE

Often caused by gonococcal and chlamydial infection, pelvic inflammatory disease (PID) may be acute or chronic. Acute PID produces very tender, bilateral adnexal areas; the patient guards and usually cannot tolerate bimanual examination. The symptoms of chronic PID are bilateral, tender, irregular, and fairly fixed adnexal areas (Fig. 18-65).

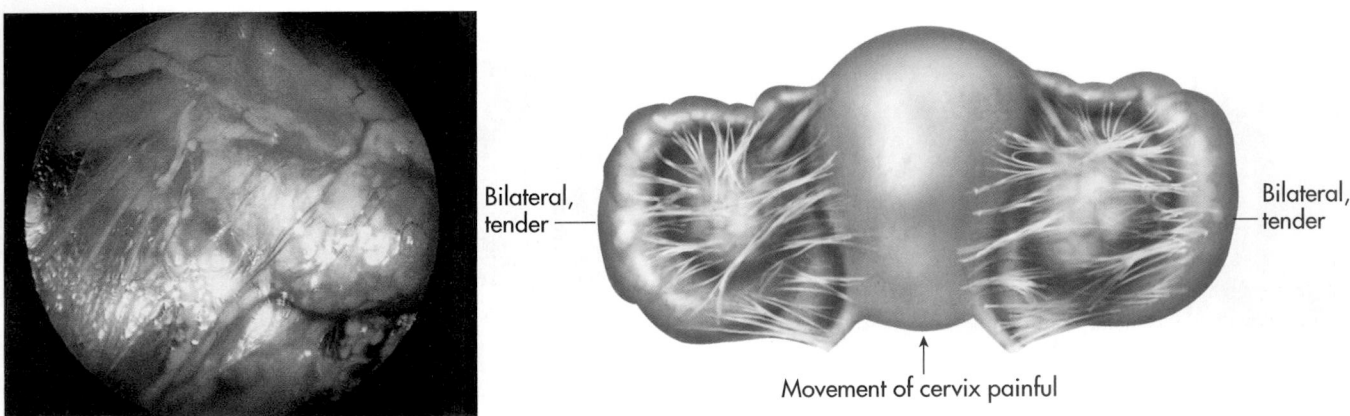

Bilateral, tender

Bilateral, tender

Movement of cervix painful

FIGURE 18-65
Pelvic inflammatory disease. Photo shows sheet of fine adhesions covering tubes and ovary, which is buried beneath the tubes.
Photo from Symonds, Macpherson, 1994.

SALPINGITIS

Inflammation or infection of the fallopian tube is often associated with PID. Salpingitis causes lower quadrant pain with tenderness on bimanual examination (Fig. 18-66).

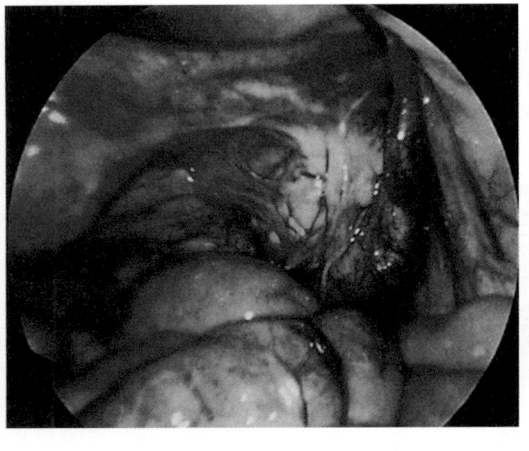
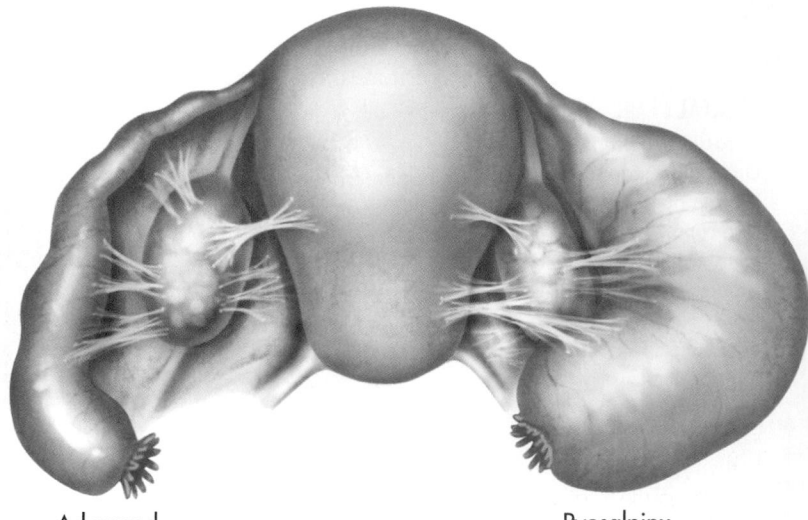

Advanced

Pyosalpinx

FIGURE 18-66
Salpingitis. Photo shows acute salpingitis with adhesions. Dye has been instilled into the grossly swollen fallopian tube on the right. Dense adhesions obscure the ovary.
Photo from Morse et al, 2003.

INFANTS AND CHILDREN

AMBIGUOUS GENITALIA

Certain conditions of the labia and clitoris may indicate ambiguous genitalia. For example, partially fused labia suggest the presence of a scrotum; a urinary meatus that is not located behind the clitoris may indicate the presence of a penis (Fig. 18-67).

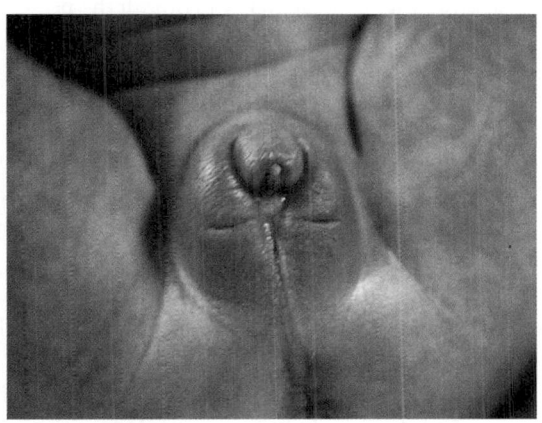

FIGURE 18-67
Ambiguous genitalia.
Courtesy Patrick C. Walsh, MD, The Johns Hopkins School of Medicine, Baltimore.

HYDROCOLPOS

Vaginal secretions can collect behind an imperforate hymen. Hydrocolpos may be manifested by a small midline lower abdominal mass or a small cystic mass between the labia. The condition may resolve spontaneously or may require surgical intervention.

VULVOVAGINITIS

Vaginal discharge that is accompanied by warm, erythematous, and swollen vulvar tissues is termed vulvovaginitis. Possible causes include sexual abuse; trichomonal, monilial, or gonococcal infection; secondary infection from a foreign body; and nonspecific infection from bubble baths, diaper irritation, urethritis, and injury (Fig. 18-68).

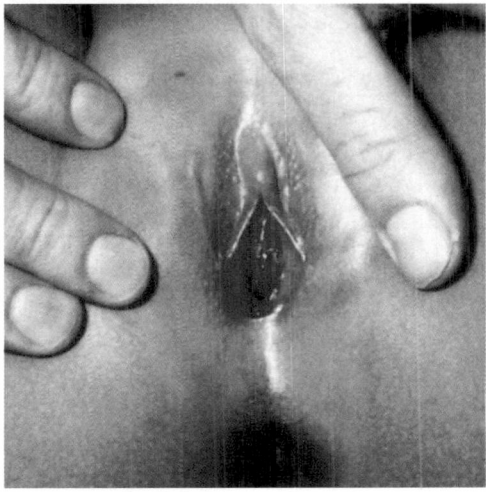

FIGURE 18-68
Nonspecific inflammation characteristic of chemical irritant vulvovaginitis.
From Zitelli, Davis, 1997.

PREGNANT WOMEN

PREMATURE RUPTURE OF MEMBRANES

The spontaneous premature rupture of the membranes (PROM) in a preterm pregnancy carries a high risk of perinatal morbidity and mortality, as well as maternal morbidity and mortality. The cause of PROM is not known; however, certain conditions such as infection and hydramnios have been implicated. Some health care professionals also consider the rupture of membranes before the onset of labor in a term pregnancy to be premature rupture if labor does not begin in 12 hours. Symptoms include the passage of fluid from the vagina. PROM should be verified with a sterile speculum exam to collect fluid for testing with Nitrazine paper and microscopic examination. Amniotic fluid has a pH of 7.15 and will turn Nitrazine paper blue-green. Amniotic fluid placed on a slide and air-dried will have a "fern" pattern. Ultrasound evaluation of fluid will reveal decreased or absent amniotic fluid. Management depends on the weeks of gestation and the condition of the mother and fetus.

PROLAPSE OF THE UMBILICAL CORD	When the presenting part of the fetus does not fill the pelvic inlet, a loop of cord may advance with the presenting part. Prolapse of the cord usually occurs with rupture of the membranes. Predisposing factors are premature labor, a fetus in breech presentation or transverse position, hydramnios, a high or floating presenting part (not engaged), and multiple pregnancy. The symptoms may be obvious, such as a loop of cord protruding from the vagina or the palpation of the pulsating cord on vaginal examination. The presence of variable decelerations in fetal heart rate is also associated with cord compression. Unless immediate measures are taken to relieve compression of the cord and deliver the fetus, death of the fetus can result.
BLEEDING	There are many causes for bleeding during pregnancy. In early pregnancy, bleeding may be due to unknown causes of little consequence or to a potentially life-threatening condition such as an ectopic pregnancy. Late in pregnancy, causes of bleeding may range from benign conditions such as cervical changes to a potentially life-threatening abruptio placentae. Whatever the cause, bleeding in pregnancy should be investigated thoroughly with a careful history and physical examination. However, women who are bleeding in labor or who have a suspected placenta previa should not be examined without preparation for emergency cesarean section.
VULVAR VARICOSITIES	Vulvar varicosities occur commonly during pregnancy. The varicosities may involve both the vulva and the rectal area. Pressure from the pregnant uterus and possibly hereditary factors contribute to the formation of the varicosities.

Older Adults

ATROPHIC VAGINITIS	Atrophy of the vagina is caused by lack of estrogen. The vaginal mucosa is dry and pale, although it may become reddened and develop petechiae and superficial erosions. The accompanying vaginal discharge may be white, gray, yellow, green, or blood-tinged. It can be thick or watery, and although it varies in amount, the discharge is rarely profuse.
URINARY INCONTINENCE	See the discussion on p. 577.

ELECTRONIC RESOURCES

For Weblinks and additional resources, go to   **evolve**

http://evolve.elsevier.com/Seidel

or to the Companion CD-ROM.

Additional information related to the content in Chapter 18 can be found on the companion website at http://evolve.elsevier.com/Seidel/ or on the interactive companion CD-ROM. Resources and activities for Chapter 18 include:
- Sound and Vision Theater
- Printouts for Your Practice
- Interactive Challenge
- Spanish Assessment Terms with Pronunciation Guide
- Instant Calculator

MALE GENITALIA

ANATOMY AND PHYSIOLOGY

The penis, testicles, epididymides, scrotum, prostate gland and seminal vesicles constitute the male genitalia (Fig. 19-1).

The physiologic function of the penis is to serve as the final excretory organ for urine and, when erect, as the means of introducing semen into the vagina. The penis consists of the two corpora cavernosa, which form the dorsum and sides, and the corpus spongiosum, which contains the urethra. The corpus spongiosum expands at its distal end to form the glans penis. The urethral orifice is a slitlike opening located approximately 2 mm ventral to the tip of the glans (Figs. 19-2 and 19-3). The skin of the penis is thin, redundant to permit erection, and free of subcutaneous fat. It is generally more darkly pigmented than body skin. Unless the patient has been circumcised, the prepuce (foreskin) covers the glans. In the uncircumcised male, smegma is formed by the secretion of sebaceous material by the glans and the desquamation of epithelial cells from the prepuce. It appears as a cheesy white material on the glans and in the fornix of the foreskin.

The scrotum, like the penis, is generally more darkly pigmented than body skin. A septum divides the scrotum into two pendulous sacs, each containing a testis, epididymis, spermatic cord, and a muscle layer, termed the cremasteric muscle, that allows the scrotum to relax or contract (Fig. 19-4). Testicular temperature is controlled by altering the distance of the testes from the body through muscular action. Spermatogenesis requires maintenance of temperatures lower than 37° C.

The testicles are responsible for the production of both spermatozoa and testosterone. The adult testis is ovoid and measures approximately $4 \times 3 \times 2$ cm. The epididymis is a soft, comma-shaped structure located on the posterolateral and upper aspect of the testis in 90% of males. It provides for storage, maturation, and transit of sperm. The vas deferens begins at the tail of the epididymis, ascends the spermatic cord, travels through the inguinal canal, and unites with the seminal vesicle to form the ejaculatory duct.

The prostate gland, which resembles a large chestnut and is approximately the size of a testis, surrounds the urethra at the bladder neck. The physiologic function of the prostate and its secretions is not completely understood. It produces the major volume of ejaculatory fluid, which contains fibrinolysin. This enzyme liquefies the coagulated semen, a process that may be important for satisfactory sperm motility. The seminal vesicles extend from the prostate onto the posterior surface of the bladder.

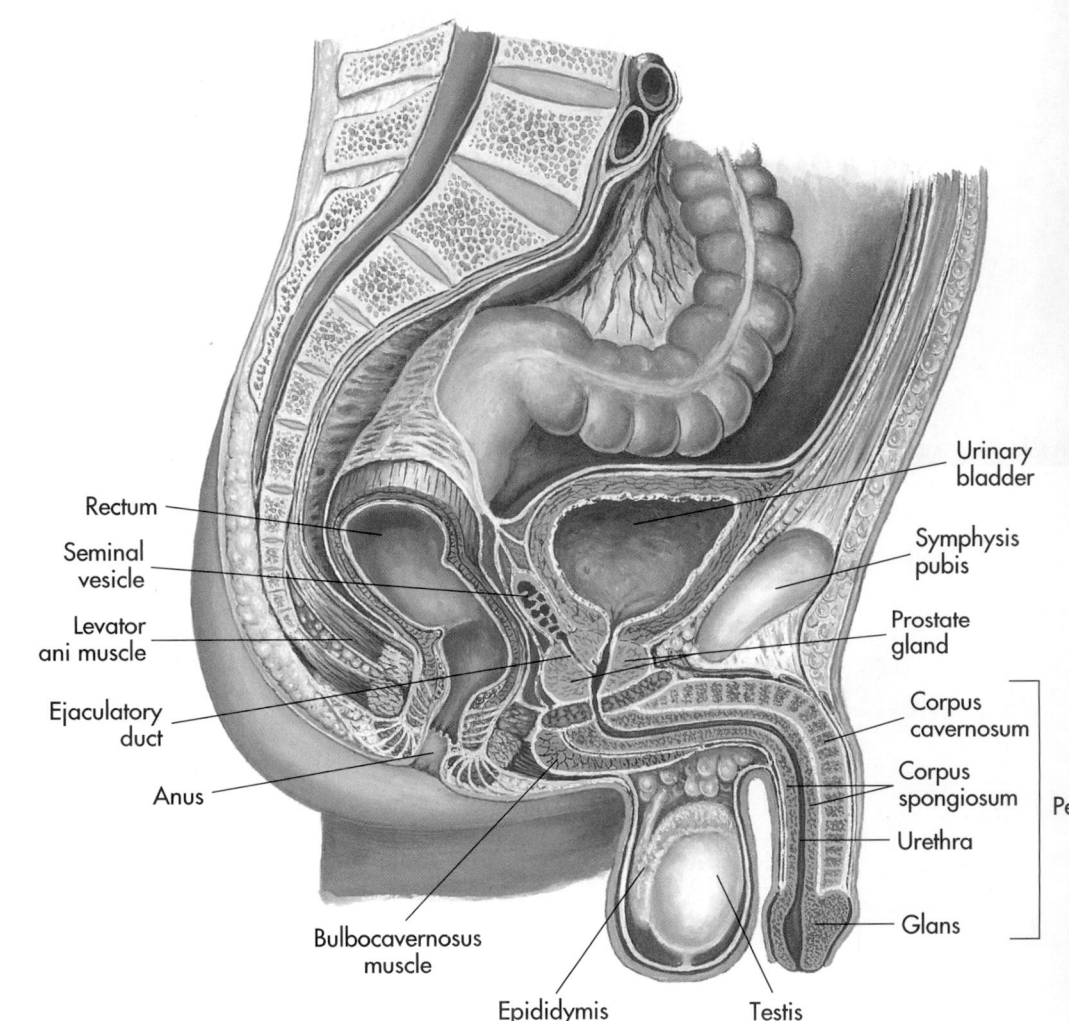

Rectum

Seminal vesicle

Levator ani muscle

Ejaculatory duct

Anus

Bulbocavernosus muscle

Urinary bladder

Symphysis pubis

Prostate gland

Corpus cavernosum

Corpus spongiosum

Urethra

Glans

Penis

Epididymis

Testis

FIGURE 19-1
Male pelvic organs.

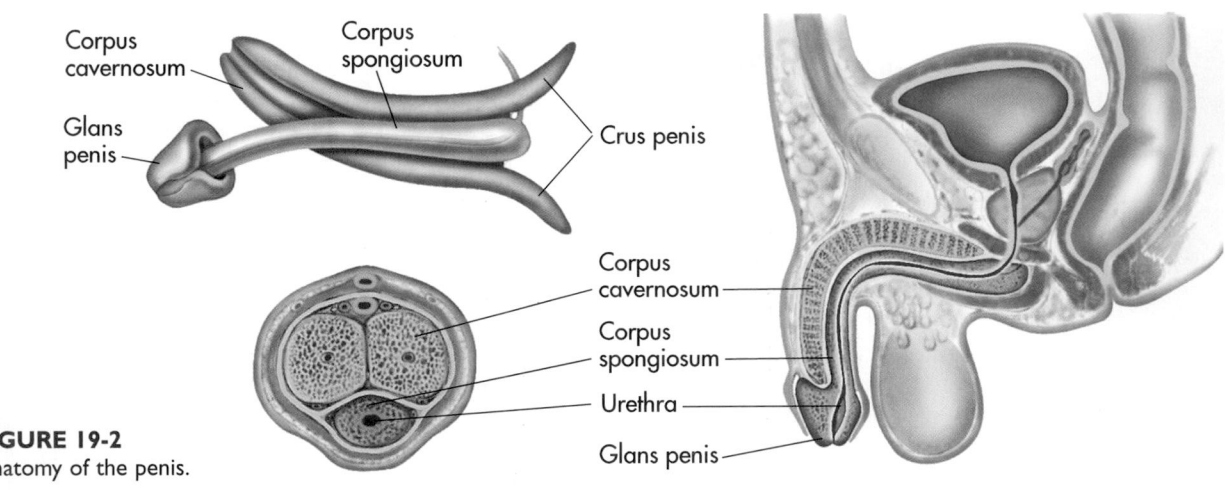

Corpus cavernosum

Corpus spongiosum

Glans penis

Crus penis

Corpus cavernosum

Corpus spongiosum

Urethra

Glans penis

FIGURE 19-2
Anatomy of the penis.

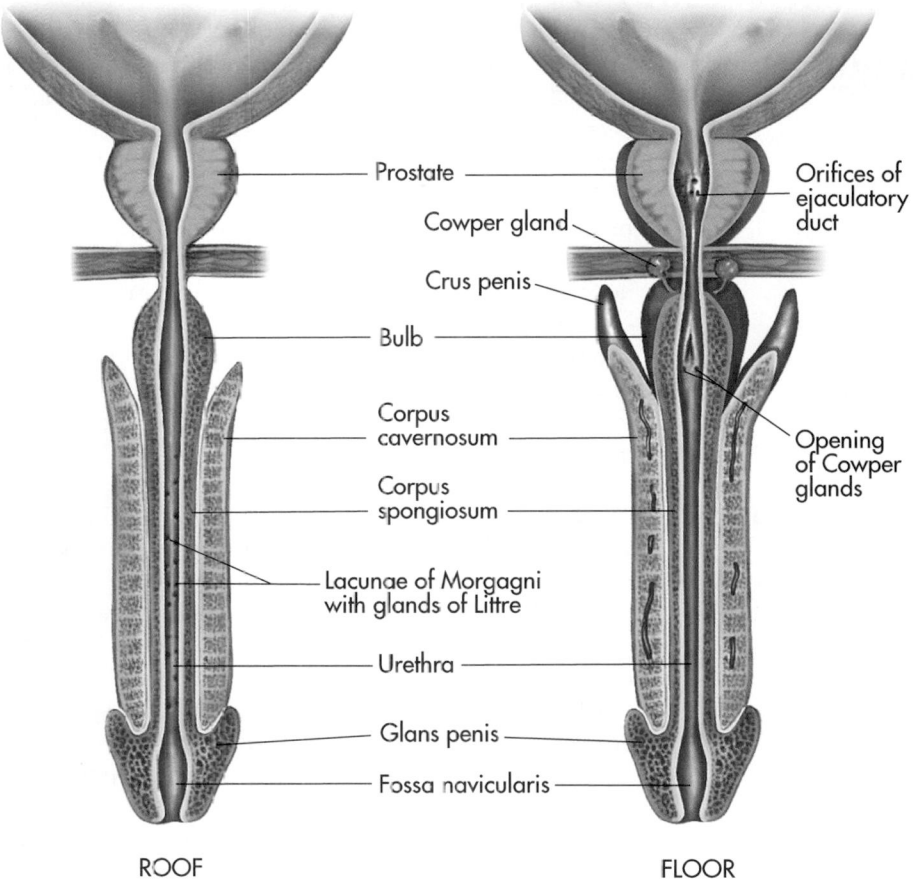

FIGURE 19-3
Anatomy of urethra and penis.
From Lowdermilk, Perry, Bobak, 1997.

ROOF   FLOOR

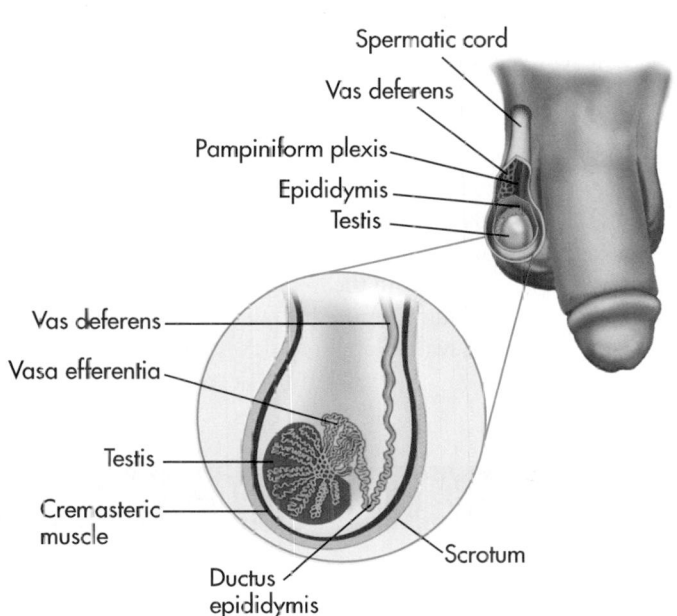

FIGURE 19-4
Scrotum and its contents.

SEXUAL PHYSIOLOGY

ERECTION

Erection of the penis occurs when the two corpora cavernosa become engorged with blood, generally 20 to 50 mL. Increased blood supply is produced by increased arterial dilation and decreased venous outflow; both processes are under the control of the autonomic nervous system and occur because of the local synthesis of nitric oxide.

Erection is a neurovascular reflex that can be induced by psychogenic and local reflex mechanisms. Local reflex mechanisms involve spinal reflex arcs that are initiated by tactile stimuli. Psychogenic erection can be initiated by any type of sensory input—auditory, visual, tactile, or imaginative stimuli. Cortical input can also serve to suppress sexual arousal.

ORGASM

Orgasm is a complex, pleasurable sensation accompanying ejaculation, which is the emission of secretions from the vas deferens, epididymides, prostate, and seminal vesicles. Orgasm is followed by constriction of the vessels supplying blood to the corpora cavernosa and gradual detumescence.

INFANTS AND CHILDREN

The external genitalia are identical for males and females at 8 weeks of gestation, but by 12 weeks of gestation sexual differentiation has occurred. Any fetal insult during 8 or 9 weeks of gestation may lead to major anomalies of the external genitalia. Minor morphologic abnormalities arise from injury after that period of development.

During the third trimester, the testes descend from the retroperitoneal space through the inguinal canal to the scrotum. At full term, one or both testes may still lie within the inguinal canal, with the final descent into the scrotum occurring in the early postnatal period. Descent of the testicles may be arrested at any point, however, or they may follow an abnormal path.

Small separations between the glans and the inner preputial epithelium begin during the third trimester. Separation of the prepuce from the glans is usually incomplete at birth and often remains so until the age of 3 to 4 years in uncircumcised males.

ADOLESCENTS

With the onset of puberty, testicular growth begins and the scrotal skin reddens, thins, and becomes increasingly pendulous. Then sparse, downy, straight hair appears at the base of the penis. Finally the penis begins enlarging. As maturation continues, the pubic hair darkens and extends over the entire pubic area, and the prostate gland enlarges. By the completion of puberty, the pubic hair is curly, dense, and coarse and forms a diamond-shaped pattern from the umbilicus to the anus. The growth and development of the testes and scrotum are complete. The penis is enlarged in length and breadth (see Chapter 5).

OLDER ADULTS

Pubic hair becomes finer and less abundant with aging, and pubic alopecia may occur.

No change in the length of time necessary for the production of mature spermatozoa occurs with aging. The viability of the sperm, however, probably decreases in that the rate of conception declines with age. The ejaculatory volume may actually increase with age, perhaps because of decreased frequency of intercourse. The scrotum becomes more pendulous with aging, and the patient may complain about it.

Frequency of sexual activity usually declines with aging, although the rate of decline correlates most strongly with the frequency of sexual activity in youth—that is, the man who was highly active in youth is more likely to maintain a higher level of sexual activity during later years. Erection may develop more slowly, and orgasm may be less intense.

REVIEW OF RELATED HISTORY

For each of the conditions discussed in this section, targeted topics to include in the history of the present illness are listed. Responses to questions about these topics help fully assess the patient's condition and provide clues for focusing the physical examination.

HISTORY OF PRESENT ILLNESS

- Difficulty achieving or maintaining erection
  - Pain with erection, prolonged painful erection
  - Constant or intermittent, with one or more sexual partners
  - Associated with alcohol ingestion or medication
  - Medications: prescription, nonprescription drugs, complementary, or alternative therapies that might interfere with sexual performance (diuretics, sedatives, antihypertensive agents, tranquilizers, estrogens inhibitors of androgen synthesis, antidepressants)
- Persistent erections unrelated to sexual stimulation
- Curvature of penis in any direction with erection
- Difficulty with ejaculation
  - Painful or premature, efforts to treat the problem
  - Ejaculate color, consistency, odor, and amount
  - Medications: prescription, nonprescription, complementary, or alternative therapies
- Discharge or lesion on the penis
  - Character: lumps, sores, rash
  - Discharge: color, consistency, odor, tendency to stain underwear
  - Symptoms: itching, burning, stinging
  - Exposure to sexually transmitted infection (STI): multiple partners, infection in partners, failure to use condom, history of prior STI
  - Medications: prescription, nonprescription, complementary, or alternative therapies
- Infertility
  - Lifestyle factors that may increase temperature of scrotum: tight clothing, briefs, hot baths, employment in high-temperature environment (e.g., a steel mill) or requiring prolonged sitting (e.g., truck driving), varicocele
  - Length of time attempting pregnancy, sexual activity pattern, knowledge of fertile period of woman's reproductive cycle
  - History of undescended testes
  - Diagnostic evaluation to date: semen analysis, physical examination, sperm antibody titers
  - Medications: prescription (testosterone, glucocorticoids, hypothalamic releasing hormone) or nonprescription, alternative, or complementary therapies
- Enlargement in inguinal area
  - Intermittent or constant, association with straining or lifting, duration, presence of pain
  - Change in size or character of mass; ability to reduce the mass; if unable to reduce it, how long since it could be reduced
  - Pain in the groin: character (tearing, sudden, searing, or cutting pain), associated activity (lifting heavy object, coughing, or straining at stool)
  - Use of truss or other treatment
  - Medications: for pain; prescription, nonprescription, alternative, or complementary therapies

RISK FACTORS

CARCINOMA OF THE MALE GENITALIA

Penile
- Lack of circumcision with failure to maintain good hygiene
- Condyloma acuminatum infection

Testicular
- Cryptorchidism with elevated testicular temperature (Elevated temperature cannot be the complete explanation because the descended testicle is also at increased risk of developing cancer.)

- Testicular pain or mass
  - Change in testicular size
  - Events surrounding onset: noted casually while bathing, after trauma, during a sporting event
  - Irregular lumps, soreness, or heaviness of testes
  - Medications: for pain; antibiotics; prescription, nonprescription, alternative, or complementary therapies

PAST MEDICAL HISTORY

- Surgery of genitourinary tract: undescended testes, hypospadias, epispadias, hydrocele, varicocele, hernia, prostate, sterilization
- STIs: single or multiple infections, specific organism (gonorrhea, syphilis, herpes, warts, chlamydia), treatment, effectiveness, residual problems
- Chronic illness: testicular or prostatic cancer, neurologic or vascular impairment, diabetes mellitus, arthritis, cardiac or respiratory disease

FAMILY HISTORY

- Infertility in siblings
- History of prostate, testicular, or penile cancer
- Hernias

PERSONAL AND SOCIAL HISTORY

- Employment risk of trauma to suprapubic region or genitalia, exposure to radiation or toxins
- Exercise: use of a protective device with contact sports or bicycle riding
- Concerns about genitalia: size, shape, surface characteristics, texture
- Testicular self-examination practices
- Concerns about sexual practices: sexual partners (single or multiple), sexual lifestyle (heterosexual, homosexual, bisexual)
- Reproductive function: number of children, form of contraception used, frequency of ejaculation (Frequent ejaculation has been associated with a lower risk of carcinoma of the prostate.)
- Use of alcohol
- Use of street drugs

INFANTS AND CHILDREN
- Maternal use of sex hormones or birth control pills during pregnancy
- Circumcised boy: complications from procedure
- Uncircumcised boy: hygiene measures, retractability of foreskin, interference with urinary stream
- Scrotal swelling with crying or bowel movement
- Congenital anomalies: hypospadias, epispadias, undescended testes, ambiguous genitalia
- Parental concerns with masturbation, sexual exploration
- Swelling, discoloration, or sores on the penis or scrotum, pain in the genitalia
- Concern of sexual abuse

ADOLESCENTS
- Knowledge of reproductive function, source of information about sexual activity and function
- Presence of nocturnal emissions, pubic hair, enlargement of genitalia, age at time of each occurrence
- Concern of sexual abuse
- Sexual activity, contraception used

OLDER ADULTS

♦ Change in frequency of sexual activity or desire: related to loss of spouse or other sexual partner; no sexual partner; sexually restrictive environment; depression; physical illness resulting in fatigue, weakness, or pain

♦ Change in sexual response: Longer time required to achieve full erection, less forceful ejaculation, more rapid detumescence, longer interval between erections, prostate surgery

EXAMINATION AND FINDINGS

EQUIPMENT

♦ Gloves
♦ Penlight for transillumination of any mass
♦ Drapes

Examination of the genitalia involves inspection, palpation, and transillumination of any mass found. The patient may be anxious about examination of his genitalia, so it is important to examine the genitalia carefully and completely but also expeditiously (Box 19-1). The patient may be lying or standing for this part of the examination (Fig. 19-5).

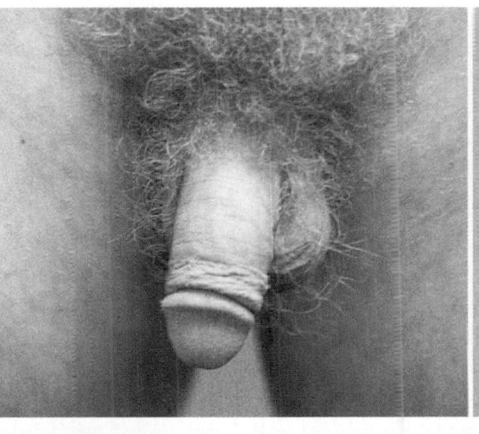 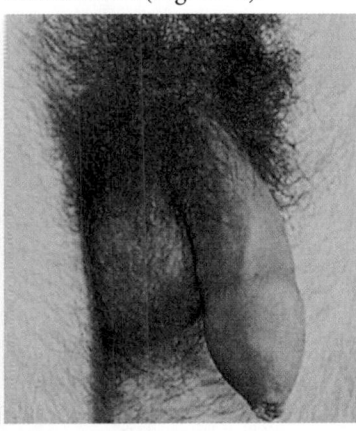

A   B

FIGURE 19-5
Appearance of male genitalia.
A, Circumcised. **B,** Uncircumcised.

BOX 19-1

MINIMIZING THE PATIENT'S ANXIETY

The physical examination is laden with anxiety-provoking elements for most people, but no part of the body is likely to arouse as much psychic discomfort for the male patient as examination of his genitals. Adolescents and men are often fearful of having an erection during the examination. Boys and adolescents may worry about whether their genitals are "normal," and misinformation on sexual matters (such as "the evils of masturbation") can add to their concerns. Your attitude and ability to communicate can reassure the apprehensive patient. Some important elements to remember:

• Know the language. It is inappropriate to talk down to anyone, but you and the patient must understand each other. You may not be entirely comfortable with some of the common words and phrases you hear from the patients, but the common language may be appropriate in certain circumstances. You will not lose your dignity if you maintain your composure and succeed in communicating effectively. Know the language and use it effectively, without apology, and in an undemeaning fashion.

• Never make jokes. Light, casual talk or jokes about the genitalia or sexual function are always inappropriate, no matter how well you know the patient. Feelings about one's own sexuality run deep and are often well masked. Do not pull at the edges of a mask you may not suspect is there.

• Remember that your face is easily seen by the patient when you are examining the genitalia. An unexpected finding may cause a sudden change in your expression. You must guard against what you communicate by the unspoken.

• You need not be defensive if you are a woman examining a man, any more than if you are a man examining a woman—an ordinary event, historically. Here again, you communicate much by demeanor and hesitancy in speech. Do not be apologetic in any obvious or subtle way. Remember that you are a professional, fulfilling the responsibility of a professional.

INSPECTION AND PALPATION

GENITAL HAIR DISTRIBUTION

First inspect the genital hair distribution. Genital hair is coarser than scalp hair. It should be abundant in the pubic region and may continue in a narrowing midline pattern to the umbilicus (the male escutcheon pattern). Depending on how the patient is positioned, it may be possible to note that the distribution continues around the scrotum to the anal orifice. The penis itself is not covered with hair, and the scrotum generally has a scant amount.

PENIS

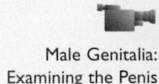

Male Genitalia: Examining the Penis

Examine the penis. The dorsal vein should be apparent on inspection. If the patient is uncircumcised, retract the foreskin or ask the patient to do so. It should retract easily, and a bit of white, cheesy smegma may be seen over the glans. Occasionally the foreskin is tight and cannot be retracted. This condition is called phimosis (Fig. 19-6) and may occur during the first 6 years of life. It is usually congenital but may result from recurrent infections or balanoposthitis (inflammation of the glans penis and prepuce). It may also be caused by previous unsuccessful efforts to retract the foreskin that have caused radial tearing of the preputial ring, resulting in adhesions of the foreskin to the glans. Balanitis, inflammation of the glans (Fig. 19-7), occurs only in uncircumcised individuals and is often associated with phimosis. It may be caused by either bacterial or fungal infections and is most commonly seen in men with poorly controlled diabetes mellitus and a candidal infection.

If the patient is circumcised, the glans is exposed and appears erythematous and dry. No smegma will be present.

URETHRAL MEATUS

Examine the external meatus of the urethra. The orifice should appear slitlike and be located on the ventral surface just millimeters from the tip of the glans. Press the glans between thumb and forefinger to open the urethral orifice (Fig. 19-8). You can certainly ask the patient to perform this procedure for you. The opening should be glistening and pink. Bright erythema or a discharge indicates inflammatory disease, whereas a pinpoint or round opening may result from meatal stenosis.

PENILE SHAFT

Palpate the shaft of the penis for tenderness and induration. Strip the urethra for any discharge by firmly compressing the base of the penis with your thumb and forefinger and moving them toward the glans. The presence of a discharge may indicate a venereal infection. The texture of the flaccid penis should be soft and free of nodularity. Reposition the foreskin after performing these maneuvers.

Rarely, you may see a patient with a prolonged penile erection, called priapism (Fig. 19-9). It is often painful. Although in the majority of cases the condition is idiopathic, it can occur in patients with leukemia or hemoglobinopathies such as sickle cell disease.

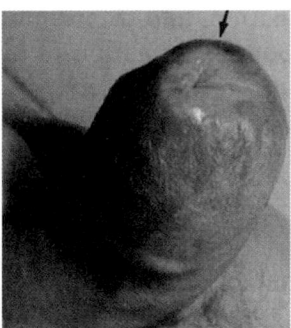

FIGURE 19-6
Phimosis.
From 400 Self-assessment picture tests in clinical medicine, 1984. By permission of Mosby International.

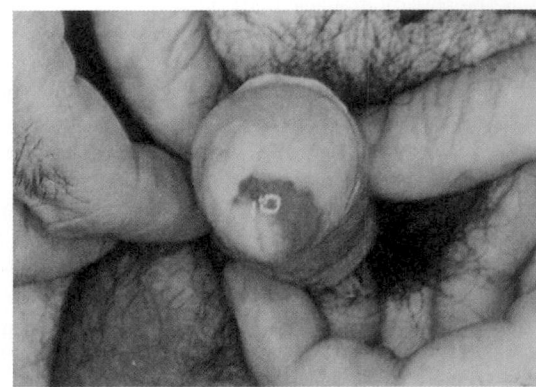

FIGURE 19-7
Balanitis.
From Lloyd-Davies et al, 1994.

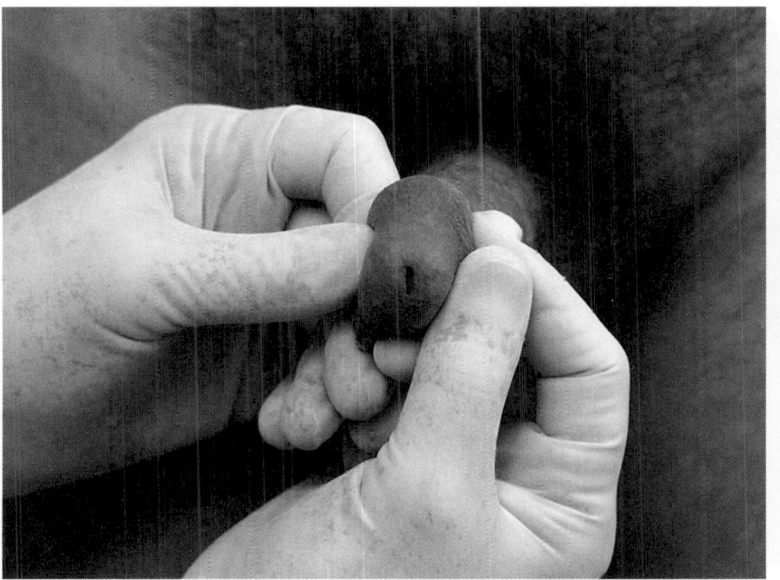

FIGURE 19-8
Examination of urethral orifice.

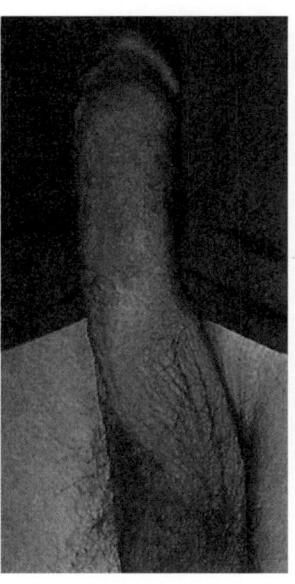

FIGURE 19-9
Priapism.
From Lloyd-Davies et al, 1994.

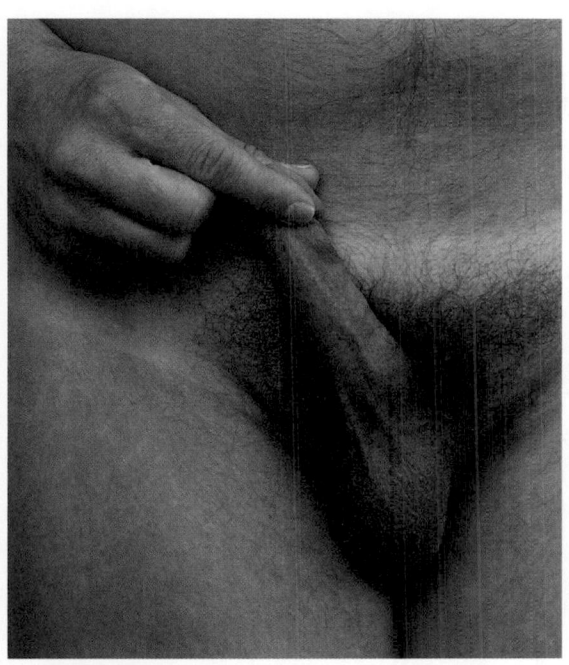

FIGURE 19-10
Inspection of scrotum and ventral surface of penis as
the patient positions his penis.

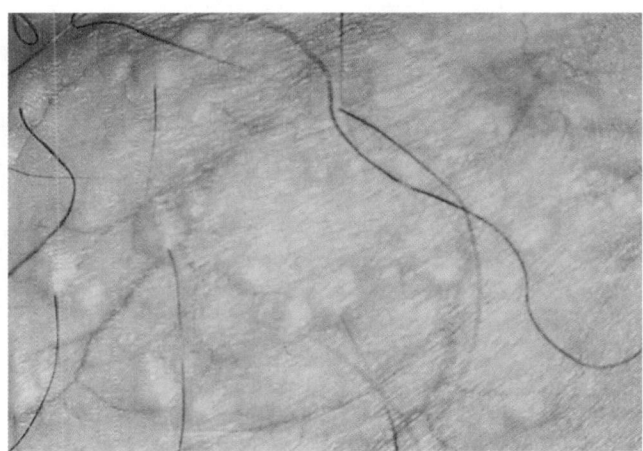

FIGURE 19-11
Sebaceous glands on the scrotum.
From Morse et al, 2003.

SCROTUM

Inspect the scrotum (Fig. 19-10). It may appear more deeply pigmented than the body skin, and the surface may be coarse. The scrotal skin is often reddened in red-haired individuals; however, reddened skin in other individuals may indicate an infectious process. The scrotum usually appears asymmetric because the left testicle has a longer spermatic cord and therefore is often lower. The thickness of the scrotum definitely varies with temperature and age, and perhaps with emotional state. Lumps in the scrotal skin are commonly caused by sebaceous cysts, also called epidermoid cysts. They appear as small lumps on the scrotum, but they may enlarge and discharge oily material (Fig. 19-11).

Occasionally you may observe unusual thickening of the scrotum caused by edema, often with pitting. This does not generally imply disease related to the genitalia, but is more likely a consequence of general fluid retention associated with cardiac, renal, or hepatic disease.

HERNIA

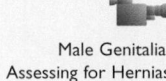

Male Genitalia:
Assessing for Hernias

Examine for evidence of a hernia. Figure 19-16 shows the anatomy of the region and the three common types of hernias. With the patient standing, ask him to bear down as if having a bowel movement. While he is straining, inspect the area of the inguinal canal and the region of the fossa ovalis. After asking the patient to relax again, insert your examining finger into the lower part of the scrotum and carry it upward along the vas deferens into the inguinal canal (Fig. 19-12).

Which finger you use depends on the size of the patient. In the young child, the little finger is appropriate; in the adult the index or middle finger is generally used. You should be able to feel the oval external ring. Ask the patient to cough. If a hernia is present, you should feel the sudden presence of a viscus against your finger. The hernia is described as indirect if it lies within the inguinal canal. It may also come through the external canal and even pass into the scrotum. This type of hernia occurs more commonly in young men and is the most common of the abdominal hernias. Since an indirect hernia on one side strongly suggests the possibility of bilateral herniation, be sure to examine both sides thoroughly. If the viscus is felt medial to the external canal, it probably represents a direct inguinal hernia.

Although inguinal hernias are more common in males, they do occur in females as well. The pathway for testicular descent is present in the female in utero; if it remains open, a hernia can develop at a later date. A femoral hernia, caused by the protrusion of viscus through the site of exit of the femoral vessels from the abdomen, is infrequent and is more common in women than in men.

TESTES

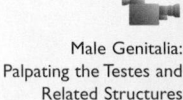

Male Genitalia:
Palpating the Testes and
Related Structures

The testes should be palpated using the thumb and first two fingers. The testis should be sensitive to gentle compression but not tender, and they should feel smooth and rubbery and be free of nodules (Fig. 19-13). In some diseases (e.g., syphilis and diabetic neuropathy), a testis may be totally insensitive to painful stimuli. Irregularities in texture or size may indicate an infection, cyst, or tumor.

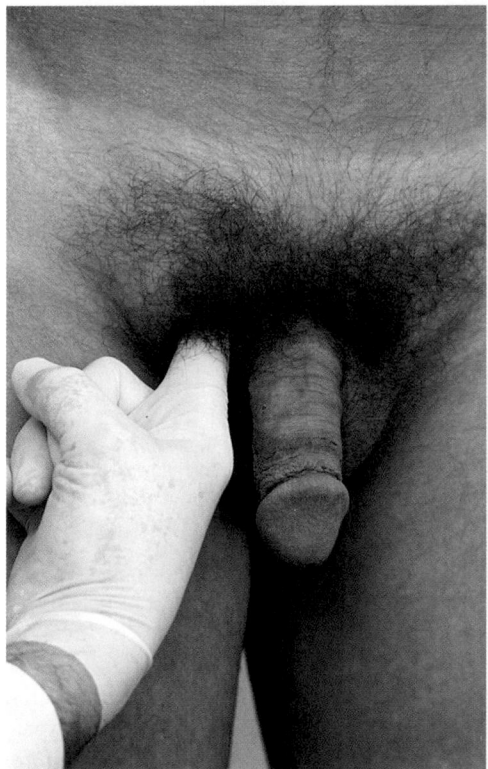

FIGURE 19-12
Checking for inguinal hernia; gloved finger inserted through inguinal canal.

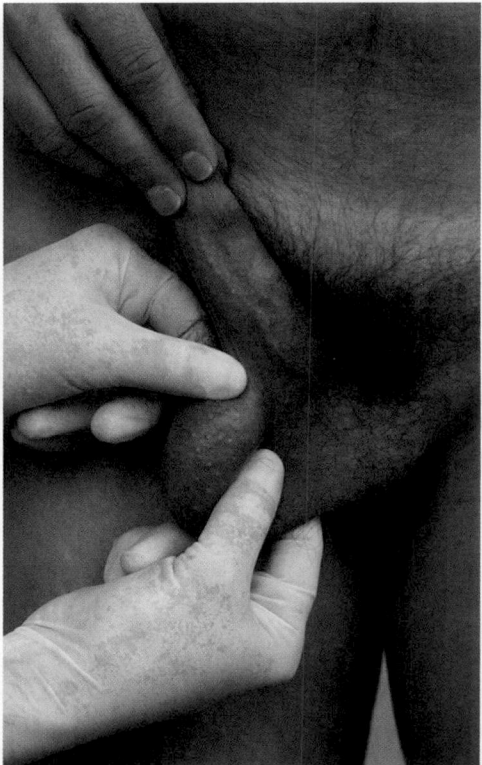

FIGURE 19-13
Palpating contents of the scrotal sac.

The epididymis, located on the posterolateral surface of the testis, should be smooth, discrete, larger cephalad, and nontender. You may be able to feel the appendix epididymidis as an irregularity on the cephalad surface.

Next palpate the vas deferens. It has accompanying arteries and veins, but they cannot be precisely identified by palpation. The vas deferens itself feels smooth and discrete; it should not be beaded or lumpy in its course as you palpate from the testicle to the inguinal ring. The presence of such unexpected findings might indicate diabetes or old inflammatory changes, especially tuberculosis.

All patients, but especially boys and young men, should be taught the techniques of self-examination of the genitalia (see the Staying Well box below).

STAYING WELL
GENITAL SELF-EXAMINATION FOR MEN

Because testicular tumors are the most common cancer occurring in young men, all male patients should be instructed in the technique of genital self-examination (GSE). Obviously the patient should be made aware of the rationale. GSE is also recommended for anyone who is at risk for contracting a sexually transmitted infection (STI). This includes sexually active persons who have had more than one sexual partner or whose partner has had other partners. In these cases, the purpose of GSE is to detect any signs or symptoms that might indicate the presence of an STI. Many people who have an STI do not know they have one, and some STIs can remain undetected for years. GSE should become a part of routine self-health care practices.

You should explain and demonstrate the following procedure to your patients and give them the opportunity to perform a GSE with your guidance.

Instruct the patient to hold the penis in his hand and examine the head. If not circumcised, he should pull back the foreskin to expose the glans. Inspection and palpation of the entire head of the penis should be performed in a clockwise motion, while the patient carefully looks for any bumps, sores, or blisters on the skin. Bumps and blisters may be red or light colored, or may resemble pimples. Have the patient also look for genital warts, which may look similar to warts on other

parts of the body. They may be small bumpy spots at first; left untreated, they could develop a fleshy, cauliflower-like appearance. The urethral meatus should also be examined for any discharge.

Next the patient will examine the entire shaft and look for the same signs. Instruct him to separate the pubic hair at the base of the penis and carefully examine the skin underneath. Make sure he includes the underside of the shaft in the examination; a mirror may be helpful.

Instruct the patient to move on to the scrotum and examine it. He should hold each testicle gently and inspect and palpate the skin including the underneath of the scrotum, for the same signs. The patient should also be alert to any lump, swelling, soreness, or irregularities in the testicle. (Suggest to the patient that self-examination of the scrotum at home be performed while bathing, because the warmth is likely to make the scrotal skin less thick.)

Educate the patient about other symptoms associated with STIs: specifically, pain or burning on urination or discharge from the penis. The discharge may vary in color, consistency, and amount.

If the patient has any of the above signs or symptoms, he should see a health care provider.

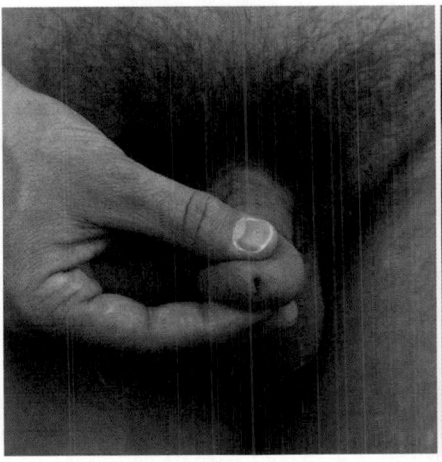

Self-examination of penis.
Modified from Burroughs Wellcome, 1989.

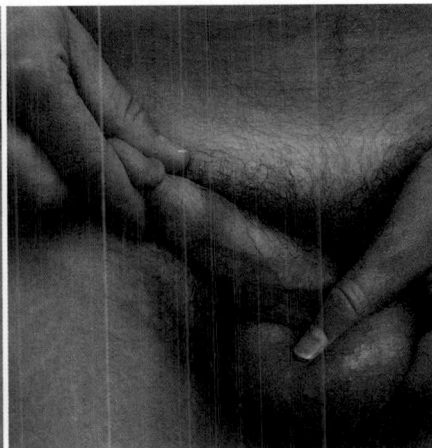

Self-examination of scrotum and testicle.

CREMASTERIC REFLEX

Finally, evaluate the cremasteric reflex. Stroke the inner thigh with a blunt instrument such as the handle of the reflex hammer, or for a child, with your finger. The testicle and scrotum should rise on the stroked side (see Chapter 22).

Examination of the prostate is detailed in Chapter 20.

INFANTS

Examine the genitalia of the newborn for congenital anomalies, incomplete development, and sexual ambiguity. Inspect the penis for size, placement of the urethral opening, and any anomalies. The nonerect length of the penis at birth is 2 to 3 cm. Transitory erection of the penis during infancy is common, and the penis should have a straight projection. A small penis (microphallus) may indicate other organ anomalies. The small penis must also be differentiated from the unusually large clitoris found in pseudohermaphroditism. A hooked, downward bowing of the penis suggests a chordee.

INSPECTION AND PALPATION

Inspect the glans penis of the neonate. The foreskin in the uncircumcised infant is commonly tight, but it should retract enough to permit a good urinary stream. Do not retract the foreskin more than necessary to see the urethra, especially if the neonate will not be circumcised. Do not force, because this can tear the prepuce from the glans, causing binding adhesions to form between the prepuce and the glans. Mobility of the foreskin increases with time, and it should be fully retractable by 3 or 4 years of age. The slitlike urethral meatus should be located near the tip. Inspect the glans of the circumcised infant for ulcerations, bleeding, and inflammation (Box 19-2). The urinary stream should be strong with good caliber. Dribbling or a reduced force or caliber of the urinary stream may indicate stenosis of the urethral meatus. On occasion, hypospadias may be associated with a sex chromosomal abnormality 47XXY or 47XYY.

Inspect the scrotum for size, shape, rugae, the presence of testicles, and any anomalies (Fig. 19-14). The scrotum of the premature infant may appear underdeveloped, without rugae, and without testes; whereas the full-term neonate should have a loose, pendulous scrotum with rugae and a midline raphe. The proximal end of the scrotum should be the widest area. The scrotum in infants usually appears large compared with the rest of the genitalia. Edema of the external genitalia is common, especially after a breech delivery. A deep cleft in the scrotum (bifid scrotum) is usually associated with other genitourinary anomalies or ambiguous genitalia.

When examining the scrotum, particularly in the young, make certain that your hands are warm and your touch is gentle. The cremasteric reflex (known as the yo-yo reflex), in which the scrotal contents retract, is a response to cold hands and abrupt handling. Before you palpate the scrotum, place the thumb and index finger of one hand over the inguinal canals at the upper part of the scrotal sac. This maneuver helps prevent retraction of the testes into the inguinal canal or abdomen. Palpate each side of the scrotum to detect the presence of the testes or other masses. The testicle of the newborn is approximately 1 cm in diameter.

BOX 19-2

CIRCUMCISION

There has been much discussion about the appropriateness of routine circumcision; some believe it is not medically indicated (American College of Pediatrics Policy Statement, 1999). However, attitudes vary and are highly personal, often reflecting the personal opinion of the pediatrician. Recent evidence suggesting that circumcision prevents urinary tract infections in infants has received much attention. So has the appreciation that infants do perceive pain even in the newborn state. Parents should be reminded of the importance of careful hygiene and the importance of not retracting the foreskin (see p. 653). Although a definitive answer may not yet be available, circumcision will continue to be performed on many children, often on the basis of religious prescription.

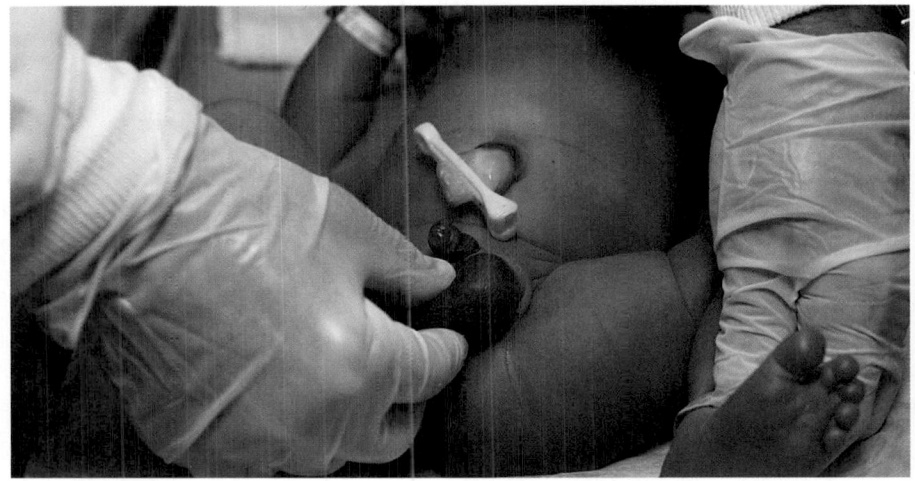

FIGURE 19-14
Palpating the scrotum of an infant.

If either of the testicles is not palpable, place a finger over the upper inguinal ring and gently push toward the scrotum. You may feel a soft mass in the inguinal canal. Try to push it toward the scrotum and palpate it with your thumb and index finger. If the testicle can be pushed into the scrotum, it is considered a descended testicle, even though it retracts to the inguinal canal. A testicle that is either palpable in the inguinal canal but cannot be pushed into the scrotum or not palpable at all is considered an undescended testicle.

Palpate over the internal inguinal canal with the flat part of your fingers. Roll the spermatic cord beneath the fingers to feel the solid structure going through the ring. If the feeling of smoothness disappears as you palpate, the peritoneum is passing through the ring, indicating an invisible hernia. An apparent bulge in the inguinal area suggests a visible hernia. Palpation may elicit a sensation of crepitus.

TRANSILLUMINATION

When any mass other than the testicle or spermatic cord is palpated in the scrotum, determine whether it is filled with fluid, gas, or solid material. It will most likely be a hernia or hydrocele. Attempt to reduce the size of the mass by pushing it back through the external inguinal canal. If a bright penlight transilluminates the mass, and there is no change in size when reduction is attempted, it most likely contains fluid (hydrocele with a closed tunica vaginalis). A mass that does not transilluminate but does change in size when reduction is attempted is probably a hernia. A mass that neither changes in size nor transilluminates may represent an incarcerated hernia, which is a surgical emergency.

CHILDREN

The external genitalia of the toddler and preschooler are examined as described for infants. Preschoolers may have developed a sense of modesty, so you should explain what you are doing and quickly complete the examination. Reassure the child that he is developing appropriately whenever such reassurance is possible.

INSPECTION AND PALPATION

Inspect the penis for size, lesions, swelling, inflammation, and malformation. Retract the foreskin in the uncircumcised boy without forcing it, and inspect the glans for lesions, discharge, and the location and appearance of the urethral meatus. It is important not to force the retraction of the foreskin, because forced retraction may contribute to the formation of binding adhesions. Some adherence of the prepuce to the glans may continue even until 6 years of age. The penis may appear relatively small if obscured by fat in obese boys. If the penis appears swollen, tender, or if ecchymotic lesions are present, be concerned about the possibility of sexual abuse.

The scrotum is inspected for size, shape, color, and the presence of testicles or other masses. Well-formed rugae indicate that the testes have descended during infancy, even if the testes are not apparent in the scrotum. Palpate the scrotum to identify the testes and epididymides. The testes should be about 1 cm in size. Again bruises on the scrotum or in the groin area raise the specter of sexual abuse.

Some testes are very retractile and therefore hard to find. Warm hands, a warm room, and a gentle approach will help. If the patient is old enough to cooperate, ask him to sit in tailor position with legs crossed, or have the child sit on a chair with the heels of his feet on the chair seat and his hands on his knees. Either position places pressure on the abdominal wall that will help push the testicles into the scrotum. If an inguinal hernia exists, this maneuver is also useful in eliciting that finding (Fig. 19-15). A scrotum that remains small, flat, and undeveloped is a good indication of cryptorchidism (undescended testes).

A hard, enlarged, painless testicle may indicate a tumor. Acute swelling in the scrotum with discoloration can result from torsion of the spermatic cord or orchitis. Acute, painful swelling without discoloration and a thickened or nodular epididymis suggests epididymitis. An enlarged penis without enlargement of the testes occurs with precocious puberty, adrenal hyperplasia, and some central nervous system lesions.

ADOLESCENTS

The examination of older children and adolescents is the same as for adults. Because of their modesty and great sensitivity to development, this portion of the physical examination is usually performed last. The degree of maturation should be classified for the pubic hair, penile size, and the development of testes and scrotum according to the stages described by Tanner (see Chapter 5).

CLINICAL PEARL

Concerns of Adolescence
The adolescent male may need to be reassured that his genital development is proceeding as expected. If he has an erection during the examination, explain that this is a common response to touch and that it is not a problem.

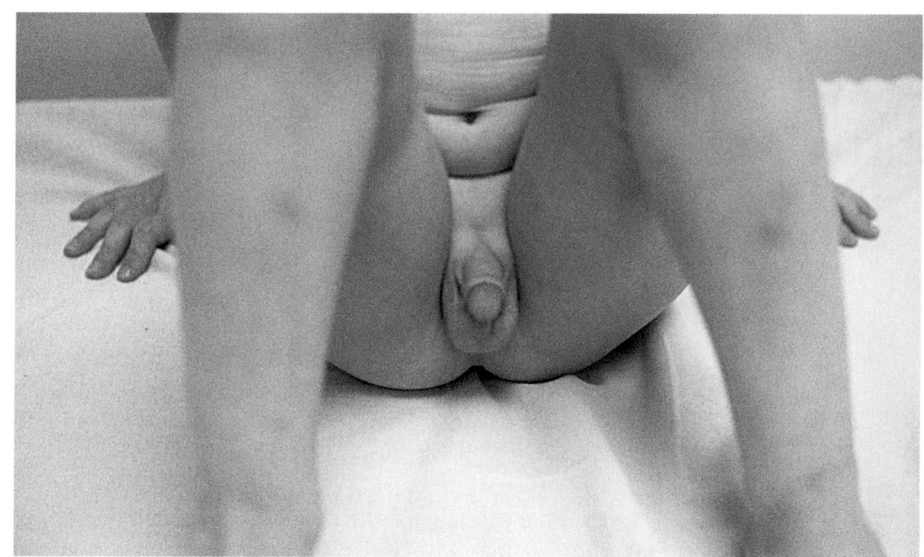

FIGURE 19-15
Position of child to push testicles into the scrotum. An alternative maneuver is to seat the child in tailor position.

SAMPLE DOCUMENTATION

HISTORY AND PHYSICAL EXAMINATION

Subjective

Two days ago, a 19-year-old male noted the onset of dysuria, staining of his underwear, and urethral discharge that is more severe today. He reports sexual intercourse with a new partner about a week ago without the use of a condom. No pain in testes. No prior sexually transmitted infections.

For additional sample documentation, see Chapter 26.

Objective

Yellow, thick urethral discharge upon expression of the urethra. No tenderness along the course of the spermatic cords, no testicular tenderness, no inguinal lymphadenopathy.

SUMMARY OF EXAMINATION

MALE GENITALIA

The following steps are performed with the patient lying or standing:

1. Inspect the pubic hair characteristics and distribution (p. 648).
2. Retract the foreskin if the patient is uncircumcised (p. 648).
3. Inspect the glans of the penis with foreskin retracted, noting the following (p. 648):
   - Color
   - Smegma
   - External meatus of urethra
   - Urethral discharge
4. Palpate the penis, noting the following (p. 648):
   - Tenderness
   - Induration
5. Strip the urethra for discharge (p. 648).
6. Inspect the scrotum and ventral surface of the penis for the following (p. 649):
   - Color
   - Texture
   - Asymmetry
   - Unusual thickening
   - Presence of hernia
7. Transilluminate any masses in the scrotum (p. 653).
8. Palpate the inguinal canal for a direct or indirect hernia (p. 650).
9. Palpate the testes, epididymides, and vasa deferentia for the following (pp. 650-651):
   - Consistency
   - Size
   - Tenderness
   - Bleeding, lumpiness, or nodules
10. Palpate for inguinal lymph nodes (pp. 247-248).
11. Elicit the cremasteric reflex bilaterally (p. 652).

COMMON ABNORMALITIES

HERNIA

An abdominal hernia is the protrusion of a peritoneal-lined sac through some defect in the abdominal wall. Fig. 19-16 shows the anatomy of the region and the three common types of pelvic hernias. The Differential Diagnosis box on p. 657 explains their distinguishing characteristics. Hernias occur because there is a potential space for protrusion of some abdominal organ, commonly the bowel but occasionally the omentum. These hernias arise along the course that the testicle traveled as it exited the abdomen and entered the scrotum during intrauterine life. Femoral hernias occur at the fossa ovalis, where the femoral artery exits the abdomen, and are more common in females than males. A strangulated hernia is a nonreducible hernia in which the blood supply to the protruded tissue is compromised; this condition requires prompt surgical intervention.

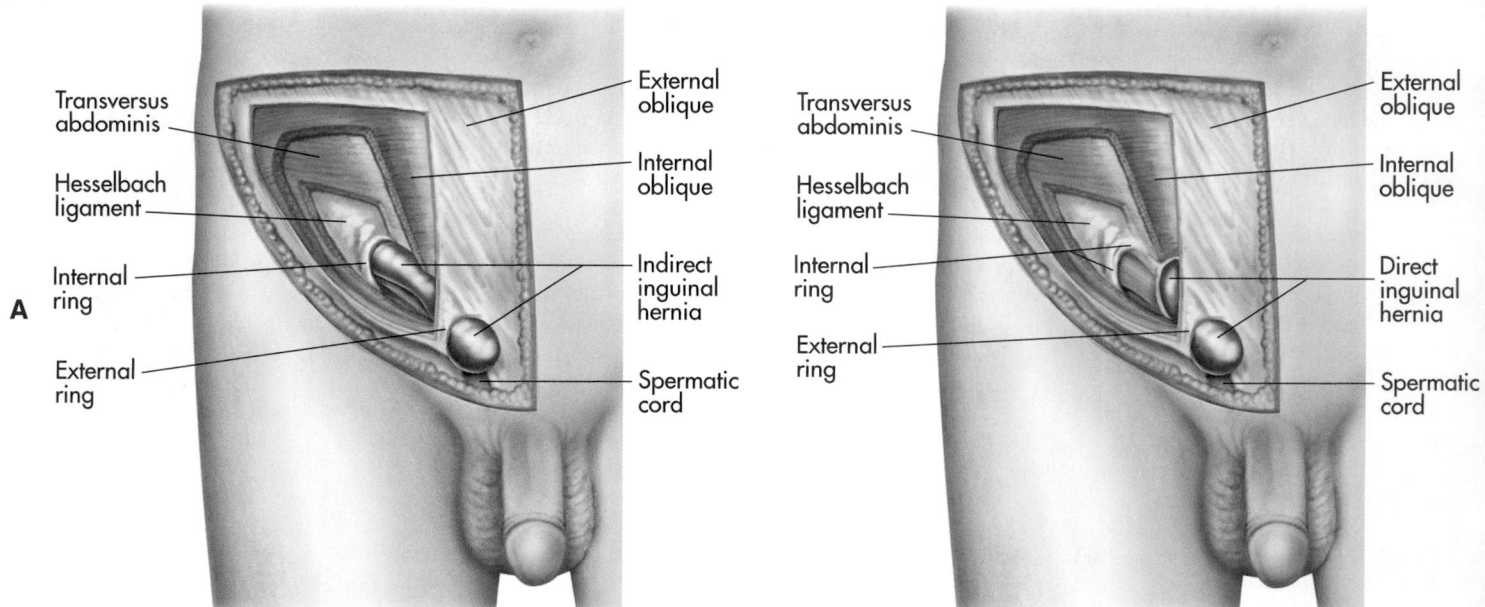

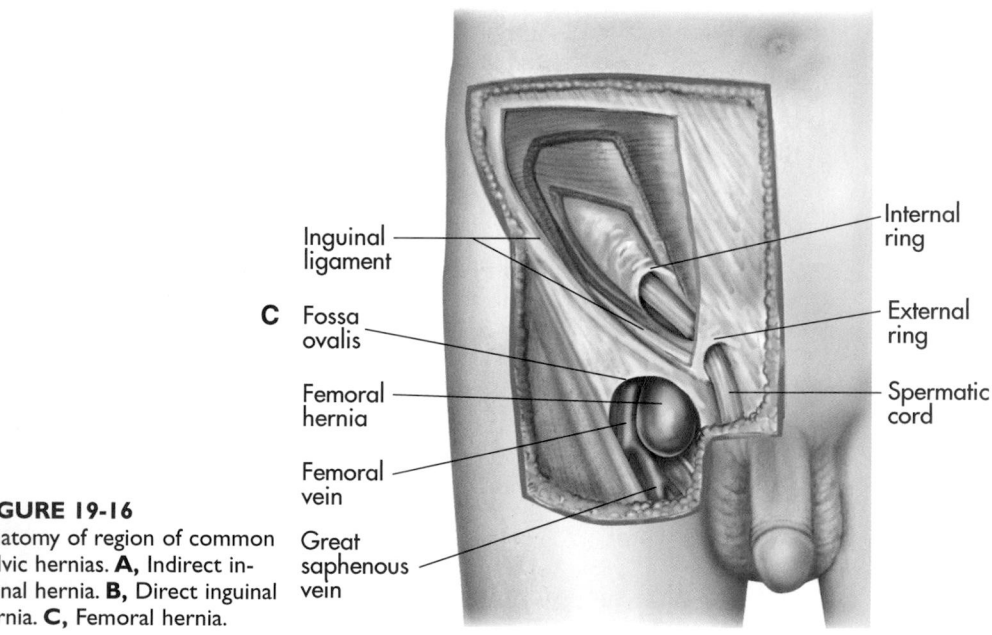

FIGURE 19-16
Anatomy of region of common pelvic hernias. **A,** Indirect inguinal hernia. **B,** Direct inguinal hernia. **C,** Femoral hernia.

DIFFERENTIAL DIAGNOSIS

DISTINGUISHING CHARACTERISTICS OF HERNIAS

	Indirect Inguinal	Direct Inguinal	Femoral
Incidence	Most common type of hernia; both genders are affected; often patients are children and young males	Less common than indirect inguinal; occurs more often in males than females; more common in those older than 40 years of age	Least common type of hernia; occurs more often in females than males; rare in children
Occurrence	Through internal inguinal ring; can remain in canal, exit the external ring, and pass into scrotum; may be bilateral	Through external inguinal ring; located in region of the Hesselbach triangle; rarely enters scrotum	Through femoral ring, femoral canal, and fossa ovalis
Presentation	Soft swelling in area of internal ring; pain on straining; hernia comes down canal and touches fingertip on examination	Bulge in area of Hesselbach triangle; usually painless; easily reduced; hernia bulges anteriorly, pushes against side of finger on examination	Right side presentation more common than left; pain may be severe; inguinal canal empty on examination

PENIS

PARAPHIMOSIS

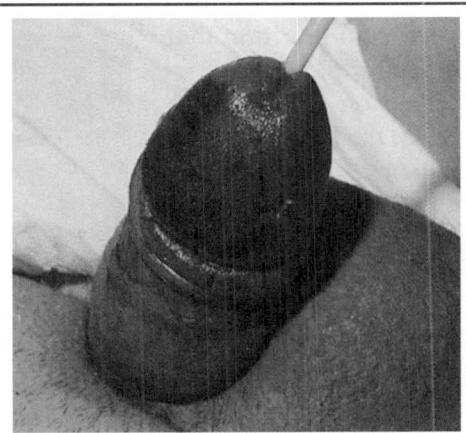

FIGURE 19-17
Paraphimosis.
Courtesy Patrick C. Walsh, MD, The Johns Hopkins University School of Medicine, Baltimore.

Paraphimosis is the inability to replace the foreskin to its usual position after it has been retracted behind the glans. Impairment of local circulation can lead to edema or gangrene of the glans (Fig. 19-17).

HYPOSPADIAS

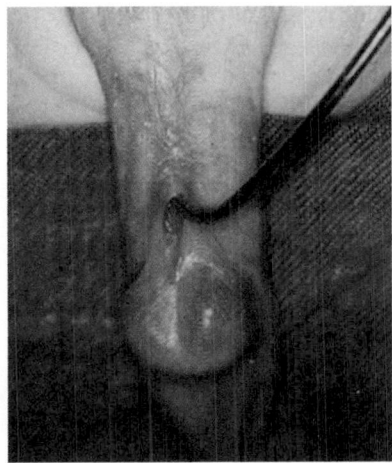

FIGURE 19-18
Hypospadias.
From 400 Self-assessment picture tests in clinical medicine, 1984. By permission of Mosby International.

Hypospadias is a congenital defect in which the urethral meatus is located on the ventral surface of the glans, penile shaft, or the perineal area. If the orifice is ventral but within the substance of the glans, it is termed *primary hypospadias*; an orifice along the ventral shaft of the penis is termed *secondary hypospadias*; and one located at the base of the penis is termed *tertiary hypospadias* (Fig. 19-18). The presence of hypospadias does put the infant at greater risk of having undescended testicles. Rarely, the orifice may appear on the dorsal surface, a condition called *epispadias*.

SYPHILITIC CHANCRE The lesion of primary syphilis generally occurs 2 weeks after exposure. It is most commonly located on the glans, but can be located on the foreskin. Painless, the lesion has indurated borders with a clear base. Scrapings from the ulcer, when examined microscopically, show spirochetes (Fig. 19-19).

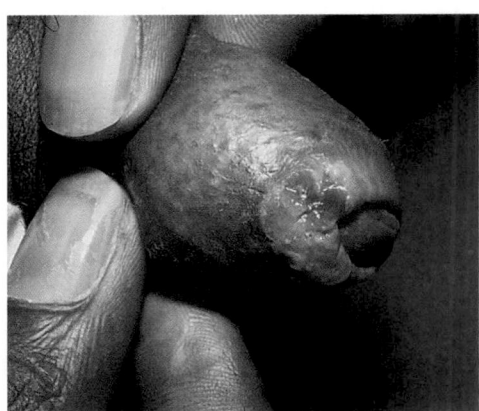

FIGURE 19-19
Syphilitic chancre.
Courtesy Antoinette Hood, MD, Indiana University School of Medicine, Indianapolis.

HERPES Venereal herpes is a viral infection that appears as superficial vesicles. The lesions may be located on the glans, on the penile shaft, or at the base of the penis. They are commonly quite painful, and at the time of primary infection are often associated with inguinal lymphadenopathy and systemic symptoms including fever (Fig. 19-20).

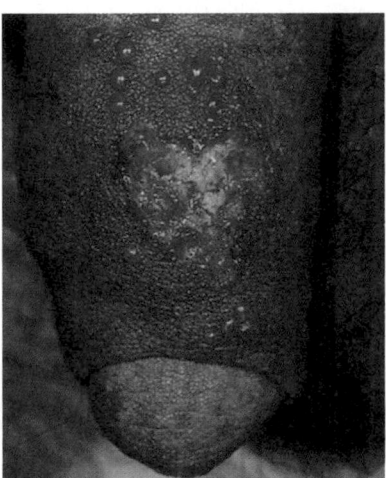

FIGURE 19-20
Genital herpes.
From Habif, 2004.

CONDYLOMA ACUMINATUM (GENITAL WARTS)

A soft, reddish lesion that arises because of infection with a papovavirus is called condyloma acuminatum. The lesions are commonly present on the prepuce, glans penis, and penile shaft; but they may be present within the urethra as well. The lesions may undergo malignant degeneration to squamous cell carcinoma (Fig. 19-21).

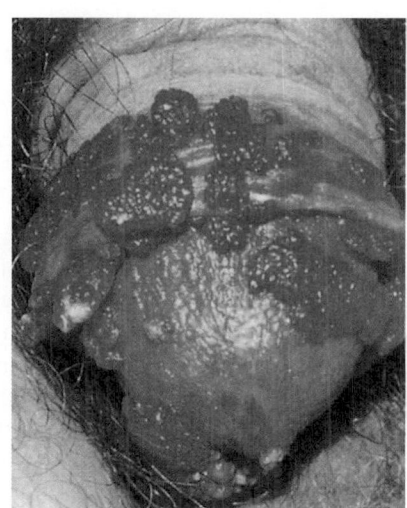

FIGURE 19-21
Condyloma acuminatum (genital warts).
From 400 self-assessment picture tests in clinical medicine, *1984. By permission of Mosby International.*

LYMPHOGRANULOMA VENEREUM

Lymphogranuloma venereum is an STI caused by a chlamydial organism. Although the lesions appear on the genitalia, symptoms may be systemic. The initial lesion is a painless erosion at or near the coronal sulcus (Fig. 19-22). Subsequently, local lymph nodes become involved; unless the infection is treated, draining sinus tracts may form. If lymphatic drainage is blocked, penile and scrotal lymphedema may ensue.

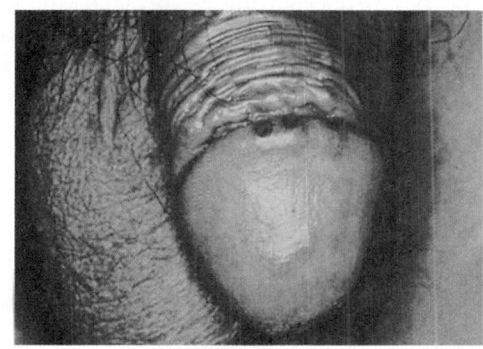

FIGURE 19-22
Lymphogranuloma venereum.
From Meheus, Ursi: Sexually transmitted diseases, *Kalamazoo, Michigan, 1982, The Upjohn Company.*

MOLLUSCUM CONTAGIOSUM

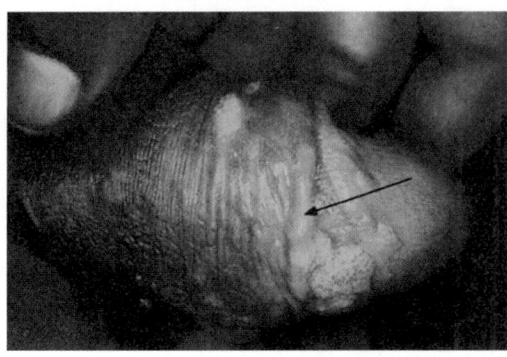

FIGURE 19-23
Molluscum contagiosum *(arrow)* with condyloma acuminatum (genital warts).
Reprinted with permission from Meheus, Ursi, 1982.

Molluscum contagiosum is an STI caused by a poxvirus. The lesions are pearly gray, often umbilicated, smooth, dome shaped, and with discrete margins. They occur most commonly on the glans penis (Fig. 19-23).

PEYRONIE DISEASE

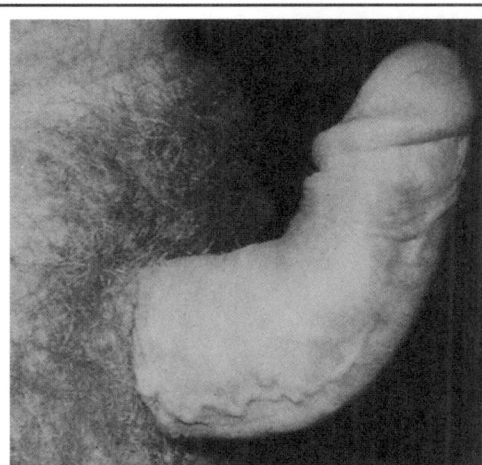

FIGURE 19-24
Peyronie disease.
Courtesy Patrick C. Walsh, MD, The Johns Hopkins University School of Medicine, Baltimore.

A disorder of unknown cause, Peyronie disease is characterized by a fibrous band in the corpus cavernosum. It is generally unilateral and results in deviation of the penis during erection. Depending on the extent of the fibrous band, the condition may make erection painful and intromission impossible. No treatment has been altogether successful. Vitamin E therapy has recently become popular, and corticosteroid injection has also been used. Occasionally, surgery is required to remove the fibrous band (Fig. 19-24).

PENILE CARCINOMA

Cancer of the penis is generally squamous and tends to occur in uncircumcised men who practice poor hygiene. It often appears as a painless ulceration that, unlike a syphilitic chancre, fails to heal. The lesions are often extensive by the time help is sought, either because of fear or because the lesion is unnoticed under the foreskin (Fig. 19-25).

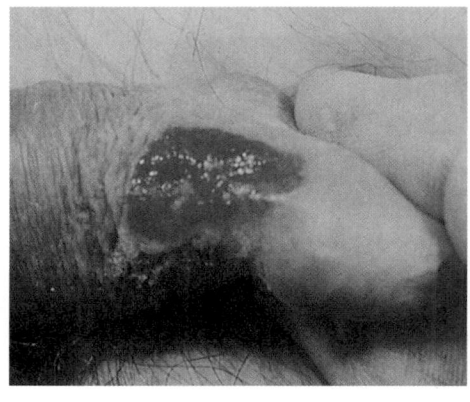

FIGURE 19-25
Carcinoma of the penis.
Courtesy Patrick C. Walsh, MD, The Johns Hopkins University School of Medicine, Baltimore.

SCROTUM

HYDROCELE	The nontender, smooth, firm mass of the hydrocele results from fluid accumulation in the tunica vaginalis. Unless it has been present for a long time and is very large and taut, palpation of a hydrocele should reveal that it is confined to the scrotum and does not enter the inguinal canal. The mass will transilluminate. This condition is common in infancy. If the tunica vaginalis is not patent, the hydrocele will generally disappear spontaneously in the first 6 months of life (Fig. 19-26).

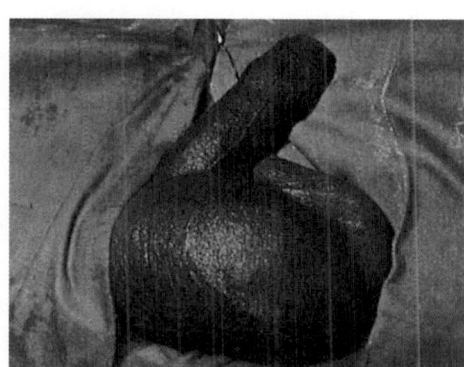

FIGURE 19-26
Hydrocele.
From Lloyd-Davies et al, 1994.

SPERMATOCELE	A spermatocele is a cystic swelling occurring on the epididymis. It is not as large as a hydrocele, but it does transilluminate (Fig. 19-27).

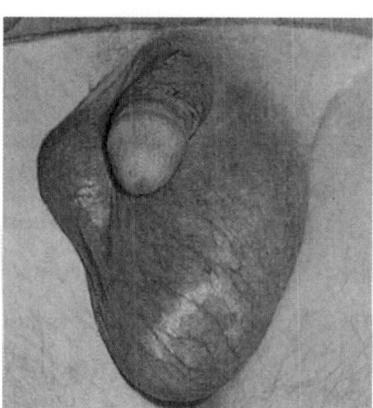

FIGURE 19-27
Spermatocele.
From Lloyd-Davies et al, 1994.

VARICOCELE

An abnormal tortuosity and dilation of veins of the pampiniform plexus within the spermatic cord is termed a *varicocele*. It is most common on the left side and may be painful. It occurs in boys and young men and may be associated with reduced fertility, probably from increased venous pressure and elevated testicular temperature. The condition, often visible only when the patient is standing, is classically described as "bag of worms" (Fig. 19-28). Varicoceles are graded as small (palpated only during Valsalva maneuver), moderate (easily palpated without Valsalva maneuver, and large (causing visible bulging of the scrotal skin).

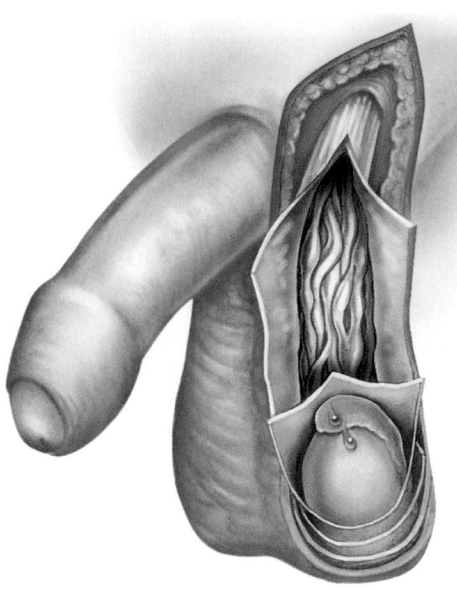

FIGURE 19-28
Varicocele.

ORCHITIS

An acute inflammation of the testis, orchitis is uncommon except as a complication of mumps in the adolescent or adult. It is generally unilateral and results in testicular atrophy in 50% of the cases. In older adults it may result from bacterial migration from a prostatic infection (Fig. 19-29).

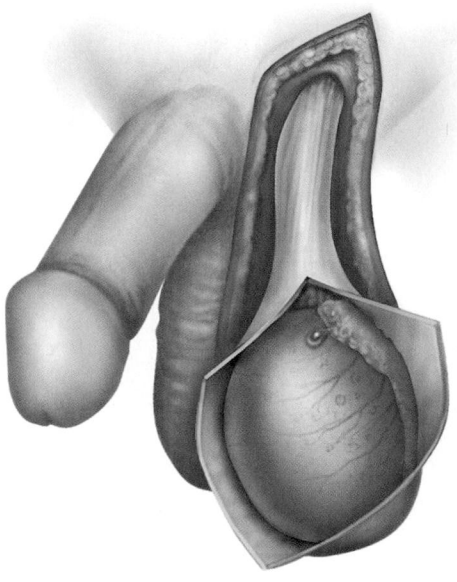

FIGURE 19-29
Orchitis.

EPIDIDYMITIS

Inflammation of the epididymis is often seen in association with a urinary tract infection. It may also occur as a result of an STI. The epididymis is exquisitely tender, and the overlying scrotum may be markedly erythematous. Scrotal elevation may relieve the pain. A major consideration in the differential diagnosis is testicular torsion, a surgical emergency (see the Differential Diagnosis box). Systemic symptoms such as fever and examination of the urine for white blood cells and bacteria may help distinguish between these two conditions. Occasionally, chronic epididymitis may occur as a consequence of tuberculosis. In the chronic form, the epididymis feels firm and lumpy and may be slightly tender, and the vasa deferentia may be beaded (Fig. 19-30).

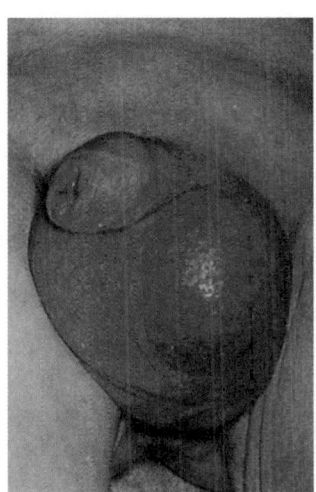

FIGURE 19-30
Epididymitis.
From Lloyd-Davies et al, 1994.

TESTICULAR TORSION

Testicular torsion is a surgical emergency occurring most commonly in adolescents. It has an acute onset and is often accompanied by nausea and vomiting. On examination, the testicle is exquisitely tender, and scrotal discoloration is often present (see the Differential Diagnosis box below).

DIFFERENTIAL DIAGNOSIS
ACUTE TESTICULAR SWELLING

	Torsion	Epididymitis
Cause	Twisting of testis on spermatic cord	Bacterial infection (STI or UTI)
Age	Newborn to adolescence	Adolescence to adulthood
Onset of pain	Acute	Gradual
Vomiting	Common	Uncommon
Anorexia	Common	Uncommon
Fever	Uncommon	Possible
Dysuria	Uncommon	Possible
Supporting findings	Absence of cremasteric reflex on side of acute swelling Scrotal discoloration	Urethral discharge History of recent sexual activity Fever Pyuria Thickened or nodular epididymis

STI, Sexually transmitted infection; *UTI,* urinary tract infection.

TESTICULAR TUMOR

A neoplasm arising from the testicle appears as an irregular, nontender mass fixed on the testis. It does not transilluminate. It may be associated with inguinal lymphadenopathy; often it is not, because lymphatic drainage is to the retroperitoneal nodes (see Chapter 9). Testicular tumor tends to occur in young men and is the most common tumor in males 15 to 30 years of age. Most testicular tumors are malignant (Fig. 19-31).

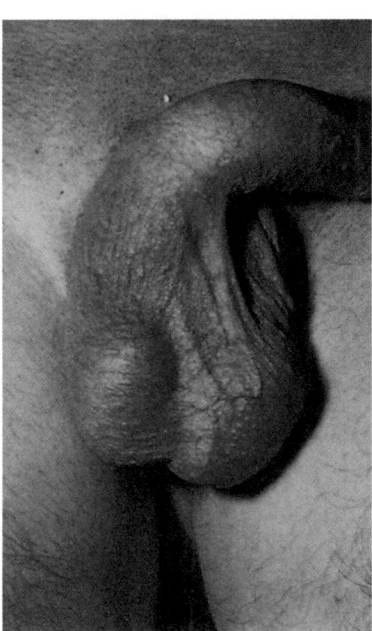

FIGURE 19-31
Testicular tumor.
From 400 Self-assessment picture tests in clinical medicine, 1984. By permission of Mosby International.

KLINEFELTER SYNDROME

Klinefelter syndrome is a congenital anomaly associated with XXY chromosomal inheritance. It is associated with hypogonadism, including a small scrotum; female distribution of pubic hair; and, in some cases, gynecomastia (Fig. 19-32).

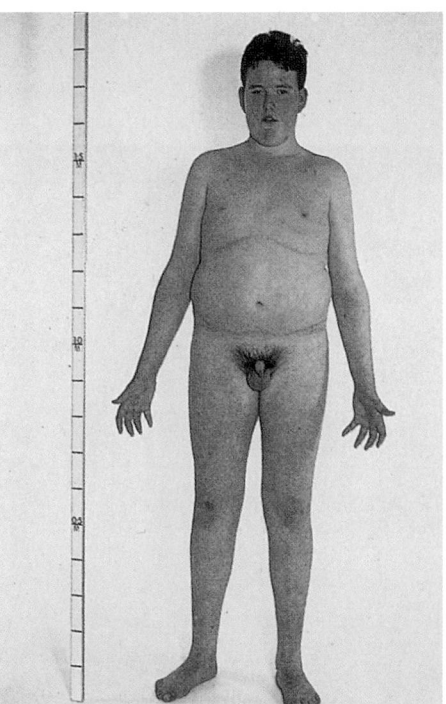

FIGURE 19-32
Klinefelter syndrome.
From Thibodeau, Patton, 2003.

INFANTS

AMBIGUOUS GENITALIA

This is a condition in which the examiner is uncertain whether the newborn has a very small penis with hypospadias or an enlarged clitoris. There may be partial fusion of the labioscrotal fold or a bifid scrotum. Testes cannot be palpated. The infant should have chromosomal studies performed promptly (Fig. 19-33).

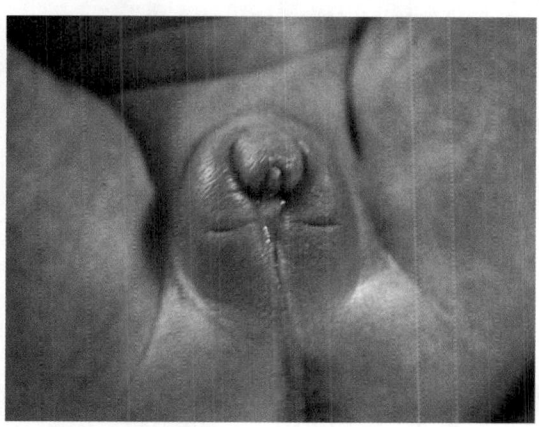

FIGURE 19-33
Ambiguous genitalia in infant.
Courtesy Patrick C. Walsh, MD, The Johns Hopkins University School of Medicine, Baltimore.

ELECTRONIC RESOURCES

For Weblinks and additional resources, go to   evolve

http://evolve.elsevier.com/Seidel

or to the Companion CD-ROM.

Additional information related to the content in Chapter 19 can be found on the companion website at http://evolve.elsevier.com/Seidel/ or on the interactive companion CD-ROM. Resources and activities for Chapter 19 include:
- Sound and Vision Theater
- Printouts for Your Practice
- Interactive Challenge
- Spanish Assessment Terms with Pronunciation Guide
- Instant Calculator

ANUS, RECTUM, AND PROSTATE

ANATOMY AND PHYSIOLOGY

The rectum and anus form the terminal portions of the gastrointestinal (GI) tract (Fig. 20-1). The anal canal is approximately 2.5 to 4 cm long and opens onto the perineum. The tissue visible at the external margin of the anus is moist, hairless mucosa. Juncture with the perianal skin is characterized by increased pigmentation and, in the adult, the presence of hair.

The anal canal is normally kept securely closed by concentric rings of muscle, the internal and external sphincters. The internal ring of smooth muscle is under involuntary autonomic control. The urge to defecate occurs when the rectum fills with feces, which causes reflexive stimulation that relaxes the internal sphincter. Defecation is controlled by the striated external sphincter, which is under voluntary control. The lower half of the canal is supplied with somatic sensory nerves, making it sensitive to painful stimuli, whereas the upper half is under autonomic control and is relatively insensitive. Therefore conditions of the lower anus cause pain, whereas those of the upper anus may not.

Internally the anal canal is lined by columns of mucosal tissue (columns of Morgagni) that fuse to form the anorectal junction. The spaces between the columns are called *crypts*, into which anal glands empty. Inflammation of the crypts can result in fistula or fissure formation. Anastomosing veins cross the columns, forming a ring called the *zona hemorrhoidalis*. Internal hemorrhoids result from dilation of these veins. The lower segment of the anal canal contains a venous plexus that drains into the inferior rectal veins. Dilation of this plexus results in external hemorrhoids.

The rectum lies superior to the anus and is approximately 12 cm long. Its proximal end is continuous with the sigmoid colon. The distal end, the anorectal junction, is visible on proctoscopic examination as a sawtooth-like edge, but it is not palpable. Above the anorectal junction, the rectum dilates and turns posteriorly into the hollow of the coccyx and sacrum, forming the rectal ampulla, which stores flatus and feces. The rectal wall contains three semilunar transverse folds (Houston valves) with as yet poorly defined function. The lowest of these folds can be palpated by the examiner.

In males the prostate gland is located at the base of the bladder and surrounds the urethra. It is composed of muscular and glandular tissue and is approximately $4 \times 3 \times 2$ cm. The posterior surface of the prostate gland is in close contact with the anterior rectal wall and is accessible by digital examination. It is convex and is divided by a shallow median sulcus into right and left lateral lobes. A third or median lobe, not palpable on examination, is composed of glandular tissue and lies between the ejaculatory duct and the urethra. It contains active se-

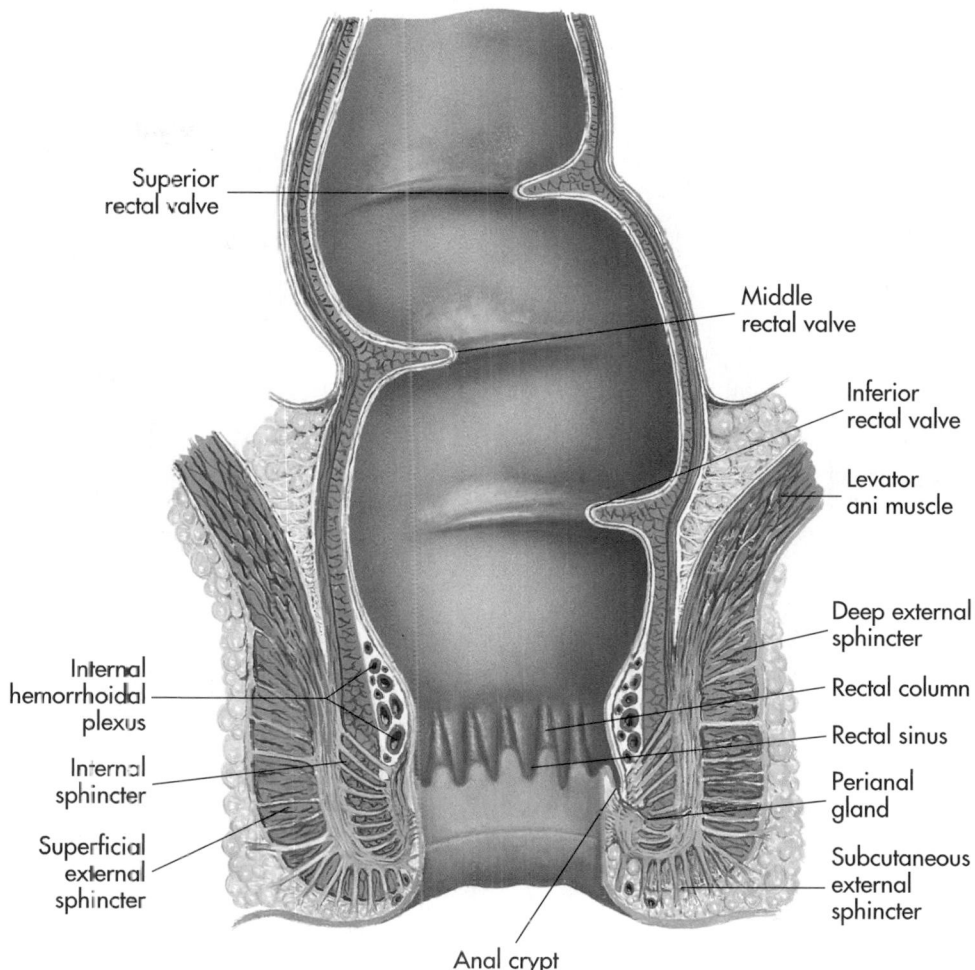

Superior
rectal valve

Middle
rectal valve

Inferior
rectal valve

Levator
ani muscle

Deep external
sphincter

Rectal column

Rectal sinus

Perianal
gland

Subcutaneous
external
sphincter

Internal
hemorrhoidal
plexus

Internal
sphincter

Superficial
external
sphincter

Anal crypt

FIGURE 20-1
Anatomy of the anus and
rectum.

cretory alveoli that contribute to ejaculatory fluid. The seminal vesicles extend outward from
the prostate (Fig. 20-2).

In females the anterior rectal wall lies in contact with the vagina and is separated from it
by the rectovaginal septum. See Chapter 18 for a more detailed discussion.

INFANTS

At 7 weeks of gestation a portion of the caudal hindgut is divided by an anorectal septum into
a urogenital sinus and a rectum. The urogenital sinus is covered by a membrane that develops
into the anal opening by 8 weeks of gestation. Most anorectal malformations result from abnormalities in this partitioning process.

The first meconium stool is ordinarily passed within the first 24 to 48 hours after birth and
indicates anal patency. Thereafter, it is common for newborns to have a stool after each feeding (the gastrocolic reflex). Both the internal and external sphincters are under involuntary reflexive control because myelination of the spinal cord is incomplete.

By the end of the first year, the infant may have one or two bowel movements daily. Control of the external anal sphincter is gradually achieved between the ages of 18 and 24 months.

In males the prostate is undeveloped, small, inactive, and not palpable on rectal examination. The prostate remains undeveloped until puberty, at which time androgenic influences
prompt its growth and maturation. The initially minimal glandular component develops active secretory alveoli, and the prostate becomes functional.

PREGNANT WOMEN

In pregnancy, pressure in the veins below the enlarged uterus increases, as does blood flow. Dietary habits and hormonal changes that decrease GI tract tone and motility produce constipation. These factors predispose pregnant women to the development of hemorrhoids. Labor,
which results in pressure on the pelvic floor by the presenting part of the fetus and expulsive

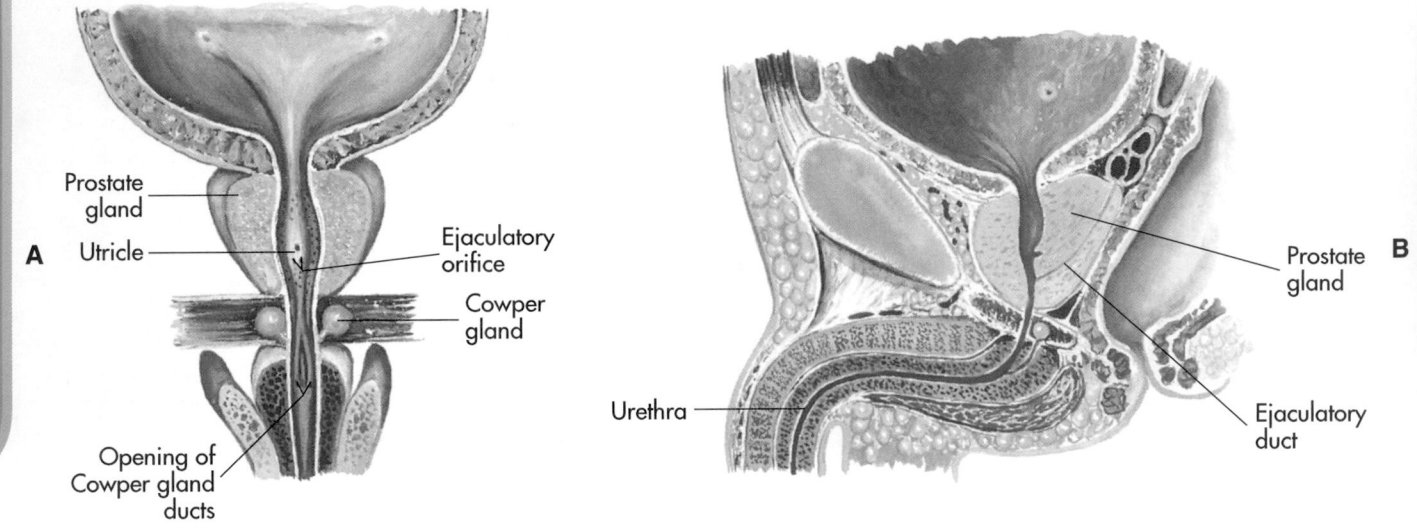

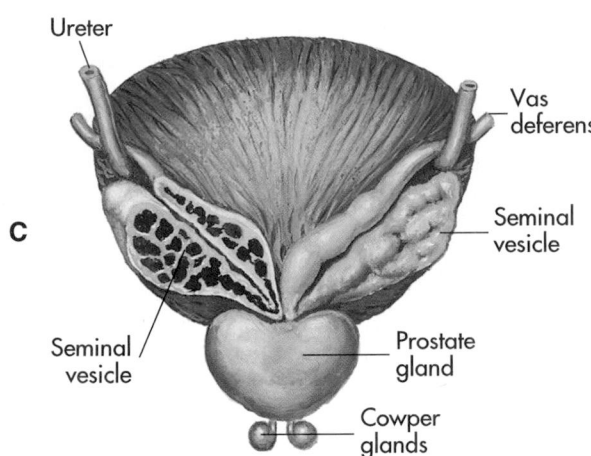

FIGURE 20-2
Anatomy of the prostate gland and seminal vesicles. **A,** Cross section. **B,** Lateral view. **C,** Posterior view.

efforts of the woman, may also aggravate the condition, causing protrusion and inflammation of hemorrhoids.

OLDER ADULTS

Degeneration of afferent neurons in the rectal wall interferes with the process of relaxation of the internal sphincter in response to distention of the rectum. This can result in an elevated pressure threshold for the sensation of rectal distention in the older adult, with consequent retention of stool. Conversely, as the autonomically controlled internal sphincter loses tone, the external sphincter cannot by itself control the bowels, and the older adult may experience fecal incontinence.

In men the fibromuscular structures of the prostate gland atrophy, with loss of function of the secretory alveoli; however, the atrophy of aging is often obscured by benign hyperplasia of the glandular tissue. The muscular component of the prostate is progressively replaced by collagen.

REVIEW OF RELATED HISTORY

For each of the conditions discussed in this section, targeted topics to include in the history of the present illness are listed. Responses to questions about these topics help fully assess the patient's condition and provide clues for focusing the physical examination.

HISTORY OF PRESENT ILLNESS

- ◆ Changes in bowel function
  - ◆ Character: number, frequency, consistency of stools; presence of mucus or blood; color (dark, bright red, black, light, or clay-colored); odor
  - ◆ Onset and duration: sudden or gradual, relation to dietary change, relation to stressful events
  - ◆ Accompanying symptoms: incontinence, flatus, pain, fever, nausea, vomiting, cramping, abdominal distention
  - ◆ Medications: iron, laxatives, stool softeners; prescription or nonprescription
- ◆ Anal discomfort: itching, pain, stinging, burning
  - ◆ Relation to body position and defecation
  - ◆ Straining at stool
  - ◆ Presence of mucus or blood
  - ◆ Interference with activities of daily living or sleep
  - ◆ Medications: hemorrhoid preparations; prescription or nonprescription
- ◆ Rectal bleeding
  - ◆ Color: bright or dark red, black
  - ◆ Relation to defecation
  - ◆ Amount: spotting on toilet paper versus active bleeding
  - ◆ Accompanying changes in stool: color, frequency, consistency, shape, odor, presence of mucus
  - ◆ Associated symptoms: incontinence, flatus, rectal pain, abdominal pain or cramping, abdominal distention, weight loss
  - ◆ Medications: iron; prescription or nonprescription medications (e.g., fiber additives)
- ◆ Males: changes in urinary function
  - ◆ History of enlarged prostate or prostatitis
  - ◆ Symptoms: hesitancy, urgency, nocturia, dysuria, change in force or caliber of stream, dribbling, urethral discharge

PAST MEDICAL HISTORY

- ◆ Hemorrhoids
- ◆ Spinal cord injury
- ◆ Males: prostatic hypertrophy or carcinoma
- ◆ Females: episiotomy or fourth-degree laceration during delivery
- ◆ Colorectal cancer or related cancers: breast, ovarian, endometrial

FAMILY HISTORY

- ◆ Rectal polyps
- ◆ Colon cancer or familial cancer syndromes (see the Risk Factors box on p. 670)
- ◆ Prostatic cancer (see the Risk Factors box on p. 670)

RISK FACTORS
COLORECTAL CANCER

- Older than 50 years of age
- Family history of colon cancer, familial adenomatous polyposis (FAP), familial hereditary nonpolyposis colorectal cancer (HNPCC), Gardner syndrome
- Personal history of colorectal cancer, intestinal polyps, chronic inflammatory bowel disease (Crohn disease, ulcerative colitis), Gardner syndrome
- Personal history of ovarian, endometrial or breast cancer
- Ethnic background: Ashkenazi Jewish descent
- Diet high in beef and animal fats, low in fiber
- Obesity
- Smoking
- Physical inactivity (regular physical activity reduces risk)
- Alcohol intake: risk increases with increased amounts

RISK FACTORS
PROSTATE CANCER

- Older than 50 years of age
- Race: black (two times the risk compared to that of white men)
- Nationality: common in North America and northwestern Europe; less common in Asia, Africa, Central America, and South America
- Family history of prostate cancer (twice the risk with one first-degree relative; risk increases with more than one first-degree relative)
- Diet high in animal fat
- Hormones: cumulative exposure of the prostate to high levels of androgens
- Physical inactivity (regular physical activity reduces risk)

PERSONAL AND SOCIAL HISTORY

- Bowel habits and characteristics: timing, frequency, number, consistency, shape, color, odor
- Travel history: areas with high incidence of parasitic infestation, including zones in the United States
- Diet: inclusion of fiber foods (cereals, breads, nuts, fruits, vegetables) and concentrated high-fiber foods; amount of animal fat
- Risk factors for colorectal or prostatic cancer
- Use of alcohol

INFANTS AND CHILDREN

- Newborns: characteristics of stool
- Bowel movements accompanied by crying, straining, bleeding
- Feeding habits: types of foods, milk (bottle or breast for infants), appetite
- Age at which bowel control and toilet training were achieved
- Associated symptoms: episodes of diarrhea or constipation; tenderness when cleaning after a stool; perianal irritations; weight loss; nausea, vomiting; incontinence in toilet-trained child (association with convulsions)
- Congenital anomaly: imperforate anus, myelomeningocele, aganglionic megacolon

PREGNANT WOMEN

- Weeks of gestation and estimated date of delivery
- Exercise
- Fluid intake and dietary habits

- Medications: prenatal vitamins, iron
- Use of complementary or alternative therapies

OLDER ADULTS
- Changes in bowel habits or character: frequency, number, color, consistency, shape, odor
- Associated symptoms: weight loss, rectal or abdominal pain, incontinence, flatus, episodes of constipation or diarrhea, abdominal distention, rectal bleeding
- Dietary changes: intolerance for certain foods, inclusion of high-fiber foods, regularity of eating habits, appetite
- Males: history of enlarged prostate, urinary symptoms (hesitancy, urgency, nocturia, dysuria, force and caliber of urinary stream, dribbling)

EXAMINATION AND FINDINGS

EQUIPMENT

- Gloves
- Water-soluble lubricant
- Penlight
- Drapes
- Fecal occult blood testing materials

PREPARATION

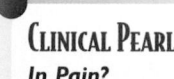

CLINICAL PEARL

In Pain?
The patient with a really acute problem will often shift uncomfortably from side to side when sitting.

Although the rectal examination is generally uncomfortable and sometimes embarrassing for the patient, it provides such important information that it is a mandatory part of every thorough examination. Be calm, slowly paced, and gentle in your touch. Explain what will happen step by step and let the patient know what to expect. A hurried or rough examination can cause unnecessary pain and sphincter spasm, and you can easily lose the trust and cooperation of the patient.

POSITIONING

The rectal examination can be performed with the patient in any of these positions: knee-chest; left lateral with hips and knees flexed; or standing with the hips flexed and the upper body supported by the examining table. In adult males, the latter two positions are satisfactory for most purposes and allow adequate visualization of the perianal and sacrococcygeal areas. In women, the rectal examination is most often performed as part of the rectovaginal examination while the woman is in the lithotomy position (see Chapter 18).

Ask the patient to assume one of the examining positions, guiding gently with your hands when necessary. Use drapes but retain good visualization of the area. Glove one or both hands.

SACROCOCCYGEAL AND PERIANAL AREAS

Inspect the sacrococcygeal (pilonidal) and perianal areas. The skin should be smooth and uninterrupted. Inspect for lumps, rashes, inflammation, excoriation, scars, pilonidal dimpling, and tufts of hair at the pilonidal area. Fungal infection and pinworm infestation can cause perianal irritation. Fungal infection is more common in adults with diabetes, and pinworms are more common in children. Palpate the area. The discovery of tenderness and inflammation should alert you to the possibility of a perianal abscess, anorectal fistula or fissure, pilonidal cyst, or pruritus ani.

ANUS

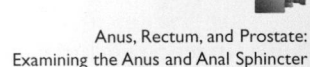

Anus, Rectum, and Prostate:
Examining the Anus and Anal Sphincter

Spread the patient's buttocks apart and inspect the anus. The use of a penlight or gooseneck lamp can assist in visualization. The skin around the anus will appear coarser and more darkly pigmented. Look for skin lesions, skin tags or warts, external hemorrhoids, fissures, and fistulas. Ask the patient to bear down. This will make fistulas, fissures, rectal prolapse, polyps, and internal hemorrhoids more readily apparent. Clock referents are used to describe the location of anal and rectal findings: 12 o'clock is in the ventral midline and 6 o'clock is in the dorsal midline.

SPHINCTER

Lubricate your index finger and press the pad of it against the anal opening (Fig. 20-3, *A*). Ask the patient to bear down to relax the external sphincter. As relaxation occurs, slip the tip of the finger into the anal canal (Fig. 20-3, *B*). Warn the patient that there may be a feeling of urgency for a bowel movement, and assure him or her that this will not happen. Ask the patient to tighten the external sphincter around your finger (Fig. 20-4, *A*), noting its tone; it should tighten evenly with no discomfort to the patient. A lax sphincter may indicate neurologic deficit. An extremely tight sphincter can result from scarring, spasticity caused by a fissure or other lesion, inflammation, or anxiety about the examination.

An anal fistula or fissure may produce such extreme tenderness that you are not able to complete the examination without local anesthesia. Rectal pain is almost always indicative of a local disease. Look for irritation, rock hard constipation, rectal fissures, or thrombosed hemorrhoids. Always inquire about previous episodes of pain.

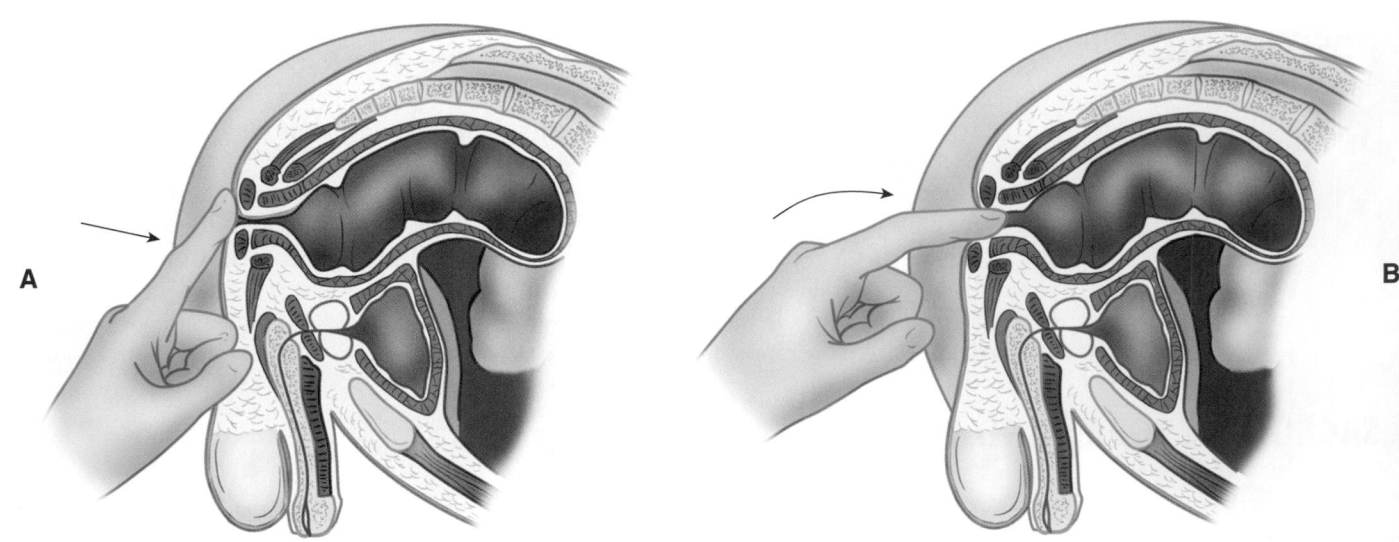

FIGURE 20-3
A, Correct procedure for introducing finger into rectum. Press pad of finger against the anal opening. **B,** As external sphincter relaxes, slip the fingertip into the anal canal. Note that patient is in the hips-flexed position.

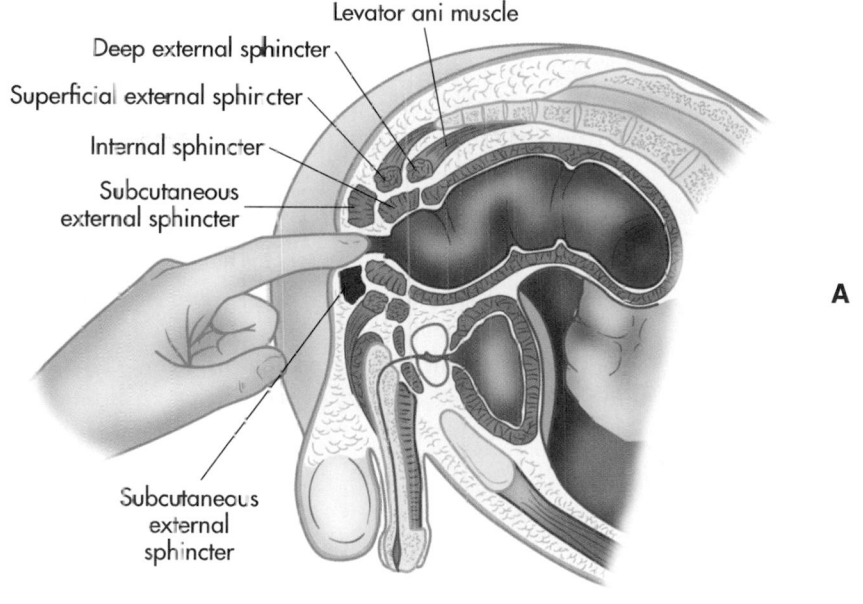

Levator ani muscle
Deep external sphincter
Superficial external sphincter
Internal sphincter
Subcutaneous external sphincter

Subcutaneous external sphincter

A

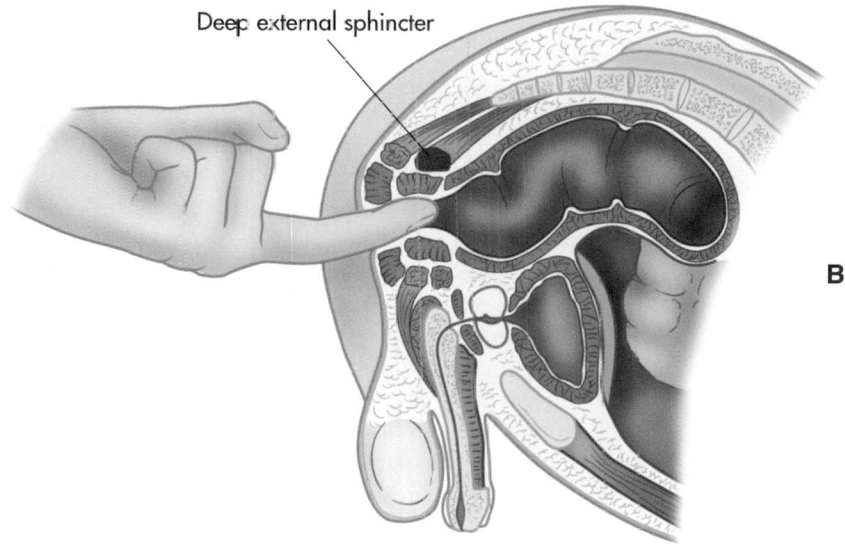

Deep external sphincter

B

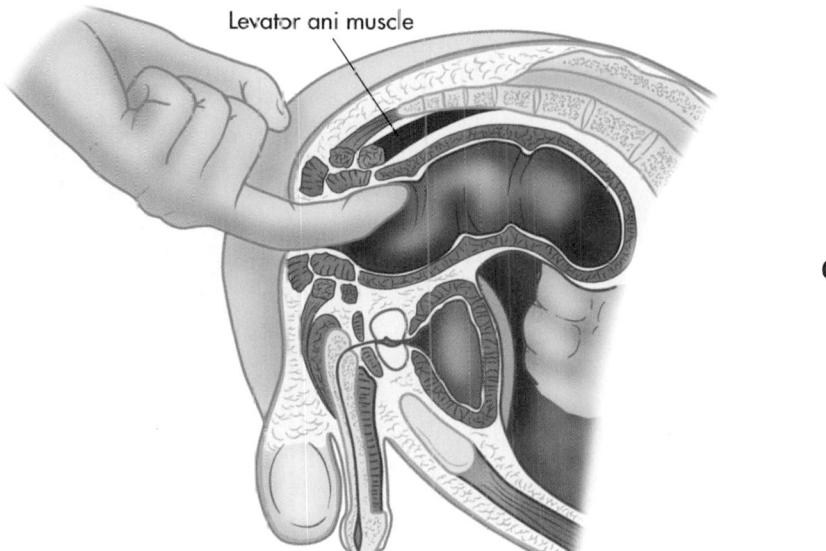

Levator ani muscle

C

FIGURE 20-4
A, Palpation of subcutaneous external sphincter. Feel it tighten around the examining finger. **B,** Palpation of deep external sphincter. **C,** Palpation of the posterior rectal wall.

ANAL RING

Rotate your finger to examine the muscular anal ring (Fig. 20-4, *B*). It should feel smooth and exert even pressure on the finger. Note any nodules or irregularities.

LATERAL AND POSTERIOR RECTAL WALLS

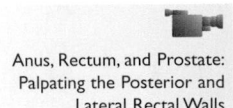

Anus, Rectum, and Prostate:
Palpating the Posterior and
Lateral Rectal Walls

Insert your finger farther and palpate in sequence the lateral and posterior rectal walls, noting any nodules, masses, irregularities, polyps, or tenderness (Fig. 20-4, *C*). The walls should feel smooth, even, and uninterrupted. Internal hemorrhoids are not ordinarily felt unless they are thrombosed. The examining finger can palpate a distance of about 6 to 10 cm into the rectum.

BIDIGITAL PALPATION

Bidigital palpation with the thumb and index finger can sometimes reveal more information than palpating with the index finger alone. To perform bidigital palpation, lightly press your thumb against the perianal tissue and bring your index finger toward the thumb. This technique is particularly useful for detecting a perianal abscess.

ANTERIOR RECTAL WALL AND PROSTATE

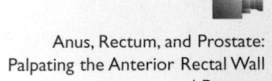

Anus, Rectum, and Prostate:
Palpating the Anterior Rectal Wall
and Prostate

Rotate the index finger to palpate the anterior rectal wall as above. In males, you can palpate the posterior surface of the prostate gland (Fig. 20-5). Tell the patient that he may feel the urge to urinate but that he will not. Note the size, contour, consistency, and mobility of the prostate. The gland should feel like a pencil eraser—firm, smooth, and slightly movable—and it should be nontender. A healthy prostate has a diameter of about 4 cm, with less than 1 cm protrusion into the rectum. Greater protrusion denotes prostatic enlargement, which should be noted and the amount of protrusion recorded (Box 20-1). The sulcus may be obliterated when the lobes are hypertrophied or neoplastic. A rubbery or boggy consistency is indicative of benign hypertrophy, whereas stony hard nodularity may indicate carcinoma, prostatic calculi, or chronic fibrosis. Fluctuant softness suggests prostatic abscess. Identify the lateral lobes and the median sulcus. The prostatic lobes should feel symmetric. The seminal vesicles are not palpable unless they are inflamed. Box 20-2 and the Evidence-Based Practice box on p. 676 discuss screening for prostate cancer.

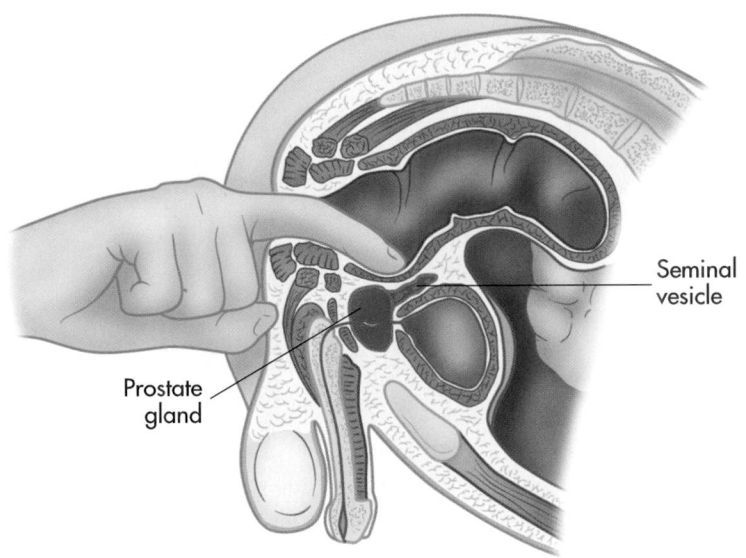

Seminal
vesicle

Prostate
gland

FIGURE 20-5
Palpation of the posterior surface of the prostate gland. Feel for the lateral lobes and median sulcus.

BOX 20-1

PROSTATE ENLARGEMENT

Prostate enlargement is classified by the amount of protrusion into the rectum:
Grade I: 1 to 2 cm
Grade II: 2 to 3 cm
Grade III: 3 to 4 cm
Grade IV: more than 4 cm

BOX 20-2

SCREENING FOR PROSTATE CANCER: THE TOOLS

Screening for prostate cancer is controversial, with recommendations varying among the major authorities (see the Evidence-Based Practice box on p. 676). The following summarizes some of the various recommendations.

Digital Rectal Examination (DRE)
Although most authorities agree on using DRE as part of periodic health screening for men older than 50 years of age, its role in screening for prostate cancer is not clear. Those authorities that do advocate DRE recommend it (in conjunction with prostate-specific antigen [PSA] testing) as part of the periodic health examination in men older than 50 years of age who are at average risk and in men older than 40 years of age who are at higher risk (e.g., black, family history of prostate cancer).

Prostate-Specific Antigen (PSA)
PSA is a glycoprotein that is specific to the prostate but not to prostate cancer. It is produced by all types of prostate tissue whether healthy, hyperplastic, or malignant; therefore whether to screen asymptomatic men for prostate cancer with PSA testing is controversial. Screening can detect tumors at a more favorable stage, but there are no data indicating that PSA screening decreases mortality from prostate cancer.

Some authorities do not recommend use of PSA for routine screening; those that do, recommend it in conjunction with DRE as described previously (i.e., older than 50 years of age for average-risk men; older than 40 years of age for high-risk men).

PSA results less than 4 ng/mL are usually considered normal; results greater than 10 ng/mL are considered high; results between 4 and 10 ng/mL are considered borderline. The higher the PSA level, the more likely the presence of prostatic cancer; however, men with prostate cancer can have a negative or borderline PSA level. A negative PSA and a negative DRE make the presence of cancer unlikely.

New types of PSA tests have been developed that may be useful when the usual PSA result is borderline:
- PSA density (PSAD) is calculated by dividing the PSA number by the prostate volume (measured by transurethral ultrasonography [TRUS]).
- Age-specific ranges maybe useful because older men have higher PSA levels than younger men, even in the absence of cancer.
- PSA velocity measures how quickly the PSA level rises over time. Serial testing may be appropriate for managing borderline results.
- Free PSA ratio indicates how much PSA circulates unbound and how much is bound. For PSA results in the borderline range, a low free PSA ratio increases the chance that prostate cancer is present and suggests the need for biopsy.

Biopsy
Biopsy of the prostate tissue is recommended when the PSA level is high. Results in the borderline range may be an indication for biopsy if the DRE is abnormal. Biopsy also may be used when the free PSA ratio is low, in the presence of borderline PSA results.

Transurethral Ultrasonography (TRUS)
TRUS is used when the PSA is borderline and the DRE is normal. TRUS may be able to indicate areas of the prostate that require biopsy. It can also be used to determine prostate volume, which can be used in the calculation of PSA density.

EVIDENCE-BASED PRACTICE IN PHYSICAL EXAMINATION
SCREENING FOR PROSTATE CANCER: THE CONTROVERSY

In the only systematic review to date, the U.S. Preventive Services Task Force (USPSTF) found insufficient evidence to recommend for or against routine screening for prostate cancer using digital rectal examination (DRE) or prostate specific antigen (PSA) testing. (Harris et al, 2001). A protocol for prostate cancer screening is currently under review by the Cochrane Prostatic Diseases and Urologic Cancer Group (Ilic et al, 2004) to determine efficacy of screening. Use of the DRE as a screening tool is limited due to its inability to palpate the entire prostate gland, and the PSA test can be compromised due to the high false-negative and false-positive results produced.

Medical experts who encourage regular screening believe current scientific evidence shows that finding and treating prostate cancer early, when treatment might be more effective, may save lives. Advocates of routine testing claim that PSA testing has the potential to detect tumors at an early stage, hopefully before they spread outside of the prostate. Studies have demonstrated a reduced death rate from prostate cancer in populations that have had prostate cancer screening as a public program. The American Cancer Society and the American Urological Association recommend that all men who have a life expectancy of at least 10 years should be offered the PSA test and DRE annually beginning at age 50. They also recommend offering screening tests earlier to black men and to men who have a father or brother with prostate cancer (Gambert 2001; Smith et al, 1997).

Medical experts who do not recommend regular screening want convincing evidence that finding early stage prostate cancer, and treating it, saves live. Causes for concern include the cost of follow-up tests and the potentially invasive nature of these tests, the potentially false sense of security following false-negative test results, and the use of potentially harmful treatment regimens that may not provide any improvement in health outcomes. Treatment for prostate cancer is not risk-free and may cause impotence or urinary incontinence. Although a man's risk of prostate cancer diagnosis increases with age, many men will live with prostate cancer only to die of another disorder, as has been confirmed in unselected autopsies. The National Cancer Institute, The USPSTF, the American College of Physicians, the Academy of Family Physicians, and the Centers for Disease Control and Prevention do not recommend routine screening (CDC, 2004; Harris & Lohr, 2002; NCI, 2003; Zoorob et al, 2001).

The experts do agree that every man needs balanced information on the pros and cons of prostate cancer screening to help him make an informed decision. Many clinicians currently use a shared decision-making model. Shared decision making is a process carried out between a patient and his health care professional in the clinical setting where both parties share information and the patient understands the nature and risks of prostate cancer; understands the risks, benefits, and alternatives to screening; participates in decision making at a level he desires; and makes a decision consistent with his preferences and values, or defers the decision to a later time.

Palpation of the prostate can force secretions through the urethral orifice. Any secretions that appear on the meatus should be cultured and examined microscopically. Specimen preparation techniques are described in Chapter 18.

UTERUS AND CERVIX

In females a retroflexed or retroverted uterus is usually palpable through rectal examination. The cervix may be palpable through the anterior rectal wall (see Chapter 18). Do not mistake these structures for a tampon or a tumor.

After palpating the anterior wall in females and the prostate in males, ask the patient to bear down. This allows you to reach a few centimeters farther into the rectum. Because the anterior rectal wall is in contact with the peritoneum, you may be able to detect the tenderness of peritoneal inflammation and the nodularity of peritoneal metastases. The nodules, called *shelf lesions*, are palpable just above the prostate in males and in the cul-de-sac of females.

STOOL

Slowly withdraw your finger and examine it for any fecal material, which should be soft and brown (Box 20-3). Note any blood or pus. Very light tan or gray stool could indicate obstructive jaundice, whereas tarry black stool should make you suspect upper intestinal tract bleeding. A more subtle blood loss can result in a virtually unchanged color of the stool, but even a small amount will yield a positive test for occult blood (Box 20-4). If indicated, fecal material can be tested for blood using a chemical guaiac procedure.

BOX 20-3

STOOL CHARACTERISTICS IN DISEASE

Changes in the shape, content, or consistency of stool suggest that some disease process is present. Stool characteristics can sometimes point to the type of disorder present; therefore you should be familiar with the following characteristics and associated disorders:

- Intermittent, pencil-like stools suggest a spasmodic contraction in the rectal area.
- Persistent, pencil-like stools indicate permanent stenosis from scarring or from pressure of a malignancy.
- Pipestem stools and ribbon stools indicate lower rectal stricture.
- A large amount of mucus in the fecal matter is characteristic of intestinal inflammation and mucous colitis.
- Small flecks of blood-stained mucus in liquid feces are indicative of amebiasis.
- Fatty stools are seen in patients with pancreatic disorders and malabsorption syndromes.
- Stools the color of aluminum (caused by a mixture of melena and fat) occur in tropical sprue, carcinoma of the hepatopancreatic ampulla, and children treated with sulfonamides for diarrhea.

BOX 20-4

COMMON CAUSES OF RECTAL BLEEDING

There are numerous reasons that blood can appear in the feces, ranging from benign, self-limiting events to serious, life-threatening disease. Following are some common causes:

- Anal fissures
- Anaphylactoid purpura
- Aspirin-containing medications
- Bleeding disorders
- Coagulation disorders
- Colitis
- Dysentery, acute and amebic
- Esophageal varices
- Familial telangiectasia
- Foreign body trauma
- Hemorrhoids
- Hiatal hernia
- Hookworm
- Intussusception
- Iron poisoning
- Meckel diverticulum
- Neoplasms of any type
- Oral steroids
- Peptic ulcers, acute and chronic
- Polyps, single or multiple
- Regional enteritis
- Strangulated hernia
- Swallowed blood
- Thrombocytopenia
- Volvulus

Further evaluation is indicated if there is persistent anal or rectal bleeding; any interruption in the smooth contour of the rectal wall on palpation; persistent pain with negative findings on rectal examination; or unexplained, persistent stool changes.

INFANTS AND CHILDREN Rectal examination is not always performed on infants and children unless there is a particular problem. An examination is required whenever there is any symptom that suggests an intraabdominal or pelvic problem, a mass or tenderness, bladder distention, bleeding, or rectal or bowel abnormalities. Deviation from the expected stool pattern in infants demands investigation (Table 20-1).

It is imperative that you respect the child's modesty and apprehension. Careful explanation of each step in the process is necessary for the child who is old enough to understand.

Routinely inspect the anal region and perineum, examining the surrounding buttocks for redness, masses, and evidence of change in firmness. Inspect for swollen, tender perirectal protrusion, abscesses, and possibly rectal fistulas. A variety of problems can be discovered by this inspection. Shrunken buttocks suggests a chronic debilitating disease. Asymmetric creases occur with congenital dislocation of the hips. Perirectal redness and irritation are suggestive of pinworms, *Candida*, or other irritants of the diaper area. Rectal prolapse results from constipation, diarrhea, or sometimes severe coughing or straining. Hemorrhoids are rare in children, and their presence suggests a serious underlying problem such as portal hypertension. Small flat flaps of skin around the rectum (condylomas) may be syphilitic in origin. Sinuses, tufts of hair, and dimpling in the pilonidal area may indicate lower spinal deformities.

Lightly touch the anal opening, which should produce anal contraction (described by clinicians as an "anal wink"). Lack of contraction may indicate a lower spinal cord lesion.

Examine the patency of the anus and its position in all newborn infants. To determine patency, insert a lubricated catheter no more than 1 cm into the rectum. Patency is usually confirmed by passage of meconium. Occasionally a perianal fistula may be confused with an anal orifice. Be careful in making this judgment. Sometimes the anal orifice can seem appropriate, yet there may be atresia just inside or a few centimeters within the rectum. Rectal examination or insertion of a catheter does not always provide definitive assessment, and radiologic studies may be necessary. If there is no evidence of stool in the newborn, suspect rectal atresia, Hirschsprung disease (congenital megacolon), or cystic fibrosis.

Perform the rectal examination in infants and young children with the child lying on his or her back. You may hold the child's feet together and flex the knees and hips on the abdomen with one hand, using the gloved index finger of your other hand for the examination (Fig. 20-6). Some examiners are reluctant to use the index finger because of its size, choosing instead the fifth finger; however, even with the smallest of adult fingers, some bleeding and tran-

> **CLINICAL PEARL**
>
> **Newborn Rectal Examination**
> When attempting to perform a digital rectal examination on a newborn, use your pinky finger and don't force.

TABLE 20-1	Sequence and Description of Stools in Infants
Infants	**Type of Stool**
Newborn meconium:	Greenish-black, viscous, contains occult blood; first stool is sterile
3 to 6 days old	Transitional: thin, slimy, brown to green
Breast-fed	Mushy, loose, golden yellow; frequency varies from after each feeding to every few days; nonirritating to skin
Formula-fed	Light yellow, characteristic odor, irritating to skin

Data from Lowdermilk & Perry, 2004.

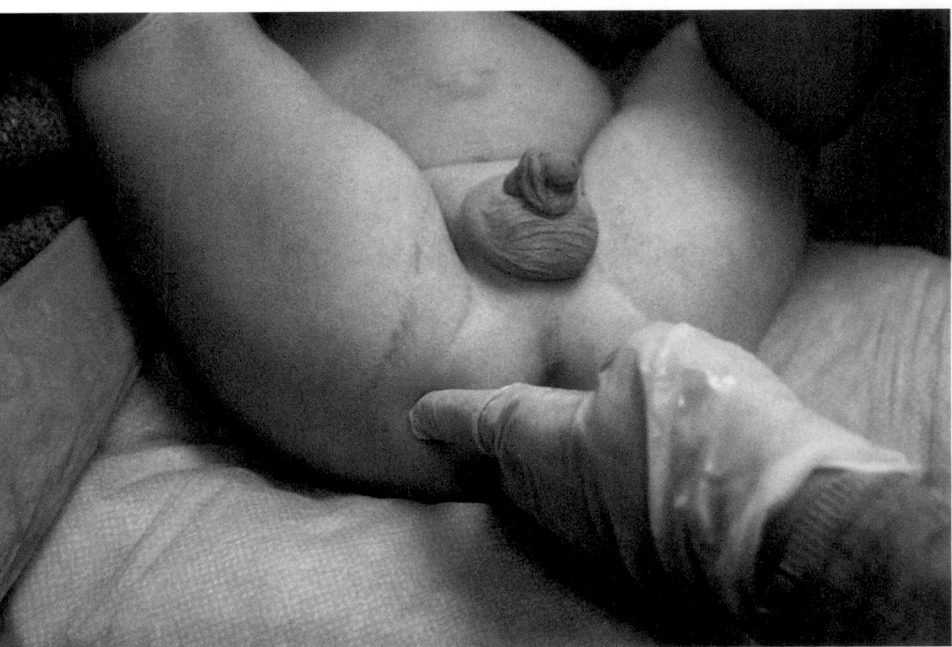

FIGURE 20-6
Positioning the infant or child for rectal examination.

sient prolapse of the rectum often occur right after examination. Always warn the parents of this possibility.

Assess the tone of the rectal sphincter. It should feel snug but neither too tight nor too loose. A very tight sphincter can cause enough tension to produce a stenosis, which leads to stool retention and pain during a bowel movement. A lax sphincter is associated with lesions of the peripheral spinal nerves or spinal cord, *Shigella* infection, and previous fecal impactions. The presence of bruises around the anus, scars, anal tears (especially those that extend into the surrounding perianal skin), and anal dilation may be evidence of sexual abuse.

Feel for feces in the rectum. Chronic constipation in children with mental deficiency or emotional problems is often associated with a rectum distended with feces. A consistently empty rectum in the presence of constipation is a clue to the diagnosis of Hirschsprung disease. A fecal mass in the rectum accompanying diarrhea suggests overflow diarrhea. Stool recovered on the examining finger should be tested for occult blood.

A rectal examination in the young female gives good access to information about the cervix and uterus (see Chapter 18). The ovaries are not usually palpable on rectal examination.

In boys the prostate is usually not felt. A palpable prostate in preadolescent boys suggests precocious puberty or some virilizing disease, which should be apparent from examination of the genitalia.

The rectum can be further evaluated for suspected fissures, fistulas, or polyps by using a small proctoscope or even a wide-mouth speculum on the otoscope.

Rectal examination should be part of the physical examination for adolescents who have symptoms related to the lower intestinal tract. The same procedures and guidelines that are used for adults apply to adolescents. Be especially sensitive to a first examination, and spend additional time explaining what to expect. Illustrations and models can be helpful.

PREGNANT WOMEN

The examination of the rectum provides information about rectovaginal musculature and more specific information about the cervix and uterus (see Chapter 18). During pregnancy the stool color may be dark green or black due to the consumption of iron preparations. Iron may also cause diarrhea or constipation. Assessment for hemorrhoids should include both external and internal evaluation. Hemorrhoids are usually not found early in pregnancy; however, they may be an expected variation late in pregnancy. Evaluate hemorrhoids for size, extent, location (internal or external), discomfort to the patient, and signs of infection or bleeding.

OLDER ADULTS

The examination procedure and findings for the older adult are much the same as those for the younger adult. The older patient may be more limited in ability to assume a position other than the left lateral. Sphincter tone may be somewhat decreased. Older adults commonly experience fecal impaction resulting from constipation. Older males are far more likely to have an enlarged prostate, which will be felt as smooth, rubbery, and symmetric. The median sulcus may or may not be obliterated. Older adults are more likely to have polyps and are at higher risk for carcinoma, making the rectal examination particularly important in this age group.

SAMPLE DOCUMENTATION
HISTORY AND PHYSICAL EXAMINATION

Subjective

A 57-year-old man complains of nighttime urination for past several months, at least twice per night. Restricts fluid intake after 8 PM. Notices difficulty in starting stream. No pain or bleeding on urination. No change in caliber of stream. Denies change in bowel habits or stool characteristics. No history of prostatitis or enlarged prostate.

Objective

Perianal area intact without lesions or visible hemorrhoids. An external skin tag is visible at the 6-o'clock position. No fissures or fistulas. Sphincter tightens evenly. Prostate is symmetric, smooth, boggy, with 1-cm protrusion into rectum. Median sulcus present. Nontender, no nodules. Rectal walls free of masses. Moderate amount of soft stool present.

For additional sample documentation, see Chapter 26.

SUMMARY OF EXAMINATION

ANUS, RECTUM, AND PROSTATE

1. Inspect the sacrococcygeal and perianal area for the following (p. 671):
   - Skin characteristics
   - Lesions
   - Pilonidal dimpling and/or tufts of hair
   - Inflammation
   - Excoriation
2. Inspect the anus for the following (p. 672):
   - Skin characteristics and tags
   - Lesions, fissures, hemorrhoids, or polyps
   - Fistulas
   - Prolapse
3. Insert finger and assess sphincter tone (p. 672).
4. Palpate the muscular ring for the following (p. 674):
   - Smoothness
   - Evenness
5. Palpate the lateral, posterior, and anterior rectal walls for the following (p. 674):
   - Nodules, masses, or polyps
   - Tenderness
   - Irregularities
6. In males, palpate the posterior surface of the prostate gland through the anterior rectal wall for the following (p. 674):
   - Size
   - Contour
   - Consistency
   - Mobility
7. In females, palpate the cervix and uterus through the anterior rectal wall for the following (p. 676):
   - Size
   - Shape
   - Position
   - Smoothness
   - Mobility
8. Have the patient bear down and palpate deeper for the following (p. 676):
   - Tenderness
   - Nodules
9. Withdraw the finger and examine fecal material for the following (p. 676):
   - Color
   - Consistency
   - Blood or pus
   - Occult blood by chemical test if indicated

STAYING WELL

SEXUALLY TRANSMITTED INFECTIONS

Infected persons may spread sexually transmitted infections (STIs) through anal sex practices in which blood, semen, or fluid is shared. Practicing safer sex can prevent STIs in men and women. STIs that affect the anus include the following:
- Herpes simplex virus (HSV) infection of the skin and mucosa causing recurring sores and pain
- Gonorrheal infection of the mucosa, producing an infectious discharge
- Human papillomavirus (HPV), causing anal warts
- Parasites that affect the entire gastrointestinal tract
- Syphilis, early infection causing a painless lesion

Hepatitis and human immunodeficiency virus (HIV) are two STIs whose symptoms do not appear on the anus but can be transmitted through anal sex practices.

It is possible to acquire an STI without penetration. Oral-to-anal contact, whether from kissing or from oral contact with fingers that have been touching the anus can spread bacteria and cause infection. The use of sex toys may transmit certain infections.

COMMON ABNORMALITIES

ANUS, RECTUM, AND SURROUNDING SKIN

PILONIDAL CYSTS

Most pilonidal cysts and sinuses are first diagnosed in young adults, although they are usually a congenital anomaly. Located in the midline, superficial to the coccyx and lower sacrum, the cyst or sinus is seen as a dimple with a sinus tract opening. The opening may contain a tuft of hair and be surrounded by erythema (Fig. 20-7). A cyst may be palpable. The condition is usually asymptomatic, but it is sometimes complicated by an abscess, secondary infection, or fistula.

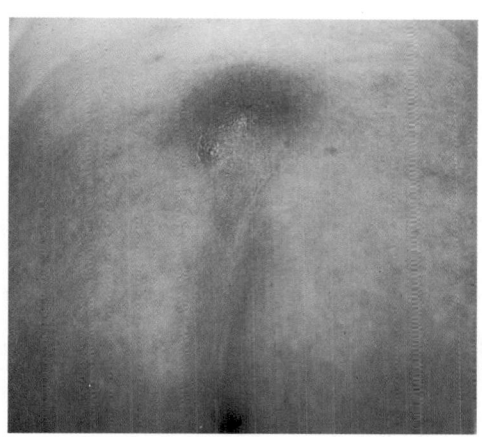

FIGURE 20-7
Pilonidal cyst.
From Zitelli, Davis, 1997.

ANAL WARTS

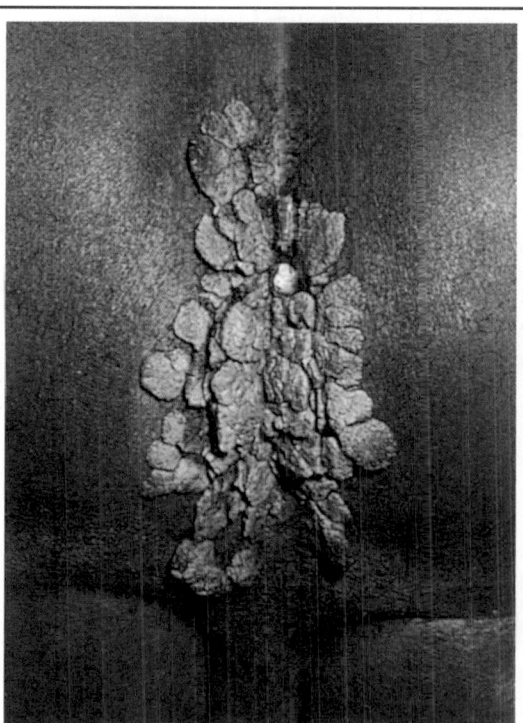

FIGURE 20-8
Anal warts (condyloma acuminata).
From Morse et al, 2003.

Anal warts, condyloma acuminata, are pink to whitish growths that occur on the anus and genitalia as a result of infection with the papilloma virus. They first appear as tiny blemishes that cause no pain or discomfort. As a result, patients may be unaware that the warts are present. The virus can be transmitted from person to person, almost always by direct sexual contact. The warts generally grow larger and become more and more numerous if left untreated. Though genital warts can be treated, none of the available treatments are a cure for HPV, which can remain in nearby skin after treatment. In some cases warts can return months or even years after treatment. In other cases, warts never recur. HPV infection is associated with anal cancer (Fig. 20-8).

ANAL CANCER	Anal cancer is an uncommon, often curable cancer that produces slow-growing tumors and lesions in the anus and nearby anal anatomy. Anal cancers are skin cancers. The majority of anal cancers are squamous cell carcinomas, which are associated with HPV infection. About 15% of anal cancers are adenocarcinomas, which originate in the glands near the anus. The remaining anal cancers are basal cell carcinoma and malignant melanoma. Melanoma in the anus is difficult to see and is often discovered at a late stage, after the cancer has spread through layers of tissue.

PERIANAL AND PERIRECTAL ABSCESSES	These abscesses appear as an area of swelling with variable degrees of erythema of the anus, both internally and externally. The abscess is painful and tender, and usually the patient has a fever (Fig. 20-9). These abscesses are truly hidden and the search for an unexplained fever should always include the rectal examination.

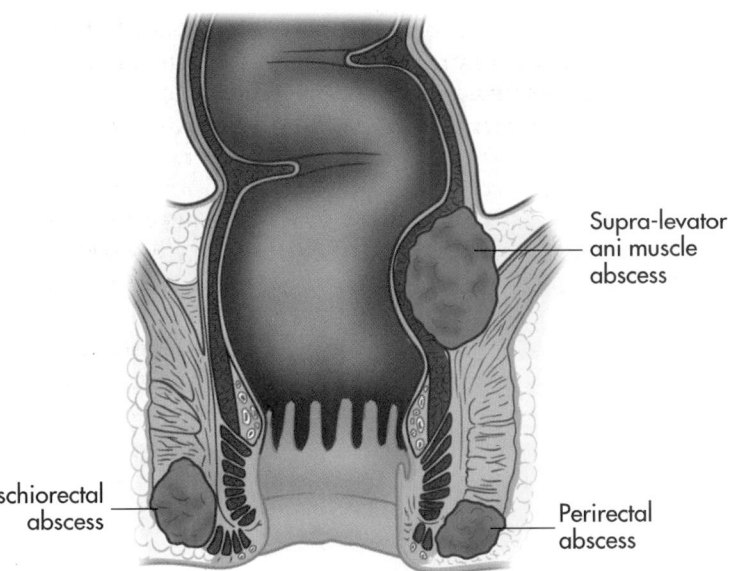

FIGURE 20-9
Perianal and perirectal abscesses. Common sites of abscess formation.

ANORECTAL FISSURE AND FISTULA

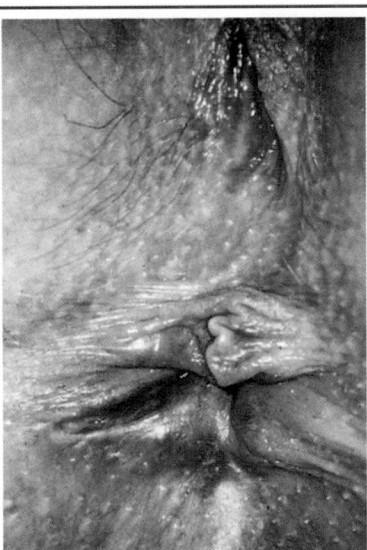

FIGURE 20-10
Lateral anal fissure in adult.
Courtesy Gershon Efron, MD, Sinai Hospital of Baltimore.

A tear in the anal mucosa (fissure) appears most often in the posterior midline, although it can also occur in the anterior midline. The fissure is usually caused by traumatic passage of large, hard stools. A sentinel skin tag may be seen at the lower edge of the fissure. There may be ulceration through which muscles of the internal sphincter are seen. The patient may have symptoms of pain, itching, or bleeding. The internal sphincter is spastic. Examination is painful and may require local anesthesia (Fig. 20-10).

An anorectal fistula is an inflammatory tract that runs from the anus or rectum and opens onto the surface of the perianal skin or other tissue. It is caused by drainage of a perianal or perirectal abscess. Serosanguineous or purulent drainage may appear with compression of the area. The external opening is usually seen as elevated red granular tissue.

PRURITUS ANI

Chronic inflammation of perianal skin results in excoriation, thickening, and pigmentation. The patient complains of burning or itching that may interfere with sleep. It is commonly caused by fungal infection in adults and by parasites in children.

HEMORRHOIDS

External hemorrhoids are varicose veins that originate below the anorectal line and are covered by anal skin. They may cause itching and bleeding with defecation. Usually not visible at rest, they can protrude on standing and on straining at stool. If not reduced, they can become edematous and thrombosed and may require surgical removal. Thrombosed hemorrhoids appear as blue, shiny masses at the anus. Hemorrhoidal skin tags, which can appear at the site of resolved hemorrhoids, are fibrotic or flaccid and painless (Fig. 20-11, A).

Internal hemorrhoids are varicose veins that originate above the anorectal junction and are covered by rectal mucosa. They produce soft swellings that are not palpable on rectal examination and are not visible unless they prolapse through the anus. They do not cause discomfort unless they are thrombosed, prolapsed, or infected. Bleeding may occur with or without defecation. Daily bleeding may be sufficient to cause anemia. Proctoscopy is usually required for diagnosis (Fig. 20-11, B).

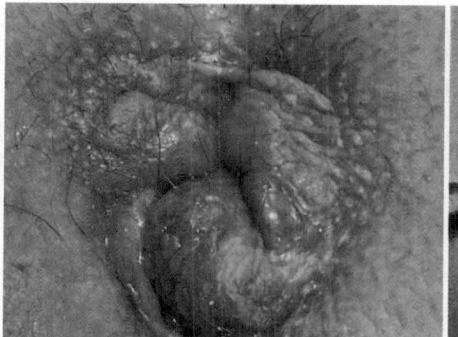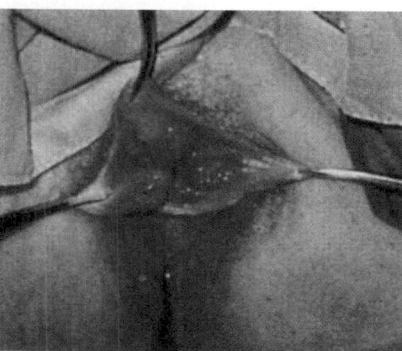

A   B

FIGURE 20-11
A, Prolapsed hemorrhoids.
B, Primary internal hemorrhoids.
Courtesy Gershon Efron, MD, Sinai Hospital of Baltimore.

POLYPS

Occurring anywhere in the intestinal tract, polyps are a relatively common finding. They may be adenomas or inflammatory in origin and can occur singly or in profusion. Polyps are usually evidenced by rectal bleeding, and it is not uncommon to find a polyp protruding through the rectum. They are sometimes palpable on rectal examination as soft nodules and can be either pedunculated (on a stalk) or sessile (closely adhering to the mucosal wall). However, because of their soft consistency, polyps may be difficult to feel on palpation. Proctoscopy is usually required for diagnosis, and biopsy is necessary to distinguish them from carcinoma (Fig. 20-12).

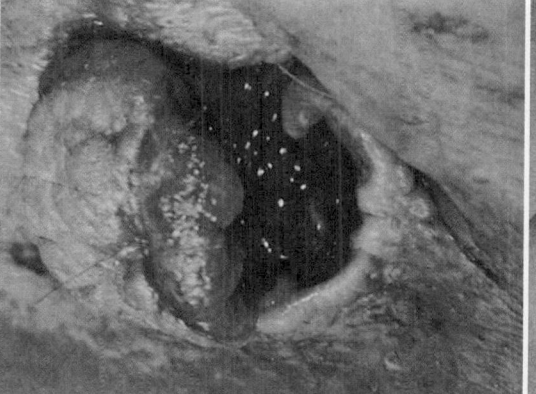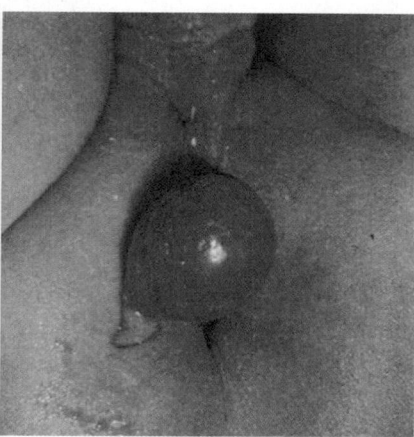

A   B

FIGURE 20-12
A, Fibroepithelial polyp of the rectum. **B,** Infant with prolapsed rectal polyp.
Courtesy Gershon Efron, MD, Sinai Hospital of Baltimore.

RECTAL CARCINOMA	Cancer of the rectum is usually felt as a sessile polypoid mass with nodular raised edges and areas of ulceration. The consistency is often stony, and the contour is irregular. Adenocarcinomas comprise the large majority of rectal cancers. Bleeding is the most common symptom, but rectal carcinoma is often asymptomatic, so routine digital rectal examination is essential for adults.
INTRAPERITONEAL METASTASES	Malignant metastases may develop in the pelvis anterior to the rectum. These can be felt as a hard, nodular shelf at the tip of the examining finger.
RECTAL PROLAPSE	The rectal mucosa, with or without the muscular wall, prolapses through the anal ring as the patient strains at stool. A prolapse of the mucosa is pink and looks like a doughnut or rosette. Complete prolapse involving the muscular wall is larger, red, and has circular folds. Rectal prolapse in children is associated with cystic fibrosis (Fig. 20-13).

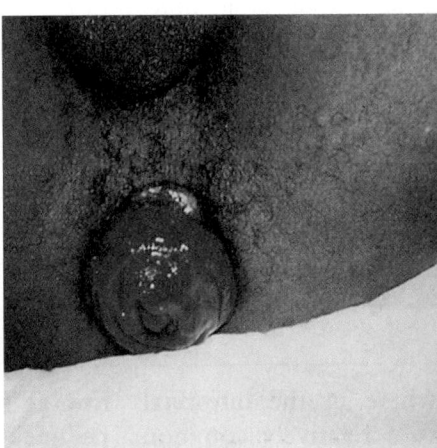
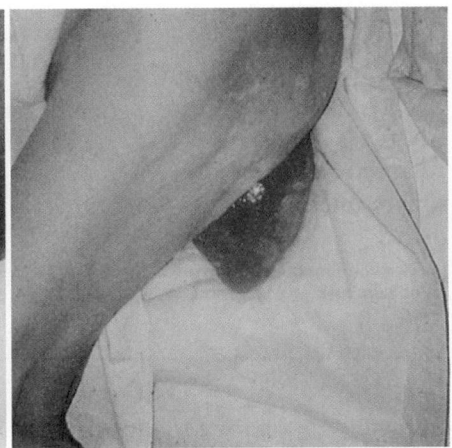

FIGURE 20-13
Prolapse of the rectum.
A, Complete prolapse. **B,** Complete prolapse in an older patient.
Courtesy Gershon Efron, MD, Sinai Hospital of Baltimore.

PROSTATE

PROSTATITIS

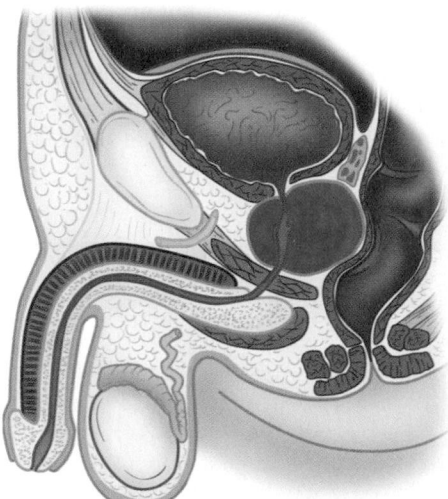

FIGURE 20-14
Prostatitis.

In acute prostatitis, the prostate is enlarged, acutely tender, and often asymmetric. The patient may also have urethral discharge and fever. An abscess may develop, which is felt as a fluctuant mass in the prostate. The seminal vesicles are often involved and may be dilated and tender on palpation (Fig. 20-14).

Chronic prostatitis is usually asymptomatic; however, the prostate may feel boggy, enlarged, and tender or have palpable areas of fibrosis that simulate neoplasm.

CHILDREN

ENTEROBIASIS (ROUNDWORM, PINWORM)	The adult nematode (parasite) lives in the rectum or colon and emerges onto perianal skin to lay eggs while the child sleeps. The patient experiences intense itching of the perianal area, and perianal irritation often results from scratching. The parents often describe unexplained irritability in the infant or child, especially at night. The nematodes can be seen on microscopic examination. To obtain a specimen, press the sticky side of cellulose tape against the perianal folds and then press the tape on a glass slide.
IMPERFORATE ANUS	A variety of anorectal malformations can occur during fetal development (Fig. 20-15). The rectum may end blindly, be stenosed, or have a fistulous connection to the perineum, urinary tract, or, in females, the vagina. The condition is usually diagnosed by rectal examination and confirmed by lack of passage of stool within the first 48 hours of life (Figs. 20-16 and 20-17). Radiographic confirmation may be necessary. Be aware that the imperforation may be just out of the reach of the examining finger on infrequent occasion. The absence of stooling should provoke further studies.

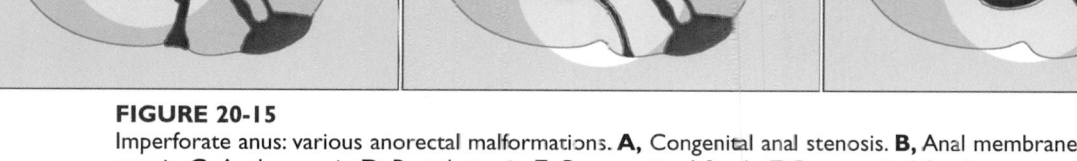

FIGURE 20-15
Imperforate anus: various anorectal malformations. **A,** Congenital anal stenosis. **B,** Anal membrane atresia. **C,** Anal agenesis. **D,** Rectal atresia. **E,** Retroperineal fistula. **F,** Rectovaginal fistula.

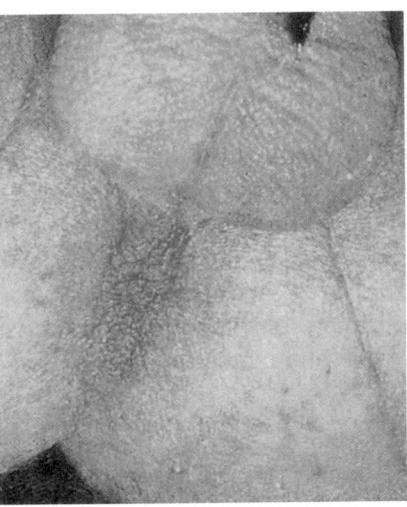

FIGURE 20-16
Imperforate anus.
From 400 self-assessment picture tests in clinical medicine, *1984. By permission of Mosby International.*

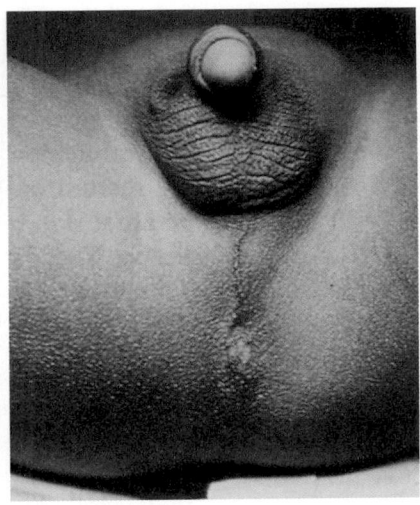

FIGURE 20-17
Rectal atresia.
Courtesy Gershon Efron, MD, Sinai Hospital of Baltimore.

OLDER ADULTS

BENIGN PROSTATIC HYPERTROPHY

> **MNEMONICS**
>
> ***Benign Prostatic Hypertrophy: NUTS***
> **N** Nocturia
> **U** Urine dribbles
> **T** Tried to void, but can't
> **S** Small stream

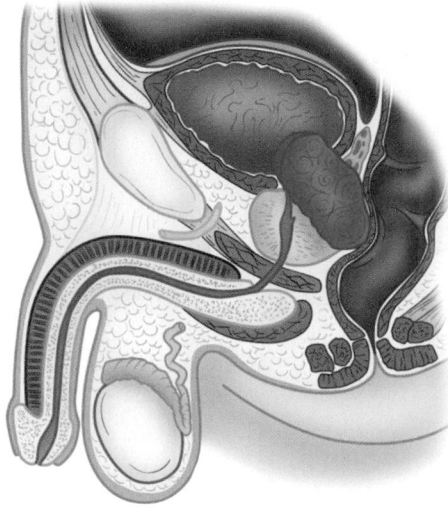

FIGURE 20-18
Benign prostatic hypertrophy.

Benign prostatic hypertrophy (BPH) is common in men older than 50 years of age. The gland begins to grow at adolescence, continuing to enlarge with advancing age. Growth of the prostate parallels the increased incidence of BPH. Urinary symptoms include hesitancy, decreased force and caliber of stream, dribbling, incomplete emptying of the bladder, frequency, urgency, nocturia, and dysuria. On rectal examination, the prostate feels smooth, rubbery, symmetric, and enlarged. The median sulcus may or may not be obliterated (Fig. 20-18).

PROSTATIC CARCINOMA

The incidence of prostatic cancer increases with age and is less frequent in men younger than 50 years of age. Early carcinoma is asymptomatic. As the malignancy advances, symptoms of urinary obstruction occur. On rectal examination, a hard, irregular nodule may be palpable. The prostate feels asymmetric, and the median sulcus is obliterated as the carcinoma enlarges. Prostatic calculi and chronic inflammation produce similar findings, and biopsy is required for differential diagnosis (Fig. 20-19).

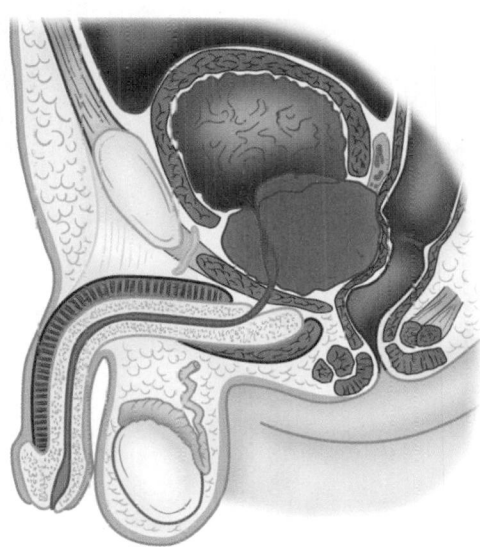

FIGURE 20-19
Carcinoma of prostate.

ELECTRONIC RESOURCES

For Weblinks and additional resources, go to
http://evolve.elsevier.com/Seidel

or to the Companion CD-ROM.

Additional information related to the content in Chapter 20 can be found on the companion website at http://evolve.elsevier.com/Seidel/ or on the interactive companion CD-ROM. Resources and activities for Chapter 20 include:
- Sound and Vision Theater
- Printouts for Your Practice
- Interactive Challenge
- Spanish Assessment Terms with Pronunciation Guide
- Instant Calculator

MUSCULOSKELETAL SYSTEM

The musculoskeletal system provides the stability and mobility necessary for physical activity. Physical performance requires bones, muscles, and joints that function smoothly and effortlessly. Because the musculoskeletal system serves as the body's main line of defense against external forces, injuries are common, and all have the potential for producing permanent disability. Numerous disease processes, including metabolic disorders, affect the musculoskeletal system and can ultimately cause disability.

Disorders that affect the musculoskeletal system may also arise from the neurologic system. For example, delay in an expected muscle response can be caused by pain from a bone or muscle injury, or it may be the result of a cerebellar defect. A careful neurologic examination will help differentiate the cause.

ANATOMY AND PHYSIOLOGY

The musculoskeletal system is a bony structure with its joints held together by ligaments, attached to muscles by tendons, and cushioned by cartilage (Figs. 21-1 and 21-2). In addition to giving structure to the soft tissues of the body and allowing movement, the functions of the musculoskeletal system include protecting vital organs, providing storage space for minerals, producing blood cells (hematopoiesis), and resorbing and reforming itself.

Most joints are diarthrodial—freely moving articulations that are enclosed by a capsule of fibrous articular cartilage, ligaments, and cartilage covering the ends of the opposing bones. A synovial membrane lines the articular cavity and secretes the serous lubricating synovial fluid. Bursae develop in the spaces of connective tissue between tendons, ligaments, and bones to promote ease of motion at points where friction would otherwise occur. Table 21-1 describes the classification of joints.

The variability in size and strength of muscles among individuals is influenced by genetic constitution, nutrition, and exercise. At all ages, muscles increase in size with use and shrink with inactivity. Individual muscles must have intact neurologic innervation to function and to move joints through their full range of motion.

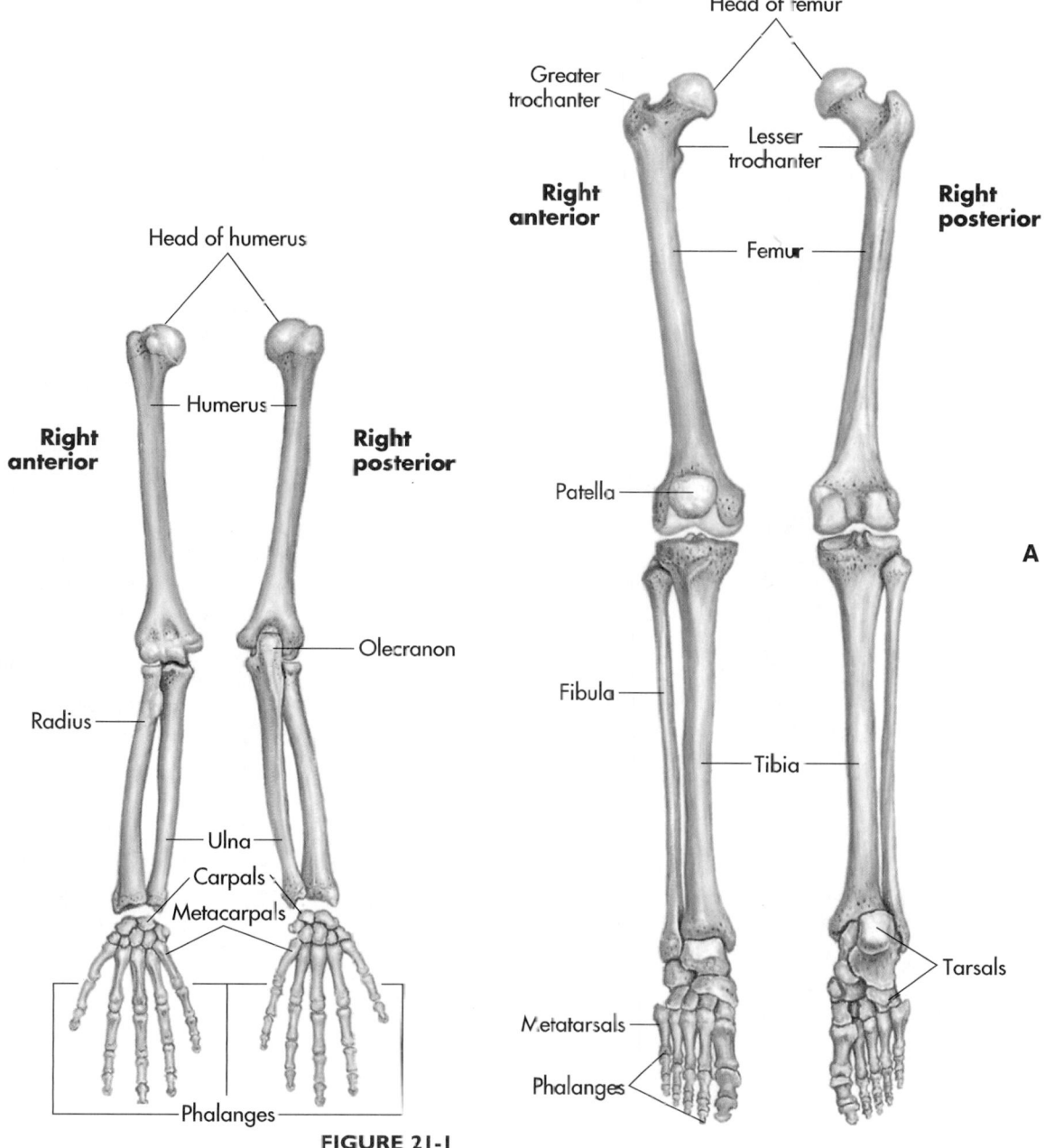

FIGURE 21-1
A, Bones of the upper and lower extremities.   *Continued*

Anterior

Posterior

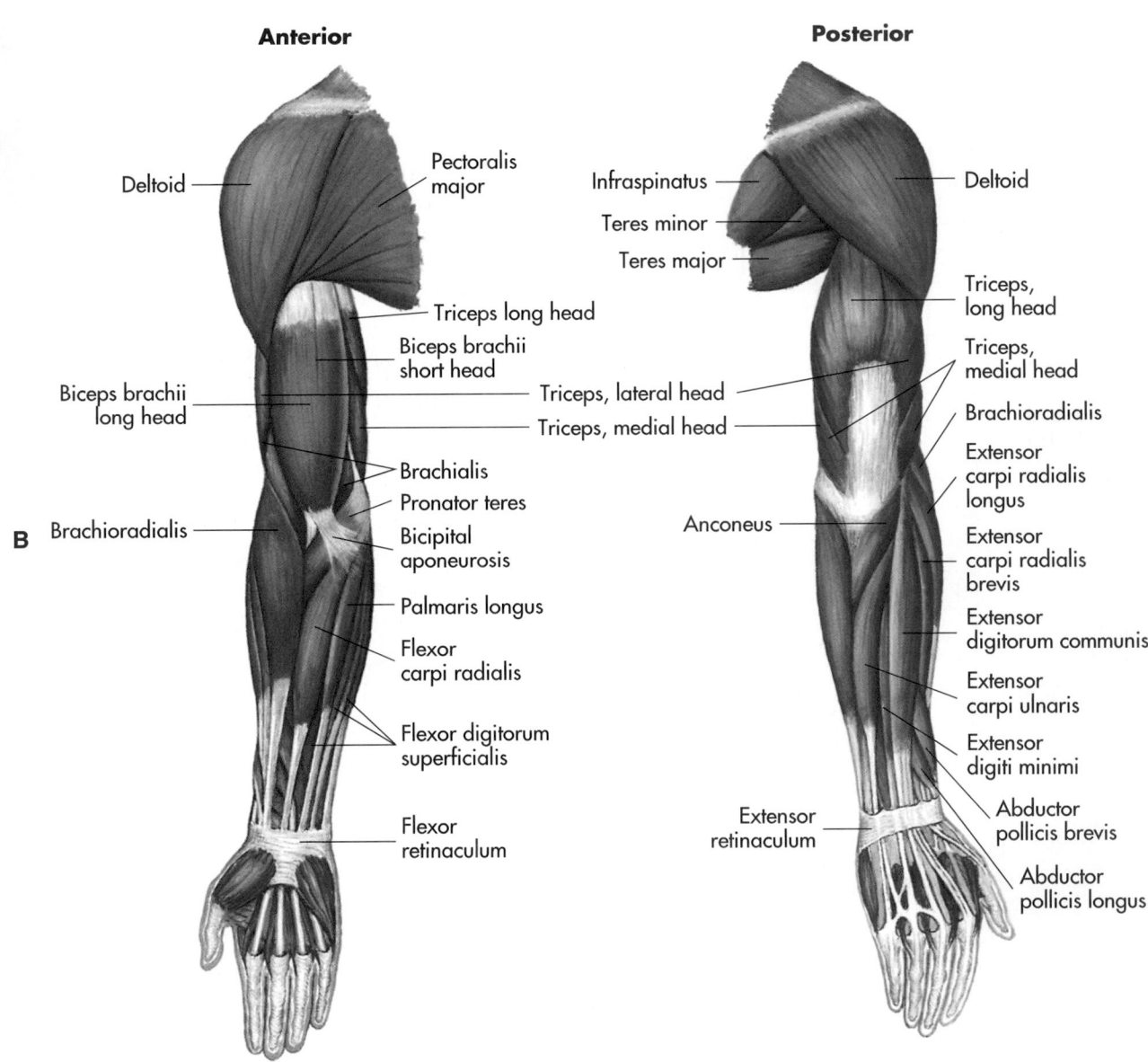

Deltoid

Pectoralis major

Triceps long head

Biceps brachii short head

Biceps brachii long head

Triceps, lateral head

Triceps, medial head

Brachialis

Pronator teres

B Brachioradialis

Bicipital aponeurosis

Palmaris longus

Flexor carpi radialis

Flexor digitorum superficialis

Flexor retinaculum

Infraspinatus

Teres minor

Teres major

Deltoid

Triceps, long head

Triceps, medial head

Brachioradialis

Extensor carpi radialis longus

Anconeus

Extensor carpi radialis brevis

Extensor digitorum communis

Extensor carpi ulnaris

Extensor digiti minimi

Abductor pollicis brevis

Extensor retinaculum

Abductor pollicis longus

FIGURE 21-1, cont'd
B, Muscles of the upper extremities.

Anterior

Posterior

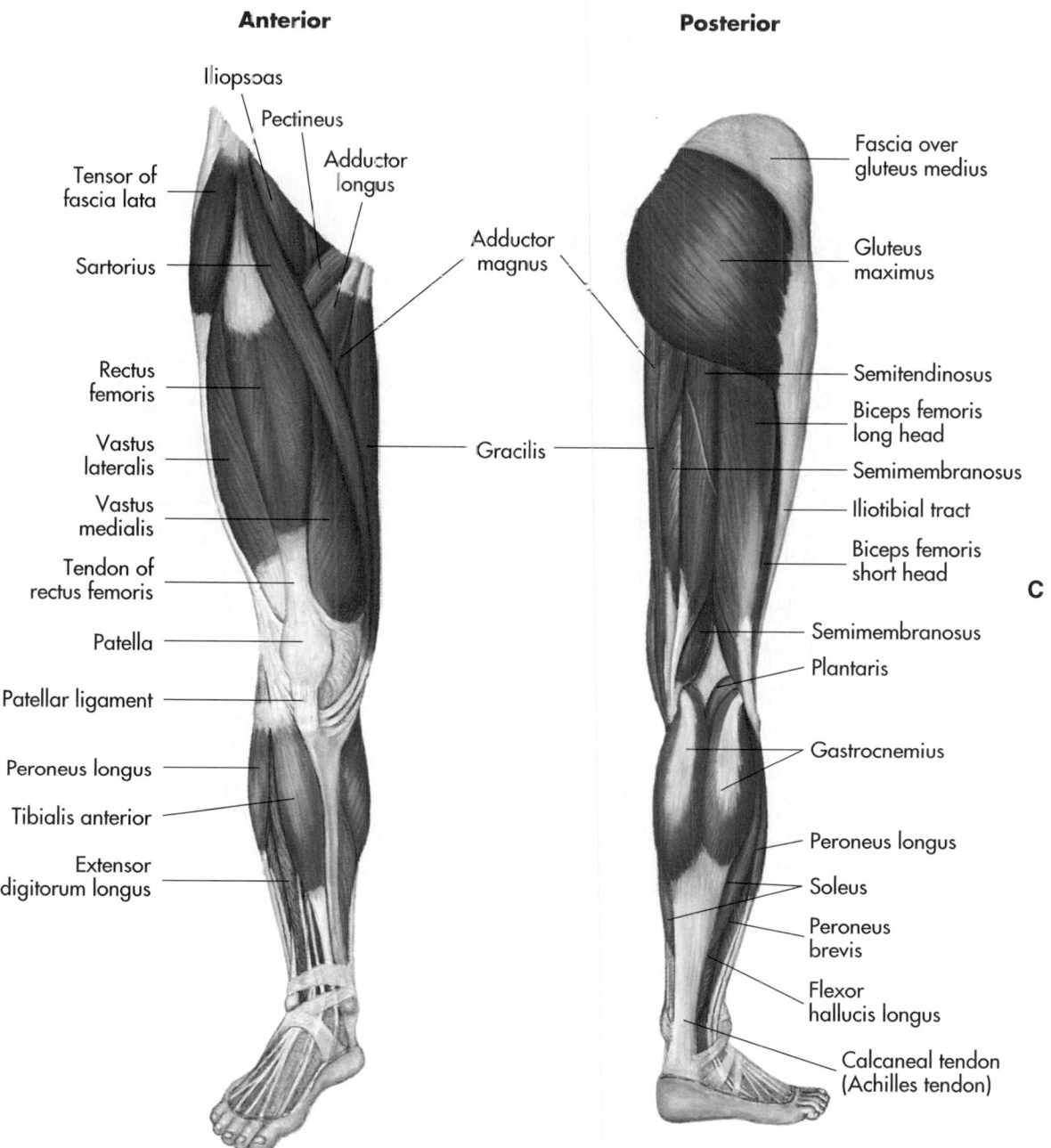

Iliopsoas

Pectineus

Adductor longus

Tensor of fascia lata

Sartorius

Rectus femoris

Vastus lateralis

Vastus medialis

Tendon of rectus femoris

Patella

Patellar ligament

Peroneus longus

Tibialis anterior

Extensor digitorum longus

Adductor magnus

Gracilis

Fascia over gluteus medius

Gluteus maximus

Semitendinosus

Biceps femoris long head

Semimembranosus

Iliotibial tract

Biceps femoris short head

Semimembranosus

Plantaris

Gastrocnemius

Peroneus longus

Soleus

Peroneus brevis

Flexor hallucis longus

Calcaneal tendon (Achilles tendon)

C

FIGURE 21-1, cont'd
C, Muscles of the lower extremities.

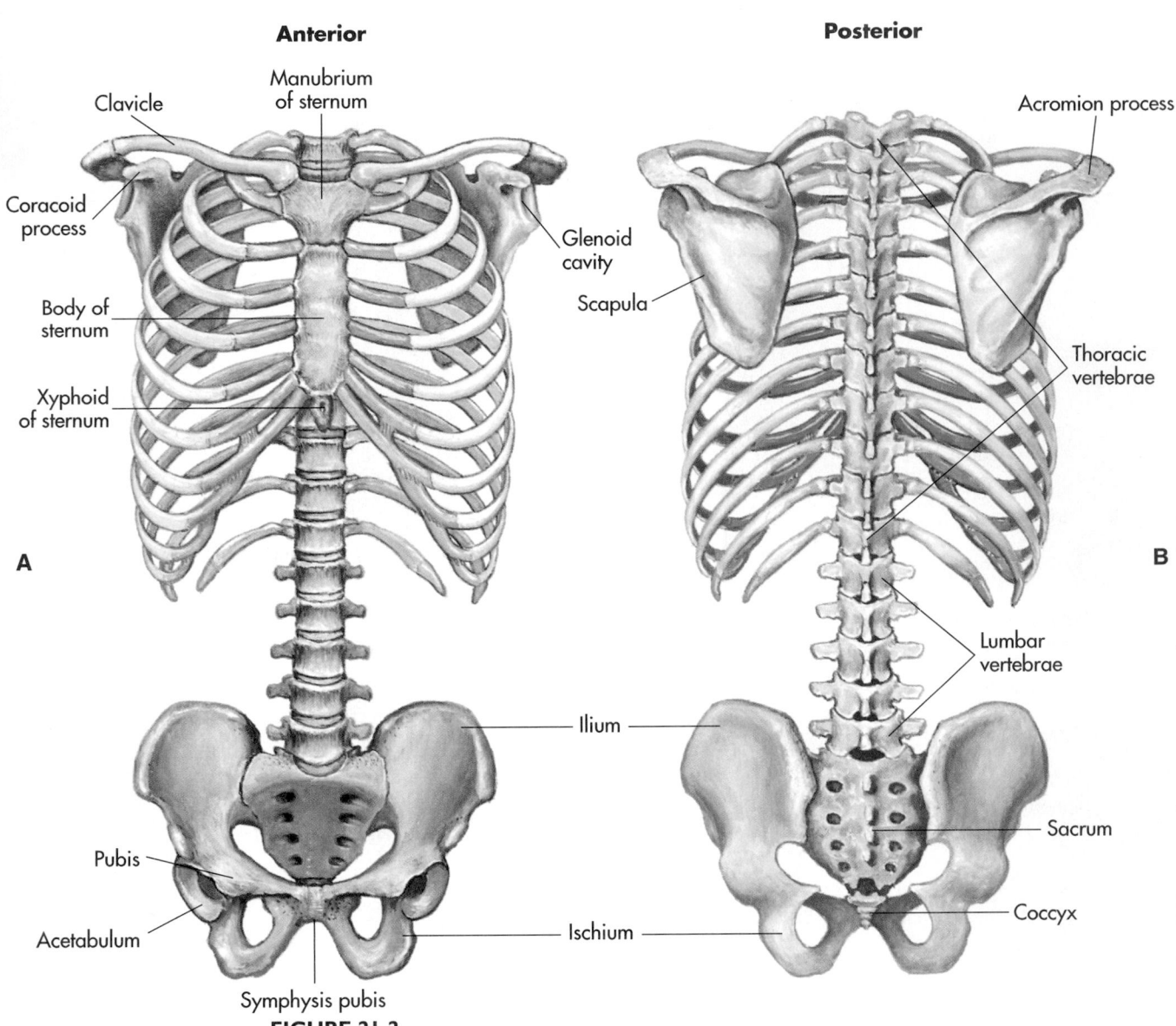

FIGURE 21-2
A, Bones of the trunk, anterior view. **B,** Bones of the trunk, posterior view.

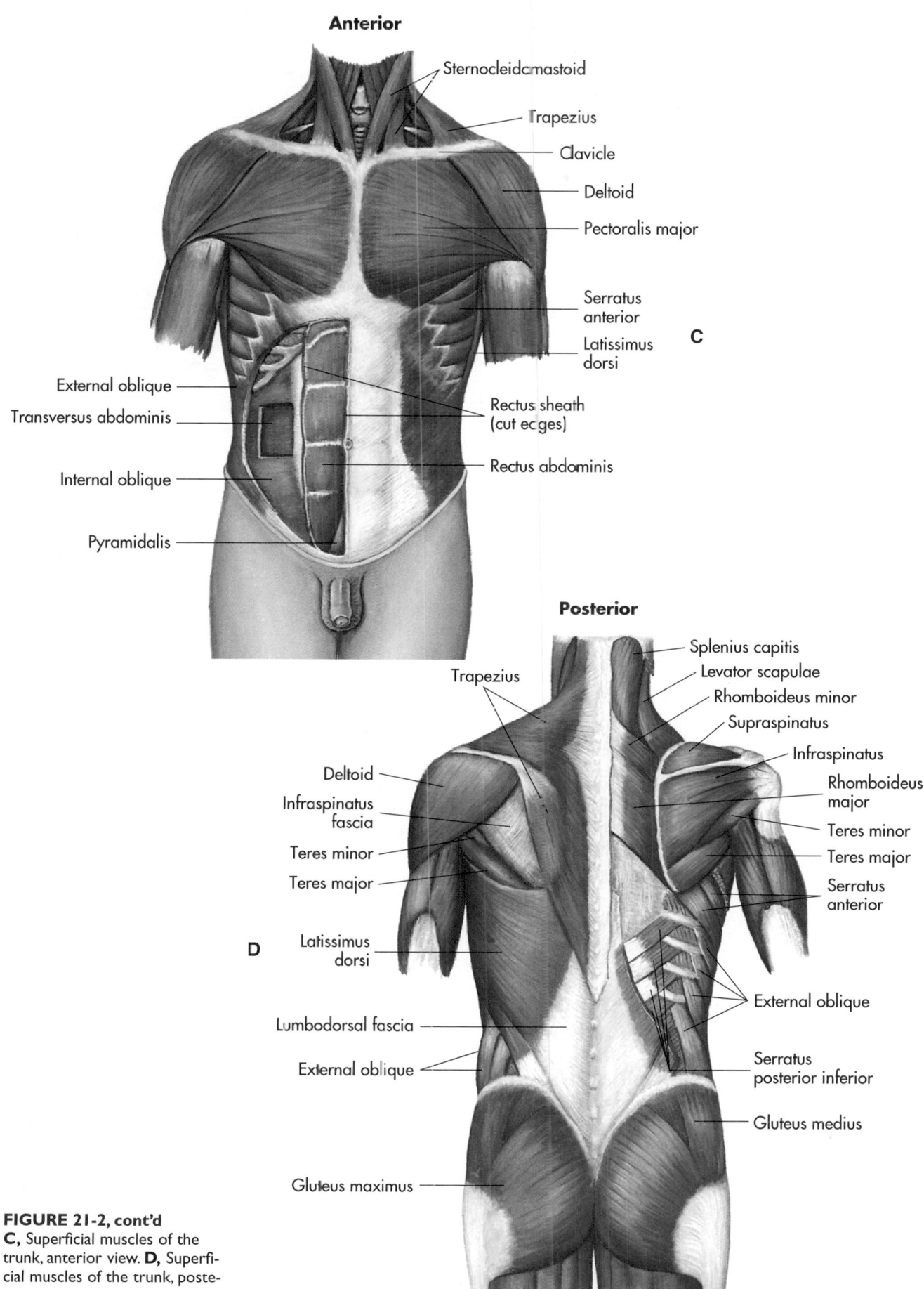

Anterior

Sternocleidomastoid
Trapezius
Clavicle
Deltoid
Pectoralis major
Serratus anterior
Latissimus dorsi
External oblique
Transversus abdominis
Rectus sheath (cut edges)
Internal oblique
Rectus abdominis
Pyramidalis

C

Posterior

Splenius capitis
Levator scapulae
Rhomboideus minor
Supraspinatus
Infraspinatus
Rhomboideus major
Teres minor
Teres major
Serratus anterior
External oblique
Serratus posterior inferior
Gluteus medius
Trapezius
Deltoid
Infraspinatus fascia
Teres minor
Teres major
Latissimus dorsi
Lumbodorsal fascia
External oblique
Gluteus maximus

D

FIGURE 21-2, cont'd
C, Superficial muscles of the trunk, anterior view. **D,** Superficial muscles of the trunk, posterior view.

TABLE 21-1	Classification of Joints	
Type of Joint	**Example**	**Description**
Synarthrosis		No movement is permitted
Suture	Cranial sutures	United by thin layer of fibrous tissue
Synchondrosis	Joint between the epiphysis and diaphysis of long bones	A temporary joint in which the cartilage is replaced by bone later in life
Amphiarthrosis		Slightly movable joint
Symphysis	Symphysis pubis	Bones are connected by a fibrocartilage disk
Syndesmosis	Radius-ulna articulation	Bones are connected by ligaments
Diarthrosis (Synovial)		Freely movable; enclosed by joint capsule, lined with synovial membrane
Ball and socket	Hip	Widest range of motion, movement in all planes
Hinge	Elbow	Motion limited to flexion and extension in a single plane
Pivot	Atlantoaxial	Motion limited to rotation
Condyloid	Wrist between radius and carpals	Motion in two planes at right angles to each other, but no radial rotation
Saddle	Thumb at carpal-metacarpal joint	Motion in two planes at right angles to each other, but no axial rotation
Gliding	Intervertebral	Motion limited to gliding

HEAD AND SPINE

The temporomandibular joint consists of the articulation between the mandible and the temporal bone in the cranium. Each is located in the depression just anterior to the tragus of the ear. The hinge action of the joint opens and closes the mouth, whereas the gliding action permits lateral movement, protrusion, and retraction of the mandible (Figs. 21-3 and 21-4). See Chapter 10 for a description of the fused bones of the cranium.

The spine is composed of cervical, thoracic, lumbar, and sacral vertebrae. Except for the sacral vertebrae, they are separated from each other by fibrocartilaginous disks. Each disk has a nucleus of fibrogelatinous material that cushions the vertebral bodies (Fig. 21-5). The vertebrae form a series of joints that glide slightly over each other's surfaces, permitting movement on several axes. The cervical vertebrae are the most mobile. Flexion and extension occur between the skull and C1, whereas rotation occurs between C1 and C2. The sacral vertebrae are fused and, with the coccyx, form the posterior portion of the pelvis.

UPPER EXTREMITIES

The glenohumeral joint (shoulder) consists of the articulation between the humerus and the glenoid fossa of the scapula. The acromion and coracoid processes and the ligament between them form the arch surrounding and protecting the joint (Fig. 21-6, *A*). Four muscles (supraspinatus, infraspinatus, teres minor, and subscapularis) and their tendons comprise the rotator cuff, reinforcing the glenohumeral joint to stabilize the shoulder and the position of the humeral head within the joint (Fig. 21-6, *B*). The shoulder is a ball-and-socket joint that permits movement of the humerus in many axes.

Two additional joints adjacent to the glenohumeral joint complete the articulation of the shoulder girdle. The acromioclavicular joint consists of the articulation between the acromion process and the clavicle, and the sternoclavicular joint consists of the articulation between the manubrium of the sternum and the clavicle.

The elbow consists of the articulation of the humerus, radius, and ulna. Its three contiguous surfaces are enclosed in a single synovial cavity, with the ligaments of the radius and ulna protecting the joint. A bursa lies between the olecranon and the skin (Fig. 21-7). The elbow is a hinge joint, permitting movement of the humerus and ulna in one plane (flexion and extension).

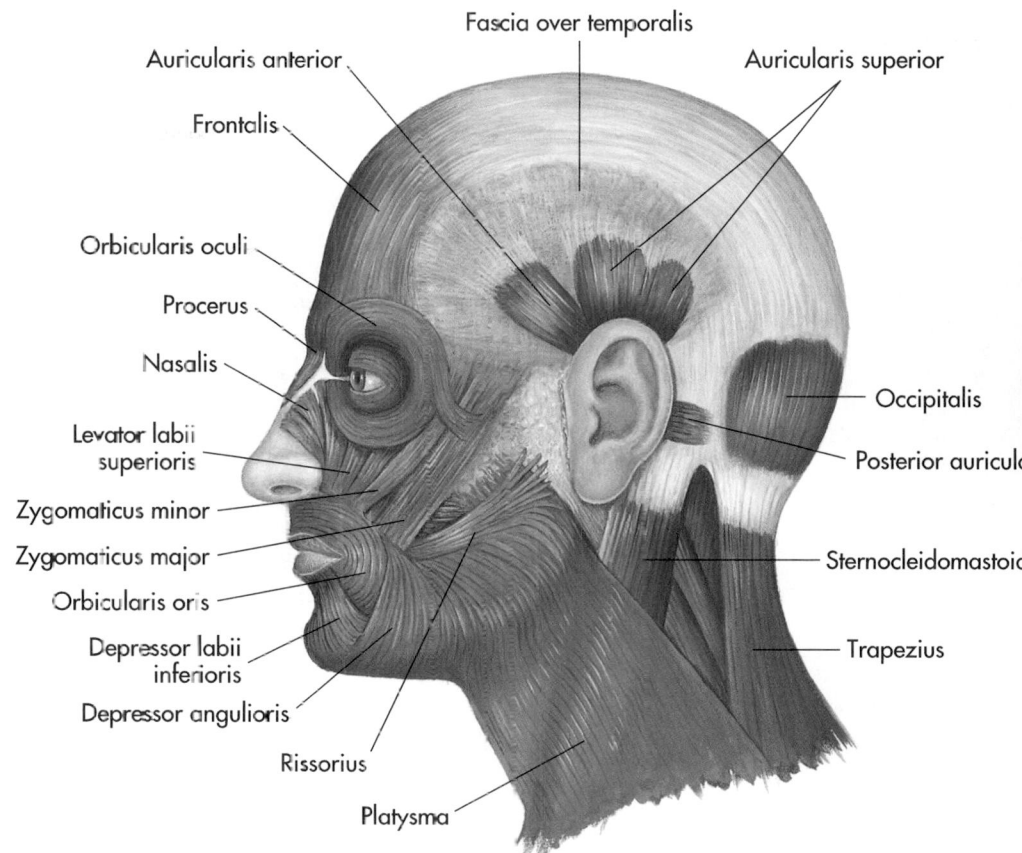

Fascia over temporalis

Auricularis anterior

Auricularis superior

Frontalis

Orbicularis oculi

Procerus

Nasalis

Levator labii
superioris

Zygomaticus minor

Zygomaticus major

Orbicularis oris

Depressor labii
inferioris

Depressor angulioris

Rissorius

Platysma

Occipitalis

Posterior auricular

Sternocleidomastoid

Trapezius

FIGURE 21-3
Muscles of the face and head,
left lateral view.

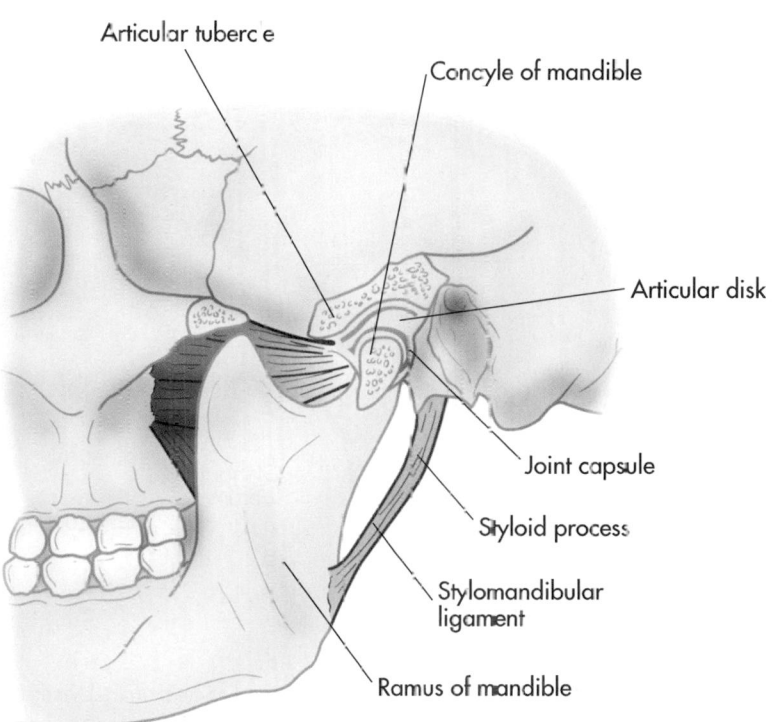

Articular tubercle

Concyle of mandible

Articular disk

Joint capsule

Styloid process

Stylomandibular
ligament

Ramus of mandible

FIGURE 21-4
Structures of the temporomandibular joint.

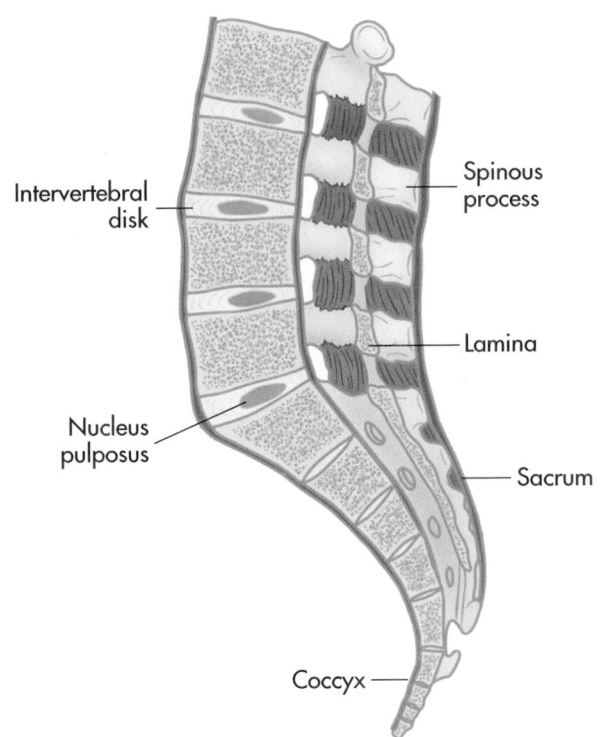

FIGURE 21-5
Structures of vertebral joints.

Intervertebral disk

Spinous process

Lamina

Nucleus pulposus

Sacrum

Coccyx

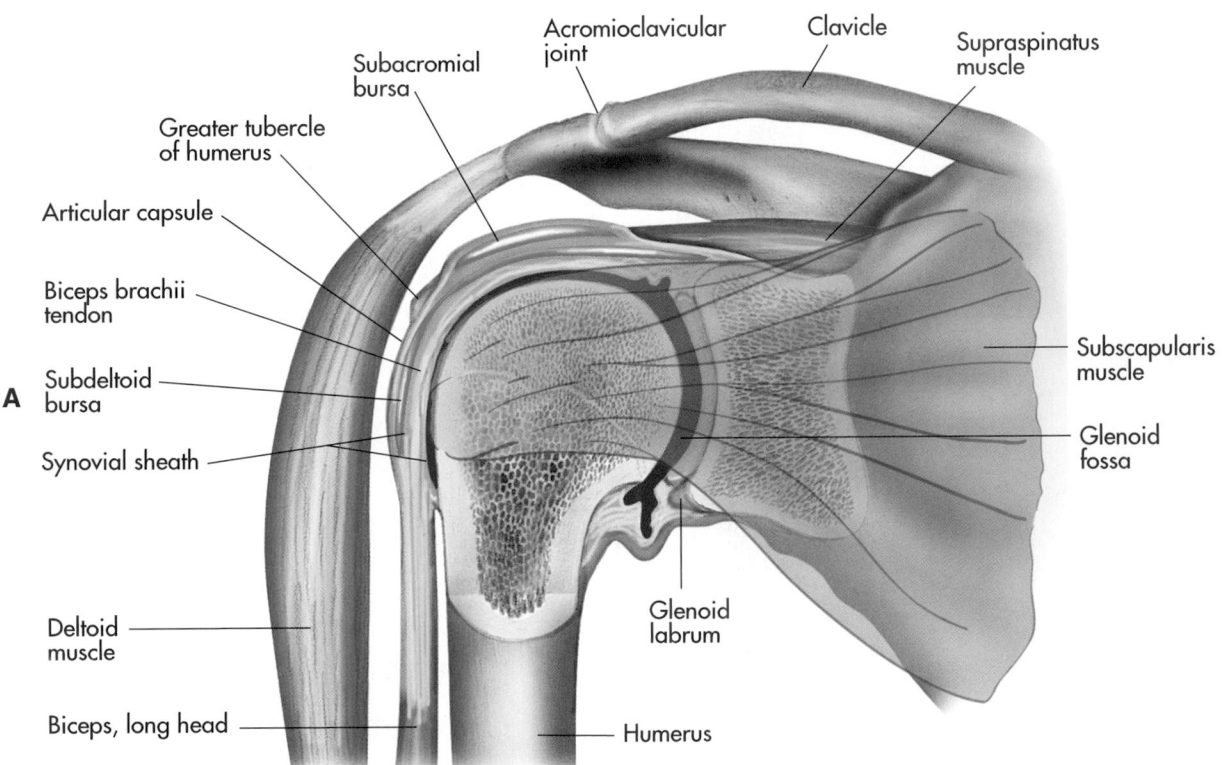

Subacromial bursa

Acromioclavicular joint

Clavicle

Supraspinatus muscle

Greater tubercle of humerus

Articular capsule

Biceps brachii tendon

Subdeltoid bursa

Synovial sheath

Subscapularis muscle

Glenoid fossa

Glenoid labrum

Deltoid muscle

Biceps, long head

Humerus

A

FIGURE 21-6
Structures of the shoulder. **A,** Structures of glenohumeral and acromioclavicular joints, anterior view.

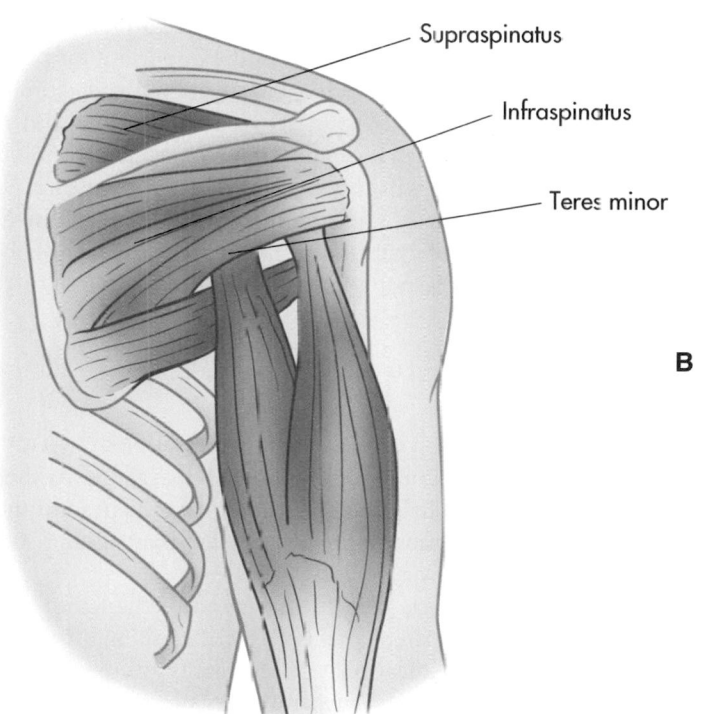

Supraspinatus

Infraspinatus

Teres minor

B

FIGURE 21-6, cont'd
B, Rotator cuff muscles of
shoulder, posterior view.

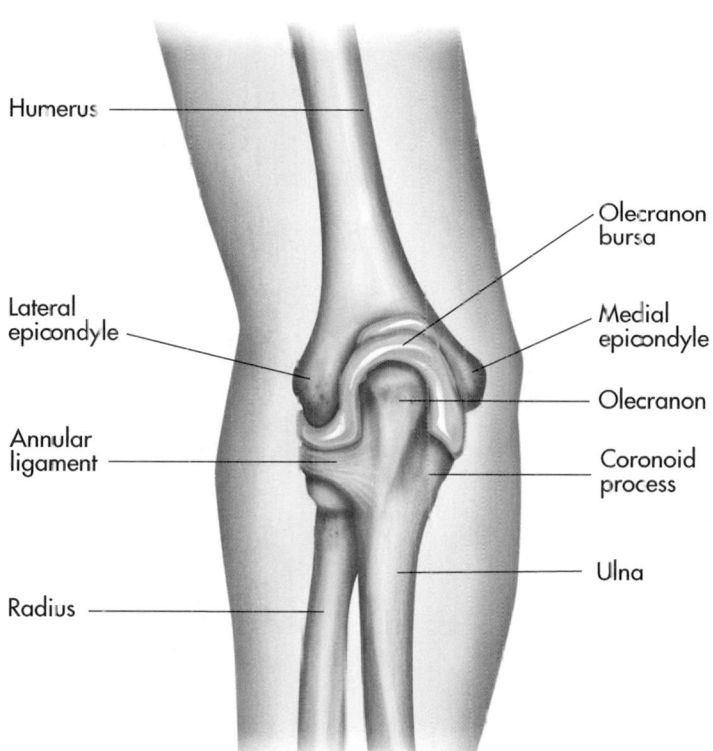

Humerus

Lateral
epicondyle

Annular
ligament

Radius

Olecranon
bursa

Medial
epicondyle

Olecranon

Coronoid
process

Ulna

FIGURE 21-7
Structures of the left elbow
joint, posterior view.

The forearm joints consist of the articulations between the radius and ulna at both the proximal and distal locations. They are important for pronation and supination.

The radiocarpal joint (wrist) consists of the articulation of the radius and the carpal bones. Additional articulations occur between the proximal and distal row of carpal bones. An articular disk separates the ulna and carpal bones, and the joint is protected by ligaments and a fibrous capsule. The wrist is a condyloid joint, permitting movement in two planes (flexion and extension movement; radial and ulnar movement). The hand has articulations between the carpals and metacarpals, metacarpals and proximal phalanges, and middle and distal phalanges. The metacarpophalangeal joints are condyloid (Fig. 21-8).

LOWER EXTREMITIES

The joint of the hip consists of the articulation between the acetabulum and the femur. The depth of the acetabulum in the pelvic bone, as well as the joint, which is supported by three strong ligaments, help stabilize and protect the head of the femur in the joint capsule. Three bursae reduce friction in the hip. The hip is a ball-and-socket joint, permitting movement of the femur on many axes (Fig. 21-9).

The knee consists of the articulation of the femur, tibia, and patella. Fibrocartilaginous disks (medial and lateral menisci), which cushion the tibia and femur, are attached to the tibia and the joint capsule. Collateral ligaments give medial and lateral stability to the knee, protecting the knee from valgus and varus stress. Two cruciate ligaments cross obliquely within the knee, adding anterior and posterior stability. The anterior cruciate ligament protects the knee from hyperextension. Several bursae reduce friction. The suprapatellar bursa separates the patella, quadriceps tendon, and muscle from the femur. The knee is a hinge joint, permitting movement (flexion and extension) between the femur and tibia on one plane (Fig. 21-10).

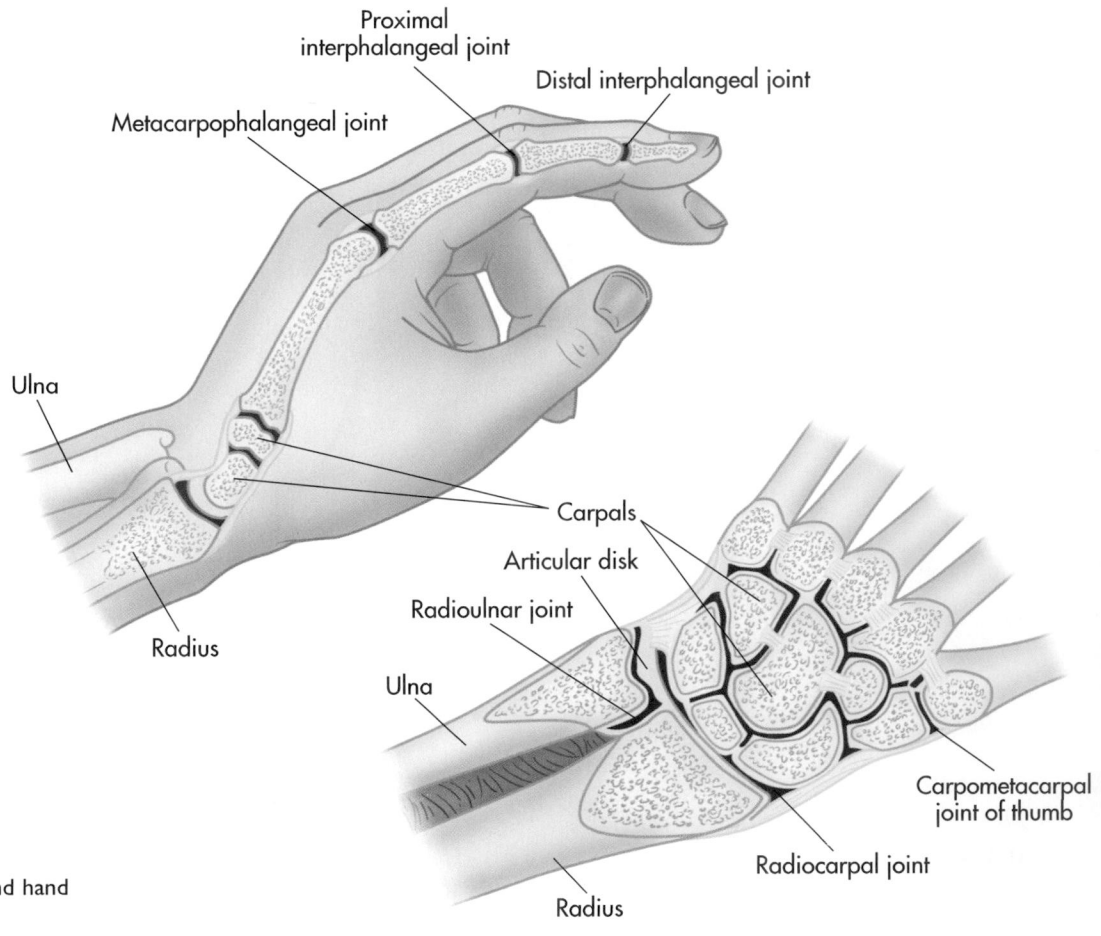

FIGURE 21-8
Structures of the wrist and hand joints.

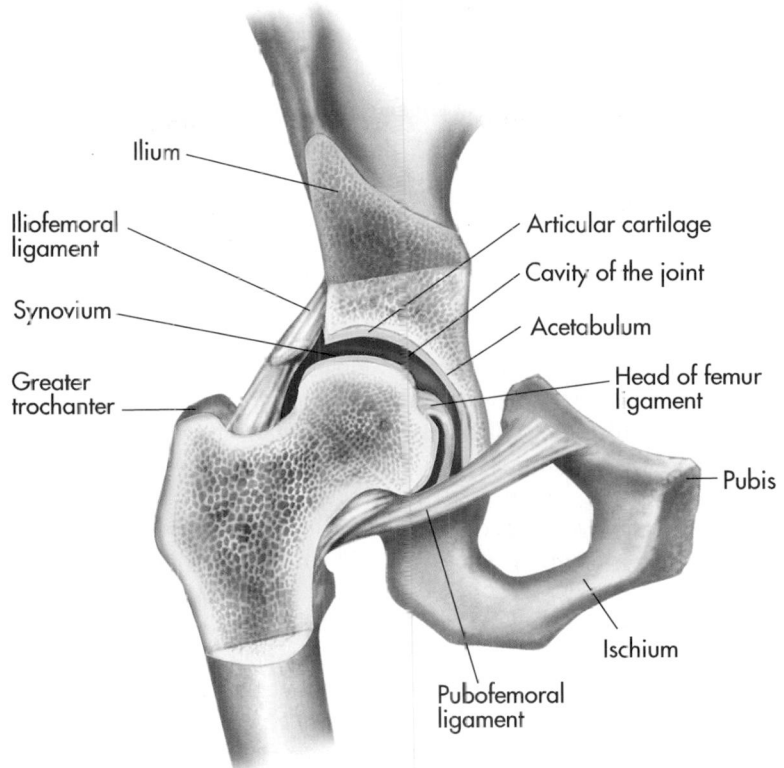

FIGURE 21-9
Structures of the hip.
From Thompson et al, 1997.

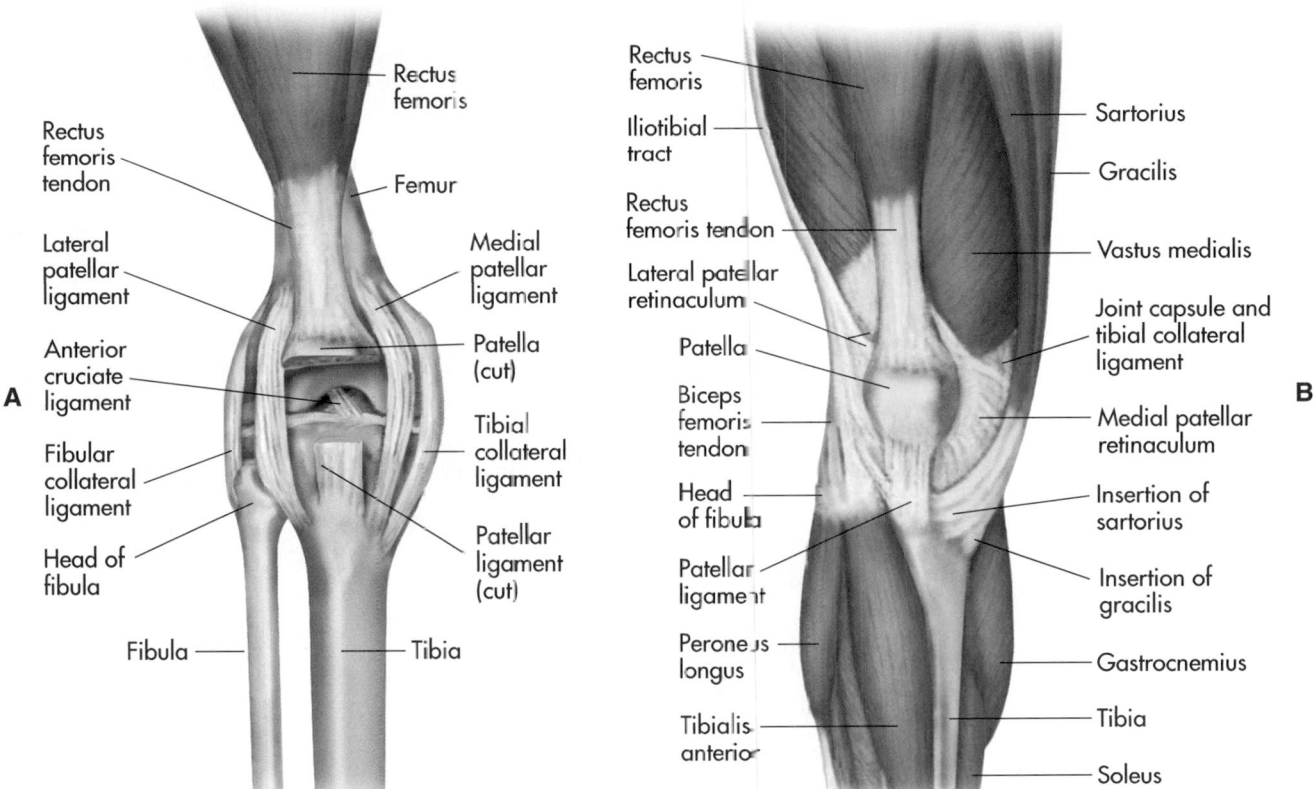

FIGURE 21-10
Structures of the knee, anterior view. **A,** Bones and ligaments of the joint. **B,** Muscles attaching at the knee.

The tibiotalar joint (ankle) consists of the articulation of the tibia, fibula, and talus. It is protected by ligaments on the medial and lateral surfaces. The tibiotalar joint is a hinge joint that permits flexion and extension (dorsiflexion and plantar flexion) in one plane. Additional joints in the ankle, the talocalcaneal joint (subtalar) and transverse tarsal joint, permit a pivot or rotation movement (pronation and supination) of the joint. Articulations of the foot between the tarsals and metatarsals, the metatarsal and proximal phalanges, and the middle and distal phalanges are condyloid (Fig. 21-11).

INFANTS AND CHILDREN

During fetal development the skeletal system emerges from embryologic connective tissues to form cartilage that calcifies and eventually becomes true bone. Throughout infancy and childhood, long bones increase in diameter by the apposition of new bone tissue around the bone shaft. Increased length of long bones results from the proliferation of cartilage at the growth plates (epiphyses). In the smaller bones, such as the carpals, ossification centers form in calcified cartilage. There is a specific sequence and timing of bone growth and ossification during childhood. Ligaments are stronger than bone until adolescence, therefore injuries to long bones and joints are more likely to result in fractures than in sprains.

The number of muscle fibers an individual ultimately develops is established during fetal life. Muscle fibers lengthen during childhood as the skeletal system grows.

ADOLESCENTS

Rapid growth during Tanner stage 3 (pp. 125-130) results in decreased strength in the epiphyses, as well as general decreased strength and flexibility, leading to greater potential for injury. Bone growth is completed at about age 20 years, when the last epiphysis closes and becomes firmly fused to the shaft. Once bone growth stops, bone density and strength continue to increase; however, peak bone mass is not achieved in either gender until about 35 years of age.

PREGNANT WOMEN

Increased levels of circulating hormones contribute to the elasticity of ligaments and softening of the cartilage in the pelvis at about 12 to 20 weeks of gestation. This results in increased mobility of the sacroiliac, sacrococcygeal, and symphysis pubis joints.

To compensate for the enlargement of the uterus during later pregnancy, progressive lordosis occurs in an effort to shift the center of gravity back over the lower extremities. The ligaments and muscles of the lower spine may become stressed, leading to lower back pain in 40% to 50% of patients.

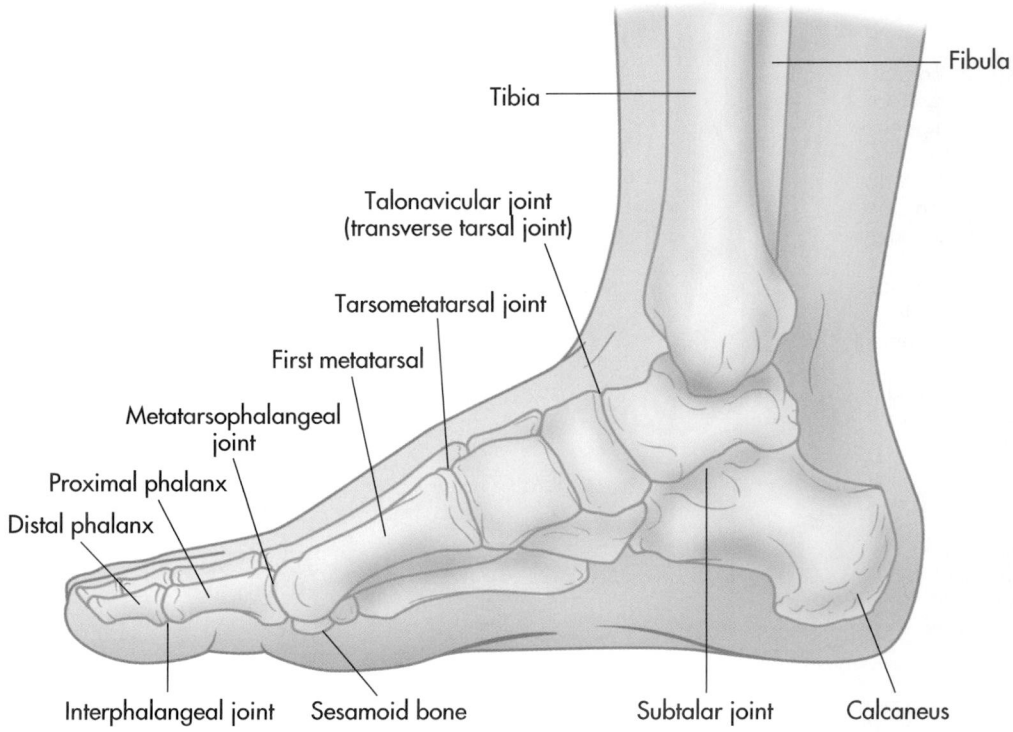

FIGURE 21-11
Bones and joints of the ankle and foot.

Painful muscle cramps, usually in the gastrocnemius, thigh, or gluteal muscles, occur during the second half of pregnancy in more than 25% of pregnant women. They are more likely to occur at night or after awakening and initiating muscle activity. The cause is unknown.

OLDER ADULTS

With aging, the skeletal system undergoes an alteration in the equilibrium between bone deposition and bone resorption, and resorption dominates. For menopausal women, decreased estrogen increases bone resorption and decreases calcium deposition, resulting in bone loss and decreased bone density. By 80 years of age, a woman can lose up to 30% of her bone mass. The loss of bone density affects the entire skeleton, but the long bones and the vertebrae are particularly vulnerable. Weight-bearing bones may become predisposed to fractures. Bony prominences become more apparent with the loss of subcutaneous fat. Cartilage around joints deteriorates.

The muscle mass also undergoes alteration as increased amounts of collagen collect in the tissues initially, followed by fibrosis of connective tissue. Tendons become less elastic. This results in a reduction of total muscle mass, tone, and strength. A progressive decrease in reaction time, speed of movements, agility, and endurance also occurs.

PHYSICAL VARIATIONS
Bone Density
Women's bones are less dense than those of men, and black women have denser bones than white, Asian, Mexican American, and Native American/American Indian women; consequently, serious osteoporosis occurs less frequently in black women.

STAYING WELL
SLOWING MUSCULOSKELETAL CHANGES WITH AGING

A sedentary lifestyle and any health problems that contribute to reduced physical activity promote and hasten the musculoskeletal changes associated with aging. Routine exercise and a well-balanced diet at all ages, including calcium and vitamin D supplementation, help slow the progression of the musculoskeletal changes.

REVIEW OF RELATED HISTORY

For each of the conditions discussed in this section, targeted topics to include in the history of the present illness are listed. Responses to questions about these topics help fully assess the patient's condition and provide clues for focusing the physical examination.

HISTORY OF PRESENT ILLNESS

- ◆ Joint complaints
  - ◆ Character: stiffness or limitation of movement, change in size or contour, swelling or redness, constant pain or pain with particular motion, unilateral or bilateral involvement, interference with daily activities, joint locking or giving way
  - ◆ Associated events: time of day, activity, specific movements, injury, strenuous activity, weather
  - ◆ Temporal factors: change in frequency or character of episodes, better or worse as day progresses, nature of onset (slow versus rapid)
  - ◆ Efforts to treat: exercise, rest, weight reduction, physical therapy, heat, ice, braces or splints
  - ◆ Medications: nonsteroidal antiinflammatory drugs, acetaminophen, antirheumatics, corticosteroids, topical analgesics; prescription or nonprescription; alternative or complementary therapies, such as glucosamine, chondroitin, hyaluronic acid
- ◆ Muscular complaints
  - ◆ Character: limitation of movement, weakness or fatigue, paralysis, tremor, tic, spasms, clumsiness, wasting, aching or pain
  - ◆ Precipitating factors: injury, strenuous activity, sudden movement, stress
  - ◆ Efforts to treat: heat, ice, splints, rest, massage

- Medications: muscle relaxants, salicylates, nonsteroidal antiinflammatory drugs; prescription or nonprescription, alternative or complementary therapies
- Skeletal complaints
  - Character: difficulty with gait or limping; numbness, tingling, or pressure sensation; pain with movement, crepitus; deformity or change in skeletal contour
  - Associated event: injury, recent fractures, strenuous activity, sudden movement, stress; postmenopause
  - Efforts to treat: rest, splints, chiropractic, acupuncture
  - Medications: hormone replacement therapy, calcium; calcitonin; prescription or nonprescription, alternative or complementary therapies
- Injury
  - Sensation at time of injury: click, pop, tearing, numbness, tingling, catching, locking, grating, snapping, warmth or coldness, ability to bear weight
  - Mechanism of injury: direct trauma, overuse, sudden change of direction, forceful contraction, overstretch
  - Pain: location, type, onset (sudden or gradual), aggravating or alleviating factors, position of comfort
  - Swelling: location, timing (with activity or injury)
  - Efforts to treat: rest, ice, heat, splints
- Back pain
  - Abrupt or gradual onset
  - Character of pain and sensation: tearing, burning, or steady ache; tingling or numbness; location and distribution (unilateral or bilateral), radiation to buttocks, groin, or legs; triggered by coughing or sneezing and sudden movements
  - Associated event: trauma, occupational and nonoccupational lifting of heavy weights, long distance driving, sports activities, change in posture or deformity
  - Efforts to treat: rest, avoid standing or sudden movements, chiropractic
  - Medications: muscle relaxants, analgesics, alternative or complementary therapies

PAST MEDICAL HISTORY

- Trauma: Nerves, soft tissue, bones, joints; residual problems; bone infection
- Surgery on joint or bone; amputation, arthroscopy
- Chronic illness: Cancer, arthritis, sickle cell anemia, hemophilia, osteoporosis, renal or neurologic disorder
- Skeletal deformities or congenital anomalies

FAMILY HISTORY

- Congenital abnormalities of hip or foot
- Scoliosis or back problems
- Arthritis: rheumatoid, osteoarthritis, ankylosing spondylitis, gout
- Genetic disorders: osteogenesis imperfecta, dwarfing syndrome, rickets, hypophosphatemia, hypercalciuria

PERSONAL AND SOCIAL HISTORY

- Employment: past and current, lifting and potential for unintentional injury, repetitive overhead motions, safety precautions, use of spinal support, chronic stress on joints, other repetitive motions
- Exercise: extent, type, and frequency; weight-bearing; stress on specific joints; overall conditioning; sport (level of competition, type of shoes and athletic gear); warm-up and cool down routines with exercise

- Functional abilities: personal care (eating, bathing, dressing, grooming, elimination); other activities (housework, walking, climbing stairs, caring for pet); use of prosthesis
- Weight: recent gain, overweight or underweight for body frame
- Height: maximum height achieved, any changes
- Nutrition: amount of calcium, vitamin D, calories, and protein
- Tobacco use
- Alcohol use

INFANTS AND CHILDREN
- Birth history
  - Presentation, large for gestational age, birth injuries (may result in fractures or nerve damage)
  - Low birth weight, premature, resuscitated, required special ventilator support (may result in anoxia leading to muscle tone disorders)

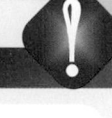

RISK FACTORS
SPORTS INJURY

- Poor physical conditioning
- Failure to warm up muscles adequately
- Intensity of competition
- Collision and contact sports participation
- Rapid growth
- Overuse of joints

RISK FACTORS
OSTEOPOROSIS

- Race (white, Asian, Native American/American Indian); northwestern European descent; blonde or red hair, freckles
- Light body frame, thin
- Family history of osteoporosis, gene for decreased bone density
- Nulliparous
- Amenorrhea or menopause before 45 years of age, postmenopausal
- Sedentary lifestyle; lack of aerobic or weight-bearing exercise
- Constant dieting; inadequate calcium and vitamin D intake; excessive carbonated soft drinks per day
- Scoliosis, rheumatoid arthritis, cancer, multiple sclerosis, chronic illness
- Metabolic disorders (e.g., diabetes, hypercortisolism, hyperthyroidism)
- Drugs that decrease bone density (e.g., thyroxine, corticosteroids, heparin, lithium, anticonvulsants, antacids with aluminum)
- Poor teeth; previous fractures
- Cigarette smoking or heavy alcohol use

RISK FACTORS
OSTEOARTHRITIS

- Obesity
- Family history of osteoarthritis
- Hypermobility syndromes
- Aging (older than 40 years of age)
- Injury, high level of sports activities
- Occupation requiring overuse of joints

- Fine and gross motor developmental milestones, appropriate for chronologic age
- Quality of movement: spasticity, flaccidity, cog wheel rigidity
- Arm or leg pain
  - Character: localized or generalized; in muscle or joint; limitation of movement; associated with movement, trauma, or growth spurt
  - Onset: age, sudden or gradual, at night with rest, after activity
  - Participation in organized sports

Pregnant Women

- Muscle cramps: nature of onset, frequency and time of occurrence, muscles involved, efforts to treat
- Back pain
  - Weeks of gestation, associated with multiple pregnancy, efforts to treat
  - Associated symptoms: uterine tightening, nausea, vomiting, fever, malaise (could signify musculoskeletal discomfort if not from another condition)
  - Type of shoes (heels may increase lordosis)

Older Adults

- Weakness
  - Onset: sudden or gradual, localized or generalized, occurred with activity or after sustained activity
  - Associated symptoms: stiffness of joints, muscle spasms or tension, any particular activity, dyspnea
- Increases in minor injuries: stumbling, falls, limited agility; association with poor vision
- Change in ease of movement: loss of ability to perform sudden movements, change in exercise endurance, pain, stiffness, localized to particular joints or generalized
- Nocturnal muscle spasm: frequency, associated back pain, numbness or coldness of extremities
- History of injuries or excessive use of a joint or group of joints, claudication, known joint abnormalities
- Previous fractures, bone mineral density screening
- Medications

EXAMINATION AND FINDINGS

EQUIPMENT

- Skin-marking pencil
- Goniometer
- Tape measure
- Reflex hammer

Begin your examination of the musculoskeletal system by observing the gait and posture when the patient enters the examining room. Note how the patient walks, sits, rises from sitting position, takes off a coat, and responds to other directions given during the examination.

As you give specific attention to bones, joints, and muscles, the body surface must be exposed and viewed under good lighting. Position the patient to provide the greatest stability to the joints. Examine each region of the body for limb and trunk stability, muscular strength and function, and joint function. Position the extremities uniformly as you examine and look for asymmetry.

INSPECTION

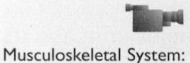

Musculoskeletal System:
Observing Gait and Posture

Inspect the anterior, posterior, and lateral aspects of the patient's posture (Fig. 21-12). Observe the patient's ability to stand erect, the symmetry of the body parts, and the alignment of extremities. Note any lordosis, kyphosis, or scoliosis.

Inspect the skin and subcutaneous tissues overlying the muscles, cartilage, bones, and joints for discoloration, swelling, and masses.

Observe the extremities for overall size, gross deformity, bony enlargement, alignment, contour, and symmetry of length and position. Expect to find bilateral symmetry in length, circumference, alignment, and the position and number of skinfolds.

Inspect the muscles for gross hypertrophy or atrophy, fasciculations, and spasms. Muscle size should approximate symmetry bilaterally, without atrophy or hypertrophy. Bilateral symmetry should not be defined as absolute, because there is no perfect symmetry. For example, the dominant forearm is expected to be larger in athletes who play racquet sports and in manual laborers. Fasciculation occurs after injury to a muscle's motor neuron. Muscle wasting occurs after injury as a result of pain, disease of the muscle, or damage to the motor neuron.

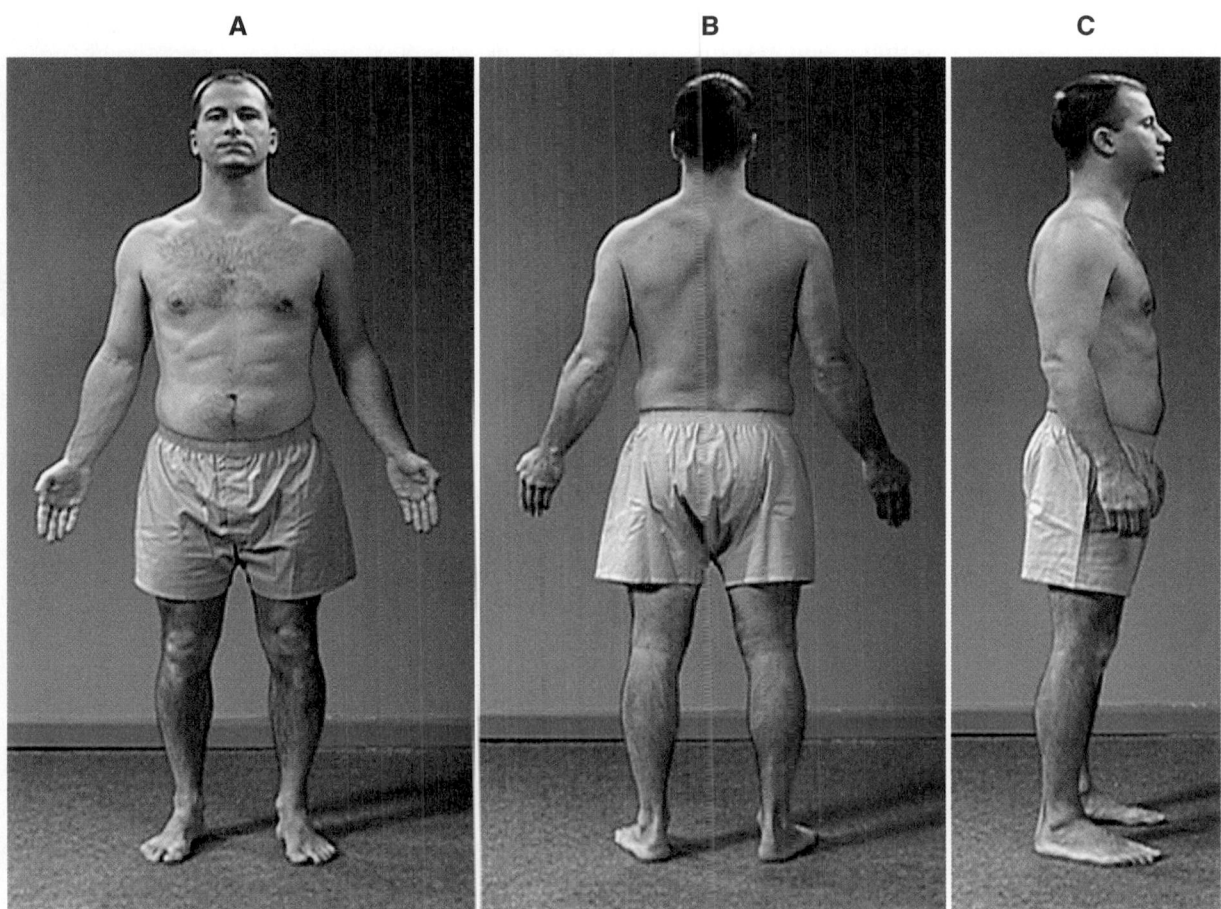

A   **B**   **C**

FIGURE 21-12
Inspection of overall body posture. Note the even contour of the shoulders, level scapulae and iliac crests, alignment of the head over the gluteal folds, and symmetry and alignment of extremities. **A,** Anterior view. **B,** Posterior view. **C,** Lateral view. The occiput, shoulders, buttocks, and heels should be able to touch the wall the patient stands against.

PALPATION

Palpate all bones, joints, and surrounding muscles. Note any heat, tenderness, swelling, fluctuation of a joint (associated with effusion), crepitus, pain, and resistance to pressure. No discomfort should occur when you apply pressure to bones or joints. Muscle tone should be firm, not hard or doughy. Spasticity is an increase in muscle tone. Palpate inflamed joints last. Synovial thickening can sometimes be felt in joints that are close to the skin surface when the synovium is edematous or hypertrophied because of inflammation. Crepitus can be felt when two irregular bony surfaces rub together as a joint moves, when two rough edges of a broken bone rub together, or with the movement of a tendon inside the tendon sheath when tenosynovitis is present.

RANGE OF MOTION

Examine both the active and passive range of motion for each major joint and its related muscle groups. Muscle tone is often evaluated simultaneously. Adequate space for the patient to move each muscle group and joint through its full range is necessary and may be provided by pulling the examining table away from the wall if appropriate. Instruct the patient in moving each joint through its range of motion as detailed under examination of specific joints and muscles. When the patient has full range of motion, muscle tone is good. Pain, limitation of motion, spastic movement, joint instability, deformity, and contracture suggest a problem with the joint, related muscle group, or nerve supply.

Ask the patient to relax and allow you to passively move the same joints until the end of the range is felt. Do not force the joint if there is pain or muscle spasm. Muscle tone may be assessed by feeling the resistance to passive stretch. During passive range of motion, the muscles should have slight tension. Passive range of motion often exceeds active range of motion by 5 degrees. Range of motion with active and passive maneuvers should be equal between contralateral joints. Discrepancies between active and passive range of motion may indicate true muscle weakness or a joint disorder. No crepitation or tenderness with movement should be apparent. Note the specific location of tenderness when present. Spastic muscles are harder to put through the range of motion. Measurements may vary if the muscle tested relaxes with gentle persistence.

When a joint appears to have an increase or limitation in its range of motion, a goniometer is used to precisely measure the angle. Begin with the joint in the fully extended or neutral position, and then flex the joint as far as possible. Measure the angles of greatest flexion and extension, comparing these with the expected flexion and extension values (Fig. 21-13).

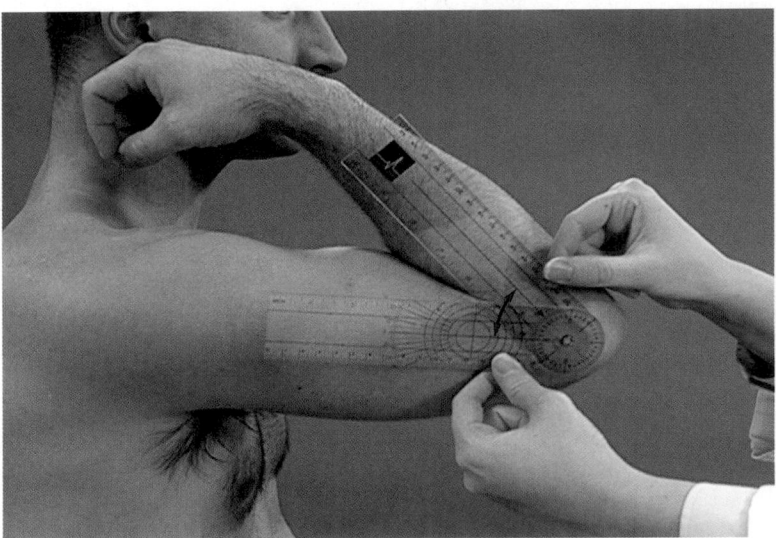

FIGURE 21-13
Use of goniometer to measure joint range of motion.

TABLE 21-2	Assessing Muscle Strength	
Muscle Function Level		**Grade**
No evidence of movement		0
Trace of movement		1
Full range of motion, but not against gravity*		2
Full range of motion against gravity but not against resistance		3
Full range of motion against gravity and some resistance, but weak		4
Full range of motion against gravity, full resistance		5

From Jacobson, 1998.
*Passive movement.

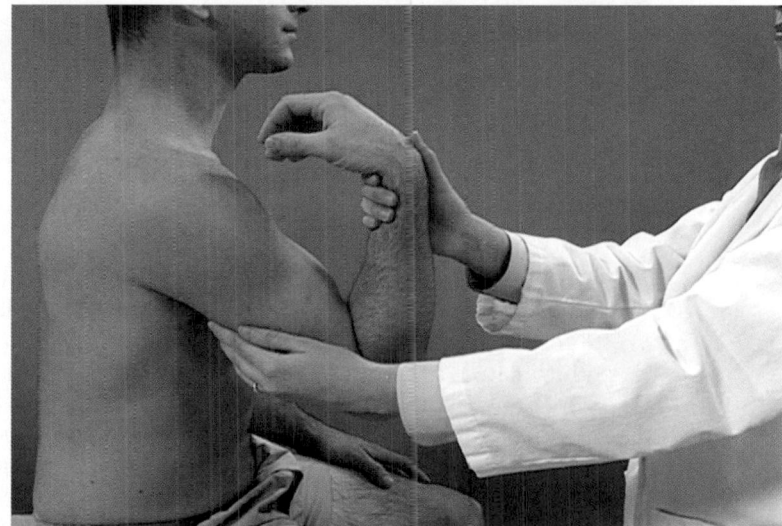

FIGURE 21-14
Evaluation of muscle strength: flexion of the elbow against opposing force.

MUSCLE STRENGTH

Evaluating the strength of each muscle group, also considered part of the neurologic examination, is usually integrated with examination of the associated joint for range of motion. Ask the patient first to contract the muscle you indicate by extending or flexing the joint; and then to resist as you apply force against that muscle contraction (Fig. 21-14). Do not allow the patient to move the joint. Alternatively, tell the patient to push against your hand to feel the resistance. Compare the muscle strength bilaterally. Expect muscle strength to be bilaterally symmetric with full resistance to opposition. Full muscle strength requires complete active range of motion.

Variations in muscle strength are graded from no voluntary contraction to full muscle strength, using the scale in Table 21-2. When muscle strength is grade 3 or less, disability is present; activity cannot be accomplished in a gravity field, and external support is necessary to perform movements. Weakness may result from disuse atrophy, pain, fatigue, or overstretching.

SPECIFIC JOINTS AND MUSCLES

TEMPORO-MANDIBULAR JOINT

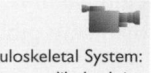

Musculoskeletal System:
Assessing the Temporomandibular Joint

Locate the temporomandibular joints by placing your fingertips just anterior to the tragus of each ear. Allow your fingertips to slip into the joint space as the patient's mouth opens, and gently palpate the joint space (Fig. 21-15). An audible or palpable snapping or clicking in the temporomandibular joints is not unusual; but pain, crepitus, locking, or popping may indicate temporomandibular joint dysfunction.

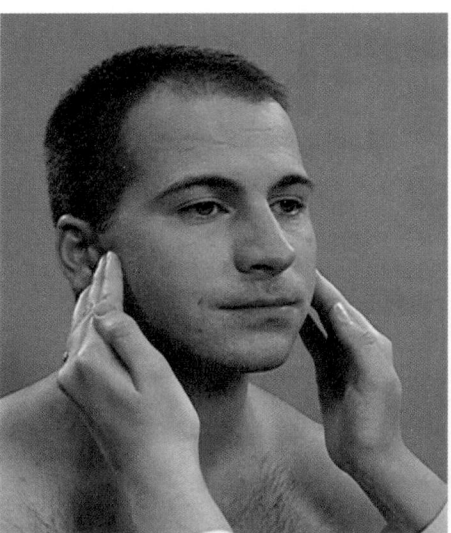

FIGURE 21-15
Palpation of the temporomandibular joint.

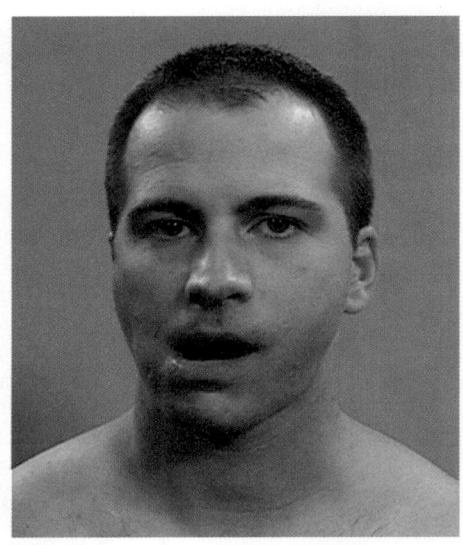

FIGURE 21-16
Lateral range of motion in the temporomandibular joint.

Range of motion is examined by asking the patient to perform the following movements:
* Open and close the mouth. Expect a space of 3 to 6 cm between the upper and lower teeth when the jaw is open.
* Laterally move the lower jaw to each side. The mandible should move 1 to 2 cm in each direction (Fig. 21-16).
* Protrude and retract the chin. Both movements should be possible.

Strength of the temporalis and masseter muscles is evaluated by asking the patient to clench the teeth while you palpate the contracted muscles and apply opposing force. Cranial nerve V is simultaneously tested with this maneuver.

CERVICAL SPINE

Inspect the patient's neck from both an anterior and a posterior position, observing for alignment of the head with the shoulders and symmetry of the skinfolds and muscles. Expect the cervical spine curve to be concave with the head erect and in appropriate alignment. No asymmetric skinfolds should be apparent.

Palpate the posterior neck; cervical spine; and paravertebral, trapezius, and sternocleidomastoid muscles. The muscles should have good tone and be symmetric in size, with no palpable tenderness or muscle spasm.

Evaluate range of motion in the cervical spine by asking the patient to perform the following movements (Fig. 21-17):
* Bend the head forward, chin to the chest. Expect flexion of 45 degrees.
* Bend the head backward, chin toward the ceiling. Expect extension of 45 degrees.
* Bend the head to each side, ear to each shoulder. Expect lateral bending of 40 degrees.
* Turn the head to each side, chin to shoulder. Expect rotation of 70 degrees.

The strength of the sternocleidomastoid and trapezius muscles is evaluated with the patient maintaining each of the above positions while you apply opposing force. With rotation, cranial nerve XI is simultaneously tested (Fig. 21-18).

THORACIC AND LUMBAR SPINE

Major landmarks of the back include each spinal process of the vertebrae (C7 and T1 are usually most prominent), the scapulae, iliac crests, and paravertebral muscles (Fig. 21-19). Expect the head to be positioned directly over the gluteal cleft and the vertebrae to be straight as indicated by symmetric shoulder, scapular, and iliac crest heights. The curve of the thoracic spine should be convex. The curve of the lumbar spine should be concave. The knees and feet should be in alignment with the trunk, pointing directly forward.

Lordosis is common in patients who are markedly obese or pregnant. The appearance of lordosis in black women may result from their more prominent gluteal muscle. Kyphosis may be observed in aging adults (Fig. 21-20). A sharp angular deformity, a gibbus, is associated with a collapsed vertebra from osteoporosis.

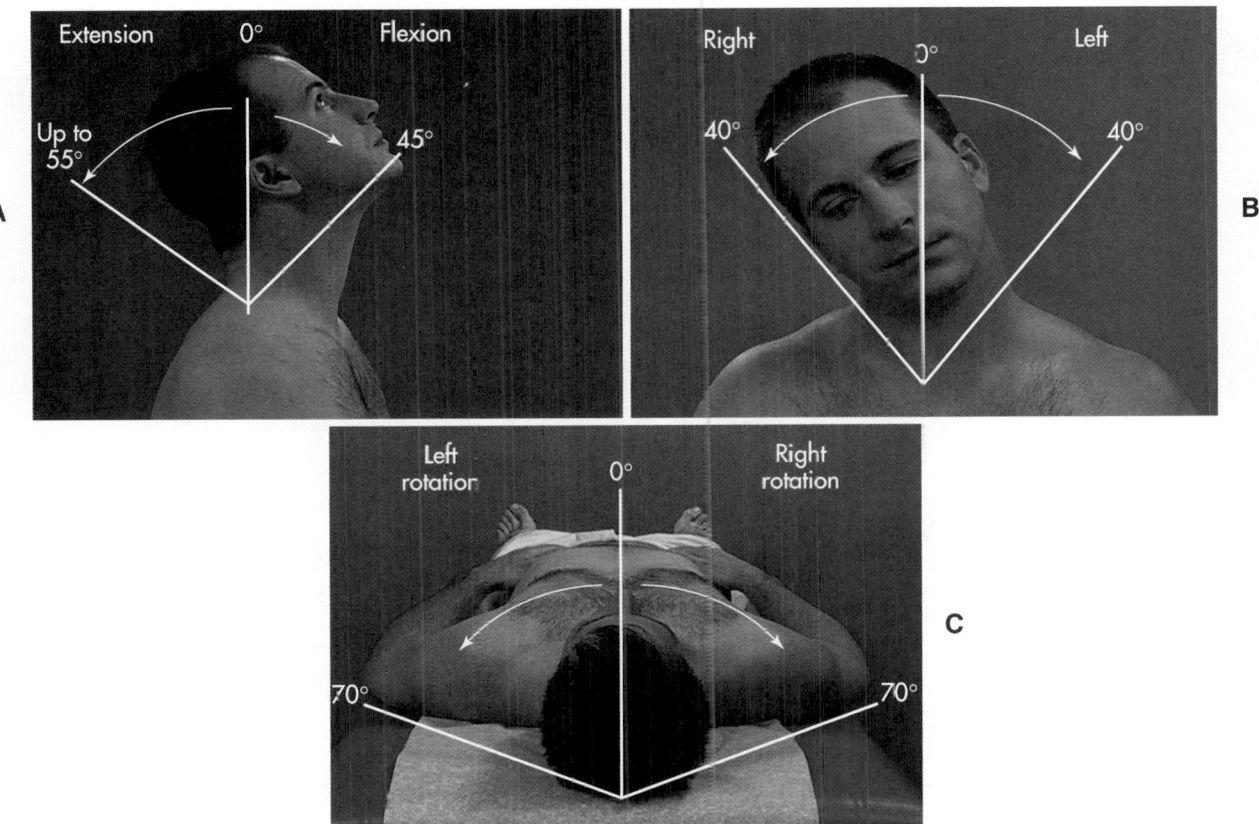

FIGURE 21-17
Range of motion of the cervical spine. **A,** Flexion and hyperextension. **B,** Lateral bending.
C, Rotation.

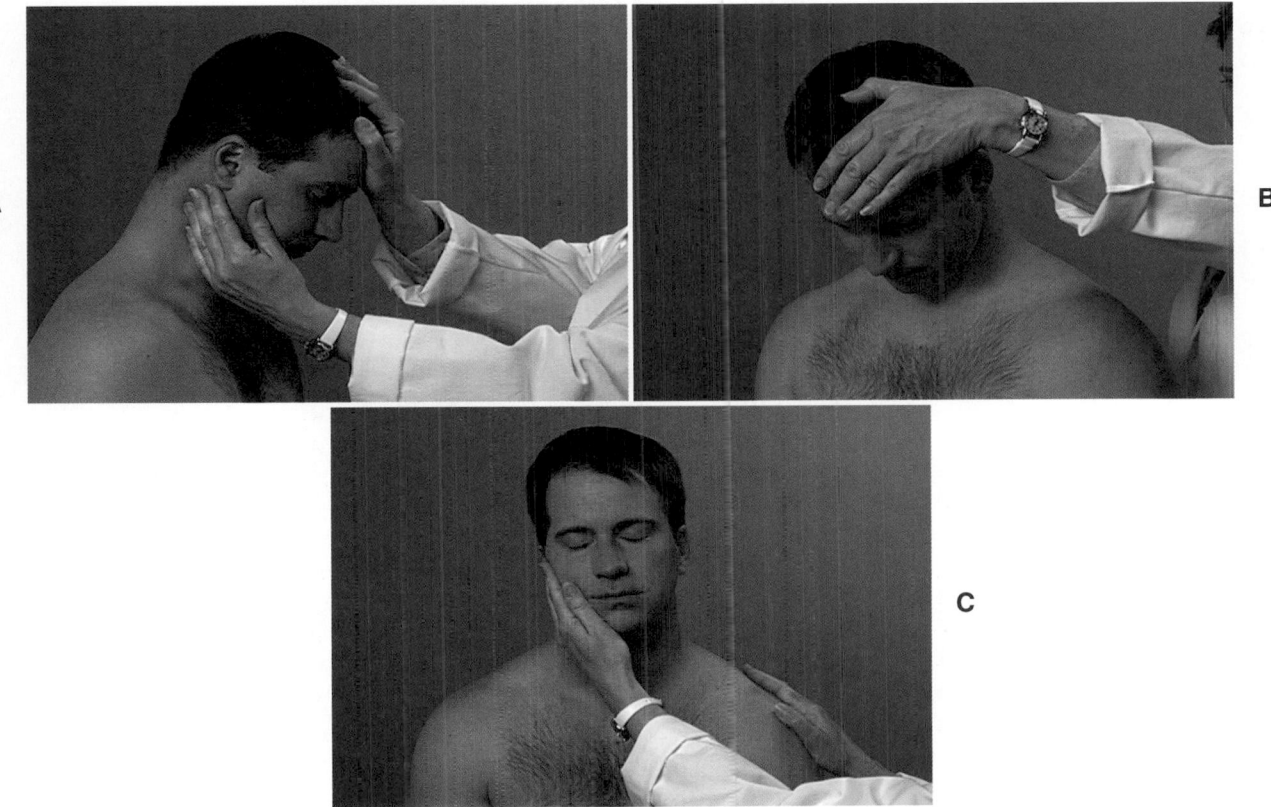

FIGURE 21-18
Examining the strength of the sternocleidomastoid and trapezius muscles. **A,** Flexion with palpation
of the sternocleidomastoid muscle. **B,** Extension against resistance. **C,** Rotation against resistance.

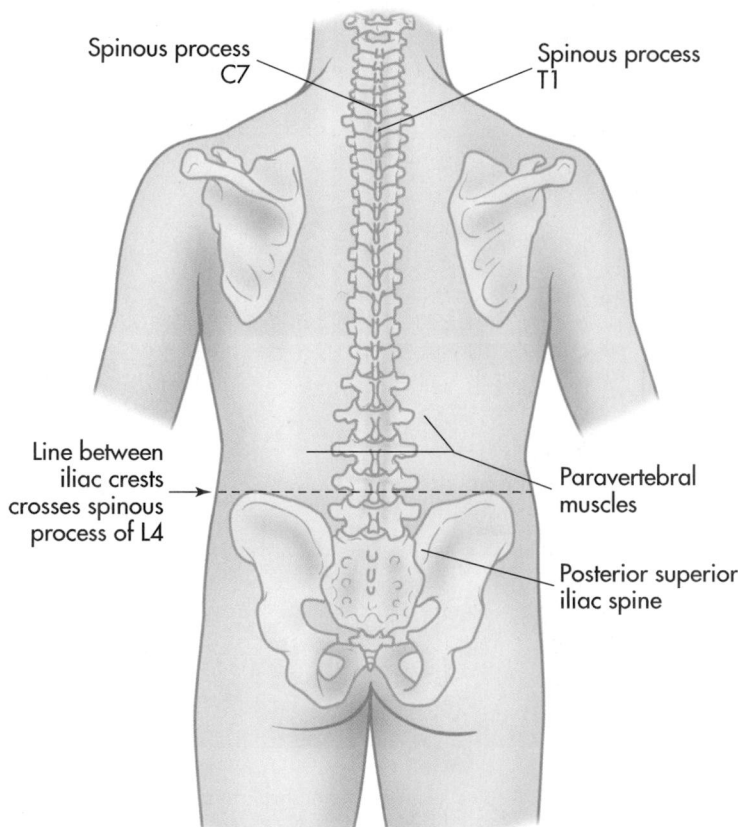

FIGURE 21-19
Landmarks of the back.

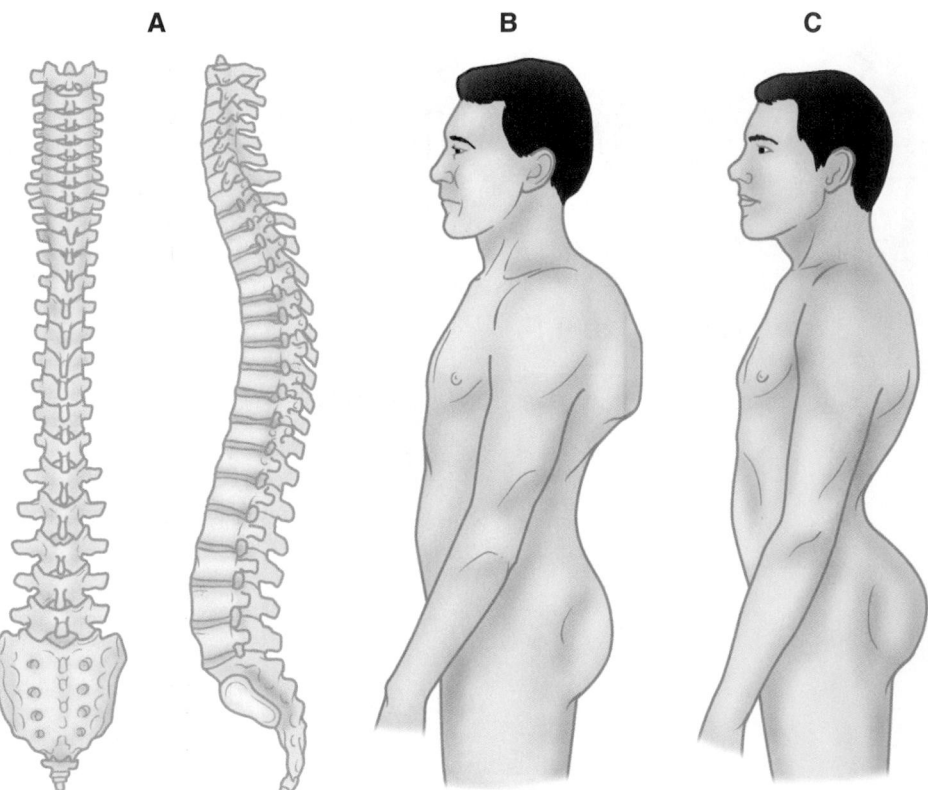

FIGURE 21-20
Deviations in spinal column
curvatures. **A,** Expected spine
curvatures. **B,** Kyphosis.
C, Lordosis.

With the patient standing erect, palpate along the spinal processes and paravertebral muscles (Fig. 21-21). No muscle spasms or spinal tenderness should be noted. Percuss for spinal tenderness, first by tapping each spinal process with one finger, and then by rapping each side of the spine along the paravertebral muscles with the ulnar aspect of your fist. No muscle spasm or spinal tenderness with palpation or percussion should be elicited.

Ask the patient to bend forward slowly and touch the toes while you observe from behind. Inspect the spine for unexpected curvature. (A mark with the skin pencil on each spinal process will enhance the inspection, especially if a curvature is suspected.) The patient's back should remain symmetrically flat as the concave curve of the lumbar spine becomes convex with forward flexion. A lateral curvature or rib hump should make you suspect scoliosis (Fig. 21-22). Then have the patient rise but remain bent at the waist to fully extend the back. Reversal of the lumbar curve should be apparent.

Range of motion is evaluated by asking the patient to perform the following movements:

* Bend forward at the waist and try to touch the toes. Expect flexion of 75 to 90 degrees (Fig. 21-23, *A*).
* Bend back at the waist as far as possible. Expect hyperextension of 30 degrees (Fig. 21-23, *B*).
* Bend to each side as far as possible. Expect lateral bending of 35 degrees bilaterally (Fig. 21-23, *C*).
* Swing the upper trunk from the waist in a circular motion front to side to back to side, while you stabilize the pelvis. Expect rotation of the upper trunk 30 degrees forward and backward (Fig. 21-23, *D*).

STAYING WELL
REDUCING THE RISK FOR LOWER BACK PAIN

Use appropriate techniques to lift heavy objects to reduce the risk for injury to the lower back. Rather than bend over to pick up a heavy object, keep the back straight and flex the knees to get closer to the object. Keep the object close to the body and lift with the knees. Avoid twisting the back during the lift.

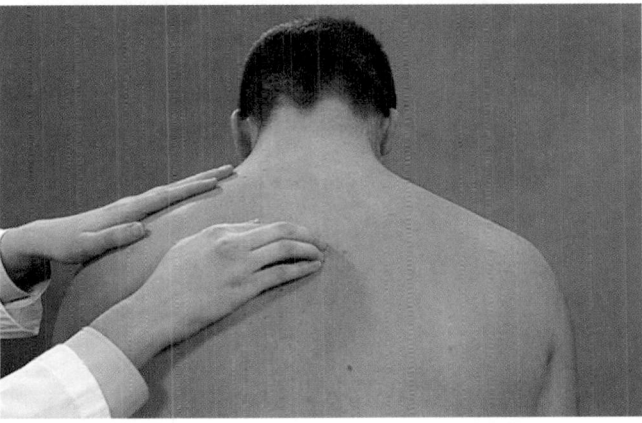

FIGURE 21-21
Palpation of the spinal processes of the vertebrae.

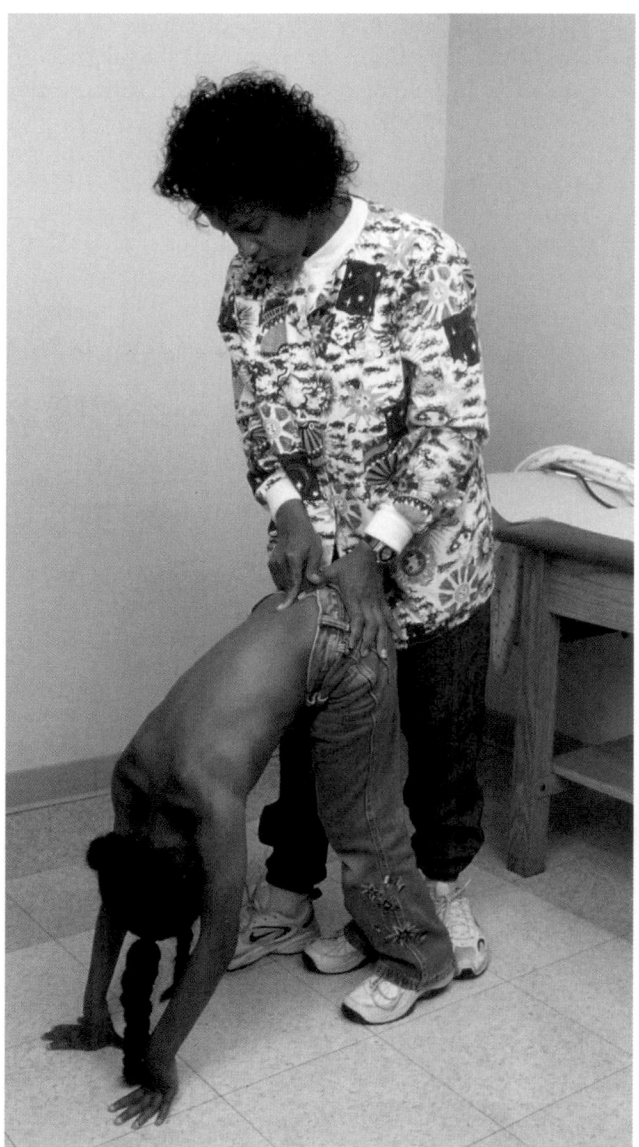

FIGURE 21-22
Inspection of the spine for lateral curvature and lumbar convexity.

SHOULDERS

Inspect the contour of the shoulders, the shoulder girdle, the clavicles and scapulae, and the area muscles. There should be symmetry of size and contour of all shoulder structures. When the shoulder contour is asymmetric and one shoulder has hollows in the rounding contour, suspect a shoulder dislocation. Ask the patient to stand close to a wall and push against it with both hands. Observe for a winged scapula, an outward prominence of the scapula, indicating injury to the nerve of the anterior serratus muscle (Fig. 21-24).

Palpate the sternoclavicular joint, clavicle, acromioclavicular joint, scapula, coracoid process, greater tubercle of the humerus, biceps groove, and area muscles. To palpate the biceps groove, rotate the arm and forearm externally. Locate the biceps muscle near the elbow and follow the muscle and its tendon into the biceps groove along the anterior aspect of the humerus. Palpate the muscle insertions of the supraspinatus, infraspinatus, and teres minor near the greater tuberosity of the humerus by lifting the elbow posteriorly to extend the shoulder. No tenderness should be noted over the muscle insertions. See p. 727 for rotator cuff assessment.

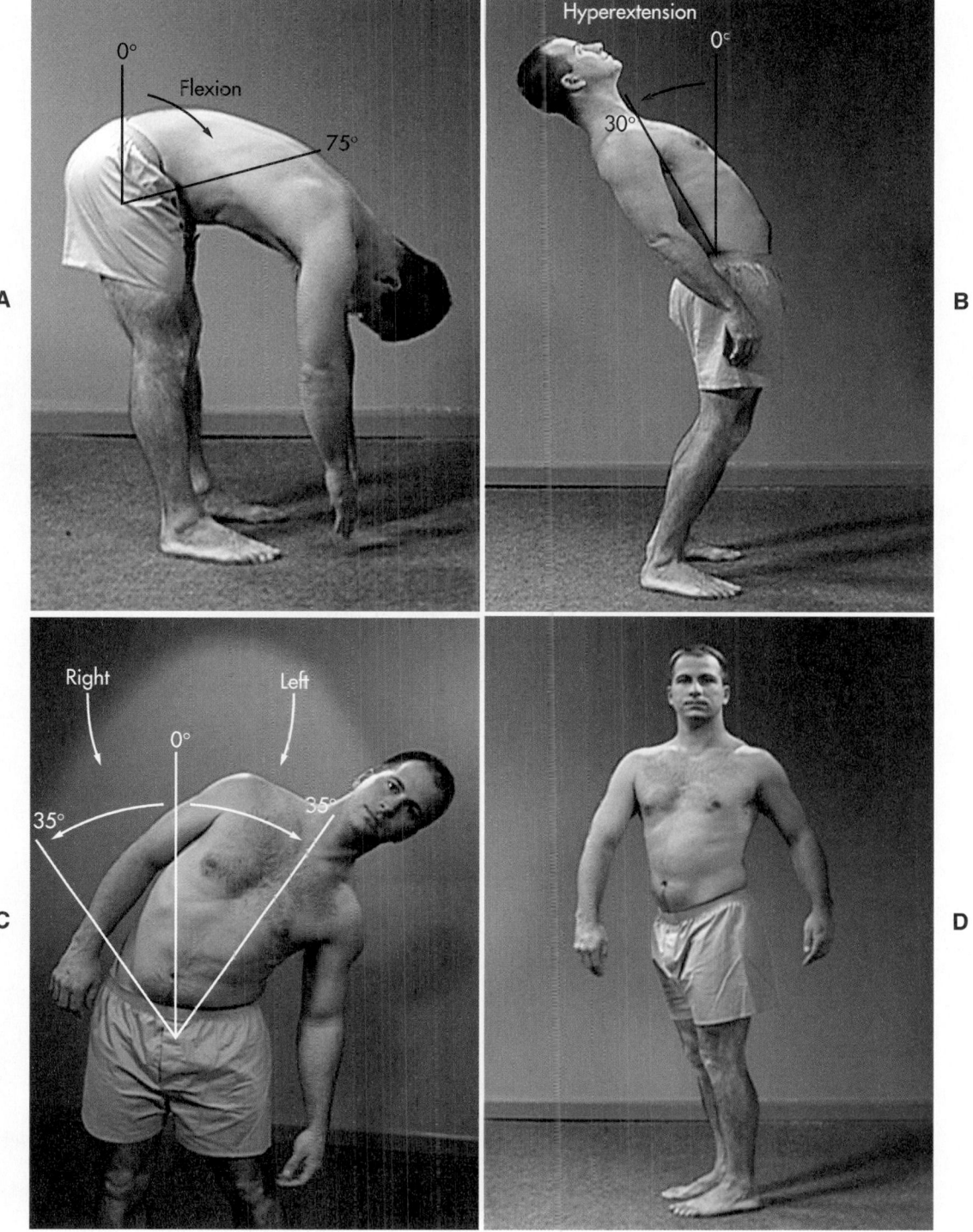

FIGURE 21-23
Range of motion of the thoracic and lumbar spine. **A,** Flexion. **B,** Hyperextension. **C,** Lateral bending. **D,** Rotation of the upper trunk.

Examine the range of motion by asking the patient to perform the following movements:
- Shrug the shoulders. Expect the shoulders to rise symmetrically.
- Raise both arms forward and straight up over the head. Expect forward flexion of 180 degrees.
- Extend and stretch both arms behind the back. Expect hyperextension of 50 degrees (Fig. 21-25, *A*).

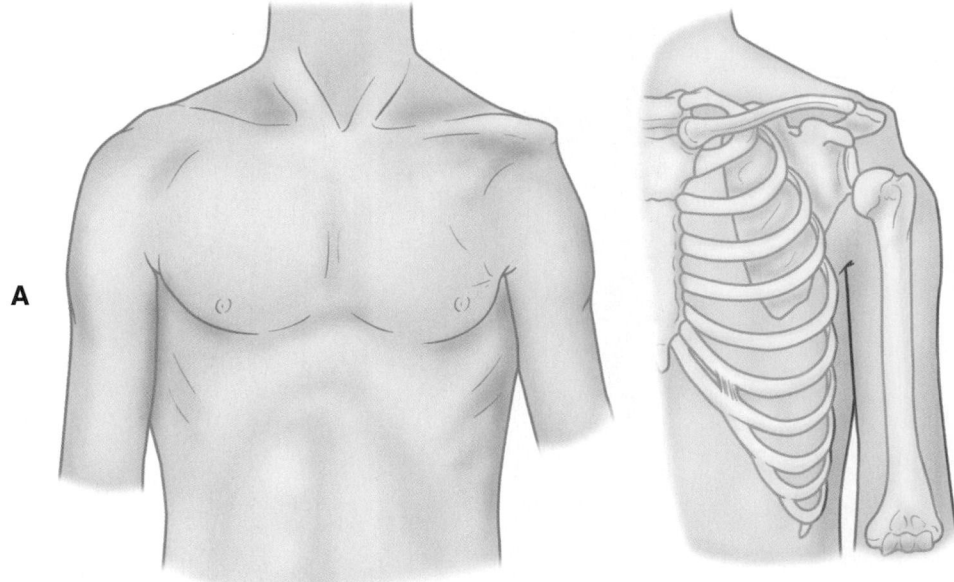

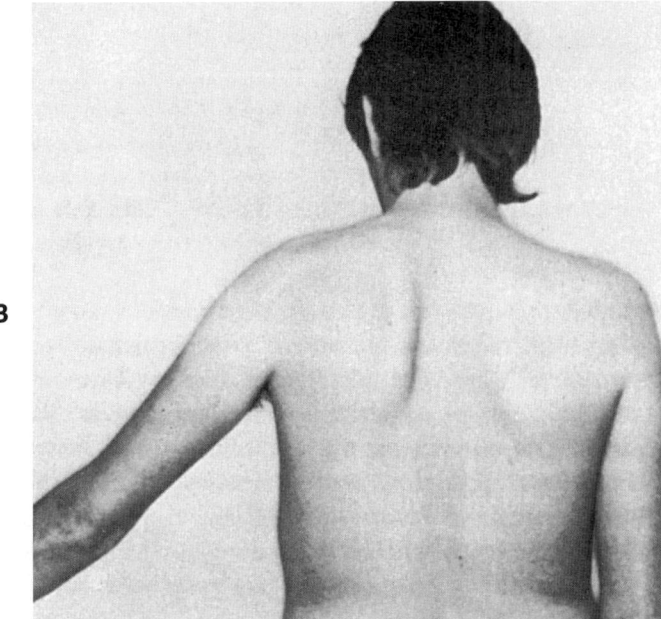

FIGURE 21-24
Contour changes of the shoulder. **A,** With dislocation. **B,** Winging of the scapula with abduction of the arm.
B from DePalma, 1983.

◆ Lift both arms laterally and straight up over the head. Expect shoulder abduction of 180 degrees.
◆ Swing each arm across the front of the body. Expect adduction of 50 degrees (Fig. 21-25, *B*).
◆ Place both arms behind the hips, elbows out. Expect internal rotation of 90 degrees (Fig. 21-25, *C*).
◆ Place both arms behind the head, elbows out. Expect external rotation of 90 degrees (Fig. 21-25, *D*).

Have the patient maintain shrugged shoulders while you apply opposing force to evaluate the strength of the shoulder girdle muscles. Cranial nerve XI is simultaneously evaluated with the shrugged shoulders maneuver (Fig. 21-25, *E*).

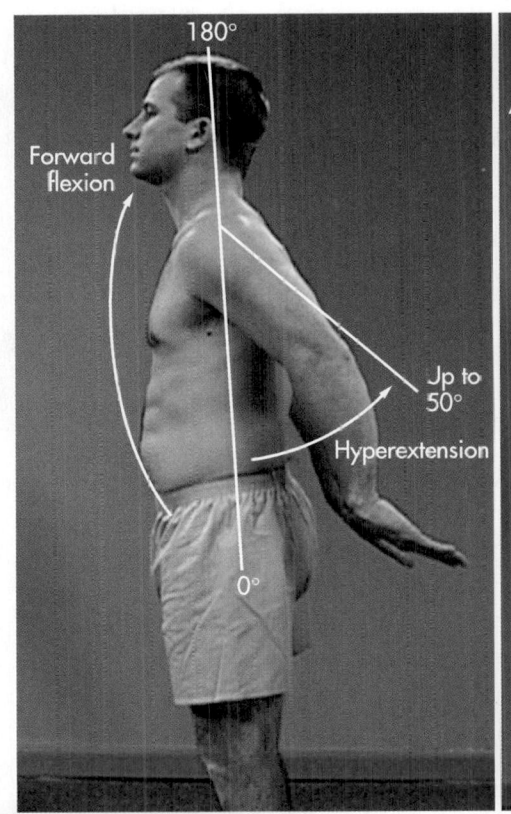

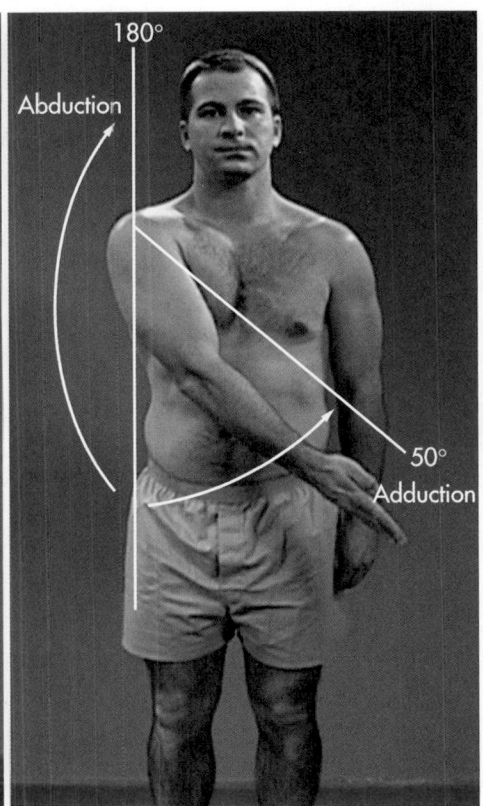

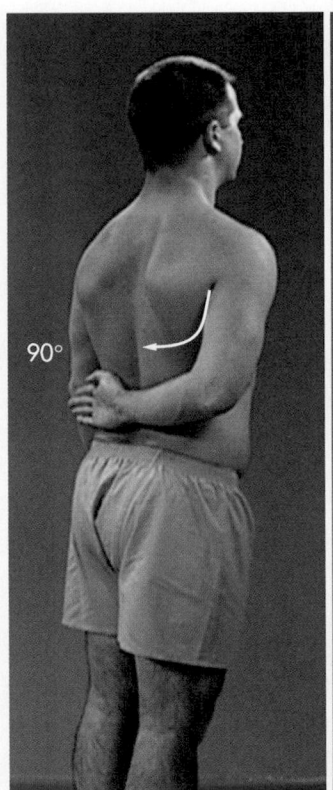

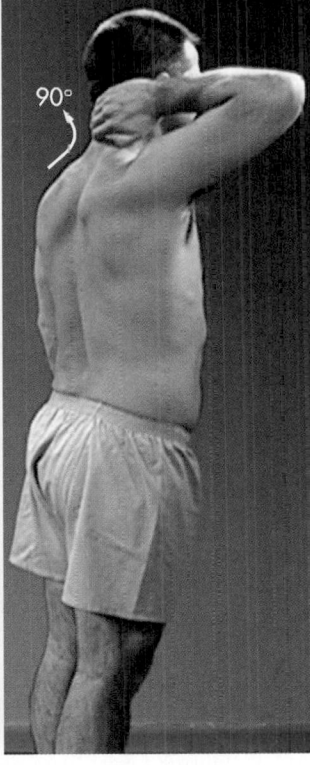

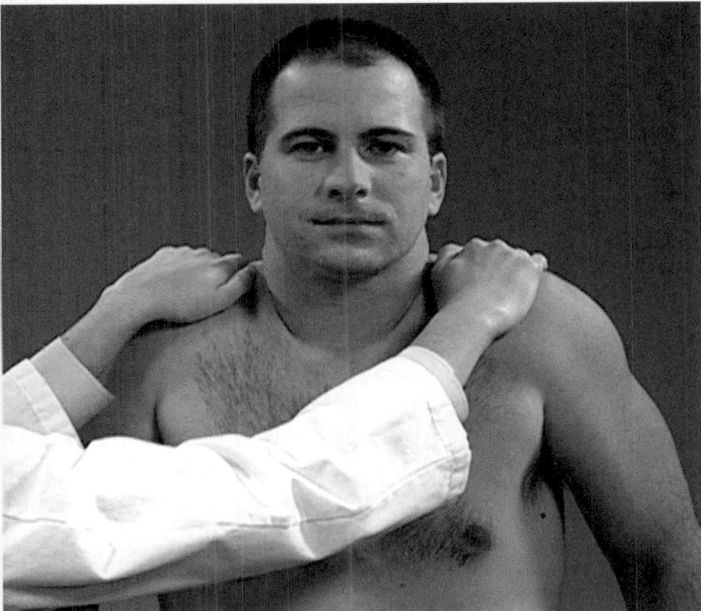

FIGURE 21-25
Range of motion of the shoulder. **A,** Forward flexion and hyperextension. **B,** Abduction and adduction. **C,** Internal rotation. **D,** External rotation. **E,** Shrugged shoulders.

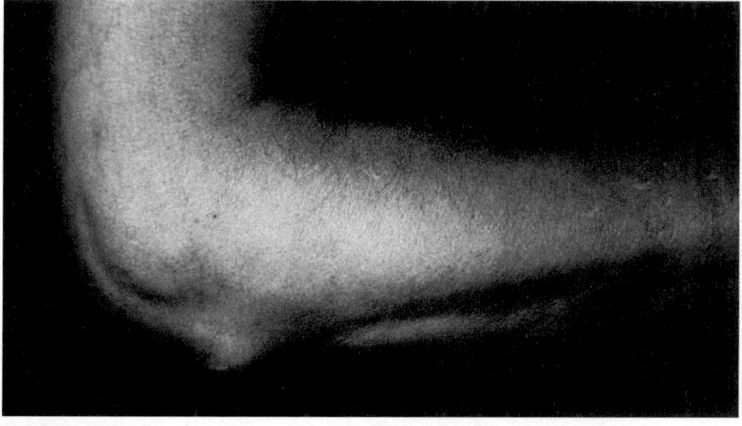

FIGURE 21-26
Subcutaneous nodules on the extensor surface of the forearm near the elbow.
Reprinted from the Clinical Slide Collection of the Rheumatic Diseases, copyright 1991. Used by permission of the American College of Rheumatology.

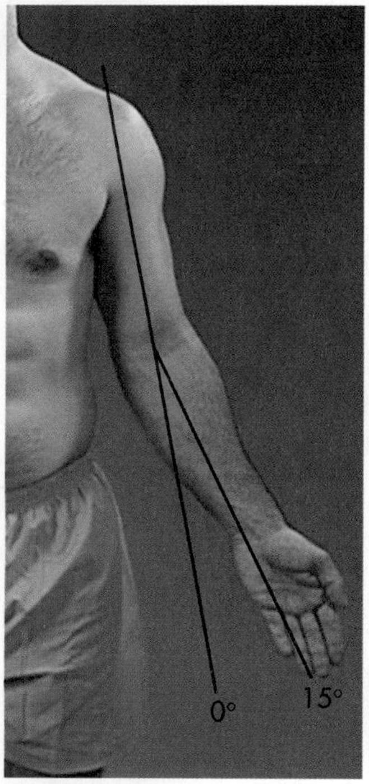

FIGURE 21-27
Expected carrying angle of the arm, at 5 to 15 degrees.

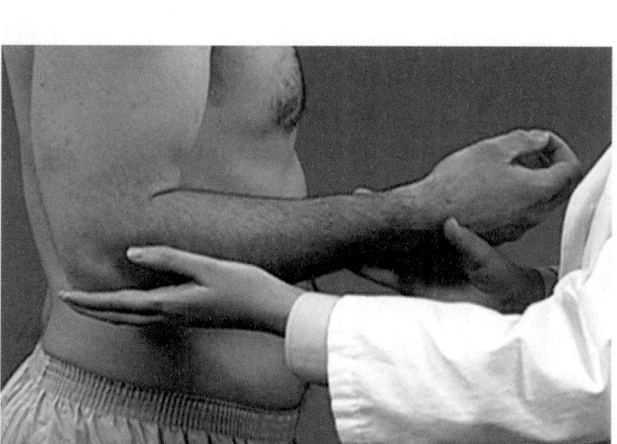

FIGURE 21-28
Palpation of the olecranon process grooves.

ELBOWS

Inspect the contour of the patient's elbows in both flexed and extended positions. Subcutaneous nodules along pressure points of the ulnar surface may indicate rheumatoid arthritis (Fig. 21-26).

Note any deviations in the carrying angle between the humerus and radius while the arm is passively extended, palm forward. The carrying angle is usually 5 to 15 degrees laterally. Variations in carrying angle are cubitus valgus, a lateral angle exceeding 15 degrees; and cubitus varus, a medial carrying angle (Fig. 21-27).

Flex the patient's elbow 70 degrees and palpate the extensor surface of the ulna, the olecranon process, and the medial and lateral epicondyles of the humerus. Then palpate the groove on each side of the olecranon process for tenderness, swelling, and thickening of the synovial membrane (Fig. 21-28). A boggy, soft, or fluctuant swelling; point tenderness at the lateral epicondyle or along the grooves of the olecranon process and epicondyles; and increased pain with pronation and supination of the elbow should cause you to suspect epicondylitis or tendinitis.

The elbow's range of motion is examined by asking the patient to perform the following movements:

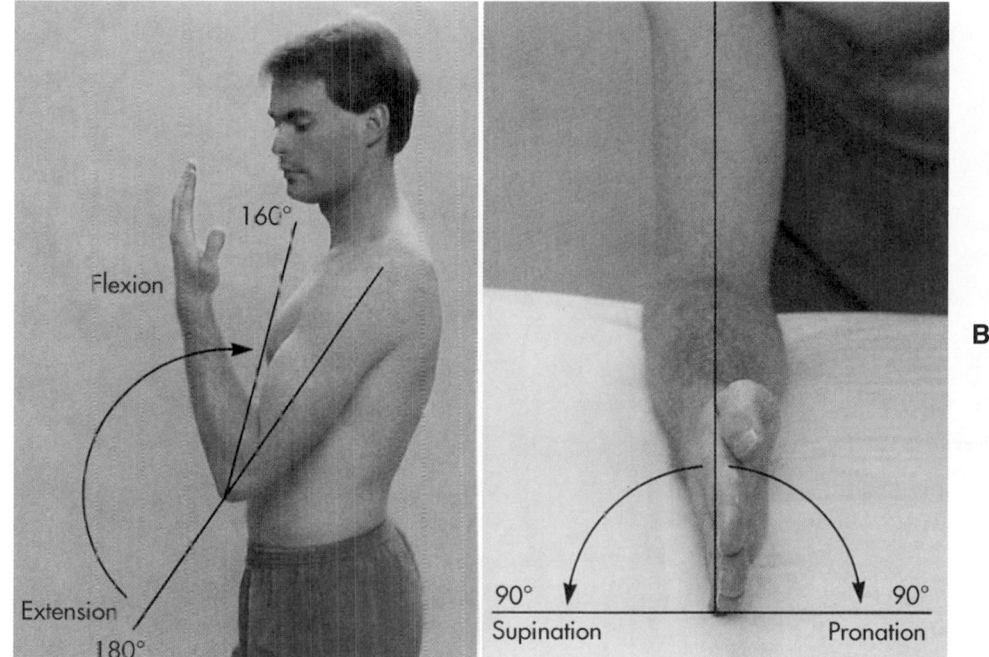

FIGURE 21-29
Range of motion of the elbow.
A, Flexion and extension.
B, Pronation and supination.

- With the elbow fully extended at 0 degrees, bend and straighten the elbow. Expect flexion of 160 degrees and extension returning to 0 degrees or 180 degrees of full extension (Fig. 21-29, *A*).
- With the elbow flexed at a right angle, rotate the hand from palm side down to palm side up. Expect pronation of 90 degrees and supination of 90 degrees (Fig. 21-29, *B*).

Have the patient maintain flexion and extension while you apply opposing force to evaluate the strength of the elbow muscles.

HANDS AND WRISTS

Inspect the dorsal and palmar aspects of the hands, noting the contour, position, shape, number, and completeness of digits. Note the presence of palmar and phalangeal creases. The palmar surface of each hand should have a central depression with a prominent, rounded mound (thenar eminence) on the thumb side of the hand and a less prominent hypothenar eminence on the little finger side of the hand. Expect the fingers to fully extend when in close approximation to each other and to be aligned with the forearm. The lateral finger surfaces should gradually taper from the proximal to the distal aspects (Fig. 21-30).

Deviation of the fingers to the ulnar side, and swan neck or boutonniere deformities of the fingers usually indicates rheumatoid arthritis (Fig. 21-31).

Palpate each joint in the hand and wrist. Palpate the interphalangeal joints with your thumb and index finger. The metacarpophalangeal joints are palpated with both thumbs. Palpate the wrist and radiocarpal groove with your thumbs on the dorsal surface and your fingers on the palmar aspect of the wrist (Fig. 21-32). Joint surfaces should be smooth and without nodules, swelling, bogginess, or tenderness. A firm mass over the dorsum of the wrist may be a ganglion.

Bony overgrowths in the distal interphalangeal joints, which are felt as hard, nontender nodules usually 2 to 3 mm in diameter but sometimes encompassing the entire joint, are associated with osteoarthritis. When located along the distal interphalangeal joints, they are called *Heberden nodes;* those along the proximal interphalangeal joints are called *Bouchard nodes.* Painful, fusiform swelling of the proximal interphalangeal joints causes spindle-shaped fingers, which are associated with the acute stage of rheumatoid arthritis (Fig. 21-33). Cystic, round, nontender swellings along tendon sheaths or joint capsules that are more prominent with flexion may indicate ganglia.

Examine the range of motion of the hand and wrist by asking the patient to perform these movements:

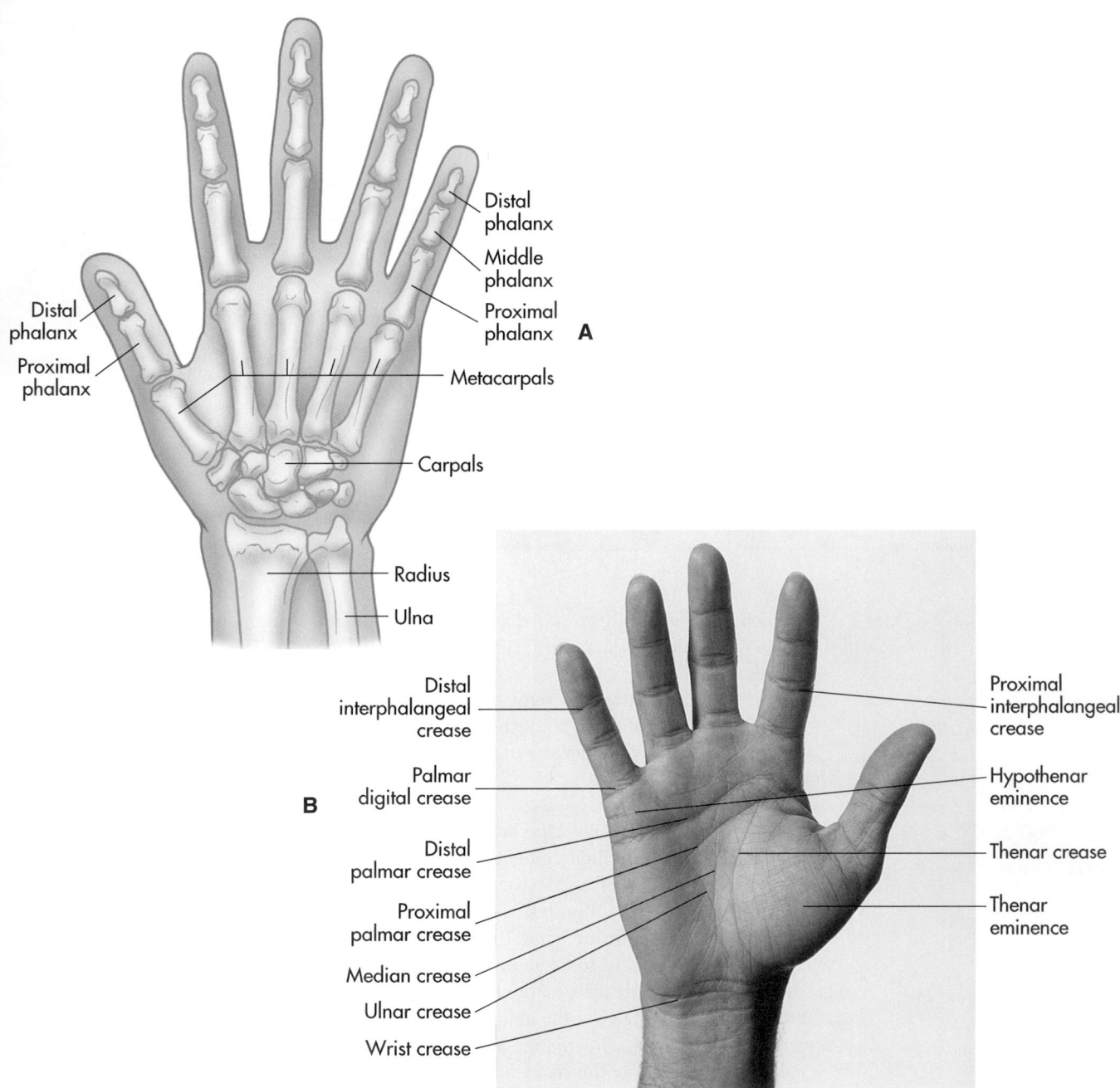

FIGURE 21-30
A, Bony structure of the right hand and wrist; note the alignment of the fingers with the radius.
B, Features of the palmar aspect of the hand; note creases, thenar eminence and hypothenar eminence, and gradual tapering of the fingers.

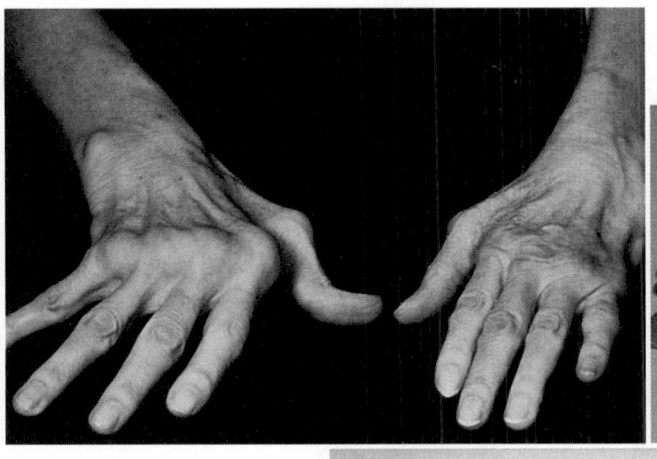
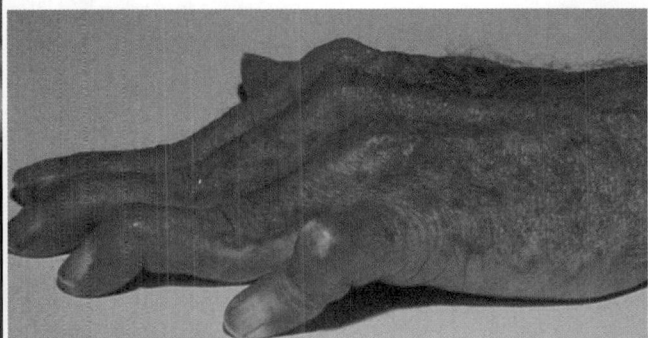
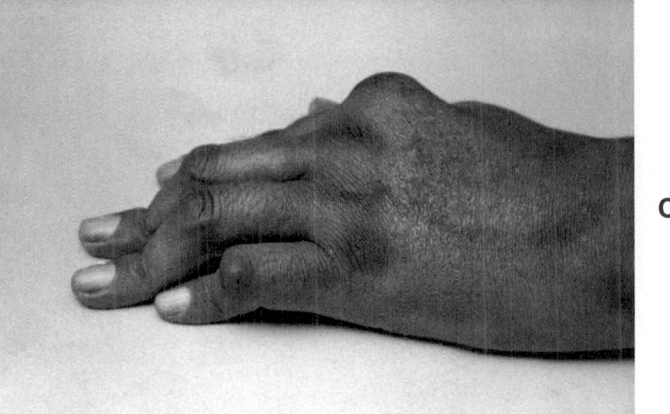

FIGURE 21-31
Unexpected findings of the hand. **A,** Ulnar deviation and subluxation of metacarpophalangeal joints.
B, Swan neck deformities. **C,** Boutonniere deformity.

A, B reprinted from the Clinical Slide Collection of the Rheumatic Diseases, copyright 1991. Used by permission of the American College of Rheumatology; C from the Arthritis Teaching Slide Collection, copyright 1980. Used by permission of the Arthritis Foundation.

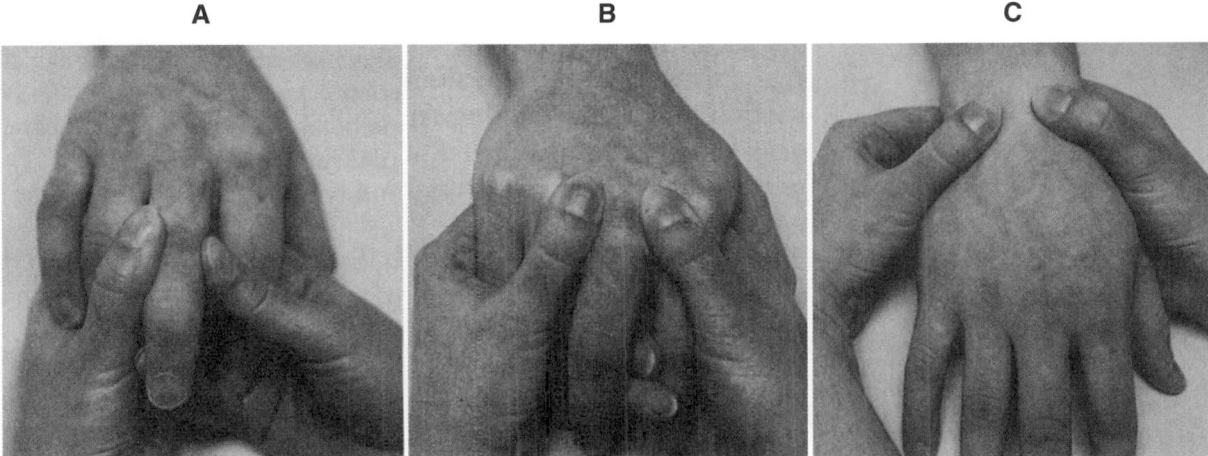

FIGURE 21-32
Palpation of joints of the hand and wrist. **A,** Interphalangeal joints. **B,** Metacarpophalangeal joints.
C, Radiocarpal groove and wrist.

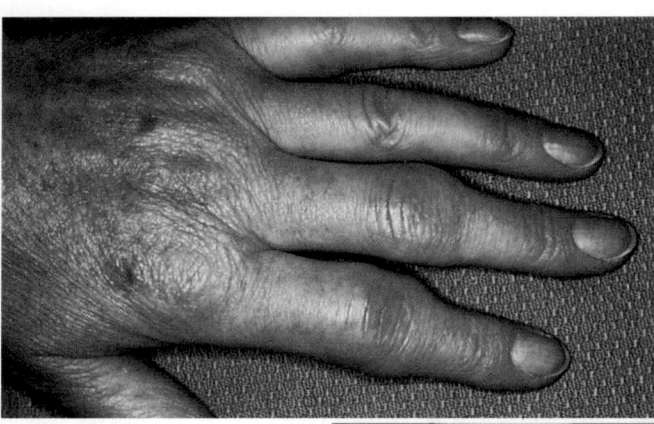 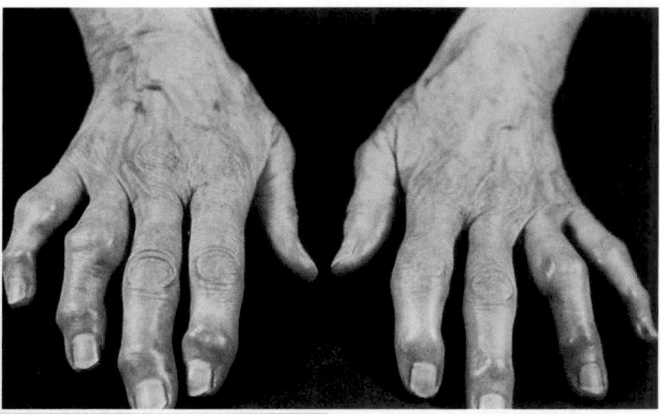

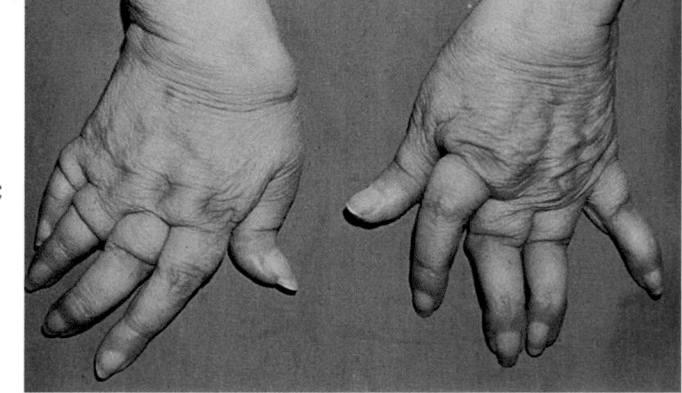

FIGURE 21-33
Unexpected findings of the fingers. **A,** Fusiform swelling or spindle-shaped enlargement of the proximal interphalangeal joints. **B,** Degenerative joint disease; Heberden nodes at the distal interphalangeal joints and Bouchard nodes at the proximal interphalangeal joints. **C,** Telescoping digits with hypermobile joints.
Reprinted from the Clinical Slide Collection of the Rheumatic Diseases, copyright 1991. Used by permission of the American College of Rheumatology.

- Bend the fingers forward at the metacarpophalangeal joint; then stretch the fingers up and back at the knuckle. Expect metacarpophalangeal flexion of 90 degrees and hyperextension up to 30 degrees (Fig. 21-34, *A*).
- Touch the thumb to each fingertip and to the base of the little finger; make a fist. All movements should be possible (Fig. 21-34, *B* and *C*).
- Spread the fingers apart and then touch them together. Both movements should be possible (Fig. 21-34, *D*).
- Bend the hand at the wrist up and down. Expect flexion of 90 degrees and hyperextension of 70 degrees (Fig. 21-34, *E*).
- With the palm side down, turn each hand to the right and left. Expect radial motion of 20 degrees and ulnar motion of 55 degrees (Fig. 21-34, *F*).

Have the patient maintain wrist flexion and hyperextension while you apply opposing force to evaluate strength of the wrist muscles. To evaluate hand strength, have the patient grip two of your fingers tightly. To avoid painful compression from an overzealous squeeze, offer your two fingers of one hand side by side in the handshake position. Finger extension, abduction, adduction, and thumb opposition may also be used to evaluate hand strength.

HIPS

Inspect the hips anteriorly and posteriorly while the patient stands. Using the major landmarks of the iliac crest and the greater trochanter of the femur, note any asymmetry in the iliac crest height, the size of the buttocks, or the number and level of gluteal folds.

Palpate the hips and pelvis with the patient supine (Fig. 21-35). No instability, tenderness, or crepitus is expected.

Examine the range of motion of the hips by asking the patient to perform the following movements:

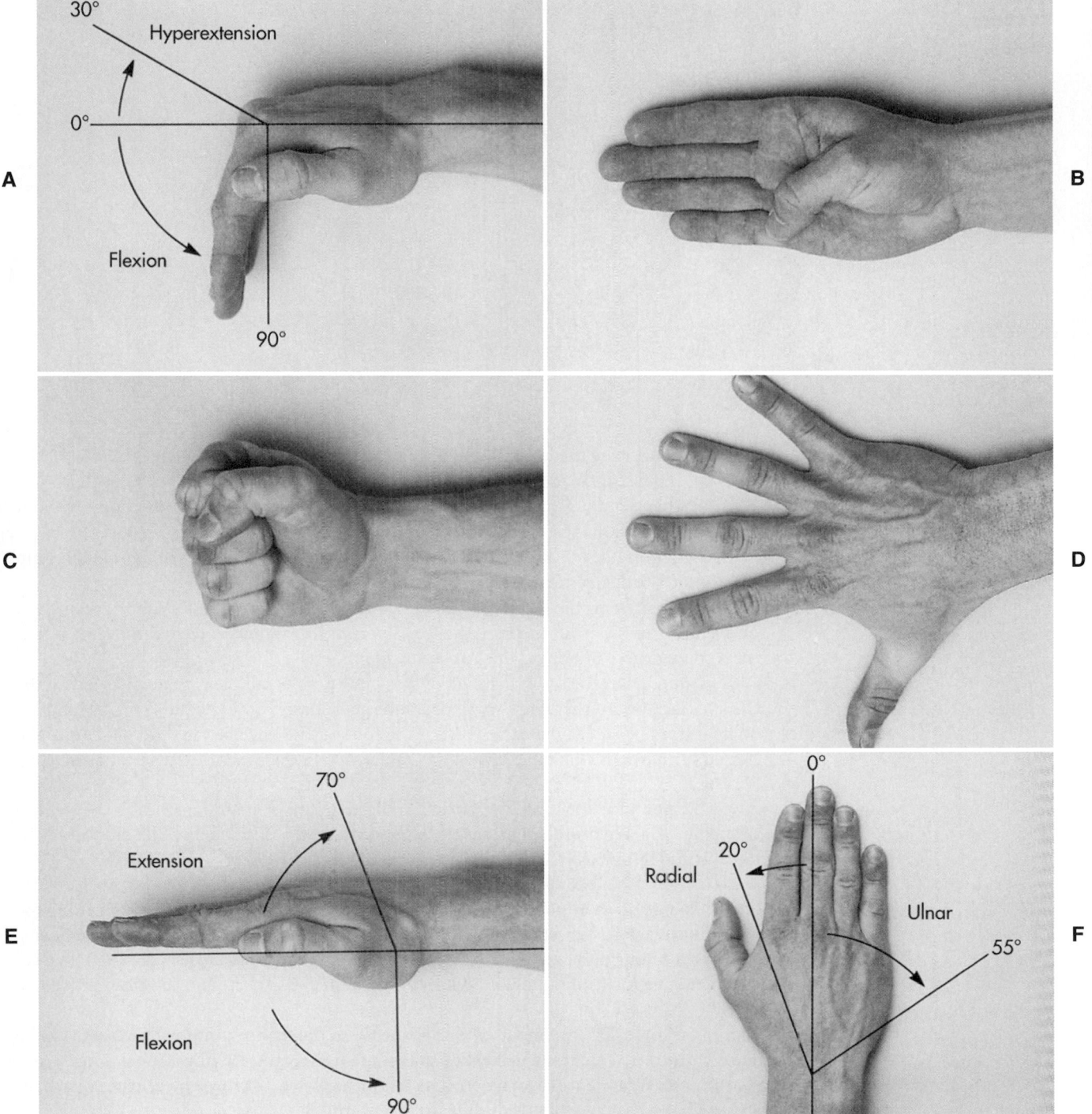

FIGURE 21-34
Range of motion of the hand and wrist. **A,** Metacarpophalangeal flexion and hyperextension. **B,** Finger flexion: thumb to each fingertip and to the base of the little finger. **C,** Finger flexion: fist formation. **D,** Finger abduction. **E,** Wrist flexion and hyperextension. **F,** Wrist radial and ulnar movement.

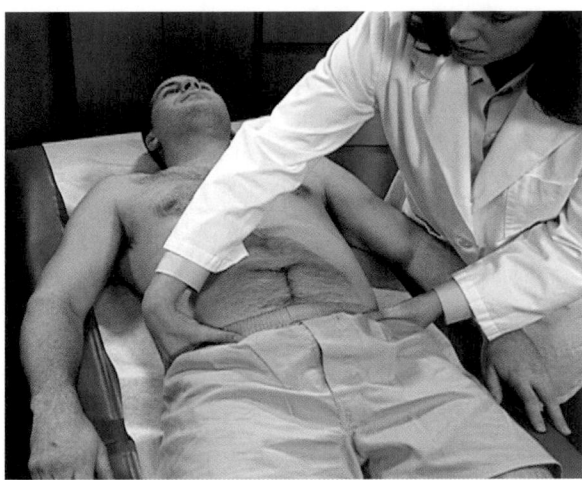

FIGURE 21-35
Palpating the pelvis for stability.

- While supine, raise the leg with the knee extended above the body. Expect up to 90 degrees of hip flexion (Fig. 21-36, *A*).
- While either standing or prone, swing the straightened leg behind the body without arching the back. Expect hip hyperextension of 30 degrees or less (Fig. 21-36, *B*).
- While supine, raise one knee to the chest while keeping the other leg straight. Expect hip flexion of 120 degrees (Fig. 21-36, *C*).
- While supine, swing the leg laterally and medially with knee straight. With the adduction movement, passively lift the opposite leg to permit the examined leg full movement. Expect some degree of both abduction and adduction (Fig. 21-36, *D*).
- While supine, flex the knee keeping the foot on the table and then rotate the leg with the flexed knee toward the other leg. Expect internal rotation of 40 degrees (Fig. 21-36, *E*).
- While supine, place the lateral aspect of the foot on the knee of the other leg; move the flexed knee toward the table (Patrick test). Expect 45 degrees of external rotation (Fig. 21-36, *F*).

To test hip flexion strength, apply resistance while the patient maintains flexion of the hip when the knee is flexed and then extended. Muscle strength can also be evaluated during abduction and adduction, as well as by resistance to uncrossing the legs while seated.

LEGS AND KNEES

PHYSICAL VARIATIONS

Leg Alignment
There are two expected variations in leg alignment: femoral torsion (rotation of the proximal end) and femoral curvature. Whites have more femoral torsion than blacks do. Femurs of Native Americans/American Indians are often quite convex anteriorly, whereas femurs of blacks are usually straight. Femurs in whites are generally intermediate. Obesity increases femoral curvature.

Inspect the knees and their popliteal spaces in both flexed and extended positions, noting the major landmarks: tibial tuberosity, medial and lateral tibial condyles, medial and lateral epicondyles of the femur, adductor tubercle of the femur, and the patella (see Fig. 21-10). Inspect the extended knee for its natural concavities on the anterior aspect, on each side, and above the patella.

Observe the lower leg alignment. The angle between the femur and tibia is expected to be less than 15 degrees. Variations in lower leg alignment are genu valgum (knock-knees) and genu varum (bowlegs). Excessive hyperextension of the knee with weight bearing (genu recurvatum) may indicate weakness of the quadriceps muscles.

An effusion of the knee fills the suprapatellar pouch. The usual indentation above the patella is filled out to be convex rather than concave.

Palpate the popliteal space, noting any swelling or tenderness. Then palpate the tibiofemoral joint space, identifying the patella, the suprapatellar pouch, and the infrapatellar fat pad. The joint should feel smooth and firm, without tenderness, swelling, bogginess, nodules, or crepitus. See p. 731 for additional assessment procedures.

Examine the knees' range of motion by asking the patient to perform the following movements (Fig. 21-37):

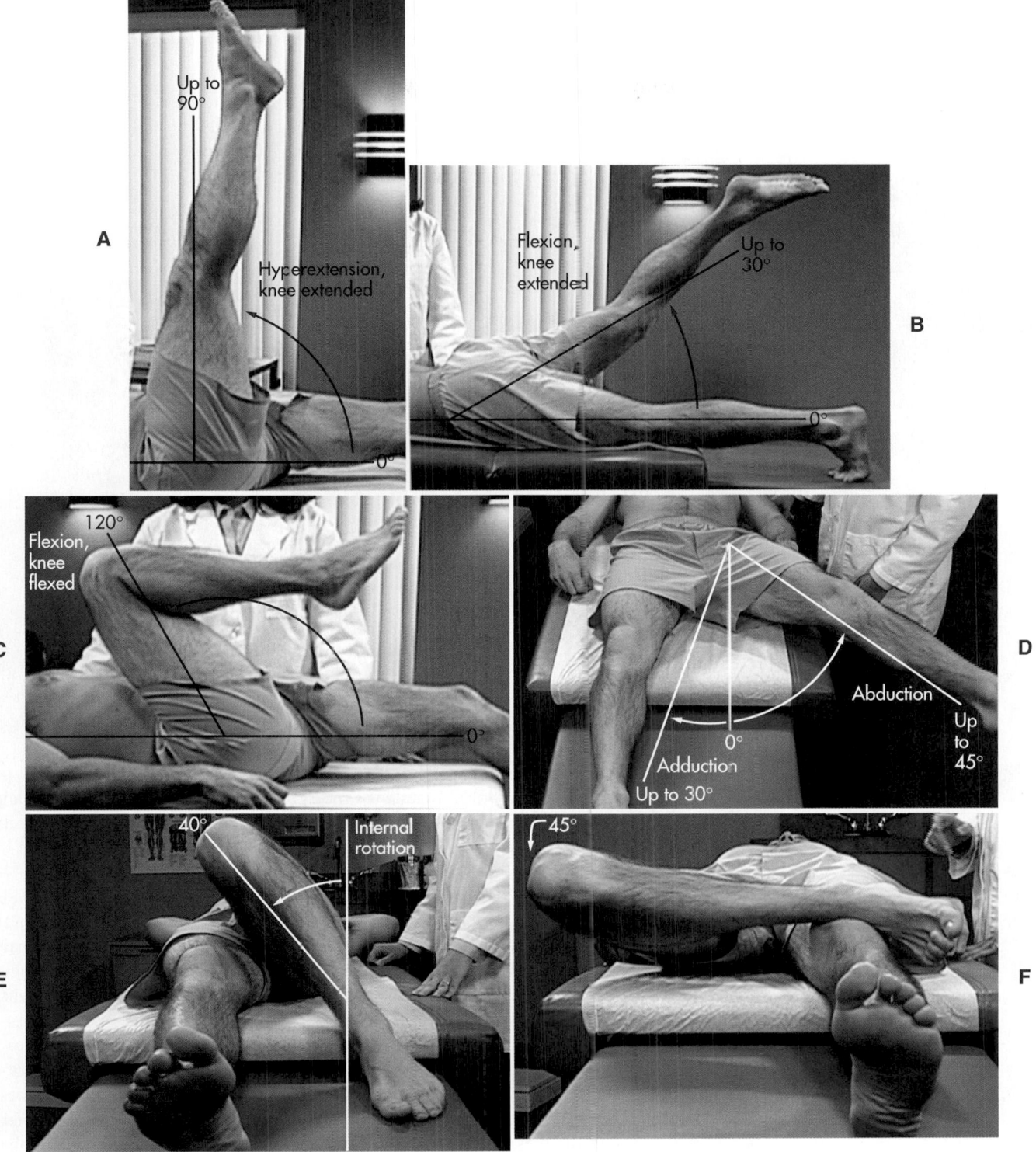

FIGURE 21-36
Range of motion of the hip. **A,** Hip flexion, knee extended. **B,** Hip extension, knee extended. **C,** Hip flexion, knee flexed. **D,** Abduction. **E,** Internal rotation. **F,** External rotation.

♦ Bend each knee. Expect 130 degrees of flexion.
♦ Straighten the leg and stretch it. Expect full extension and up to 15 degrees of hyperextension.

The strength of the knee muscles is evaluated with the patient maintaining flexion and extension while you apply opposing force. The patient may be sitting or standing for this assessment.

Musculoskeletal System:
Examining the Legs and Knees

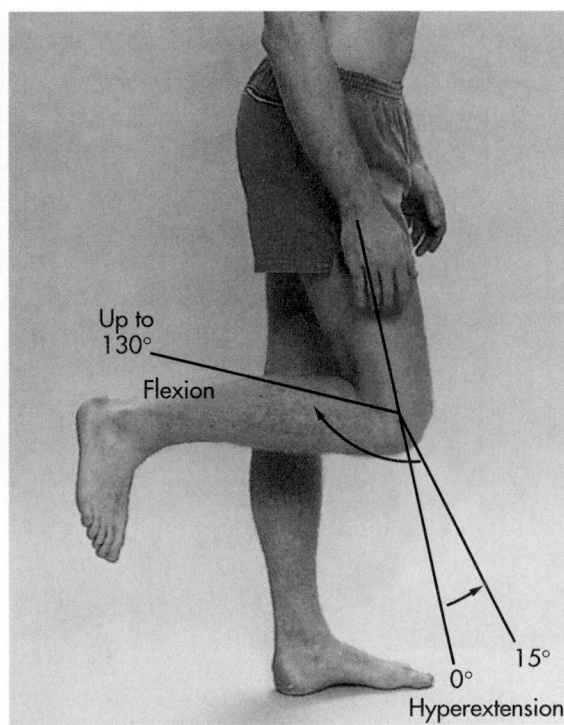

FIGURE 21-37
Range of motion of the knee: flexion and extension.

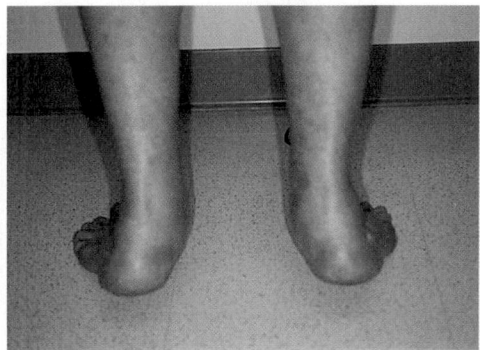

FIGURE 21-38
Pronation of heel. Notice that weight bearing is not through the midline of the foot.
Courtesy Charles W. Bradley, DPM, MPA, and Caroline Harvey, DPM, California College of Podiatric Medicine.

FEET AND ANKLES

Inspect the feet and ankles while the patient is bearing weight (i.e., standing and walking) and while sitting. Landmarks of the ankle include the medial malleolus, the lateral malleolus, and the Achilles tendon. Expect smooth and rounded malleolar prominences, prominent heels, and prominent metatarsophalangeal joints. Calluses and corns indicate chronic pressure or irritation.

Observe the contour of the feet and the position, size, and number of toes. The feet should be in alignment with the tibias. Pes varus (in-toeing) and pes valgus (out-toeing) are common alignment variations. Weight bearing should be on the midline of the foot, on an imaginary line from the heel midline to between the second and third toes. Deviations in forefoot alignment (metatarsus varus or metatarsus valgus), heel pronation, and pain or injury often cause a shift in weight-bearing position (Fig. 21-38).

Expect the foot to have a longitudinal arch, although the foot may flatten with weight-bearing. Common variations include pes planus, a foot that remains flat even when not bearing weight; and pes cavus, a high instep (Fig. 21-39). Pes cavus may be associated with claw toes.

The toes should be straight forward, flat, and in alignment with each other. Several unexpected deviations of the toes can occur (Fig. 21-40). Hyperextension of the metatarsophalangeal joint with flexion of the toe's proximal joint is called hammer toe. A flexion deformity at the distal interphalangeal joint is called a mallet toe. Claw toe is hyperextension of the metatarsophalangeal joint with flexion of the toe's proximal and distal joints. Hallux valgus is lateral deviation of the great toe, which may cause overlapping with the second toe. A bursa often forms at the pressure point and, if it becomes inflamed, forms a painful bunion.

Heat, redness, swelling, and tenderness are signs of an inflamed joint, possibly caused by rheumatoid arthritis, septic joint, fracture, or tendonitis. An inflamed metatarsophalangeal joint of the great toe should make you suspect gouty arthritis. A draining tophus may occasionally be present.

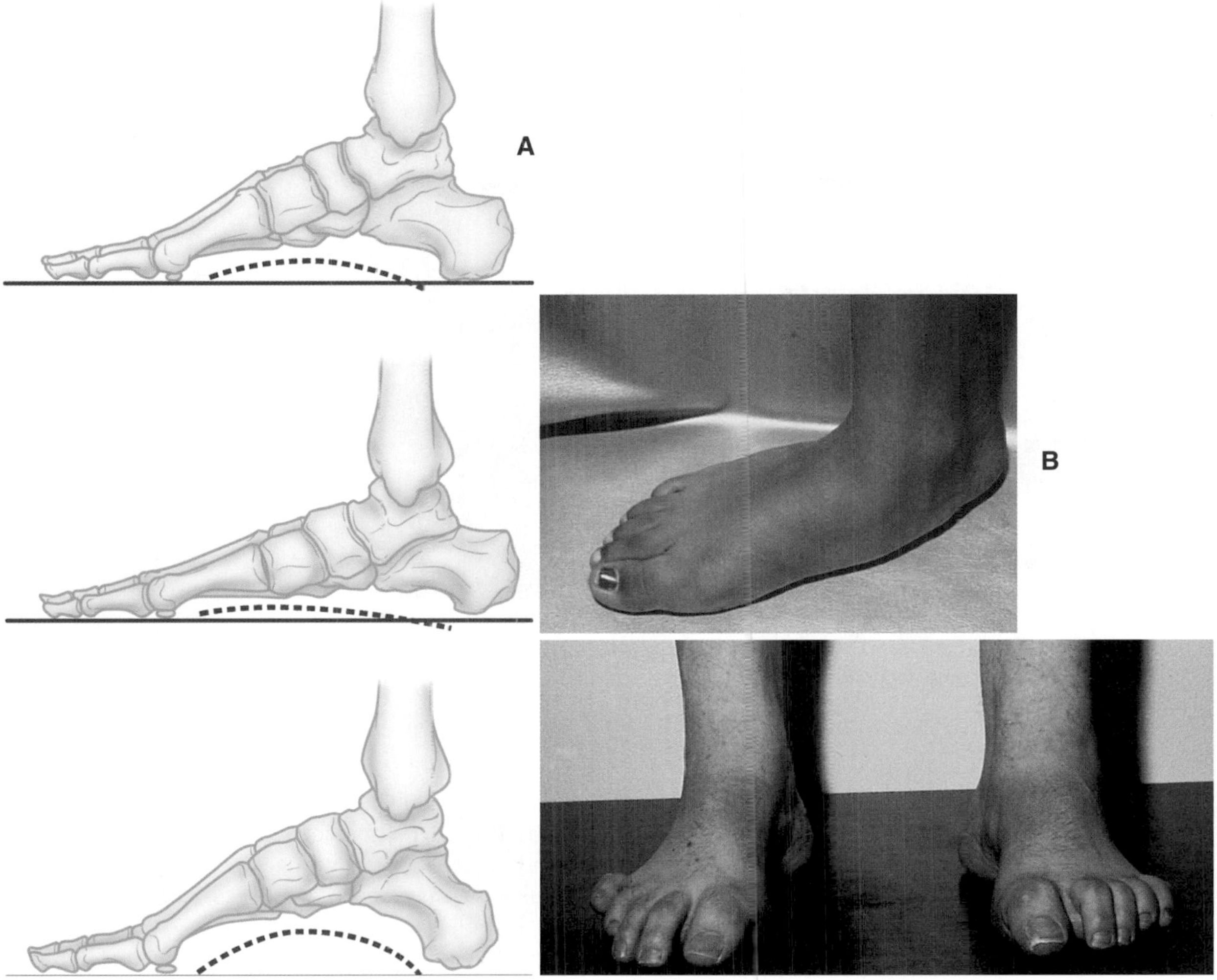

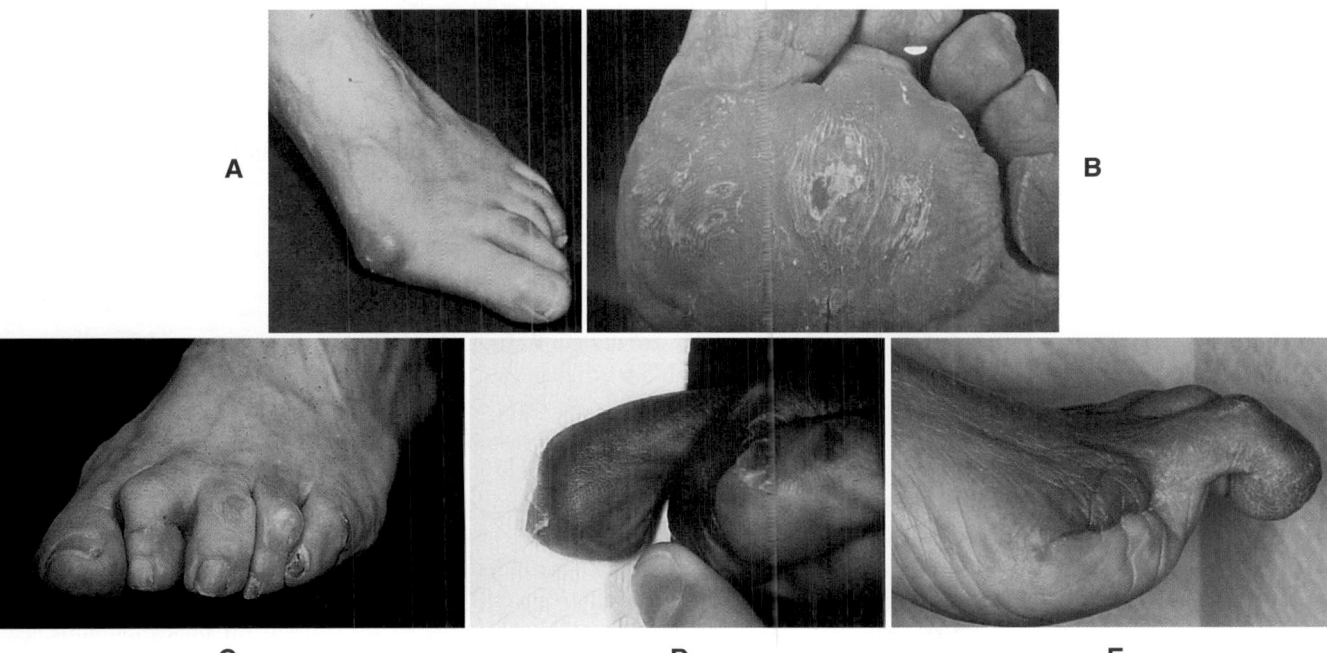

FIGURE 21-39

Variations in the longitudinal arch of the foot. **A,** Commonly expected arch. **B,** Pes planus (flatfoot). **C,** Pes cavus (high instep).

B, C courtesy Charles W. Bradley, DPM, MFA, and Caroline Harvey, DPM, California College of Podiatric Medicine.

FIGURE 21-40

Unexpected findings of the feet. **A,** Hallux valgus with bunion. **B,** Protruding metatarsal heads with callosities. **C,** Hammer toes. **D,** Mallet toe. **E,** Claw toes.

Courtesy Charles W. Bradley, DPM, MPA, and Caroline Harvey, DPM, California College of Podiatric Medicine.

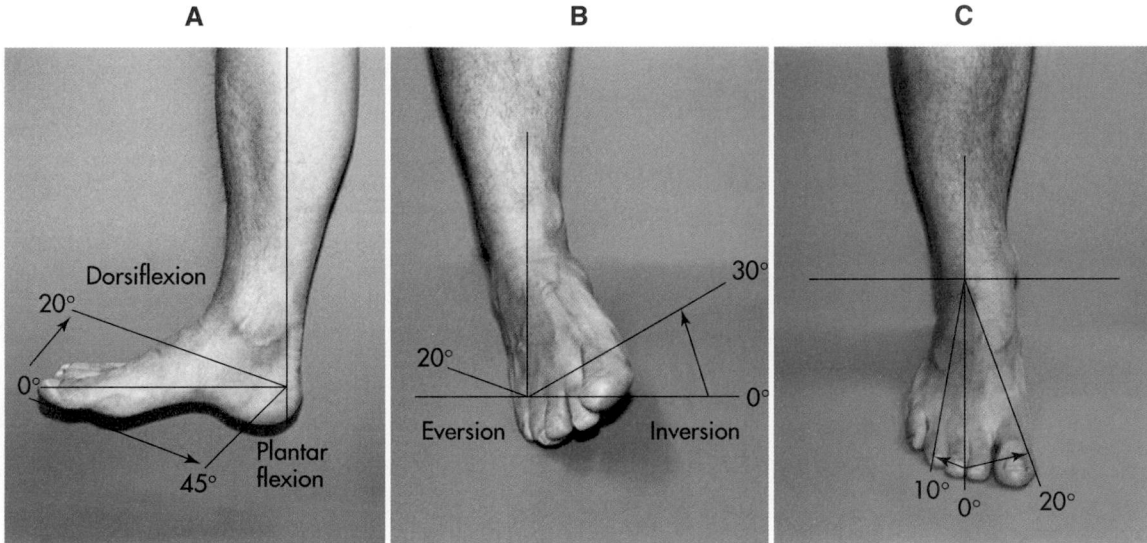

FIGURE 21-41
Range of motion of the foot and ankle. **A,** Dorsiflexion and plantar flexion. **B,** Inversion and eversion. **C,** Abduction and adduction.

Palpate the Achilles tendon, the anterior surface of the ankle, and the medial and lateral malleoli. A thickened Achilles tendon may indicate hyperlipidemia. Use the thumb and fingers of both hands to compress the forefoot and to palpate each metatarsophalangeal joint.

The range of motion of the foot and ankle is assessed by asking the patient to perform the following movements while sitting:

- Point the foot toward the ceiling. Expect dorsiflexion of 20 degrees (Fig. 21-41, *A*).
- Point the foot toward the floor. Expect plantar flexion of 45 degrees.
- Bending the foot at the ankle, turn the sole of the foot toward and then away from the other foot. Expect inversion of 30 degrees and eversion of 20 degrees (Fig. 21-41, *B*).
- Rotating the ankle, turn the foot away from and then toward the other foot while the examiner stabilizes the leg. Expect abduction of 10 degrees and adduction of 20 degrees (Fig. 21-41, *C*).
- Bend and straighten the toes. Expect flexion and extension, especially of the great toes.

Have the patient maintain dorsiflexion and plantar flexion while you apply opposing force to evaluate strength of the ankle muscles. Abduction and adduction of the ankle and flexion and extension of the great toe may also be used to evaluate muscle strength.

For the assessment of gait, see the Chapter 22.

ADDITIONAL PROCEDURES

Various other procedures for further evaluation of specific joints of the musculoskeletal system are performed when problems are detected with routine procedures (Table 21-3).

LIMB MEASUREMENT

When a difference in length or circumference of matching extremities is suspected, measure and compare the size of both extremities. Leg length is measured from the anterior superior iliac spine to the medial malleolus of the ankle, crossing the knee on the medial side (Fig. 21-42, *A*). Arm length is measured from the acromion process through the olecranon process to the distal ulnar prominence. The circumference of the extremities is measured in centimeters at the same distance on each limb from a major landmark (Fig. 21-42, *B*). Serious athletes who use the dominant arm almost exclusively in their activities (e.g., pitchers and tennis players) may have some discrepancy in circumference. For most people, no more than a 1-cm discrepancy in length and circumference between matching extremities should be found.

TABLE 21-3	Special Procedures for Assessment of the Musculoskeletal System
Procedure	**Condition Detected**
Limb measurement	Asymmetry in limb size
Neer test	Shoulder rotator cuff impingement or tear
Hawkins test	Shoulder rotator cuff impingement or tear
Katz hand diagram	Median nerve integrity
Thumb abduction test	Median nerve integrity
Tinel sign	Median nerve integrity
Phalen test	Median nerve integrity
Straight leg raising	L4, L5, S1 nerve root irritation
Bragard stretch test	L4, L5, S1 nerve root irritation
Femoral stretch test	L1, L2, L3, L4 nerve root irritation
Ballottement	Effusion or excess fluid in knee
Bulge sign	Excess fluid in knee
McMurray test	Torn meniscus in knee
Anterior and posterior drawer test	Anterior and posterior cruciate ligament integrity
Varus/valgus stress test	Mediolateral collateral ligament instability in knee
Lachman test	Anterior cruciate ligament integrity
Apley test	Torn meniscus in knee
Thomas test	Flexion contracture of hip
Trendelenburg sign	Weak hip abductor muscles

A 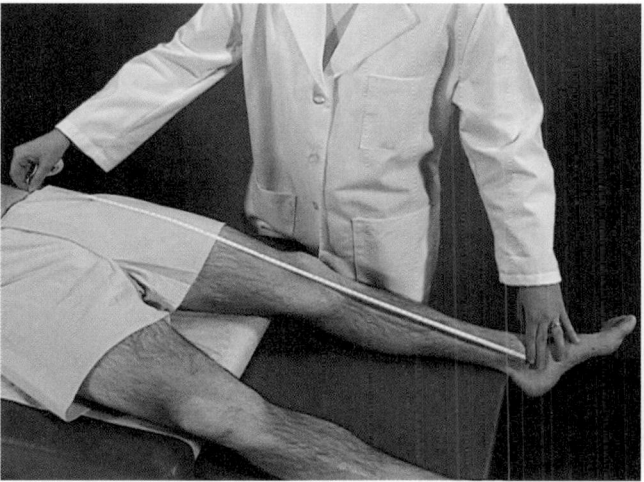 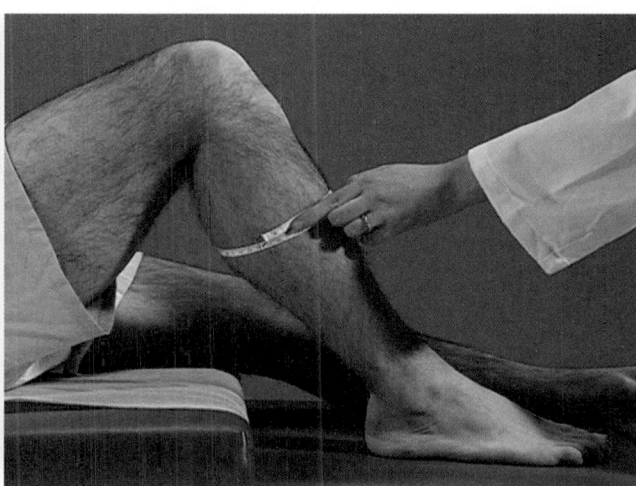 B

FIGURE 21-42
Measuring **(A)** limb length and **(B)** leg circumference.

SHOULDER ASSESSMENT

Several procedures are used to evaluate the rotator cuff for impingement (tendinitis or overuse injury from repetitive overhead activities) or a tear.

The *Neer test* is performed by having the patient internally rotate the shoulder while the examiner forward flexes the arm up to 150 degrees. This presses the supraspinatus muscle against the anteroinferior acromion. Increased shoulder pain is associated with rotator cuff inflammation or a tear (Fig. 21-43, *A*).

The Hawkins test is performed by forward flexing the shoulder to 90 degrees, flexing the elbow to 90 degrees, and then internally rotating the arm to its limit. Increased shoulder pain is associated with rotator cuff inflammation or a tear (Fig. 21-43, *B*).

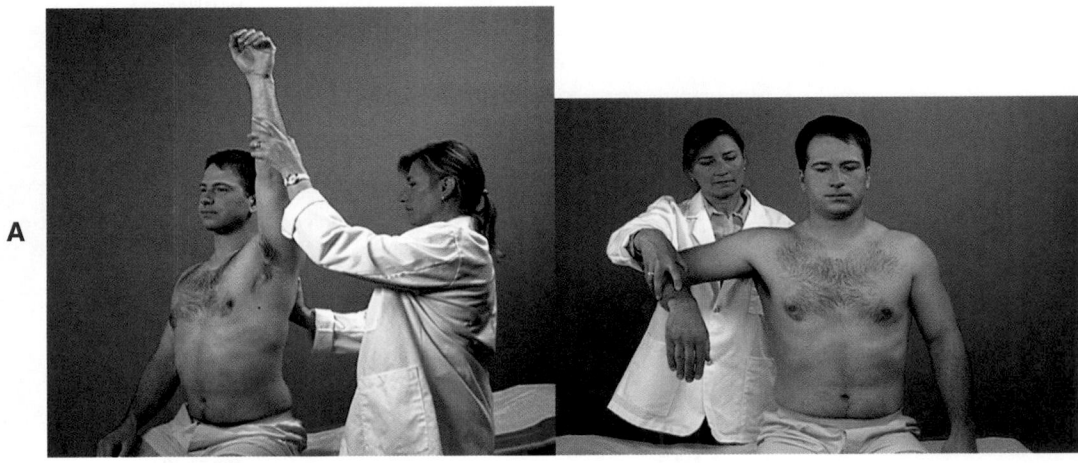

FIGURE 21-43
Assessment for rotator cuff inflammation or tear. **A,** Neer test. **B,** Hawkins test.

EVIDENCE-BASED PRACTICE IN PHYSICAL EXAMINATION
CARPAL TUNNEL SYNDROME

The likelihood that a patient will have a positive electrodiagnostic study for carpal tunnel syndrome is increased by the following: a positive flick test; a classic or probable distribution of symptoms on the Katz hand diagram (see p. 729); hypalgesia (decreased pain sensation along the thumb and median nerve distribution when compared to the little finger on the same hand); and weak thumb abduction. The Tinel and Phelan tests are less accurate.

Data from D'Arcy, McGee, 2000.

To test the strength of the rotator cuff muscles, perform the following maneuvers. Pain and weakness with opposing force is an unexpected finding and may be associated with inflammation or a tear.

For the supraspinatus muscle of the rotator cuff, have the patient abduct the arms 90 degrees and flex the shoulders forward 30 degrees. Apply downward pressure on the distal humerus when the arms are rotated so that thumbs point down or up.

For the subscapularis muscle, have the patient hold the arm at the side, elbow flexed 90 degrees, and rotate the forearm medially against resistance.

For the infraspinatus and teres minor muscles, have the patient hold the arm at the side, elbow flexed 90 degrees, and rotate the arm laterally against resistance.

HAND AND WRIST ASSESSMENT

Several procedures are used to evaluate the integrity of the median nerve, which innervates the palm of the hand and the palmar surface of the thumb, index and middle fingers, and half of the ring finger. Ask the patient to mark the specific locations of pain, numbness, and tingling on the Katz hand diagram (Fig. 21-44). Certain patterns of pain, numbness, and tingling are associated with carpal tunnel syndrome.

The *flick test* is performed by asking the patient what maneuver is used when symptoms of hand pain, numbness, and tingling are at their worst. If the patient demonstrates a flicking movement of the wrist and hand, similar to that used in shaking down a thermometer, it is a positive sign.

The *thumb abduction test* isolates the strength of the abductor pollicis brevis muscle, innervated only by the median nerve. Have the patient place the hand palm up and raise the thumb perpendicular to it. Apply downward pressure on the thumb to test muscle strength (Fig. 21-45, *A*). Full resistance to pressure is expected. Weakness is associated with carpal tunnel syndrome.

Classic pattern
Symptoms affect at least two of digits 1, 2, or 3. The classic pattern permits symptoms in the fourth and fifth digits, wrist pain, and radiation of pain proximal to the wrist, but it does not allow symptoms on the palm or dorsum of the hand.

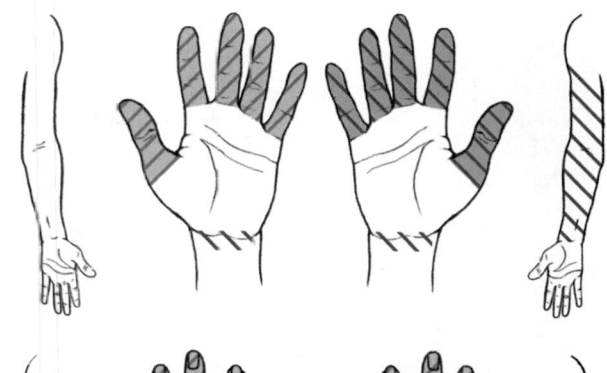
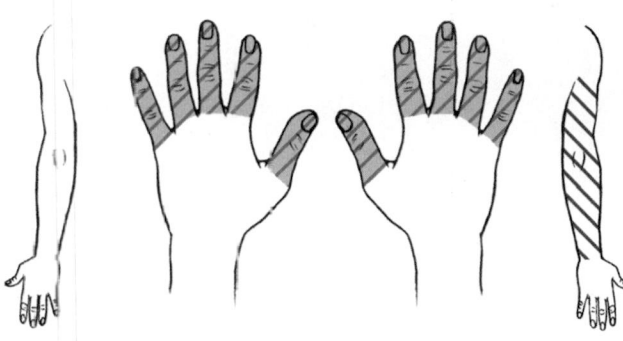

Probable pattern
Same symptom pattern as classic, except palmar symptoms are allowed unless confined solely to the ulnar aspect. In the **possible pattern,** not shown, symptoms involve only 1 of digits 1, 2, or 3.

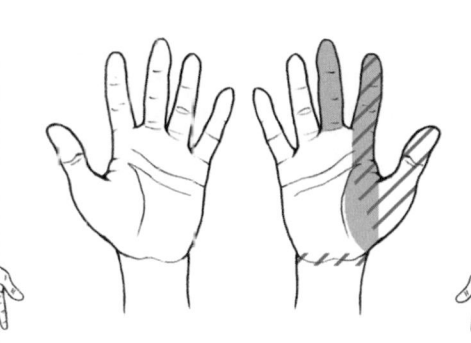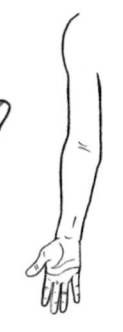

B

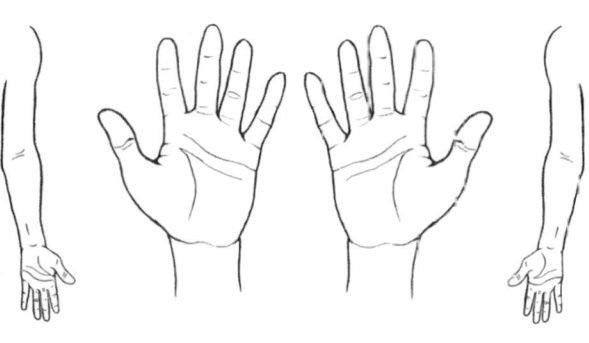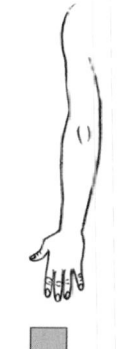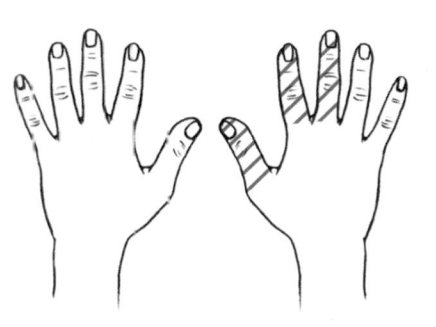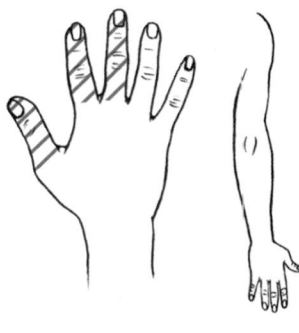

Numbness   Pain   Tingling   Decreased sensation

A

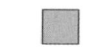
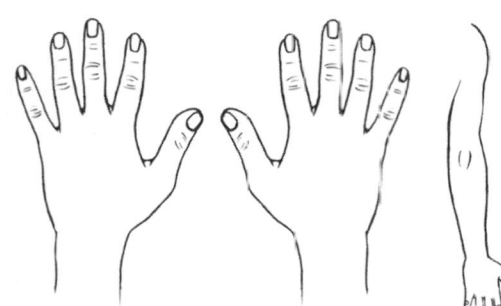

FIGURE 21-44
Assessment for carpal tunnel syndrome. **A,** Katz hand diagram. **B,** Classic and probable patterns of pain, tingling, and numbness using the Katz hand diagram.
From D'Arcy, McGee, 2000.

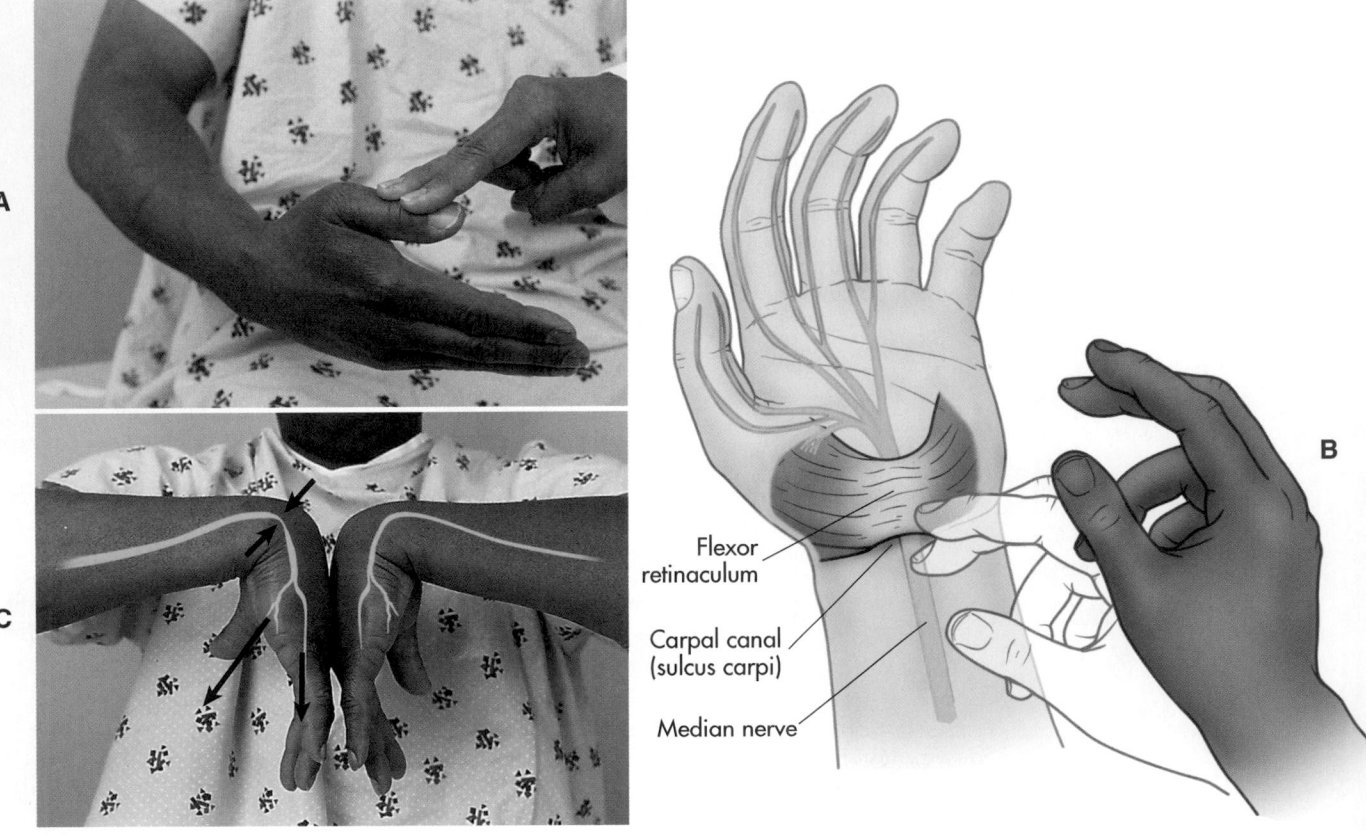

FIGURE 21-45
Additional procedures for assessment of carpal tunnel syndrome. **A,** Thumb abduction test. **B,** Elicitation of Tinel sign. **C,** Phalen test.

Tinel sign is tested by striking the patient's wrist with your index or middle finger where the median nerve passes under the flexor retinaculum and volar carpal ligament (Fig. 21-45, *B*). A tingling sensation radiating from the wrist to the hand in the distribution of the median nerve is a positive Tinel sign and is suggestive of carpal tunnel syndrome.

To evaluate *Phalen test,* ask the patient to hold both wrists in a fully palmar-flexed position with the dorsal surfaces pressed together for 1 minute (Fig. 21-45, *C*). Numbness and paresthesia in the distribution of the median nerve is suggestive of carpal tunnel syndrome.

LOWER SPINE ASSESSMENT

The *straight leg raising test* is used to test for nerve root irritation or lumbar disk herniation at the L4, L5, and S1 levels. Have the patient lie supine with the neck slightly flexed. Ask the patient to raise the leg, keeping the knee extended (see Fig. 21-36, *A*). No pain should be felt below the knee with leg raising. Pain below the knee in a dermatome pattern may be associated with disk herniation. *Lasègue sign* is positive when the patient is unable to raise the leg more than 30 degrees without pain. Flexion of the knee often eliminates the pain with leg raising. Repeat the procedure on the unaffected leg. Crossover pain in the affected leg with this maneuver is more supportive of the finding of tension on the nerve roots.

The *Bragard stretch test* also tests for lumbar disk herniation at the L4, L5, and S1 levels. Have the patient lie supine with the neck slightly flexed. Hold the patient's lower leg and raise it slowly with the knee extended until the patient feels pain. Lower the leg slightly and briskly dorsiflex the foot and internally rotate the leg. Ask the patient to locate the most distal point of pain. Pain below the knee when the leg is raised less than 70 degrees and aggravated by dorsiflexion and internal rotation of the hip is associated with a herniated disk at the L5 or S1 level (Fig. 21-46). With the patient sitting and leaning slightly forward, ask the patient to extend the leg at the knee while you apply resistance. Pain with extension or resistance, and attempts to lean backward to reduce tension on the nerve is a positive sign of sciatic nerve tenderness.

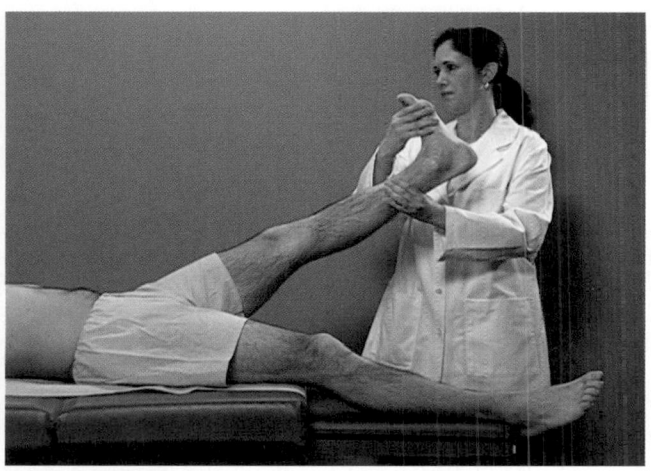

FIGURE 21-46
Bragard stretch test for lumbar nerve root irritation.

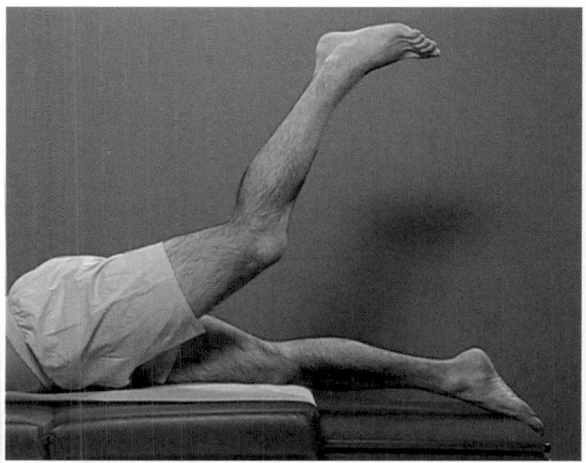

FIGURE 21-47
Femoral stretch test for high lumbar nerve root irritation.

EVIDENCE-BASED PRACTICE IN PHYSICAL EXAMINATION

HERNIATED DISK

When a straight leg raising test performed on the affected extremity reproduces or worsens the patient's radiating pain below the knee, the positive finding is 80% sensitive, but only 40% specific for a herniated disk. When the straight leg raising test is performed on the contralateral unsymptomatic extremity and sciatic pain is elicited in the affected leg, this positive finding is only 25% sensitive but 90% specific. The two maneuvers used together increases the accuracy of the herniated disk diagnosis (Defer, 2004).

The *femoral stretch test* or hip extension test is used to detect inflammation of the nerve root at the L1, L2, L3, and sometimes L4 level. Have the patient lie prone and extend the hip. No pain is expected. The presence of pain on extension is a positive sign of nerve root irritation (Fig. 21-47).

KNEE ASSESSMENT

Ballottement is used to determine the presence of excess fluid or an effusion in the knee. With the knee extended, apply downward pressure on the suprapatellar pouch with the web or the thumb and forefinger of one hand, and then push the patella sharply downward against the femur with a finger of your other hand. If an effusion is present, a tapping or clicking will be sensed when the patella is pushed against the femur. Release the pressure against the patella, but keep your finger lightly touching it. If an effusion is present, the patella will float out as if a fluid wave were pushing it (Fig. 21-48).

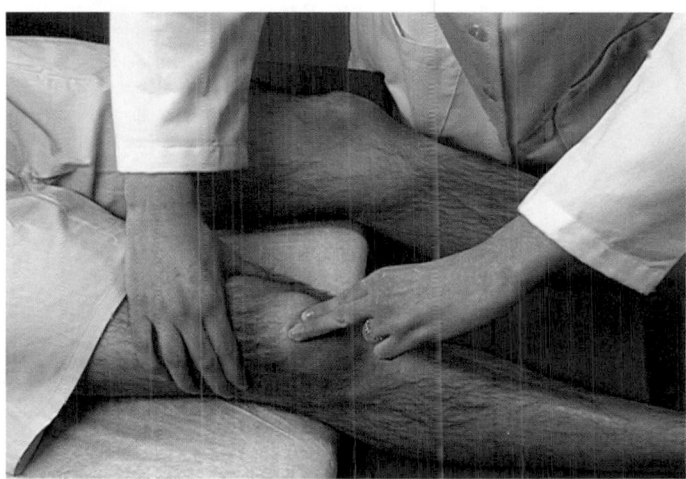

FIGURE 21-48
Procedure for ballottement examination of the knee.

Examination for the *bulge sign* is also used to determine the presence of excess fluid in the knee. With the patient's knee extended, milk the medial aspect of the knee upward two or three times, and then tap the lateral side of the patella. Observe for a bulge of returning fluid to the hollow area medial to the patella (Fig. 21-49).

The *McMurray test* is used to detect a torn medial or lateral meniscus. Have the patient lie supine and flex one knee. Position your thumb and fingers on either side of the joint space. Hold the heel with your other hand, fully flexing the knee, and rotate the foot and knee outward (valgus stress) to a lateral position. Extend and flex the patient's knee. Any palpable or audible click, grinding, pain, or limited extension of the knee is a positive sign of a torn medial meniscus. Repeat the procedure, rotating the foot and knee inward (varus stress) (Fig. 21-50). A palpable or audible click, pain, grinding, or lack of extension is a positive sign of a torn lateral meniscus.

The anterior and posterior *drawer test* is used to identify instability of the anterior and posterior cruciate ligaments. Have the patient lie supine and flex the knee 45 to 90 degrees, placing the foot flat on the table. Place both hands on the lower leg with the thumbs on the ridge of the anterior tibia just distal to the tibial tuberosity. Draw the tibia forward, forcing the tibia to slide forward of the femur. Then push the tibia backward (Fig. 21-51). Anterior or posterior movement of the knee greater than 5 mm in either direction is an unexpected finding.

A 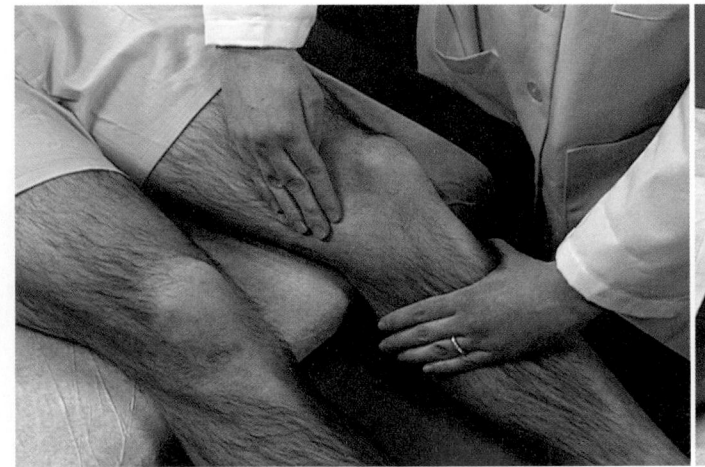 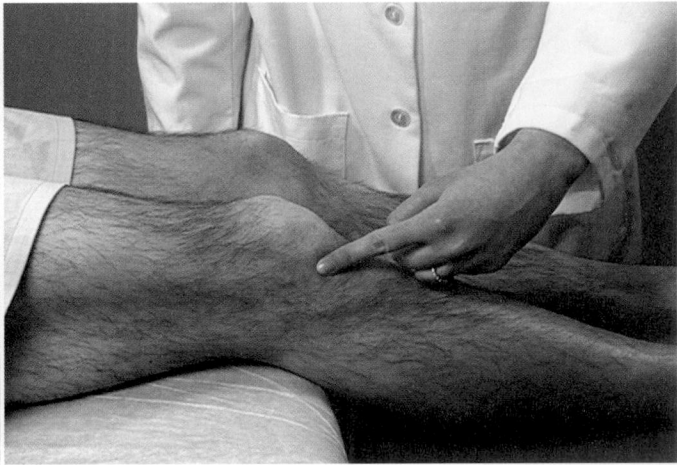 B

FIGURE 21-49
Testing for the bulge sign in examination of the knee. **A,** Milk the medial aspect of the knee two or three times. **B,** Tap the lateral side of the patella.

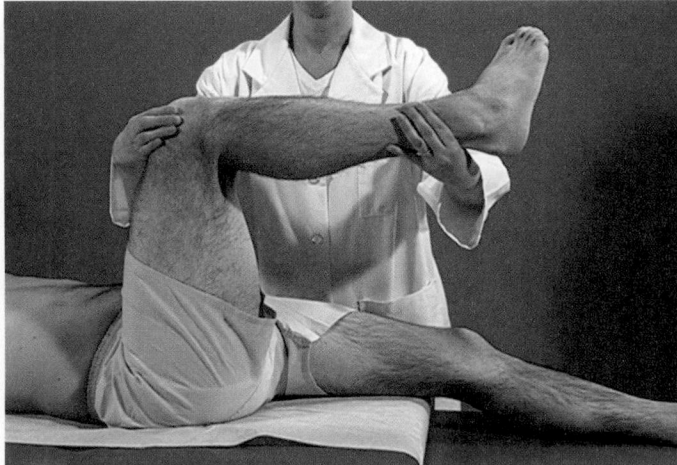

FIGURE 21-50
Procedure for examination of the knee with the McMurray test. Knee is flexed after lower leg was rotated to medial position.

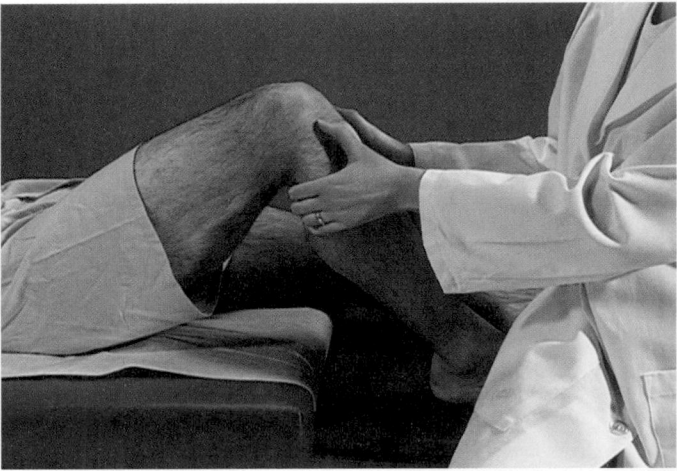

FIGURE 21-51
Examination of the knee with the drawer test for anterior and posterior stability.

The *Lachman test* is used to evaluate anterior cruciate ligament integrity. With the patient supine, flex the knee 10 to 15 degrees with the heel on the table. Place one hand above the knee to stabilize the femur and place the other hand around the proximal tibia. While stabilizing the femur, pull the tibia anteriorly. Attempt to have the patient relax the hamstring muscles for an optimal test. Increased laxity, greater than 5 mm compared to the uninjured side, indicates injury to the ligament.

The *varus (abduction) and valgus (adduction) stress test* is used to identify instability of the lateral and medial collateral ligaments. Have the patient lie supine and extend the knee. Stabilize the femur with one hand and hold the ankle with your other hand. Apply varus force against the ankle (toward the midline) and internal rotation. Excessive laxity is felt as joint opening. Laxity in this position indicates injury to the lateral collateral ligament. Then apply valgus force against the ankle (away from the midline) and external rotation. Laxity in this position indicates injury to the medial collateral ligament (Fig. 21-52). Repeat the movements with the patient's knee flexed to 30 degrees. No excessive medial or lateral movement of the knee is expected.

When the patient complains of a knee locking, use the *Apley test* to detect a meniscal tear. Have the patient lie prone and flex the knee to 90 degrees. Place your hand on the heel of the foot and press firmly, opposing the tibia to the femur. Then rotate the lower leg externally and internally (Fig. 21-53). Be cautious and do not cause the patient excess pain. Any clicks, locking, or pain in the knee is a positive Apley sign.

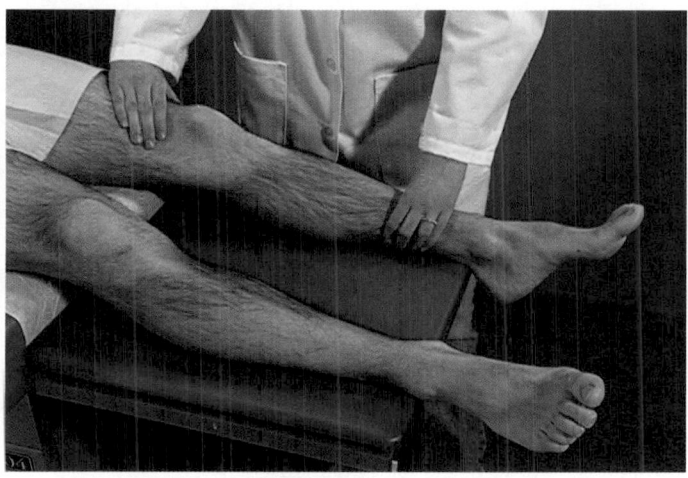

FIGURE 21-52
Valgus stress test of the knee with knee extended.

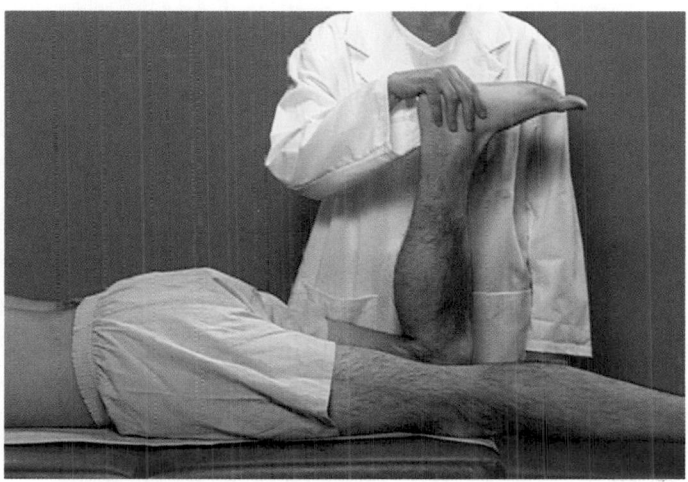

FIGURE 21-53
Examination of the knee with the Apley test.

HIP ASSESSMENT

The *Thomas test* is used to detect flexion contractures of the hip that may be masked by excessive lumbar lordosis. Have the patient lie supine; fully extend one leg flat on the examining table and flex the other leg with the knee to the chest. Observe the patient's ability to keep the extended leg flat on the examining table (Fig. 21-54). Lifting the extended leg off the examining table indicates a hip flexion contracture in the extended leg.

The *Trendelenburg test* is a maneuver to detect weak hip abductor muscles. Ask the patient to stand and balance first on one foot and then the other. Observing from behind, note any asymmetry or change in the level of the iliac crests. When the iliac crest drops on the side of the lifted leg, the hip abductor muscles on the weight-bearing side are weak (Fig. 21-55).

INFANTS

Genetic and fetal insults can produce musculoskeletal anomalies. The fetus is exposed to various postural pressures that can be manifested in the infant as reduced extension of extremities and torsions of various bones.

Fully undress the infant and observe the posture and spontaneous generalized movements. (Use a warming table when examining a newborn.) No localized or generalized muscular twitching is expected. Inspect the back for tufts of hair, dimples, discolorations, cysts, or masses near the spine. A mass near the spine that transilluminates should cause you to suspect a meningocele or myelomeningocele.

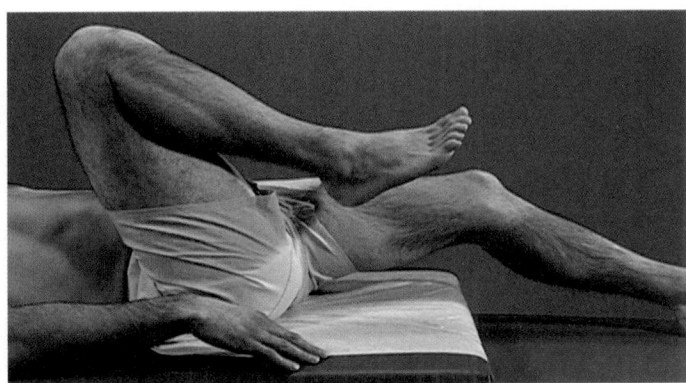

FIGURE 21-54
Procedures for examination of the hip with the Thomas test. Note the elevation of the extended leg off the examining table.

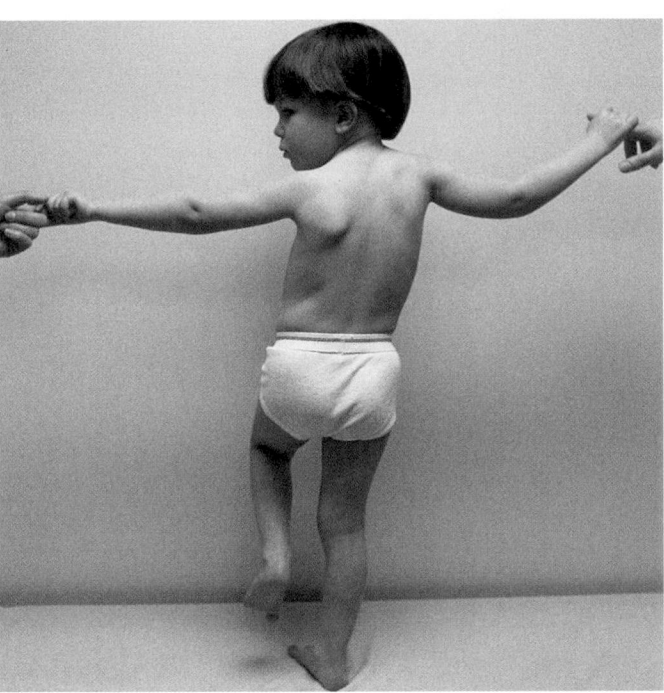

FIGURE 21-55
Test for the Trendelenburg sign. Note any asymmetry in the level of the iliac crests with weight bearing.

From about age 2 months the infant should be able to lift the head and trunk from the prone position, giving you an indication of forearm strength. Assess the curvature of the spine and the strength of the paravertebral muscles with the infant in sitting position. Kyphosis of the thoracic and lumbar spine will be apparent in sitting position until the infant can sit without support (Fig. 21-56).

Inspect the extremities, noting symmetric flexion of arms and legs. The axillary, gluteal, femoral, and popliteal creases should be symmetric, and the limbs should be freely movable. No unusual proportions or asymmetry of limb length or circumference, constricted annular bands, or other deformities should be noted. Unequal limb length and circumference have been associated with intraabdominal neoplasms.

Place the newborn in a fetal position to observe how that may have contributed to any asymmetry of flexion, position, or shape of the extremities. Newborns have some resistance to full extension of the elbows, hips, and knees. Movements should be symmetric.

All infants are flat-footed, and many newborns have a slight varus curvature of the tibias (tibial torsion) or forefoot adduction (metatarsus adductus) from fetal positioning. The midline of the foot may bisect the third and fourth toes, rather than the second and third toes. The forefoot should be flexible, straightening with abduction. It is necessary to follow apparent problems carefully, but it is seldom necessary to intervene. As growth and development take place, the expected body habitus is usually achieved.

The hands should open periodically with the fingers fully extended. When the hand is fisted, the thumb should be positioned inside the fingers. Open the fist and observe the dermatoglyphic features, noting the palmar and phalangeal creases on each hand. A Simian crease—a single crease extending across the entire palm—is associated with Down syndrome. Count the fingers and toes, noting polydactyly or syndactyly (Fig. 21-57).

Palpate the clavicles and long bones for fractures, dislocations, crepitus, masses, and tenderness. One of the most easily missed findings in the newborn is a fractured clavicle. It is embarrassing to have a parent ask what that lump is on the baby's collarbone. It is the callus that forms as the healing clavicle shapes and remolds itself. The telltale bony irregularity and crepitus is better detected during the neonatal examination.

Position the baby with the trunk flexed and palpate each spinal process. Feel the shape of each, noting whether it is thin and well formed, as expected, or whether it is split, possibly indicating a bifid defect (Fig. 21-58).

Palpate the muscles to evaluate muscle tone, grasping the muscle to estimate its firmness. Observe for spasticity or flaccidity and, when detected, determine whether it is localized or generalized. Use passive range of motion to examine joint mobility.

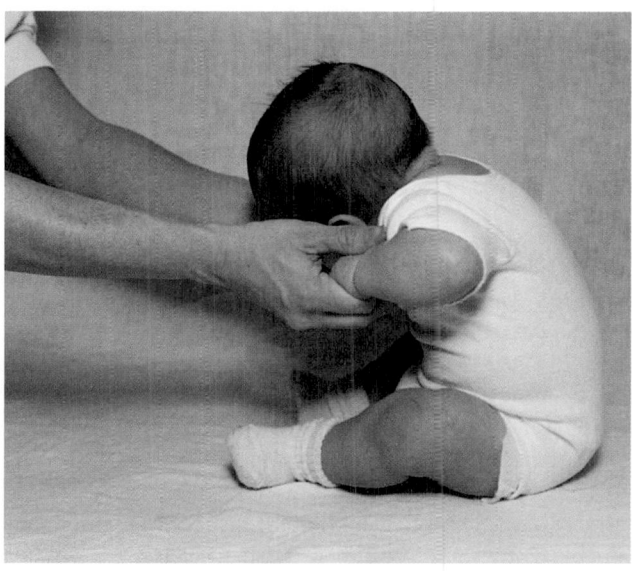

FIGURE 21-56
Kyphosis, expected convex curvature of the newborn's thoracic and lumbar spine.

A   B   C

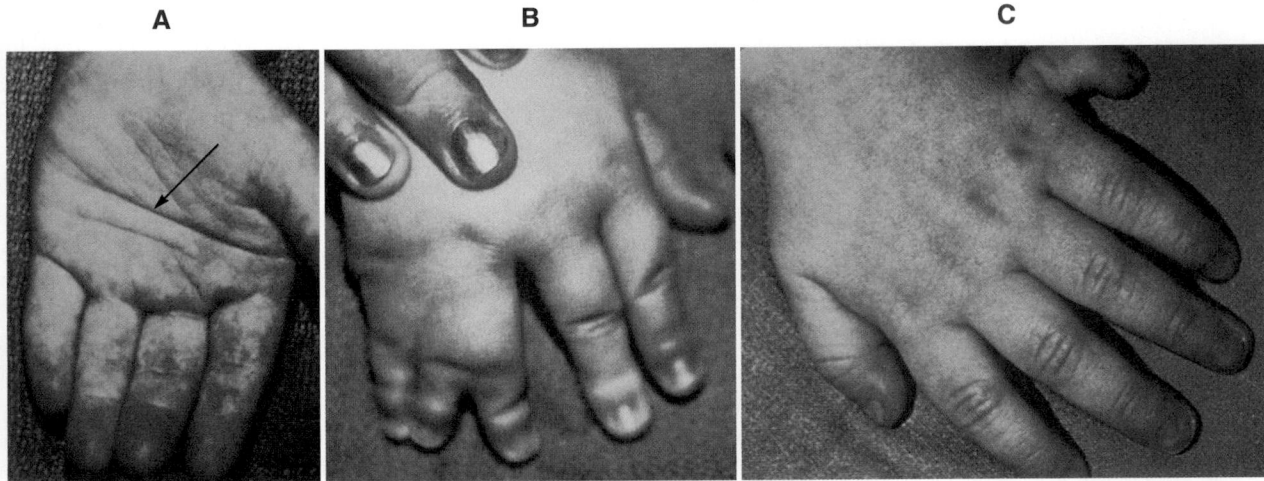

FIGURE 21-57
Anomalies of the newborn's hand. **A,** Simian crease. **B,** Syndactyly. **C,** Polydactyly.
Courtesy Mead Johnson, Evansville, IN.

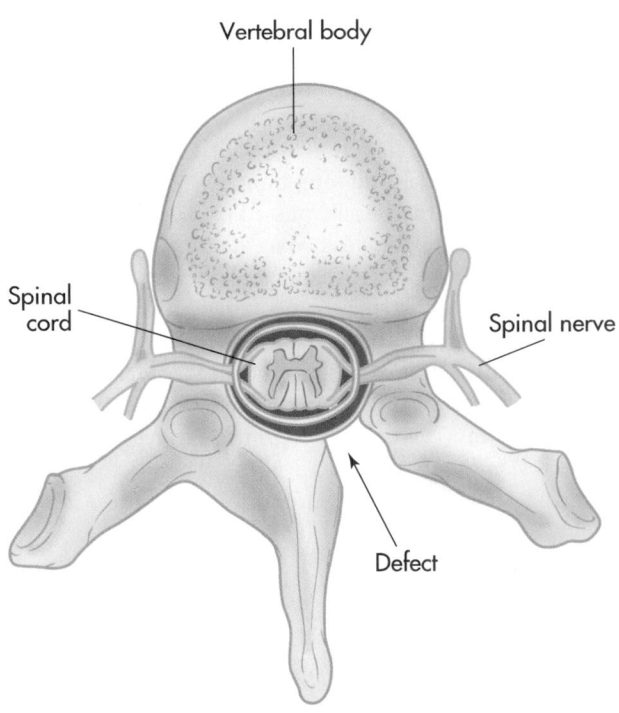

Vertebral body

Spinal
cord

Spinal nerve

Defect

FIGURE 21-58
Bifid defect of the vertebra
identified by palpation.

The *Barlow-Ortolani maneuver* to detect hip dislocation or subluxation should be performed each time you examine the infant during the first year of life. Using little force, test one hip at a time, stabilizing the pelvis with the other hand. Position yourself at the supine infant's feet, and flex the hip and knee to 90 degrees. For the Barlow maneuver, grasp the leg with your thumb on the inside of the thigh, the base of the thumb on the knee, and your fingers gripping the outer thigh with fingertips resting on the greater trochanter (Fig. 21-59). Adduct the thigh and gently apply downward pressure on the femur in an attempt to disengage the femoral head from the acetabulum. A clunk or sensation may be felt if the femoral head exits the acetabulum posteriorly, a positive sign. For the Ortolani maneuver, slowly abduct the thigh while maintaining axial pressure. With the fingertips on the greater trochanter, exert a lever movement in the opposite direction so that your fingertips press the head of the femur back toward the acetabulum center. If the head of the femur slips back into the acetabulum with a palpable clunk when pressure is exerted, suspect hip subluxation or dislocation. High-pitched clicks are common and expected. By 3 months of age, muscles and ligaments tighten, and lim-

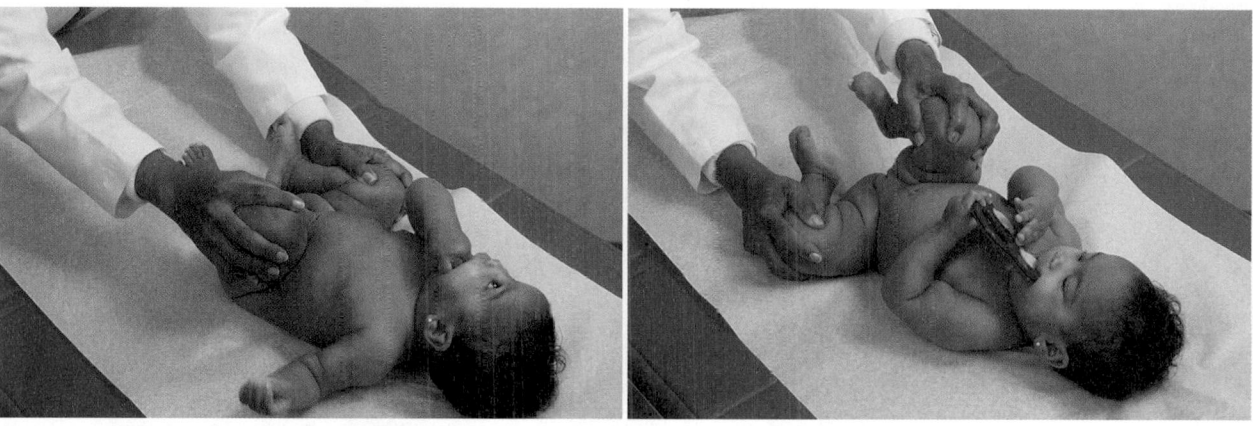

FIGURE 21-59
Barlow-Ortolani maneuver to detect hip dislocation. **A,** Phase I, adduction. **B,** Phase II, abduction.

FIGURE 21-60
Signs of hip dislocation: limitation of abduction and asymmetric gluteal folds.

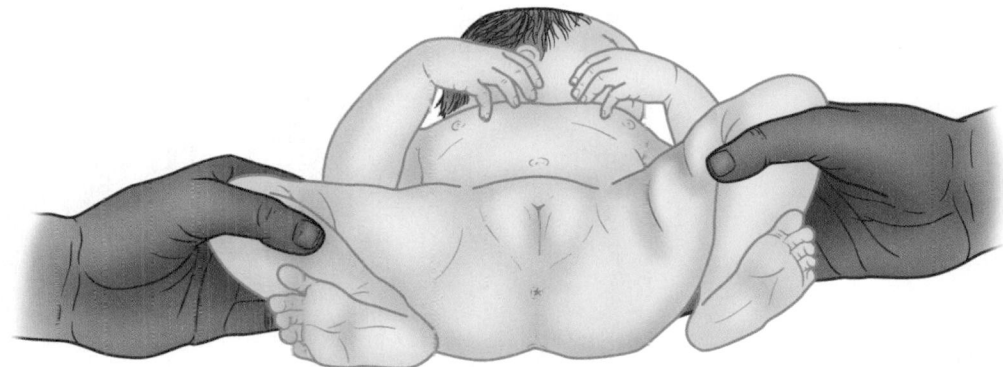

FIGURE 21-61
Examination for the Allis sign. Unequal upper leg length would indicate a positive sign.

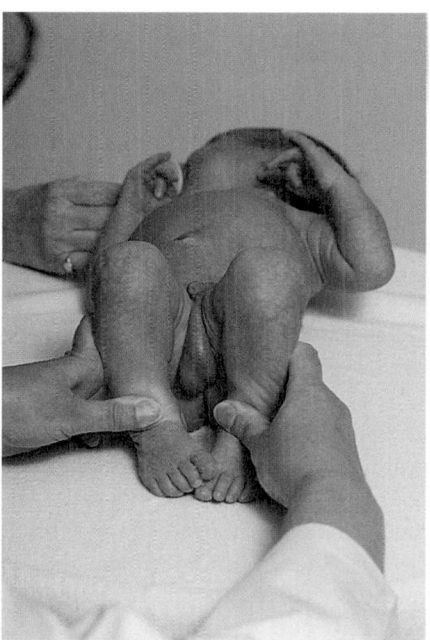

ited abduction of the hips becomes the most reliable sign of hip subluxation or dislocation (Fig. 21-60).

The test for the *Allis sign* is also used to detect hip dislocation or a shortened femur. With the infant supine on the examining table, flex both knees, keeping the feet flat on the table and the femurs aligned with each other. Position yourself at the child's feet, and observe the height of the knees (Fig. 21-61). When one knee appears lower than the other, the Allis sign is positive.

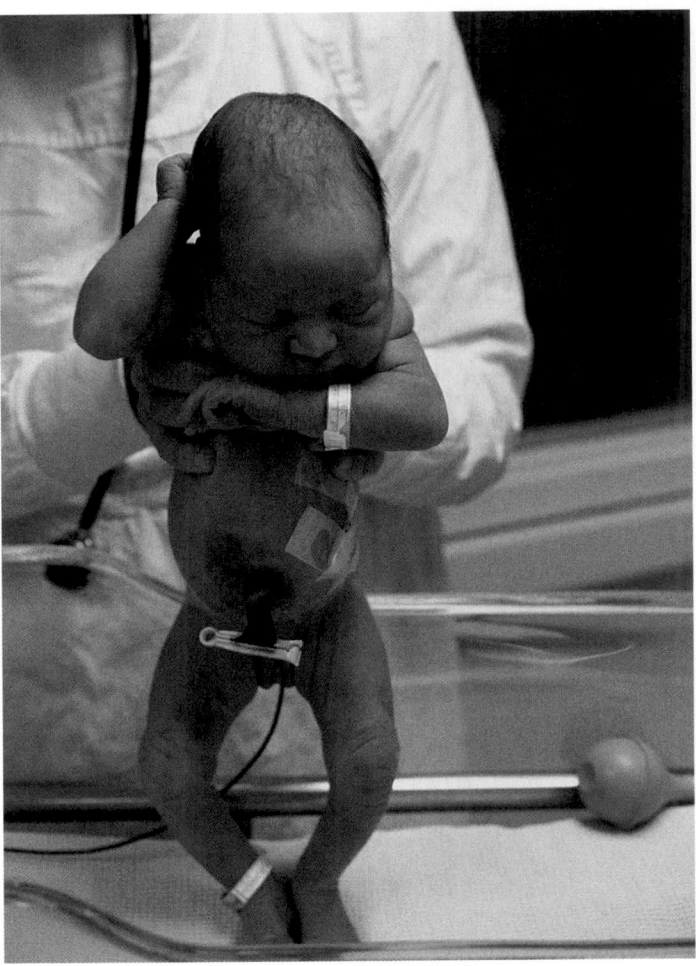

FIGURE 21-62
Evaluation of shoulder muscle strength in the newborn.

Muscle strength is evaluated by holding the infant upright with your hands under the axillae (Fig. 21-62). Adequate shoulder muscle strength is present if the infant maintains the upright position. If the infant begins to slip through your fingers, muscle weakness is present.

Tibial torsion is evaluated with the child prone on the examining table. Flex one knee 90 degrees and align the midline of the foot parallel to the femur. Using the thumb and index finger of one hand, grasp the medial and lateral malleoli of the ankle; grasp the knee, placing your thumb and index finger on the same side of the leg (Fig. 21-63). If your thumbs are not parallel to each other, tibial torsion is present. Tibial torsion, a residual effect of fetal positioning, is expected to resolve after 6 months of weight bearing.

CHILDREN

Watching young children during play or while they are with the parent as the history is taken can provide a great deal of information about the child's musculoskeletal system. If the child has been able to pick up and play with toys, moving in unconstrained fashion without evidence of limitation, the laying on of hands—though still necessary—may not reveal any additional information. Suggest activities that will enhance your observations. The function of joints, range of motion, bone stability, and muscle strength can be adequately evaluated by observing the child climb, jump, hop, rise from a sitting position, and manipulate toys or other objects.

Position the young child to observe motor development and musculoskeletal function. Inspect the spine of the child while he or she is standing. Young children will have a lumbar curvature of the spine and a protuberant abdomen (Fig. 21-64). Observe the toddler's ability to sit, creep, and grasp and release objects during play. Knowledge of the expected sequence of motor development (Table 21-4) will facilitate your examination.

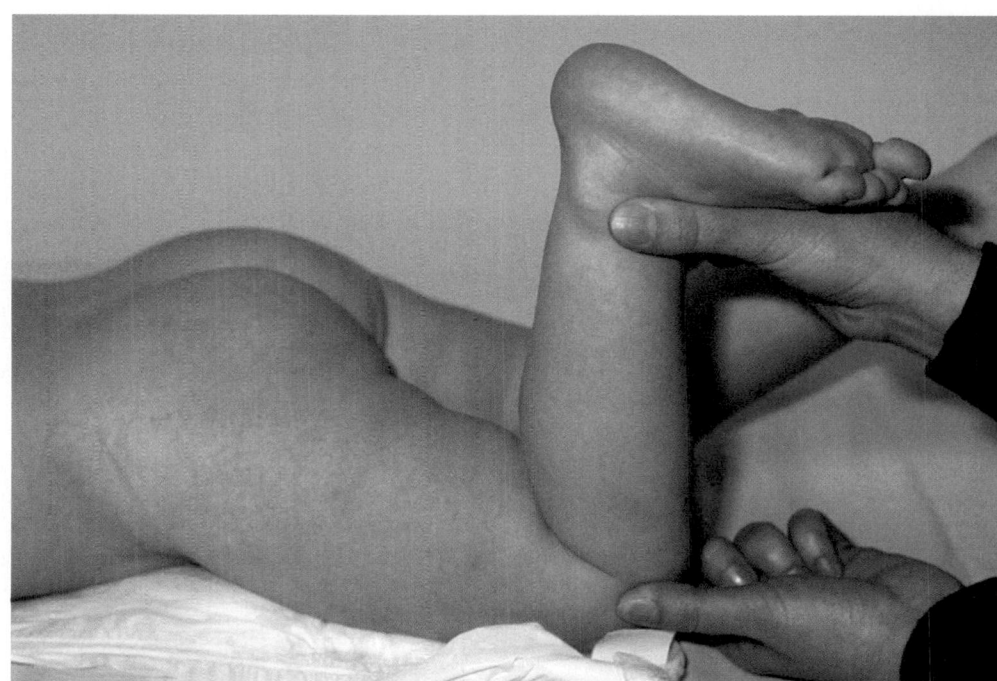

FIGURE 21-63
Examination for tibial torsion.

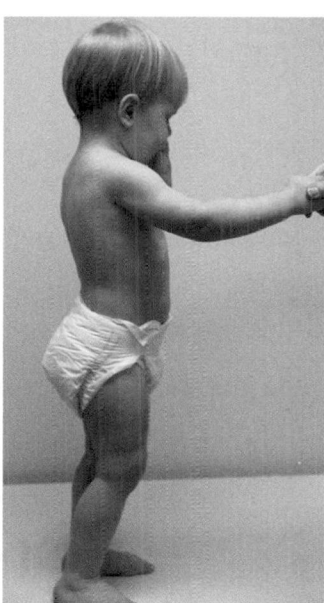

FIGURE 21-64
Lumbar curvature of the toddler's spine.

The motor development of black infants is often advanced over that of white infants; thus black children younger than 3 years of age may reach the milestones outlined in Table 21-4 before white children. White children start to catch up with black children around 3 years of age. As you inspect the bones, joints, and muscles, pay particular attention to the alignment of the legs and feet because developmental stresses are placed on the musculoskeletal system. Remember to observe the wear of the child's shoes and ask about his or her favorite sitting posture. The W or reverse tailor position places stress on the joints of the hips, knees, and ankles. It is commonly seen in children with intoeing associated with femoral anteversion (Fig. 21-65).

Inspect the longitudinal arch of the foot and the position of the feet with weight bearing. A fat pad obscures the longitudinal arch of the foot until about 3 years of age; after that time it should be apparent when the foot is not bearing weight. Metatarsus adductus should be resolved. The feet of the toddler will often pronate slightly inward until about 30 months of age. After that time, weight bearing should shift to the midline of the feet.

TABLE 21-4	Expected Motor Development Sequence in Children, Birth to 9 Years of Age	
Age	**Fine Motor Development**	**Gross Motor Development**
1 month		Turns head to side; keeps knees tucked under abdomen; gross head lag and rounded back when pulled to sitting position
2 months		Holds head in same plane as rest of body; can raise head and hold position
3 months	When supine, puts hands together; holds hands in front of face	Raises head to 45 degrees; may turn from prone to side position; slight head lag when pulled to sitting position
4 months	Grasps rattle; hands held together	Actively lifts head, looks around; rolls from prone to supine position; no head lag when pulled to sitting position; attempts to bear weight when held standing up
5 months	Can reach and pick up object; plays with toes	Able to push up from prone position with forearms and maintain position; rolls over prone to supine to prone; back straight when sitting
6 months	Drops object to reach for another offered; holds rattle or spoon	Sits, posture shaky, uses tripod position; raises abdomen off table when prone; when standing, supports almost full weight
7 months	Transfers object between hands; holds object in each hand	Uses hands for support; bounces in standing position; pulls feet to mouth
8 months	Begins thumb-finger grasping	Sits without support
9 months	Bangs objects together	Begins creeping, abdomen off floor; stands holding on when placed in position
10 months	Points with one finger; picks up small objects	Pulls self to standing position, unable to let self down; walks holding on to stable objects
11 months		Walks around room holding on to objects; stands securely, holding on with one hand
12 months	Feeds self with cup and spoon fairly well; offers toy and releases it	Sits from standing posture; twists and turns, maintaining posture; stands without support momentarily
15 months	Puts raisin into bottle; takes off shoes; pulls toys	Walks alone well; seats self in chair
18 months	Holds crayon, scribbles spontaneously	Walks up and down steps holding one hand, some running ability
2 years	Turns doorknob; takes off shoes and socks; builds 2-block tower	Walks up stairs alone, two feet on each step; walks backward; kicks ball
30 months	Builds 4-block tower; feeds self more neatly; dumps raisin from bottle	Jumps from object; throws ball overhand; walking more stable
3 years	Unbuttons front buttons; copies vertical line within 30 degrees; copies circle; builds 8-block tower	Walks up stairs alternating feet; walks down steps two feet on each step; pedals tricycle; jumps in one place; performs broad jump
4 years	Copies cross; buttons large buttons	Walks down stairs alternating feet; balances on one foot for 5 seconds
5 years	Dresses self with minimal assistance; colors within lines; draws 3-part human	Hops on one foot; catches bounced ball 2 of 3 times; heel-toe walking
6 years	Copies square; draws 6-part human	Jumps, tumbles, skips, hops; walks straight line; skips rope with practice; rides bicycle; heel-toe walking backward
7 years	Prints well, begins to write script	Skips and plays hopscotch; running and climbing more coordinated
8 years	Mature handwriting skill	Movements more graceful
9 years		Eye-hand coordination developed

Bowleg (genu varum) is evaluated with the child standing, facing you, knees at your eye level. Measure the distance between the knees when the medial malleoli of the ankles are together. Genu varum is present if a space of 2.5 cm (1 inch) exists between the knees. The expected 10- to 15-degree angle at the tibiofemoral articulation increases with genu varum but remains bilaterally symmetric. On future examinations, note any increase in the angle or increased space between the knees. Genu varum is a common finding of toddlers until 18 months of age. Asymmetry of the tibiofemoral articulation angle or space between the knees should not exceed 4 cm ($1\frac{1}{2}$ inches).

Knock-knee (genu valgum) is also evaluated with the child standing, facing you, knees at your eye level. With the knees together, measure the distance between the medial malleoli of

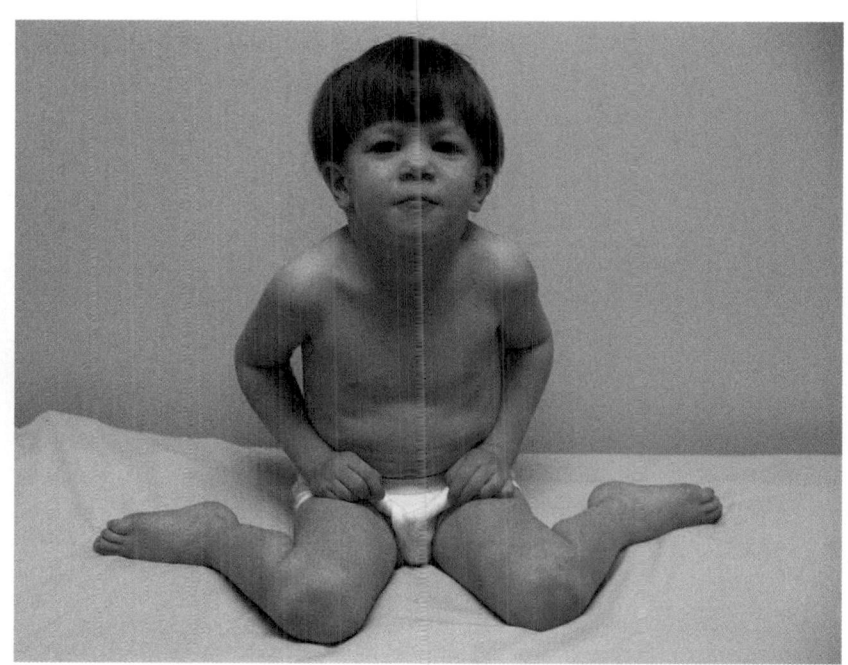

FIGURE 21-65
Reverse tailor sitting position.

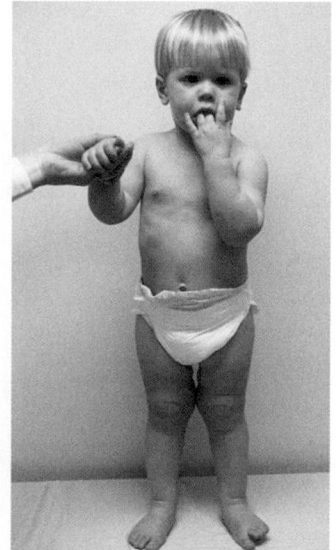

FIGURE 21-66
Genu valgum (knock-knee) in the young child.

the ankles. Genu valgum is present if a space of 2.5 cm (1 inch) exists between the medial malleoli. As with genu varum, the tibiofemoral articulation angle will increase with genu valgum. On future examinations, note any increase in the angle or increased space between the ankles. Genu valgum is a common finding of children between 2 and 4 years of age (Fig. 21-66). Asymmetry of the tibiofemoral articulation angle or a space between the medial malleoli should not exceed 5 cm (2 inches).

Palpate the bones, muscles, and joints, paying particular attention to asymmetric body parts. Use passive range of motion to examine a joint and muscle group if some limitation of movement is noted while the child is playing.

Ask the child to stand, rising from a supine position. The child with good muscle strength will rise to a standing position without using the arms for leverage. Generalized muscle weakness is indicated by the *Gower sign* in which the child rises from a sitting position by placing hands on the legs and pushing the trunk up (Fig. 21-67).

ADOLESCENTS

Examine older children and adolescents with the same procedures used for adults. Specific procedures for the musculoskeletal examination for sports participation are found in Chapter 23.

The spine should be smooth with balanced concave and convex curves. No lateral curvature or rib hump with forward flexion should be apparent. The shoulders and scapulae should be level with each other within ½ inch, and a distance between the scapulae of 3 to 5 inches is usual (see Fig. 21-12, *B*). Adolescents may have slight kyphosis and rounded shoulders with an interscapular space of 5 or 6 inches.

PREGNANT WOMEN

Postural changes with pregnancy are common. The growing fetus shifts the woman's center of gravity forward, leading to increased lordosis and a compensatory forward cervical flexion (Fig. 21-68). Stooped shoulders and large breasts exaggerate the spinal curvature. Increased mobility and instability of the sacroiliac joints and symphysis pubis as the ligaments become

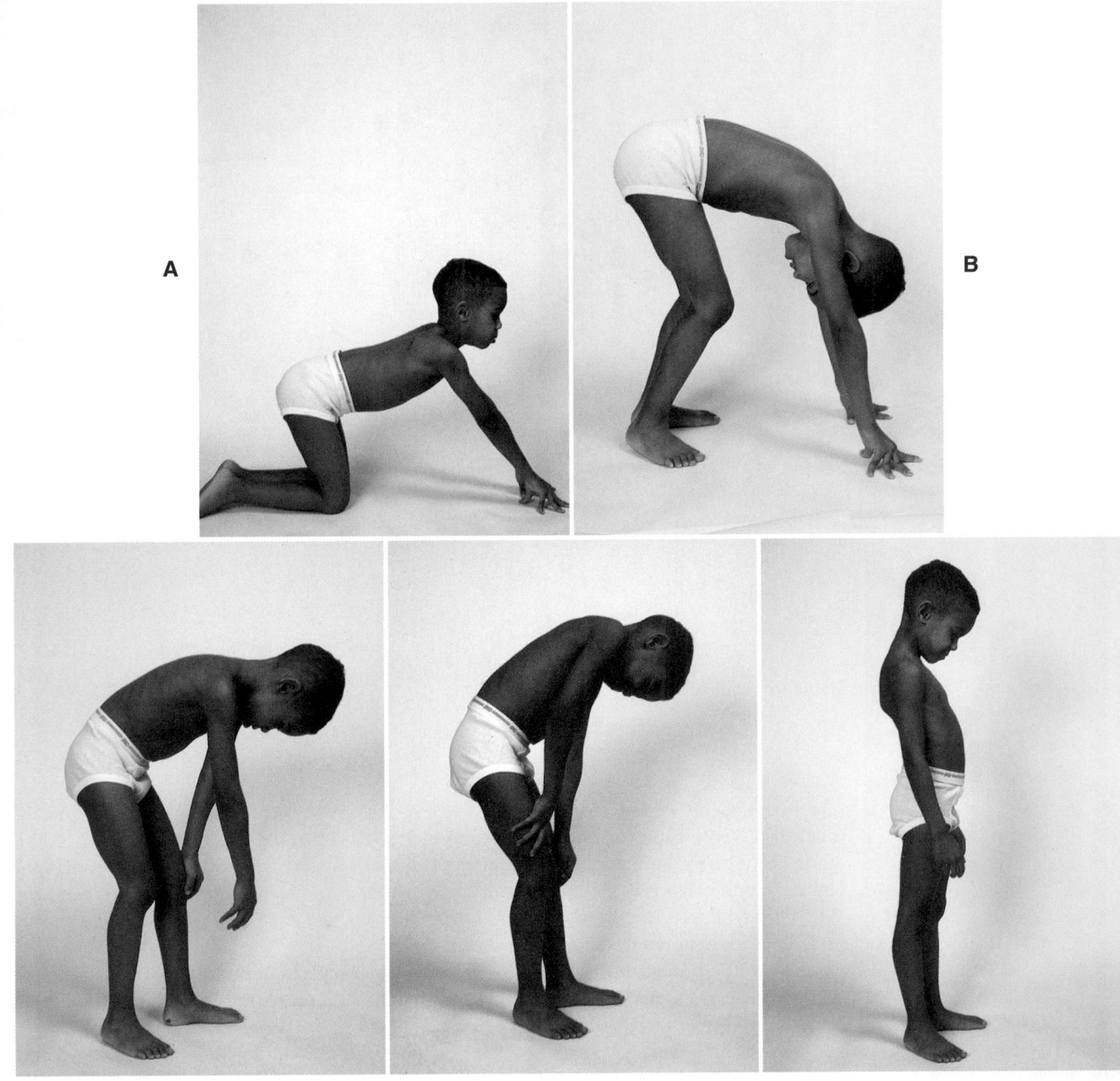

FIGURE 21-67
Gower sign of generalized muscle weakness. **A-B,** The child maneuvers to a position supported by both the arms and legs. **C-D,** The child pushes off the floor, rests the hand on the knee, and pushes self up with the hands and arms on the legs. **E,** The child stands upright.
From Ball, Bindler, 2003.

less tense contribute to the "waddling" gait of late pregnancy. The pregnant woman can experience pain from the pubic symphysis down into the inner thigh when standing and may have a feeling that the bones are moving or snapping when walking. This may be due to the effect of the hormone relaxin on the pubic symphysis and sacroiliac joints (Gordon, 2002).

During pregnancy, expected increases in the lumbosacral curve and anterior flexion of the head in the cervicodorsal region become apparent. To assess for lumbosacral hyperextension, ask the woman to bend forward at the waist toward her toes. Palpate the distance between the L4 and S1 spinal processes. As the woman rises to standing, from full flexion to full extension,

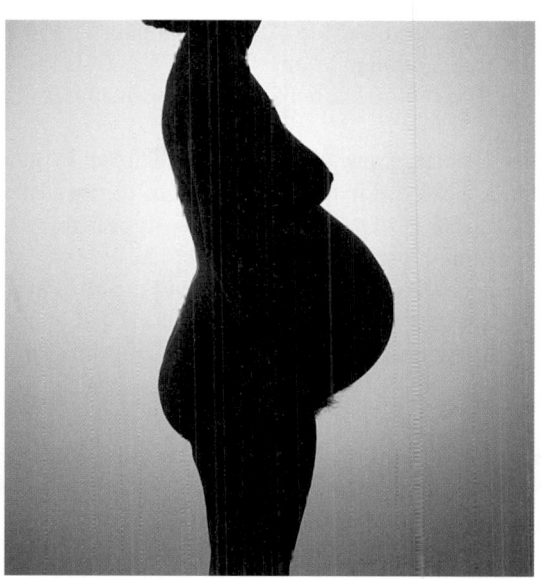

FIGURE 21-68
Postural changes with pregnancy.

FIGURE 21-69
Agility in the older adult. Note the flexibility and ability to balance of this 83-year-old woman.

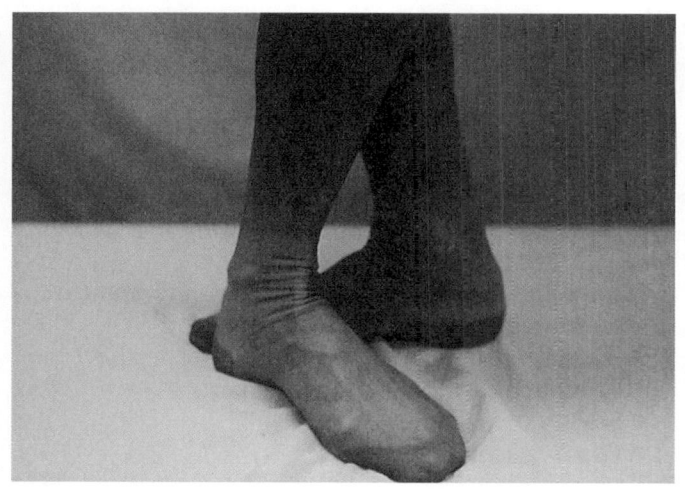

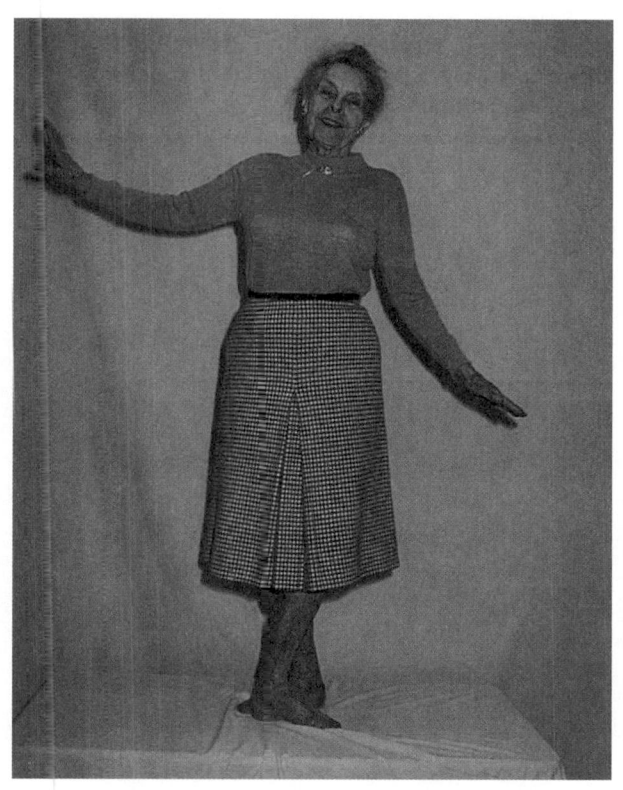

note when the distance between L4 and S1 becomes fixed. If it becomes fixed before the spine is fully extended, the woman will be hyperextended when walking, possibly resulting in lower back pain. Most back pain resolves within 6 months after delivery.

Carpal tunnel syndrome is experienced by some women during the last trimester because of the associated fluid retention during pregnancy. The symptoms abate after delivery.

OLDER ADULTS

The older adult should be able to participate in the physical examination as described for the adult, but the response to your requests may be more slow and deliberate. Fine and gross motor skills required to perform activities of daily living such as dressing, grooming, climbing steps, and writing will provide an evaluation of the patient's joint muscle agility (see the Functional Assessment box on p. 744). Joint and muscle agility have tremendous extremes among older adults (Fig. 21-69).

Identify the patient's risk for osteoporosis based upon risk factors and make referral for bone density measurement as appropriate. The Osteoporosis Risk Assessment Instrument (Table 21-5) is one tool suggested for screening purposes (U.S. Preventive Services Task Force, 2003).

The patient's posture may display increased dorsal kyphosis, accompanied by flexion of the hips and knees. The head may tilt backward to compensate for the increased thoracic curvature (see Fig. 21-20, *B*). The extremities may appear to be relatively long if the trunk has diminished in length due to vertebral collapse. The base of support may be broader with the feet more widely spaced, and the patient may hold the arms away from the body to aid balancing.

The reduction in total muscle mass is often related to atrophy, either from disuse, as in patients with arthritis; or from loss of nerve innervation, as in patients with diabetic neuropathy.

FUNCTIONAL ASSESSMENT

MUSCULOSKELETAL ASSESSMENT

Activity to Observe	Indicators of Weakened Muscle Groups
Rising from lying to sitting position	Rolling to one side and pushing with arms to raise to elbows; grabbing a siderail or table to pull to sitting
Rising from chair to standing	Pushing with arms to supplement weak leg muscles; upper torso thrusts forward before body rises
Walking	Lifting leg farther off floor with each step; shortened swing phase; foot may fall or slide forward; arms held out for balance or move in rowing motion
Climbing steps	Holding handrail for balance; pulling body up and forward with arms; uses stronger leg
Descending steps	Lowering weakened leg first; often descends sideways holding rail with both hands; may watch feet
Picking up item from floor	Leaning on furniture for support; bending over at waist to avoid bending knees; uses one hand on thigh to assist with lowering and raising torso
Tying shoes	Using footstool to decrease spinal flexion
Putting on and pulling up trousers or stockings	Difficulty may indicate decreased shoulder and upper arm strength; these activities often performed in sitting position until clothing is pulled up
Putting on sweater	Putting sleeve on weaker arm or shoulder first; uses internal or external shoulder rotation to get remaining arm in sleeve
Zipping dress in back	Difficulty with this indicates weakened shoulder rotation
Combing hair	Difficulty indicates problems with grasp, wrist flexion, pronation and supination of forearm, and elbow rotation
Pushing chair away from table while seated	Standing and easing chair back with torso; difficulty indicates problems with upper arm, shoulder, lower arm strength, and wrist motion
Buttoning button or writing name	Difficulty indicates problem with manual dexterity and finger-thumb opposition

Modified from Wilson, Giddens, 2005.

SAMPLE DOCUMENTATION

HISTORY AND PHYSICAL EXAMINATION

Subjective
A 13-year-old female referred by school nurse because of uneven shoulder and hip heights. Active in sports, good strength, no back pain or stiffness.

Objective
Spine straight without obvious deformities when erect, but mild right curvature of thoracic spine with forward flexion. No rib hump. Right shoulder and iliac crest slightly higher than left. Muscles and extremities symmetric; muscle strength appropriate and equal bilaterally; active range of motion without pain, locking, clicking, or limitation in all joints.

For additional sample documentation, see Chapter 26.

TABLE 21-5	Osteoporosis Risk Assessment Instrument (ORAI)
Variable	**Score**
AGE (YEAR)	
75 or older	15
64 to 74	9
55 to 64	6
45 to 54	0
WEIGHT (KG)	
Under 60	9
60 to 69	3
70 or more	0
CURRENT ESTROGEN USE	
No	2
Yes	0

Calculate the sum of the score for the three variables. Refer the patient for bone density measurement when the total score is 9 or greater.

From Cadarette et al, 2000.

SUMMARY OF EXAMINATION
MUSCULOSKELETAL SYSTEM

The following steps are performed with the patient standing, sitting, and walking:

1. Inspect the skeleton and extremities and compare sides for the following (p. 705):
   - Alignment
   - Contour and symmetry of body parts
   - Size
   - Gross deformity
2. Inspect the skin and subcutaneous tissues over muscles and joints for the following (p. 705):
   - Color
   - Number of skinfolds
   - Swelling
   - Masses
3. Inspect muscles and compare contralateral sides for the following (p. 705):
   - Size
   - Symmetry
   - Fasciculations or spasms
4. Palpate all bones, joints, and surrounding muscles for the following (p. 706):
   - Muscle tone
   - Heat
   - Tenderness
   - Swelling
   - Crepitus
5. Test each major joint for active and passive range of motion and compare contralateral sides (p. 706).
6. Test major muscle groups for strength and compare contralateral sides (p. 707).

Joints that deserve particular attention include the following:

Temporomandibular Joint
1. Palpate the joint space for clicking, popping, and pain (p. 707).
2. Test range of motion by having the patient perform the following (p. 708):
   - Opening and closing mouth
   - Moving jaw laterally to each side
   - Protruding and retracting jaw
3. Test strength of temporalis muscles with the patient's teeth clenched (p. 708).

Cervical Spine
1. Inspect the neck for the following (p. 708):
   - Alignment
   - Symmetry of skinfolds and muscles
2. Test range of motion by the following maneuvers (p. 708):
   - Forward flexion (45 degrees)
   - Hyperextension (55 degrees)
   - Lateral bending (40 degrees)
   - Rotation (70 degrees)
3. Test strength of sternocleidomastoid and trapezius muscles (cranial nerve XI, spinal accessory) (p. 708).

Thoracic and Lumbar Spine
1. Inspect the spine for alignment (p. 708).
2. Palpate the spinal processes and paravertebral muscles (p. 711).
3. Percuss for spinal tenderness (p. 711).
4. Test range of motion by the following maneuvers (p. 711):
   - Forward flexion (75 degrees)
   - Hyperextension (30 degrees)
   - Lateral bending (35 degrees)
   - Rotation

Continued

SUMMARY OF EXAMINATION

MUSCULOSKELETAL SYSTEM—cont'd

Shoulders

1. Inspect shoulders and shoulder girdle for contour (p. 712).
2. Palpate the joint spaces and bones of the shoulders (p. 712).
3. Test range of motion by the following maneuvers (pp. 713-715):
   - Shrugging the shoulders
   - Forward flexion (180 degrees) and hyperextension (up to 50 degrees)
   - Abduction (180 degrees) and adduction (50 degrees)
   - Internal and external rotation (90 degrees)
4. Test muscle strength by the following maneuvers (p. 714):
   - Shrugged shoulders
   - Abduction with forward flexion
   - Medial rotation
   - Lateral rotation

Elbows

1. Inspect the elbows in flexed and extended position for the following (p. 716):
   - Contour
   - Carrying angle (5 to 15 degrees)
2. Palpate the extensor surface of the ulna, olecranon process, and the medial and lateral epicondyles of the humerus (p. 716).
3. Test range of motion by the following maneuvers (pp. 716-717):
   - Flexion (160 degrees)
   - Extension (180 degrees)
   - Pronation and supination (90 degrees)

Hands and Wrists

1. Inspect the dorsum and palm of hands for the following (p. 717):
   - Contour
   - Position
   - Shape
   - Number and completeness of digits
2. Palpate each joint in the hand and wrist (p. 717).
3. Test range of motion by the following maneuvers (pp. 717-720):
   - Metacarpophalangeal flexion (90 degrees) and hyperextension (30 degrees)
   - Thumb opposition
   - Forming a fist
   - Finger adduction and abduction
   - Wrist extension, hyperextension (70 degrees), and flexion (90 degrees)
   - Radial (20 degrees) and ulnar motion (55 degrees)
4. Test muscle strength by the following maneuvers (p. 720):
   - Wrist extension and hyperextension
   - Hand grip

Hips

1. Inspect the hips for symmetry and level of gluteal folds (p. 720).
2. Palpate hips and pelvis for the following (p. 720):
   - Instability
   - Tenderness
   - Crepitus
3. Test range of motion by the following maneuvers (pp. 720-722):
   - Flexion (120 degrees), extension (90 degrees) and hyperextension (30 degrees)
   - Adduction (30 degrees) and abduction (45 degrees)
   - Internal rotation (40 degrees)
   - External rotation (45 degrees)
4. Test muscle strength of hips with the following maneuvers (p. 722):
   - Knee in flexion and extension
   - Abduction and adduction

Legs and Knees

1. Inspect the knees for natural concavities (p. 722).
2. Palpate the popliteal space and joint space (p. 722).
3. Test range of motion by flexion (130 degrees) and extension (0 to 15 degrees) (pp. 722-723).
4. Test the strength of muscles in flexion and extension (p. 723).

Feet and Ankles

1. Inspect the feet and ankles during weight bearing and non-weight bearing for the following (p. 724):
   - Contour
   - Alignment with tibias
   - Size
   - Number of toes
2. Palpate the Achilles tendon and each metatarsal joint (p. 726).
3. Test range of motion by the following maneuvers (p. 726):
   - Dorsiflexion (20 degrees) and plantar flexion (45 degrees)
   - Inversion (30 degrees) and eversion (20 degrees)
   - Flexion and extension of the toes
4. Test strength of muscles in plantar flexion and dorsiflexion (p. 726).

Additional procedures include the following:

Limb Measurement (pp. 726-727)

Lower Spine Assessment (pp. 730-731)
Straight leg raising test
Bragard stretch test
Sitting knee extension test
Femoral stretch test

Shoulder Assessment (pp. 727-728)
Neer test
Hawkins test

Hand and Wrist Assessment (pp. 728-730)
Katz hand diagram
Thumb abduction test
Tinel sign
Phalen test

Knee Assessment (pp. 731-733)
Ballottement
Bulge sign
McMurray test
Anterior and posterior drawer test
Lachman test
Varus and valgus stress test
Apley test

Hip Assessment (p. 734)
Thomas test
Trendelenburg test

COMMON ABNORMALITIES

ANKYLOSING SPONDYLITIS

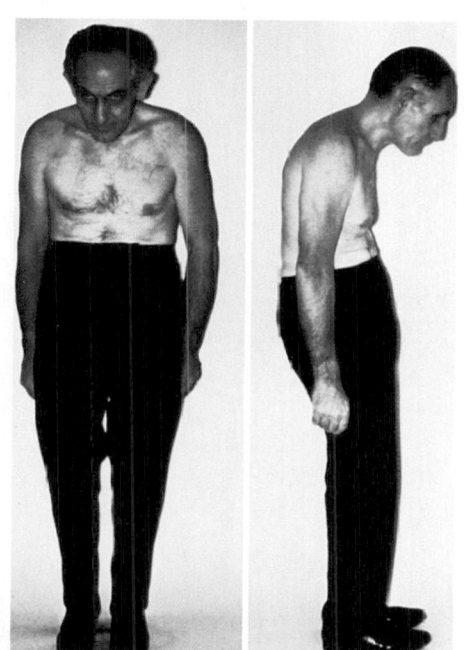

FIGURE 21-70
Gross postural changes in man affected by ankylosing spondylitis.
Reprinted from the Clinical Slide Collection of the Rheumatic Diseases, copyright 1991. Used by permission of the American College of Rheumatology.

A hereditary, chronic inflammatory disease, ankylosing spondylitis initially affects the lumbar spine and sacroiliac joints. Larger joints of the shoulders, hips, and knees may be affected later. The inflamed intervertebral disks become infiltrated with vascular connective tissue that ossifies, leading to eventual fusion and severe deformity of the vertebral column. The disease begins insidiously with low back pain and progresses to reduced spinal mobility. Uveitis may be present. The disease develops predominantly in males between 20 and 40 years of age (Fig. 21-70).

LUMBOSACRAL RADICULOPATHY (HERNIATED LUMBAR DISK)

Lumbosacral radiculopathy is herniation of a lumbar disk that irritates the corresponding nerve root and results in muscle weakness, paresthesia, and pain in the distribution of the nerve root dermatome. Disk herniation is generally caused by degenerative changes of the disk, most commonly occurring at the L4, L5, and S1 nerve roots. The greatest incidence occurs between 31 and 50 years of age. The condition is commonly associated with lifting heavy objects while the arms are extended and the spine is flexed, such as occurs when bending to lift a child weighing more than 25 pounds. Common symptoms include low back pain with radiation to the buttocks and posterior thigh or down the leg in the distribution of the dermatome of the nerve root. Numbness, tingling, or weakness may occur in the involved extremity. Spasm and tenderness over the paraspinal musculature may also be present. The patient may have difficulty with heel walking (L4 and L5) or toe walking (S1). Pain in the lower extremity, often described as burning, may be unilateral, bilateral, or on alternating sides. Sneezing and coughing or bending toward the affected side often induce or aggravate the pain. Pain relief is often achieved by lying down (Fig. 21-71).

Nerve root	L4	L5	S1
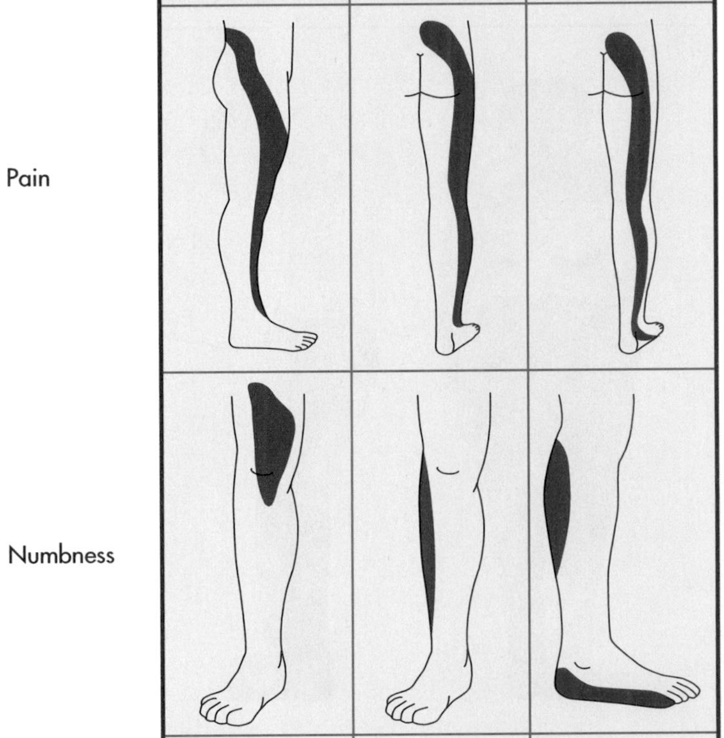 Pain			
Numbness			
Motor weakness	Extension of quadriceps	Dorsiflexion of great toe and foot	Plantar flexion of great toe and foot
Screening examination	Squat and rise	Heel walking	Walking on toes
Reflexes	Knee jerk diminished	None reliable	Ankle jerk diminished

FIGURE 21-71
Distribution of paresthesia and radiating pain associated with herniated disks at the L4, L5, and S1 nerve roots.
From Thompson et al, 1997.

LUMBAR STENOSIS	Spinal stenosis is usually caused by hypertrophy of the ligamentum flavum and facet joints that results in narrowing of the spinal canal. Narrowing may lead to entrapment of the nerve roots as they traverse the spinal canal. Signs and symptoms include pain with walking or standing that often seems to originate in the buttocks and may then radiate down the legs, followed by pain relief with sitting. Pain in the lower extremities may be worsened by prolonged standing, walking, bending, or hyperextending the back. The pain is generally relieved by sitting down.
CARPAL TUNNEL SYNDROME	Compression on the median nerve caused by thickening of its flexor tendon sheath often results from microtrauma, repetitive motion of the arms and hands, or vibration. It is also associated with rheumatoid arthritis, gout, hypothyroidism, and the hormonal changes of pregnancy and menopause. The symptoms of numbness, burning, and tingling in the hands often occur at night, but they can also be elicited by rotational movements of the wrist. Pain may radiate to the arms. Weakness of the hand and flattening of the thenar eminence of the palm may result. The disorder is three times more common in women. For a discussion of assessment procedures, see pp. 728-730.

GOUT

Gout, a form of arthritis, is a disorder of purine metabolism that results from an elevated serum uric acid level. The formation of monosodium urate crystal deposits in joints and surrounding tissues results in acute attacks of arthritis. The joint classically affected is the proximal phalanx of the great toe, although other joints of the wrists, hands, ankles, and knees are sometimes affected. Symptoms include sudden onset of a hot, swollen joint; exquisite pain; limited range of motion; and mild fever. The skin over the swollen joint may be shiny and red or purple. Uric acid crystals may form as tophi under the skin with chronic gout. The disease primarily affects men older than 40 years of age and some postmenopausal women. It is strongly associated with obesity, hypertension, hyperlipidemia, and diabetes. (Fig. 21-72).

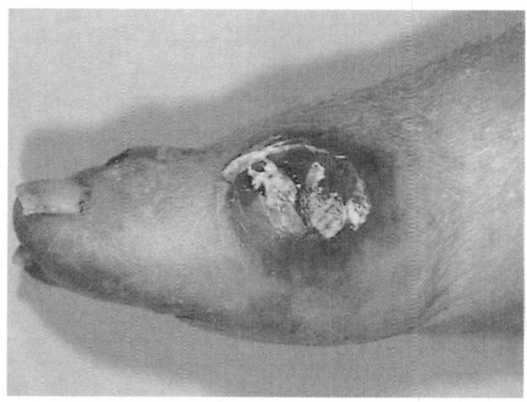

FIGURE 21-72
Gouty tophus on right foot.
From Dieppe et al, 1991.

TEMPOROMANDIBULAR JOINT SYNDROME

Temporomandibular joint (TMJ) syndrome is painful jaw movement caused by congenital anomalies, malocclusion, trauma, arthritis, and other joint diseases. There is unilateral facial pain that usually worsens with joint movement and may be referred to any point on the face or neck. Most patients have a muscle spasm, and many have clicking, popping, or crepitus in the affected joint.

OSTEOMYELITIS

Osteomyelitis, an infection in the bone, usually results from an open wound or systemic infection. Purulent matter spreads through the cortex of the bone and into the soft tissues. Blood flow to the affected bone may become blocked, causing necrosis. Signs of infection include edema; erythema; warmth at the site; tenderness; pain with movement; and generalized signs such as spiking fevers, headache, and nausea.

BURSITIS

Bursitis is an inflammation of a bursa resulting from constant friction between the skin and tissues around the joint. Common sites include the shoulder, elbow, hip, and knee. Signs include limitation of motion caused by swelling; pain on movement; point tenderness; and an erythematous, warm site. Soreness may radiate to tendons at the site (Fig. 21-73).

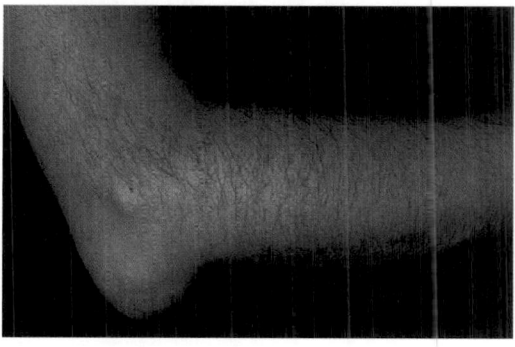

FIGURE 21-73
Olecranon bursitis.
Reprinted from the Clinical Slide Collection of the Rheumatic Diseases, copyright 1991. Used by permission of the American College of Rheumatology.

PAGET DISEASE (OSTEITIS DEFORMANS)	A metabolic focal disorder of the bone, Paget disease appears in persons older than 45 years of age. Excessive bone resorption and excessive bone formation produce a mosaic pattern of lamellar bone. Bowed tibias, misshapen pelvis or skull, shortened thorax, and frequent fractures occur. The bones of the skull are often affected, which can produce symptoms of vertigo, headache, and progressive deafness from involvement of the ossicles or neural elements. While the cause is unknown, a genetic component and a slow-acting virus are suspected.
FIBROMYALGIA	Fibromyalgia is a painful, nonarticular condition that primarily affects the muscles. Symptoms include widespread pain and aching, persistent fatigue, generalized morning stiffness, multiple tender points (11 or more) at nine bilateral sites (i.e., occiput, low cervical spine, trapezius, supraspinatus, second rib, lateral epicondyle, gluteus, greater trochanter, and knee). The condition may also be accompanied by headaches, irritable bowel, dysmenorrhea, cold sensitivity, Raynaud phenomenon, restless legs, atypical patterns of numbness and tingling, and exercise intolerance and weakness. It more commonly affects women older than 50 years of age.
OSTEOARTHRITIS	Osteoarthritis is the deterioration of the articular cartilage covering the ends of bone in synovial joints from inflammatory and noninflammatory causes. The resulting abrasion, pitting, and thinning of the cartilage surface eventually exposes the bone. The bones begin to grind against each other, leading to remodeling of the bone surface and formation of bone spurs. The joint becomes swollen due to soft tissue swelling and joint effusion. The hands, feet, hips, knees, and cervical or lumbar spine are most commonly affected. Onset usually begins after 40 years of age and develops slowly over many years. The incidence increases as people age, with nearly 100% of people older than 75 years of age being affected.
RHEUMATOID ARTHRITIS	Rheumatoid arthritis is a chronic, systemic, inflammatory, progressive disorder of joints that can occur between 3 and 80 years of age and affects 1% of the population. The cause is unknown but may be associated with infection, autoimmunity, trauma, stress, or familial pre-

DIFFERENTIAL DIAGNOSIS

COMPARISON OF OSTEOARTHRITIS AND RHEUMATOID ARTHRITIS

Signs and Symptoms	Osteoarthritis	Rheumatoid Arthritis
Onset	Insidious, over many years	Gradual or sudden (24 to 48 hours), sometimes weeks to months
Duration of stiffness	Few minutes, localized, but short "gelling" after prolonged rest	At least 1 hour, often longer, most pronounced after rest
Pain	On motion, with prolonged activity, relieved by rest	Even at rest, may disturb sleep
Weakness	Usually localized and not severe	Often pronounced, out of proportion with muscle atrophy
Fatigue	Unusual	Often severe, with onset 4 to 5 hours after rising
Emotional depression and lability	Unusual	Common, coinciding with fatigue and disease activity, often relieved if in remission
Tenderness localized over afflicted joint	Common	Almost always, most sensitive indicator of inflammation
Swelling	Effusion common, little synovial reaction, swelling rare	Fusiform soft tissue enlargement, effusion common, synovial proliferation and thickening, often symmetric, rheumatoid nodules
Heat, erythema	Unusual, minimal if present	Sometimes present
Crepitus, crackling	Coarse to medium on motion	Medium to fine
Joint enlargement	Mild with firm consistency	Moderate to severe

Modified from McCarty, 1993.

disposition. One recent theory is that the immune system is prematurely exhausted, and the existing immune cells clone themselves and begin attacking the body rather than defending it. Joint inflammation results from infiltration of the joint synovial fluid by immune cells. Cytokinins are released that inhibit bone formation, induce bone resorption, and stimulate the secretion of enzymes that destroy cartilage and the joint. Articular surfaces are then remodeled by muscular mechanical forces. Disease onset is characterized by an unremitting fever, maculopapular rash, and arthritis. Although it is progressive, the disease has unpredictable flares and remissions. Joints most commonly affected include the wrists, hips, knees, ankles, and cervical spine. Predilection by gender is 3:1, females to males, and it occurs in all ethnic groups. The Differential Diagnosis box on p. 750 contrasts rheumatoid arthritis and osteoarthritis.

SPORTS INJURIES

Trauma to the musculoskeletal system results in a variety of injuries to muscles, bones, and supportive joint structures. The injury may be the result of an acute incident or overuse and repetitive trauma. Often a neurovascular assessment is performed to detect nerve damage or circulatory impairment (Box 21-1).

MUSCLE STRAIN

A muscle can become strained from excessive stretching or by forceful contraction beyond its functional capacity. Muscle strain is often associated with improper exercise warm-up, fatigue, or previous injury. Severity ranges from a mild intrafibrinous tear to a total rupture of a single muscle. Signs include temporary weakness, spasm, pain, and contusion.

SPRAIN

Stretching or tearing a supporting ligament of a joint by forced movement beyond its normal range can cause a sprain. Severe sprains may result in total rupture of ligaments and permanent joint instability if not treated. Signs include pain, marked swelling, hemorrhage, and loss of function.

DISLOCATION

Dislocation is the complete separation of the contact between two bones in a joint, often caused by pressure or force pushing the bone out of the joint. Signs include deformity and inability to use the extremity or joint as usual.

FRACTURE

A fracture is a partial or complete break in the continuity of a bone resulting from trauma (direct, indirect, twisting, or crushing). Muscle contractions and spasms lead to shortening of tissues around the bone, thus causing deformity. Other signs include edema, pain, loss of function, color changes, and paresthesia.

BOX 21-1

NEUROVASCULAR ASSESSMENT

Assessment of circulation and nerve sensation is important when an extremity is injured. Perform the following steps to complete a neurovascular assessment distal to the injury. Use the contralateral extremity for comparison.

Assessment	Unexpected Findings
Color	Pallor or cyanosis
Temperature	Cool or cold
Capillary refill time	Greater than 4 seconds
Swelling	Significantly swollen
Pain	Presence of moderate to severe pain
Sensation	Numbness, tingling, pins and needles sensation
Movement	Decreased or no movement

Consider all the findings simultaneously to complete the neurovascular assessment. Presence of most or all of these unexpected findings indicates significantly impaired circulation and pressure or injury to the nerve that needs emergency intervention.

EVIDENCE-BASED PRACTICE IN PHYSICAL EXAMINATION
ACUTE ANKLE INJURY

In cases of acute ankle injury, the Ottawa Ankle Rules help identify the characteristics of patients needing an ankle x-ray series. There must be pain in the malleolar zone and one of the following:
- Bone tenderness along the distal 6 cm of the posterior edge of the fibula or tip of the lateral malleolus
- Bone tenderness along the distal 6 cm of the posterior edge of the tibia or tip of the medial malleolus
- Inability to bear weight for 4 steps both immediately after the injury and in the emergency department.

Absolute *exclusion* criteria for an ankle x-ray series include the following: age younger than 18, intoxication, multiple painful (distracting) injuries, pregnancy, head injury, and neurologic deficit.

The Ottawa Ankle Rules have a 99% to 100% sensitivity and a 50% specificity for detecting an ankle fracture that is present on x-ray.

Data from Stiell et al, 1993.

EVIDENCE-BASED PRACTICE IN PHYSICAL EXAMINATION
ACUTE KNEE INJURY

In cases of acute knee injury, the Ottawa Knee Rules identify the characteristics of patients who should have an x-ray of the knee. The rules include any of the following findings:
- Age older than 55
- Tenderness at head of fibula
- Isolated tenderness of the patella
- Inability to flex the knee to 90 degrees

Data from Stiell et al, 1996.

TENOSYNOVITIS (TENDONITIS)	An inflammation of the synovium-lined sheath around a tendon, tenosynovitis results from repetitive actions associated with occupational or sports activities. Common sites include the shoulder, knee, heel, and wrist. Signs include point tenderness over the involved tendon, pain with active movement, and some limitation of movement in the affected joint.
ROTATOR CUFF TEAR	Microtrauma to the rotator cuff muscles, most often the supraspinatus, occurs with repeated overhead lifting as the muscle and tendon are compressed under the acromion. The repetitive trauma weakens the rotator cuff and may result in a partial or complete tear. An acute tear may also result from a fall on an outstretched arm. Signs and symptoms of an acute injury include severe pain in the shoulder and deltoid area, inability to raise the arm sideways due to pain or an inability to maintain a lateral raised arm against resistance, inability to shrug shoulders, tenderness over the acromioclavicular joint, grating sound upon movement, crepitus, and weakness in external shoulder rotation.

INFANTS AND CHILDREN

MYELOMENINGOCELE, SPINA BIFIDA

Congenital neural tube defects, with incomplete closure of the vertebral column, permit the meninges and sometimes the spinal cord to protrude into a saclike structure (Fig. 21-74). Significant sensory and motor impairment results below the level of the myelomeningocele. The supplementation with folic acid of the diets of women who are pregnant and those not yet pregnant but intending pregnancy has reduced the incidence of this serious deformity significantly.

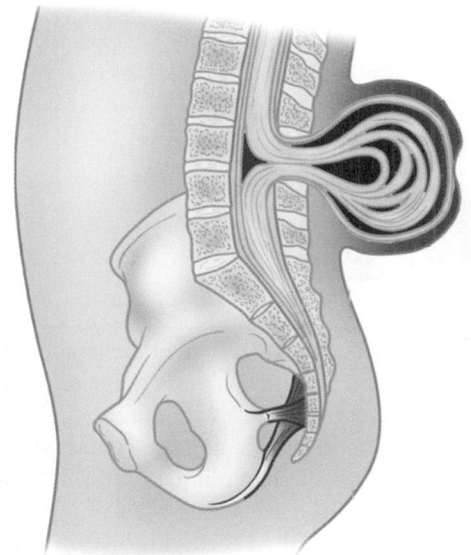
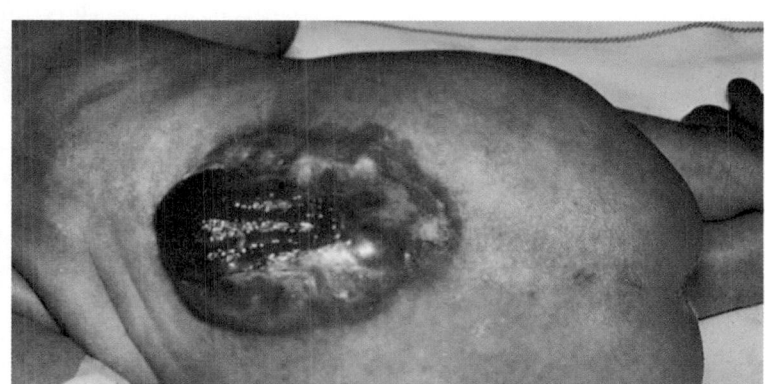

FIGURE 21-74
Myelomeningocele.
Photo from Zitelli, Davis, 1997; courtesy Christine L. Williams, New York Medical College.

CLUBFOOT (TALIPES EQUINOVARUS)

Clubfoot is a fixed congenital defect of the ankle and foot. The most common combination of position deformities includes inversion of the foot at the ankle and plantar flexion, with the toes lower than the heel (Fig. 21-75).

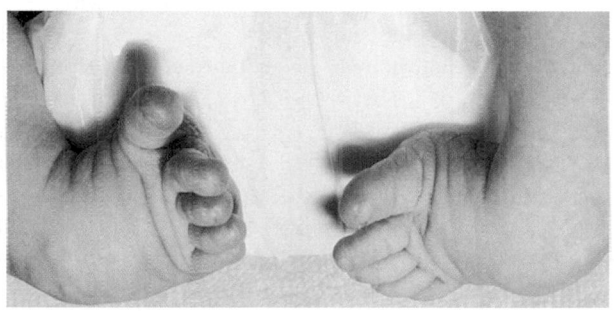

FIGURE 21-75
Clubfoot deformity, talipes equinovarus (bilateral deviation).
From Zitelli, Davis, 1997.

METATARSUS ADDUCTUS (METATARSUS VARUS)

The most common congenital foot deformity, metatarsus adductus can be either fixed or flexible. This defect is caused by intrauterine positioning. Medial adduction of the toes and forefoot results from angulation at the tarsometatarsal joint. The lateral border of the foot is convex, and a crease is sometimes apparent on the medial border of the foot. The heel and ankle are uninvolved. The deformity generally resolves within 6 months of birth, and fewer than 10% of children require casting or surgery for treatment (Fig. 21-76).

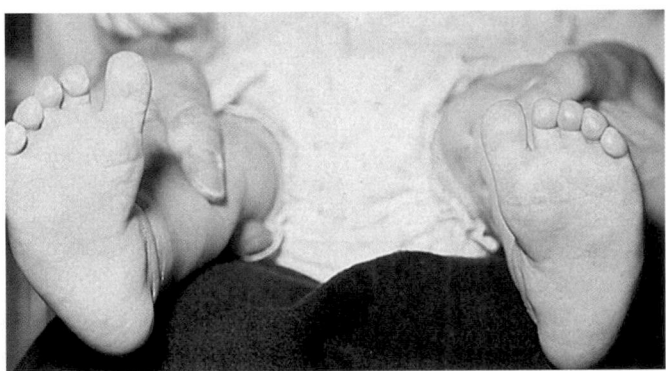

FIGURE 21-76
Bilateral metatarsus adductus. Viewed from plantar aspect showing rounding of the lateral border of the feet.
From Zitelli, Davis, 1997.

DEVELOPMENTAL DYSPLASIA OF THE HIP

Developmental dysplasia of the hip is a condition present at birth in which the femoral head has an inappropriate relationship with the acetabulum. This term covers a range of severity: frank dislocation, in which the femoral head loses contact completely with the acetabular capsule; subluxation or partial dislocation, in which the femoral head remains in contact with the acetabulum but the joint ligaments allow displacement of the femoral head; and instability. Females are affected more than males. The incidence of hip dislocations is 1 to 1.5 per 1000 live births, and the left hip is involved three times more often than the right.

LEGG-CALVÉ-PERTHES DISEASE

Legg-Calvé-Perthes disease is avascular necrosis of the femoral head resulting from a decreased blood supply to the femoral head. The cause is unknown. It is most commonly seen in males between 3 and 11 years of age. The child may have a limp that is painless or antalgic (painful limp with shortened time on extremity); a loss of internal rotation; a loss of abduction; and decreased range of motion on the affected side. Pain is often referred to the medial thigh, knee, or groin. Muscle weakness of the upper leg may be present if symptoms have been present for a prolonged period. There may be bilateral involvement in 10% of cases.

OSGOOD-SCHLATTER DISEASE

Osgood-Schlatter disease is a traction apophysitis (inflammation of a bony outgrowth) of the anterior aspect of the tibial tubercle in association with inflammation of the anterior patellar tendon. The child presents with a limp, knee pain, and swelling that is aggravated by strenuous activity, especially activity involving the quadriceps muscle. This self-limiting disorder is most common in males between 9 and 15 years of age.

SLIPPED CAPITAL FEMORAL EPIPHYSIS

Slipped capital femoral epiphysis is a disorder in which the capital femoral epiphysis slips over the neck of the femur. The child or adolescent presents with knee pain, an antalgic limp, leg weakness, and reduced internal hip rotation. The affected child is commonly obese, taller than most, and between 8 and 16 years of age. Affected girls are often younger than boys. The majority of cases (75%) are unilateral, and the left side is involved more often than the right.

MUSCULAR DYSTROPHY

Muscular dystrophy is a group of genetic disorders involving gradual degeneration of the muscle fibers. The disorders are characterized by progressive symmetric weakness and muscle atrophy or pseudohypertrophy from fatty infiltrates. Both skeletal muscles and those of organs such as the heart may be involved. Some forms cause mild disability, and these patients can expect a normal life span. Other types produce severe disability, deformity, and death. Early signs may include clumsiness, difficulty climbing stairs, frequent falls, waddling gait, and a positive Gower sign (see Fig. 21-67).

SCOLIOSIS

Structural scoliosis is a physical deformity with a concave curvature of the anterior vertebral bodies, convex posterior curves, and lateral rotation of the thoracic spine. Lateral curvature is greater than 10 degrees, but curves often vary from 20 to 60 degrees. In severe deformities the patient has uneven shoulder and hip levels, and the rotational deformity causes a rib hump and flank asymmetry on forward flexion. Physiologic alterations occur in the spine, chest, and pelvis (Fig. 21-77). Structural scoliosis most commonly affects girls and progresses during early adolescence and has no known cause. In functional scoliosis the spine has a lateral curve, no spinal rotation, and no trunk asymmetry. The spine straightens when the child reclines. It is often associated with a leg length discrepancy.

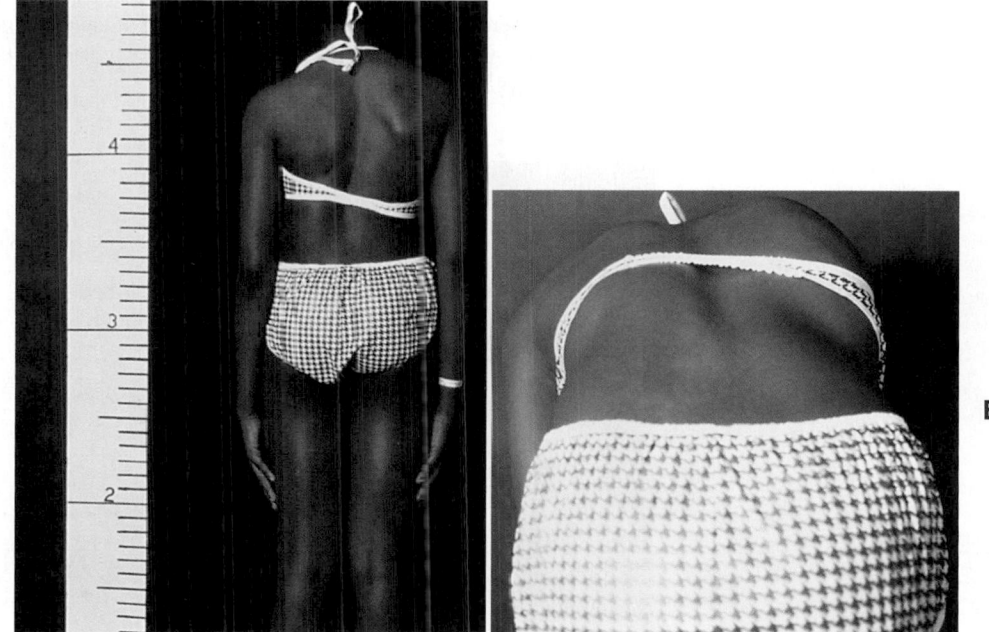

A

B

FIGURE 21-77
Scoliosis, lateral curvature of the spine, with increased convexity to the right. **A,** Scapular asymmetry is easily discernible in the upright position. **B,** Forward flexion reveals a mild rib hump deformity.
From Zitelli, Davis, 1997.

RADIAL HEAD SUBLUXATION

Radial head subluxation, also known as nursemaid's elbow, is a dislocation injury caused by jerking the arm upward while the elbow is extended. The jerking pulls apart the elbow joint and tears the margin of the annular ligament around the radial head into the joint and allows the torn ligament to become trapped in the joint. This injury is common in children 1 to 4 years of age. The child complains of pain in the elbow and wrist, refuses to move the arm, and holds it slightly flexed and pronated. Supination motion is resisted.

OLDER ADULTS

OSTEOPOROSIS

Osteoporosis is a silent progressive disease in which a decrease in bone mass occurs because bone resorption is more rapid than bone deposition. The bones become fragile and susceptible to spontaneous fractures; the presenting symptom is usually loss of height or an acute, painful fracture. The most common fracture sites are hip, vertebrae, and wrist. In the spine, vertebral compression fractures lead to kyphosis or scoliosis of the spine. Vertebral fractures may occur spontaneously, without trauma or tumors. Affected persons lose height and the waistline, have decreased abdominothoracic space, and appear to sink into their hips (Fig. 21-78). Women are more commonly affected than men by a 4:1 ratio because men have a 30% greater bone mass than women. It is most commonly seen in postmenopausal women, but its presence in persons taking corticosteroids for disease management is increasing. Older men treated for prostate cancer with medications that halt testosterone production or by surgical removal of the testes have an accelerated loss of bone mass.

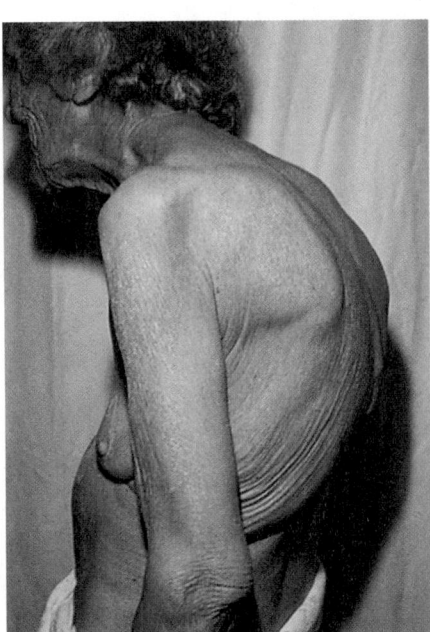

FIGURE 21-78
Hallmark of osteoporosis: dowager hump.
From Kamal, 1992.

DUPUYTREN CONTRACTURE

Dupuytren contracture affects the palmar fascia of one or more fingers and tends to be bilateral. Although the cause is unknown, there appears to be a hereditary component. A gradual increase in incidence occurs with age. It is also seen with increased frequency in patients with diabetes, alcoholic liver disease, and epilepsy (Fig. 21-79).

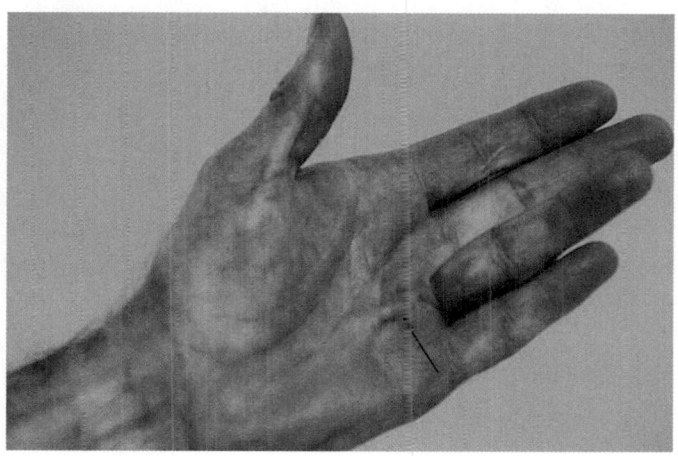

FIGURE 21-79
Dupuytren contracture.

ELECTRONIC RESOURCES

For Weblinks and additional resources, go to   **evolve**

http://evolve.elsevier.com/Seidel

or to the Companion CD-ROM.

Additional information related to the content in Chapter 21 can be found on the companion website at http://evolve.elsevier.com/Seidel/ or on the interactive companion CD-ROM. Resources and activities for Chapter 21 include:
- Sound and Vision Theater
- Printouts for Your Practice
- Interactive Challenge
- Spanish Assessment Terms with Pronunciation Guide
- Instant Calculators

NEUROLOGIC SYSTEM

The nervous system, with its central and peripheral divisions, maintains and controls all body functions by its voluntary and autonomic responses. The evaluation of motor, sensory, autonomic, cognitive, and behavioral elements makes neurologic assessment one of the most complex portions of the physical examination.

ANATOMY AND PHYSIOLOGY

The central nervous system (brain and spinal cord) is the main network of coordination and control for the body (Fig. 22-1). The peripheral nervous system, comprising motor and sensory nerves and ganglia outside the central nervous system, carries information to and from the central nervous system. The autonomic nervous system regulates the internal environment of the body, functions over which a person has no voluntary control. It has two divisions, each tending to balance the impulses of the other. The sympathetic division prods the body into action during times of physiologic and psychologic stress; the parasympathetic division functions in a complementary and a counterbalancing manner to conserve body resources and maintain day-to-day body functions such as digestion and elimination.

The intricate interrelationship of the nervous system permits the body to perform the following:
- Receive sensory stimuli from the environment
- Identify and integrate the adaptive processes needed to maintain current body functions
- Orchestrate body function changes required for adaptation and survival
- Integrate the rapid responsiveness of the central nervous system with the more gradual responsiveness of the endocrine system
- Control cognitive and voluntary behavioral processes
- Control subconscious and involuntary body functions

The brain and spinal cord are protected by the skull and vertebrae, the meninges, and the cerebrospinal fluid. Three layers of meninges surround the brain and spinal cord, assisting in the production and drainage of cerebrospinal fluid (Fig. 22-2). Cerebrospinal fluid circulates between an interconnecting system of ventricles in the brain and around the brain and spinal cord, serving as a shock absorber.

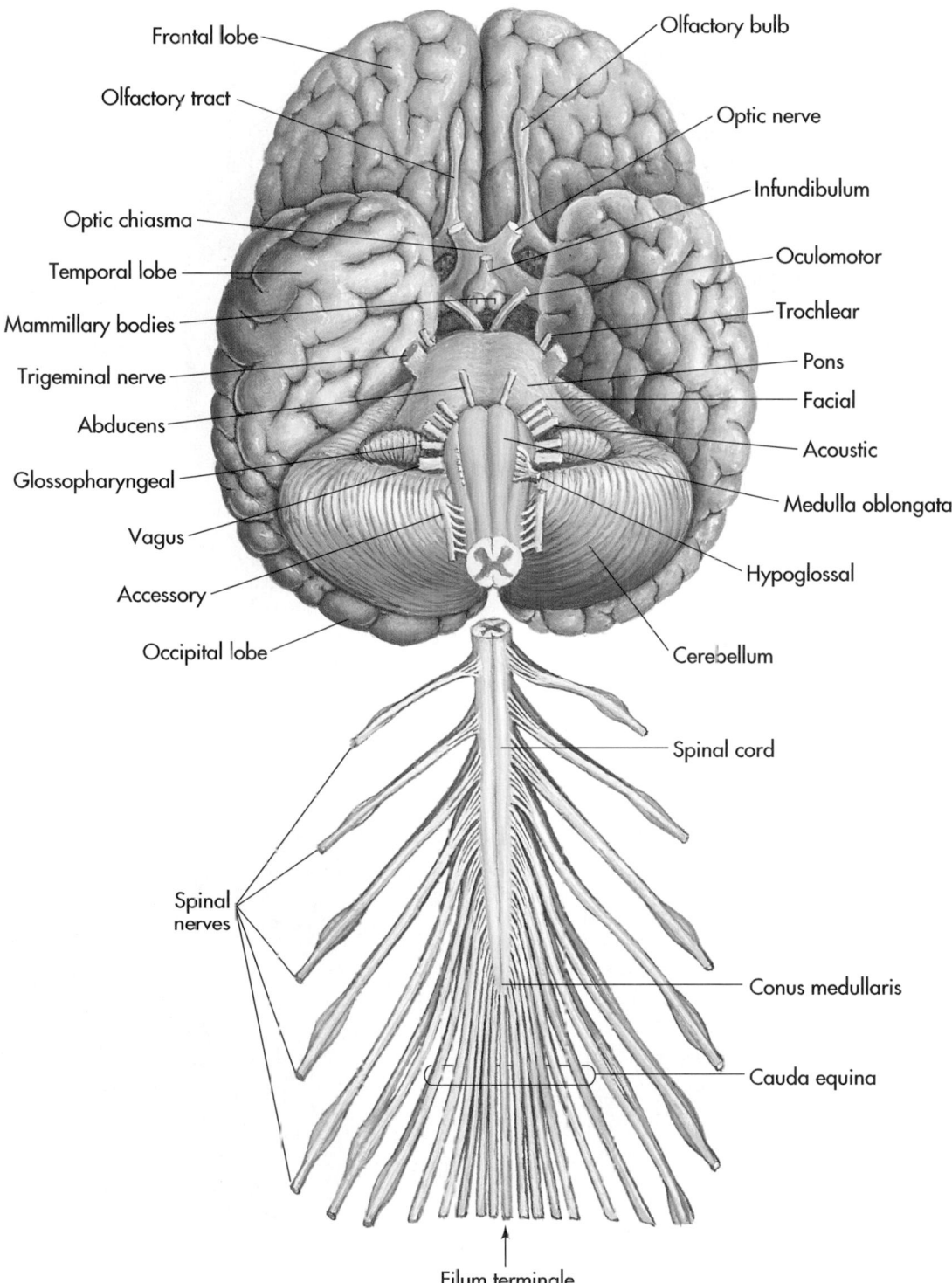

Frontal lobe

Olfactory tract

Optic chiasma

Temporal lobe

Mammillary bodies

Trigeminal nerve

Abducens

Glossopharyngeal

Vagus

Accessory

Occipital lobe

Olfactory bulb

Optic nerve

Infundibulum

Oculomotor

Trochlear

Pons

Facial

Acoustic

Medulla oblongata

Hypoglossal

Cerebellum

Spinal cord

Spinal nerves

Conus medullaris

Cauda equina

Filum terminale

FIGURE 22-1
Base view of brain and cross-sectional view of spinal cord.

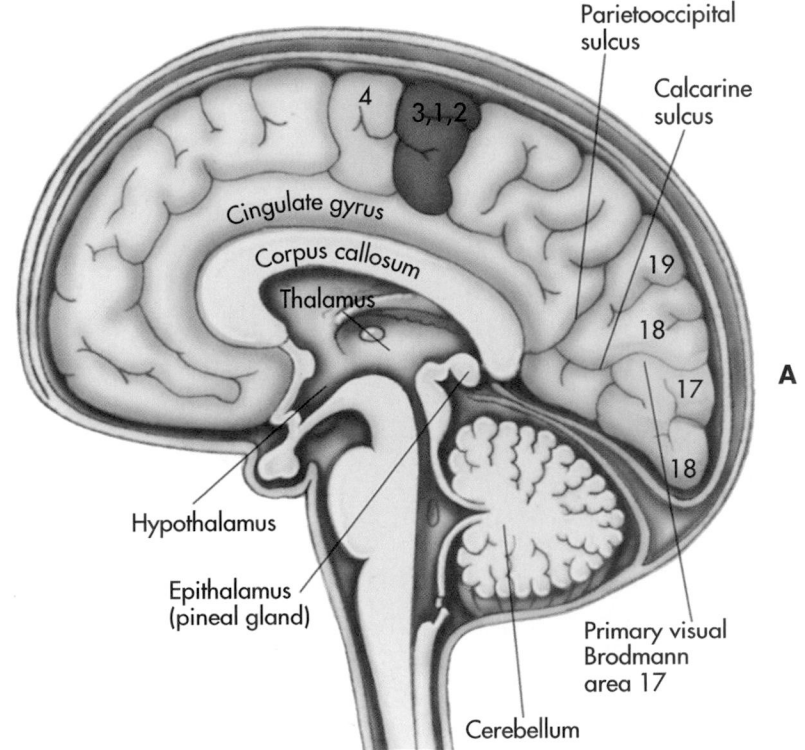

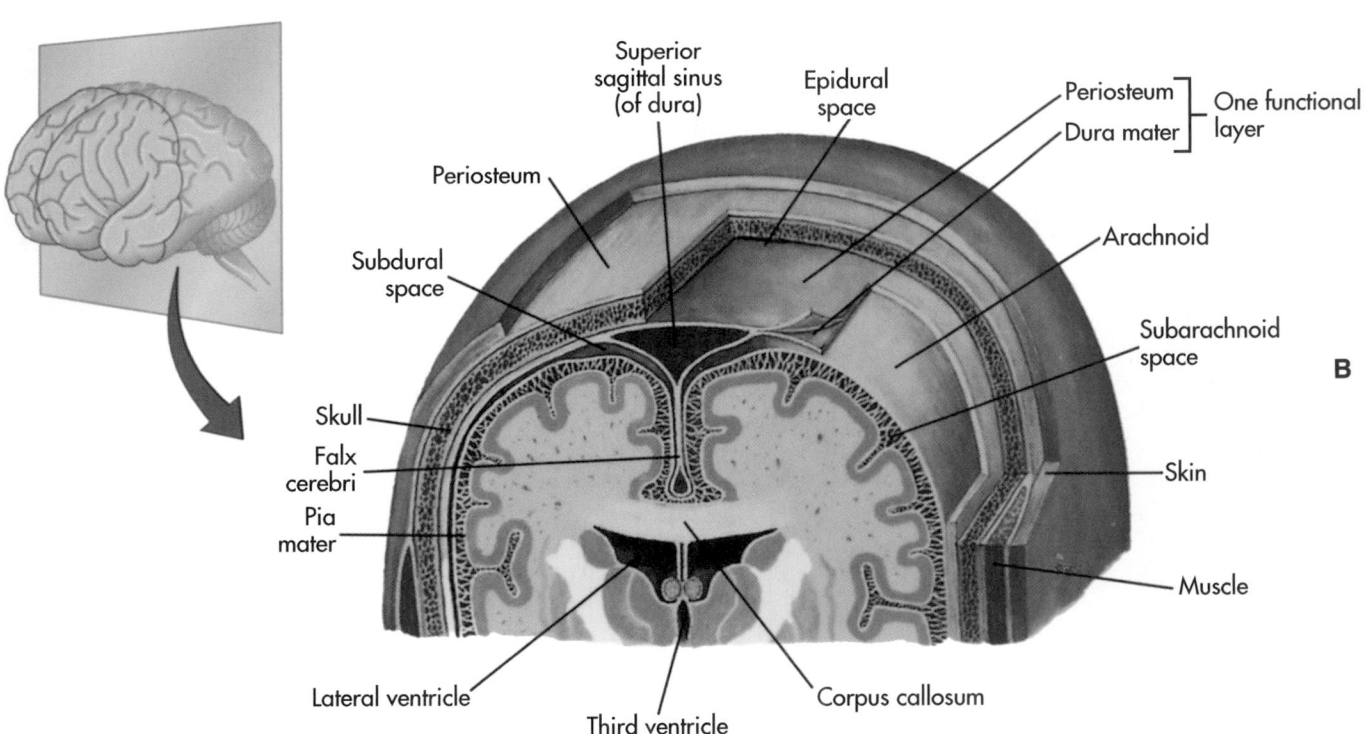

FIGURE 22-2

Cross-sectional view of brain and meningeal layers. **A,** Functional areas of the cerebral cortex, mid-sagittal view. **B,** Frontal section of the superior portion of the head, as viewed from the front. Both bony and membranous coverings of the brain can be seen.

A from McCance, Huether, 2002; B from Thibodeau, Patton, 2003.

BRAIN

The brain receives its blood supply (approximately 15% to 20% of the total cardiac output) from the two internal carotid arteries and two vertebral arteries that join to form the basilar artery (Fig. 22-3). Blood drains from the brain through venous plexuses and dural sinuses that empty into the internal jugular veins. The three major units of the brain are the cerebrum, the cerebellum, and the brainstem.

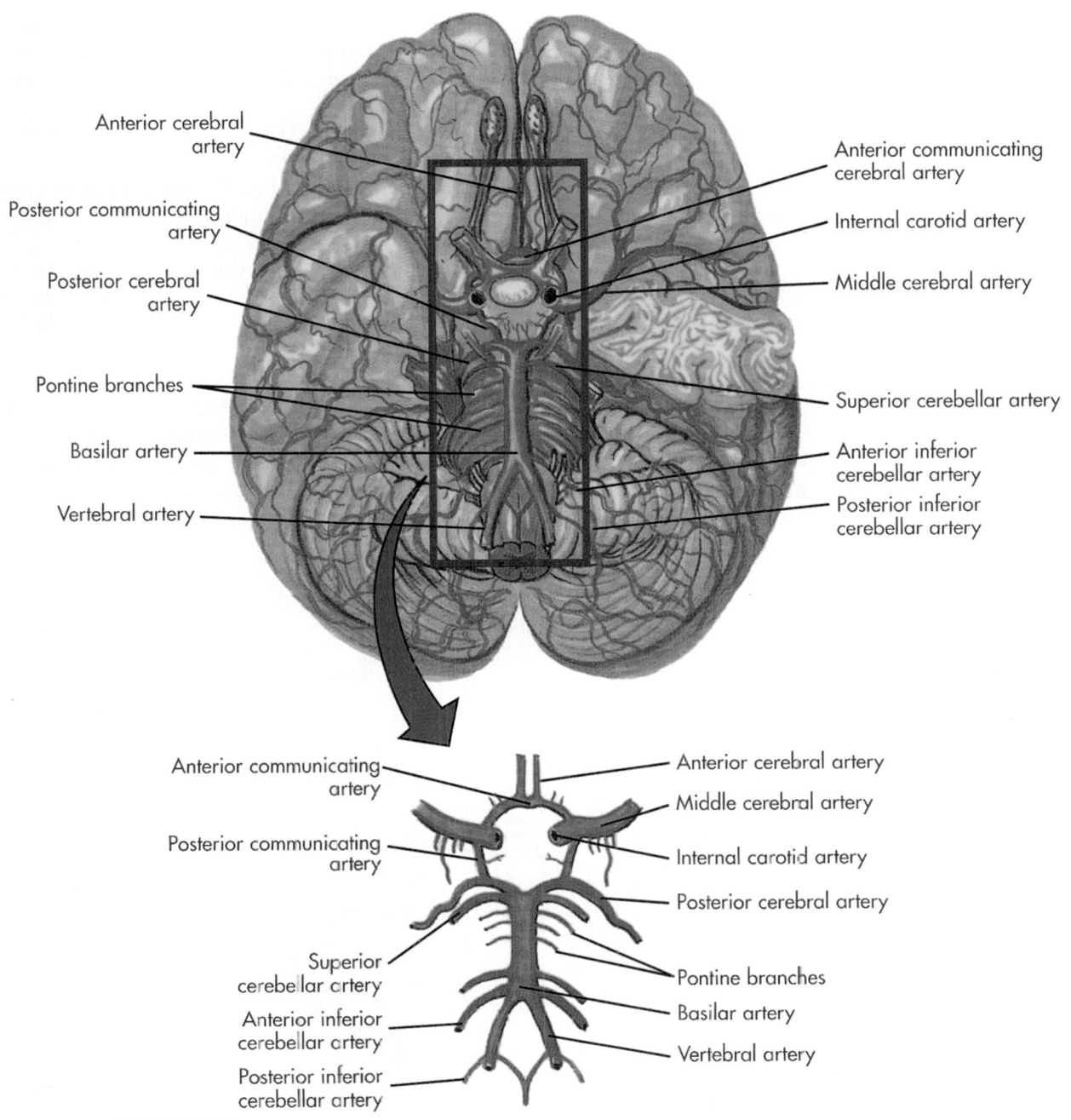

FIGURE 22-3
Arterial blood supply to the brain. The internal carotid arteries supply 80% and the vertebral basilar arteries supply 20%.
From Thibodeau, Patton, 2003.

CEREBRUM

Two cerebral hemispheres, each divided into lobes, form the cerebrum. The gray outer layer, the cerebral cortex, houses the higher mental functions and is responsible for general movement, visceral functions, perception, behavior, and the integration of these functions. Commissural fibers (corpus callosum) interconnect the counterpart areas in each hemisphere, unifying the cerebrum's higher sensory and motor functions (Fig. 22-4; see also Fig. 4-1).

The *frontal lobe* contains the motor cortex associated with voluntary skeletal movement and fine repetitive motor movements, as well as the control of eye movements. Specific areas in the primary motor area are associated with the movement of specific parts of the body. The corticospinal tracts extend from the primary motor area into the spinal cord.

The *parietal lobe* is primarily responsible for processing sensory data as it is received. It assists with the interpretation of tactile sensations (i.e., temperature, pressure, pain, size, shape, texture, and two-point discrimination), as well as visual, gustatory, olfactory, and auditory sensations. Recognition of body parts and awareness of body position (proprioception) are dependent on the parietal lobe. Association fibers provide communication between the sensory and motor areas of the brain.

The *occipital lobe* contains the primary vision center and provides interpretation of visual data.

The *temporal lobe* is responsible for the perception and interpretation of sounds and determination of their source. It is also involved in the integration of taste, smell, and balance. The reception of speech and interpretation of speech is located in Wernicke area.

The *limbic system* mediates the sense of smell and certain patterns of behavior (primitive behaviors, visceral response to emotional and biologic rhythms) that determine survival, such as mating, aggression, fear, and affection. Interference with the physiology of the limbic system results in distorted perception and inappropriate behavior.

CEREBELLUM

The cerebellum aids the motor cortex of the cerebrum in the integration of voluntary movement. It processes sensory information from the eyes, ears, touch receptors, and musculoskeleton. Integrated with the vestibular system, the cerebellum uses the sensory data for reflexive control of muscle tone, equilibrium, and posture to produce steady and precise movements.

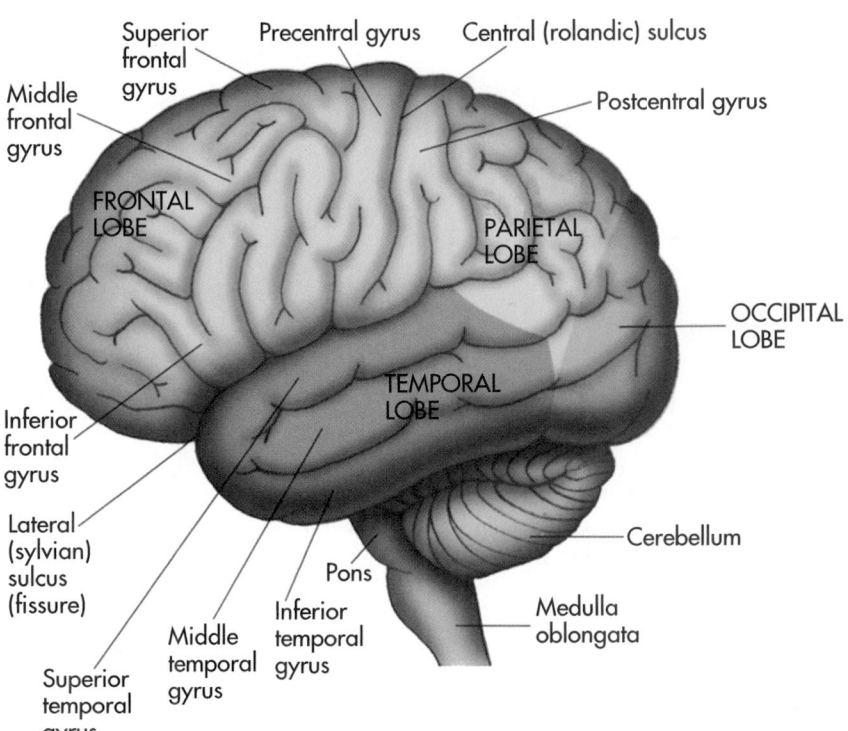

FIGURE 22-4
Lobes and principal fissures of the cerebral cortex, cerebellum, and brainstem (left hemisphere, lateral view).
From McCance, Huether, 2002.

BRAINSTEM

The brainstem is the pathway between the cerebral cortex and the spinal cord, and it controls many involuntary functions. Its structures include the medulla oblongata, pons, midbrain, and diencephalon. The nuclei of the 12 cranial nerves arise from these structures (Fig. 22-5; Table 22-1). The reticular formation contains a network that provides constant muscle stimulation to counteract gravitational forces and regulates cardiovascular functioning and respiration. The reticular formation has fibers that conduct impulses from below the brainstem and up into the cerebral cortex called the reticular activating system. This system must function for an individual to maintain consciousness. The thalamus is the major integrating center for perception of various sensations such as pain and temperature (along with the cortical processing for interpretation), serving as the relay center between the basal ganglia and cerebellum. The pons transmits information between the brainstem and the cerebellum, relaying motor information from the cerebral cortex to the contralateral cerebellar hemisphere. The medulla oblongata is the site where the descending corticospinal tracts decussate (cross to the contralateral side).

CRANIAL NERVES

Cranial nerves are peripheral nerves that arise from the brain rather than the spinal cord. Each nerve has motor or sensory functions, and four cranial nerves have parasympathetic functions (Table 22-2).

BASAL GANGLIA

The basal ganglia or cerebral nuclei function as the extrapyramidal system pathway and processing station between the cerebral motor cortex and the upper brainstem. They contribute input from visual, labyrinthine, and proprioceptive sources that allow gross intentional movement without conscious thought by exerting a fine tuning effect on motor movements.

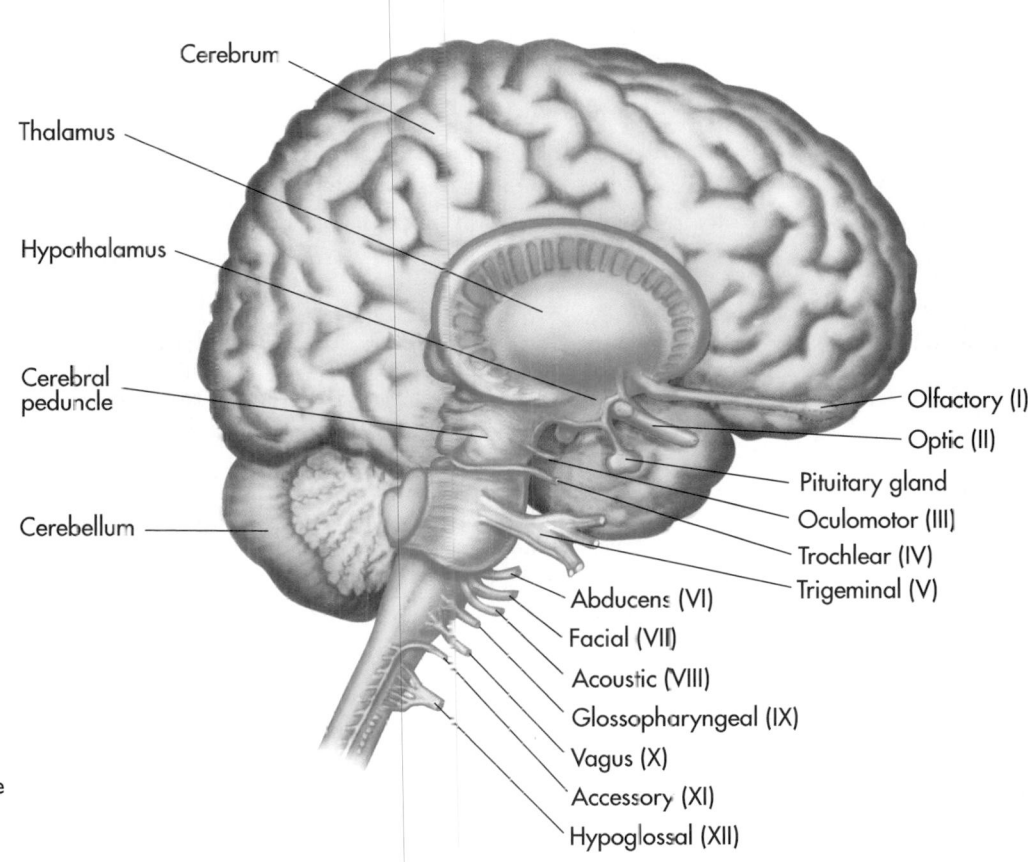

FIGURE 22-5
Structures of the diencephalon and location of the cranial nerve roots.
Modified from Rudy, 1984.

TABLE 22-1	Structures of the Brainstem and Their Functions

Structure	Function
Medulla oblongata CN IX-XII	Respiratory, circulatory, and vasomotor activities; houses respiratory center Reflexes of swallowing, coughing, vomiting, sneezing, and hiccupping Relay center for major ascending and descending spinal tracts that decussate at the pyramid
Pons CN V-VIII	Reflexes of pupillary action and eye movement Regulates respiration; houses a portion of the respiratory center Controls voluntary muscle action with corticospinal tract pathway
Midbrain CN III-IV	Reflex center for eye and head movement Auditory relay pathway Corticospinal tract pathway
Diencephalon CN I-II Thalamus	Relays impulses between cerebrum, cerebellum, pons, and medulla (see Fig. 22-5) Conveys all sensory impulses (except olfaction) to and from cerebrum before their distribution to appropriate associative sensory areas Integrates impulses between motor cortex and cerebrum, influencing voluntary movements and motor response Controls state of consciousness, conscious perceptions of sensations, and abstract feelings
Epithalamus	Houses the pineal body Sexual development and behavior
Hypothalamus	Major processing center of internal stimuli for autonomic nervous system Maintains temperature control, water metabolism, body fluid osmolarity, feeding behavior, and neuroendocrine activity
Pituitary gland	Hormonal control of growth, lactation, vasoconstriction, and metabolism

TABLE 22-2	The Cranial Nerves and Their Functions

Cranial Nerves	Function
Olfactory (I)	Sensory: smell reception and interpretation
Optic (II)	Sensory: visual acuity and visual fields
Oculomotor (III)	Motor: raise eyelids, most extraocular movements Parasympathetic: pupillary constriction, change lens shape
Trochlear (IV)	Motor: downward, inward eye movement
Trigeminal (V)	Motor: jaw opening and clenching, chewing and mastication Sensory: sensation to cornea, iris, lacrimal glands, conjunctiva, eyelids, forehead, nose, nasal and mouth mucosa, teeth, tongue, ear, facial skin
Abducens (VI)	Motor: lateral eye movement
Facial (VII)	Motor: movement of facial expression muscles except jaw, close eyelids, labial speech sounds (b, m, w, and rounded vowels) Sensory: taste—anterior two thirds of tongue, sensation to pharynx Parasympathetic: secretion of saliva and tears
Acoustic (VIII)	Sensory: hearing and equilibrium
Glossopharyngeal (IX)	Motor: voluntary muscles for swallowing and phonation Sensory: sensation of nasopharynx, gag reflex, taste—posterior one third of tongue Parasympathetic: secretion of salivary glands, carotid reflex Motor: voluntary muscles of phonation (guttural speech sounds) and swallowing
Vagus (X)	Sensory: sensation behind ear and part of external ear canal Parasympathetic: secretion of digestive enzymes; peristalsis; carotid reflex; involuntary action of heart, lungs, and digestive tract
Spinal accessory (XI)	Motor: turn head, shrug shoulders, some actions for phonation
Hypoglossal (XII)	Motor: tongue movement for speech sound articulation (l, t, d, n) and swallowing

Modified from Rudy, 1984.

SPINAL CORD AND SPINAL TRACTS

The spinal cord, 40 to 50 cm long, begins at the foramen magnum as a continuation of the medulla oblongata and terminates at L1 or L2 of the vertebral column. Fibers, grouped into tracts, run through the spinal cord carrying sensory, motor, and autonomic impulses between higher centers in the brain and the body. The myelin-coated white matter of the spinal cord contains the ascending and descending tracts (Fig. 22-6). The gray matter, which contains the nerve cell bodies, is arranged in a butterfly shape with anterior and posterior horns.

The *descending spinal tracts* (corticospinal, reticulospinal, vestibulospinal) originate in the brain and convey impulses to various muscle groups by inhibiting or exciting spinal activity. They also have a role in the control of muscle tone, posture, and precise motor movements. The corticospinal (pyramidal) tract permits skilled, delicate, and purposeful movements. The vestibulospinal tract causes the extensor muscles of the body to suddenly contract when an individual starts to fall. The corticobulbar tract arising from the brainstem innervates the motor functions of the cranial nerves.

The *ascending spinal tracts* (spinothalamic, spinocerebellar) mediate various sensations. They facilitate the sensory signals necessary for complex discrimination tasks and are capable of transmitting precise information about the type of stimulus and its location. The posterior (dorsal) column spinal tract (fasciculus gracilis and fasciculus cuneatus) carries the fibers for the discriminatory sensations of touch, deep pressure, vibration, position of the joints, stereognosis, and two-point discrimination. The spinothalamic tracts carry the fibers for the sensations of light and crude touch, pressure, temperature, and pain.

Upper motor neurons are motor pathways that all originate and terminate within the central nervous system. They comprise the descending pathways from the brain to the spinal cord. Their primary role is influencing, directing, and modifying spinal reflex arcs and circuits. The upper motor neurons can affect movement only through the lower motor neurons. The *lower motor neurons,* cranial and spinal motor neurons, originate in the anterior horn of the spinal cord and extend into the peripheral nervous system. They transmit neural signals directly to the muscles to permit movement. Injury to the upper motor neurons results in initial paralysis followed by partial recovery over an extended period. Injury to the lower motor neurons often results in permanent paralysis (Sugarman, 2002).

SPINAL NERVES

Thirty-one pairs of spinal nerves arise from the spinal cord and exit at each intervertebral foramen (Fig. 22-7). The sensory and motor fibers of each spinal nerve supply and receive information in a specific body distribution called a *dermatome* (Fig. 22-8). The anterior branches of several spinal nerves combine to form nerve plexi, so that a spinal nerve may lose its individuality to some extent. The spinal nerve may also complement the effort of an anatomically related nerve or even help compensate for some loss of function. A multitude of peripheral nerves originate from these nerve plexi (Fig. 22-9).

Within the spinal cord, each spinal nerve separates into ventral and dorsal roots. The motor or efferent fibers of the anterior (ventral) root carry impulses from the spinal cord to the muscles and glands of the body. The sensory or afferent fibers of the posterior (dorsal) root carry impulses from sensory receptors of the body to the spinal cord. From here the impulses travel to the brain for interpretation by the cerebral sensory cortex.

An impulse may alternatively initiate a reflex action when it synapses immediately with the motor fiber after a stimulus such as a tap on a stretched muscle tendon. In this case, the impulse is transmitted outward by the motor neuron in the anterior horn of the spinal cord via the spinal nerve and peripheral nerve of the skeletal muscle, stimulating a brisk contraction (Fig. 22-10). Such a reflex is dependent on intact afferent nerve fibers, functional synapses in the spinal cord, intact motor nerve fibers, functional neuromuscular junctions, and competent muscle fibers.

INFANTS AND CHILDREN

The major portion of brain growth occurs in the first year of life, along with myelinization of the brain and nervous system. Any intruding event (e.g., infection, biochemical imbalance, or trauma) that upsets brain development and growth during this period can have profound effects on eventual brain function.

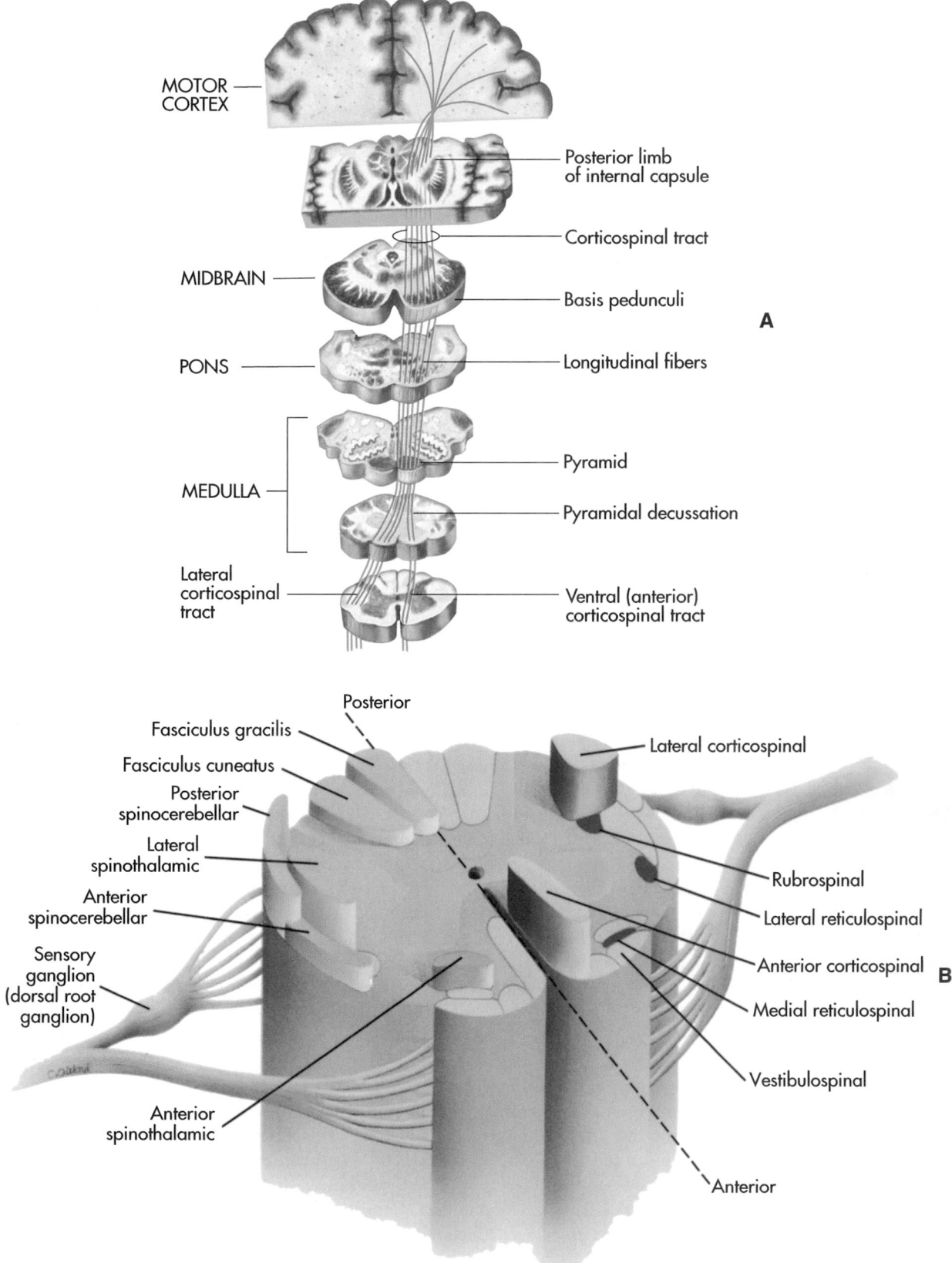

MOTOR CORTEX

Posterior limb of internal capsule

Corticospinal tract

MIDBRAIN

Basis pedunculi

A

PONS

Longitudinal fibers

MEDULLA

Pyramid

Pyramidal decussation

Lateral corticospinal tract

Ventral (anterior) corticospinal tract

Posterior

Fasciculus gracilis

Lateral corticospinal

Fasciculus cuneatus

Posterior spinocerebellar

Lateral spinothalamic

Rubrospinal

Anterior spinocerebellar

Lateral reticulospinal

Sensory ganglion (dorsal root ganglion)

Anterior corticospinal

B

Medial reticulospinal

Vestibulospinal

Anterior spinothalamic

Anterior

FIGURE 22-6
Tracts of the spinal cord. **A,** Pathway of spinal tracts from spinal cord to motor cortex. Note decussation of the pyramids at the level of the medulla. **B,** Major ascending (sensory) tracts, shown here only on the left, are highlighted in blue. Major descending (motor) tracts, shown here only on the right, are highlighted in red.
A modified from Rudy, 1984; B from Thibodeau, Patton, 2003.

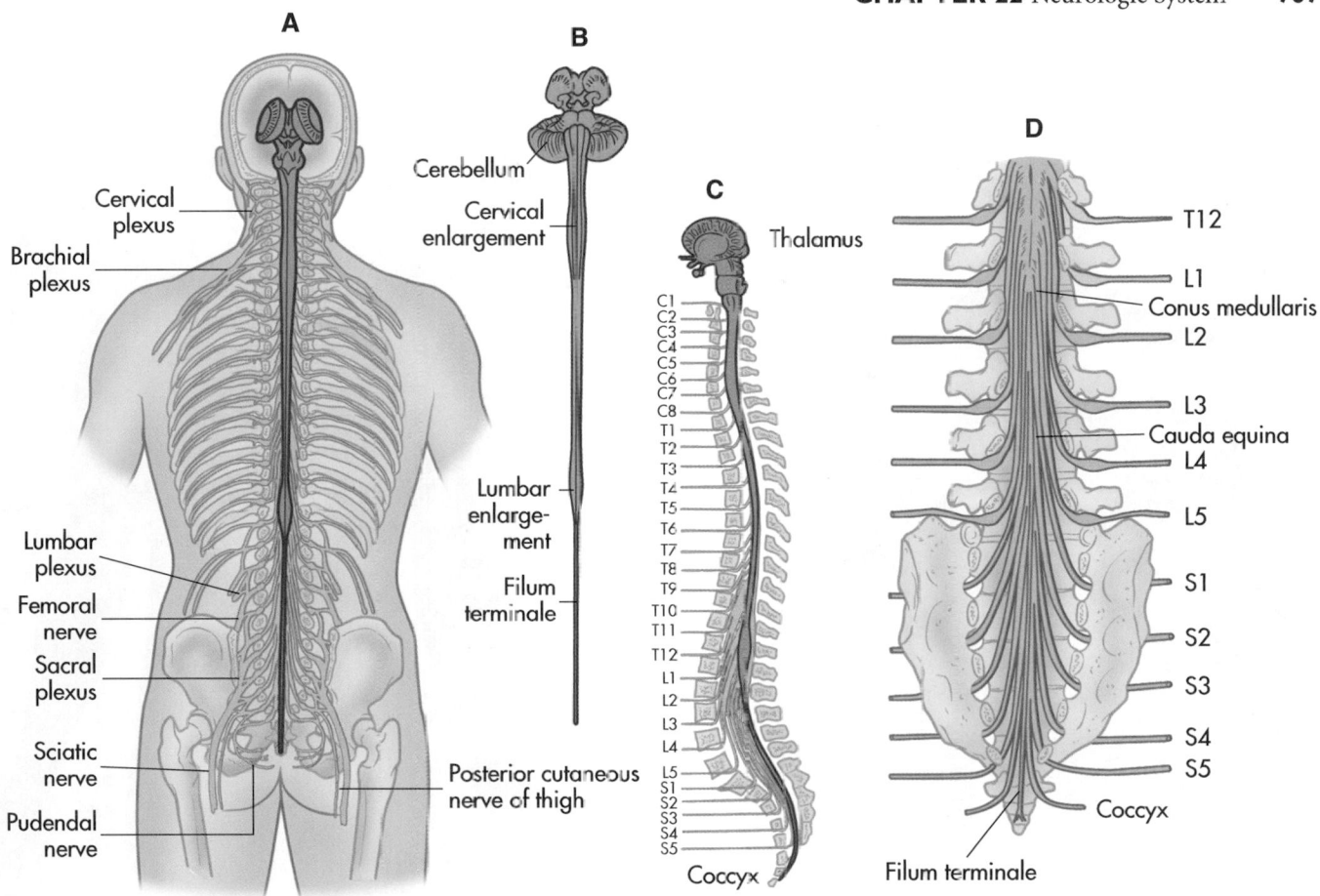

FIGURE 22-7
Location of exiting spinal nerves in relation to the vertebrae. **A,** Posterior view. **B,** Anterior view of brainstem and spinal cord. **C,** Lateral view showing relationship of spinal cord to vertebrae. **D,** Enlargement of caudal area with group of nerve fibers composing the cauda equina.
Modified from Rudy, 1984.

PHYSICAL VARIATIONS

Motor Development
The timing of motor development varies considerably in children. Black children generally are more advanced than white children, at least until the age of 3 years.

The following primitive reflexes are present in the newborn: yawn, sneeze, hiccup, blink at bright light and loud sound, pupillary constriction with light, and withdrawal from painful stimuli. As the brain develops, some primitive reflexes are inhibited when more advanced cortical functions and voluntary control take over.

Motor maturation proceeds in a cephalocaudal direction. Motor control of the head and neck develops first, followed by the trunk and extremities. Motor development is a succession of integrated milestones, each leading to more complex and independent function (see Table 21-4). There is an orderly sequence to development, but considerable variation in timing exists in children. Many capabilities may be developing simultaneously in any one child.

Brain growth continues until 12 to 15 years of age.

PREGNANT WOMEN

Hypothalamic-pituitary neurohormonal changes occur with pregnancy; however, specific alterations in the neurologic system are not well identified. More common physiologic alterations that may occur during pregnancy are contraction or tension headaches (worsened by postural changes and new situational problems); and acroparesthesia (numbness and tingling of the hands) due to postural kinking of blood vessels at the thoracic outlet. This may be confused with carpal tunnel syndrome. Acroparesthesia can be worse in the supine position and severely interrupt or disrupt sleep. During the first trimester, women increase their nap time and sleep time, but they may not feel rested even with increased sleep. Late in pregnancy women have more frequent night awakenings and less sleep time.

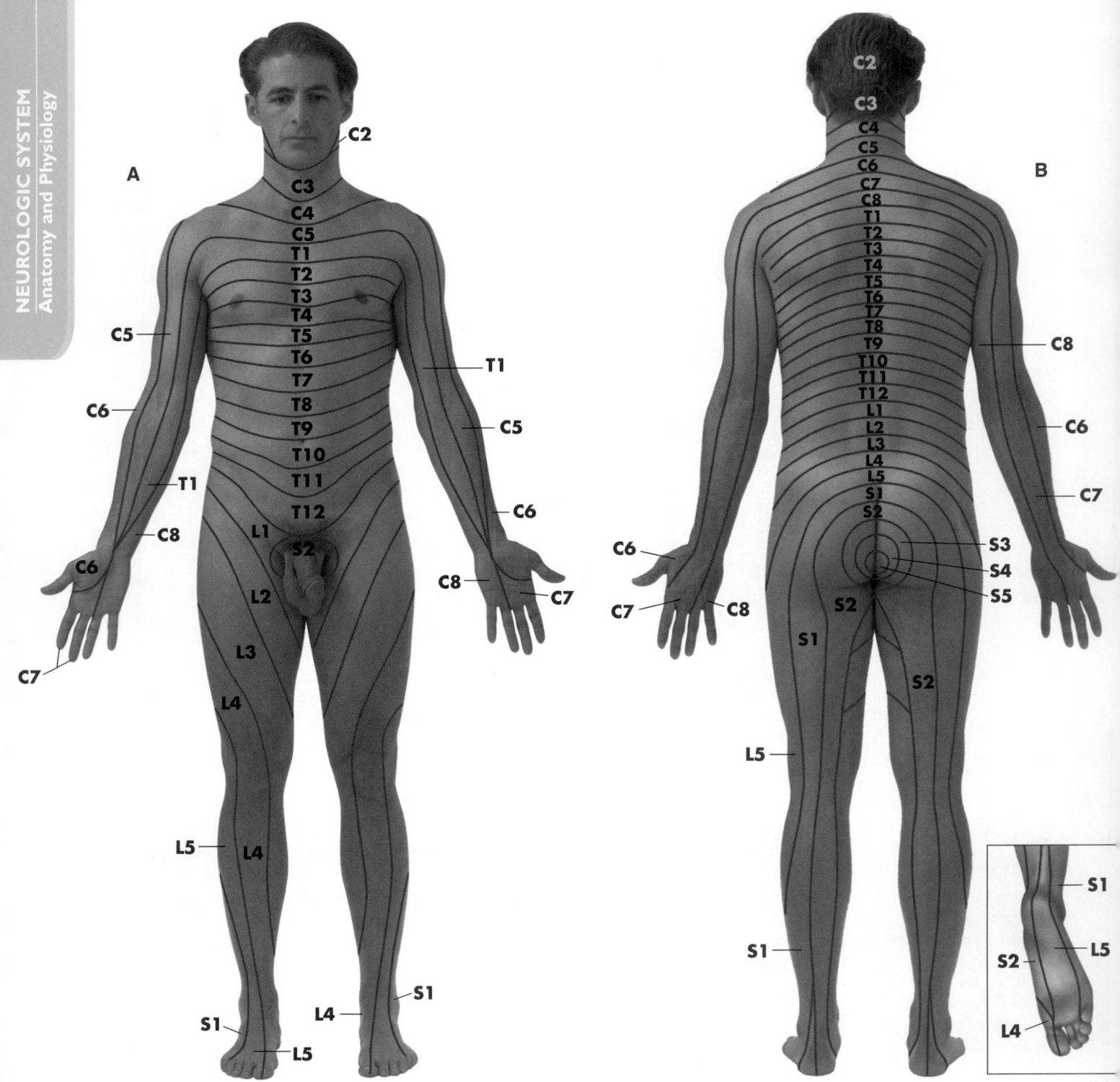

FIGURE 22-8
Dermatomes of the body, the area of body surface innervated by particular spinal nerves; CI usually has no cutaneous distribution. **A,** Anterior view. **B,** Posterior view. It appears that there is a distinct separation of surface area controlled by each dermatome, but there is almost always overlap between spinal nerves.

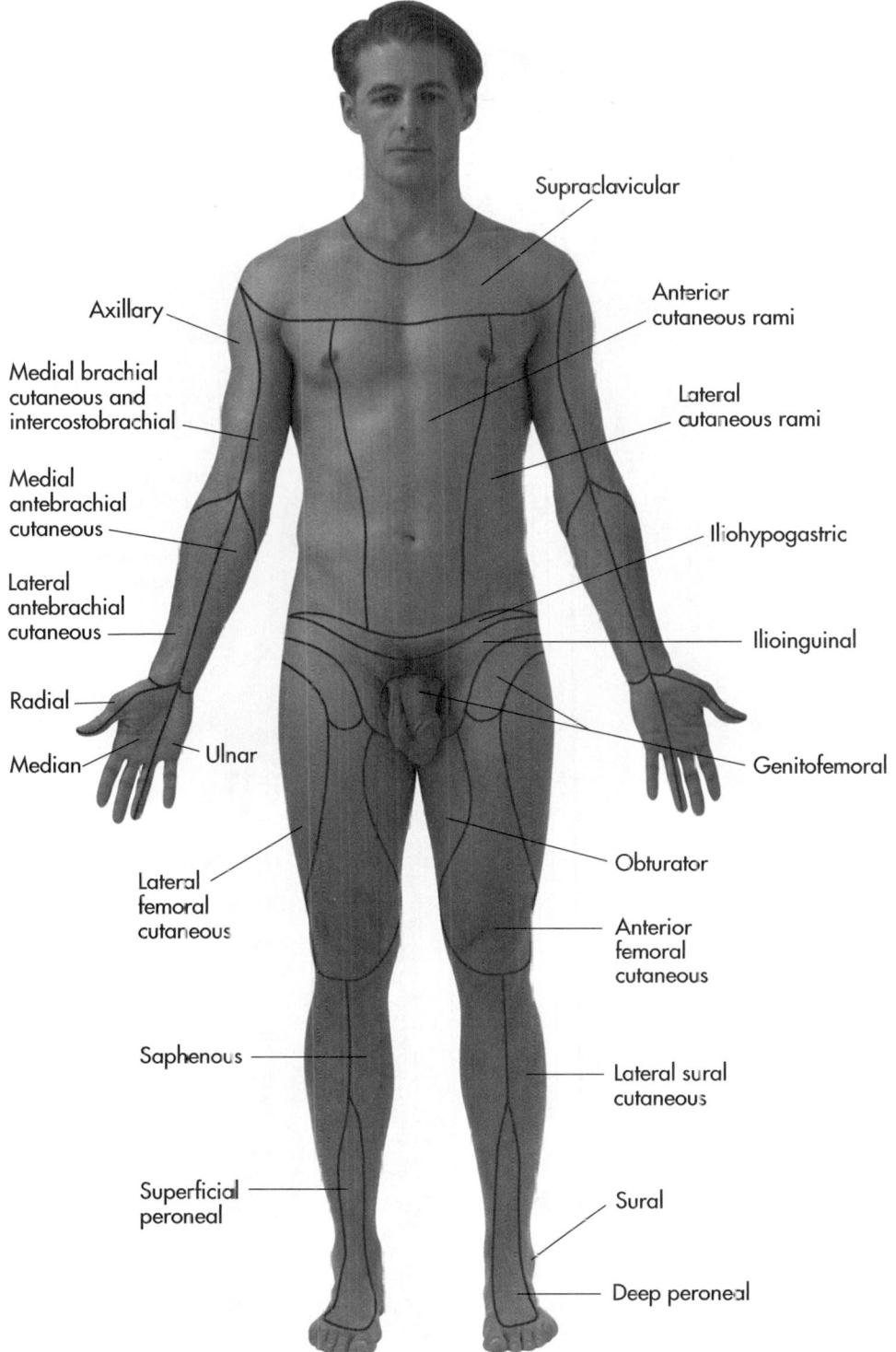

Supraclavicular

Axillary

Medial brachial
cutaneous and
intercostobrachial

Medial
antebrachial
cutaneous

Lateral
antebrachial
cutaneous

Radial

Median

Ulnar

Anterior
cutaneous rami

Lateral
cutaneous rami

Iliohypogastric

Ilioinguinal

Genitofemoral

Lateral
femoral
cutaneous

Saphenous

Superficial
peroneal

Obturator

Anterior
femoral
cutaneous

Lateral sural
cutaneous

Sural

Deep peroneal

FIGURE 22-9
Area of sensory innervation by certain peripheral nerves. **A,** Anterior view.

Continued

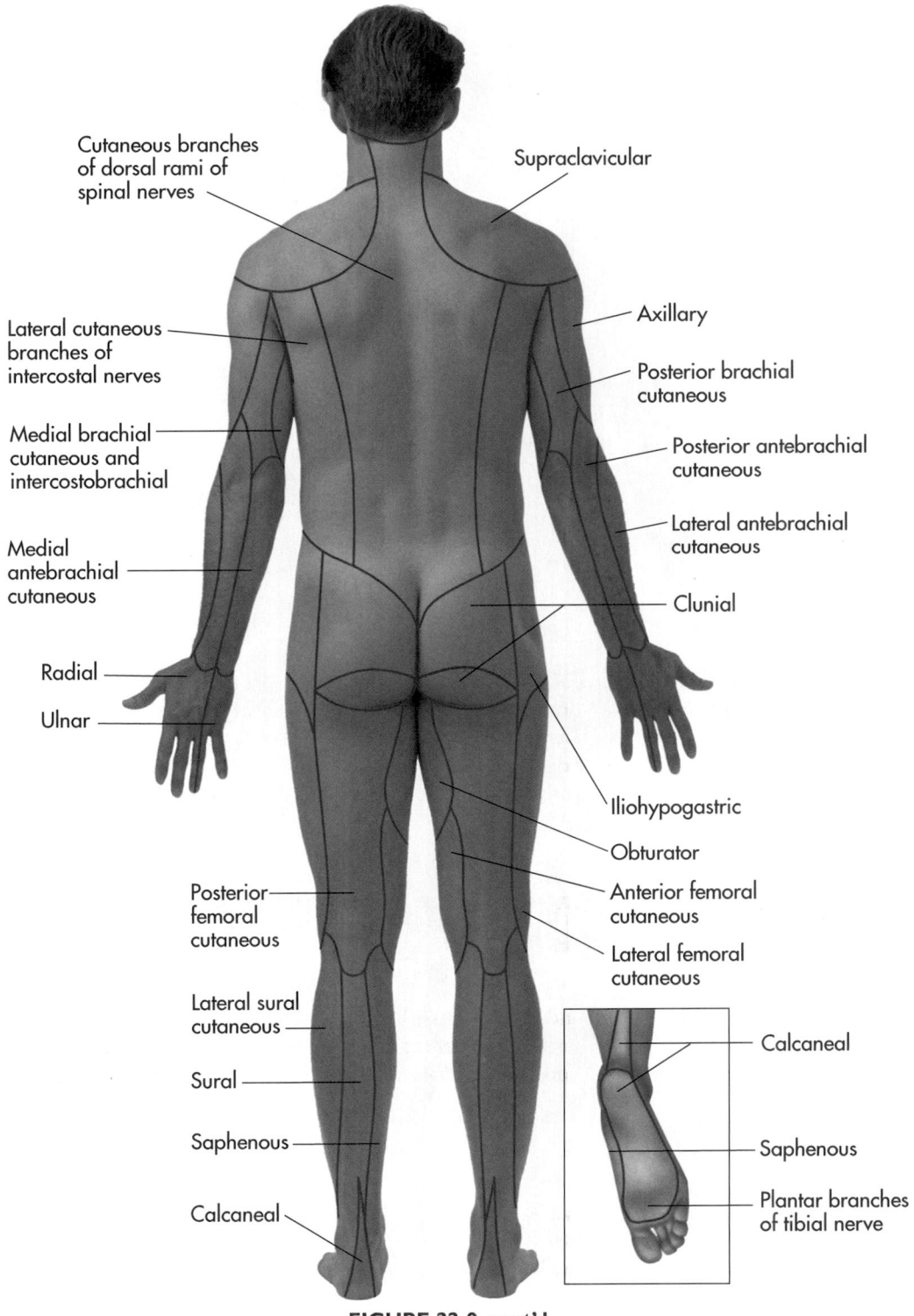

Cutaneous branches
of dorsal rami of
spinal nerves

Supraclavicular

Lateral cutaneous
branches of
intercostal nerves

Axillary

Posterior brachial
cutaneous

Medial brachial
cutaneous and
intercostobrachial

Posterior antebrachial
cutaneous

Medial
antebrachial
cutaneous

Lateral antebrachial
cutaneous

Clunial

Radial

Ulnar

Iliohypogastric

Obturator

Anterior femoral
cutaneous

Posterior
femoral
cutaneous

Lateral femoral
cutaneous

Lateral sural
cutaneous

Calcaneal

Sural

Saphenous

Saphenous

Calcaneal

Plantar branches
of tibial nerve

FIGURE 22-9, cont'd
B, Posterior view.

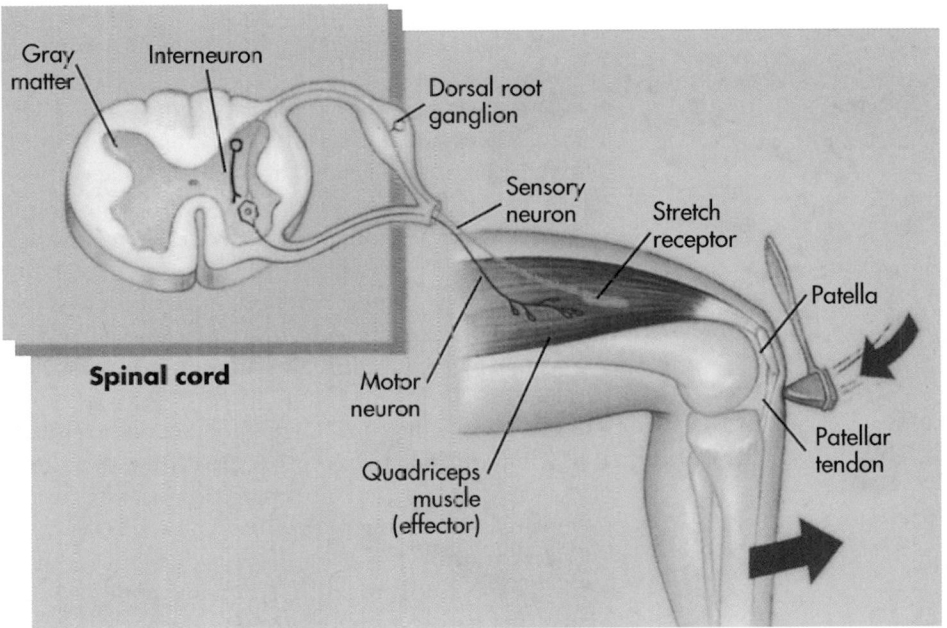

FIGURE 22-10
Cross section of spinal cord
showing simple reflex arc.
From Thibodeau, Patton, 1996.

OLDER ADULTS

The changes that occur with aging are more physiologic than anatomic. The number of cerebral neurons is thought to decrease by 1% a year beginning at 50 years of age; however, the vast number of reserve cells inhibits the appearance of clinical signs. The velocity of nerve impulse conduction declines 10% between 30 and 90 years of age, so responses to various stimuli take longer. Sensory perceptions of touch and pain stimuli may also be diminished.

REVIEW OF RELATED HISTORY

For each of the conditions discussed in this section, targeted topics to include in the history of the present illness are listed. Responses to questions about these topics help fully assess the patient's condition and provide clues for focusing the physical examination.

HISTORY OF PRESENT ILLNESS

- Seizures or convulsions
  - Sequence of events (independent observer's report): aura, fall to ground, shrill cry, motor activity, transition phase, change in color of face or lips, pupil changes or eye deviations, loss of consciousness, postictal phase, total length of seizure activity
  - Character of symptoms
  - Aura: irritability, tension, confusion, blurred vision, mood changes, focal motor seizure activity, gastrointestinal distress
  - Level of consciousness: loss, impairment, duration
  - Automatism: eyelid fluttering, chewing, lip smacking, swallowing
  - Muscle tone: flaccid, stiff, tense, twitching; where spasm began and moved through the body; change in character of motor activity during seizure
  - Postictal behavior: weakness, paralysis, confusion, drowsiness, headaches, muscle aching, time sleeping after seizure; any lateralization of signs

- Relationship of seizure to time of day, meals, fatigue, emotional stress, excitement, menses, and discontinuing medications or poor compliance with medications; activity before attack
- Frequency of seizures; age at first seizure
- Medications: anticonvulsant; prescription and nonprescription; initiation of medication that hastens catabolism of anticonvulsant; alternative or complementary therapies

- Pain: see Chapter 7 for general topics, but consider "neurologic-specific" pain such as headaches associated with meningitis or encephalitis, neck pain, sciatica, or trigeminal neuralgia
  - Onset: sudden or progressive, associated with fever or injury
  - Quality and intensity: deep or superficial; aching, boring, throbbing, sharp or stabbing, burning, pressing, stinging, cramping, gnawing, prickling, shooting; duration and constancy
  - Location or path: along distribution of one or more peripheral nerves or a more general distribution; radiating from one part to another
  - Associated manifestations: crying, decreased activities, sweating, muscle rigidity, tremor, impaired mental processes or concentration, weakness
  - Efforts to treat
  - Medications: opioids and nonsteroidal antiinflammatories; prescription, nonprescription, alternative, or complementary therapies

- Gait coordination
  - Balance: sensation of listing when walking to doorway; unsteadiness when walking
  - Falling: fall one way, backward, forward, consistent direction; associated with looking up
  - Legs simply give way; stiffness of limbs
  - Associated problems: rheumatoid arthritis of cervical spine, ataxia, stroke, seizure, arthritis in knees, arrhythmias, sensory changes
  - Medications: phenytoin, pyrimethamine, etoposide, vinblastine; prescription, nonprescription, alternative, or complementary therapies

- Weakness or paresthesia
  - Onset: sudden, or with initiation of or following sustained activity, time before symptoms begin, rapid or slow
  - Character: generalized or specific body area affected (face, extremity); progressively ascending or transient; proximal or distal extremities, unilateral, bilateral, or asymmetrical; difficulty walking; loss of balance or coordination; hypersensitivity to touch or burning sensation
  - Associated symptoms: tingling or numbness; confusion, trouble speaking or understanding speech; severe headache; impaired vision in one or both eyes; limb feels encased in tight bandage, pain, shortness of breath, stiffness of joints, spasms, muscle tension, sensory deficits; loss of urinary or bowel control
  - Concurrent chronic illness such as infection with human immunodeficiency virus (HIV), nutritional or vitamin deficiency, or recent acute illness
  - Medications: zidovudine, diaminodiphenylsulfone, dideoxyinosine, amphotericin B; prescription, nonprescription, alternative, or complementary therapies

- Tremor
  - Onset: sudden or gradual
  - Character: worse with rest, intentional movement, anxiety; unilateral or bilateral; body location (distal extremities, head); interference with daily activities
  - Associated problems: hyperthyroidism, familial tremor, liver or kidney disorder, consumption of alcohol, multiple sclerosis
  - Relieved by: rest, activity, alcohol
  - Medications: neuroleptics, valproate, phenytoin, albuterol, pseudoephedrine, antiarrhythmics, corticosteroids, caffeine (all may cause essential tremor)

PAST MEDICAL HISTORY

- Trauma: head, spinal cord, or localized injury; central nervous system insult; birth trauma; cerebrovascular accident or stroke
- Meningitis, encephalitis, plumbism, poliomyelitis
- Deformities, congenital anomalies
- Cardiovascular, circulatory problem: hypertension, aneurysm, stroke
- Neurologic disorder, brain surgery, residual effects

FAMILY HISTORY

- Hereditary disorders: neurofibromatosis, Huntington chorea, muscular dystrophy, Tay-Sachs disease
- Alcoholism
- Mental retardation
- Epilepsy or seizure disorder, headaches
- Alzheimer disease
- Learning disorders
- Weakness or gait disorders
- Medical or metabolic disorder: thyroid disease, hypertension, diabetes mellitus

PERSONAL AND SOCIAL HISTORY

- Environmental or occupational hazards: exposure to lead, arsenic, insecticides, organic solvents, other chemicals; operate farm or other dangerous equipment; work at heights or in water
- Hand, eye, and foot dominance; family patterns of dexterity and dominance
- Ability to care for self: hygiene, activities of daily living, finances, communication, shopping; ability to fulfill work expectations
- Sleeping or eating patterns; weight loss or gain; anxiety
- Use of alcohol
- Use of street drugs, especially mood-altering drugs

INFANTS

- Prenatal history: mother's health, medications taken, infections, exposure to TORCH (toxoplasmosis, other [syphilis, tuberculosis], rubella, cytomegalovirus, herpes) infections, feelings of well-being, toxemia, bleeding, history of trauma or stress, persistent vomiting, hypertension, drug or alcohol use
- Birth history: Apgar score, gestational age, birth weight, presentation, use of instruments, prolonged or precipitate labor, fetal distress
- Respiratory status at birth: breathed immediately, need for oxygen, continuous apnea, cyanosis, resuscitative efforts, need for ventilator
- Neonatal health: jaundice (from blood type incompatibility or breast-feeding), infections, seizures, irritability, sucking and swallowing poorly coordinated
- Congenital anomalies, multiple handicapping conditions
- Hypotonia or hypertonia in infancy, developmental delay

CHILDREN

- Developmental milestones
  - Age attained: smiling, head control in prone position, grasping, transferring objects between hands, rolling over, sitting, crawling, independent walking, toilet trained, similar pattern in siblings
  - Loss of previously achieved function: change in the child's rate of development; progress occurred as expected until a certain age with slow progress after that; or has always been slow to do things

- ◆ Performance of self-care activities: dressing, toileting, feeding
- ◆ Impulsive behavior; problems with schedule changes, sitting for entire meal; poor organizational skills, unable to handle more than one instruction at a time, uncontrolled anger, poor social skills; school problems
- ◆ Health problems
  - ◆ Headaches, unexplained vomiting, lethargy, personality changes
  - ◆ Seizure activity: association with fever, frequency, duration, character of movement
  - ◆ Any clumsiness, unsteady gait, progressive muscular weakness, unexplained falling, problems going up and down stairs, problems getting up after lying down on floor

PREGNANT WOMEN

- ◆ Weeks of gestation or estimated date of delivery
- ◆ Convulsions
- ◆ Seizure activity: past history of seizures or pregnancy-induced hypertension; frequency, duration, character of movement
- ◆ Headache: onset, character, frequency, association with hypertension; visual changes
- ◆ Nutritional status: Dietary supplements such as prenatal vitamins, calcium; salt depletion

OLDER ADULTS

- ◆ Pattern of increased stumbling, falls, unsteadiness, or decreased agility; worse in the dark; safety modifications in home
- ◆ Interference with performance of daily living tasks, social withdrawal, feelings about symptoms
- ◆ Hearing loss, vision deficit, or anosmia—transient or longer term
- ◆ Fecal or urinary incontinence
- ◆ Transient neurologic deficits (may indicate transient ischemic attacks)

RISK FACTORS
CEREBROVASCULAR ACCIDENTS (BRAIN ATTACK OR STROKE)

- Hypertension
- Obesity
- Sedentary lifestyle
- Smoking tobacco products
- Stress
- Increased levels of serum cholesterol, lipoproteins, and triglycerides
- Use of oral contraceptives in high-risk women
- Sickle cell anemia
- Family history of diabetes mellitus, cardiovascular disease, hypertension, and increased serum cholesterol levels
- Congenital cerebrovascular anomalies

EXAMINATION AND FINDINGS

EQUIPMENT

- ◆ Penlight
- ◆ Tongue blade
- ◆ Sterile needles
- ◆ Tuning forks, 200 to 400 Hz and 500 to 1000 Hz
- ◆ Familiar objects—coins, keys, paper clip
- ◆ Cotton wisp
- ◆ 5.07 Monofilament

◆ Reflex hammer
◆ Vials of aromatic substances—coffee, orange, peppermint extract, oil of cloves
◆ Vials of solutions—glucose, salt, lemon or vinegar, and quinine—with applicators
◆ Test tubes of hot and cold water for temperature sensation testing
◆ Denver Developmental Screening Test (for infants and children)

Because the neurologic examination is complex, the discussion is divided into four sections to give an organized approach. These sections include cranial nerves, proprioception and cerebellar function, sensory function, and reflex function. Assessment of mental status is detailed in Chapter 4. Evaluation of muscle tone and strength, an integral part of the neurologic examination, is detailed in Chapter 21.

The neurologic system can be examined almost constantly while the rest of the body is explored. In fact, when the patient enters the room and you offer some suggestion as to where he or she might sit, the patient's response tells you a good deal about the functioning of the neurologic system. Your observation throughout the history and physical examination completes many aspects of the neurologic examination. Information from the musculoskeletal examination, particularly muscle tone and strength, are important in interpreting much of the neurologic examination as the systems are interdependent. By the time you begin to examine the neurologic status specifically, you should already be armed with clues to the system's state of health. When the history and examination findings have not yet revealed a potential neurologic problem, a neurologic screening examination may be performed (Box 22-1).

CRANIAL NERVES

An evaluation of the cranial nerves is an integral part of the neurologic examination. Ordinarily, taste and smell are not evaluated unless a problem is suspected. Often, patients will not recognize that they have lost hearing in some ranges, certain taste sensations, or some visual aspects. When a sensory loss is suspected, it is necessary to be compulsive about determining the extent of loss when testing the relevant cranial nerve.

Examination of some cranial nerves is described in detail in other chapters, associated with the body system in which they are most commonly evaluated. Testing of the optic (II), oculomotor (III), trochlear (IV), and abducens (VI) nerves is described in Chapter 11; the acoustic (VIII) and hypoglossal (XII) nerves in Chapter 12; and the spinal accessory nerve (XI) in Chapters 10 and 21. Table 22-3 describes a review of all cranial nerve examination procedures.

MNEMONICS
Cranial Nerves
Names of Cranial Nerves: On Old Olympus' Towering Tops A Finn And German Viewed Some Hops
Classification of Cranial Nerves by Function— Sensory, Motor, or Both: Some Say Marry Money But My Brother Says Bad Business Marry Money
O Olfactory (S)
O Optic (S)
O Oculomotor (M)
T Trochlear (M)
T Trigeminal (B)
A Abducens (M)
F Facial (B)
A Acoustic (S)
G Glossopharyngeal (B)
V Vagus (B)
S Spinal accessory (M)
H Hypoglossal (M)

BOX 22-1

PROCEDURE FOR THE NEUROLOGIC SCREENING EXAMINATION

The shorter screening examination is commonly used for health visits when no known neurologic problem is apparent.

Cranial Nerves
Cranial nerves II through XII are routinely tested; however, taste and smell are not tested unless some aberration is found (pp. 775-780).

Proprioception and Cerebellar Function
One test is administered for each of the following: rapid rhythmic alternating movements, accuracy of movements, balance (Romberg test is given), and gait and heel-toe walking (pp. 780-785).

Sensory Function
Superficial pain and touch at a distal point in each extremity are tested; vibration and position senses are assessed by testing the great toe (pp. 785-788).

Deep Tendon Reflexes
All deep tendon reflexes are tested, excluding the plantar reflex and the test for clonus (pp. 789-791).

TABLE 22-3	Procedure for Cranial Nerve Examination
Cranial Nerve (CN)	**Procedure**
CN I (olfactory)	Test ability to identify familiar aromatic odors, one naris at a time with eyes closed.
CN II (optic)	Test vision with Snellen chart and Rosenbaum near vision chart. Perform ophthalmoscopic examination of fundi.
CN III (oculomotor), IV (trochlear), and VI (abducens)	Test visual fields by confrontation and extinction of vision. Inspect eyelids for drooping. Inspect pupils' size for equality and their direct and consensual response to light and accommodation. Test extraocular eye movements.
CN V (trigeminal)	Inspect face for muscle atrophy and tremors. Palpate jaw muscles for tone and strength when patient clenches teeth. Test superficial pain and touch sensation in each branch (test temperature sensation if there are unexpected findings to pain or touch). Test corneal reflex.
CN VII (facial)	Inspect symmetry of facial features with various expressions (e.g., smile, frown, puffed cheeks, wrinkled forehead). Test ability to identify sweet and salty tastes on each side of tongue.
CN VIII (acoustic)	Test sense of hearing with whisper screening tests or by audiometry. Compare bone and air conduction of sound. Test for lateralization of sound.
CN IX (glossopharyngeal)	Test ability to identify sour and bitter tastes. Test gag reflex and ability to swallow.
CN X (vagus)	Inspect palate and uvula for symmetry with speech sounds and gag reflex. Observe for swallowing difficulty. Evaluate quality of guttural speech sounds (presence of nasal or hoarse quality to voice).
CN XI (spinal accessory)	Test trapezius muscle strength (shrug shoulders against resistance). Test sternocleidomastoid muscle strength (turn head to each side against resistance).
CN XII (hypoglossal)	Inspect tongue in mouth and while protruded for symmetry, tremors, and atrophy. Inspect tongue movement toward nose and chin. Test tongue strength with index finger when tongue is pressed against cheek. Evaluate quality of lingual speech sounds (l, t, d, n).

Modified from Rudy, 1984.

Cranial nerve function is expected to be intact, as described in Table 22-2 for each individual nerve. Unexpected findings indicate trauma or a lesion in the cerebral hemisphere or local injury to the nerve.

OLFACTORY (I)

Have available two or three vials of familiar aromatic odors. Use the least irritating aromatic substance (e.g., orange or peppermint extract) first so that the patient's perception of weaker odors is not impaired. To make sure the patient's nasal passages are patent, you should alternately occlude each naris as the patient inspires and expires.

The patient's eyes should be closed and one naris occluded. As you hold an opened vial under the nose, the patient should take a deep inspiration for the odor to reach the upper nose and swirl around the olfactory mucosa (Fig. 22-11). Ask the patient to identify the odor. Repeat the process with the other naris occluded and using a different odor. Continue the process, comparing the patient's sensitivity and discriminatory ability from side to side, alternating the two or three odors. It is important to allow periods of rest between the offerings of different odors. Offering one odor after the other too quickly can confuse the olfactory sense.

The patient should be able to perceive an odor on each side, and usually identify it. Inflammation of the mucous membranes, allergic rhinitis, and excessive tobacco smoking may all interfere with the ability to distinguish odors. The sense of smell may diminish with age. Anosmia, the loss of sense of smell or an inability to discriminate odors, can be caused by trauma to the cribriform plate or by an olfactory tract lesion.

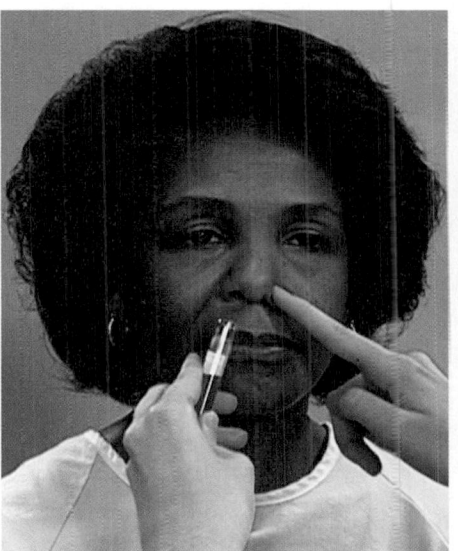

FIGURE 22-11
Examination of the olfactory cranial nerve. Occlude one naris, hold the vial with aromatic substance under the nose, and ask the patient to deeply inspire. If the patient's eyes are open, make sure there are no visual cues to odors. The patient should discriminate between odors.

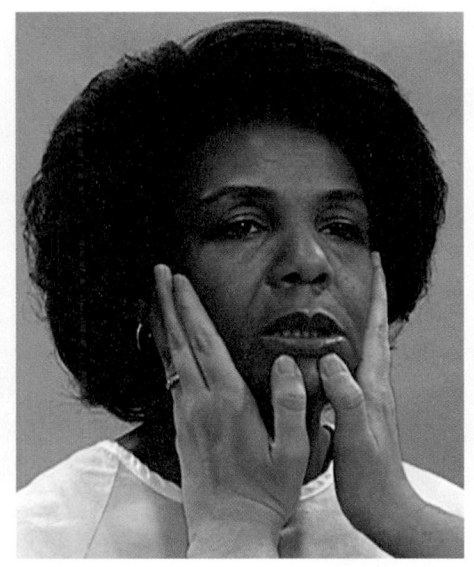

FIGURE 22-12
Examination of the trigeminal cranial nerve for motor function. Have the patient tightly clench the teeth, and then palpate the muscles over the jaw for tone.

OPTIC (II)	Visual acuity and visual fields are evaluated as in Chapter 11.

OCULOMOTOR, TROCHLEAR, AND ABDUCENS (III, IV, AND VI)

Movement of the eyes through the six cardinal points of gaze, pupil size, shape, response to light and accommodation, and opening of the upper eyelids are all described in Chapter 11.

When assessing patients with severe, unremitting headaches, the experienced examiner evaluates movement of the eyes for the presence or absence of lateral (temporal) gaze. The sixth cranial nerve is commonly one of the first to lose function in the presence of increased intracranial pressure.

TRIGEMINAL (V)

Motor function is evaluated by observing the face for muscle atrophy, deviation of the jaw to one side, and fasciculations. Have the patient tightly clench the teeth as you palpate the muscles over the jaw, evaluating tone (Fig. 22-12). Muscle tone over the face should be symmetric without fasciculations.

Three divisions of the nerve are evaluated for sharp, dull, and light touch sensation (Fig. 22-13). With the patient's eyes closed, touch each side of the face at the scalp, cheek, and chin areas, alternately using the sharp and smooth edges of a broken tongue blade or a paper clip. Make sure you do not use a predictable pattern. Ask the patient to report whether each sensation is sharp or dull. Then stroke the face in the same six areas with a cotton wisp or brush, asking the patient to tell when the stimulus is felt. A wooden applicator is used to test sensation over the buccal mucosa. There should be symmetric sensory discrimination over the face to all stimuli.

If sensation is impaired, use test tubes filled with hot and cold water to evaluate temperature sensation. Ask the patient to tell you if hot or cold is felt as you touch the same six areas of the face. Contrast the sensory discrimination of temperature with the other primary sensations.

To test the corneal reflex, have the patient look up and away from you as you approach from the side (contact lenses, if used, should be removed). Avoiding the eyelashes and the conjunctiva, lightly touch the cornea of one eye with a cotton wisp. Repeat the procedure on the other cornea. A symmetric blink reflex to corneal stimulation should occur. Patients who wear contact lenses may have a diminished or absent reflex.

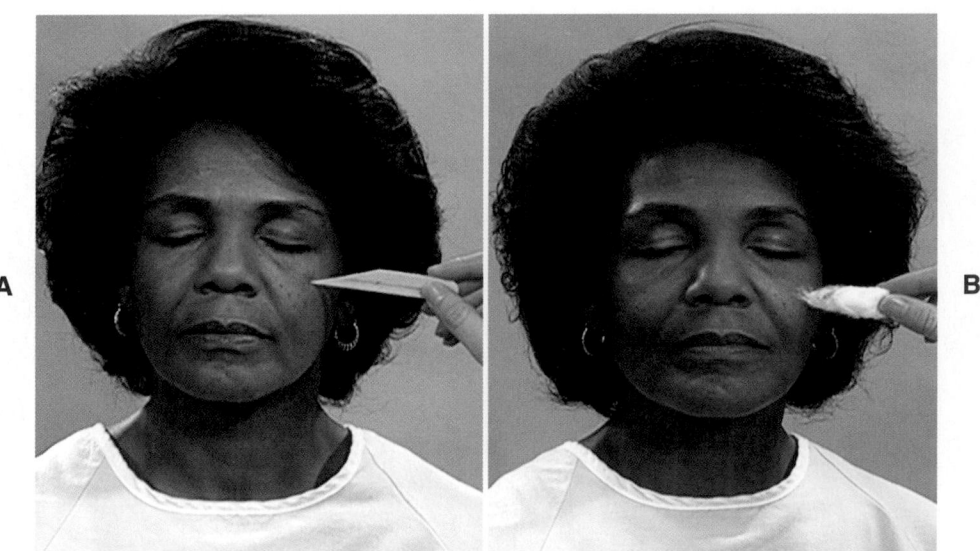

FIGURE 22-13
Examination of the trigeminal cranial nerve for sensory function. Touch each side of the face at the scalp, cheek, and chin areas alternately using no predictable pattern (**A**) with the point and rounded edge of a paper clip or broken tongue blade and (**B**) with a brush or cotton wisp. Ask the patient to discriminate between sensations.

FACIAL (VII)

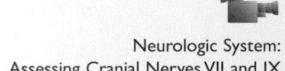

Neurologic System:
Assessing Cranial Nerves VII and IX

Motor function is evaluated by observing a series of expressions you ask the patient to make: raise the eyebrows, squeeze the eyes shut, wrinkle the forehead, frown, smile, show the teeth, purse the lips to whistle, and puff out the cheeks (Fig. 22-14). Observe for tics, unusual facial movements, and asymmetry of expression. Listen to the patient's speech and note any difficulties with enunciating labial sounds (b, m, and p). Muscle weakness is evidenced by one side of the mouth drooping, a flattened nasolabial fold, and lower eyelid sagging.

When evaluating taste, a sensory function of cranial nerves VII and IX, have available the four solutions, applicators, and a card listing the tastes. Make sure the patient cannot see the labels on the vials. Ask the patient to keep the tongue protruded and to point out the taste perceived on the card. Apply one solution at a time to the lateral side of the tongue in the appropriate taste bud region (Fig. 22-15). Alternate the solutions, using a different applicator for each. Offer a sip of water after each stimulus. Each solution is used on both sides of the tongue to identify taste discrimination. The patient should identify each taste bilaterally when placed correctly on the tongue surface.

ACOUSTIC (VIII)

Hearing is evaluated with an audiometer or the simple screening tests described in Chapter 12. Vestibular function is tested by the Romberg test (see p. 781). Other vestibular function tests are not routinely performed.

GLOSSOPHARYN-GEAL (IX)

The sensory function of taste over the posterior third of the tongue is tested during cranial nerve VII evaluation. The glossopharyngeal nerve is simultaneously tested during evaluation of the vagus nerve for nasopharyngeal sensation (gag reflex) and the motor function of swallowing.

VAGUS (X)

To evaluate nasopharyngeal sensation, tell the patient you will be testing the gag reflex. Touch the posterior wall of the patient's pharynx with an applicator as you observe for upward movement of the palate and contraction of the pharyngeal muscles. The uvula should remain in the midline, and no drooping or absence of an arch on either side of the soft palate should be noted.

Motor function is evaluated by inspection of the soft palate for symmetry. Have the patient say "ah," and observe the movement of the soft palate and uvula for asymmetry. If the vagus or glossopharyngeal nerve is damaged and the palate fails to rise, the uvula will deviate from the midline.

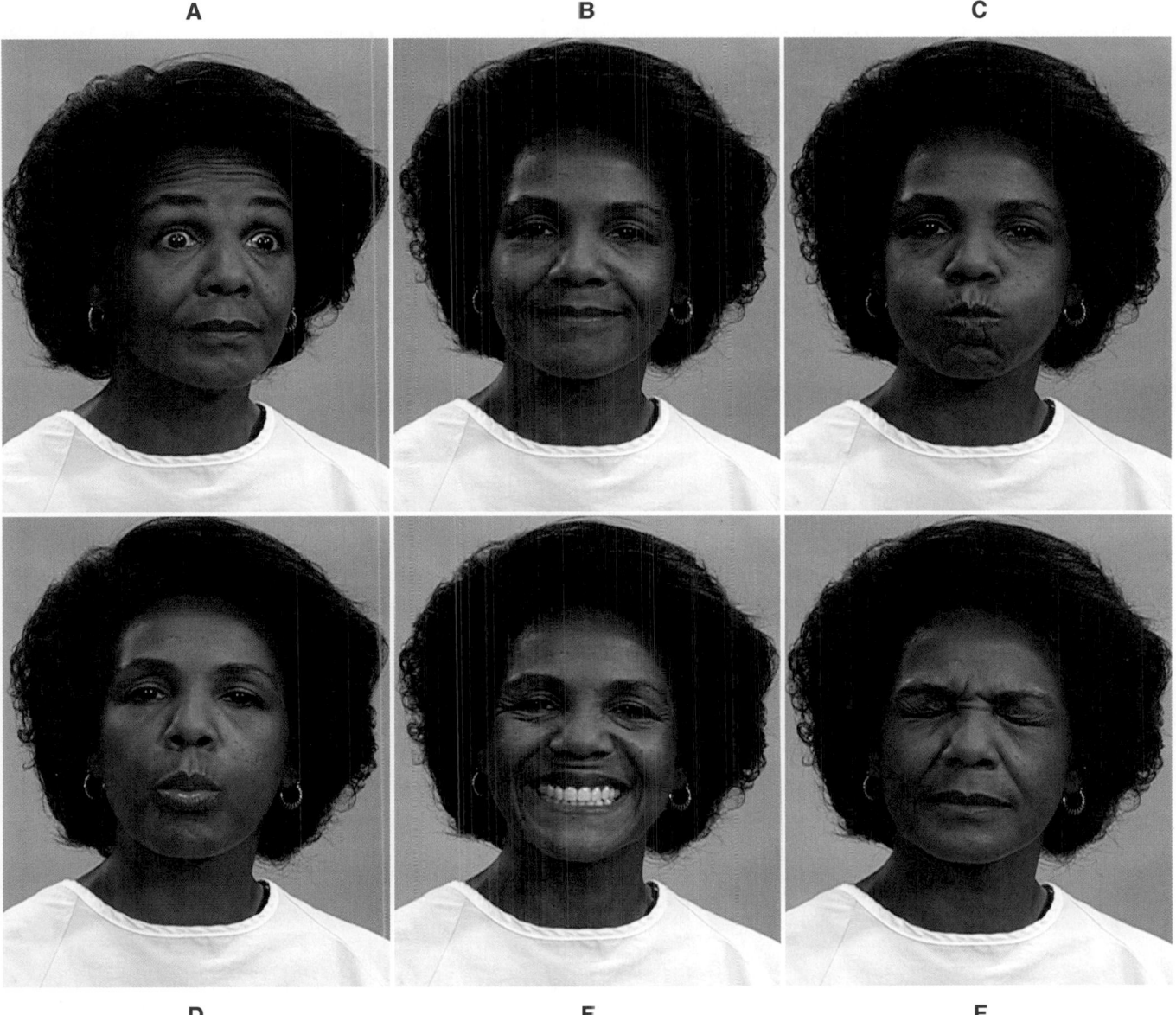

FIGURE 22-14
Examination of the facial cranial nerve for motor function. Ask the patient to (**A**) wrinkle the forehead by raising the eyebrows; (**B**) smile; (**C**) puff out the cheeks; (**D**) purse the lips and blow out; (**E**) show the teeth; and (**F**) squeeze the eyes shut.

Have the patient sip and swallow water. This observation can be made while examining the thyroid gland (see Chapter 10). The patient should swallow easily, having no retrograde passage of water through the nose after the nasopharynx has closed off. Listen to the patient's speech, noting any hoarseness, nasal quality, or difficulty with guttural sounds.

SPINAL ACCESSORY (XI)	Evaluation of the size, shape, and strength of the trapezius and sternocleidomastoid muscles is described in Chapters 10 and 21, respectively.
HYPOGLOSSAL (XII)	Inspect the patient's tongue while at rest on the floor of the mouth and while protruded from the mouth (Fig. 22-16). Note any fasciculations, asymmetry, atrophy, or deviation from the midline. Ask the patient to move the tongue in and out of the mouth, from side to side, curled

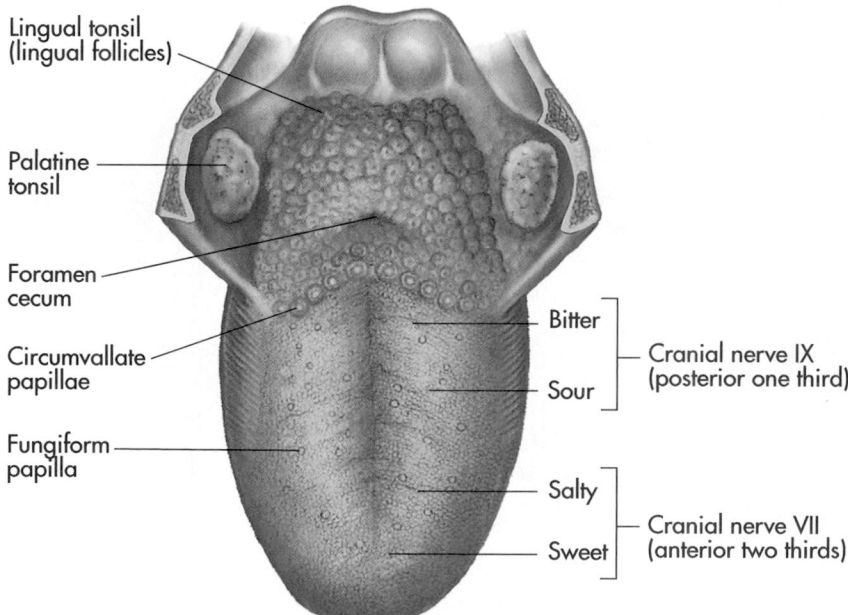

FIGURE 22-15
Location of the taste bud regions tested for the sensory function of the facial and glossopharyngeal cranial nerves.

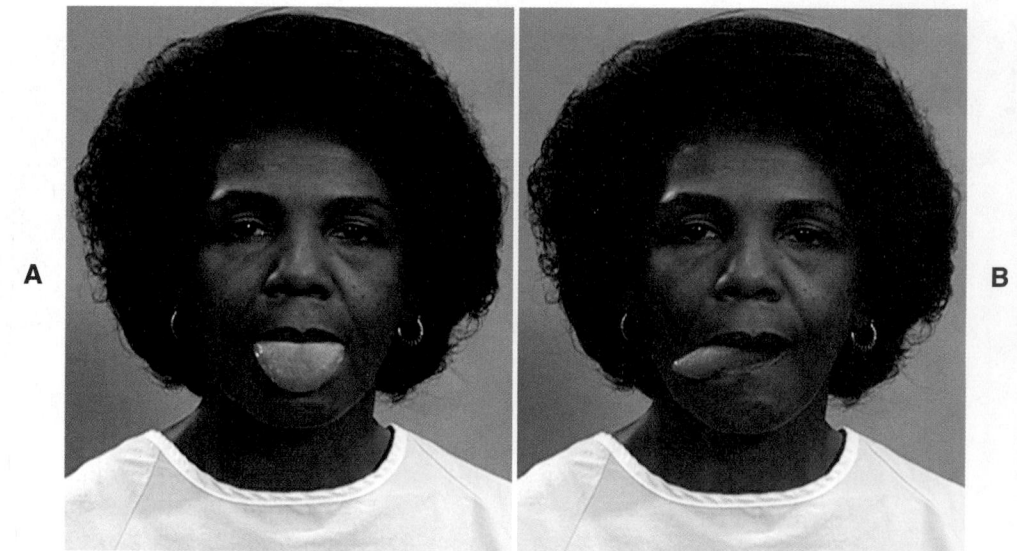

FIGURE 22-16
Examination of the hypoglossal cranial nerve. **A,** Inspect the protruded tongue for size, shape, symmetry, and fasciculation. **B,** Observe movement of the tongue from side to side.

upward as if to touch the nose, and curled downward as if to lick the chin. Test the tongue's muscle strength by asking the patient to push the tongue against the cheek as you apply resistance with an index finger. When listening to the patient's speech, no problems with lingual speech sounds (l, t, d, n) should be apparent.

PROPRIOCEPTION AND CEREBELLAR FUNCTION

COORDINATION AND FINE MOTOR SKILLS

Rapid Rhythmic Alternating Movements. Ask the seated patient to pat his or her knees with both hands, alternately turning up the palm and back of the hands and increasing the rate gradually (Fig. 22-17, *A* and *B*). As an alternate procedure, have the patient touch the thumb to each finger on the same hand, sequentially from the index finger to the little finger and back. Test one hand at a time, increasing speed gradually (Fig. 22-17, *C*).

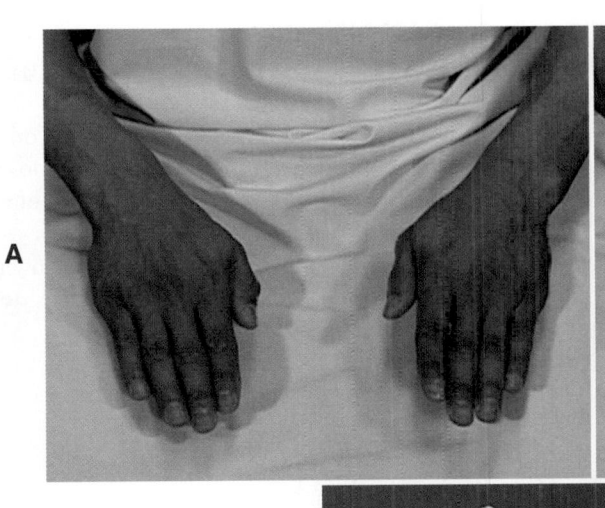
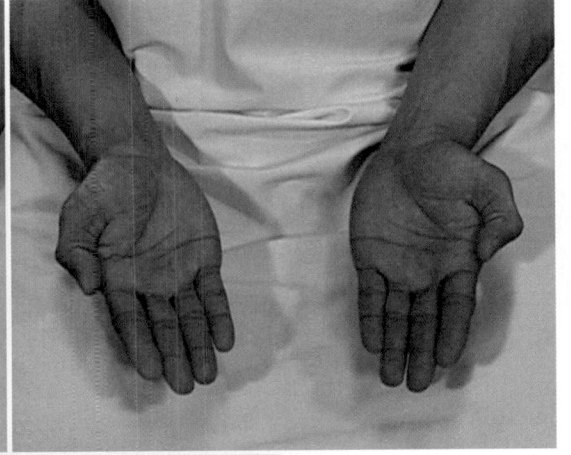
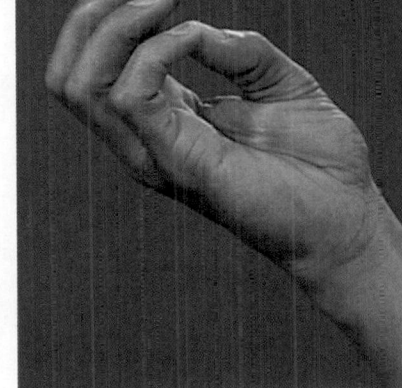

FIGURE 22-17
Examination of coordination with rapid alternating movements. **A** and **B,** Pat the knees with both hands, alternately using the palm and back of the hand. **C,** Touch the thumb to each finger of the hand in sequence from index finger to small finger and back.

Neurologic System:
Testing Accuracy of Movements

Observe for stiff, slowed, nonrhythmic, or jerky clonic movements. The patient should smoothly execute these movements, maintaining rhythm with increasing speed.

Accuracy of Movements. The finger-to-finger test is performed with the patient's eyes open. Ask the patient to use the index finger and alternately touch his or her nose and your index finger (Fig. 22-18, *A* and *B*). Position your index finger about 18 inches from the patient and change the location of your finger several times during the test. Repeat the procedure with the other hand. The movements should be rapid, smooth, and accurate. Consistent past pointing (i.e., missing the examiner's index finger) may indicate cerebellar disease.

To perform the finger-to-nose test, ask the patient to close both eyes and touch his or her nose with the index finger of each hand. Alternate the hands used and increase speed gradually (Fig. 22-18, *C*). Movement should be smooth, rapid, and accurate, even with increasing speed.

The heel-to-shin test is performed with the patient standing, sitting, or supine. Ask the patient to run the heel of one foot up and down the shin (from knee to ankle) of the opposite leg (Fig. 22-18, *D*). Repeat the procedure with the other heel. The patient should move the heel up and down the shin in a straight line, without irregular deviations to the side.

BALANCE

Equilibrium. Balance is initially evaluated with the Romberg test. Ask the patient (with eyes open and then closed) to stand, feet together and arms at the sides (Fig. 22-19). Stand close, prepared to catch the patient if he or she starts to fall. Slight swaying movement of the body is expected, but not to the extent that there is danger of falling. Loss of balance, a positive Romberg sign, indicates cerebellar ataxia, vestibular dysfunction, or sensory loss. If the patient staggers or loses balance with the Romberg test, postpone other tests of cerebellar function requiring balance.

To further evaluate balance, have the patient stand with feet slightly apart. Push the shoulders with enough effort to throw him or her off balance. Be ready to catch the patient if necessary. Recovery of balance should occur quickly.

Balance may also be tested with the patient standing on one foot. The patient's eyes should be closed, with arms held straight at the sides. Repeat the test on the opposite foot. Balance on each foot should be maintained for 5 seconds, but slight swaying is expected.

Have the patient (eyes open) hop in place first on one foot and then on the other (Fig. 22-20). Note any instability, a need to continually touch the floor with the opposite foot, or a tendency to fall. The patient should hop on each foot for 5 seconds without loss of balance.

Gait. Observe the patient walk without shoes around the examining room or down a hallway, first with the eyes open and then closed. Observe the expected gait sequence, noting simultaneous arm movements and upright posture (Fig. 22-21):

1. The first heel strikes the floor and then moves to full contact with the floor.
2. The second heel pushes off, leaving the ground.

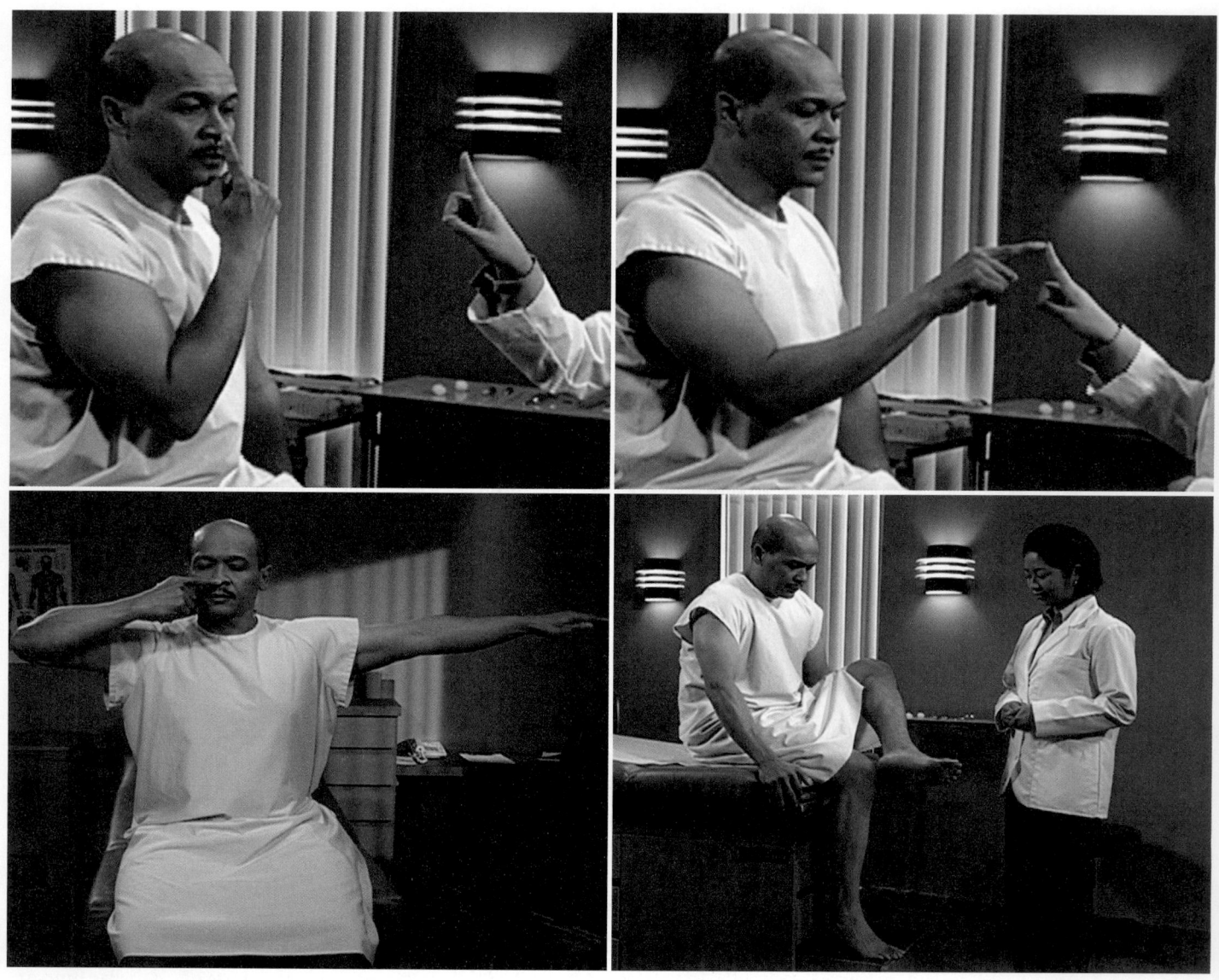

A

C

FIGURE 22-18
Examination of fine motor function. The patient alternately touches own nose and the examiner's index finger with the index finger of one hand (**A** and **B**); alternately touches own nose with the index finger of each hand (**C**); and runs the heel of one foot down the shin or tibia of the other leg (**D**).

3. Body weight is transferred from the first heel to the ball of its foot.
4. The leg swing is accelerated as weight is removed from the second foot.
5. The second foot is lifted and travels ahead of the weight-bearing first foot, swinging through.
6. The second foot slows in preparation for heel strike.

Note any shuffling, widely placed feet, toe walking, foot flop, leg lag, scissoring, loss of arm swing, staggering, or reeling. The patient should continuously sequence both stance and swing, step after step. The gait should have a smooth, regular rhythm and symmetric stride length. The trunk posture should sway with the gait phase, and arm swing should be smooth and symmetric. Fig. 22-22 and Table 22-4 describe unexpected gait patterns.

Heel-toe walking will exaggerate any unexpected finding in gait evaluation. Have the patient walk a straight line, first forward and then backward, with eyes open and arms at the sides. Direct the patient to touch the toe of one foot with the heel of the other foot (Fig. 22-23). Note any extension of the arms for balance, instability, a tendency to fall, or lateral staggering and reeling. Consistent contact between the heel and toe should occur, although slight swaying is expected.

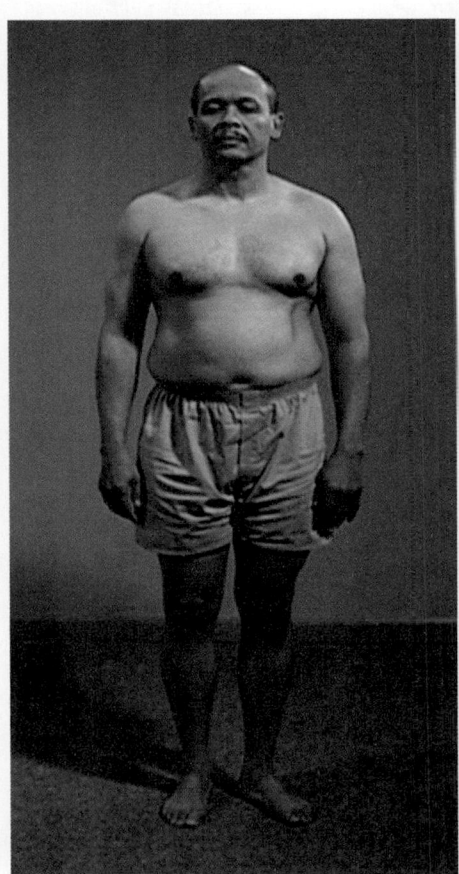

FIGURE 22-19
Evaluation of balance with the Romberg test.

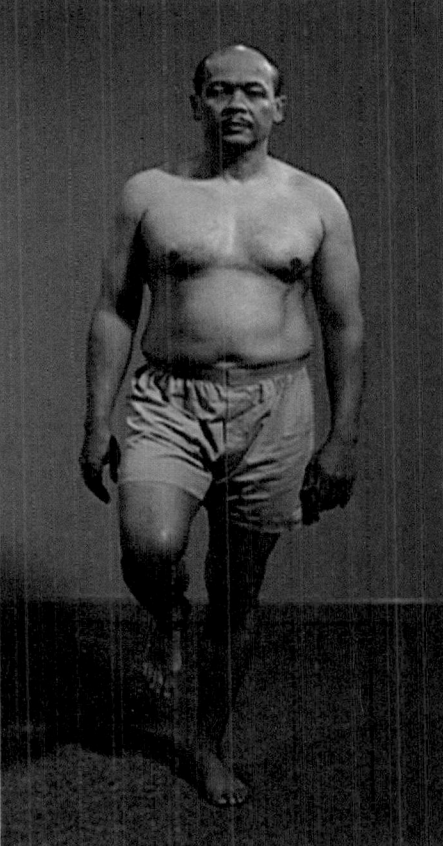

FIGURE 22-20
Evaluation of balance with the patient hopping in place on one foot.

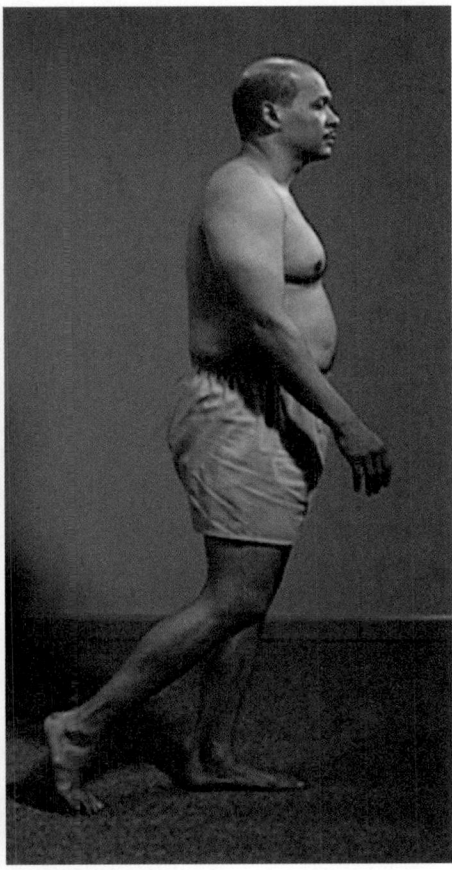

FIGURE 22-21
Evaluation of gait. Note the expected gait sequence and arm movements.

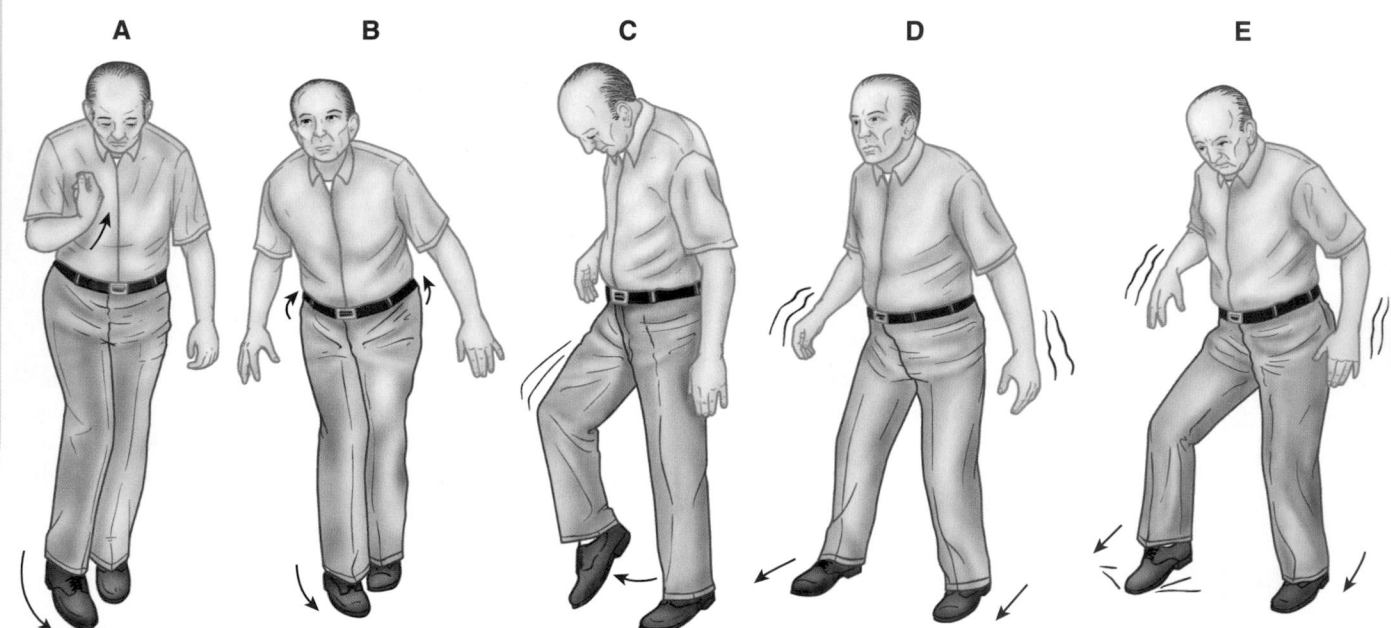

FIGURE 22-22
Unexpected gait patterns. **A,** Spastic hemiparesis. **B,** Spastic diplegia (scissoring). **C,** Steppage gait.
D, Cerebellar ataxia. **E,** Sensory ataxia.

TABLE 22-4	Characteristics of Unexpected Gait Patterns
Gait Pattern	**Characteristics**
Spastic hemiparesis	The affected leg is stiff and extended with plantar flexion of the foot; movement of the foot results from pelvic tilting upward on the involved side; the foot is dragged, often scraping the toe, or it is circled stiffly outward and forward (circumduction); the affected arm remains flexed and adducted and does not swing (see Fig. 22-22, A).
Spastic diplegia (scissoring)	The patient uses short steps, dragging the ball of the foot across the floor; the legs are extended, and the thighs tend to cross forward on each other at each step, due to injury to the pyramidal system (see Fig. 22-22, B).
Steppage	The hip and knee are elevated excessively high to lift the plantar flexed foot off the ground; the foot is brought down to the floor with a slap; the patient is unable to walk on the heels (see Fig. 22-22, C).
Dystrophic (waddling)	The legs are kept apart, and weight is shifted from side to side in a waddling motion due to weak hip abductor muscles; the abdomen often protrudes, and lordosis is common.
Tabetic	The legs are positioned far apart, lifted high and forcibly brought down with each step; the heel stamps on the ground.
Cerebellar gait (cerebellar ataxia)	The patient's feet are wide-based; staggering and lurching from side to side is often accompanied by swaying of the trunk (see Fig. 22-22, D).
Sensory ataxia	The patient's gait is wide-based; the feet are thrown forward and outward, bringing them down first on heels, then on toes; the patient watches the ground to guide his or her steps; a positive Romberg sign is present (see Fig. 22-22, E).
Parkinsonian gait	The patient's posture is stooped and the body is held rigid; steps are short and shuffling, with hesitation on starting and difficulty stopping (see Fig. 22-36 C).
Dystonia	Jerky, dancing movements appear nondirectional.
Ataxia	Uncontrolled falling occurs.
Antalgic limp	The patient limits the time of weight bearing on the affected leg to limit pain.

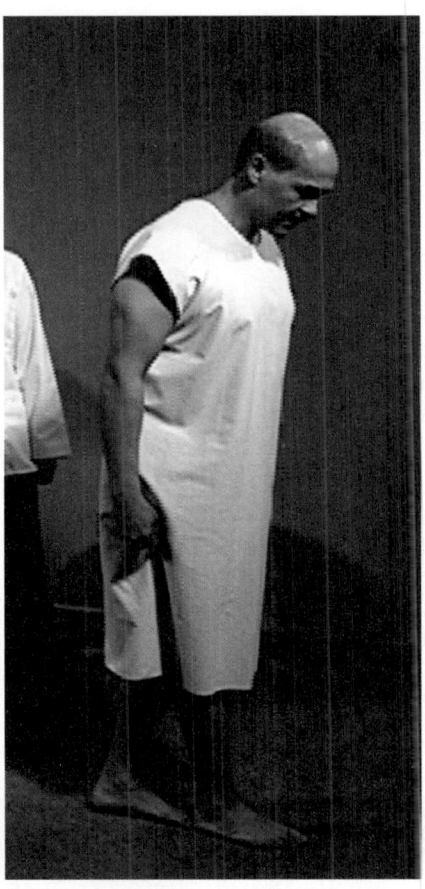

FIGURE 22-23
Evaluation of balance with heel-toe walking on a straight line.

SENSORY FUNCTION

Both primary and cortical discriminatory sensation are evaluated by having the patient identify various sensory stimuli. For the complete neurologic examination, each sense is tested in each major peripheral nerve. These sites should be routinely evaluated during the physical examination: hands, lower arms, abdomen, feet, and lower legs. Sensory discrimination of the face is determined with cranial nerve V evaluation.

Each sensory discrimination procedure is tested with the patient's eyes closed. Use minimal stimulation initially, increasing it gradually until the patient becomes aware of it. A stronger stimulus is needed over the back, buttocks, and heavily cornified areas, where there are lower levels of sensitivity. Test contralateral areas of the body, and ask the patient to compare perceived sensations, side to side. With each type of sensory stimulus, there should be:

- Minimal differences side to side
- Correct interpretation of sensations (e.g., hot/cold, sharp/dull)
- Discrimination of the side of the body tested
- Location of sensation and whether proximal or distal to the previous stimuli

If evidence of sensory impairment is found, map the boundaries of the impairment by the distribution of major peripheral nerves or dermatomes (see Figs. 22-8 and 22-9). Loss of sensation can indicate spinal tract, brainstem, or cerebral lesions.

PRIMARY SENSORY FUNCTIONS

Superficial Touch. Touch the skin with a cotton wisp or with your fingertip, using light strokes. Do not depress the skin, and avoid stroking areas with hair (Fig. 22-24, *A*). Have the patient point to the area touched or tell you when the sensation is felt.

Superficial Pain. Alternating the sharp and smooth edges of a broken tongue blade or the point and hub of a sterile needle, touch the patient's skin in an unpredictable pattern. Allow 2 seconds between each stimulus to avoid a summative effect (see Fig. 22-24, *B*). Ask the patient to identify each sensation as sharp or dull and where it is felt. It is possible to combine evaluation of superficial pain and touch. Alternate the use of the tongue blade or sterile needle with strokes of your fingertip to determine whether the patient can identify the change in sensation.

Temperature and Deep Pressure. Only when superficial pain sensation is not intact are temperature and deep pressure sensation tests performed. Roll test tubes of hot and cold water alternately against the skin, again in an unpredictable pattern, to evaluate temperature sensation. Ask the patient to indicate which temperature is perceived and where it is felt. Deep pressure sensation is tested by squeezing the trapezius, calf, or biceps muscle. The patient should experience discomfort.

Vibration. Place the stem of a vibrating tuning fork (the tuning fork with lower Hz has slower reduction of vibration) against several bony prominences, beginning at the most distal joints. The sternum, shoulder, elbow, wrist, finger joints, shin, ankle, and toes may all be tested (see Fig. 22-24, *C*). A buzzing or tingling sensation should be felt. Ask the patient to tell you when and where the vibration is felt. Occasionally dampen the tines before application to determine whether the patient distinguishes a difference.

Position of Joints. Hold the joint to be tested (e.g., great toe or finger) by the lateral aspects to avoid giving a clue about the direction moved. Beginning with the joint in neutral position, raise or lower the digit, and ask the patient to tell you which way it was moved. Return the digit to the neutral position before moving it in another direction (see Fig. 22-24, *D*). Repeat the procedure so that the great toe of each foot and a finger on each hand are tested.

Loss of sensory modalities may indicate peripheral neuropathy. Symmetric sensory loss indicates a polyneuropathy.

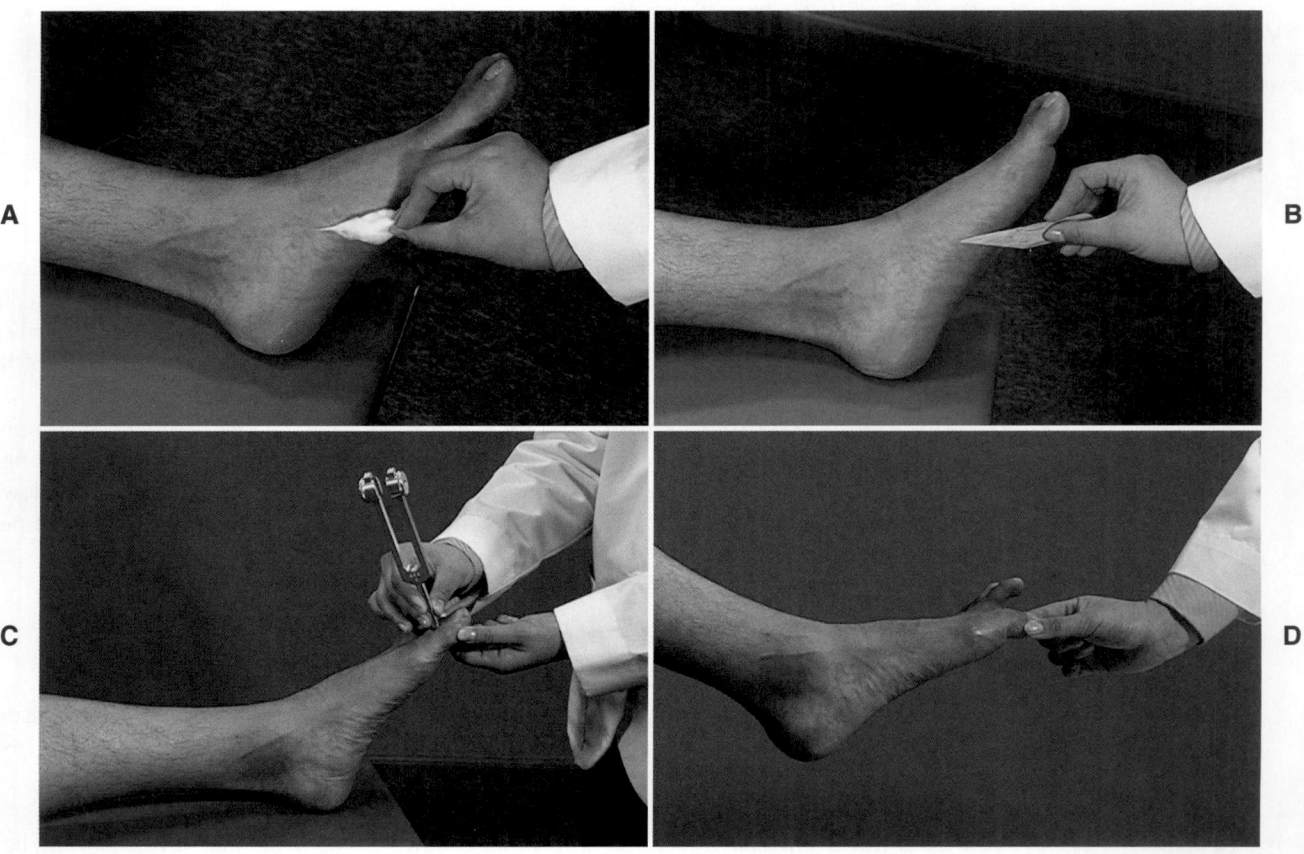

FIGURE 22-24
Evaluation of primary sensory function. **A,** Superficial tactile sensation; use a light stroke to touch the skin with a cotton wisp or brush. **B,** Superficial pain sensation; use the sharp and rounded edge of a broken tongue blade in a nonpredictable alternate pattern. **C,** Vibratory sensation; place the stem of a vibrating tuning fork against several bony prominences. **D,** Position sense of joints; hold the toe or finger by the lateral aspects while raising and lowering the toe.

CORTICAL SENSORY FUNCTIONS

Cortical or discriminatory sensory functions test cognitive ability to interpret sensations. Inability to perform these tests should make you suspect a lesion in the sensory cortex or the posterior columns of the spinal cord. The patient's eyes should be closed for these procedures.

Stereognosis. Hand the patient a familiar object (e.g., key, coin) to identify by touch and manipulation (Fig. 22-25, *A*). Tactile agnosia, an inability to recognize objects by touch, suggests a parietal lobe lesion.

Two-Point Discrimination. Use two sterile needles and alternate touching the patient's skin with one point or both points simultaneously at various locations over the body (see Fig. 22-25, *B*). Find the distance at which the patient can no longer distinguish two points. Table 22-5 lists the minimal distances at which adults can discriminate two points on various parts of the body.

Extinction Phenomenon. Simultaneously touch the cheek, hand, or other area on each side of the body with a sterile needle. Ask the patient to tell you how many stimuli there are and where they are. Similar sensations should be felt bilaterally.

Graphesthesia. With a blunt pen or an applicator stick, draw a letter or number on the palm of the patient's hand (see Fig. 22-25, *C*). Other body locations may also be used. Ask the patient to identify the figure. Repeat the procedure with a different figure on the other hand. The letter or number should be readily recognized.

TABLE 22-5	Minimal Distances for Discriminating Two Points
Body Part	**Minimal Distance (mm)**
Tongue	1
Fingertips	2 to 8
Toes	3 to 8
Palms of hands	8 to 12
Chest and forearms	40
Back	40 to 70
Upper arms and thighs	75

From Barkauskas et al, 2002.

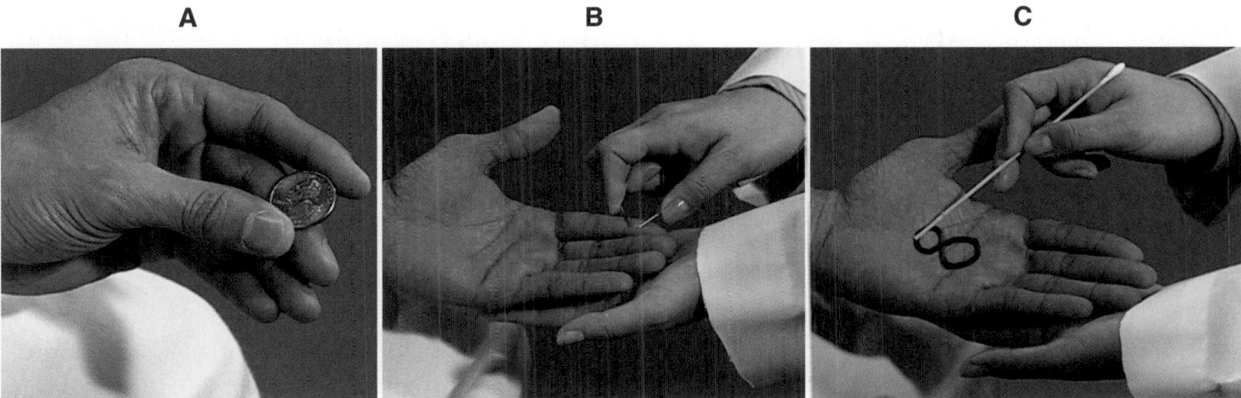

A   B   C

FIGURE 22-25
Evaluation of cortical sensory function. **A,** Stereognosis; patient identifies a familiar object by touch. **B,** Two-point discrimination; using two sterile needles or two points of a paper clip, alternately place one or two points simultaneously on the skin, and ask the patient to determine whether one or two sensations are felt. **C,** Graphesthesia; draw a letter or number on the body (without actually marking skin) and ask the patient to identify it.

Point Location. Touch an area on the patient's skin and withdraw the stimulus. Ask the patient to point to the area touched. No difficulty localizing the stimulus should be noted. This procedure is often performed simultaneously with superficial tactile sensation.

Table 22-6 provides a summary of procedures used to test the integrity of spinal tracts. Patterns of sensory loss are described in Box 22-2.

TABLE 22-6	Procedures for Testing the Integrity of Individual Spinal Tracts for Upper and Lower Motor Neuron Disorders
Spinal Tracts	**Neurologic Tests**
ASCENDING TRACTS—FOR LOWER MOTOR NEURON DISORDERS	
Lateral spinothalamic	Superficial pain
	Temperature
Anterior spinothalamic	Superficial touch
	Deep pressure
Posterior column	Vibration
	Deep pressure
	Position sense
	Stereognosis
	Point location
	Two-point discrimination
Anterior and dorsal spinocerebellar	Proprioception
DESCENDING TRACTS—FOR UPPER MOTOR NEURON DISORDERS	
Lateral and anterior corticospinal	Rapid rhythmic alternating movements
	Voluntary movement
	Deep tendon reflexes
	Plantar reflex
Medial and lateral reticulospinal	Posture and Romberg
	Gait
	Instinctual motor reactions

BOX 22-2

PATTERNS OF SENSORY LOSS

Injury or Defect and Description of Findings

Single Peripheral Nerve
Sensory loss generally less than anatomic distribution of nerve; lost sensation in central portion with a zone of partial loss due to overlap with adjacent nerves; may lose all or selected modalities of sensation.

Multiple Peripheral Nerves (Polyneuropathy)
Sensory loss most severe over legs and feet or over hands (i.e., glove and stocking anesthesia); change from expected to impaired sensation is gradual; usually involves all modalities of sensation.

Multiple Spinal Nerve Roots
Usually incomplete loss of sensation in any area of the skin when one nerve root affected; when two or more nerve roots are completely divided, there is a zone of sensory loss surrounded by partial loss; tendon reflexes may also be lost.

Complete Transverse Lesion of the Spinal Cord
All forms of sensation are lost below the level of the lesion; loss of pain, temperature, and touch sensation occurs one to two dermatomes below the lesion.

Partial Spinal Sensory Syndrome (Brown-Séquard Syndrome)
Pain and temperature sensation occur one to two dermatomes below the lesion on the opposite side of the body from the lesion; proprioceptive loss and motor paralysis occur on the lesion side of the body.

REFLEXES

Both superficial and deep tendon reflexes are used to evaluate the function of specific spine segmental levels (Table 22-7).

SUPERFICIAL REFLEXES

With the patient supine, stroke each quadrant of the abdomen with the end of a reflex hammer or tongue blade edge (see Chapter 17). A slight movement of the umbilicus toward each area of stimulation should be bilaterally equal. When abdominal reflexes are absent, either an upper or lower motor neuron disorder should be suspected.

Stroke the inner thigh of the male patient (proximal to distal) to elicit the cremasteric reflex. The testicle and scrotum should rise on the stroked side.

To elicit the plantar reflex, use a pointed object; stroke the lateral side of the foot from the heel to the ball; then curve across the ball of the foot to the medial side (Fig. 22-26). Observe for plantar flexion, fanning of the toes, or dorsiflexion of the great toe with or without fanning of the other toes.

The patient should have plantar flexion of all toes. The Babinski sign is present when there is dorsiflexion of the great toe with or without fanning of the other toes. This is an expected response in children younger than 2 years of age, but it indicates pyramidal tract disease in other individuals. The ticklish patient may respond with some degree of Babinski sign, but this can be avoided with a firm touch.

DEEP TENDON REFLEXES

Evaluation of deep tendon reflexes is performed with the patient relaxed, either sitting or lying down. Focus the patient's attention on an alternate muscle contraction (e.g., pulling clenched hands apart). Position the limb with slight tension on the tendon to be tapped. Palpate the tendon to locate the correct point for stimulation, rather than randomly tapping in the area. Hold the reflex hammer loosely between your thumb and index finger and briskly tap the tendon with a flick of the wrist. At first you may strike too forcefully, but with practice you will learn to be more gentle.

Test each reflex, comparing responses on corresponding sides. Symmetric visible or palpable responses should be noted. Scoring of deep tendon reflex responses is shown in Table 22-8. Documentation of findings on a stick figure is illustrated in Chapter 26. Absent reflexes may indicate neuropathy or lower motor neuron disorder, whereas hyperactive reflexes suggest an upper motor neuron disorder. The characteristics of upper and lower motor neuron disorders are listed in the Differential Diagnosis box on p. 790.

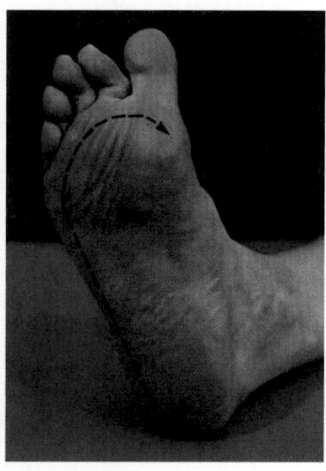

FIGURE 22-26
Plantar reflex indicating the direction of the stroke and the Babinski sign—dorsiflexion of the great toe with or without fanning of the toes.

TABLE 22-7	Superficial and Deep Tendon Reflexes
Reflex	**Spinal Level Evaluated**
SUPERFICIAL	
Upper abdominal	T7, T8, and T9
Lower abdominal	T10 and T11
Cremasteric	T12, L1, and L2
Plantar	L4, L5, S1, and S2
DEEP TENDON	
Biceps	C5 and C6
Brachioradial	C5 and C6
Triceps	C6, C7, and C8
Patellar	L2, L3, and L4
Achilles	S1 and S2

Modified from Rudy, 1984.

TABLE 22-8	Scoring Deep Tendon Reflexes
Grade	**Deep Tendon Reflex Response**
0	No response
1+	Sluggish or diminished
2+	Active or expected response
3+	More brisk than expected, slightly hyperactive
4+	Brisk, hyperactive, with intermittent or transient clonus

DIFFERENTIAL DIAGNOSIS

CHARACTERISTICS OF UPPER AND LOWER MOTOR NEURON DISORDERS

Assessment Parameters	Upper Motor Neuron	Lower Motor Neuron
Muscle tone	Increased tone, muscle spasticity, risk for contractures	Decreased tone, muscle flaccidity
Muscle atrophy	Little or no muscle atrophy, but decreased strength	Loss of muscle strength; muscle atrophy or wasting
Sensation	Sensation loss may affect entire limb	Sensory loss following distribution of dermatomes or peripheral nerves
Reflexes	Hyperactive deep tendon and abdominal reflexes; positive Babinski sign	Weak or absent deep tendon, plantar, and abdominal reflexes, absent Babinski sign, no pathologic reflexes
Fasciculation	No fasciculations	Fasciculations
Motor effect	Paralysis of voluntary movements	Paralysis of muscles
Location of insult	Damage above level of brainstem affects contralateral side of body, damage below the brainstem affects the ipsilateral side of the body	Damage affects muscle on ipsilateral side of body

CLINICAL PEARL

Upper and Lower Neuron Disease

To distinguish between upper and lower neuron disease affecting the face, inspect the face with emotional expression (laughing or crying). When the upper motor neurons are affected, as in a stroke or brain attack, voluntary movements are paralyzed, but emotional movements are spared. In a lower motor neuron disorder, such as Bell palsy, all facial movements on the affected side are paralyzed.

Neurologic System: Assessing the Patellar and Achilles Reflexes

Biceps Reflex. Flex the patient's arm to 45 degrees at the elbow. Palpate the biceps tendon in the antecubital fossa (Fig. 22-27, *A*). Place your thumb over the tendon and your fingers under the elbow. Strike your thumb, rather than the tendon directly, with the reflex hammer. Contraction of the biceps muscle causes visible or palpable flexion of the elbow.

Brachioradial Reflex. Flex the patient's arm up to 45 degrees and rest his or her forearm on your arm with the hand slightly pronated (see Fig. 22-27, *B*). Strike the brachioradial tendon (about 1 to 2 inches above the wrist) directly with the reflex hammer. Pronation of the forearm and flexion of the elbow should occur.

Triceps Reflex. Flex the patient's arm at the elbow up to 90 degrees, supporting the arm proximal to the antecubital fossa. Palpate the triceps tendon and strike it directly with the reflex hammer, just above the elbow (see Fig. 22-27, *C*). Contraction of the triceps muscle causes visible or palpable extension of the elbow.

Patellar Reflex. Flex the patient's knee to 90 degrees, allowing the lower leg to hang loosely. Support the upper leg with your hand, not allowing it to rest against the edge of the examining table. Strike the patellar tendon just below the patella (see Fig. 22-27, *D*). Contraction of the quadriceps muscle causes extension of the lower leg.

Achilles Reflex. With the patient sitting, flex the knee to 90 degrees and keep the ankle in neutral position, holding the foot in your hand. (Alternatively, the patient may kneel on a chair with the toes pointing toward the floor.) Strike the Achilles tendon at the level of the ankle malleoli (see Fig. 22-27, *E*). Contraction of the gastrocnemius muscle causes plantar flexion of the foot.

Clonus. Test for ankle clonus, especially if the reflexes are hyperactive. Support the patient's knee in partially flexed position and briskly dorsiflex the foot with your other hand, main-

A   B   C

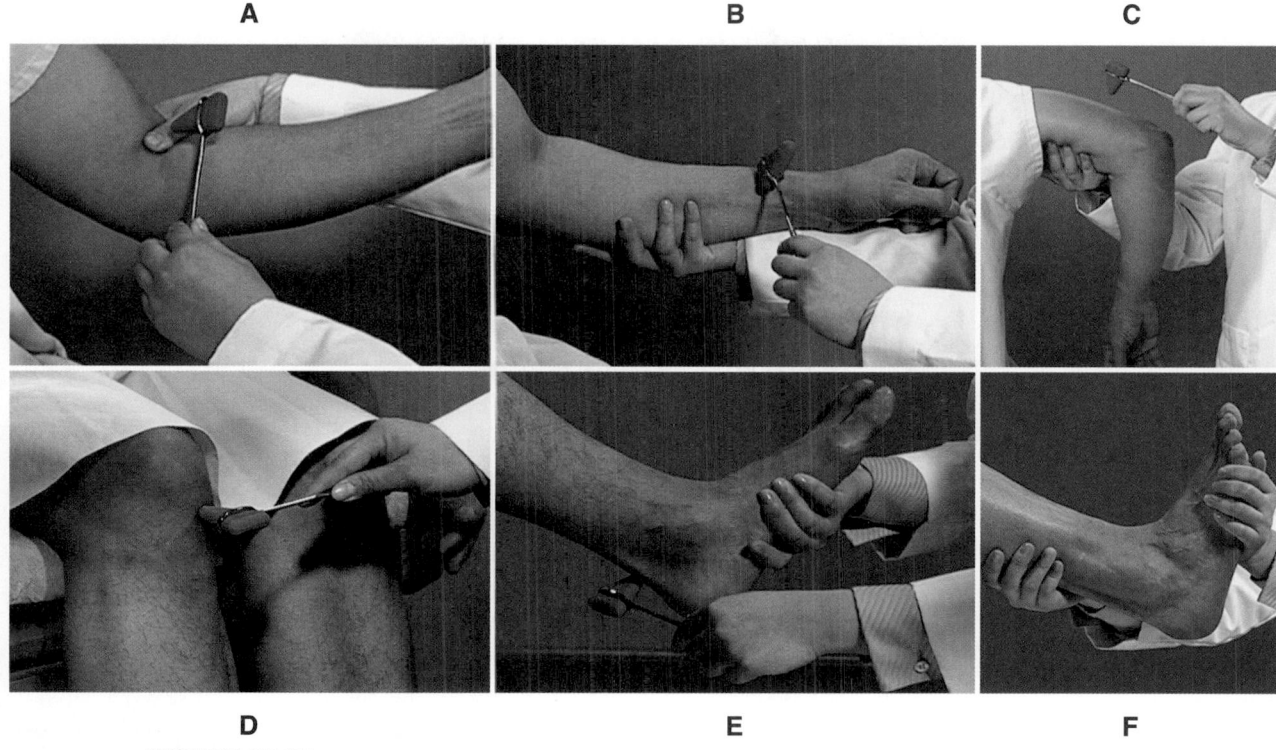

D   E   F

FIGURE 22-27
Location of tendons for evaluation of deep tendon reflexes. **A,** Biceps. **B,** Brachioradial. **C,** Triceps.
D, Patellar. **E,** Achilles. **F,** Evaluation of ankle clonus.

taining the foot in flexion (see Fig. 22-27, *F*). No rhythmic oscillating movements between dorsiflexion and plantar flexion should be palpated. Sustained clonus is associated with upper motor neuron disease.

ADDITIONAL PROCEDURES

Various other procedures for further evaluation of the neurologic system are performed when problems are detected with routine examination.

5.07 MONOFILAMENT

Use the 5.07 monofilament to test for protective sensation on several sites of the foot in all patients with diabetes mellitus and peripheral neuropathy (Fig. 22-28). While the patient's eyes are closed, apply the monofilament in a random pattern in several sites on the plantar surface of the foot and on one site of the dorsal surface. Do not test over calluses or broken skin. Do not repeat a test site. The monofilament should be applied to each site for 1.5 seconds. When the filament bends, adequate pressure is applied. Patients should feel the sensation in all sites. Loss of sensation to the touch of the monofilament is an indication of peripheral neuropathy, and the loss of protective pain sensation that alerts patients to skin breakdown and injury.

MENINGEAL SIGNS

A stiff neck or *nuchal rigidity* is a sign associated with meningitis and intracranial hemorrhage. With the patient supine, slip your hand under the head and raise it, flexing the neck. Try to make the patient's chin touch the sternum, but do not force it. Placing your hand under the shoulders when the patient is supine and raising the shoulders slightly will help relax the neck, making the determination of true stiffness more accurate. Patients generally do not resist or complain of pain. Pain and a resistance to neck motion are associated with nuchal rigidity. Occasionally, painful swollen lymph nodes in the neck and superficial trauma may also cause pain and resistance to neck motion.

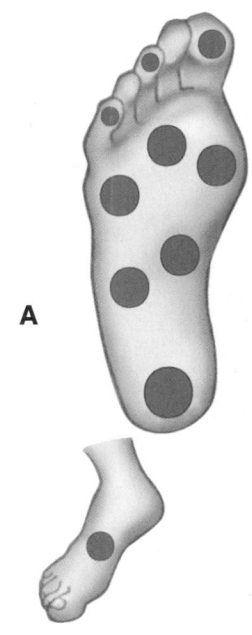

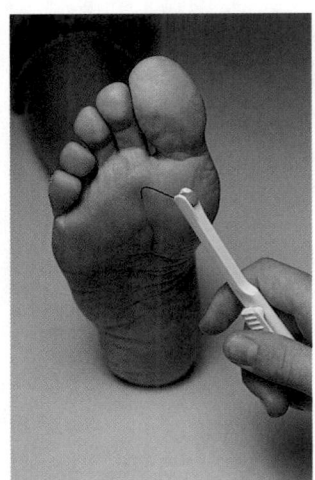

FIGURE 22-28
A, Sites for application of the 5.07 monofilament to test for sensation. Indicate presence (+) or absence (−) of sensory perception. **B,** Apply the monofilament to the patient's foot with just enough pressure to bend the monofilament.

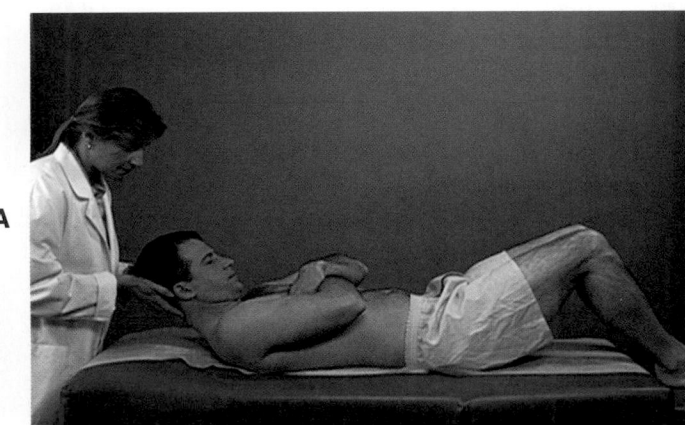

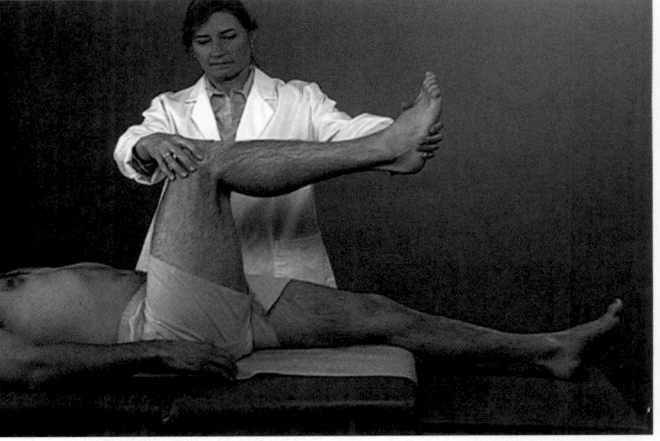

FIGURE 22-29
A, Brudzinski sign, flex the neck and observe for involuntary flexion of the hips and knees. **B,** Kernig sign, flex the leg at the knee and hip when the patient is supine, and then attempt to straighten the leg. Observe for pain in the lower back and resistance to straightening the leg.

The *Brudzinski sign* may also be present when neck stiffness is assessed. Involuntary flexion of the hips and knees when flexing the neck is a positive Brudzinski sign for meningeal irritation (Fig. 22-29, *A*).

The *Kernig sign* is evaluated by flexing the leg at the knee and hip when the patient is supine, then attempting to straighten the leg. Pain in the lower back and resistance to straightening the leg at the knee constitute a positive Kernig sign, indicating meningeal irritation (see Fig. 22-29, *B*).

INFANTS

We ordinarily begin to suspect neurologic problems in the young when they are not doing something we expect them to do, rather than because we find a problem on physical examination. As in so much else, the major clues are discovered with an accurate and painstaking history. Observe for odd facies that may be suggestive of congenital conditions that include neurologic problems (e.g., low-set ears or port wine stain).

TABLE 22-9	Indirect Cranial Nerve Evaluation in Newborns and Infants
Cranial Nerves (CN)	**Procedures and Observations**
CN II, III, IV, and VI	Optical blink reflex: shine a light at the infants open eyes; observe the quick closure of the eyes and dorsal flexion of the infant's head; no response may indicate poor light perception. Gazes intensely at close object or face. Focuses on and tracks an object with both eyes. Doll's eye maneuver: (see CN VIII).
CN V	Rooting reflex: touch one corner of the infant's mouth; the infant should open its mouth and turn its head in the direction of stimulation; if the infant has been recently fed, minimal or no response is expected (see Fig. 22-31). Sucking reflex: place your finger in the infant's mouth, feeling the sucking action; the tongue should push up against your finger with good strength; note the pressure, strength, and pattern of sucking.
CN VII	Observe the infant's facial expression when crying; note the infant's ability to wrinkle the forehead and the symmetry of the smile.
CN VIII	Acoustic blink reflex: loudly clap your hands about 30 cm from the infant's head; avoid producing an air current; note the blink in response to the sound; no response after 2 to 3 days of age may indicate hearing problems; infant will habituate to repeated testing. Moves eyes in direction of sound; freezes position with high-pitched sound. Doll's eye maneuver: hold the infant under the axilla in an upright position, head held steady, facing you; rotate the infant first in one direction and then in the other; the infant's eyes should turn in the direction of rotation and then the opposite direction when rotation stops; if the eyes do not move in the expected direction, suspect a vestibular problem or eye muscle paralysis.
CN IX and X	Swallowing and gag reflex.
CN XII	Coordinated sucking and swallowing ability. Pinch infant's nose; mouth will open and tip of tongue will rise in a midline position.

Modified from Thompson et al, 1997.

CLINICAL PEARL

New Age Range for Rolling Over

Change in sleep position from prone to the back as currently advised to reduce the risk of sudden infant death syndrome has an effect on the age at which infants roll over. Infants roll over at a later age than those that sleep in a prone position.

Data from Jantz, Blosser, Freuchting, 1997.

The cranial nerves are not directly tested, but several observations made during the physical examination provide indirect evaluation (Table 22-9).

Observe the infant's spontaneous activity for symmetry and smoothness of movement (Fig. 22-30). Coordinated sucking and swallowing is also a function of the cerebellum. Hands are usually held in fists for the first 3 months of life, but not constantly; after 3 months they begin to open for longer periods. Purposeful movement (e.g., reaching and grasping for objects) begins at about 2 months of age. This progresses to taking objects with one hand at 6 months, transferring objects hand to hand at 7 months, and purposefully releasing objects by 10 months of age. There should be no tremors or constant overshooting of movements.

A withdrawal of all limbs from a painful stimulus provides a measure of sensory integrity. Other sensory function is not routinely tested.

The patellar tendon reflexes are present at birth, and the Achilles and brachioradial tendon reflexes appear at 6 months of age. When deep tendon reflexes are tested, the examiner should use a finger, rather than the reflex hammer, to tap the tendon. In each case, the muscle attached to the tendon struck should contract. Interpret findings as for adults; however, one or two beats of ankle clonus are common.

The plantar reflex is routinely performed as described in the adult examination. A positive Babinski sign, fanning of the toes and dorsiflexion of the great toe, is found until the infant is 16 to 24 months of age.

The posture and movement of the developing infant are routinely evaluated by primitive reflexes (Table 22-10) and are shown in Figs. 22-31 and 22-32. Less commonly evaluated primitive reflexes are listed in Table 22-11. These reflexes appear and disappear in a sequence corresponding with central nervous system development. Symmetry and smoothness of response are important observations. Posture and movement should also be inspected for any rhythmic twitching of the facial, extremity, and trunk musculature, as well as for any sustained asymmetric posturing. These signs, especially in paroxysmal episodes, are associated with seizure activity.

A

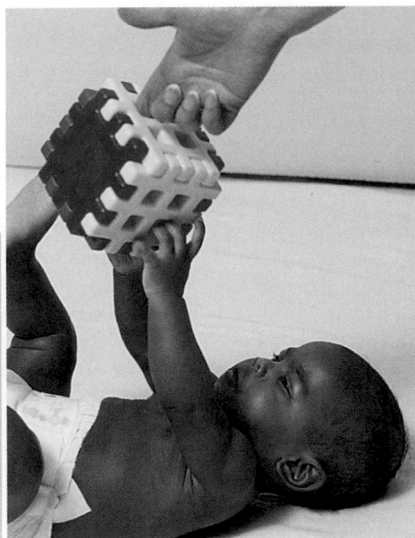

B

FIGURE 22-30
A, Note this infant's beginning effort to roll over. The asymmetric tonic neck reflex has disappeared (p. 795). **B,** Observe purposeful movement such as reaching for the block.

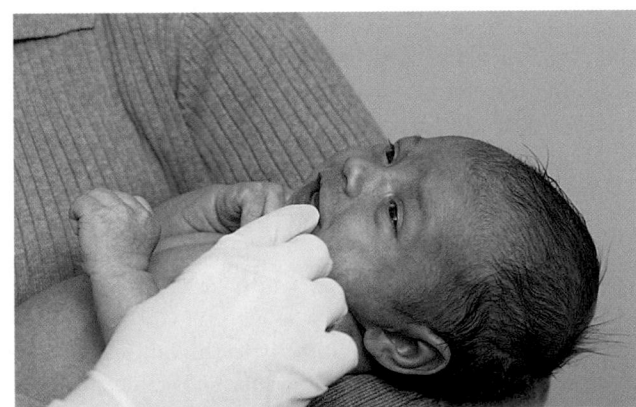

FIGURE 22-31
Demonstration of technique to elicit rooting reflex. Touch the corner of the infant's mouth and observe for movement of the head and opening of the mouth on the side of the stimulation.

TABLE 22-10	Primitive Reflexes Routinely Evaluated in Infants
Reflex (Appearance)	**Procedure and Findings**
Palmar grasp (birth)	Making sure the infant's head is in midline, touch the palm of the infant's hand from the ulnar side (opposite the thumb); note the strong grasp of your finger; sucking facilitates the grasp; it should be strongest between 1 and 2 months of age and disappear by 3 months (see Fig. 22-32, A).
Plantar grasp (birth)	Touch the plantar surface of the infant's feet at the base of the toes; the toes should curl downward; the reflex should be strong up to 8 months of age (see Fig. 22-32, B).
Moro (birth)	With the infant supported in semisitting position, allow the head and trunk to drop back to a 30-degree angle; observe symmetric abduction and extension of the arms; fingers fan out and thumb and index finger form a C; the arms then adduct in an embracing motion followed by relaxed flexion; the legs may follow a similar pattern of response; the reflex diminishes in strength by 3 to 4 months and disappears by 6 months (see Fig. 22-32, C).
Placing (4 days of age)	Hold the infant upright under the arms next to a table or chair; touch the dorsal side of the foot to the table or chair edge; observe flexion of the hips and knees and lifting of the foot as if stepping up on the table; age of disappearance varies (see Fig. 22-32, D).
Stepping (between birth and 8 weeks)	Hold the infant upright under the arms and allow the soles of the feet to touch the surface of the table; observe for alternate flexion and extension of the legs, simulating walking; it disappears before voluntary walking (see Fig. 22-32, E).
Asymmetric tonic neck or "fencing" (by 2 to 3 months)	With the infant lying supine and relaxed or sleeping, turn its head to one side so the jaw is over the shoulder; observe for extension of the arm and leg on the side to which the head is turned and for flexion of the opposite arm and leg; turn the infant's head to the other side, observing the reversal of the extremities' posture; this reflex diminishes at 3 to 4 months of age and disappears by 6 months; be concerned if the infant never exhibits the reflex or seems locked in the fencing position; this reflex must disappear before the infant can roll over or bring its hands to its face (see Fig. 22-32, F).

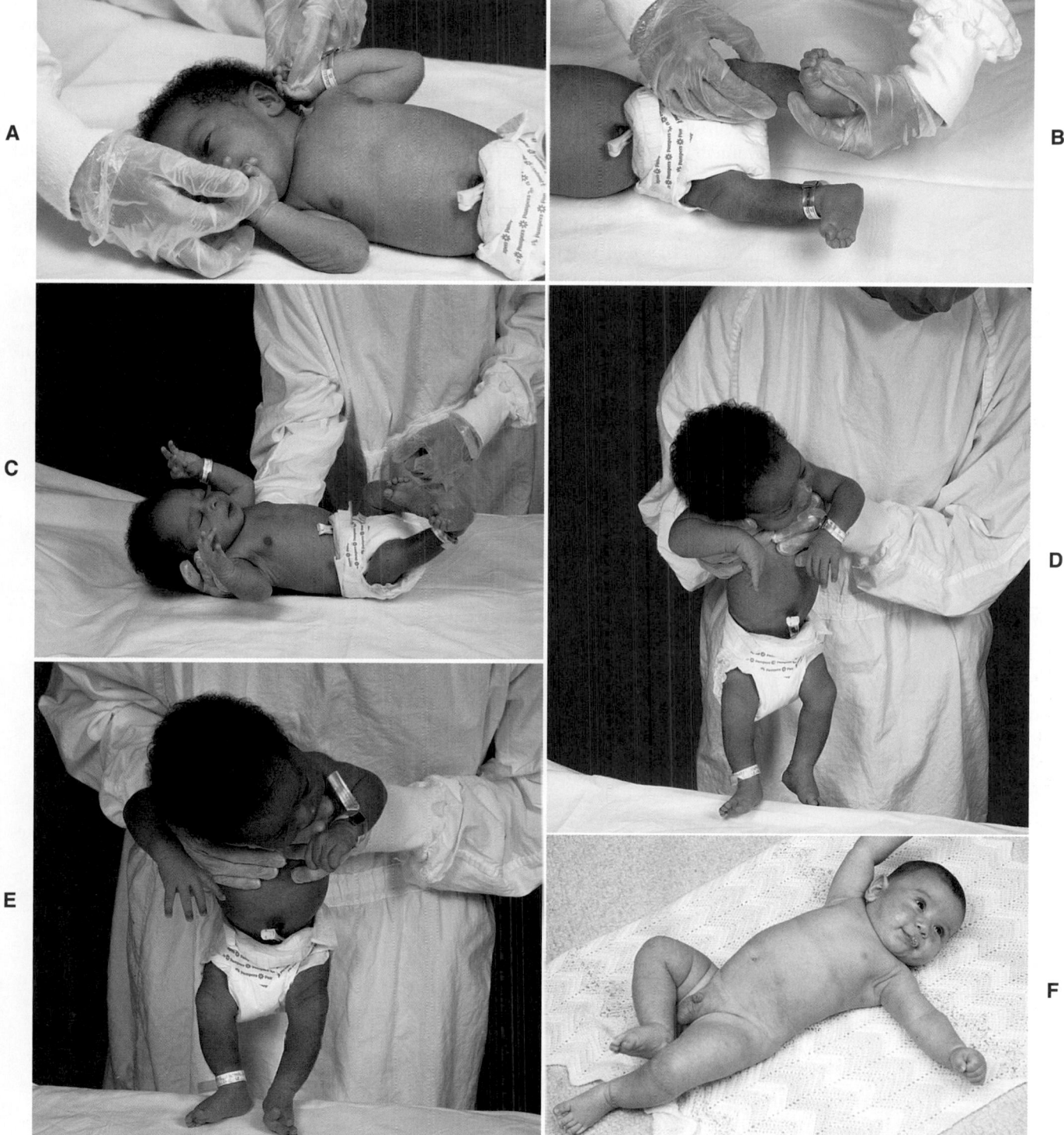

FIGURE 22-32
The preferred state of the infant for testing primitive reflexes is "quiet alert," neither hungry nor drowsy. Elicitation of the primitive reflexes. **A,** Palmar grasp. **B,** Plantar grasp. **C,** Moro reflex. **D,** Placing reflex. **E,** Stepping reflex. **F,** Asymmetric tonic neck reflex.

Muscle strength and tone are especially important to evaluate in the newborn and infant. Chapter 21 provides details related to this portion of the examination. The infant's neuromuscular development at the time of birth should be evaluated with the Ballard Clinical Assessment for gestational age (see Chapter 5).

CHILDREN

The neurologic examination of the young child is done by observing the neuromuscular developmental progress and skills displayed during the examination. The Denver II is a useful tool to determine whether the child is developing as expected with fine and gross motor skills, language, and personal-social skills (see Appendix D).

Direct examination of cranial nerves requires some modifications in procedure according to the age of the child. Often a game is played to elicit the response. Table 22-12 describes these procedures.

Observe the young child at play, noting gait and fine motor coordination. The beginning walker exhibits a wide-based gait; whereas the older child walks with feet closer together, has better balance, and recovers more easily when unbalanced. Observe the child's skill in reaching for, grasping, and releasing toys. No tremors or constant overshooting movements should be apparent.

Heel-to-toe walking, hopping, and jumping are all coordination skills that develop in the young child. They can be evaluated by modifying the skill tested into a game for the child. The Denver II provides guidance for the ages at which you can expect these maneuvers to be accomplished, and this tool is standardized for most cultural groups.

TABLE 22-11 Primitive Reflexes Less Commonly Evaluated in Infants

Reflex (Appearance)	Procedure and Findings
Glabella (birth)	With your index finger, briskly tap the bridge of the infant's nose between the eyes (glabella) when its eyes are open; observe the sudden symmetric blinking of the eyes; the infant will blink for the first four to five taps.
Galant or trunk incurvature (birth to 4 weeks)	Suspend the infant in prone position on one of your hands or on a flat surface; stroke one side of the infant's back between the shoulders to the buttocks, about 4 to 5 cm from the spinal cord; observe for the curvature of the trunk toward the side stroked; repeat on the other side.
Landau (birth to 6 months)	Suspend the infant in prone position on both of your hands so that the infant's legs and arms are extending over both sides of your hand; observe the infant's ability to lift its head and extend its spine on a horizontal plane; the reflex diminishes by 18 months of age and disappears by 3 years.
Parachute (4 to 6 months)	Hold the infant suspended in prone position and slowly lower it head first toward a surface; observe the infant extend its arms and legs as if to protect itself; this reflex should not disappear.
Neck righting (3 months, after tonic neck disappears)	With the infant supine, turn its head to the side; observe the infant turning its whole body in the direction the head is turned.

TABLE 22-12 Cranial Nerve Examination Procedures for Young Children

Cranial Nerves (CN)	Procedures and Observations
CN II	If the child cooperates, the Snellen E, HOTV, or Picture Chart may be used to test vision. Visual fields may be tested, but the child may need the head immobilized.
CN III, IV, and VI	Have the child follow an object with the eyes, immobilizing the head if necessary. Move the object through the cardinal points of gaze to test extraocular muscle movement.
CN V	Observe the child chewing a cookie or cracker, noting bilateral jaw strength. Touch the child's forehead and cheeks with cotton or string and watch the child bat it away.
CN VII	Observe the child's face when smiling, frowning, and crying. Ask the child to show his or her teeth. Demonstrate puffed cheeks and ask the child to imitate.
CN VIII	Observe the child turn to sounds such as a bell or whisper. Whisper a commonly used word behind the child's back and have him or her repeat the word. Perform audiometric testing.
CN IX, X	Elicit gag reflex.
CN XI, XII	Instruct older child to stick out the tongue and shrug the shoulders or raise the arms.

Modified from Bowers, Thompson, 1992.

Three pennies can be used to evaluate several aspects of the neurologic system, including vision, extraocular movements, and hearing (coin dropped on floor). Ask the child who is standing to pick up a penny off of the floor (tests vision and balance). Stick a moistened coin to the child's nose and ask the child to walk across the room (allows you to observe gait and any posturing). Have the child balance a penny on the nose and dorsum of each extended hand (tests the Romberg) (Freeman, 1997).

Many of the techniques used in the adult neurologic examination are used for children, with some modifications for the child's level of understanding.

Deep tendon reflexes are not routinely tested in a child who demonstrates appropriate development, because poor cooperation is often a problem. When reflexes are tested, use the same techniques described for adults; responses should be the same. Your index finger may also take the place of a reflex hammer, and may be less threatening to a child.

Evaluate light touch sensation by asking the child to close his or her eyes and point to where you touch or tickle. Have the child discriminate between rough and soft textures as an alternate procedure. Use the tuning fork to evaluate vibration sensation, asking the child to point to the area where the buzzing sensation is felt. Superficial pain sensation is not routinely tested in young children because of their fear of needles and sharp objects.

When checking cortical sensory integration, use geometric figures rather than numbers to evaluate graphesthesia. Draw each figure twice and ask the child if the figures are the same or different. (Make sure the child understands the terms same and different.) Some children will need a practice session with their eyes open to get good compliance with the examination.

There may be some unexpected findings in the school-age child that would be normal in younger children. These neurologic soft signs are nonfocal, functional neurologic findings that often provide subtle clues to an underlying central nervous system deficit or a neurologic maturation delay. Soft signs can be found in gross motor, fine motor, sensory, and reflex functional areas. Table 22-13 describes neurologic soft sign findings and the age at which you should become concerned if still present. Children with multiple soft signs are often found to have learning problems.

TABLE 22-13   Activities for Evaluating Neurologic Soft Signs in Children

Activity	Soft Sign Findings	Latest Expected Age of Disappearance (yr)
Walking, running gait	Stiff-legged with a foot slapping quality, unusual posturing of the arms	3
Heel walking	Difficulty remaining on heels for a distance of 10 feet	7
Tiptoe walking	Difficulty remaining on toes for a distance of 10 feet	7
Tandem gait	Difficulty walking heel-to-toe, unusual posturing of arms	7
One-foot standing	Unable to remain standing on one foot longer than 5 to 10 seconds	5
Hopping in place	Unable to rhythmically hop on each foot	6
Motor stance	Difficulty maintaining stance (arms extended in front, feet together, and eyes closed), drifting of arms, mild writhing movements of hands or fingers	3
Visual tracking	Difficulty following object with eyes when keeping the head still; nystagmus	5
Rapid thumb-to-finger test	Rapid touching thumb to fingers in sequence is uncoordinated; unable to suppress mirror movements in contralateral hand	8
Rapid alternating movements of hands	Irregular speed and rhythm with pronation and supination of hands patting the knees	10
Finger-nose test	Unable to alternately touch examiner's finger and own nose consecutively	7
Right-left discrimination	Unable to identify right and left sides of own body	5
Two-point discrimination	Difficulty in localizing and discriminating when touched in one or two places	6
Graphesthesia	Unable to identify geometric shapes drawn in child's open hand	8
Stereognosis	Unable to identify common objects placed in own hand	5

PREGNANT WOMEN

Examination of the pregnant woman is the same as for the adult. Assessment of deep tendon reflexes during the initial examination can serve as a baseline evaluation.

OLDER ADULTS

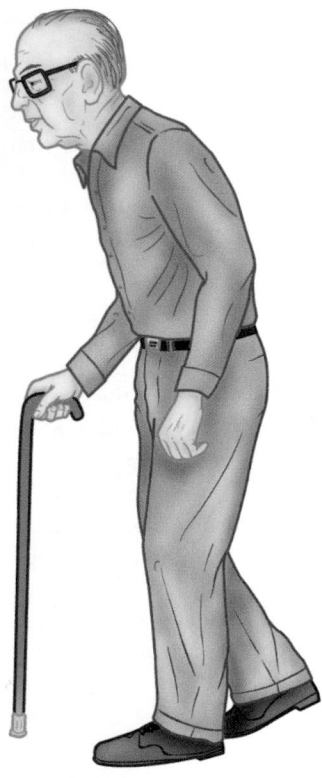

Examination of the neurologic system of the older adult is identical to that of the adult. You may need to allow more time for performing maneuvers that require coordination and movement.

Medications can impair central nervous system function and cause slowed reaction time, tremors, and anxiety. Problems may develop because of the dosage, number, or interaction of prescription or nonprescription medications.

The older adult may have markedly diminished senses of smell and taste. Sweet and salty tastes are usually impaired first. Other common cranial nerve changes include a reduced ability to differentiate colors, reduced upward gaze, slower adjustment to lighting changes, decreased corneal reflex, middle to high-frequency hearing loss, and a reduced gag reflex (Crigger, Forbes, 1997).

Gait with advancing age is characterized by short, uncertain steps as proprioception declines. Shuffling may occur as speed, balance, and grace decrease with age. Legs may be flexed at the hips and knees (Fig. 22-33). The Tinetti Balance and Gait Assessment Tool can be used for any older adult thought to be at risk for falls or for people who have difficulty performing daily activities (e.g., rising from a chair or performing a task that involves unsupported standing).

Tactile and vibratory sensation, as well as position sense, are often impaired in the older adult. These patients may need stronger stimuli to detect sensation.

Changes in deep tendon reflexes occur with aging. The older adult usually has less brisk or even absent reflexes, with response diminishing in the lower extremities before the upper extremities are affected. The Achilles and plantar reflexes may be absent or difficult to elicit in some older adults. The superficial reflexes may also disappear. There is typically an increase in benign essential tremor with aging. Fine motor coordination and agility may be impaired.

FIGURE 22-33
Short, uncertain steps are characteristic of gait with advancing age.

FUNCTIONAL ASSESSMENT

TINETTI BALANCE AND GAIT ASSESSMENT TOOL

Balance Tests

Eight positions and position changes are evaluated.
Instructions: The patient is seated in a hard, armless chair. The following maneuvers are tested.

1. Sitting balance	Leans or slides in chair	= 0
	Steady, safe	= 1 _____
2. Arises (ask patient to rise without using arms)	Unable without help	= 0
	Able, uses arms to help	= 1
	Able without using arms	= 2 _____
3. Attempts to arise	Unable without help	= 0
	Able, requires more than one attempt	= 1
	Able to arise, one attempt	= 2 _____
4. Immediate standing balance (first 5 seconds)	Unsteady (swaggers, moves feet, trunk sways)	= 0
	Steady but uses walker or other support	= 1
	Steady without walker or other support	= 2 _____
5. Standing balance (once stance balances)	Unsteady	= 0
	Steady but wide stance (medial heels more than 4 inches apart) or uses cane or other support	= 1
	Narrow stance without support	= 2 _____

From Tinetti, 1986.

FUNCTIONAL ASSESSMENT

TINETTI BALANCE AND GAIT ASSESSMENT TOOL—cont'd

Balance Tests—cont'd

6. Nudged (subject at maximum position with feet as close together as possible, examiner pushes lightly on subject's sternum with palm of hand three times)	Begins to fall	= 0
	Staggers, grabs, catches self	= 1
	Steady	= 2 _____
7. Eyes closed (at maximum position, as in 6)	Unsteady	= 0
	Steady	= 1 _____
8. Turning 360 degrees	Discontinuous steps	= 0
	Continuous steps	= 1 _____
	Unsteady (grabs, staggers)	= 0
	Steady	= 1 _____
9. Sitting down	Unsafe (misjudges distance, falls into chair)	= 0
	Uses arm or not a smooth motion	= 1
	Safe, smooth motion	= 2 _____

Balance Score: _____ of 16

Gait Tests

Eight components of gait are observed.

Initial instructions: The patient stands with examiner, walks down hallway or across room for at least 10 feet, first at "usual" pace, then back at "rapid but safe" pace (using usual walking aids).

10. Initiation of gait (immediately after being told "go")	Any hesitancy or multiple attempts to start	= 0
	No hesitancy	= 1 _____
11. Step length and height	Right swing foot does not pass left foot with stance	= 0
	Passes left stance foot	= 1 _____
	Right foot does not clear floor completely with step	= 0
	Right foot completely clears floor	= 1 _____
	Left swing foot does not pass right stance foot with step	= 0
	Passes right stance foot	= 1 _____
	Left foot does not clear floor completely with step	= 0
	Left foot completely clears floor	= 1 _____
12. Step symmetry	Right and left step length not equal (estimate)	= 0
	Right and left step length appear equal	= 1 _____
13. Step continuity	Stopping or discontinuity between steps	= 0
	Steps appear continuous	= 1 _____
14. Path (estimated in relation to floor tiles, 12 inches square; observe excursion of one of the subject's feet over about 10 feet of the course)	Marked deviation	= 0
	Mild/moderate deviation or uses walking aid	= 1
	Straight without walking aid	= 2 _____
15. Trunk	Marked sway or uses walking aid	= 0
	No sway, but flexion of knees or back, or spreads arms out while walking	= 1
	No sway, no flexion, no use of arms, and no use of walking aid	= 2 _____
16. Walking stance	Heels apart	= 0
	Heels almost touching while walking	= 1 _____

Gait Score: _____ of 12

Balance and Gait Score: _____ of 28

A score below 19 indicates a high risk for falls. A score of 19 to 24 suggests there is a greater chance of falls, but not a high risk.

SAMPLE DOCUMENTATION
HISTORY AND PHYSICAL EXAMINATION

Subjective

A 48-year-old man presents for his annual physical examination. No complaints of poor balance, loss of sensation, unsteady gait. History of diabetes mellitus type I for 30 years, well-controlled.

For additional sample documentation, see Chapter 26.

Objective

Cranial nerves I to XII grossly intact. Gait is coordinated and even. Romberg negative. Rapid alternating movements are coordinated and smooth. Superficial touch, pain, and vibratory sensation are intact bilaterally. Deep tendon reflexes 2+ bilaterally in all extremities. Babinski (plantar) reflex produces expected plantar flexion of toes. No ankle clonus. Monofilament test reveals decreased sensation on plantar surfaces of both feet.

SUMMARY OF EXAMINATION
NEUROLOGIC SYSTEM

Test cranial nerves I through XII (pp. 775-780).
Cerebellar Function and Proprioception
1. Evaluate coordination and fine motor skills by the following (pp. 780-781):
   - Rapid rhythmic alternating movements
   - Accuracy of upper and lower extremity movements
2. Evaluate balance using the Romberg test (p. 781).
3. Observe the patient's gait (pp. 782-785).
   - Posture
   - Rhythm and sequence of stride and arm movements

Sensory Function
1. Test primary sensory responses to the following (pp. 785-786):
   - Superficial touch
   - Superficial pain
2. Test vibratory response to tuning fork over joints or bony prominences on upper and lower extremities (p. 786).
3. Evaluate perception of position sense with movement of the great toes or a finger on each hand (p. 786).

4. Assess ability to identify familiar object by touch and manipulation (p. 787).
5. Assess two-point discrimination (p. 787).
6. Assess ability to identify letter or number "drawn" on palm of hand (p. 787).
7. Assess ability to identify body area when touched (p. 788).

Superficial and Deep Tendon Reflexes
1. Test abdominal reflexes (p. 789).
2. Test the cremasteric reflex in male patients (p. 789).
3. Test the plantar reflex (p. 789).
4. Test the following deep tendon reflexes (pp. 789-791):
   - Biceps
   - Brachioradial
   - Triceps
   - Patellar
   - Achilles
5. Test for ankle clonus (pp. 790-791).

COMMON ABNORMALITIES

Disorders of the central and peripheral nervous systems often fall into groups. A *static* problem may develop at any age and not get better or worse (e.g., nerve deafness and some trauma). An individual may have been well until function is lost with a *degenerative* condition, and it progressively worsens. Some problems are *intermittent*, and others are *genetic* or related to a *metabolic disorder*.

DISORDERS OF THE CENTRAL NERVOUS SYSTEM

HIV ENCEPHALOPATHY (AIDS DEMENTIA COMPLEX)	A progressive dementia that is likely related to direct HIV infection of the brain tissue, HIV encephalopathy may be difficult to distinguish from clinical depression in early stages. Insidious onset occurs, with headaches, loss of short-term memory and concentration, and inability to follow complex instructions. Eventually global cognitive impairment occurs. Behavior changes include irritability, apathy related to work and recreation, social withdrawal, and emotional lability. Motor findings include hyperreflexia; increased tone; slowed, rapid rhythmic movements; clumsiness and weakness in the arms and legs; and gait ataxia that mimics Huntington chorea and Parkinson disease. Fecal and urinary incontinence may also occur.
MULTIPLE SCLEROSIS	Multiple sclerosis is a debilitating, degenerative disorder in which the blood-brain barrier breaks down and permits immune cells to pass into the myelinated white matter of the brain or spinal cord tissue. With attacks, the myelin of the brain's white matter is destroyed, and axons no longer permit nerve impulse transmission. Brain mass decreases. Progression of the disorder is gradual, with or without remissions, unpredictable and variable among patients. Between remissions, acute episodes occur, with varying types and severity of symptoms. The primary symptoms include fatigue, bowel and bladder dysfunction, sexual dysfunction, sensory changes, muscle weakness, ataxia, blurred vision, diplopia, loss of vision, hyperactive deep tendon reflexes, paresthesias, and cognitive and emotional changes. Symptoms are variable, depending on the site of the lesions. The onset of symptoms occurs between 20 and 40 years of age, and the disease affects women twice as often as men.
GENERALIZED SEIZURE DISORDER	A generalized seizure disorder is characterized by episodic, sudden, involuntary contractions of a group of muscles, resulting from excessive discharge of cerebral neurons. The disorder may be caused by systemic disease, head trauma, toxins, stroke, or hypoxic syndromes. Disturbances in consciousness, behavior, sensation, and autonomic functioning often occur. Urinary and fecal incontinence may also accompany seizures. As many as 1% of the population have seizures, and 75% of new cases develop during childhood and adolescence.
ENCEPHALITIS	Encephalitis is an acute inflammation of the brain and spinal cord, involving the meninges that is often viral in origin. An arthropod or mosquito may be the vector for the virus, such as in West Nile virus. The onset is often a mild, febrile viral illness with malaise. A quiescent stage may precede the disturbance in central nervous system function, or there can be sudden onset of mental confusion, lethargy, and coma. Signs of meningitis (photophobia, headache, and stiff neck) may also be present. Motor functions and muscle weakness may be impaired with severe paralysis or ataxia.

MENINGITIS

An inflammatory process in the meninges, meningitis is caused by bacteria and viruses. Signs and symptoms include fever, chills, nuchal rigidity, headache, seizures, and vomiting, followed by alterations in level of consciousness. Young infants do not demonstrate nuchal rigidity until about 6 to 9 months of age. Those infants affected will generally be very irritable and inconsolable and have fever, diarrhea, poor appetite, and toxic appearance. Bacterial meningitis is a life-threatening illness if not rapidly treated with appropriate antibiotics.

CLINICAL PEARL

Smell the Cerebrospinal Fluid

When a lumbar puncture is done for suspected meningitis, the odor of alcohol can indicate a cryptococcal infection.

STAYING WELL

VACCINES TO REDUCE MENINGITIS RISK

Vaccines are available to reduce the risk of developing meningitis caused by various organisms. Infants and young children are protected by the Haemophilus *influenzae* type b (Hib) and 7-valent pneumococcal vaccines (PCV7) administered as routine immunizations. Adolescents, college students, military recruits, and others living in dormitories or other residential facilities can be protected against four strains of *Neisseria meningitides* by the meningococcal vaccine. Older adults and other individuals with chronic medical conditions can be protected against many strains of pneumococci with the 23-valent pneumococcal vaccine (PPV) (American Academy of Pediatrics, 2003, Centers for Disease Control and Prevention National Immunization Program, 2005).

LYME DISEASE

Lyme disease is a multisystem infection caused by the *Borrelia burgdorferi* spirochete, which is carried by ticks. The disease has three stages of progression, with varying signs and symptoms in each patient. It often presents with a characteristic skin circular red rash that continues to grow with central clearing, giving the appearance of a bulls-eye (Fig. 22-34). Neurologic signs may include headache, meningitis, encephalitis, polyneuritis, unilateral or bilateral facial paralysis, choreic movements, spastic paralysis, and ataxia. These signs may occur during early or late stages of the disease. Arthritis and acrodermatitis are signs associated with the third stage of the infection. Treatment with appropriate antibiotics generally cures the infection, but some neurologic signs may be unresolved.

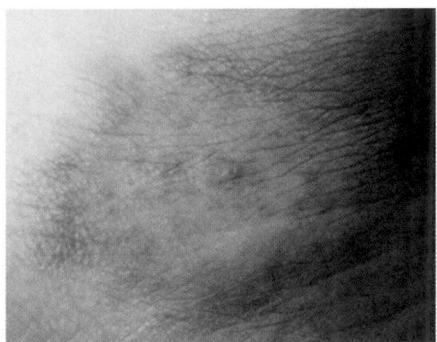

FIGURE 22-34
The rash of Lyme disease.
From Lookingbill, Marks, 2000.

SPACE-OCCUPYING LESIONS (INTRACRANIAL TUMORS)

A space-occupying lesion is an abnormal growth of neural or nonneural tissue within the cranial cavity that may be primary or metastatic cancer. The lesion causes displacement of tissue and pressure on the cerebrospinal fluid circulation and may threaten function through the compression and destruction of tissues. Early signs and symptoms vary by the location of the tumor but often include headaches, papilledema, vomiting, change in cognition, motor dysfunction, unsteady gait, seizures, and behavioral or personality changes. Peak ages of incidence are 3 to 12 years and 50 to 70 years.

CEREBROVASCULAR ACCIDENT (BRAIN ATTACK OR STROKE)

A sudden, focal neurologic deficit resulting from impaired circulation of the brain, cerebrovascular accident (CVA) is associated with cardiovascular disease. A thrombosis, embolism, or hemorrhage causes the circulation impairment. The most common site of lesions is within the distribution of the anterior circulation of the brain (Fig. 22-35). Five major warning signs of a brain attack include the following:

- Sudden weakness, numbness, or paralysis of face, arms or legs, especially one side
- Sudden trouble seeing in one or both eyes, diplopia, monocular blindness
- Sudden confusion, difficulty speaking or understanding speech (dysarthria, aphasia)
- Sudden severe headache without apparent reason
- Sudden trouble walking, loss of balance or falling without apparent reason, loss of coordination

General signs and symptoms include headache, progressive sudden neurologic deficits (e.g., restlessness, lethargy, changes in level of consciousness); vital sign and pupil changes; nausea and vomiting; impaired communication; shock; and cardiac arrest. Disability severity varies in survivors. Table 22-14 lists neurologic signs associated with CVA by location of lesion.

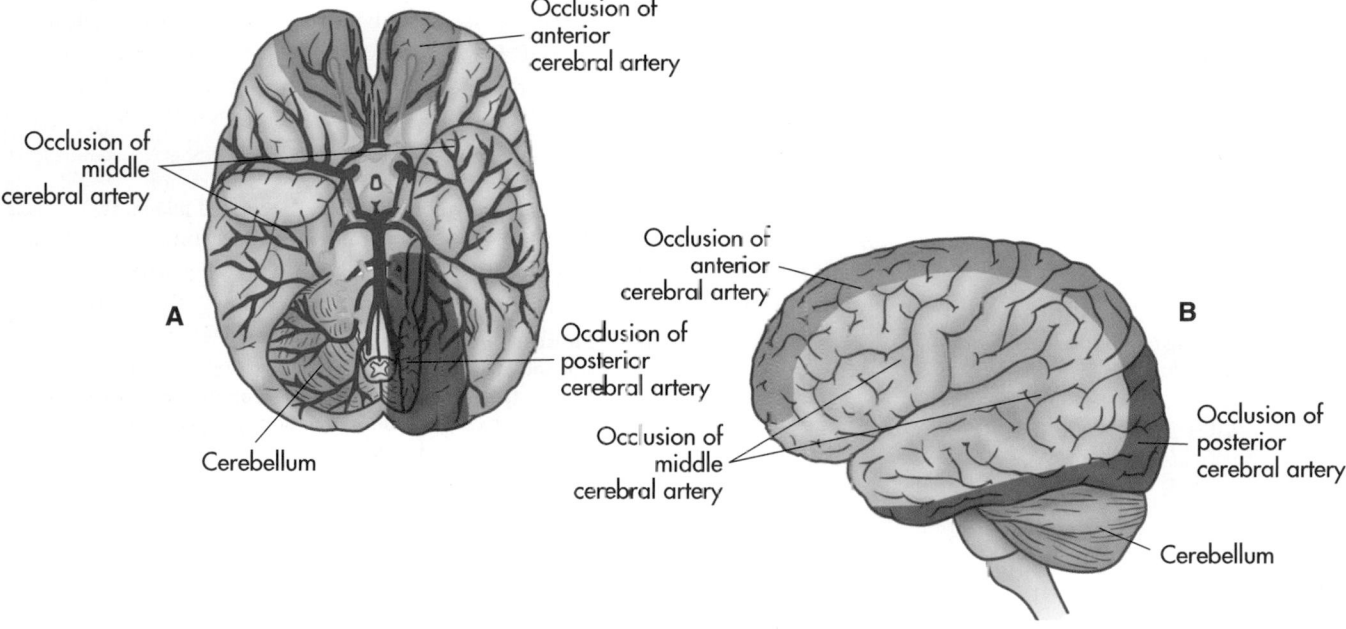

FIGURE 22-35
Areas of the brain affected by occlusion of the anterior, middle, and posterior cerebral artery branches. **A,** Inferior view. **B,** Lateral view.
Modified from Rudy, 1984.

TABLE 22-14 Neurologic Signs Associated with CVA by Location

Artery Affected	Neurologic Signs
INTERNAL CAROTID ARTERY Supplies the cerebral hemispheres and diencephalon by the ophthalmic and ipsilateral hemisphere arteries	Unilateral blindness Severe contralateral hemiplegia and hemianesthesia Profound aphasia
MIDDLE CEREBRAL ARTERY Supplies frontal lobe, parietal lobe, cortical surfaces of temporal lobe (affecting structures of higher cerebral processes of communication; language interpretation; perception and interpretation of space, sensation, form, and voluntary movement)	Alterations in communication, cognition, mobility, and sensation Contralateral homonymous hemianopia (see Chapter 11) Contralateral hemiplegia or hemiparesis, motor and sensory loss, greater in face and arm than the leg
ANTERIOR CEREBRAL ARTERY Supplies superior surfaces of frontal and parietal lobes and medial surface of cerebral hemispheres (includes motor and somesthetic cortex serving the legs), basal ganglia, corpus callosum	Emotional lability Confusion, amnesia, personality changes Urinary incontinence Contralateral hemiplegia or hemiparesis, greater in lower than upper extremities
POSTERIOR CEREBRAL ARTERY Supplies medial and inferior temporal lobes, medial occipital lobe, thalamus, posterior hypothalamus, and visual receptive area	Hemianesthesia Contralateral hemiplegia, greater in face and upper extremities than in lower extremities, cerebellar ataxia, tremor Visual loss—homonymous hemianopia, cortical blindness Receptive aphasia Memory deficits
VERTEBRAL OR BASILAR ARTERIES Supply the brainstem and cerebellum Incomplete occlusion	Transient ischemic attacks Unilateral and bilateral weakness of extremities; upper motor neuron weakness involving face, tongue, and throat; loss of vibratory sense, two-point discrimination, and position sense Diplopia, homonymous hemianopia Nausea, vertigo, tinnitus, and syncope Dysphagia Dysarthria Sometimes confusion and drowsiness
Anterior portion of pons	"Locked-in" syndrome—no movement except eyelids; sensation and consciousness preserved
Complete occlusion or hemorrhage	Coma Miotic pupils Decerebrate rigidity Respiratory and circulatory abnormalities Death
POSTERIOR INFERIOR CEREBELLAR ARTERY Supplies the lateral and posterior portion of the medulla	Wallenberg syndrome Dysphagia, dysphonia Ipsilateral anesthesia of face and cornea for pain and temperature (touch preserved) Ipsilateral Horner syndrome (see Chapter 11) Contralateral loss of pain and temperature sensation in trunk and extremities Ipsilateral decompensation of movement
ANTERIOR INFERIOR AND SUPERIOR CEREBELLAR ARTERIES Supply the cerebellum	Difficulty in articulation, swallowing, gross movements of limbs; nystagmus
ANTERIOR SPINAL ARTERY Supplies the anterior spinal cord	Flaccid paralysis, below level of lesion Loss of pain, touch, temperature sensation (proprioception preserved)
POSTERIOR SPINAL ARTERY Supplies the posterior spinal cord	Sensory loss, particularly proprioception, vibration, touch, and pressure (movement preserved)

DISORDERS OF THE PERIPHERAL NERVOUS SYSTEM

MYASTHENIA GRAVIS	Myasthenia gravis is a chronic autoimmune neuromuscular disease involving the lower motor neurons and muscle fibers. The disorder is characterized by an insidious, muscle fatigue and progressive weakness of the voluntary muscles with repetitive activity. The immune system attacks the synaptic junction between the nerve and muscle fibers. Acetylcholine receptor antibodies block the acetylcholine receptor sites and block the binding of acetylcholine needed for transmission of nerve impulses across the neuromuscular junction and effective muscle contraction. Initial muscle weakness of the eyes, face, mouth, throat, and neck occurs, so that chewing, swallowing, and speech are affected. The muscles of the neck, shoulder girdle, and hip flexors may also be involved. The respiratory muscles may also become weak, impairing ventilation. Fatigue and loss of strength are worse toward the end of the day. Weakness is improved with rest. Patients may have a rapid decline in respiratory muscle function, resulting in a life-threatening crisis.
GUILLAIN-BARRÉ SYNDROME	Guillain-Barré syndrome (acute idiopathic polyneuritis) is an acute polyradiculoneuropathy that commonly follows a nonspecific infection that occurred 10 to 14 days earlier. It primarily affects the motor and autonomic peripheral nerves. Widespread inflammation or demyelination of the ascending or descending peripheral nerves leads to impaired conduction of nerve impulses between the nodes of Ranvier. It is characterized by ascending symmetric weakness (with sensation preserved) that increases in severity over days or weeks. Decreased or absent strength and sensory loss, as well as hyporeflexia or areflexia may also occur. Motor paralysis and respiratory muscle failure may result, requiring life support; however, 85% of patients eventually have full functional recovery after a recovery period lasting several weeks. Signs and symptoms may differ depending upon the variant forms of the disorder.
TRIGEMINAL NEURALGIA (TIC DOULOUREUX)	Trigeminal neuralgia is a recurrent paroxysmal sharp pain that radiates into one or more of the branches of cranial nerve V. Potential causes of the disorder include chronic compression of the trigeminal nerve by a small artery that wears away the nerve's myelin or irritation of the afferent portion of the trigeminal nerve. Sharp jabs of pain on one side of the face are most common. Painful episodes last seconds to minutes, during which the patient grimaces, and the patient is pain free between episodes. Attack frequency may vary from several times a day to several times a month. Triggers of pain may include chewing, swallowing, talking, washing the face, brushing the teeth, exposure to cold, and even a breeze across the face. The usual age of onset is 40 to 60 years, and women are more commonly affected than men.
PERIPHERAL NEUROPATHY	Peripheral neuropathy is a disorder of the peripheral nervous system that results in motor and sensory loss in the distribution of one or more nerves, most commonly in the hands and feet. Patients may have sensation of numbness, tingling, burning, and cramping. The most common cause is diabetes mellitus, but it may also be caused by toxins, such as kerosene, or vitamin B_{12} deficiency. In moderate to severe diabetic neuropathy, there is wasting of the foot muscles, absent ankle and knee reflexes, decreased or no vibratory sensation below the knees, and loss of pain or sharp touch sensation to the mid-calf level. Temperature sensation may be less impaired. The loss of pain, pressure, and temperature sensations decrease the patient's awareness of an injury. Loss of skin integrity can lead to ulceration and infection. Muscle atrophy can lead to foot deformities. In diabetes mellitus, this condition is compounded by impaired circulation that results in poor healing of skin ulcers.

MNEMONICS

Causes of Peripheral Neuropathy: I'M DISTAL

I Idiopathic, Inherited
M Metabolic, Mechanical
D Drugs
I Infections
S Sarcoidosis
T Tumors
A Autoimmune, Allergy
L Lack of vitamins

From Shipman, 1984.

CHILDREN

CEREBRAL PALSY	Cerebral palsy is a group of brain damage syndromes in which a static and nonprogressive cerebral lesion causes significant motor delay and abnormal neuromuscular findings. Cerebral palsy occurs in an estimated 2 to 3 per 1000 births. Signs include delayed gross motor development; alterations in muscle tone (spasticity, hypotonia); and abnormalities of posture, motor performance, and reflexes, as well as sensory impairment. Mental retardation occurs in 60% of cases. Severity is determined by the degree of motor impairment. Some patients can expect near-normal levels of functioning.
SHAKEN BABY SYNDROME	Shaken baby syndrome is a severe form of child abuse resulting from violent shaking that is most commonly seen in infants younger than 1 year of age. The violent shaking causes shearing injuries to the brain through acceleration, deceleration, and rotational forces as the brain moves within the skull. The forces stretch and tear blood vessels in the brain. The spinal cord may also be damaged as the head rocks back and forth. The infant may be thrown into the crib or bed causing a cerebral contusion or skull fracture. Often no external signs of injury are apparent. Characteristic signs include retinal hemorrhages, altered consciousness with axonal injury, as well as subdural or subarachnoid hemorrhage.
HIV ENCEPHALOPATHY	Progressive encephalopathy associated with acquired immunodeficiency syndrome in children is generally an advanced feature of the disease. It is associated with impaired brain growth due to cerebral atrophy, progressive motor dysfunction, regression or a plateau in developmental milestones, and generalized weakness with upper motor neuron signs. Less common findings include dysphagia, gait ataxia, and seizures.
RETT SYNDROME	Rett syndrome is a progressive encephalopathy of unknown cause that develops in girls between 6 and 18 months of age after normal neurologic and mental development. Head growth decelerates between 5 and 48 months of age. Characteristic signs include loss of voluntary hand movement, loss of previously acquired hand skills, hand wringing movements, gradual development of ataxia and rigidity of the legs, growth retardation, seizures, loss of facial expression, and autistic behavior. Neurologic regression slows and plateaus after a period, but autistic behavior persists. The disorder is believed to account for substantial numbers of children with mental retardation. Children can survive several years in a helpless state.

PREGNANT WOMEN

MATERNAL OBSTETRIC PALSY	A number of different neuropathies result in weakness in the lower extremities because of mechanical compression of nerves during delivery. Femoral neuropathy results from compression of the lumbosacral plexus and peripheral nerves in the pelvic wall by the fetal head or forceps. Postpartum footdrop may result from compression of nerves in the lumbosacral trunk when the fetal brow presses against the mother's sacral ala. Compression of the common peroneal nerve between the leg holders and the fibula during delivery can also cause unilateral footdrop. If the axons are not crushed and degeneration of the nerves does not occur, these disorders are reversible.

OLDER ADULTS

PARKINSON DISEASE

Parkinson disease is a slowly progressive, degenerative neurologic disorder of the brain's dopamine neuronal systems. Deficiency of dopamine neurotransmitter results in poor communication between parts of the brain that coordinate and control movement and balance. Patients may have a history of encephalitis, drug use, or cerebrovascular disease. There may be genetic, environmental, viral, vascular, toxic, or other factors associated with disease onset. Patients older than 50 years of age are most often affected, but it sometimes occurs in young adults. Symptoms (often unilateral initially) begin with tremors at rest and with fatigue, disappearing with intended movement and sleep, respectively. The disorder progresses with tremor of the head, slowing of voluntary and automatic movements (bradykinesia), and bilateral pillrolling of the fingers. Motor impairment causes delays in execution of movement, masked facial expression, and poor blink reflex. Muscular rigidity interferes with walking, leading to a gait of short, shuffling steps with the trunk in a forward flexion posture. Speech becomes slowed, slurred, and monotonous. Postural instability occurs late in the disease. Sensory symptoms such as numbness, aching, tingling, and muscle soreness occur in many patients. Behavioral change and dementia occur in about 10% to 15% of patients (Fig. 22-36).

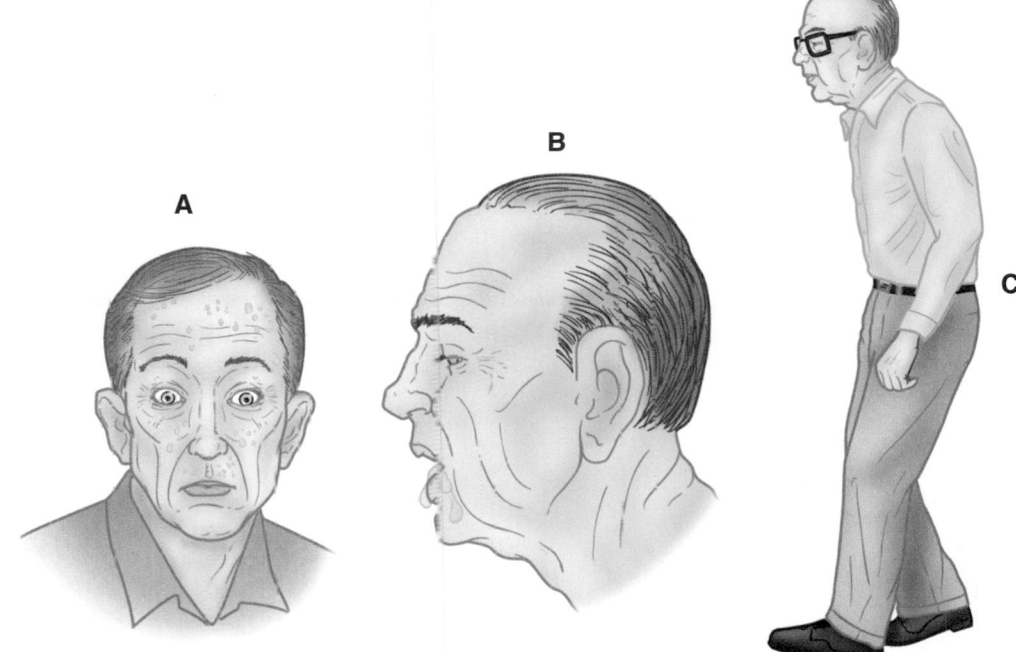

FIGURE 22-36
Characteristic features of Parkinson disease. **A,** Excessive sweating. **B,** Drooling with excess saliva. **C,** Gait with rapid, short, shuffling steps and reduced arm swinging.
Modified from Rudy, 1984.

NORMAL PRESSURE HYDROCEPHALUS

Normal pressure hydrocephalus is a syndrome caused by noncommunicating hydrocephalus (i.e., dilated ventricles, but intracranial pressure is within expected ranges) that simulates degenerative diseases. Patients have a triad of signs including a gait disorder, psychomotor slowing, and incontinence. Patients may have progressive dementia with memory loss, mild bilateral upper motor neuron signs, and fecal and urinary incontinence. Some patients have a history of subarachnoid hemorrhage, traumatic brain injury, or meningitis. The condition is often correctable by a ventriculoperitoneal shunt.

NEUROLOGIC SYSTEM
Common Abnormalities

POSTPOLIO SYNDROME

Postpolio syndrome is the reappearance of neurologic signs in survivors of the polio epidemics of the 1950s. The cause is unknown, but it is thought to be caused by the inability of surviving neurons from the primary case of polio to continue developing axon sprouts because of age or overuse. Patients feel profoundly fatigued with minimal exertion. New weakness develops in previously affected or unaffected muscles leaving them at greater risk for falls. Other symptoms include muscle and joint pain, dyspnea, dysphagia, and cold intolerance. The disorder results in progressive loss of muscle strength, including the muscles for ventilation. Men and women are affected equally.

ELECTRONIC RESOURCES

For Weblinks and additional resources, go to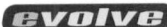

http://evolve.elsevier.com/Seidel

or to the Companion CD-ROM.

Additional information related to the content in Chapter 22 can be found on the companion website at http://evolve.elsevier.com/Seidel/ or on the interactive companion CD-ROM. Resources and activities for Chapter 22 include:
- Sound and Vision Theater
- Printouts for Your Practice
- Interactive Challenge
- Spanish Assessment Terms with Pronunciation Guide
- Instant Calculator

CHAPTER 23

SPORTS PARTICIPATION EVALUATION

Each year millions of children and youth who participate in organized sports seek a health care provider's signature on a preparticipation evaluation (PPE) (American Academy of Pediatrics, 1991). States and local school districts require young athletes to obtain medical clearance before participation in sports. Moreover, rare high-profile cases of death and serious injury on the playing field, usually among big-time college and professional athletes, keep concerns about the risks of sports participation in the public eye.

Whether athletes receive the PPE in the context of an ongoing primary care relationship or as a focused preseason checkup, certain goals of the evaluation are universal:

+ To identify conditions that may interfere with a person's ability to participate in a sport
+ To identify health problems that increase the risk of injury or death during sports participation
+ To help select an appropriate sport for a person's particular abilities and physical status

The ultimate goal of the PPE is to ensure safe participation in an appropriate physical activity. Sports and disciplined physical effort enhance fitness and coordination, increase self-esteem, and provide positive social experiences. Ultimately, relatively few persons undergoing PPEs have conditions that might limit participation, and most of these conditions are known before the PPE takes place (Box 23-1).

A PPE may be performed in many settings, but ideally it occurs in the office of a regular provider in the context of an ongoing primary care relationship. This takes advantage of a medical history that may already exist in the provider's records. It is individualized and tailored to the specific needs of the particular patient, and discussion of important issues that may be unrelated to sports participation is feasible and expected. Coordination of follow-up care should be efficient.

Another approach to the PPE is the *stations method,* in which a large number of patients are evaluated in a single session by providers from many disciplines, including physicians, nurses, trainers, and physical therapists. Each provider takes responsibility for a specific aspect of the evaluation at a station dedicated to that purpose. Athletes move from one station to the next, accumulating historical and objective information on a standard form. A checkout station is critical to the success of this approach. The person in charge of this station reviews the data collected during the evaluation and coordinates any necessary follow-up action, communicating directly with the athlete (and parents if appropriate) and generating a written re-

---

NOTE: This chapter was originally prepared in large part by Dr. John Andrews. We have continued to rely on him for this edition.

port. If the PPE is not itself a comprehensive service that addresses issues unrelated to sports participation, the need for routine primary care remains. This point should be emphasized at the checkout station.

The PPE should be completed well enough in advance of the projected sports participation so that rehabilitation or therapy of any problems identified can be completed before participation begins. As a rule, 6 weeks before participation is appropriate. Once an initial, thorough PPE has been completed, subsequent PPEs can be more brief and attention can be given to interim problems.

The physical examination component of the PPE should center on high-yield areas, particularly those related to sports participation and those identified by the history. Items such as auscultation of the lung fields and otoscopy are low-yield—unless the patient is symptomatic at the time of the evaluation—and can distract from more fruitful areas such as the cardiac and orthopedic examinations.

Recommended components of the PPE are shown in Box 23-2. It lists elements of the history and physical examination organized by system, with physical examination items in italics. The orthopedic component of the physical examination is the one with which most pri-

CLINICAL PEARL

Brain Injury

Some 20% of high school and 40% of college football players sustain some kind of brain injury during their playing days; once they do, the chances that they will sustain another increase by two to four times. A preparticipation evaluation may not predict a brain injury and concussion, but it can help you learn the "normal" neuropsychologic status in the person involved before the injury so that you might better judge the return to "normal" neuropsychologic status after injury. Comparing self with self is best.

BOX 23-1

SPECIAL OLYMPICS

Special Olympics offers an opportunity for year-round sports training and athletic competition for persons with "mental retardation or a closely related developmental disability that results in functional limitations in both general learning and adaptive skills" (Lively, 2003). The official sports include aquatics, track and field, basketball, golf, gymnastics, softball, tennis, and volleyball among others. Participants must be at least 8 years old. A preparticipation physical examination (PPE) is require for admission to the program.

Significantly, the risk of injury or other need for medical attention during Special Olympics events is less than in the similar activities of nondisabled athletes and most injuries sustained are minor. Past experience indicates that there is some risk of eye injury in badminton, basketball, floor hockey, handball, soccer, softball, and tennis; and an increased risk for those with atlantoaxial instability in Alpine skiing, diving, equestrian sports, gymnastics, high jump, soccer, and swimming.

The variety of sports is clearly impressive but you need not hesitate to validate participation for one of your patients based on mental retardation alone. The results of your PPE performed as outlined in this chapter, of course, may add findings that preclude participation just as it might for the nondisabled patient.

The same care is due for persons seeking to join in *Paralympic Games*, an opportunity offered by a different organizing group for athletes with a physical disability of a serious nature, such as amputation, cerebral palsy, spinal cord impairment, or visual impairment. These athletes, however, need not have mental retardation or a developmental disability.

EVIDENCE-BASED PRACTICE IN PHYSICAL EXAMINATION

THE PARTICULAR VALUE OF A CAREFUL HISTORY

The only proven benefit of the PPE is recognition of athletes at risk for later orthopedic injury by identifying recent or poorly rehabilitated injuries that can become worse with sports participation (American Medical Association, 1994). Most of these injuries are detected by a careful history. In fact, the majority of all problems affecting athletes are detected by history alone (American Medical Association, 1994). It is the highest yield component of the PPE. Asthma is a good example. Unless a patient is in respiratory distress at the time of the evaluation, physical examination is unlikely to lead to recognition of this condition; however, a history should lead quickly to the diagnosis. Sudden cardiac death on the playing field is a source of great concern. It accounts for the greatest number of sudden deaths in young athletes; the remainder are caused by blunt chest trauma, drug abuse, asthma, heat stroke, and drowning. Conditions leading to these uncommon events are rarely associated with detectable physical findings. They may, however, be associated with symptoms revealed by a careful family history at the time of the PPE.

CLINICAL PEARL

Atlantoaxial Instability

Atlantoaxial instability is a particular problem for as many as 1 to 2 in every 10 patients with Down syndrome. The atlantoaxial joint is excessively mobile. There may be no neurologic complications at first but the risk of subluxation and spinal cord compression with neck pain, increasing weakness, and even ultimate loss of bladder or bowel control is real. On careful neurologic examination, you may find increased deep tendon reflexes, a positive Babinski sign, and ankle clonus. That demands action. Neurologic consultation and cervical x-rays become necessary.

mary care providers are unfamiliar. Garrick has developed a "2-minute" screening orthopedic examination that is useful for this purpose (Fig. 23-1) (Garrick, 1977). Having undergone several revisions since its publication in 1977, this 14-step musculoskeletal examination consists of observing the athlete in a variety of positions and postures that highlight asymmetries in range of motion, strength, and muscle bulk. These differences serve to identify acute or old, poorly rehabilitated injuries. The steps pictured in Fig. 23-1 help in assessing most of the following:

- ◆ Posture and general muscle contour bilaterally
- ◆ Patient's duck walk, four steps with knees completely bent
- ◆ Spine for curvature and lumbar extension, fingers touching toes with knees straight
- ◆ Shoulder and clavicle for dislocation
- ◆ Neck, shoulder, elbow, forearm, hand, fingers, and hips for range of motion
- ◆ Knee ligaments for drawer sign

You should also assess the following:

- ◆ Gait
- ◆ Patient's ability to hop on each foot
- ◆ Patient's ability to walk on tiptoes and heels

Once a PPE has been completed, the information gathered must be used to guide sport selection; to plan therapy or rehabilitation of illnesses or injuries detected during the valuation; and, in rare instances, to limit participation or disqualify a child (Figs. 23-2, 23-3, and 23-4). These decisions are individual, but there are resources available to guide them (Tables 23-1, 23-2, and 23-3). There is nothing legally binding about a health care provider's recommendation to limit participation.

BOX 23-2

RECOMMENDED COMPONENTS OF THE PPE*

Medical History
- Illnesses or injuries since the last checkup or PPE
- Hospitalizations or surgeries
- Medications used by the athlete (including those he or she may be taking to enhance performance)
- Use of any special equipment or protective devices during sports participation
- Allergies, particularly those associated with anaphylaxis or respiratory compromise and those provoked by exercise
- Immunization status including hepatitis B and varicella
- *Height and weight*

Cardiac
- Symptoms of syncope, dizziness, shortness of breath, fatigue, or chest pain during exercise
- History of high blood pressure, heart murmurs, arrhythmias
- Family history of heart disease (e.g., cardiomyopathies, long QT syndrome, Marfan syndrome, arrhythmias)
- Previous history of disqualification or limited participation in sports because of a cardiac problem
- *Blood pressure (sitting position, appropriate size cuff, repeated readings)*
- *Heart rate and rhythm*
- *Pulses*
- *Auscultation for murmurs*

Respiratory
- Asthma, coughing, wheezing, or dyspnea with exercise

Neurology
- History of a significant brain injury or concussion
- Numbness or tingling in the extremities
- Severe headaches

Vision
- Visual problems
- Corrective lenses
- *Visual acuity*

Orthopedic
- Previous injuries that have limited sports participation
- Injuries that have been associated with pain, swelling, or the need for medical intervention
- *Screening orthopedic examination*

Psychosocial
- Weight control and body image
- Dietary habits; calcium intake
- Stresses at home or in school
- Use or abuse of drugs and alcohol
- *Attention to signs of eating disorders including oral ulcerations, decreased tooth enamel, calcium intake, edema*

Genitourinary
- Age at menarche, last menstrual period, regularity of menstrual periods, number of periods in the last year, and longest interval between periods (athletic girls tend to experience menarche at a later age than nonathletic girls).
- *Palpation of the abdomen*
- *Palpation of the testicles*
- *Examination of inguinal canals*

From Andrews, 1997.
*Italics indicate physical examination items.

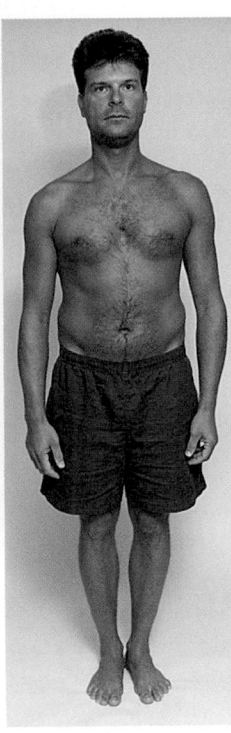
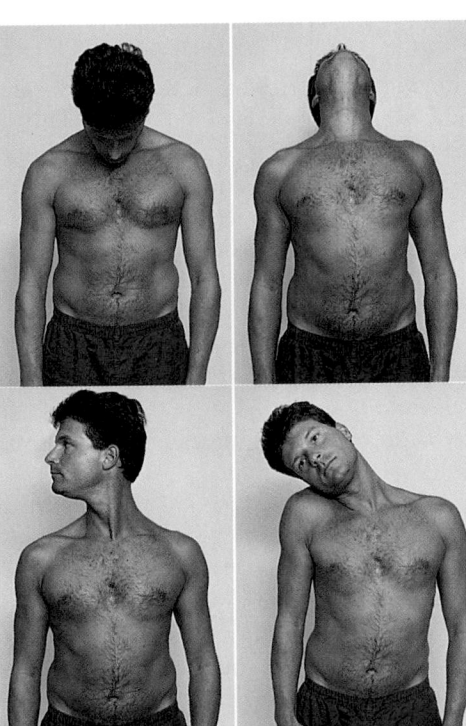
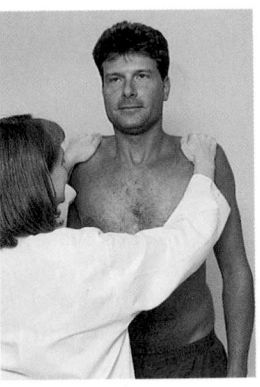
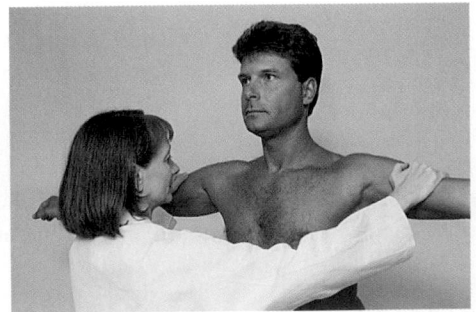

Step 3: Have the athlete shrug the shoulders against resistance from the examiner to evaluate trapezius strength.

Step 1: Observe the standing athlete from the front for symmetry of trunk, shoulders, and extremities.

Step 2: Observe neck flexion, extension, lateral flexion on each side, and rotation to evaluate range of motion and the cervical spine.

Step 4: Have the athlete perform shoulder abduction against resistance from the examiner to assess deltoid strength.

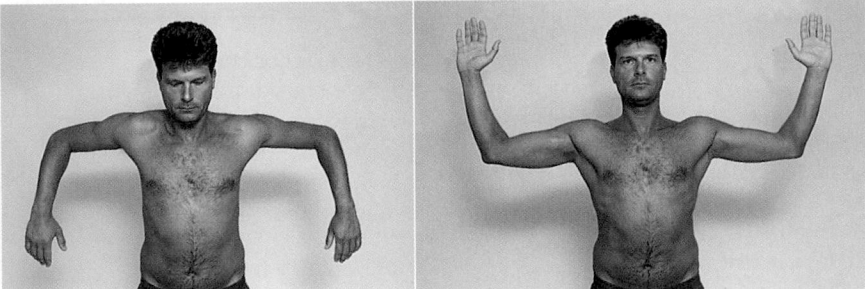

Step 5: Observe internal and external rotation of the shoulder to evaluate range of motion of the glenohumeral joint.

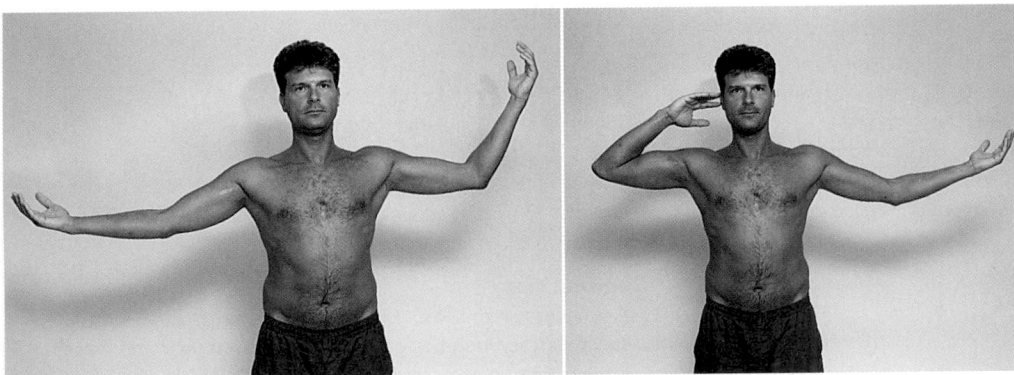

Step 6: Observe extension and flexion of the elbow to assess range of motion.

FIGURE 23-1
The 14-step screening orthopedic examination. The athlete should be dressed so that the joints and muscle groups included in the examination are easily visible—usually gym shorts for males, gym shorts and a T-shirt for females. Keep in mind that one of the most important points to look for in the orthopedic screening examination is symmetry.
From Andrews, 1997.

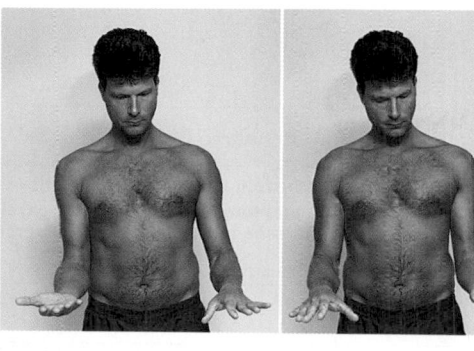

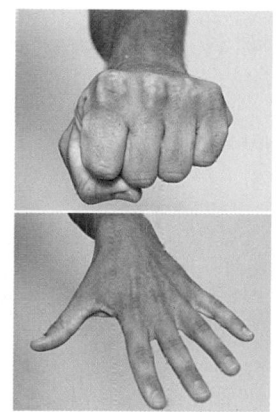

Step 7: Observe pronation and supination of the forearm to evaluate elbow and wrist range of motion.

Step 8: Have the athlete clench the fist, then spread the fingers to assess range of motion in the hand and fingers.

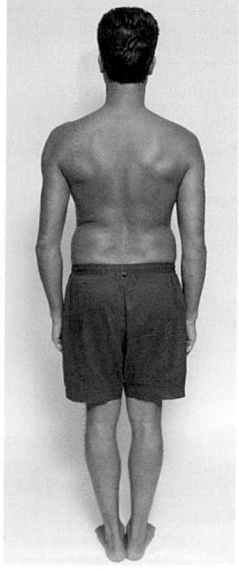

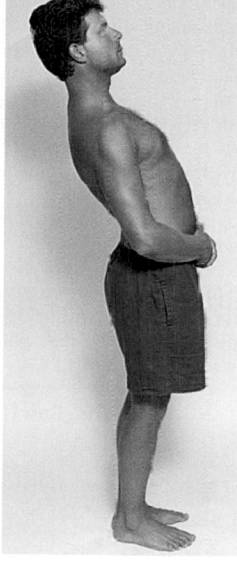

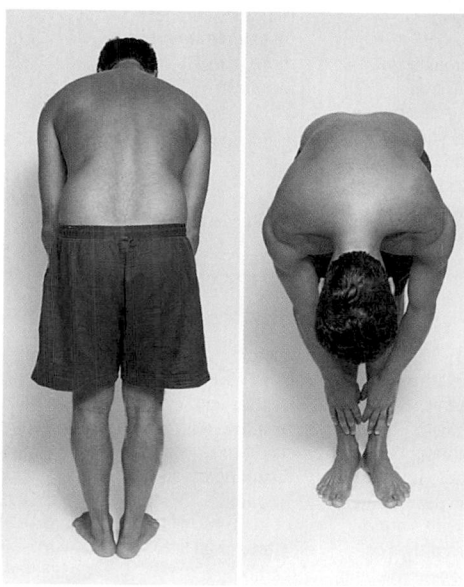

Step 9: Observe the standing athlete from the rear for symmetry of truck, shoulders, and extremities.

Step 10: Have the athlete stand with the knees straight and bend backward from the waist. Discomfort with extension of the lumbar spine may be associated with spondylolysis and spondylolisthesis.

Step 11: Have the athlete stand with the knees straight and flex forward at the waist, first away from the examiner, then toward the examiner, to assess for scoliosis, spine range of motion, and hamstring flexibility.

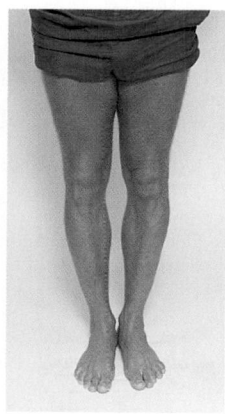

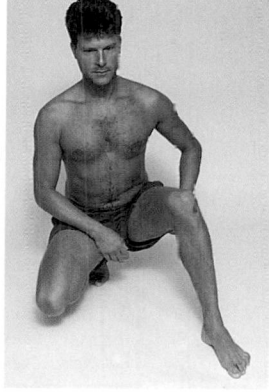

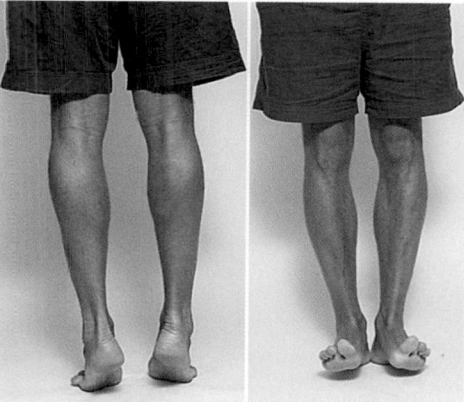

Step 12: Have the athlete stand facing the examiner with quadriceps flexed to observe symmetry of leg musculature.

Step 13: Have the athlete duck walk four steps to assess hip, knee, and ankle range of motion, strength, and balance.

Step 14: Have the athlete stand on the toes, then the heels to evaluate calf strength, symmetry, and balance.

FIGURE 23-1—cont'd
The 14-step screening orthopedic examination. The athlete should be dressed so that the joints and muscle groups included in the examination are easily visible—usually gym shorts for males, gym shorts and a T-shirt for females. Keep in mind that one of the most important points to look for in the orthopedic screening examination is symmetry.
From Andrews, 1997.

Management of Concussion in Sports

Grades of Concussion

Grade 1:
1. Transient confusion (inattention, inability to maintain a coherent stream of thought and carry out goal-directed movements)
2. No loss of consciousness
3. Concussion symptoms or mental status abnormalities on examination resolve in less than 15 minutes

Grade 2:
1. Transient confusion
2. No loss of consciousness
3. Concussion symptoms or mental status abnormalities (including amnesia) on examination last more than 15 minutes

Grade 3:
1. Any loss of consciousness
   a) Brief (seconds)
   b) Prolonged (minutes)

Management Recommendations

Grade 1:
1. Remove from contest
2. Examine immediately and at 5-minute intervals for the development of mental status abnormalities or postconcussive symptoms at rest and with exertion
3. May return to contest if mental status abnormalities or postconcussive symptoms clear within 15 minutes

Grade 2:
1. Remove from contest and disallow return that day
2. Examine on-site frequently for signs of evolving intracranial pathology
3. A trained person should reexamine the athlete the following day
4. A physician should perform a neurologic examination to clear the athlete for return to play after 1 full asymptomatic week at rest and with exertion

Grade 3:
1. Transport the athlete from the field to the nearest emergency department by ambulance if still unconscious or if worrisome signs are detected (with cervical spine immobilization, if indicated)
2. A thorough neurologic evaluation should be performed emergently, including appropriate neuroimaging procedures when indicated
3. Hospital admission is indicated if any signs of pathology are detected, or if the mental status of the athlete remains abnormal

When to Return to Play

Grade of concussion:	Return to Play Only After Being Asymptomatic with Normal Neurologic Assessment at Rest and with Exercise:
Grade 1 Concussion	15 minutes or less
Multiple Grade 1 Concussions	1 week
Grade 2 Concussion	1 week
Multiple Grade 2 Concussions	2 weeks
Grade 3—Brief Loss of Consciousness (seconds)	1 week
Grade 3—Prolonged Loss of Consciousness (minutes)	2 weeks
Multiple Grade 3 Concussions	1 month or longer, based on decision of evaluating physician

Features of Concussion Frequently Observed

1. Vacant stare (befuddled facial expression)
2. Delayed verbal and motor responses (slow to answer questions or follow instructions)
3. Confusion and inability to focus attention (easily distracted and unable to follow through with normal activities)
4. Disorientation (walking in the wrong direction; unaware of time, date and place)
5. Slurred or incoherent speech (making disjointed or incomprehensible statements)
6. Gross observable incoordination (stumbling, inability to walk tandem/straight line)
7. Emotions out of proportion to circumstances (distraught, crying for no apparent reason)
8. Memory deficits (exhibited by the athlete repeatedly asking the same question that has already been answered, or inability to memorize and recall 3 of 3 words or 3 of 3 objects in 5 minutes)
9. Any period of loss of consciousness (paralytic coma, unresponsiveness to arousal)

Sideline Evaluation

Mental Status Testing

Orientation: Time, place, person, and situation (circumstances of injury).

Concentration: Digits backward (i.e., 3-1-7, 4-6-8-2, 5-3-0-7-4). Months of the year in reverse order.

Memory: Names of teams in prior contest. Recall of 3 words and 3 objects at 0 and 5 minutes. Recent newsworthy events. Details of the contest (plays, moves, strategies, etc.)

Exertional Provocative Tests

40 yard sprint
5 push-ups
5 sit-ups
5 knee-bends

Neurological Tests

Strength
Coordination and Agility
Sensation

Any appearance of associated symptoms is abnormal, e.g., headaches, dizziness, nausea, unsteadiness, photophobia, blurred or double vision, emotional lability, or mental status changes.

FIGURE 23-2
Sports participation evaluation guidelines.
Modified from Preparticipation Physical Evaluation, ed 2. Reprinted with permission from the American Academy of Neurology, 1997.

Preparticipation Physical Evaluation

PHYSICAL EXAMINATION

Name _____ Date of birth _____

Height _____ Weight _____ % Body fat (optional) _____ Pulse _____ BP ___/___ (___/___ , ___/___)

Vision R 20/ _____ L 20/ _____   Corrected: Y N   Pupils: Equal _____ Unequal _____

	NORMAL	ABNORMAL FINDINGS	INITIALS*
MEDICAL			
Appearance			
Eyes/Ears/Nose/Throat			
Lymph Nodes			
Heart			
Pulses			
Lungs			
Abdomen			
Genitalia (males only)			
Skin			
MUSCULOSKELETAL			
Neck			
Back			
Shoulder/arm			
Elbow/forearm			
Wrist/hand			
Hip/thigh			
Knee			
Leg/ankle			
Foot			

* Station-based examination only

CLEARANCE

❑ **Cleared**

❑ **Cleared after completing evaluation/rehabilitation for:** _____

_____

_____

_____

❑ **Not cleared for:** _____ **Reason:** _____

Recommendations: _____

_____

_____

_____

Name of physician (print/type) _____ **Date** _____

Address _____ **Phone** _____

Signature of physician _____, **MD or DO**

FIGURE 23-3
Preparticipation physical evaluation form.
Modified from the American Academy of Family Physicians, American Academy of Pediatrics, American Medical Society for Sports Medicine, American Orthopaedic Society for Sports Medicine, and American Osteopathic Academy of Sports Medicine, 1997.   *Continued*

Preparticipation Physical Evaluation

HISTORY   DATE OF EXAM _____

Name _____ Sex _____ Age _____ Date of birth _____

Grade ____ School _____ Sport(s) _____

Address _____ Phone _____

Personal physician _____

In case of emergency, contact

Name _____ Relationship _____ Phone (H) _____ (W) _____

Explain "Yes" answers below.
Circle questions you don't know the answers to.

	Yes	No
1. Have you had a medical illness or injury since your last check up or sports physical?	☐	☐
Do you have an ongoing or chronic illness?	☐	☐
2. Have you ever been hospitalized overnight?	☐	☐
Have you ever had surgery?	☐	☐
3. Are you currently taking any prescription or nonprescription (over-the-counter) medications or pills or using an inhaler?	☐	☐
Have you ever taken any supplements or vitamins to help you gain or lose weight or improve your performance?	☐	☐
4. Do you have any allergies (for example, to pollen, medicine, food, or stinging insects)?	☐	☐
Have you ever had a rash or hives develop during or after exercise?	☐	☐
5. Have you ever passed out during or after exercise?	☐	☐
Have you ever been dizzy during or after exercise?	☐	☐
Have you ever had chest pain during or after exercise?	☐	☐
Do you get tired more quickly than your friends do during exercise?	☐	☐
Have you ever had racing of your heart or skipped heartbeats?	☐	☐
Have you had high blood pressure or high cholesterol?	☐	☐
Have you ever been told you have a heart murmur?	☐	☐
Has any family member or relative died of heart problems or of sudden death before age 50?	☐	☐
Have you had a severe viral infection (for example, myocarditis or mononucleosis) within the last month?	☐	☐
Has a physician ever denied or restricted your participation in sports for any heart problems?	☐	☐
6. Do you have any current skin problems (for example, itching, rashes, acne, warts, fungus, or blisters)?	☐	☐
7. Have you ever had a head injury or concussion?	☐	☐
Have you ever been knocked out, become unconscious, or lost your memory?	☐	☐
Have you ever had a seizure?	☐	☐
Do you have frequent or severe headaches?	☐	☐
Have you ever had numbness or tingling in your arms, hands, legs, or feet?	☐	☐
Have you ever had a stinger, burner, or pinched nerve?	☐	☐
8. Have you ever become ill from exercising in the heat?	☐	☐
9. Do you cough, wheeze, or have trouble breathing during or after activity?	☐	☐
Do you have asthma?	☐	☐
Do you have seasonal allergies that require medical treatment?	☐	☐

	Yes	No
10. Do you use any special protective or corrective equipment or devices that aren't usually used for your sport or position (for example, knee brace, special neck roll, foot orthotics, retainer on your teeth, hearing aid)?	☐	☐
11. Have you had any problems with your eyes or vision?	☐	☐
Do you wear glasses, contacts, or protective eyewear?	☐	☐
12. Have you ever had a sprain, strain, or swelling after injury?	☐	☐
Have you broken or fractured any bones or dislocated any joints?	☐	☐
Have you had any other problems with pain or swelling in muscles, tendons, bones, or joints?	☐	☐

If yes, check appropriate box and explain below.

☐ Head   ☐ Elbow   ☐ Hip
☐ Neck   ☐ Forearm   ☐ Thigh
☐ Back   ☐ Wrist   ☐ Knee
☐ Chest   ☐ Hand   ☐ Shin/calf
☐ Shoulder   ☐ Finger   ☐ Ankle
☐ Upper arm   ☐ Foot

	Yes	No
13. Do you want to weigh more or less than you do now?	☐	☐
Do you lose weight regularly to meet weight requirements for your sport?	☐	☐
14. Do you feel stressed out?	☐	☐

15. Record the dates of your most recent immunizations (shots) for:

Tetanus _____ Measles _____
Hepatitis B _____ Chickenpox _____

FEMALES ONLY

16. When was your first menstrual period? _____
When was your most recent menstrual period? _____
How much time do you usually have from the start of one period to the start of another? _____
How many periods have you had in the last year? _____
What was the longest time between periods in the last year? _____

Explain "Yes" answers here: _____

_____
_____
_____
_____
_____
_____
_____
_____
_____

I hereby state that, to the best of my knowledge, my answers to the above questions are complete and correct.

Signature of athlete _____ Signature of parent/guardian _____ Date _____

FIGURE 23-3—cont'd
Preparticipation physical evaluation form.
Modified from the American Academy of Family Physicians, American Academy of Pediatrics, American Medical Society for Sports Medicine, American Orthopaedic Society for Sports Medicine, and American Osteopathic Academy of Sports Medicine, 1997.

Preparticipation Physical Evaluation

CLEARANCE FORM

❏ **Cleared**

❏ **Cleared after completing evaluation/rehabilitation for:** _____

_____

_____

_____

❏ **Not cleared for:** _____   **Reason:** _____

Recommendations: _____

_____

_____

_____

Name of physician (print/type) _____   **Date** _____

Address _____   **Phone** _____

Signature of physician _____ **, MD or DO**

FIGURE 23-4

Preparticipation physical evaluation clearance form.
Modified from the American Academy of Family Physicians, American Academy of Pediatrics, American Medical Society for Sports Medicine, American Orthopaedic Society for Sports Medicine, and American Osteopathic Academy of Sports Medicine, 1997.

STAYING WELL

THE FEMALE ATHLETE TRIAD

A trio of problems, *disordered eating, amenorrhea, and osteoporosis*, define the female athlete triad. The greatest risk is for athletes whose sport stresses the need to be lean (gymnastics, figure skating, diving, ballet) or to be able to endure (distance running, swimming, cross-country skiing). Early recognition of a possible problem is essential and the sports preparticipation evaluation is the right time to begin. A review of diet, exercise, and menstrual history should be routine:

An energy deficit occurs when calorie expenditure exceeds calorie intake, sometimes unintentionally but at other times intentionally (such as binging and purging, using laxatives, diuretics, and diet pills inappropriately). The body may adapt at first so that the problem may have a subtle onset.

Primary amenorrhea (no onset of menses by 16 years of age), secondary amenorrhea (no periods for 3 to 6 months), or oligomenorrhea (intervals between periods longer than 35 days) are all possibilities in the triad. These findings are *not* a normal response to exercise. Amenorrhea occurs in as many

as 2% to 5% of the general female population and, among athletes, depending on the sport, from 3.4% to 66%.

The teenage years, when more than half of adult bone calcium is deposited, are a particularly sensitive time. A too thin body encourages a hypoestrogenic state and the possibility of menstrual dysfunction and a resultant osteopenia or osteoporosis. The risk of stress fracture increases. The problem may be irreversible if discovered too late; it needs *early* recognition.

The history then is a compulsive necessity if female athletes are to be kept healthy or, when necessary, treated early and thus more effectively. Amenorrhea suggests pregnancy or thyroid disease and must be considered but, particularly when your patient is a committed, frequently performing athlete in sports demanding endurance and slenderness, the triad must also be considered. A stress fracture offers another important clue. The issues are sensitive and a rewarding history will evolve only if your relationship with the athlete is based on trust.

TABLE 23-1	Classification of Sports by Contact	
Contact or Collision	**Limited Contact**	**Noncontact**
Basketball	Baseball	Archery
Boxing*	Bicycling	Badminton
Diving	Cheerleading	Body building
Field hockey	Canoeing or kayaking	Bowling
Football	(white water)	Canoeing or kayaking
Tackle	Fencing	(flat water)
Ice hockey†	Field events	Crew or rowing
Lacrosse	High jump	Curling
Martial arts	Pole vault	Dancing§
Rodeo	Floor hockey	Ballet
Rugby	Football	Modern
Ski jumping	Flag	Jazz
Soccer	Gymnastics	Field events
Team handball	Handball	Discus
Water polo	Horseback riding	Javelin
Wrestling	Racquetball	Shot put
	Skating	Golf
	Ice	Orienteering¶
	In-line	Power lifting
	Roller	Race walking
	Skiing	Riflery
	Cross-country	Rope jumping
	Downhill	Running
	Water	Sailing
	Skateboarding	Scuba diving
	Snowboarding‡	Swimming
	Softball	Table tennis
	Squash	Tennis
	Ultimate Frisbee	Track
	Volleyball	Weight lifting
	Windsurfing or surfing	

*Participation not recommended by the American Academy of Pediatrics.
†The American Academy of Pediatrics recommends limiting the amount of body checking allowed for hockey players 15 years and younger to reduce injuries.
‡Snowboarding has been added since previous statement was published.
§Dancing has been further classified into ballet, modern, and jazz since previous statement was published.
¶A race (contest) in which competitors use a map and compass to find their way through unfamiliar territory.

TABLE 23-2	Medical Conditions and Sports Participation

This table is designed to be understood by clinical and nonclinical personnel. In the explanation section below, "Needs evaluation" means that a clinician with appropriate knowledge and experience should assess the safety of a given sport for an athlete with the listed medical condition. Unless otherwise noted, this is because of the variability of the severity of the disease, the risk of injury among the specific sports in Table 23-3, or both. A good rule: Do not suggest that an athlete "play through" an injury or problem.

Condition	May Participate
Atlantoaxial instability (instability of the joint between cervical vertebra 1 and 2) *Explanation:* Athlete needs evaluation to assess risk of spinal cord injury during sports participation.	Qualified yes
Bleeding disorder *Explanation:* Athlete needs evaluation.	Qualified yes
Cardiovascular disease	
Carditis (inflammation of the heart) *Explanation:* Carditis may result in sudden death with exertion.	No

Congenital heart disease (structural heart defects present at birth)
     Explanation: Those with mild forms may participate fully; those with moderate or severe forms or who
     have undergone surgery need evaluation.
	Qualified yes

Dysrhythmia (irregular heart rhythm)
     Explanation: Those with symptoms (chest pain, syncope, dizziness, shortness of breath, or other
     symptoms of possible dysrhythmia) or evidence of mitral regurgitation (leaking) on physical examination
     need evaluation. All others may participate fully.
	Qualified yes

Heart murmur
     Explanation: If the murmur is innocent (does not indicate heart disease), full participation is permitted.
     Otherwise, the athlete needs evaluation (see congenital heart disease and mitral valve prolapse).
	Qualified yes

Hypertension (high blood pressure)
     Explanation: Those with significant essential (unexplained) hypertension should avoid weight and power
     lifting, body building, and strength training. Those with secondary hypertension (hypertension caused by
     a previously identified disease) or severe essential hypertension need evaluation.
	Qualified yes

Cerebral palsy *Explanation:* Athlete needs evaluation.	Yes

Diabetes mellitus
   Explanation: All sports can be played with proper attention to diet, blood glucose concentration, hydration,
   and insulin therapy. Blood glucose concentration should be monitored every 30 minutes during continu-
   ous exercise and 15 minutes after completion of exercise.
	Qualified yes

Diarrhea
   Explanation: Unless disease is mild, no participation is permitted, because diarrhea may increase the risk of
   dehydration and heat illness. See fever.
	Qualified yes

Eating disorders
   Anorexia nervosa
   Bulimia nervosa
     Explanation: Patients with these disorders need medical and psychiatric assessment before participation.
	Qualified yes

Eyes
   Functionally one-eyed athlete
   Loss of an eye
   Detached retina
   Previous eye surgery or serious eye injury
     Explanation: A functionally one-eyed athlete has a best-corrected visual acuity of less than 20/40 in the
     eye with worse acuity. These athletes would suffer significant disability if the better eye were seriously
     injured, as would those with loss of an eye. Some athletes who previously have undergone eye surgery
     or had a serious eye injury may have an increased risk of injury because of weakened eye tissue. Avail-
     ability of eye guards approved by the American Society for Testing and Materials and other protective
     equipment may allow participation in most sports, but this must be judged on an individual basis.
	Qualified yes

Fever
   Explanation: Fever can increase cardiopulmonary effort, reduce maximum exercise capacity, make heat
   illness more likely, and increase orthostatic hypertension during exercise. Fever may rarely accompany
   myocarditis or other infections that may make exercise dangerous.
	No

Heat illness, history of
   Explanation: Because of the increased likelihood of recurrence, the athlete needs individual assessment to
   determine the presence of predisposing conditions and to arrange a prevention strategy.
	Qualified yes

Continued

TABLE 23-2	Medical Conditions and Sports Participation—cont'd	
Condition		**May Participate**
Hepatitis		Yes
Explanation: Because of the apparent minimal risk to others, all sports may be played that the athlete's state of health allows. In all athletes, skin lesions should be covered properly, and athletic personnel should use universal precautions when handling blood or body fluids with visible blood.		
Human immunodeficiency virus infection		Yes
Explanation: Because of the apparent minimal risk to others, all sports may be played that the athlete's state of health allows. In all athletes, skin lesions should be covered properly, and athletic personnel should use universal precautions when handling blood or body fluids with visible blood.		
Kidney, absence of one		Qualified yes
Explanation: Athlete needs individual assessment for contact, collision, and limited-contact sports.		
Liver, enlarged		Qualified yes
Explanation: If the liver is acutely enlarged, participation should be avoided because of risk of rupture. If the liver is chronically enlarged, individual assessment is needed before collision, contact, or limited-contact sports are played.		
Malignant neoplasm		Qualified yes
Explanation: Athlete needs individual assessment.		
Musculoskeletal disorders		Qualified yes
Explanation: Athlete needs individual assessment.		
Neurologic disorders		Qualified yes
History of serious brain or spine trauma, severe or repeated concussions, or craniotomy.		
Explanation: Athlete needs individual assessment for collision, contact, or limited-contact sports and for noncontact sports if deficits in judgment or cognition are present. Research supports a conservative approach to management of concussion.		
Seizure disorder, well-controlled		Yes
Explanation: Risk of seizure during participation is minimal		
Seizure disorder, poorly controlled		Qualified yes
Explanation: Athlete needs individual assessment for collision, contact, or limited-contact sports. The following noncontact sports should be avoided: archery, riflery, swimming, weight or power lifting, strength training, or sports involving heights. In these sports, occurrence of a seizure may pose a risk to self or others.		
Obesity		Qualified yes
Explanation: Because of the risk of heat illness, obese persons need careful acclimatization and hydration.		
Organ transplant recipient		Qualified yes
Explanation: Athlete needs individual assessment.		
Ovary, absence of		Yes
Explanation: Risk of severe injury to remaining ovary is minimal.		
Respiratory conditions		
Pulmonary compromise, including cystic fibrosis		Qualified yes
Explanation: Athlete needs individual assessment, but generally, all sports may be played if oxygenation remains satisfactory during a graded exercise test. Patients with cystic fibrosis need acclimatization and good hydration to reduce the risk of heat illness.		
Asthma		Yes
Explanation: With proper medication and education, only athletes with the most severe asthma will need to modify their participation.		
Acute upper respiratory infection		Qualified yes
Explanation: Upper respiratory obstruction may affect pulmonary function. Athlete needs individual assessment for all but mild disease. See fever.		
Sickle cell disease		Qualified yes
Explanation: Athlete needs individual assessment. In general, if status of the illness permits, all but high exertion, collision, and contact sports may be played. Overheating, dehydration, and chilling must be avoided.		
Sickle cell trait		Yes
Explanation: It is unlikely that persons with sickle cell trait have an increased risk of sudden death or other medical problems during athletic participation, except under the most extreme conditions of heat, humidity, and possibly increased altitude. These persons, like all athletes, should be carefully conditioned, acclimatized, and hydrated to reduce any possible risk.		
Skin disorders (boils, herpes simplex, impetigo, scabies, molluscum contagiosum)		Qualified yes
Explanation: While the patient is contagious, participation in gymnastics with mats; martial arts; wrestling; or other collision, contact, or limited-contact sports is not allowed.		
Spleen, enlarged		Qualified yes
Explanation: A patient with an acutely enlarged spleen should avoid all sports because of risk of rupture. A patient with a chronically enlarged spleen needs individual assessment before playing collision, contact, or limited-contact sports.		

TABLE 23-3	Classification of Sports by Strenuousness

HIGH TO MODERATE INTENSITY (THE DEGREE TO WHICH A DEMAND ON THE BODY IS MADE FOR EXCESSIVE MOVEMENT [DYNAMIC] OR FOR *RELATIVELY* LESS MOVEMENT [STATIC])

High to Moderate Dynamic and Static Demands	High to Moderate Dynamic and Low Static Demands	High to Moderate Static and Low Dynamic Demands
Boxing*	Badminton	Archery
Crew or rowing	Baseball	Auto racing
Cross-country skiing	Basketball	Diving
Cycling	Field hockey	Horseback riding (jumping)
Downhill skiing	Lacrosse	Field events (throwing)
Fencing	Orienteering	Gymnastics
Football	Race walking	Karate or judo
Ice hockey	Racquetball	Motorcycling
Rugby	Soccer	Rodeo
Running (sprint)	Squash	Sailing
Speed skating	Swimming	Ski jumping
Water polo	Table tennis	Water skiing
Wrestling	Tennis	Weight lifting
	Volleyball	

LOW-INTENSITY (LOW) DYNAMIC AND LOW STATIC DEMANDS
Bowling
Cricket
Curling
Golf
Riflery

---

*Participation not recommended by the American Academy of Pediatrics.

PUTTING IT ALL TOGETHER

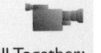

Putting It All Together:
See the complete Putting It All Together
head-to-toe physical examination video
on the Companion CD-ROM

The relationship with the patient, when well established, leads to marvelous benefit. There is a powerful therapeutic effect in really listening to what the patient is saying, in careful exploration for hidden concerns, and in using explanation in nonpatronizing, understandable terms. The enduring message is that you care and that the patient is a full partner with you in the effort. This of itself helps in the relief of suffering. If you communicate well and if you and the patient can achieve a genuine alliance, you will find that you are of service and, happily, will feel much rewarded.

We have indicated routines for history-taking and physical examination, and we have stressed your need to adopt a disciplined approach particular to your comfort. Discipline, however, does not suggest rigidity. Too great an adherence to routine may prevent the true story from emerging. That is why open-ended encouragement of the patient to speak candidly and with trust, to tell the real story, can be so rewarding (Coles, 1989). It is helpful at a first meeting, if the situation allows, to sit back comfortably and to say, "Tell me about yourself," and to listen and to hear.

As a skillfully evoked story—the history—evolves, the absolute unity of mind and body and the power of an effective alliance with the patient become manifest. The physical examination, the "laying on of hands," complements the story and is essential to the confirmation of the alliance. Words and physical acts are all invested with pragmatic need and symbolic meaning, and are all contributors to the conscious and subconscious requirements of an effective relationship. They ultimately make it possible to understand not only the objective biologic findings—the disease—but also the great variety of subjective findings that modify the experience of the disease and result in an illness being understood in human, not scientific, terms. Obviously, art and science are inextricable, and technologic expertise is a complement to, never a substitute for, skillful art. The computer cannot replace a good history and a competent physical examination.

GENERAL GUIDELINES

When you begin learning about a patient, do not expect to proceed from A to Z on a rigid pathway. The information in this book is arranged by body systems, but the actual examination should be both flexible and disciplined. The history and physical examination are so interrelated that they need not be done in a particular sequence. The artistry of your effort arises from your ability to integrate the two procedures according to the demands of the situation. Each of the steps in history taking and physical examination is an entity with its own sensitivity and specificity. You must understand the limits of each of those steps and how much information can be gained from them. Although you need to be always alert to deviations from the usual and the expected, you will learn when to omit steps that will yield information of little value. This is not being sloppy; it is using clinical judgment in adapting to circumstance. The steps blend into a fluid and comprehensible whole. The process of taking the history and performing the physical examination not only teaches you much about the patient, but also teaches the patient much about you—your personal discipline, your professional composure, and the respect you accord others (Box 24-1).

Do not forget that the patient, who usually seeks your help because of a problem, may feel dependent and may have some unease, anxiety, or even fear (Box 24-2). You can help allay these feelings simply by respecting them and by not demeaning or ignoring them. Your explanations of what you will do next will be reassuring. Always be honest about the possibility that a part of the examination may cause discomfort or pain, or you risk losing trust. If either you or the patient feels the need to have a third person in the room, you must arrange it.

Always respect the patient's modesty. This does not mean that you do not ask the patient to undress, but rather that comfortable gowns and covers be available that can be shifted from the area under examination while providing cover for other parts of the body. Age, gender, and particular circumstance (e.g., pelvic and rectal examination and/or a given patient's sensibili-

---

BOX 24-1

HOW TO ENSURE DIFFICULTY WITH PATIENTS AND RISK BEING SUED

- Make them wait a long time, without explanation, especially alone in the examining room.
- Act busy and rushed; don't give them the necessary time.
- Talk "medicalese."
- Be casual and superficial in offering reassurance, deflecting real concerns.
- Skip the extra question that might reveal an underlying problem.
- Ignore emotional responses to illness, such as anger, fear, uncertainty, guilt, and self-blame.
- Ignore the stresses in a patient's life (and yours), the day-to-day pressures, and the needs that can overwhelm.
- Convey your negative feelings or discomfort about a particular illness.

Modified from Jellinck et al, 1991.

BOX 24-2

THE PATIENT WE DEFINE AS DIFFICULT

We always want to do our best, and we always want our relationship with the patient to be positive. Sometimes, however, we find ourselves reacting negatively when patients are:

- Dependent, apparently needing insatiable, never-ending contact
- Denying, using denial to cope, being inattentive to instructions, not following through on treatment regimens
- Demanding, wanting preferential treatment, seeming always on the edge of a lawsuit, really often quite dependent, and often impressed with their self-determined status in society (the VIP)
- Rejecting, distrusting, always testing your competency and reliability

In all of these circumstances, it pays to learn what the patient's needs really are, to understand their insecurities, to learn the available family and other social resources, and to never put them down. Certainly, it is necessary to be as precise as possible, to keep all promises, to set firm limits on what you can do, and to try to retain an empathetic approach. The alliance with these patients can grow and mature, albeit sometimes painfully. It will not happen instantly. The advantage we have is that patients are, more often than not and particularly when they are vulnerable, inclined to give us the chance to gain their trust and respect.

Suggested by Jellinck et al, 1990.

ties) should govern the decision to use a chaperone. Doors and curtains should be closed, and it is best to leave the room when the patient undresses and prepares for the examination.

Early encounters with the human body generally result in some discomfort—sometimes revulsion, and often embarrassment. At times, sexual connotations cannot be ignored. There is also the thrilling privilege in taking on, at last, the responsibility for serving patients. Your comfort with the situation should never become so great that you forget that the experience may be much newer for the patient. Your own early reactions can provide insight into the patient's experience.

The invasion of a stranger's sensibilities can be most distracting to the student. You will learn a gentle and balanced demeanor. Your professional concern can be reassuring to the patient, but you must avoid inappropriate reassurance and premature expressions of concern over unexpected findings. Remember that patients are examining you while you examine them, and are titrating their anxiety by your manner, your hesitations in speech, your changes in facial expression, your lingering over a part of the examination. In fact, many patients equate the gravity of the situation with the length of time you spend on a part of the examination, whereas others equate length of time with thoroughness.

Patients should be told that you are a student and that you are apt to be slower than the more experienced practitioner. You will naturally feel some pressure and uncertainty about your level of ability, but there is a half-life to this anxiety. Time, experience, and appropriate supervision by preceptors will help build the foundation for your self-confidence.

At the beginning, when you are unaccustomed to the sequence of an examination, rely on guides such as those in this book. You should be flexible, however, in adapting the sequence to the circumstance of the moment. There is no such thing as a complete examination. The goal is an examination in which your observations are appropriate to the circumstance. This varies with the nature of the complaint and with the age and gender of the patient. Because there is no best way, you should develop an approach that is comfortable for you and ensures comfort for your patient. You need not take the history or perform the physical examination in the same sequence in which you will record them. Part of the history can be obtained while you are doing the physical examination because, as you discover certain findings, you will need more details than the earlier history may have elicited. Regardless of sequence, there are certain guidelines that should not be ignored (Box 24-3).

Once you have the basic information, you need to assess the urgency of the situation, determine whether the principal problems are new or long-standing, decide which clues are most important, determine the extent of the problems and the number of body systems involved, and decide which of the possible clinical areas concerned are dominant.

You may then need to ask more questions and return to your physical examination if you are to understand the problem. Do not assume that your initial list of clinical possibilities is all-inclusive. There may be an unusual presentation of a common problem or a common presentation of a rarity. There may be more than one disease process or a confounding emotional or social problem. There may be a new illness superimposed on an existing one. Every clue, however subtle, counts. Finally, you need to decide where first to concentrate. To do this well, you must consider the entire range of pathophysiologic and psychosocial problems and, with probabilities in mind, go beyond the obvious to the obscure, constantly challenging your conclusions by being your own devil's advocate or asking others to do so.

RELIABILITY

The health professional and the patient have responsibility for the reliability of findings and observations, but yours is greater. Take the time with open-ended questions to ensure that the patient has the opportunity to report accurately.

THE PATIENT AS HISTORIAN

There is much that can limit the patient's ability to observe well and to report accurately:

- Sensory deprivation. A partial or total loss of any of the senses (e.g., vision, hearing, touch, smell) is clearly constraining. Do not rely on the unaffected senses being heightened. This may be the case with some people, but not with all.

BOX 24-3

SOME GUIDELINES TO AN APPROPRIATE RELATIONSHIP WITH THE PATIENT

- Dress neatly; always be well groomed.
- Address the patient respectfully and with the patient's name; although a child's mother is a mother, she should not be addressed as such; she has a name.
- Patients are culturally diverse; use the patient's language if possible; it is important that the patient understand you; if you must use colloquialisms to accomplish this, do so; *do not* use complex medical terminology.
- Ensure comfort for the patient and, to the extent possible, for yourself.
- Be gentle.
- The setting should be quiet (radios and televisions should be turned off), comfortable, and well lighted (without glare).
- Avoid distraction and interruption. (The telephone should not be allowed into the history and examining room unless there is an emergency.)
- Adapt to the patient's circumstance. (A person in traction will offer a different challenge from the 7-month-old baby on the parent's lap.)
- Be flexible and avoid rigid adherence to a particular sequence; however, be certain that by the end of the examination you have made all the necessary observations.
- An examining table should allow you access to the patient from every side and be at a height that is convenient for both you and the patient; because a table against the wall is an obstacle to examining the patient from every perspective, it is preferable to have the table away from the wall.
- Have the patient free of clothing but comfortably draped, paying attention to modesty at every age.
- Always consider the need for a chaperone.
- Expose the part of the body to be examined appropriately and well, or you may lose the vital finding.
- Keep your hands and stethoscope warm.
- Avoid using too vigorous an approach when examining tender areas.
- Talk with the patient but do not chatter; explain as you go, anticipating the patient's concern about what comes next;

briefly state the reasons for examining an area and warn the patient of any discomfort it might incur.
- Never order the patient to do things; say "please" and "thank you" (but not so endlessly so that the courtesy itself becomes obsequious); occasionally ask if the patient is warm enough and comfortable enough or has any questions.
- Gather information from the patient's attitude, demeanor, speech, and body; it is worrisome, for example, to find the patient apathetic, disinterested, unable to respond socially, or so overwhelmed by the problem that a smile cannot be elicited. (This is as true for a 3-month-old baby as it is for an adult.)
- Make some assessment, at least in your own mind, about the reliability of the patient as an observer; remember that there is much in illness and in life to put constraints on the patient's ability to observe carefully and objectively; be objective and make no premature assumptions about what you find. Carefully describe first without diagnosing. (For example, a lump in the neck may be a swollen node and not a cyst. Diagnosis can usually wait until after the examination is completed.)
- Make quantitative measurements with a ruler; do not use a coin, a piece of fruit, or a nut for comparison.
- Remember that physical findings are age oriented and that their meanings will vary according to age.
- Be reassuring only when you honestly can.
- Do not jump to conclusions and share impressions before all the information has been collected; do not make promises that cannot be kept; developing the composure that allows you to be reassuring without overstating the case takes practice and time.
- Do not feel that you have to do it all in one sitting. If the situation requires it, you can allow the patient a chance for rest and return later to complete the examination; you should pace your approach according to the patient's need, guided by the sense of urgency and the recognition of fatigue and frailty.

- Emotional constraints, apparent and inapparent. Patients who are psychotic, delirious, depressed, or in any way seriously emotionally affected may confuse you. Emphasize mental status during the history when you suspect this.
- Language barriers. Patients may speak a language different from yours. Translation can be difficult in the best of circumstances. Passing messages among three persons often results in changes in meaning that might have serious importance, and confusion may be the result. Even using the same language may be a problem if the patient has a limited vocabulary, speaks English as a second language, or cannot read it very well.
- Cultural barriers. Pay attention to the possibility of cultural differences between you and the patient (see Chapter 2). Approach the variety of life experience with candor and interested, compassionate inquiry (Box 24-4).
- Unresponsive or comatose patient. Refer to the section on the unresponsive patient (see Chapter 27).

> **BOX 24-4**
>
> **CULTURAL DIFFERENCES RELATED TO LIFE EXPERIENCE**
>
> Cultural differences manifest in many ways. Whereas race and ethnicity are often obvious, there are also meaningful separations in life experiences among the fat and the thin, the gravely ill and the well, the patients accustomed to exploring complementary and alternative therapies and those who are not, the drug abuser and the nonuser, and the aged and the young. The recognition of these differences and the conscientious attempt to encourage the patient to talk of them and thus to educate you can build empathic bridges and eliminate, or at least minimize, doubts about each other. It is all right, for example, to ask how it feels to be markedly overweight in an airplane seat designed for a slender, short person (see Chapter 2).

The immediate need in these circumstances is to identify and understand the limitations and take the steps to enhance reliability. The patient with a sensory impairment deserves a response from you that facilitates communication (e.g., write questions; pay careful attention to the needs of a lip reader, such as good light, a slow pace to speech, and a constant visibility of your lips; and recognize that the blind person cannot see your gestures).

You must often rely on family, friends, or an emergency medical technician for information. The rules that guide interactions with patients guide interactions with others. If possible, the patient must be aware that you are receiving information from other historians. When possible, there must be agreement with the patient about the limits that can be placed on the sharing of information. Respect for autonomy and the rules of confidentiality remain essential.

There are patients, of course, who are "unreliable" because of life situations, limited intelligence, indifference, apathy, or personal emotional needs that lead to distortions, overstatements, or understatements of reality. Any number of variables can get in the way. All of these possibilities require skill and sensitivity in responding to the enormous variety in the human condition. You might begin by rejecting the common use of the descriptor "unreliable," because of its pejorative connotation.

THE PROFESSIONAL AS OBSERVER

We are all susceptible to human error. The same practitioner may palpate the same abdomen at different times on the same day and conclude that the liver has a somewhat different span each time. Multiple observers may palpate the same abdomen on the same day and individually decide on different liver spans. These are not unconscientious, ill-considered observations; they are demonstrations of the potential for error, as likely in each of us as in the many tests we order for our patients (Box 24-5). Every observation has a certain sensitivity (i.e., the assurance that if something is to be found, it will be found) and specificity (i.e., the assurance that if it is found, it is a true finding and not a misinterpretation or false-positive finding). No test has 100% sensitivity and specificity (see Chapter 25). So, you will not always be right. Knowing this, guarding against it, candidly questioning yourself, and seeking confirmation from others when necessary will serve to assure your reliability.

UNCERTAINTY

The likelihood of some error increases uncertainty and influences our decision making as we consider probabilities. A numeric value of probability can often be given, providing an idea of the degree of uncertainty. Many psychosocial, environmental, and physical considerations affect the perception of the same set of facts and have a variable impact on our interpretations of that figure.

Most of us are uncomfortable with uncertainty at the start. The diagnostic process may be initiated by thinking in a deterministic or mechanistic fashion, by seeking certain and fixed knowledge, and by avoiding to the extent possible anything that is subjective in a search for absolutes that are free of beliefs, attitudes, and values. However, the variables of life will not often allow this; they will not always let you express your findings in numbers.

BOX 24-5

HUMANS VERSUS MACHINES

There are a number of observations better made by you than a machine, including the following:

- All perceptions obtained through watching, listening, touching, and smelling
- The appearance of the patient, his or her vitality, the presence or absence of apathy, and the sense of illness
- The patient's cognitive awareness

There are, however, an almost infinite variety of diagnostic procedures that enable better understanding of patients' problems. Just as with observation, these procedures are not always sensitive to potential findings or necessarily specific about them.

For example, diagnostic imaging—the use of x-ray film, nuclear medicine, ultrasonography, computed tomography (CT), and magnetic resonance imaging (MRI) —offers a powerful resource. Yet, diagnostic imaging has its limitations and penalties:

- The x-ray examination is easily available and relatively inexpensive and can give a sense of motion with the fluoroscope and cineradiograph; however, the procedure utilizes contrast agents that can be toxic, there is confusion of shadows, and the patient is exposed to radiation.

- The ultrasonograph is safe, can also provide a sense of motion, and delineates soft tissue very well; however, fat, bone, and air impede sound waves.
- CT clearly delineates anatomy, works better in the presence of obesity than does x-ray examination, and outlines soft tissues very well; however, it is expensive, does not work as well in the lean individual, and uses radiation.
- Nuclear medicine takes a step toward enhancing knowledge about the body's physiology, and it can reveal early bone infection and bone metastasis; however, it is expensive and uses radiation.
- MRI gives excellent soft tissue contrast and precise anatomic detail without the need for contrast agents. Similar to ultrasonography, it is safe, but it is also very expensive and is not always available. In addition, the machine and the process can at times intimidate patients, particularly children.

These reminders are not meant to discourage but are intended only to suggest caution and thoughtfulness in everything we do. This is particularly necessary as newer imaging techniques come into play. No procedure occurs without cost to the human body, to emotion, or to the pocketbook.

Modified from Johns, Fortuin, Wheeler, 1988; Taylor, 1989.

BOX 24-6

EUREKA!! THE WELL-DONE HISTORY AND PHYSICAL EXAMINATION

EUREKA! is a Greek word that, loosely translated, means "I found it!" or, even better, "Aha!!" It suggests the feeling of delight and appropriate self-congratulation when a discovery, a sudden realization, provides the essential key to the solution of a difficult problem. Hellman reminds us that this can come at any point in the evaluation of a patient (Hellmann, 2003). He also laments the probably increasing paucity of such moments in a time of excessive workload and, among other reasons, the substitution of increasing unselective use of technology for the proper honing of physical examination skills. We offer a ready solution. The well-taken history and well-performed physical examination burnished by your sensitivity and skill will open the way to an infinity of EUREKA! moments for you.

Even so, we often attempt to quantify data. We use scales that may require a subjective judgment of several variables and the assignment of a fixed number for each in order to arrive at a total score. That fixed number is really a pseudo quantification. Rivara and Wasserman (1984), aware of our addiction to numbers, suggested that we might give more attention to psychosocial issues in our day-to-day work with people if we were able to quantify them. Tongue in cheek and referring to the woman whose beauty launched a thousand ships, they noted that one milli-Helen equals exactly that amount of beauty it takes to launch one ship. There is false comfort in the apparent certainty of many numbers.

Because we have not yet reached an ideal state of certainty, we must continue to recognize the potential for error, the variety of interpretations of the same event, and the need to think in terms of probability. The mature observer is one who is comfortable making decisions with a certain degree of uncertainty (Box 24-6).

EXAMINATION SEQUENCE

We remind you again that there is no one right way to put together the parts of the physical examination so that the process flows smoothly, minimizes the number of times the patient has to change positions, and conserves patient energy. The following is a suggested approach. Like any other approach, it may need to be adapted for a particular setting, patient condition, or patient disability. Box 24-7 gives a list of supplies you should have on hand.

GENERAL INSPECTION

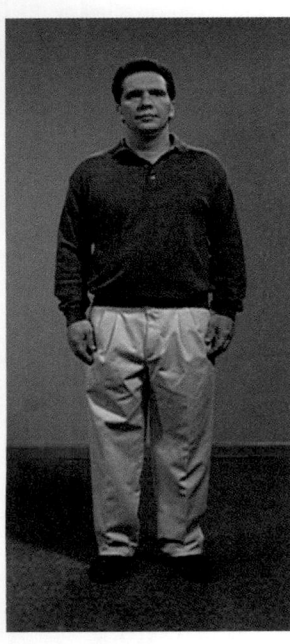

Begin the inspection as you greet the patient on entering the room, looking for signs of distress or disease. You can perform parts of your physical examination at any time as long as the patient is within your view, even in the waiting room (Fig. 24-1). If you go there to invite the patient into your examining room, take a moment to see the habitus, manner of sitting, degree of relaxation, relationship with others in the room, and degree of interest in what is happening in the room. There are no blank moments when you are with the patient. On your first greeting, you can judge the alacrity with which you are met; the moistness of the palm when you shake hands; the gait as the patient walks back to the room; and the eyes, their luster, and their expression of emotion. All of this contributes to your examination, along with assessments of the following:

- Skin color
- Facial expression
- Mobility
  - Use of assistive devices
  - Gait
  - Sitting, rising from chair
  - Taking off coat
- Dress and posture
- Speech pattern, disorders, foreign language
- Difficulty hearing, assistive devices

BOX 24-7

EQUIPMENT SUPPLIES FOR PHYSICAL EXAMINATION

Basic Materials
Cotton balls
Cotton-tipped applicator sticks
Drapes
Examining gloves
Flashlight with transilluminator
Gauze squares
Lubricant
Marking pen
Measuring tape
Nasal speculum
Odorous substances
Ophthalmoscope
Otoscope with pneumatic bulb
Penlight
Percussion hammer
Ruler
Sharp and dull testing implements
Sphygmomanometer

Stethoscope with diaphragm and bell
Taste-testing substances
Thermometer
Tongue blades
Tuning forks
Vaginal speculum
Visual acuity screening charts for near and
    far vision

Materials for Gathering Specimens
Culture media
Glass slides
KOH (potassium hydroxide)
Occult blood testing materials
Pap smear spatula and/or brush, fixative,
    and container
Saline
Sterile cotton-tipped applicators

* Stature and build
* Musculoskeletal deformities
* Vision problems, assistive devices
* Eye contact with examiner
* Orientation, mental alertness
* Nutritional state
* Respiratory problems
* Significant others accompanying patient

PREPARATION

Respecting modesty, instruct the patient to empty the bladder, remove as much clothing as is necessary, and put on a gown. Ask for a chaperone if you think it necessary. Then, continue. A suggested sequence follows.

MEASUREMENTS

* Measure height.
* Measure weight.
* Assess distance vision: Snellen chart.
* Document vital signs: temperature, pulse, respiration, and blood pressure in both arms.

PATIENT SEATED, WEARING GOWN

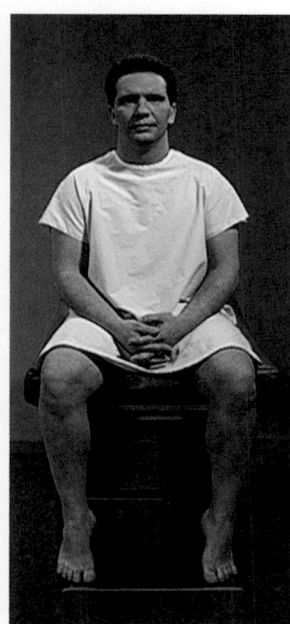

Patient is seated on examining table; examiner stands in front of patient (Fig. 24-2).

Head and Face

* Inspect skin characteristics.
* Inspect symmetry and external characteristics of eyes and ears.
* Inspect configuration of skull.
* Inspect and palpate scalp and hair for texture, distribution, and quantity.
* Palpate facial bones.
* Palpate temporomandibular joint while patient opens and closes mouth.
* Palpate and percuss sinus regions; if tender, transilluminate.
* Inspect ability to clench teeth, squeeze eyes tightly shut, wrinkle forehead, smile, stick out tongue, puff out cheeks (CN V, VII).
* Test light touch sensation of forehead, cheeks, chin (CN V).

Eyes

* External examination
  * Inspect eyelids, eyelashes, palpebral folds.
  * Determine alignment of eyebrows.
  * Inspect sclera, conjunctiva, iris.
  * Palpate lacrimal apparatus.
* Near vision screening: Rosenbaum chart (CN II)
* Eye function
  * Test pupillary response to light and accommodation.
  * Perform cover-uncover test and corneal light reflex.
  * Test extraocular eye movements (CN III, IV, VI).
  * Assess visual fields (CN II).
  * Test corneal reflexes (CN V).
* Ophthalmoscopic examination
  * Test red reflex.
  * Inspect lens.
  * Inspect disc, cup margins, vessels, retinal surface.

Ears
* Inspect alignment and placement.
* Inspect surface characteristics.
* Palpate auricle.
* Assess hearing with whisper test or ticking watch (CN VIII).
* Perform otoscopic examination.
    * Inspect canals.
    * Inspect tympanic membranes for landmarks, deformities, inflammation.
* Perform Rinne and Weber tests.

Nose
* Note structure, position of septum.
* Determine patency of each nostril.
* Inspect mucosa, septum, and turbinates with nasal speculum.
* Assess olfactory function: Test sense of smell (CN I).

Mouth and Pharynx
* Inspect lips, buccal mucosa, gums, hard and soft palates, floor of mouth for color and surface characteristics.
* Inspect oropharynx. Note anteroposterior pillars, uvula, tonsils, posterior pharynx, mouth odor.
* Inspect teeth for color, number, surface characteristics.
* Inspect tongue for color, characteristics, symmetry, movement (CN XII).
* Test gag reflex and "ah" reflex (CN IX, X).
* Perform taste test (CN VII).

Neck
* Inspect for symmetry and smoothness of neck and thyroid.
* Inspect for jugular venous distention.
* Inspect and palpate range of motion; test resistance against examiner's hand.
* Test shoulder shrug (CN IX).
* Palpate carotid pulses, one at a time.
* Palpate tracheal position.
* Palpate thyroid.
* Palpate lymph nodes: preauricular and postauricular, occipital, tonsillar, submaxillary, submental, superficial cervical chain, posterior cervical, deep cervical, supraclavicular.
* Auscultate carotid arteries and thyroid.

Upper Extremities
* Observe and palpate hands, arms, and shoulders.
    * Skin and nail characteristics
    * Muscle mass
    * Musculoskeletal deformities
    * Joint range of motion and muscle strength: fingers, wrists, elbows, shoulders
* Assess pulses: radial, brachial.
* Palpate epitrochlear nodes.

PATIENT SEATED, BACK EXPOSED

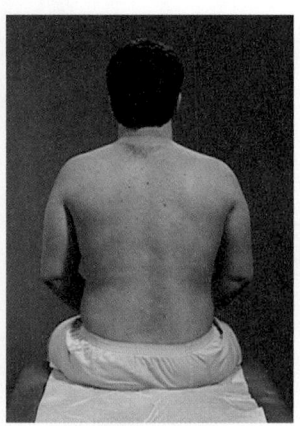

Patient is still seated on examining table. Gown is pulled down to the waist for males so the entire chest and back are exposed; for females, back is exposed, but breasts are covered (Fig. 24-3). Examiner stands behind the patient.

Back and Posterior Chest
* Inspect skin and thoracic configuration.
* Inspect symmetry of shoulders, musculoskeletal development.
* Inspect and palpate scapula and spine, and percuss spine.
* Palpate and percuss costovertebral angle.

Lungs
* Inspect respiration: excursion, depth, rhythm, pattern.
* Palpate for expansion and tactile fremitus.
* Palpate scapular and subscapular nodes.
* Percuss posterior chest and lateral walls systematically for resonance.
* Percuss for diaphragmatic excursion.
* Auscultate systematically for breath sounds. Note characteristics and adventitious sounds.

PATIENT SEATED, CHEST EXPOSED

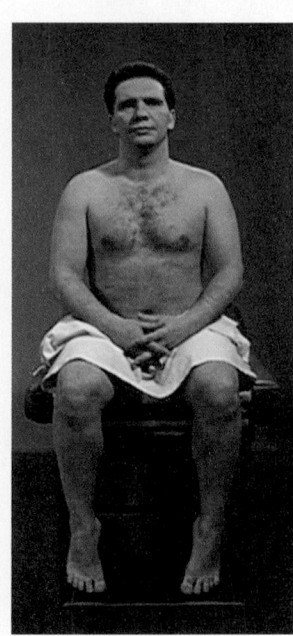

Examiner moves around to the front of the patient (Fig. 24-4). The gown is lowered in females to expose the anterior chest.

Anterior, Chest, Lungs, and Heart
* Inspect skin, musculoskeletal development, symmetry.
* Inspect respirations: patient posture, respiratory effort.
* Inspect for pulsations or heaving.
* Palpate chest wall for stability, crepitation, tenderness.
* Palpate precordium for thrills, heaves, pulsations.
* Palpate left chest to locate apical impulse.
* Palpate for tactile fremitus.
* Palpate nodes: infraclavicular, axillary.
* Percuss systematically for resonance.
* Auscultate systematically for breath sounds.
* Auscultate systematically for heart sounds: aortic area, pulmonic area, second pulmonic area, apical area.

Female Breasts
* Inspect in the following positions: patient's arms extended over head, pushing hands on hips, hands pushed together in front of chest, patient leaning forward.
* Palpate breasts in all four quadrants, tail of Spence, over areolae; if breasts are large, perform bimanual palpation.
* Palpate nipple, compress breasts to observe for discharge.

Male Breasts
* Inspect breasts and nipples for symmetry, enlargement, surface characteristics.
* Palpate breast tissue.

PATIENT RECLINING 45 DEGREES

Assist the patient to a reclining position at a 45-degree angle (Fig. 24-5). Examiner stands to the side of the patient that allows the best approach for necessary examination and comfort for patient and examiner.

- ◆ Inspect chest in recumbent position.
- ◆ Inspect jugular venous pulsations and measure jugular venous pressure.

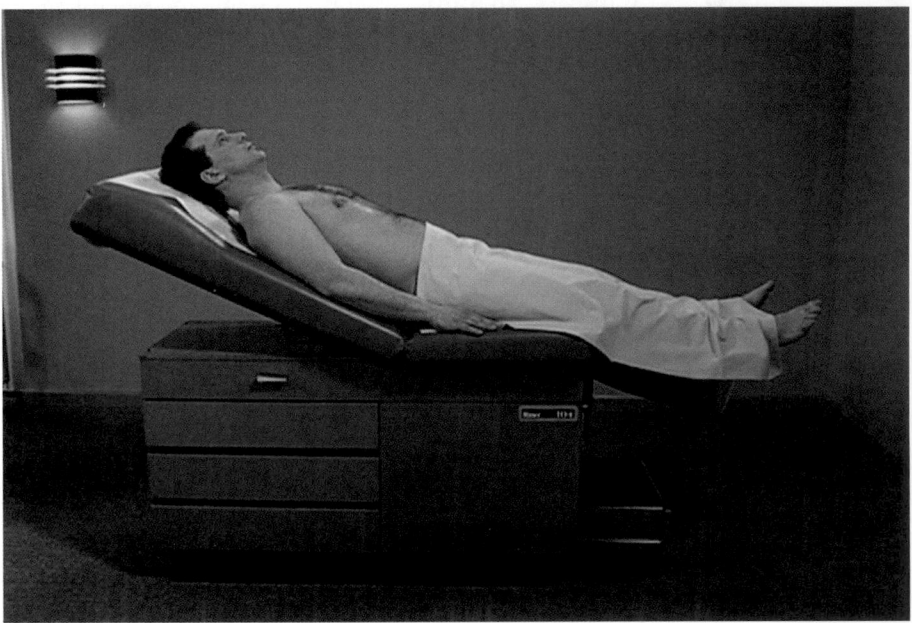

PATIENT SUPINE, CHEST EXPOSED

Assist the patient into a supine position. If the patient cannot tolerate lying flat, maintain head elevation at 30-degree angle if possible. Uncover the chest while keeping the abdomen and lower extremities draped.

Female Breasts
- ◆ Inspect and palpate using the recumbent and upright positions
- ◆ Palpate systematically with the patient's arm over her head and also with her arm at her side.

Heart
- ◆ Palpate the chest wall for thrills, heaves, pulsations.
- ◆ Auscultate systematically; you can turn the patient slightly to the left side and repeat auscultation.

PATIENT SUPINE, ABDOMEN EXPOSED

Patient remains supine. Cover the chest with the patient's gown. Arrange draping to expose the abdomen from pubis to epigastrium (Fig. 24-6).

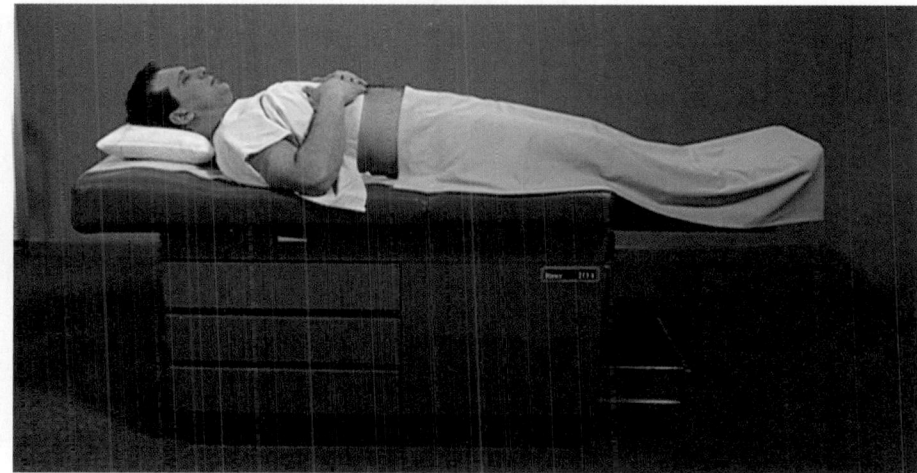

Abdomen

- Inspect skin characteristics, contour, pulsations, movement.
- Auscultate all quadrants for bowel sounds.
- Auscultate the aorta and renal, iliac, and femoral arteries for bruits or venous hums.
- Percuss all quadrants for tone.
- Percuss liver borders and estimate span.
- Percuss left midaxillary line for splenic dullness.
- Lightly palpate all quadrants.
- Deeply palpate all quadrants.
- Palpate right costal margin for liver border.
- Palpate left costal margin for spleen.
- Palpate for right and left kidneys.
- Palpate midline for aortic pulsation.
- Test abdominal reflexes.
- Have patient raise the head as you inspect the abdominal muscles.

Inguinal Area

- Palpate for lymph nodes, pulses, hernias.

External Genitalia, Males

- Inspect penis, urethral meatus, scrotum, pubic hair.
- Palpate scrotal contents.

PATIENT SUPINE, LEGS EXPOSED

Patient remains supine. Arrange drapes to cover the abdomen and pubis and to expose the lower extremities (Fig. 24-7).

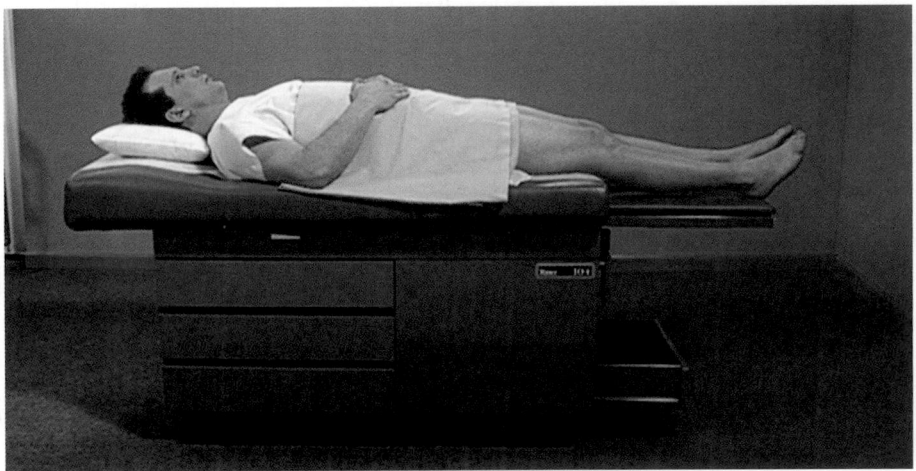

Feet and Legs
- Inspect for skin characteristics, hair distribution, muscle mass, musculoskeletal configuration.
- Palpate for temperature, texture, edema, pulses (dorsalis pedis, posterior tibial, popliteal).
- Test range of motion and strength of toes, feet, ankles, knees.

Hips
- Palpate hips for stability.
- Test range of motion and strength of hips.

PATIENT SITTING, LAP DRAPED

Assist the patient to a sitting position. The patient should have the gown on with a drape across the lap (Fig. 24-8).

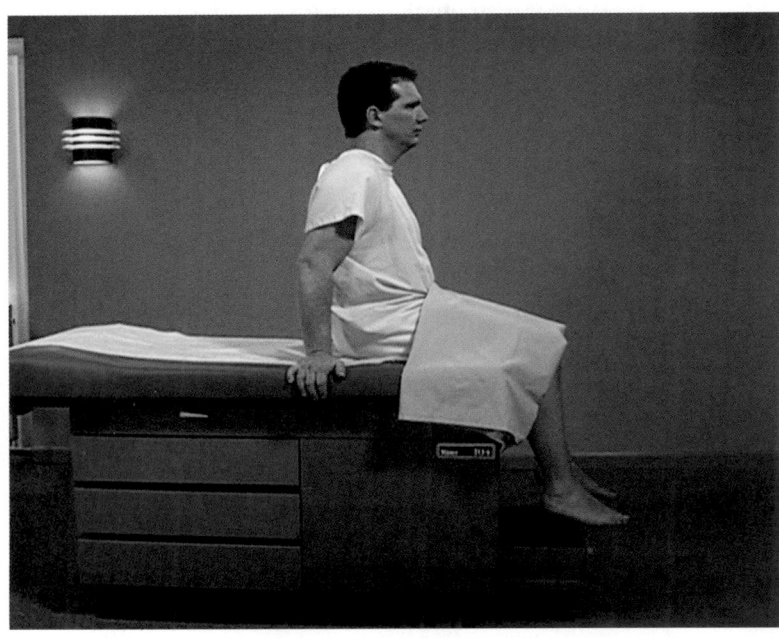

Musculoskeletal
* Observe patient moving from lying to sitting position.
* Note coordination, use of muscles, ease of movement.

Neurologic
* Test sensory function: Dull and sharp sensation of forehead, paranasal sinus area, lower arms, hands, lower legs, feet.
* Test vibratory sensation of wrists, ankles.
* Test two-point discrimination of palms, thighs, back.
* Test stereognosis, graphesthesia.
* Test fine motor function and coordination. Ask the patient to perform the following tasks:
  * Touch his or her nose with alternating index fingers
  * Rapidly alternate fingers to thumb
  * Rapidly move index finger between his or her own nose and the examiner's finger
* Test fine motor function and coordination. Ask the patient to do the following:
  * Run heel down tibia of opposite leg
  * Alternately and rapidly cross leg over opposite knee
* Test position sense of upper and lower extremities.
* Test deep tendon reflexes and compare bilaterally: biceps, triceps, brachioradial, patellar, Achilles.
* Test plantar reflex bilaterally.

PATIENT STANDING

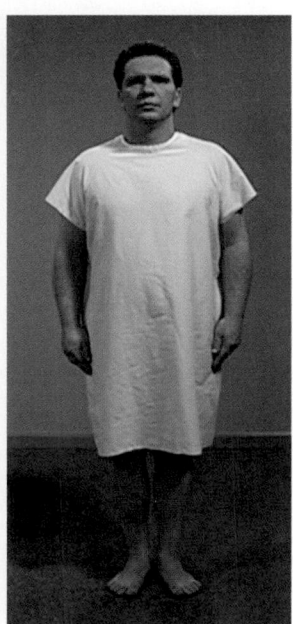

Assist patient to a standing position (Fig. 24-9). Examiner stands next to patient.

Spine
* Inspect and palpate spine as patient bends over at waist.
* Test range of motion: hyperextension, lateral bending, rotation of upper trunk.

Neurologic
* Observe gait.
* Test proprioception and cerebellar function.
  * Assess Romberg test.
  * Ask the patient to walk heel to toe.
  * Ask the patient to stand on one foot, then the other, with eyes closed.
  * Ask the patient to hop in place on one foot, then the other.
  * Ask the patient to do deep knee bends.

Abdominal/Genital
* Test for inguinal and femoral hernias.

FEMALE PATIENT, LITHOTOMY POSITION

Assist female patients into lithotomy position and drape appropriately (Fig. 24-10). Examiner is seated.

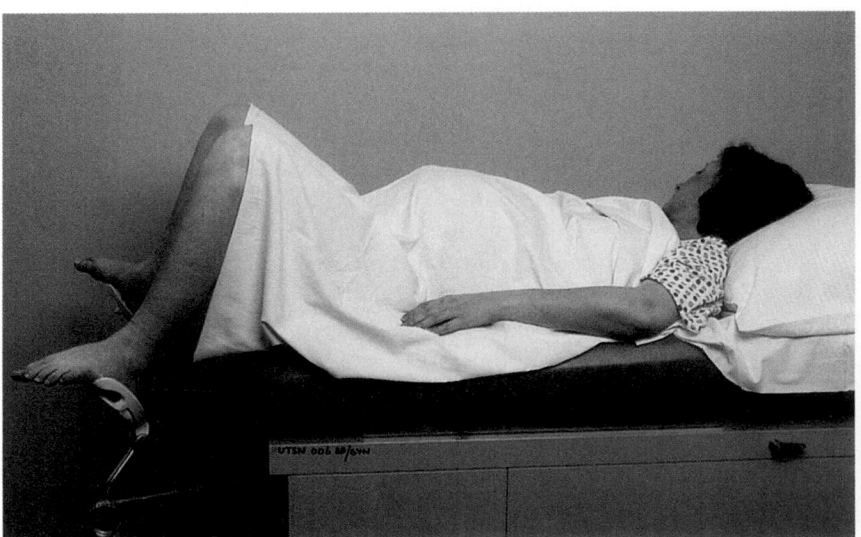

External Genitalia
* Inspect pubic hair, labia, clitoris, urethral opening, vaginal opening, perineal and perianal areas, anus.
* Palpate labia and Bartholin glands; milk Skene glands.

Internal Genitalia
* Perform speculum examination.
    * Inspect vagina and cervix.
    * Collect Pap smear and other necessary specimens.
* Perform bimanual palpation to assess for characteristics of vagina, cervix, uterus, adnexa.
* Perform rectovaginal examination to assess rectovaginal septum, broad ligaments.
* Perform rectal examination.
    * Assess anal sphincter tone and surface characteristics; palpate circumferentially for rectal mass.
    * Obtain rectal culture if needed.
    * Note characteristics of stool when gloved finger is removed.

MALE PATIENT, BENDING FORWARD

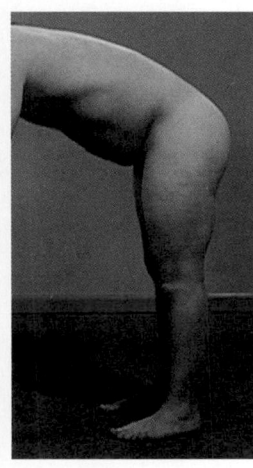

Assist male patients in leaning over examining table or into knee-chest position (Fig. 24-11). Examiner is behind patient. It is at times more relaxing for the buttocks, thus making for an easier examination, to ask the patient, unlike the illustration, to point his toes inward and to put his chest on the table.

- Inspect sacrococcygeal and perianal areas.
- Perform rectal examination.
  - Palpate sphincter tone and surface characteristics; palpate circumferentially for rectal mass.
  - Obtain rectal culture if needed.
  - Palpate prostate gland and seminal vesicles.
  - Note characteristics of stool when gloved finger is removed.

The conclusion of the examination is another time for review and reflection. It gives the patient an opportunity to hear your findings and your interpretations to the extent that you can give them, as well as to ask questions. You must be sure that the patient has a clear understanding of all aspects of the situation and, as indicated in Box 24-8, allow for possible stress.

If the patient is examined in a hospital bed, remember to put everything back in order when you are finished. Make sure the patient is comfortably settled in an appropriate manner, with side rails up if the clinical condition warrants, and buttons and buzzers within easy reach.

BOX 24-8

THE STRESSFUL MOMENT

There are times when what you have learned during the process of taking the history and performing the physical examination leads to a conclusion that will be unpleasant or even disastrous for the patient. Certain principles should guide you when something "bad" must be communicated. These principles apply to patients of all ages, and to the participation of a variety of family members and other persons.

- Arrange a setting that is quiet, as much as possible apart from a noisy ambiance.
- If you do not know the patient well, try to involve in a direct manner someone who does—and who has the patient's trust—if at all possible.
- Involve family members and others essential to the emotional and practical support of the patient. Consider their base of knowledge, experience, and understanding of the situation.
- Be specific in all details.
- Provide information in a deliberate flow that is adjusted to the needs of the patient, allowing time for questions and for frequent repetition whenever necessary.
- Use jargon-free language adapted to the patient's understanding.
- Inform the patient immediately unless, for example, the sensorium is clouded. A prolonged delay in communicating needed information to which the patient is, after all, entitled does not often help and is most often inappropriate.

INFANTS

NEWBORNS

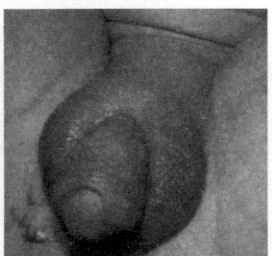

Photo from Biomedical Photography, Johns Hopkins University School of Medicine.

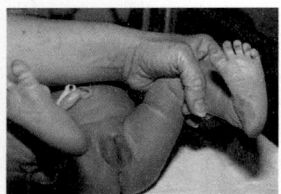

Normal infant female external genitalia.
Lowdermilk, Perry, 2004

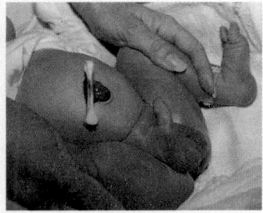

Normal infant male external genitalia.
Lowdermilk, Perry, 2004

The newborn is at greater risk but also has a better potential for health than patients of other ages. The Apgar score, taken at 1 and 5 minutes of age, provides insight to the baby's in utero, intrapartum, and immediate postnatal experience. A low score is evidence of difficulty. A depressed heart rate, respiratory difficulty, loss of muscle tone, and decreased reflex irritability all indicate trouble. Of all these observations, color is the least reliable because most new babies have blue fingers and toes. The Apgar score does not address problems that are suggested by increased irritability, tachypnea, or tachycardia. Nor should it be interpreted as an actual quantitative measure. It is liable to variations in observers' judgments. Still, it is a readily available assessment of combined objective and subjective observations and allows communication from one observer to the next over time.

Because menstrual histories are often inaccurate, more objective means of estimating gestational age are required. The following observations are helpful in determining gestational age. Before 36 weeks, only one or two transverse creases are present on the sole of the foot; the breast nodule is less than 3 mm in diameter; no cartilage is present in the helix of the ear; and the testes are seldom in the scrotum, which has few or no rugae. By 40 weeks, many creases are present on the sole; the breast nodule exceeds 4 mm; cartilage is present in the helix of the ear; and the testes have descended into the scrotum, which is covered with rugae. Increasing muscle tone with a posture of predominantly flexed extremities is another sign of increased maturity.

The premature infant often has brief periods of apnea lasting up to 20 seconds. Respiratory distress is indicated by a sustained increased rate, grunting, retraction of intercostal and subcostal spaces and suprasternal notch, seesaw sinking of the chest with rising abdomen in contrast to the normal synchronous motions, and flaring of the nostrils.

Major congenital anomalies are usually obvious, but there are exceptions. Some life-threatening problems such as diaphragmatic hernia may not be readily apparent. When examining a new baby, your index of suspicion must be high and your search for clues must extend into intrauterine life, the mother's immediate perinatal and postnatal experience, and the family history. The difficulty and mode of labor and delivery will have meaning and need exploration. If the mother has fever during or after delivery, or if she has herpetic lesions about the mouth or genitalia, the infant may be at risk. Her use of drugs—prescribed, nonprescribed, or illicit—will often have an impact on the baby. Most medications are safe, but some have teratogenic effects. Sedatives and anticonvulsants can have a worrisome impact on the baby's state of consciousness; frequent use of narcotics will cause the baby to go through withdrawal. Problems with earlier pregnancies may be relevant to the newborn's intrauterine life. The fate of siblings may suggest the fate of your present patient.

With a baby, as with patients at any age, it is important to look first. You can learn a lot before touching, without abruptly handling or invading with an instrument. Note the baby's degree of awareness or apathy; the posture, and whether unusual flaccidity, tension, or spasticity is present; skin color; and unexpected gross deformities or distortions of facies. The responsive, eager infant with a strong suck is reassuring. Note the presence or absence of spontaneity in the baby's behavior, and always keep track of the interaction between parents and between parent and child. Observing a feeding is most informative, as is simply allowing the baby to demonstrate interest in life by latching onto your gloved finger eagerly and with strength.

When you begin the physical examination, palpate the head and fontanels, then the extremities and abdomen, and finally the rest of the baby. Use a gentle touch that will not obscure unusual findings. Chest percussion is generally of little value because of the relatively small chest, especially in the premature infant, and because of the examiner's relatively large hands and fingers; however, an abdomen distended from intestinal obstruction may resonate on percussion.

OLDER INFANTS

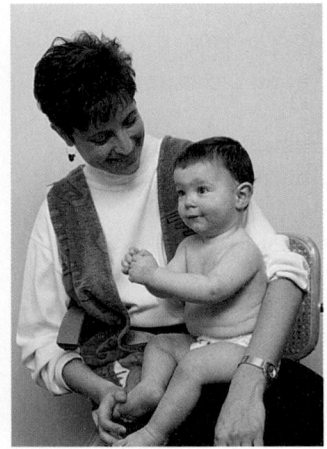

As with adults, there is no right sequence to the examination. From time to time, you will vary what you do depending on the baby's age and whether the baby is awake or asleep at the start. You want to have cooperation for as long as possible. Again, this may be achieved by observing as much as you can before touching (e.g., observe the quality and rate of respiration, flaring of the alae nasi, skin color, even the pulse [visible apical thrust]) and defer to the end anything invasive (e.g., examination of the ears, throat, and eyes) (Fig. 24-12).

Take advantage of opportunities presented throughout the examination. The sleeping infant presents a wonderful chance to auscultate the heart, lungs, and abdomen and to observe the infant's position at rest. The crying infant can be evaluated for lustiness of cry, tactile fremitus, lung excursion, and facial symmetry; the mouth and pharynx can be assessed for integrity of the soft palate and cranial nerves IX, X, and XII. Observe the infant during feeding to evaluate sucking and swallowing coordination, cranial nerve XII, and alertness and responsiveness. A crying infant may keep the eyes tightly shut, but the parent can stand and hold the infant over the shoulder while you stand behind the parent. At this point, the child will often stop crying for a moment and open the eyes. If you are poised with flashlight, you can quickly make some assessment. Similarly, the crying infant—and older children, too—will still need to take a breath, and you can be ready to listen to the heart each time a breath is taken. Over several intervals of breathing, you can hear enough of the heart and lung sounds. Seizing these advantages may mean a change in the sequence of the examination to suit the moment. Similarly, an older infant less than a year of age, given something to hold in each hand, will not always let go quickly. You may have some freedom to examine without tugs at your stethoscope.

EXAMINATION SEQUENCE

CLINICAL PEARL

Positioning the Infant
When you have finished examining, it is best to place a young infant in a supine position and to repeat instructions to the parents to always do the same. There is, contrary to long-established custom, a valid realization that the prone position is not as safe as was once thought. It is a contributor to sudden infant death syndrome (SIDS).

The following is a guideline for the examination sequence of the newborn or young infant. The infant's temperature, weight, length, and head circumference are usually measured first. Weight, length, and head circumference are plotted on a growth curve for the infant's age. Newborns may have the Dubowitz Assessment of Gestational Age done before the examination is ordered (see Chapter 5).

General Inspection

Inspect the undressed, supine newborn on a warming table; inspect the older infant preferably on a parent's lap.

- Assess positioning or posture at rest: symmetry and size of extremities, the newborn's assumption of in utero position, flexion of extremities, unusual flaccidity or spasticity, any difference in positioning between upper and lower extremities.
- Note voluntary movement of extremities.
- Inspect skin: color, meconium staining, and vernix in newborn; a cover glass pressed over a suspected telangiectasia will reveal pulsation.
- Note presence of tremors.
- Assess for any apparent anomalies.
- Inspect face: symmetry of features, spacing and position of features (e.g., intracanthal distance, presence of a philtrum).
- Inspect configuration and movement of the chest.
- Inspect shape of the abdomen, movement with respiration.

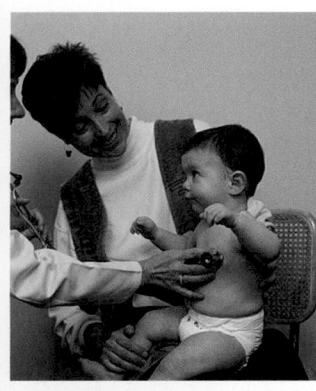

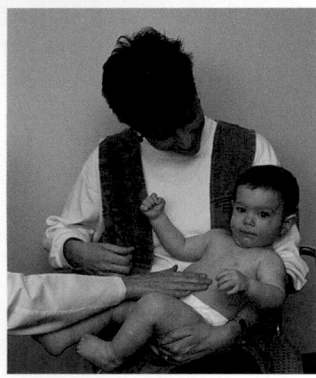

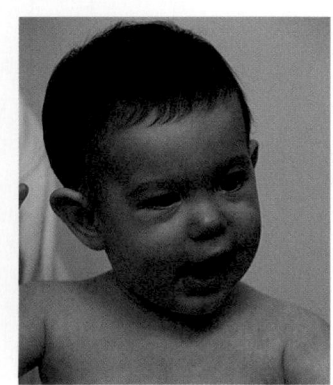

Chest, Lungs, and Heart

* Inspect the following: chest structure, symmetry of expansion with respiration; presence of retractions, heaves, or lifts (Fig. 24-13).
* Note quality of respirations, count the rate.
* Inspect the breasts for nipple and tissue development.
* Palpate the chest and precordium. Locate the apical impulse (point of maximal impulse); note any thrills; note tactile fremitus in crying infant.
* Auscultate entire anterior and lateral chest for breath sounds; note any bowel sounds.
* Auscultate each cardiac listening area for S1 and S2, splitting, murmurs.
* Count the apical pulse rate.
* Percussion may be necessary at times; it is not always performed.

Abdomen

* Inspect shape and configuration. Note scaphoid or distended appearance (Fig. 24-14).
* Inspect the umbilicus, count the vessels, note oozing of blood; if the stump has fallen off, inspect the area for lesions, erythema, drainage, foul odor.
* Auscultate each quadrant for bowel sounds.
* Lightly palpate all areas. Note size of liver, muscle tone, bladder, spleen tip.
* Palpate more deeply for kidneys, any masses, note any muscle rigidity or tenseness.
* Percuss each quadrant.
* Check skin turgor.
* Palpate the inguinal area for femoral pulses and lymph nodes.

Head and Neck

Inspection and palpation can be done preceding or simultaneously with use of invasive instruments (Fig. 24-15).

* Inspect shape of the head. Note molding, swelling, scalp electrode site, hairline.
    * Palpate the head: fontanels, sutures, areas of swelling or asymmetry. Measure fontanels in two dimensions.
    * Measure head circumference.
    * Transilluminate newborn's skull.
* Inspect ears.
    * Shape, position, and alignment of auricles; patency of auditory canals; pits, sinuses
    * Otoscopic examination
* Inspect eyes: swelling of eyelids and discharge, size, shape, position, epicanthal folds, conjunctivae, pupils.
    * Pupillary response to light
    * Corneal light reflex
    * Red reflex, ophthalmoscopic examination
    * Inspection of eye movement: nystagmus, tracking a light or following a moving picture or face
* Inspect nose: flaring, discharge, size, shape.
    * Inspect nasal mucosa, alignment of septum.
    * Check patency of choanae; observe respiratory effort while alternately occluding each naris. If any doubt about patency, pass a small feeding tube through each naris to the stomach.
* Inspect mouth: lips, gums, hard and soft palates (a very high arched palate may suggest cerebral dysfunction); size of tongue; excessive secretions in the newborn, drooling in the infant; presence of teeth, lesions.
    * Palpate mouth. Insert gloved small finger into mouth, palpate hard and soft palates with fingerpad, evaluate suck.
    * Stimulate gag reflex.
    * Stroke each side of mouth to evaluate rooting reflex.

- Lift infant's trunk, allowing head to fall back and rest against the table, slightly hyperextended.
    - Inspect and palpate the position of the trachea.
    - Inspect for alignment of head with neck.
    - Inspect for webbing, excess skinfolds.
    - Palpate for masses, thyroid, muscle tone.
    - Palpate lymph nodes: anterior and posterior cervical, preauricular, postauricular, submental, sublingual, tonsillar, supraclavicular.
    - Palpate the clavicles for integrity, crepitus.
    - Lift infant and test Moro reflex with a sudden dropping motion.
- Inspect neck with infant again supine.
    - Rotate head to each side for passive range of motion.
    - Observe tonic neck reflex for asymmetry.
    - Observe neck righting reflex in older infants.

Upper Extremities
- Inspect and palpate arms.
- Move arms through range of motion.
- Palpate brachial or radial pulses; compare quality and timing with femoral pulses.
- Open the hands: Inspect nails and palmar and phalangeal creases; count fingers.
- Place a finger in infant's palms to evaluate palmar grasp reflex.
- Keeping fingers in infant's hands, pull the infant slowly to sitting position, evaluate grasp and arm strength; evaluate head control.
- Measure blood pressure.

Lower Extremities

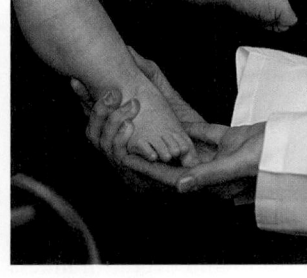

- Inspect the legs and feet for alignment and skinfolds (Fig. 24-16).
- Palpate the bones and muscles of each leg.
- Move legs through range of motion; adduct and abduct the hips.
- Palpate the dorsalis pedis pulses.
- Count the toes.
- Elicit the plantar, patellar, and Achilles reflexes.
- Measure blood pressure.

Genitals and Rectum
- Females: Inspect external genitalia, noting size of clitoris, any discharge, hymenal opening, any ambiguity of structures.
- Males
    - Inspect placement of urethral opening without fully retracting the foreskin.
    - Inspect scrotum for rugae and presence of contents; note any ambiguity of structures.
    - Palpate scrotum for the testes, presence of hernia or hydrocele.
    - Transilluminate the scrotum when a mass other than testes is noted.
    - Observe voiding for strength of stream.
- Inspect rectum; assess sphincter tone; if newborn has not passed meconium within 24 hours of birth, evaluate rectal patency with a soft catheter.

Neurologic
Hold the infant upright facing you with your hands under the axillae.
- Observe for the sunsetting sign as the baby's eyes open.
- Perform the doll's eyes maneuver.
- Evaluate general body strength. Without gripping the infant's chest, keep your hands under the infant's axillae, and note whether the baby begins to slip through your hands or maintains its position.
- Elicit the stepping reflex.
- Elicit the placing reflex.

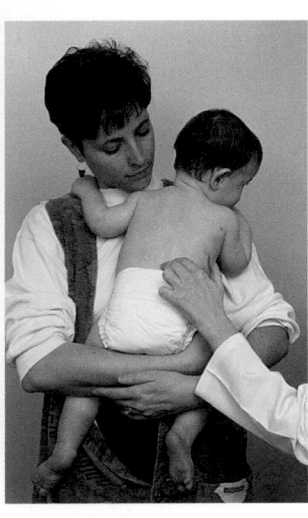

Back

Position the newborn prone on the warming table or have the parent hold the infant upright over the shoulder (Fig. 24-17).

- ◆ Inspect spine: observe for alignment, symmetry of muscle development, any masses, tufts of hair, dimples, lesions, defects over lower spine.
- ◆ Palpate each spinal process for defect.
- ◆ Auscultate posterior chest for breath sounds, any heart sounds.
- ◆ Inspect symmetry of gluteal folds.

Behavior

Throughout examination of the newborn, note the alertness, ability to be quieted or consoled, and the response to handling. With the somewhat older infant, too, note the alertness, the responsiveness to the parent, and the ability of the parent to sense the infant's need for consoling and to respond.

- ◆ Note the quality of crying, presence of stridor or hoarseness.
- ◆ Note the responses to voices or noise: quieting, stopping movement, turning toward sounds.

CHILDREN

Most infants and children will be accompanied by one or more parents or parent surrogates. For children who are small enough, the parent's lap is a splendid examining table. It is helpful when taking the history to keep the child and parent together and to observe the nature of their interaction (Box 24-9). How they feel about each other is conveyed through the parent's touching, soothing, and reassuring gestures and the child's response. Excessive parental indulgence may indicate a smothering relationship; on the other hand, if interaction is minimal and the child does not look to the parent for help, the family dynamics may be devoid of warmth and affection. Take note of the obvious and subtle ways in which children and parents communicate with each other, and record what you learn. Ask the parent to be present when you are performing procedures (e.g., venipuncture); generally it is reassuring to the child. Most parents will accept, and the reaction to your request gives you more information about the family's dynamics and emotional resources.

With the young of any age, you will often take a history and do a physical examination at the same time. These need not be in a rigid sequence, and the complaint and degree of illness can govern your approach to integration. In general, however, you may prefer to start with the history while making overtures to the child to establish some reassuring contact before you actually begin examination. A gentle pat (always with warm hands), a few pleasant words, or

---

BOX 24-9

OBSERVING YOUNG CHILDREN

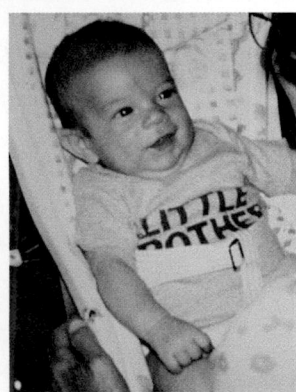

The child's ability at any age to react socially offers clues to physical and emotional well-being. It is possible to elicit responses by exploring with questions; you may also make direct observations. The classic example of a response is the "social smile"—the smile that you know is meant for you—that we learn to expect from infants by the time they are 2 to 3 months old. With the understanding that it is very hard to smile if you have meningitis, we can ask parents and, as we work with the child, we can ask ourselves the following:

- Is that smile there?
- Is the child playful, alert, and responsive?
- Or is there dullness and apparent apathy?
- If the child is fearful, does he or she respond to soothing behavior?
- Does the child move around, show interest in the immediate environment, reach for toys, and ask questions?
- These things matter fully as much as temperature, pulse, and respirations. A similar assessment of emotional well-being—with some adaptation to age—is obviously appropriate in the examination of adults.

> **BOX 24-10**
>
> **WHY ARE CHILDREN FEARFUL?**
>
> Reasons that children may be fearful include the following:
> - They have experienced medical procedures that hurt.
> - They do not want to be separated from parents or another familiar figure.
> - They have learned that perverse behavior can get a "rise" out of adults.
> - They are abused and have great inner pain and few socially acceptable means of expression.
>
> When a child is fearful, it is important, as always, to respect the child and parent; to explain what is going to happen; and to be honest, firm, unapologetic, and gently expeditious. This requires that you achieve a degree of comfort working in the presence of a sharply observant, sometimes tentative, sometimes hostile parent. Do not separate the child from the parent for the sole purpose of improving your personal comfort.

playing with the child can often win cooperation. A few relaxed moments—and patience—can break the ice. Children do not necessarily know your routine. You are often a stranger, and the environment may be frightening. Not every child will be smiling and happy about an examination (Box 24-10).

It does not often pay to rush, and sometimes it pays not to be too persistent. It is always important to be thorough, but unless the matter is urgent, you may defer some of your inquiries and observations to a time when the child is more relaxed and less afraid of you. It takes time, after all, to develop friendship and to establish trust with the young and, of course, adults as well.

General inspection of the toddler and preschooler may begin in the waiting room or as the child enters the examining room. The temperature, weight, and length are usually taken earlier. Offer toys or paper and pencil to entertain the child; to develop rapport; and to evaluate development, motor, and neurologic status. Use a developmental screening test such as the Denver II (see Chapter 5) to evaluate language, motor coordination, and social skills. Evaluate mental status as the child interacts with you and with the parent.

The following sequence is intended only as a guideline to get you started. Take advantage of opportunities the child presents during the examination to make your observations. You will find that the sequence of examination may vary with each child (Box 24-11).

CHILD PLAYING

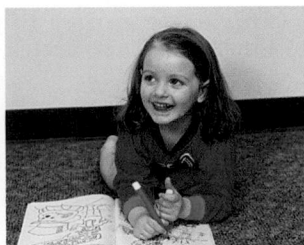

The child playing on the floor offers an opportunity to evaluate both the musculoskeletal and neurologic systems while developing a rapport with the child (Fig. 24-18).
- Observe the child's spontaneous activities.
- Ask the child to demonstrate some skills: throwing a ball, building block towers, drawing geometric figures, coloring.
- Evaluate gait, jumping, hopping, range of motion.
- Muscle strength: Observe the child climbing on the parent's lap, stooping, and recovering.

BOX 24-11

SOME TIPS FOR EXAMINING A YOUNG CHILD

- Telling the child a story or asking about the child's experience, (e.g., about school, games, or television) can help to attract attention or, at times, to distract.
- Restraining a child with wrappings and adults looming over the examining table increases the child's apprehension and decreases cooperation. If the child's arms must be restrained and the head kept still (e.g., to look at the ears) it is usually better to do this on the parent's lap, using the parents' arms for restraint.
- Postpone using the tongue blade until the end of the examination. If the tongue blade must be used, ease the tendency to gag by moistening it first with warm water.
- Allow a young child to "blow out" your flashlight as one way of gaining familiarity with your instruments. Offer your flashlight, otoscope, or stethoscope as a toy (they will not break), or draw a doll's face on a tongue blade. There are times when you might get down on the floor with the child, or use your own lap as an examining table. You will not sacrifice your dignity; anything goes (within bounds of propriety) to get the information you need.
- Enlist the help of the child if he or she is ticklish. Place your hand on top of the child's hand to gently probe the abdomen or the axilla. The diaphragm of your stethoscope can also serve as a probe.
- Take the opportunity to hold and feed a young baby. This increases your understanding and helps establish rapport.
- If the child is uncomfortable or uncooperative, be patient. You can sometimes stop and come back at a later time when calm is restored to complete the examination.
- Use specific, polite directions rather than asking the child's permission at each step in the examination. It is better to say, "Please open your mouth" rather than "Do you want to open your mouth?" After all, what will you do next if the answer is "no?"

CHILD ON PARENT'S LAP

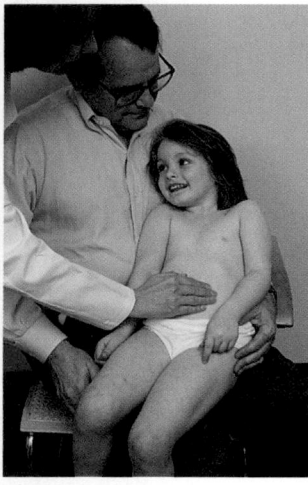

Performing the examination on the parent's lap usually enhances the child's participation. Begin with the child sitting and undressed except for the diaper or underpants (Fig. 24-19).

Upper Extremities

- Inspect arms for movement, size, shape; observe use of the hands; inspect hands for number and configuration of fingers, palmar creases.
- Palpate radial pulses.
- Elicit biceps and triceps reflexes when child cooperates.
- Take blood pressure at this point or later, depending on child's attitude.

Lower Extremities

Child may stand for much or part of the examination.

- Inspect legs for movement, size, shape, alignment, lesions.
- Inspect feet for alignment, longitudinal arch, number of toes.
- Palpate dorsalis pedis pulse.
- Elicit plantar reflex and, if cooperative, the Achilles and patellar reflexes.

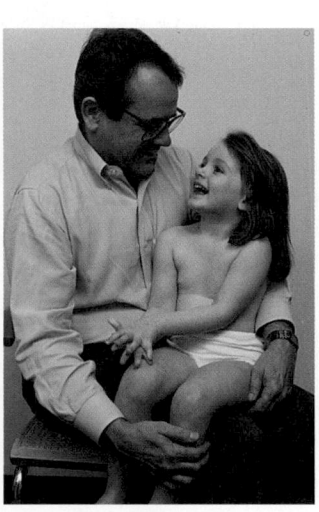

Head and Neck
- Inspect head (Fig. 24-20).
  - Inspect shape, alignment with neck, hairline, position of auricles.
  - Palpate anterior fontanel for size; head for sutures, depressions; hair for texture.
- Measure head circumference.
- Inspect neck for webbing, voluntary movement.
- Palpate neck. Position of trachea, thyroid, muscle tone, lymph nodes.

Chest, Heart, and Lungs
- Inspect the chest for respiratory movement, size, shape, precordial movement, deformity, nipple and breast development.
- Palpate the anterior chest, locate the point of maximal impulse, note tactile fremitus in the talking or crying child.
- Auscultate the anterior, lateral, and posterior chest for breath sounds; count respirations.
- Auscultate all cardiac listening areas for S1 and S2, splitting, and murmurs; count apical pulse.

CHILD RELATIVELY SUPINE, STILL ON LAP, DIAPER LOOSENED

- Inspect abdomen.
  - Auscultate for bowel sounds.
  - Palpate. Identify size of the liver and any other palpable organs or masses.
  - Percuss.
- Palpate the femoral pulses, compare to radial pulses.
- Palpate for lymph nodes.
- Inspect the external genitalia.
- Males: Palpate scrotum for descent of testes and other masses.

CHILD STANDING

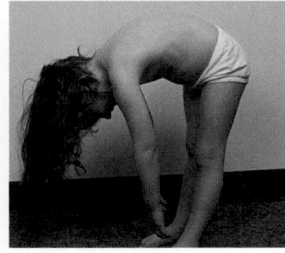

- Inspect spinal alignment as the child bends slowly forward to touch toes (Fig. 24-21).
- Observe posture from anterior, posterior, and lateral views.
- Observe gait.

CHILD RETURNS TO PARENT'S LAP

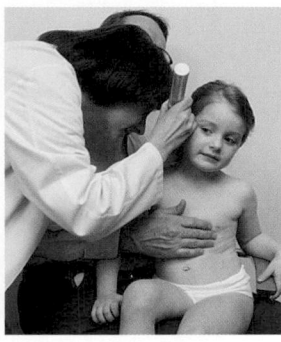

Only as a last resort should you restrain the child for the funduscopic, otoscopic, and examinations (Fig. 24-22). Lessen the fear of this aspect of the examination by permitting the child to handle the instruments, "blow out" the light, or use them on a doll or the parent. Attempt to gain the child's cooperation, even if it takes more time. It will be worth the effort because future visits will be more pleasant for the child and for you. After finishing these preliminary maneuvers, perform the following:
- Inspect eyes: pupillary light reflex, red reflex, extraocular movements, funduscopic examination.
- Perform otoscopic examination.
- Inspect nasal mucosa.
- Inspect mouth and pharynx.

By the time the child is school age, it is usually possible to use an examination sequence very similar to that for adults.

PREGNANT WOMEN

The process of physical examination is the same for the pregnant woman as for the adult, with the addition of more extensive abdominal and pelvic evaluation for pregnancy status and fetal well-being. Late in pregnancy the woman may find it difficult to assume the supine position without experiencing hypotension. Therefore have her assume this position only when necessary, and provide alternative positioning by elevating the backrest or by supplying pillows for the woman to assume the side-lying position. The abdominal assessment is both more comfortable for the woman and more accurate if the bladder is empty. Remember that during pregnancy, urinary urgency and frequency are common.

The baseline physical examination is important. A healthy woman may not have had a recent examination before becoming pregnant and non-obstetric examinations are not usually performed during pregnancy. Baseline vital signs, height, weight, and prepregnancy weight should be recorded. All physical findings that may be significant later in pregnancy should be dealt with and documented (e.g., cervical or gynecologic abnormalities, mitral valve prolapse, other heart findings, neurologic, and visual problems) (Johnson, 2002).

OLDER ADULTS

The process of physical examination is the same for older adults as it is for younger adults; however, special considerations may be necessary. Many older patients have difficulty assuming some of the positions, particularly the lithotomy and knee-chest positions. Sometimes all that is needed is a little extra assistance and patience on your part, but otherwise you may need to use alternate positioning (see Chapter 18). The quality of clinical data is not necessarily compromised by having the patient lie on the side rather than assume a knee-chest position, for example. Your skill, thoroughness, and willingness to take whatever time is necessary are far more important in yielding accurate clinical data.

Time is a central issue in examining older patients. Time may be needed to develop the patient's trust and subsequent cooperation and to allow for any apparent degree of frailty. A hurried pace or an impatient manner can create tension that may fluster or confuse an older patient. In neurologic testing, reaction time may be longer or may require more intense stimuli.

FUNCTIONAL ASSESSMENT

Functional assessment (see Chapter 1) is an important part of examining the older adult (Box 24-12). Initial observation and interaction can provide a wealth of information about the individual's independent functional capacity. Watch how the patient walks, and observe the ability to follow instructions, remove clothes, and maneuver to the examining table. In doing this, you will obtain information related to mobility, balance, fine motor skills (e.g., unbuttoning clothes), and range of motion (Box 24-13). In addition, you may gather some clues about perceptual abilities and mental status. Many older adults (and, a reminder, patients of all ages) seem to have a variety of diseases, conditions, or disorders that indicate apparent poor health (Box 24-14). Yet physical health is only one dimension of the picture and, for many, the bottom line is not what might be wrong with their bodies but what else gets in the way of successful daily living and what they are able to do and how well they are able to function.

In reality, functional assessment is simply an attempt to determine the extent to which patients can deal with the daily demands of life (i.e., how well they function). This idea is stressed earlier (see Chapter 1) where we advise that such an assessment should be a part of every older

---

BOX 24-12

ASSESSMENT OF THE OLDER ADULT

Assessment of the older adult is a comprehensive evaluation of a person who is doing well and who has the goal of maintaining that status, or of one who is not succeeding in the community environment. It includes the following:
- Comprehensive history and physical examination
- Assessment of social situation

The history should include the following:
- Detailed listing of medications, (e.g., nonprescription drugs, especially hypnotics, sedatives, and laxatives). Try the "brown bag approach," asking the patient to bring all medications, prescribed and nonprescribed, including those derived from complementary or alternative approaches.
- Extensive review of function, including gait and activities of daily living (ADLs) and evaluation of degree of independence versus need for caretaker assistance.
  - Basic ADLs: bathing, dressing, toileting, ambulation, feeding
  - Instrumental ADLs: housekeeping, grocery shopping, meal preparation, medication compliance, communication skills, money management
  - Use of assistive devices for ambulation and function: cane, walker, commode chair, hospital bed
- Systems review, particularly common geriatric problems
  - Nutritional status, evidence of malnutrition
  - Urinary incontinence
  - Early dementia
  - Depression
  - Medication-induced delirium
  - Falls, gait and balance disorders that result in fear of falling
  - Skin breakdown: decubitus ulcers

- Social situation
  - Identification of caretakers and probable caretakers, including those who maintain the home environment
  - Assessment of caretaker abilities
  - Assessment of financial resources and health insurance, with particular reference to long-term services not ordinarily covered: personal grooming, home care, medication supervision
  - Frank and open discussion of patient's wishes regarding advanced life support in the event of an irreversible condition and/or cognitive impairment, the "advance directives" in this regard (necessarily written), and the need for a Durable Power of Attorney for Health Care (the formal investment of decision-making authority for health care in a family member or other trusted person)

The physical examination should include an assessment of gait and coordination and a mental status evaluation with particular attention to the following:
- Cognition
- Memory
- Mood

All of this takes time and sensitive conversation. It cannot usually be accomplished in one visit or by one person. Multiple approaches include traditional nursing and medical processes, social and dietary interventions, and rehabilitation. Everybody who participates in care may contribute. The evaluation is complex, but it is possible to achieve it in several brief visits.

Dr. Michele F. Bellantoni of the Gerontology Research Center, Baltimore, MD, gave considerable advice regarding geriatric assessment.

BOX 24-13

EXAMINING PEOPLE WITH DISABILITIES

You may need to vary some aspects of the physical examination for persons with disabilities. Each disability affects each person differently; therefore it is important to educate yourself about relevant facets of your patient's disability. What body systems are affected? What is the degree of impairment? What assistance does the patient require? What is the patient able to do without assistance? What is the communication system used by a hearing- or speech-impaired patient (e.g., sign language interpreter, word board, or talk box)? When speaking with a disabled patient, speak directly to the patient. Often clinicians will inappropriately address a disabled person's friend, an attendant, or an interpreter instead of speaking directly to the patient.

Consider some variations that may facilitate the physical examination. It may not be necessary for the patient to undress fully, thereby conserving time and energy. Removing or rearranging the furnishings in an examination room will provide the space needed to maneuver a wheelchair. Some patient positions can be varied without compromising the quality of the examination (see, e.g., Alternative Positions for the Pelvic Examination, pp. 620-622). Some patients may require only additional time and assistance in getting positioned or performing maneuvers. Some older patients may experience limitation in joint range of motion (see, e.g., pp. 743-744). Gentleness and patience are the hallmarks of a caring and sensitive examiner.

BOX 24-14

FACTORS THAT INFLUENCE THE PERCEPTION AND INTERPRETATION OF SYMPTOMS

Innumerable subjective modifications may convert disease into illness or cause illness without disease, including the following:
- Recent termination of a significant relationship because of death, divorce, or other less obvious intrusions (e.g., moving to a new city)
- Physical or emotional illness or disability in family members or other significant individuals
- Unharmonious spousal or family relationships
- School problems and stresses
- Poor self-image
- Drug and alcohol misuse
- Poor understanding of the facts of a physical problem
- Peer pressures (e.g., trying to keep up with the Joneses or with schoolmates)
- Secondary gains from the complaints of symptoms (e.g., indulgent family response to complaints, providing extra comforts, gifts; solicitous attention from others; distraction from other intimidating problems)

At any age, circumstances such as these can modify perception and contribute to the intensity and persistence of symptoms or, quite the opposite, the denial of an insistent, objective complaint. Sometimes, as a result, the patient will be led to seek help and, at other times, to avoid it.

Modified from Green, Stuy, 1992.

---

adult's history, with attention given to self-care activities and instrumental activities such as ability to drive a car, use public transportation, and even dial a telephone.

Indeed, you will always be making this type of assessment on each patient, regardless of age. After all, an infant must be able to suck, a 6-year-old child must be able to adapt to a classroom and find the way home from school, and an adolescent must be able to come to grips with the essentials of life in determining a sense of self and of his or her future. Thus a functional assessment underlies every history, and the judgment about each individual's ability to cope with the demands and stresses of life is an essential part of your conclusions. A functional understanding will ultimately help shape your management plans, guide the level of instruc-

---

BOX 24-15

THE PATIENT WHO IS DYING

As with all patients, those who are dying need your commitment. When we are face to face with death, we often cope by attempting to avoid it. We tend not to visit with the patient who is dying as often as with the patient we know will live. We are too often reluctant to confront the fact of dying, perhaps because of our personal fears or because we subconsciously feel we have failed in our healing role. If you learn to understand your own feelings about death, you will be better equipped to care for the dying.

Learn to accept that dying patients need you as much as other patients. Talk with them, share with them. Never hesitate to participate in chit-chat, but also become comfortable with being quiet and filling the silent spaces with the touch of a hand.

Above all, do not back away from dying patients. This avoidance behavior denies them an assumptive world, the world for which they had hoped and may not have. Your attention and honest discussion offer hope without denial. This is a key to palliative care, as necessary in its time as the effort to cure.

---

tion you can provide the patient, and determine the expectation you might have about the potential fulfillment of patient needs.

ALLIANCE AND COMPLIANCE

You cannot assume that patients will behave predictably or that they will invariably respond to your suggestions and instructions. We define adherence to our instructions as compliance. There is perhaps some arrogance in the inference that when we order, the patient must respond. Still, compliance is one measure of your alliance with patients. The controlling factors include the nature of the relationship you have developed, your recognition of the patient's autonomy, your success in communicating the basics of the patient's condition, and the clarity of your instructions. Equally important factors are the patient's ability to understand the problem and the value the patient places on resolving the problem. For example, your primary concern may be a patient's hypertension, whereas the patient's main worry may be an alcoholic spouse. There are also times when a patient's refusal to comply may be appropriate. Always ask that the patient repeat the instructions to you so you can be sure he or she understands. This can also help you discover whether there may be a problem with compliance.

Most interactions with patients are unique, and you must be adaptable and flexible—particularly when your first efforts may be halting. It is not always easy! You will at times be sorely tried, particularly when you are worried, rushed, and tired. If you are to be successful, you must also understand the biases you might bring to each interaction with the patient and learn how to constrain them. Because you are human, you may respond differently to people who will live and to those who are dying (Box 24-15), to children and the aged, to men and women, to blacks and whites, to rich and poor. Important also are your interactions with family members who may be suffering emotionally (Box 24-16). You must know why and how (see Chapter 2).

Finally, you must be disciplined enough to pursue complete information, even when the solution seems obvious (because sometimes the obvious is wrong); and courageous enough to make the decision for urgency when the data are incomplete (Box 24-17).

Serving the whole patient—the physical, emotional, and social needs—is not an easy task, but you can succeed if you follow a disciplined course and learn how to be flexible within that course, guided by it, but not imprisoned by it. You are at the point of organizing the information you have assembled into a usable whole, ready for providing care, caring, and problem solving. That information must be well-documented if the ongoing service to the patient is to be competent and, a secondary but important consideration, if there should ever be a legal challenge to your effort. Contrary to the view of some, the taking of a history and the performance of a physical examination are still and will remain the heart, soul, and mind of the alliance with the patient. Technology will not overwhelm the "laying on of hands."

BOX 24-16

COMPASSION FOR THOSE WHO ARE GRIEVING

When one of our patients dies, those who were close family, friends, or significant others need our attention during the time they are grieving, not only in the immediate aftermath of death but also later on. Obviously, it is difficult to find words, and often the words we find may be clichés that do not seem quite appropriate for the moment. It is not a good idea to tell people to be strong when they are really feeling utterly empty. It is all right to tell them that it is good to cry and to share feelings, and that it is permissible to talk about what has been lost and what will not be realized for the future. It is not a good idea to assure someone that time will take care of things. Your appreciation that the present moments are long and sometimes unendurable is needed. If time does heal, that may ultimately be found out. In the settings in which so many of us work, we may find ourselves minimizing a misfortune by comparing it with the apparent or obvious misfortune of others. We should not allow ourselves to make such a judgment about another person's pain and loss. It is also better not to invoke God as a being who decided that this might have been best—"It was God's will." In a moment of acute human suffering, we cannot allow our interpretations of God to be imposed on others. Their interpretation should prevail. In sum, we should be there. If we do not have words that seem right, our simple presence may be enough. Our words should not define someone else's feelings. We should give permission for the fact that it is all right to feel bad, to say so, and to share those feelings.

BOX 24-17

ASSESSMENT OF THE STUDENT'S PERFORMANCE

Every student's effort with patients should be observed many times by a qualified instructor. Certain behaviors will help to characterize your performance:

At the Start of the Interview, Did You Do the Following?
• Say "Hello," and greet the patient appropriately.
  • Introduce yourself.
  • Give appropriate attention to everyone's comfort.
  • Eliminate noise and other distractions when possible.
  • Outline the purposes of the interview and assess the patient's understanding.
  • Begin with a comfortable, open-ended question, such as, "How can I be of help?"

During the Interview, Did You Do the Following?
• Encourage and facilitate further response (e.g., with a head nod).
  • Follow responses to open-ended questions with appropriate specific questions.
  • Consistently seek clarification when a response was in some way unclear.
  • Direct the course of the interview gently.
  • Ask one question at a time.
  • Occasionally restate what you heard to check accuracy and to ensure that you are paying attention.
  • Make smooth transitions.

At the Close of the Interview, Did You Do the Following?
• Summarize and recheck for accuracy.
  • Ask if there were any other questions or concerns.
  • Appropriately indicate next steps.
  • Say "Thank you" with appreciation and with an appropriate "Good-bye."

BOX 24-17

ASSESSMENT OF THE STUDENT'S PERFORMANCE—cont'd

Throughout the Interview, Did You Do the Following?
- Maintain appropriate eye contact.
  - Maintain a comfortable posture, invoking body language that shows attentiveness to the patient.
  - Use appropriate silence, allowing enough time for the patient's comments, expressions, thoughts, and feelings.
  - Avoid following the answer to one question with the next question.
  - Empathize when appropriate.
  - Restate your willingness to help when appropriate.
  - Confirm that you and the patient are allies, working together to find appropriate outcomes.

Did the Patient Do the Following?
- Appear comfortable, relaxed, and engaged, freely giving responses and discussing concerns.
  - Convey a sense of understanding of your remarks.

Modified from Brown University Interpersonal Skill Evaluation Instrument; Burchard, Rowland-Morin, 1990.

ELECTRONIC RESOURCES

For Weblinks and additional resources, go to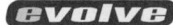

http://evolve.elsevier.com/Seidel

or to the Companion CD-ROM.

Additional information related to the content in Chapter 24 can be found on the companion website at http://evolve.elsevier.com/Seidel/ or on the interactive companion CD-ROM. Resources and activities for Chapter 24 include:
- Sound and Vision Theater
- Printouts for Your Practice
- Spanish Assessment Terms with Pronunciation Guide
- Instant Calculators

TAKING THE NEXT STEPS: CRITICAL THINKING

THE CLINICAL EXAMINATION

Thus far, we have been concerned with the initial interaction with the patient; the establishment of respectful rapport; and the processes by which we gather information about the patient (i.e., history and physical examination). These together form the clinical examination, a necessary starting point. We then organize information, integrate it, and prepare it for the next steps. This process, which might be called "critical thinking," leads to diagnoses, the setting of priorities, and the institution of management plans (Fig. 25-1). In this, we are partners with the patient all of the way.

CRITICAL THINKING

ASSESSMENT, JUDGMENT, AND EVIDENCE

Critical thinking requires that you bring to your decision making your experience and an intimate knowledge of your patient and knowledge of the current best evidence regarding the issues involved. You need to modify your judgment judiciously in the light of that evidence. That, however, does not make inconsequential your intuitive responses, but it does discipline them. The best available evidence has to be constantly sorted from the plethora of information available in books and journals, and on the Internet. Be critical of what those sources offer. The use of evidence in decision making has recently been called "evidence-based practice." That is simply a new jargon for a traditional and essential component of the critical thinking that is the responsibility of everyone who cares for patients.

The first step in critical thinking is to assess what you have learned from the patient, determining its value and significance. Then priorities are assigned as to the extent to which a particular bit of information might have an impact on your clinical judgment and on the management plans to be formulated with the patient. You arrive at clinical opinions.

Further assessment depends on your preferences and, importantly, on those of the patient, preferences influenced by feelings, attitudes, and values. Discussion with the patient should include the clear presentation of risks and probabilities and result in mutually agreed upon decisions. Your clinical opinions, then, help direct further assessment, balancing advantage and risk to the patient, increasing cost, and the use of limited resources. Given this and your presumptive diagnoses, a potential management plan for the immediate and ongoing care of the patient can be formulated with the full participation of the patient.

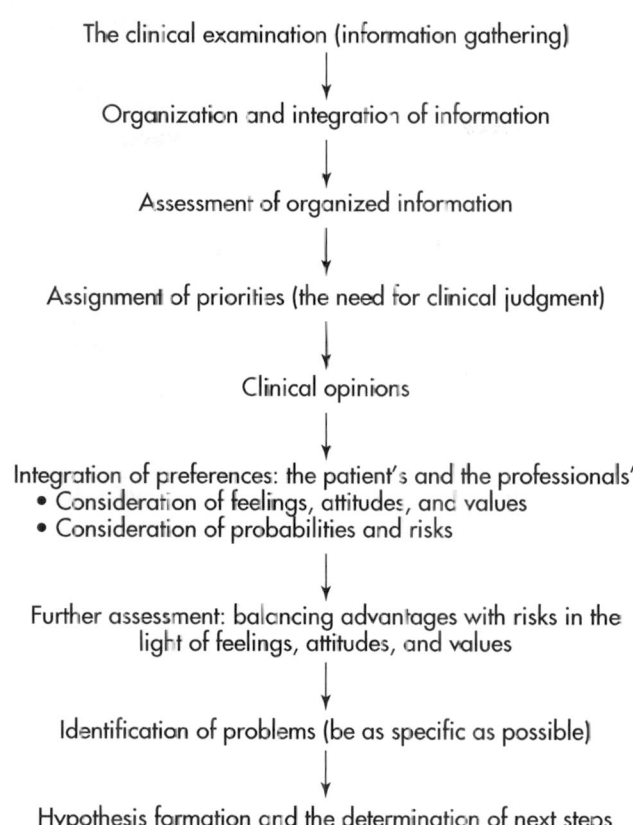

The clinical examination (information gathering)

↓

Organization and integration of information

↓

Assessment of organized information

↓

Assignment of priorities (the need for clinical judgment)

↓

Clinical opinions

↓

Integration of preferences: the patient's and the professionals'
• Consideration of feelings, attitudes, and values
• Consideration of probabilities and risks

↓

Further assessment: balancing advantages with risks in the light of feelings, attitudes, and values

↓

Identification of problems (be as specific as possible)

↓

Hypothesis formation and the determination of next steps

FIGURE 25-1
Steps for critical thinking.

PROBLEM IDENTIFICATION

A problem may be defined as anything that will need further evaluation and/or attention. It may be related to one or more of the following:

◆ An uncertain diagnosis
◆ New findings related to a previous diagnosis
◆ New findings of unknown cause
◆ Unusual findings revealed in the clinical examination or by laboratory tests
◆ Personal or social difficulties

Try to formulate problems as specifically as possible. It helps to identify and list the signs and symptoms associated with the patient's complaint. Aggregate all information, objective and subjective, related to the same body system or regions to help identify the domain of the disorder. This necessary listing of the findings, expected and unexpected, for each body system or region is a key to a clear and complete picture of a problem. Once a particular body system or region is identified, relate the signs and symptoms to a pathologic, physical, emotional, or social process. Form hypotheses based on the available information (Box 25-1). Note the absence of findings that indicate health or well-being or the absence of those that you might expect in support of your hypotheses. After all, there may be no problem to be defined. Reconsider the reason the patient sought care. Think through the patient's nonverbal communication, attempting to determine whether there are any questions you may have neglected to ask or information you did not fully understand. When possible, seek additional information from the patient to fill in these gaps. Beware of "red herrings," the bits of information that are distracting and draw your thinking away from central issues. Of course, pay attention to unexpected or unusual findings, but examine them critically and do not let them lead you astray so that you distort the full consideration of all you have learned.

After a close match between the data (both subjective and objective) and a presumed diagnosis is made, consider the laboratory tests needed to confirm the presumed diagnosis. Laboratory tests or consultation will often be needed for further evaluation before establishing the diagnosis (Box 25-2).

BOX 25-1

DECISION MAKING

There are several ways to make a diagnosis:
- Recognizing patterns (on the assumption that if he looks like Elvis, he must be Elvis)
- Sampling the universe (on the assumption that including everything precludes missing anything)
- Using algorithms (on the assumption that a rigidly defined thought process precludes error)

Although each of these may have limited use in specific situations, the broad consideration of all your findings should most often result in the development of one or more hypotheses needing a disciplined, evidence-based approach to solutions.

Guidelines to a sound decision-making process include the following:
- Always derive possibilities that are consistent with the chief complaint and your database, and with known psychosocial and pathophysiologic mechanisms.
- Remember that common problems occur commonly, and rare ones do not.
- Remember that common problems can have unusual presentations and rare ones may have a seemingly common complaint.
- Remember, too, that a rarity that has a necessary treatment available should be considered, lest harm come to a patient.
- Do not rush to a diagnosis with no available treatment, and do not pursue a line of reasoning that will not alter your course of action.
- Do not undertake procedures that are not reasonably related to your hypotheses.
- Always consider harm and cost as well as benefit when judging the need for a test or action.
- Consider whether the risk is worth the possible gain in information, invoking the ethical principle of nonmaleficence: do no harm.
- Recognize that your favorite hypotheses may not be valid. Remain open in your thinking and be ready to discard or modify your hypotheses when necessary; avoid the tendency to discount information that may invalidate your favorite thoughts.
- Try to have a single process explain all or most of your data, but do not be slavish in this regard. After all, a patient with many complaints and problems may have more than one disease; two common diseases may occur simultaneously more often than one rare disease alone.
- Probability and utility should always be your guides to sequencing your actions unless a life-threatening situation exists. A conscientious estimate of probability is the best way to define the limits of uncertainty and utility, and the best way to establish priorities.

BOX 25-2

RED HERRINGS

A patient with swollen cervical nodes and fever owned a cat, which had claws. The patient did not prove to have cat scratch disease. The too obvious apparent source of the problem, a "red herring," delayed the ultimate diagnosis of non-Hodgkin lymphoma.

VALID HYPOTHESES

Critical thinking allows you to consider and discard the variety of possible diagnoses—from the common to the rare—before settling on the best match between the patient's signs and symptoms and a specific disorder. It has been said (Kopp, 1997) that there are at least three diagnoses for every disease: the one that unifies what you have learned; the one you can't afford to miss; and the one that it actually is. Sometimes, they are all one, but usually not. As you gain experience, you will more confidently collect, analyze, evaluate, and synthesize information, relating it to the chief complaint or your initial impression of the problem. Be cautious about doing this too quickly. Do not let your first thoughts narrow the focus of your questions during the interview. In other words, do not jump to conclusions.

BOX 25-3

"A PATIENT CAN HAVE AS MANY DIAGNOSES AS HE DARN WELL PLEASES"

Hilliard and colleagues have recently reminded us that common problems happen commonly and even at the same time (Hilliard, 2004). They noted that C. F. M. Saint noted several decades ago that more than one disease may be responsible for a patient's signs and symptoms when he could find no pathophysiologic explanation for the coexistence of hiatal hernia, gallbladder disease, and diverticulosis in one of his patients. That, they added, was the same point made by Hickam's dictum: "A patient can have as many diagnoses as he darn well pleases." It was William Osler, however, who invoked the competing fourteenth century philosophy of William of Occam: "Plurality must not be posited without necessity." In other words, do not consider more than one diagnosis unless you really have to, and, "among competing hypotheses, favor the simplest one." Thus, we are given the term "Occam's razor" to signify this.

But, suppose Occam's razor doesn't always work. As Hilliard writes, "As the population continues to age—and as diagnostic studies increase in number and sophistication—the dulling of Occam's razor is certain to continue." What are you to think, then? We suggest that you not accept either Saint or Occam uncritically. They must both be held in mind and given appropriate balance as you make your clinical judgments.

Positive outcomes rely on the quality of your decisions, the soundness of your hypotheses, the actions they suggest, and the way in which those actions are implemented. One of your most important contributions is your ever-present sensitivity. As you look for the hidden clue to a problem, stay attuned to the nuances, the slightest of variations in even the more easily recognized signs and symptoms. These may have important implications that are not at first obvious. Clinical acumen develops with that sensitivity to the meaning of events and from your ability to intermingle the precise and the probable.

One of the clichés of clinical practice is that all findings should be unified into one diagnosis. This is not always true. More than one disease process can exist at one time in the same person, an acute illness can be imposed on a chronic one, and a chronic disease can cycle endlessly through remission and relapse. You must be sure that all of the information is logically explained by your ultimate conclusions. The laboratory and consultation can often help validate your observations and confirm your clinical opinions (Box 25-3).

POSSIBLE BARRIERS TO CRITICAL THINKING

Illness evolves from disease and is almost always multifaceted. You may not be able to explain all your findings on a pathophysiologic level because the physical is inseparable from the emotional. Therefore you must not be misled into believing that, given a pathophysiologic conclusion, management targeted to that finding will necessarily solve the problem. You must consider the full range of issues—from the physical to the emotional, social, and economic—that might affect the expected outcomes The pitfall is that you may allow yourself to be lost in physical detail and lose the context of the broader view, explicit or implicit in the expression of feelings, attitudes, and values.

Feelings, Attitudes, and Values. Complexity is intensified by emotions in both patient and provider. Feelings, attitudes, and values may be so strong that our opinions may be impaired or distorted by the content of those feelings and by a consequent fear, uncertainty, anxiety, and/or resentment. If these feelings are to be given a proper context, you must know yourself. The questioning must be relentless: "What is really happening?" "Have feelings overtaken logic?" "Have ethical concepts been ignored?" "What are the issues that matter?" "What should take precedence?" "Do I understand my contribution to the interaction?" "Do I understand the patient?" "How do I feel about all this?" "How does the patient feel about it?"

Mechanism and Probabilism. Mechanistic (deterministic) thinking is governed by a sense that knowledge must be certain, and that it is not subject to any of the attributes of the observer (who must be detached). Knowledge is to be free of belief, attitudes, and values. There is no room for the probable, that which is likely but uncertain; and, of course, there must be. There must be a balance between mechanism and probabilism in our decision making despite the difficulty in controlling all of the variables when we are at the patient's side. Also, we introduce variables to the decision-making process fully as much as the patient. These variables include, among others, our age, extent of our experience, occasional fatigue, and our worry about malpractice litigation. We are not in an isolated system uninfluenced by what we bring to it and what the patient brings to it; uncertainty in large part stems from that (see Chapter 24). Accepting the inevitability of probability simply recognizes that the certainty of truth, whatever that may be, is hard to achieve. Why is this so?

- ◆ Causes may act or interact differently at different times.
- ◆ The same effect may not always have the same cause.
- ◆ The effect of a given cause cannot be isolated with certainty.

Causes, effects, and our interpretations of them change probabilistically with time. They involve uncertainty, conjecture, and chance. Dependence on the purely scientific and the technical offers an unrealistic comfort; certainty can often be more apparent than real (Box 25-4). Acknowledging this may be viewed as gambling. True, but it is a gamble taken with the justification (or faith) that there is order in the world. That puts limits on uncertainty, and probability can be quantified. A high probability diminishes uncertainty; a low probability does not.

We cannot be dominated by the mechanistic assumption that there is a precise and discoverable cause for every event. That can only lead to excessive invasion of the patient. Making judgments on the basis of well-informed probabilities recognizes the complexity of the decision-making process and saves the patient pain and cost, both physical and emotional. Comfort with uncertainty and complexity permits considered judgment of the information gleaned from the history and physical examination.

Thus critical thinking does not require a compulsive listing of all of the possible options in diagnosis and management. Rather, it is dominated by hypothesis formation; asking whether a particular diagnosis should be made at all depending on its probability; or whether a test or other technical modality may be indicated, depending at least in part on the probability suggested by its sensitivity and specificity.

BOX 25-4

THE COMPUTER

The computer is a remarkable resource. It is helpful in recording and providing information. It can remind you about unrecognized possibilities in diagnosis and can place at your fingertips, if you have entered it correctly, all the information you have about the patient. Still, it is a threat. There is an unacceptable temptation at times to substitute the computer for critical thinking. The computer has no sense of the subtleties of the human dimension. It poses a serious threat to confidentiality, which can be breached by inadvertent accidental intrusion or by purposeful invasion. It is your responsibility to provide information appropriately and with the knowledge of the patient but you must be the guardian of what belongs to the patient.

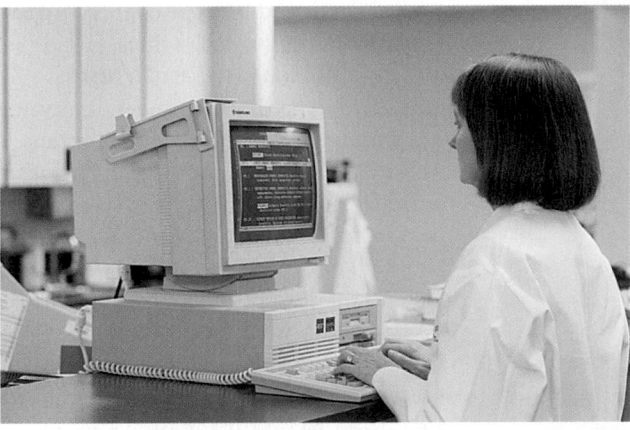

VALIDITY OF THE CLINICAL EXAMINATION

We are in a time when there is considerable effort to reduce the cost of health care. If you recognize that the great majority of diagnoses can be achieved with the information gleaned from a competent clinical examination, you can limit the indiscriminate use of expensive technology. This requires some assurance of the reliability of your observations so that, with demonstrated greater sensitivity and specificity, you can relieve potential uncertainty. Unfortunately, there is not yet a mass of information that allows widespread quantification of the information learned on clinical examination. Laboratory tests are easier to evaluate in this way. Nevertheless, with accumulating experience, you can learn more of the sensitivity and specificity of your findings and begin to assign such values.

Keep the following definitions in mind:

- Sensitivity: the ability of an observation to identify correctly those who have a disease
- Specificity: the ability of an observation to identify correctly those who do not have the disease
- True positive: an expected observation that is found when the disease characterized by that observation is present
- True negative: an expected observation that is not found when the disease characterized by that observation is not present
- False positive: an observation made that suggests a disease when that disease is not present
- False negative: a disease is present, the observation is there to be made, and it is not appreciated
- Positive predictive value: the proportion of persons with an observation characteristic of a disease who have it (e.g., when an observation is made 100 times, and on 95 of those occasions that observation proves to be consistent with the ultimate diagnosis, the positive predictive value of the observation is 95%)
- Negative predictive value: the proportion of persons with an expected observation who ultimately prove not to have the expected condition (e.g., if 100 observations are made expecting a disease, and 95 times that observation is not found and the condition proves not to have been the diagnosis, the negative predictive value of the observation is 95%)

BAYES FORMULA

As a critical thinker, you will discover that the likelihood of your diagnosis being related to your findings depends on the probability of those findings being associated with that diagnosis, and the prevalence of both that particular diagnosis and that combination of findings in the community you are serving. Patterns prevail. It is not common that just one observation ensures a diagnosis. These considerations have been formalized as Bayes formula. This juggling of probabilities is implicit during diagnostic decision making. We do not think consciously of Bayes formula most of the time, but we are using it at some level all of the time.

We have stressed that diagnostic decision making is generally best served by the development of hypotheses that will provide a disciplined approach to solutions. If you are uncertain about an observation, never hesitate to recheck its validity. That is vital to critical thinking. To limit uncertainty, the ratio of fact to conjecture must be positive, and it must be achieved within the emotional and social context of your patient. Much as you strive to be scientific and base what you do on the disciplined principles of science, at times you will make undeniable intuitive judgments. Intuition, however, must be as fully subject to critical thinking as any other aspect of your effort.

THE MANAGEMENT PLAN/SETTING PRIORITIES

You decide what you think is going on (the diagnosis) and what you are going to do about it (the management plan). You often need to investigate further, deciding on which of the available laboratory and imaging techniques you might use and who might help you with them. Having thought critically (and, always, with the patient), you can arrive at a jointly considered approach that may include some of the following:

- Laboratory studies to be obtained
- Consultation requested

- ◆ Medications or appliances prescribed
- ◆ Special care to be provided (e.g., nursing, physical therapy, respiratory therapy)
- ◆ Surgery
- ◆ Diet modification
- ◆ Activity modification
- ◆ Follow-up visit schedule
- ◆ Patient education needs

In addition, you need to decide the degree of urgency of each of these items and what it is that underlies the issues in terms of the social, economic, and pathophysiologic considerations. Priorities must be set. There is much to think about. The following is only a partial guide:

- ◆ What is the patient's physical condition?
  - ◆ Is something going on that overrides every other consideration (e.g., a problem with the central nervous system, the heart, the kidneys, a degree of pain, a distressing change in mental status)?
  - ◆ Are there abnormal laboratory values that need immediate attention?
- ◆ What is the patient's social circumstance?
  - ◆ Will a job be threatened if there is prolonged absence from work?
  - ◆ Are there small children at home for whom no other caretaker is available?
  - ◆ Is there available and convenient transportation to and from services and care?
- ◆ What is the patient's economic circumstance?
  - ◆ Is there adequate insurance coverage?
  - ◆ Is the cost of care going to compromise other areas of the patient's life?

These are but a few of the considerations. They suggest the kind of critical thinking that must address the setting of priorities and the development of a management plan that may be modified to meet a particular circumstance. Perhaps, without risk, there can be delay in tests, in treatments, in therapies; perhaps there might be a sequence of steps that meets priority needs, some needing to be done now, some that might await the information gleaned from an earlier step or the result of a first therapeutic attempt.

And, certainly, the patient's subsequent behavior is a major variable whether in a health prevention (e.g., stopping smoking) or therapeutic (e.g., taking a necessary medication) circumstance. The patient, surely, must be actively and positively involved if an optimal outcome is to be achieved. Does the patient want to take the necessary steps? What is the extent of the patient's commitment and recognition that the benefits of action outweigh any possible disadvantages? (There are, after all, risks to certain tests, procedures and medications.) Finally, given a positive action, what is the patient's ability to sustain the effort? (DiClemente, Prochaska, 1998). The depth of our understanding of the multiple factors in a patient's life is a measure of the potential of an optimal outcome (Shinitzky, Kub, 2001).

A tremendous amount of information has been offered in this text. Your need to develop a sequence for your critical thinking can be facilitated by careful attention to Chapter 26 and its consideration of the problem-oriented medical record. Careful attention to the need to record information well will suggest the discipline by which you can organize your thoughts and discipline your critical thinking, utilizing the findings in the history and physical examination.

That discipline, then, will assure that the entire process will be (as it must be) recorded thoughtfully, completely, and with ready accessibility (see Chapter 26).

CHAPTER
26

RECORDING INFORMATION

After collecting the history and completing the physical examination, the health care practitioner must condense, organize, and record the collected raw data along with the problems identified and plan of care. The information in the patient's record enables you and your colleagues to care for the patient by identifying health problems, making diagnoses and judgments of diagnostic testing needed, planning appropriate care, and monitoring the patient's responses to treatment.

Appropriate medical terminology and a traditional organizational style make the record more readily understood by your colleagues. The patient's record is only as good as the accuracy, depth, and detail provided.

Most health professionals use a customary organization of information from the interview and physical examination. Health agencies often incorporate the information in standardized forms or electronic recording systems. Following this customary outline of information enables all health professionals in the agency to find and use the patient information more efficiently. The problem-oriented medical record (POMR) with SOAP notes is one such system.

The patient's record is a legal document, and any information contained in it may be used in court and in other legal proceedings, as well as to make health care payment determinations. It is your responsibility to present the data legibly, accurately, and in a manner that is representative of the examination. Recorded information should not be erased. Make necessary changes by lining out data, leaving crossed-out data legible. Initial and date the changes. Any portion of the examination that has been deferred or omitted should be so noted, rather than neglecting to mention particular findings. It is appropriate in some circumstances to defer a portion of an examination, and stating the reason for that deferral is useful. A clear, exact record of your assessment, an analysis of the problem, and a management plan are vital to your protection in case there is ever a question relevant to your care of the patient.

Concerns about the privacy of health data have grown with the development of computer-based health data systems and the ease with which electronic data can be accessed and transferred. Indeed, beginning medical students are now commonly encouraged to use PDAs (personal digital assistants or "palm pilots") as a resource in their recording effort. The future trend is obvious. Health agencies must have policies to control access to both paper and electronic patient record databases, so that data can only be used for the legitimate purposes of direct care, utilization review, quality assessment, public health, and research.

GENERAL GUIDELINES

It is certainly permissible to take brief notes about the patient's concerns and your findings during the course of the interview and physical examination. You should record certain data as you obtain it, specifically the vital signs and any measurements. However, do not try to record all the data during the visit, because writing must not distract your attention from the patient.

New information related to a previously discussed topic may emerge later in the interview or examination. Postponement of recording will sharpen your interviewing skills, but it also enables you to gather, reflect, and organize all the data appropriately before making the record final. Your recall of information is limited, however, so complete your recording as soon as possible after the examination. Resist going on to other patients before completing the first patient's record. Although this is sometimes unavoidable, you can easily become confused about which patient had a particular finding or even forget to record an important finding.

Be concise because of the volume of information collected during the examination. Use an outline form to avoid the repetition of phrases such as, "Patient states." Abbreviations and symbols may be used judiciously and sparingly, but take care to use only those acceptable in your setting. Inappropriate abbreviations may be confusing to other health professionals (Box 26-1). Similarly, avoid the use of words such as normal, good, poor, and negative, because these words are open to various interpretations by other examiners.

Document what you observe and what the patient tells you, rather than the conclusions you interpret or infer. Use direct quotes from the patient when a description is particularly vivid. Keep subjective and symptomatic data in the history, making sure none gets woven into the physical findings. Physical examination findings should be the result of your observation and interpretation of the patient's description. For example, when a patient complains of pain (a symptom) during palpation, you should note tenderness (a sign) in the record; or report the patient's reaction to pain, such as crying, withdrawal, rigid posturing, or facial expression.

Record expected findings, both what the patient tells you and what you observe, as well as those findings that are unexpected. Describe, in its present state, any physical finding that can change with age, disease, or pathologic condition. Detectable changes can then be better compared and documented in the future. Clues about health changes over time are lost if such details are not recorded in the patient's record.

BOX 26-1

ABBREVIATIONS AND ACRONYMS: THE INITIAL CHALLENGE TO RELIABILITY

There was a time when recorded histories and physical examinations contained few, if any, acronyms. After World War II, the use of initials began to proliferate. Today, it is a compulsive problem leading to misunderstanding that is at times inconvenient and at times dangerous.

When our interprofessional languages are obscured by acronyms, communication suffers and the safety of patients may be compromised. For example, ROM has many different meanings. The obstetrician uses ROM for rupture of membranes. The pediatrician uses ROM for right otitis media. The physiatrist uses ROM for range of motion. And these days ROM tacked on to CD has an entirely different meaning.

The Joint Commission on Accreditation of Healthcare Organizations (JCAHO) has identified "improving communications among caregivers" as a patient safety goal. Certain abbreviations have been placed on a "do not use" list when an error in misreading the abbreviation could cause harm. For example, "MS" is on the "do not use" list because it could be interpreted as either morphine sulfate or magnesium sulfate and potentially cause a dangerous medication error. Two other abbreviations that should not be used include "q" for "every day" and "qod" for "every other day."

For a complete list of abbreviations on the JCAHO "do not use" list, visit the following website: http://www.jcaho.org/accredited+organizations/patient+safety/npsg.htm.

When you are tempted to use initials, abbreviations, and acronyms to get things said and written in a hurry, resist the temptation.

SUBJECTIVE DATA

Subjective data is the information, both positive and negative, that the patient offers—what the patient tells you as stated by the patient.

Describe the patient's concerns or unexpected findings by their quality or character. For example, indicating the presence of pain without providing characteristics (e.g., timing, location, severity, and quality) is not useful, either for future comparison or for determining the extent of the present problem. Record the severity of pain using the patient's response or score on a pain scale. Be sure to name the pain scale in the record. The severity of pain may also be described by its interference with activity. Note whether the patient is able to continue regular activity despite pain or whether it is necessary to decrease or stop all activity until pain subsides (see Chapter 7). Similar detail should be provided for other signs.

One way to record expected findings is to indicate the absence of symptoms (e.g., "no vomiting, diarrhea, or constipation").

OBJECTIVE DATA

Objective data are the findings resulting from direct observation—what you see, hear, and touch.

Relate physical findings to the processes of inspection, palpation, auscultation, and percussion, making clear the process of detection so confusion does not occur. For example, "no masses on palpation" may be stated when recording abdominal findings. Include details about expected objective findings, such as "tympanic membranes pearly gray, translucent, light reflex and bony landmarks present, mobility to positive and negative pressure bilaterally." Also provide an accurate description of unexpected objective findings. Suggestions for recording the character and quality of objective findings follow.

Location of Findings. Use topographic and anatomic landmarks to add precision to your description of findings. Indicating the liver span measurement at the midclavicular line enables future comparison, because measurement at this location can be replicated. The location of the apical impulse is commonly described by both a topographic landmark (the midsternal line) and an anatomic landmark (a specific intercostal space); for example, "the apical impulse is 4 cm from the midsternal line at the fifth intercostal space."

In some cases, location of a finding on or near a specific structure (e.g., tympanic membrane, rectum, vaginal vestibule) may be described by its position on a clock. It is important that others recognize the same landmarks for the 12-o'clock reference point. For rectal findings use the anterior midline, and for vaginal vestibule findings (e.g., Bartholin glands, episiotomy scar) use the clitoris.

Incremental Grading. Findings that vary by degrees are customarily graded or recorded in an incremental scale format. Pulse amplitude, heart murmur intensity, muscle strength, and deep tendon reflexes are findings often recorded in this manner. In addition, retinal vessel changes and prostate size are sometimes graded similarly. See the chapters in which these examination techniques are discussed for the grading system used to describe the findings.

Organs, Masses, and Lesions. For organs, any type of mass (e.g., an enlarged lymph node), or skin lesion, describe the following characteristics noted during inspection and palpation:

- Texture or consistency: smooth, soft, firm, nodular, granular, fibrous, matted
- Size: recorded in centimeters on two dimensions, plus height if the lesion is elevated. Future changes in the lesion size can then be accurately detected. (This is more precise than comparing the lesion's size to fruit or nuts, which have different dimensions.)
- Shape or configuration: annular, linear, tubular, elliptical
- Mobility: moves freely under skin or fixed to overlying skin or underlying tissue
- Tenderness
- Induration *- hardening of area of body as reaction to inflammation, hyperemia, neoplastic infiltration, or area of body that has undergone this reaction*
- Heat
- Color: hyperpigmentation or hypopigmentation, redness or erythema, or the specific color of the lesion
- Location
- Other characteristics, for example, oozing, bleeding, discharge, scab formation, scarring, excoriation

Discharge. Regardless of the site, describe discharge by color and consistency (e.g., clear, serous, mucoid, white, green, yellow, purulent, bloody, or sanguineous), odor, and amount (e.g., minimal, moderate, copious).

Something that generates pus → suppurative, pyogenic, purulent

Teeth. The American Dental Association sequential numbering system is used to designate missing, filled, and carious teeth (Fig. 26-1). Numbers for 1 to 32 are used, with number 1 being the third molar in the patient's right maxilla. Numbering is sequential around the entire maxilla and then continues in the left mandible third molar. Letters are used for deciduous teeth. If preferred, the tooth name may also be used for recording dental information.

Illustrations. Drawings can sometimes provide a better description than words and should be used when appropriate. You do not have to be an artist to communicate information. Illustrations are particularly useful in describing the origin of pain and where it radiates; and the size, shape, and location of a lesion (Fig. 26-2). Stick figures are useful to compare findings in extremities, such as pulse amplitude and deep tendon reflex response (Fig. 26-3).

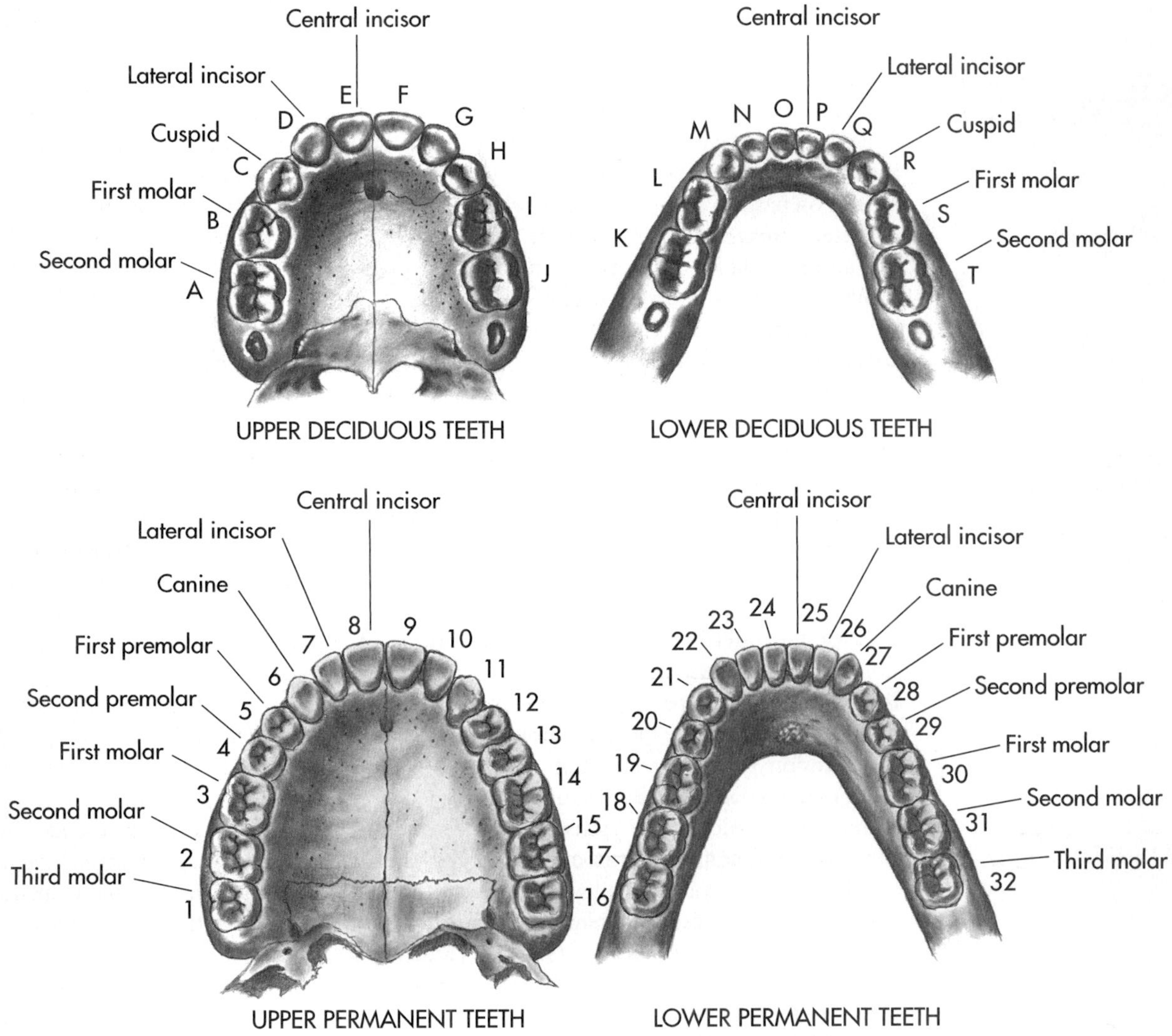

FIGURE 26-1
Tooth identification using either name or American Dental Association numbering system; letters for deciduous teeth, numbers for permanent teeth.

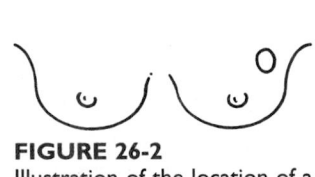

FIGURE 26-2
Illustration of the location of a breast mass.

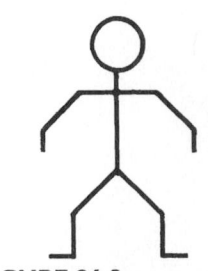

FIGURE 26-3
Illustration of a stick person.

PROBLEM-ORIENTED MEDICAL RECORD

The POMR is a commonly used process to organize patient data gained during the history and physical examination. After the history and physical examination is completed, the POMR provides a format for collecting and recording your thoughts that assists with critical thinking and clinical decision making—determining the patient's problems as well as the possible and probable diagnoses.

After the subjective data and objective data are documented, along with the problems identified, the care plan is made with the patient as a full participant to find solutions for the problems and to arrive at a diagnosis. The written record describes plans made and actions taken to address these problems, lists the information and education provided to the patient, and describes the patient's response to care provided.

The record must be well organized and written precisely, legibly, and free of excess verbiage to facilitate your thinking and the thinking of your colleagues who may need to care for the patient. The consistent recording format enables more effective communication and coordination among professionals caring for the patient.

There are six components of the POMR:

- Comprehensive health history
- Complete physical examination
- Problem list
- Assessment and plan
- Baseline and problem-directed laboratory and radiologic imaging studies
- Progress notes

COMPREHENSIVE HEALTH HISTORY AND PHYSICAL EXAMINATION

The comprehensive health history must include all data collected, both positive and negative, that contribute directly to your assessment. Arrange the history in chronologic order, starting with the current episode and then filling in relevant background information. Arrange the physical examination findings in the order and style preferred by the health agency. Follow a consistent order. This allows future readers, and you, to find specific points of information. It also enables you to quickly remember key components for assessment on each encounter.

Make your headings clear, using indentations and spacing to accentuate the organization of your documentation. Underline important points. Use short phrases for descriptions, saving time and space by omitting superfluous words. Use only those common abbreviations and symbols approved by the health care agency (see Appendix H for some commonly used abbreviations).

PROBLEM LIST

The problem list is created after the subjective and objective information has been organized. All pertinent data and positive examination findings, laboratory data, and prior diagnoses are reviewed to develop a problem list in the form of a running log with the following information: problem number, date of onset, description of problem, and date problem was resolved or became an inactive concern.

A problem may be defined as anything that will require further evaluation or attention. Problems arise in many varieties, for example, the questions regarding diagnosis, the availability of diagnostic and therapeutic resources, ethical issues and factors in the patient's life, social, emotional, monetary or insurance-related, work-related, school-related, family-related, and even the availability of caretakers. A problem may be related to any of the following:

- A firmly established diagnosis (e.g., diabetes mellitus, hypertension)
- A new symptom or physical finding of unknown etiology or significance (e.g., right knee effusion)
- Unexpected and new findings revealed by laboratory tests (e.g., cardiomegaly on chest radiograph)
- Personal or social difficulties (e.g., unemployment, homelessness)
- Risk factors for serious conditions (e.g., smoking, family history of coronary artery disease)
- Factors crucial to remember long term (e.g., allergy to penicillin)

The nature of the patient's problems determines the sequence in which you list them. You may list problems in separate lists, for example, diagnostic issues, care and therapeutic issues, and long-range issues, or you may make one list. The needs of a particular patient and the resources available to you will influence your judgment and your ultimate approach. Some controlling variables with regard to the sequencing of listed problems include the following:

- The possibility that the diagnosis is life threatening and needs immediate attention; the relative gravity of the problem
- The probability/possibility ratio: priority given to the probable diagnoses or therapeutic actions
- The likelihood of the probabilities in a differential diagnosis—the more probable taking precedence
- The availability and cost of the diagnostic, therapeutic, and care-taking resources; cost relative to need and availability
- The time sequence in which the problems arose and the time sequence dictated by their relative urgency
- The source of the problems: causative agents, care of the patient at home, money worries

This list enables all health professionals to quickly assess the patient's history by the summary presented on this list. Problems may be listed in chronologic order, listed according to the severity of problem, or listed in the order of chronologic presentation. Once problems are numbered, that numbering is not changed. When a problem is resolved, a line may be drawn through the row on the chart and the date of resolution is added to the last column. Surgical correction of a condition is one example of a resolved problem.

ASSESSMENT

The assessment section is composed of your interpretations and conclusions, their rationale, the diagnostic possibilities, present and anticipated problems, the needs of ongoing as well as present care—what you think.

Develop an assessment for each problem on the problem list. Begin the process of making a differential diagnosis by discussing and giving priority to possible causes and contributing factors for a problem or symptom. Present the rationale for the potential causes and validate the assessment from data contained in the comprehensive health history, physical examination, consultations, and any laboratory data available. When a serious potential cause is no longer under consideration, explain why.

Describe any pertinent negative information when other portions of the history or physical examination suggest that an abnormality might exist or develop in an area. Avoid the use of words such as "normal" or phrases such as "within normal limits" because they do not describe what is inspected, palpated, percussed, or auscultated. Be as objective as possible. Assessment may include anticipated potential problems such as complications or progression of the disease.

PLAN

The plan describes the need to invoke diagnostic resources, therapeutic modalities, other professional resources, and the rationale for these decisions—what you intend to do.

Develop a plan for each problem on the problem list. The plan is divided into three sections: diagnostics (Dx Tests), therapeutics (Rx), and patient education (Pt Ed):

- **Dx Tests.** List the diagnostic tests to be performed or ordered.
- **Rx.** Describe the therapeutic treatment plan. Provide a rationale for any change or addition to an established treatment plan. List any referrals initiated, with their purpose and to whom the referral is made. State the target date for reevaluating the plan.
- **Pt Ed.** Describe health education provided or planned. Include materials dispensed and evidence of the patient's understanding or lack thereof.

SOAP NOTES

The organization of the patient data within the POMR is often recorded in a series of SOAP notes. Each problem is recorded separately. Subjective and objective data relevant to each problem are clustered together, followed by the assessment and the plan. See pp. 878 to 881 as an example. Alternatively, all of the subjective and objective data can be recorded in totality. Then the list of problems with the assessment and plan for each are written. See the example on p. 882.

Carefully review all SOAP notes on a regular basis during follow-up visits to detect the emergence of a condition that accounts for many or all of the patient's complaints (Box 26-2).

BOX 26-2

GOVERNING PRINCIPLES FOR USING POMR AND SOAP

- Record legibly the information you judge is needed; you will write more early in your career but, as time goes by, you will learn to edit with experience and wisdom, especially under the time pressures you will face.
- Organize! Tell the unique story of your patient chronologically and precisely, and without flights of literary fancy, including positive as well as relevant negative information.
- Use clear headings.
- Trust your colleagues to understand the difference between relevance and irrelevance; allow them, too, to understand that you have been thorough and that you do not have to describe in full an unexceptional looking throat.
- Precision requires exact description, for example, of your judgment of the size of the liver; at times, a picture, even if crudely drawn, or a diagram may clarify your verbal description and better locate a visible lesion or a site of pain; a tape measure may provide the baseline observation for size or swelling
- Be terse. An "erythematous" throat may also be described as "red" and a bulge in an "eardrum" is as well understood as in a "tympanic membrane."
- Avoid the excessive use of acronyms and initials; not every professional involved may understand the terms the way you do.

PROGRESS NOTES

Follow-up visits for problems identified in the POMR are recorded with the progress notes. After the database has been completed through the construction of the POMR, subsequent visits are much briefer. The patient is known to you and the facility, so recording is focused primarily on updating information.

Each problem discussed during a visit is recorded by number (already assigned to it on the problem list) and name. An interval history—including subjective status of the problem, current medications, and review of systems related to the problem—is presented in the subjective portion of the note. The objective portion includes vital signs, a record of any physical examination performed at the time of the visit, and results of laboratory data or radiographic studies performed since the last visit.

The assessment section includes your assessment of the problem status. If the problem was formerly a symptom, such as shortness of breath, you may have enough data to make a diagnosis. The rationale for the diagnosis is presented in this section, and the problem list is updated accordingly.

Plans are presented in the three components: diagnostics, therapeutics, and patient education.

EPISODIC ILLNESS VISIT

Patients often seek care for acute problems such as common colds or minor injuries, which are rapidly resolved. There are three ways to incorporate these problems into the record:

- List the problem as an acute problem within the ongoing patient record and do not give it a number in the complete problem list. This avoids complicating the ongoing problem list.
- Give each acute minor problem a number and include it with the ongoing problem list. A line is drawn through each problem as it is resolved.
- Use a specially designed form for each acute problem. These forms are kept in a special section of the patient record and are not included in the problem list.

Regardless of the method chosen, a brief SOAP note is written in the chart to address each acute problem. It is not necessary to repeat the entire comprehensive health history, but do include pertinent information such as smoking, allergies, or other information that would increase your usual level of concern regarding the problem presented.

EPISODIC ILLNESS NOTES

In certain facilities, such as urgent care centers or emergency departments, you may see a patient who is new to you and the facility, so there is no POMR to refer to. An episodic illness note, which is more extensive, is then required. It includes identifying information and a complete present problem, pertinent past medical history, family history, and personal/social history, as well as a relevant review of systems. The remainder of the note follows the SOAP format.

PROBLEM-ORIENTED MEDICAL RECORD FORMAT

THE HISTORY

The patient's history, especially for an initial visit, provides a comprehensive database. Record information appropriately in specific categories and in the particular sequence preferred by the health care facility or electronic medical record template. The following organized sequence, which includes the appropriate information to record, will guide you in writing a POMR.

Identifying Information. The patient's name, date of birth, and an assigned history number are the first items of information recorded. Most health agencies have forms or electronic medical record formats with headings for each category of information to be recorded.

Problem List. Although the problem list itself is added to the record after the subjective and objective information have been organized, the printed POMR form provides space for this information at the beginning of the record where it can be reviewed at a glance by medical personnel. The problem list is an ongoing record of a patient's medical problems that is added to, as appropriate, after each visit.

Each problem is given a number. The date of onset is recorded along with a brief description of the problem, and space is also provided to record the date that the problem was resolved or became an inactive concern.

General Patient Information. Additional identifying information for each patient includes address, home and/or cell phone number, Social Security number, employer, position or title, business address and phone number, e-mail address, gender, marital status, and health insurance company name and member identification number.

Source and Reliability of Information. Document the historian's identity; that is, the patient or the person's relationship to the patient. Indicate when the old record is used. State your judgment about the reliability of the historian's information.

Chief Complaint/Presenting Problem/Reason for Seeking Care. The chief complaint or presenting problem is a brief description of the patient's main reason for seeking care. State the information verbatim in quotation marks, and include the duration of problem.

History of Present Illness. This section contains a detailed description of the problem. It includes a description of all symptoms that may be related to the chief complaint, and it describes the problem chronologically, dating events and symptoms. When describing the present illness, it is important for the examiner to record the absence of certain symptoms commonly associated with the particular area, or system, involved. Also inquire about anyone in the household with the same symptoms or possible exposure to infection or toxic agents. If pertinent to the present illness, include relevant information from the review of systems, family history, and personal/social history. When more than one problem is identified, address each problem in a separate paragraph. Include the following details of each symptom's occurrence, described in narrative form by categories:

- Onset: when the problem or symptom first started; chronologic order of events; setting and circumstances (e.g., while exercising, sleeping, working); manner of the onset (sudden vs. gradual)
- Location: exact location of pain (localized, generalized, radiation patterns)
- Duration: length of problem or episode; if intermittent, duration of each episode
- Character: nature of pain (e.g., stabbing, burning, sharp, dull, gnawing)
- Aggravating and associated factors: food, activity, rest, certain movements; nausea, vomiting, diarrhea, fever, chills
- Relieving factors and effect on the problem: food, rest, activity, position, prescribed and/or home remedies, alternative or complementary therapies
- Temporal factors: frequency of occurrence (single attack, intermittent, chronic); describe typical attack; change in symptom intensity, improvement or worsening over time
- Severity of the symptoms: 0 to 10 scale, effect on lifestyle, work performance

Past Medical History. The past medical history includes general health and strength over the patient's lifetime as well as disabilities and functional limitations, as the patient per-

---

MNEMONICS

Recording the History of the Present Illness

The OLDCARTS mnemonic helps make sure all characteristics of a problem are described in the history of present illness to assure a comprehensive presentation. The order of recording these characteristics does not need to be consistent.

O Onset
L Location
D Duration
C Character
A Aggravating/associated factors
R Relieving factors
T Temporal factors
S Severity of symptoms

ceives them. List and describe each of the following with dates of occurrence and any specific information available:

- ◆ Hospitalizations and/or surgery (including outpatient surgery): dates, hospital, diagnosis, complications, injuries, disabilities
- ◆ Major childhood illnesses: measles, mumps, whooping cough, chickenpox, scarlet fever, rheumatic fever, diphtheria, polio
- ◆ Major adult illnesses: tuberculosis, hepatitis, diabetes mellitus, hypertension, myocardial infarction, tropical or parasitic diseases, other infections
- ◆ Serious injuries: traumatic brain injury, liver laceration, spinal injury, pelvic fracture
- ◆ Immunizations: polio, diphtheria, pertussis, tetanus toxoid, hepatitis B, measles, mumps, rubella, *Haemophilus influenza*, varicella, influenza, meningococcal, pneumococcal, cholera, typhus, typhoid, anthrax, smallpox, bacille Calmette-Guérin (BCG), last PPD or other skin tests, unusual reaction to immunizations
- ◆ Medications: past, current, and recent medications (dosage, nonprescription medications, vitamins); complementary therapies, herbs
- ◆ Allergies: drugs, foods, environmental allergens
- ◆ Transfusions: reason, date, and number of units transfused; reaction
- ◆ Emotional status: mood disorders, psychiatric therapy or medications
- ◆ Recent laboratory tests: glucose, cholesterol, Pap smear, mammogram, prostate specific antigen (PSA)

Family History. Include a pedigree (with at least three generations). An example is shown in Fig. 26-4. If it is not part of the pedigree, include a family history of major health or genetic disorders (e.g., hypertension, cancer, cardiac, respiratory, kidney, strokes, or thyroid disorders;

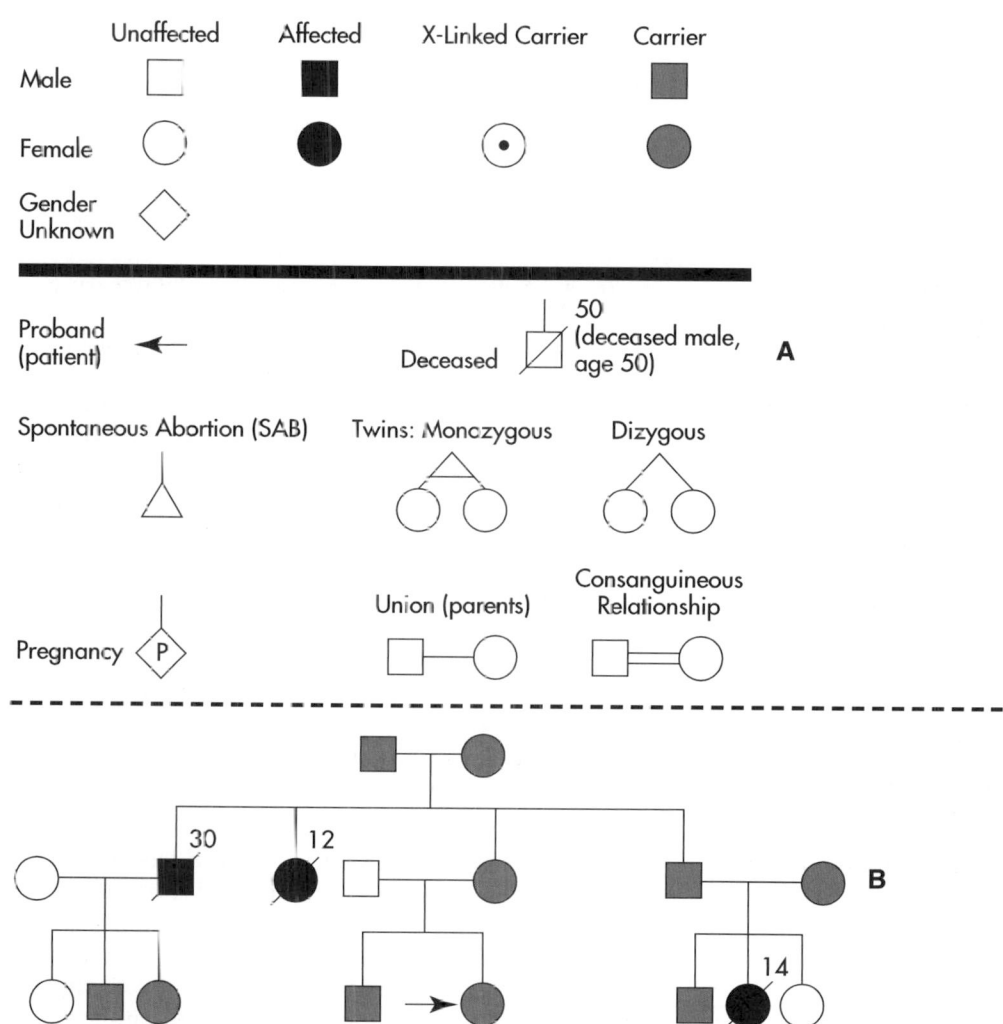

FIGURE 26-4
A, Common pedigree symbols.
B, Sample pedigree for autosomal recessive condition.

asthma or other allergic manifestations; blood dyscrasias; psychiatric difficulties; tuberculosis; rheumatologic diseases; diabetes mellitus; hepatitis; or other familial disorders). Spontaneous abortions and stillbirths suggest genetic problems. Include the age and health of the spouse and children.

Personal and Social History. The information included in this section varies according to the concerns of the patient and the influence of the health problem on the patient's life.

- Cultural background and practices, birthplace, where raised, home environment as youth, education, position in family, marital status or same-sex partner, general life satisfaction, hobbies, interests, sources of stress, religious preference (religious or cultural proscriptions concerning medical care)
- Home conditions: number in household, pets, economic condition
- Occupation: usual work and present work if different, list of job changes, work conditions and hours, physical or mental strain, duration of employment; present and past exposure to heat and cold, industrial toxins; protective devices required or used; military service
- Environment: home, school, work, structural barriers if handicapped, community services utilized; travel and other exposure to contagious diseases, residence in tropics; water and milk supply, other sources of infection when applicable
- Current health habits and/or risk factors: exercise; smoking (packs per day times duration); salt intake; obesity/weight control; alcohol intake: beer, wine, hard liquor (amount/day), duration; CAGE or TACE question responses; blackouts, seizures, or delirium tremens; drug or alcohol treatment program or support group; club/recreational drugs used (e.g., marijuana, cocaine, heroin, LSD, PCP, meth) and methods (e.g., injection, ingestion, sniffing, smoking, or use of shared needles); domestic violence HITS question responses
- Exposure to chemicals, toxins, poisons, asbestos, or radioactive material at home or work and duration; caffeine use (cups/glasses/day)
- Sexual activity: contraceptive or barrier protection method used; past sexually transmitted infection (e.g., syphilis, gonorrhea, chlamydia, pelvic inflammatory disease, herpes, warts); treatment
- Concerns about cost of care, health care coverage

REVIEW OF SYSTEMS

- General constitutional symptoms: fever, chills, malaise, easily fatigued, night sweats, weight (average, preferred, present, change)
- Skin, hair, and nails: rash or eruption, itching, pigmentation or texture change; excessive sweating, unusual nail or hair growth
- Head and neck: frequent or unusual headaches, their location, dizziness, syncope; brain injuries, concussions, loss of consciousness (momentary or prolonged)
- Eyes: visual acuity, blurring, double vision, light sensitivity, pain, change in appearance or vision; use of glasses/contacts, eye drops, other medication; history of trauma, glaucoma, familial eye disease
- Ears: hearing loss, pain, discharge, tinnitus, vertigo
- Nose: sense of smell, frequency of colds, obstruction, nosebleeds, postnasal discharge, sinus pain
- Throat and mouth: hoarseness or change in voice; frequent sore throats, bleeding or swelling of gums; recent tooth abscesses or extraction; soreness of tongue or buccal mucosa, ulcers; disturbance of taste
- Lymphatic: enlargement, tenderness, suppuration
- Chest and lungs: pain related to respiration, dyspnea, cyanosis, wheezing, cough, sputum (character and quantity), hemoptysis, night sweats, exposure to tuberculosis; last chest radiograph
- Breasts: development, pain, tenderness, discharge, lumps, galactorrhea, mammograms (screening or diagnostic), frequency of breast self-examination
- Heart and blood vessels: Chest pain or distress, precipitating causes, timing and duration, relieving factors, palpitations, dyspnea, orthopnea (number of pillows), edema, claudication, hypertension, previous myocardial infarction, exercise tolerance (flights of steps, distance walking), past electrocardiogram and cardiac tests

+ Peripheral vasculature: claudication (frequency, severity), tendency to bruise or bleed, thromboses, thrombophlebitis
+ Hematologic: anemia, any known blood cell disorder, transfusions
+ Gastrointestinal: appetite, digestion, intolerance of any foods, dysphagia, heartburn, nausea, vomiting, hematemesis, bowel regularity, constipation, diarrhea, change in stool color or contents (clay, tarry, fresh blood, mucus, undigested food), flatulence, hemorrhoids, hepatitis, jaundice, dark urine; history of ulcer, gallstones, polyps, tumor; previous radiographic studies, sigmoidoscopy, colonoscopy (where, when, findings)
+ Diet: appetite, likes and dislikes, restrictions (because of religion, allergy, or other disease), vitamins and other supplement, caffeine-containing beverages (coffee, tea, cola); food diary or daily listing of food and liquid intake as needed
+ Endocrine: thyroid enlargement or tenderness, heat or cold intolerance, unexplained weight change, polydipsia, polyuria, changes in facial or body hair, increased hat and glove size, skin striae
  + Males: puberty onset, erections, emissions, testicular pain, libido, infertility *[painful menstruation]*
  + Females: menses onset, regularity, duration, amount of flow; dysmenorrhea; last period; intermenstrual discharge or bleeding; itching; date of last Pap smear; age at menopause; libido; frequency of intercourse; sexual difficulties
  + Pregnancy: infertility; gravidity and parity (G = number of pregnancies, T = number of term pregnancies, P = number of preterm pregnancies, A = number of abortions/miscarriages, L = number of living children); number and duration of each pregnancy, delivery method; complications during any pregnancy or postpartum period; use of oral or other contraceptives
+ Genitourinary: dysuria, flank or suprapubic pain, urgency, frequency, nocturia, hematuria, polyuria, hesitancy, dribbling, loss in force of stream, passage of stone; edema of face, stress incontinence, hernias, sexually transmitted infection
+ Musculoskeletal: joint stiffness, pain, restriction of motion, swelling, redness, heat, bony deformity
+ Neurologic: syncope, seizures, weakness or paralysis, problems with sensation or coordination, tremors
+ Psychiatric: depression, mood changes, difficulty concentrating, nervousness, tension, suicidal thoughts, irritability, sleep disturbances

PHYSICAL EXAMINATION FINDINGS

Record the objective data by body systems and anatomic location. Begin with a general statement about the overall health status of the patient. All observations of physical signs should be described in the appropriate body system or region, usually organized in sequence from head to toe. Take care to describe findings in detail rather than make diagnostic statements.

List each anatomic location or body system as a separate category, using the groupings customary for your health care facility. The findings generally included in each category follow.

General Statement
+ Age, race, gender, general appearance
+ Weight, height, frame size, body mass index
+ Vital signs: temperature, pulse rate, respiratory rate, blood pressure (both arms, two positions)

Mental Status
+ Physical appearance and behavior
+ Cognitive: consciousness level, response to questions, reasoning, arithmetic ability, memory, attention span; specific mental test scores
+ Emotional stability: depression, anxiety, disturbance in thought content, hallucinations
+ Speech and language: voice quality, articulation, coherence, comprehension

Skin
+ Color, uniformity, integrity, texture, temperature, turgor, hygiene, tattoos, scars
+ Presence of edema, moisture, excessive perspiration, unusual odor, mobility
+ Presence and description of lesions (size, shape, location, configuration, blanching, inflammation, tenderness, induration, discharge), parasites, trauma
+ Hair texture, distribution, color, quality

- Nail configuration, color, texture, condition, nail base angle, ridging, beading, pitting, peeling, nail plate firmness, adherence to nail bed

Head

- Size and contour of head, scalp appearance, head position
- Symmetry and spacing of facial features, tics, characteristic facies
- Presence of edema or puffiness
- Temporal arteries: pulsations, thickening, hardness, tenderness, bruits

Eyes

- Visual acuity (near, distant), visual fields
- Appearance of orbits (edema, sagging tissue, puffiness), firmness of eyeball, conjunctivae color, sclerae, eyelids (redness, flakiness, fasciculations, ptosis), eyebrows
- Extraocular movements, corneal light reflex, cover-uncover test, nystagmus
- Pupillary shape, size, consensual response to light and accommodation, depth of anterior chamber
- Ophthalmoscopic findings of cornea, lens, retina, red reflex, optic disc and macula characteristics, retinal vessel size, caliber, and arteriovenous (AV) crossings, arteriole-venule ratio, exudates, hemorrhages

Ears

- Configuration, position, and alignment of auricles, nodules, tenderness of auricles or in mastoid area
- Otoscopic findings of canals (cerumen, lesions, discharge, foreign body) and tympanic membranes (integrity, color, bony landmarks, light reflex, mobility, bulging, retraction), fluid, air bubbles
- Hearing: Weber and Rinne tests, whispered voice, conversation

Nose

- Appearance of external nose, nasal patency
- Presence of discharge, crusting, flaring, polyp
- Appearance of turbinates, alignment of septum
- Presence of sinus tenderness, swelling
- Discrimination of odors

Throat and Mouth

- Number, occlusion, and condition of teeth; missing teeth; presence of dental appliances
- Characteristics of lips, tongue, buccal and oral mucosa, and floor of mouth (color, moisture, surface characteristics, symmetry, induration)
- Appearance of oropharynx, palate, and tonsils, tonsil size
- Symmetry and movement of tongue, soft palate, and uvula; gag reflex
- Voice quality
- Discrimination of taste

Neck

- Fullness, mobility, suppleness, and strength
- Position of trachea, tracheal tug, movement of hyoid bone and cartilages with swallowing
- Thyroid size, shape, nodules, tenderness, bruits
- Presence of masses, webbing, skinfolds

Chest

- Size and shape of chest, anteroposterior versus transverse diameter, symmetry of movement with respiration, superficial venous patterns
- Tenderness over ribs, bony prominences
- Presence of retractions, use of accessory muscles
- Diaphragmatic excursion

Lungs

- Respiratory rate, depth, regularity, quietness or ease of respiration
- Palpation findings: Symmetry and quality of tactile fremitus
- Percussion findings: quality and symmetry of percussion notes
- Auscultation findings: characteristics of breath sounds (intensity, pitch, duration, quality, vesicular, bronchial, bronchovesicular, adventitious breath sounds), phase and location where audible

* Characteristics of cough, stridor
* Presence of friction rub, egophony, bronchophony, whispered pectoriloquy, vocal resonance

Breasts

* Size, contour, symmetry, supernumerary nipples, venous patterns
* Tissue consistency, presence of masses, scars, tenderness, thickening, retractions or dimpling
* Characteristics of nipples and areolae (inversion, eversion, retraction), discharge

Heart

* Anatomic location of apical impulse, pulsations
* Heart rate, rhythm
* Palpation findings: thrills, heaves, or lifts
* Auscultation findings: characteristics of S_1 and S_2 (location, intensity, pitch, timing, splitting, systole, diastole)
* Presence of murmurs, clicks, snaps, S_3 or S_4. Description by timing, location, radiation, intensity, pitch, quality, variation with respiration

Blood Vessels

* Amplitude, symmetry of pulses in extremities
* Jugular vein pulsations and distention, pressure measurement; jugular vein and carotid artery pulse waves
* Presence of bruits over carotid, temporal, renal, iliac, and femoral arteries, abdominal aorta
* Temperature, color, hair distribution, skin texture, muscle atrophy, nail beds of lower extremities
* Presence of edema, swelling, vein distention, varicosities, circumference of extremities
* Homans sign, tenderness of lower extremities or along superficial vein

Abdomen

* Shape, contour, visible aorta pulsations, surface motion, venous patterns, scars, hernia or separation of muscles, peristalsis
* Auscultation findings: presence and character of bowel sounds in all quadrants, friction rub over liver or spleen
* Palpation findings: aorta, organs, feces, masses; location, size, contour, consistency, tenderness, muscle resistance
* Percussion findings: tone in each quadrant, areas of different percussion notes, costovertebral angle (CVA) tenderness, liver span

Male Genitalia

* Appearance of external genitalia, penis (symmetry, circumcision status, unusual thickening, smegma, color, texture, location and size of urethral opening, discharge), urethral discharge with stripping, lesions, distribution of pubic hair
* Palpation findings: penis, testes, epididymides, vasa deferentia, contour, consistency, tenderness
* Presence of hernia or scrotal swelling, transillumination findings

Female Genitalia

* Appearance of external genitalia and perineum, distribution of pubic hair, tenderness, scarring, discharge, inflammation, irritation, lesions, caruncle, polyps
* Internal examination findings: appearance of vaginal mucosa, cervix (color, position, surface characteristics, shape of os), discharge, odor
* Bimanual examination findings: size, contour, and position of uterus, tenderness and mobility of cervix, uterus, adnexa, and ovaries (size, shape, consistency, tenderness)
* Rectovaginal examination findings
* Urinary incontinence when patient bears down

Anus and Rectum

* Perianal area: appearance, presence of hemorrhoids, fissures, skin tags, pilonidal dimpling, hair tufts, inflammation, excoriation —erosion or destruction of skin by mechanical means
* Rectal wall contour, tenderness, sphincter tone and control
* Prostate size, contour, consistency, mobility
* Color and consistency of stool

Lymphatic System

- Presence of lymph nodes in head, neck, clavicular, epitrochlear, axillary, or inguinal areas
- Size, shape, warmth, tenderness, mobility, consistency (matted or discreteness of nodes)
- Redness or streaks in localized area

Musculoskeletal System

- Posture: alignment of extremities and spine, symmetry of body parts
- Symmetry of muscle mass, tone, fasciculation, spasms
- Range of motion (active and passive)
- Appearance of joints: presence of deformities, tenderness, crepitus, swelling
- Muscle strength

Neurologic System

- Cranial nerves: specific findings for each or specify those tested, if findings are recorded in head and neck sections
- Gait (posture, rhythm, sequence of stride and arm movements)
- Balance, coordination with rapid alternating motions
- Sensory function: presence and symmetry of response to pain, touch, vibration, temperature stimuli; monofilament test
- Superficial and deep tendon reflexes: symmetry, grade, plantar reflex, ankle clonus

ASSESSMENT (FOR EACH PROBLEM ON PROBLEM LIST)

The diagnosis with rationale, derived from the subjective and objective data, is stated. If a diagnosis cannot yet be made, differential diagnoses are prioritized. Assessment includes anticipated potential problems, if appropriate (e.g., complications, progression of disease, sequelae).

PLAN (FOR EACH PROBLEM ON PROBLEM LIST)

- Diagnostic tests performed or ordered
- Therapeutic treatment plan, including changes or additions to the established treatment plan with rationale
- Patient education: health education provided or planned; materials such as handouts/pamphlets dispensed; evidence of patient's understanding (or lack of understanding); counseling
- Referrals initiated (including to whom the patient is referred and the purpose)
- Target dates for reevaluating the results of the plan

INFANTS

The organizational structure for recording the history and physical examination of newborns and infants is the same as for adults. The recorded information varies from the adult's primarily because of the developmental status of the infant. With newborns the focus is on their transition to extrauterine life and the detection of any congenital anomalies. Specific additions to the history and physical examination follow.

History

Present Problem. For older infants, record information as for adults; however, for newborns include the details of the mother's pregnancy and any events occurring since birth.

Details of Pregnancy. Mother's health during pregnancy, age, specific conditions (e.g., hypertension, diabetes, seizures, bleeding, proteinuria, preeclampsia), infectious illnesses (gestational month of infection), radiation exposure, drugs taken.

Prenatal care: weight gained, planned pregnancy, attitude toward pregnancy, duration of pregnancy, use of illicit drugs.

Labor and delivery: spontaneous, induced, duration, analgesia or anesthesia, complications, presentation, forceps, vacuum extraction, vaginal or cesarean section.

Infant's Status at Birth. Birth weight, respiratory status, color, Apgar scores at 1 and 5 minutes if known; newborn's condition and duration of hospital stay, nutrition; congenital anomalies, meconium staining, bilirubin phototherapy, bleeding, convulsions, prescriptions (e.g., antibiotics).

First Month of Life. Jaundice, bleeding, convulsions, other evidence of illness.

Past Medical History. There is no past medical history for newborns. Older infants should have general health and strength, as well as prenatal and neonatal events added to this category, unless this information is directly related to the present problem.

Family History. Focus on number of miscarriages, number of deceased children, congenital anomalies, and hereditary disorders in the family.

Personal and Social History. Focus on the newborn's and infant's family structure, number of siblings, presence of both parents, stresses of new infant in family, arrangements for child care, and mother's plans to return to work.

Growth and Development. Placement of this information is variable by health care facility or according to the purpose of the examination. For the infant with no growth or development problems, it may be recorded as either history or review of systems, or it may be a separate category. When a problem with growth or development is apparent, the information will be recorded in the section for the present problem. Passing or failing of the Denver II would be recorded with objective data.

Developmental Milestones. List developmental milestones with the age at which they are attained (e.g., hold head erect while in sitting position, rolls over front to back and back to front, sits unsupported, stands and walks without support, first words, sentences, dresses self).

Current Motor and Interaction Abilities. Specify current attainments unless the Denver II is used, in which case this information is repetitive.

Injury Prevention. List parents' efforts to consistently prevent injuries.

Diet. Placement of this information varies by health care facility; it may appear in the present illness or review of systems, or it may be a separate category.

Breast-Fed Infants. Note the frequency; use of supplemental feedings and vitamins; mother's diet, fluid intake, concern with milk supply, any problems with nipple soreness, cracking, or infections; age weaned.

Formula-Fed Infants. Note the specific formula and preparation method, concentration and amount of water added, frequency of feeding, amount per feeding, total ounces per day, and whether juice, water, or vitamins are given.

Solid Foods. Note the age at which cereal and other foods were introduced; specifics about feeding methods, amount, food preparation; and the response of infant to foods.

Physical Examination Findings

General
- Age in hours, days, weeks, or months; gender; race
- Gestational age
- Length, weight, BMI, and head circumference with percentiles; for newborns, percentiles for gestational age

Mental Status
- Infant state during examination (irritable, crying, sleeping, alert, quiet)

Skin
- Color, texture, presence of lanugo or vernix, Mongolian spot, nails
- Presence of hemangiomas, nevi, telangiectasia, milia

Lymphatics
- Visible or palpable lymph nodes

Head
- Shape, molding, forceps or electrode marks
- Fontanel size, swelling
- Transillumination

Eyes
- Red reflex, corneal light reflex, follows object with eyes
- Swelling of lids, discharge

Ears
- Shape and alignment of auricles, presence of skin tags or pits
- Startle to noise or response to voice

Nose
- Patency of nares, nasal flaring, discharge

Mouth
- Palate and lip integrity
- Presence and number of teeth
- Strength of sucking, coordinated sucking and swallowing

Neck

◆ Head position, neck control
◆ Presence of masses, webbing, excess skinfolds

Chest and Lungs

◆ Symmetry of shape, circumference
◆ Breast swelling or discharge
◆ Abdominal or thoracic breathing
◆ Presence of retractions (intercostal, supraclavicular, substernal), presence of grunting or stridor
◆ Quality of cry

Heart and Blood Vessels

◆ Recording as for adults, but with peripheral vascular findings integrated in this section

Abdomen

◆ Number of umbilical arteries and veins, stump dryness, color, odor
◆ Any bulging or separation of abdominal wall
◆ Apparent peristaltic waves

Male Genitalia

◆ Appearance of penis, scrotum; position of urethra
◆ Location of testes: descended, descendable, not descended, not palpable
◆ Urinary stream
◆ Presence of hernia or hydrocele

Female Genitalia

◆ Appearance of labia, presence of discharge

Anus, Rectum

◆ Perforate, sphincter control
◆ Character of meconium or stool, if observed
◆ Presence of pilonidal dimple

Musculoskeletal System

◆ Alignment of limbs and spine
◆ Presence of joint deformity, fixed or flexible; integrity of clavicles
◆ Symmetry of movement in all extremities, hip abduction
◆ Number of fingers and toes, webbing or extra digits, palmar creases

Neurologic System

◆ Presence and symmetry of primitive reflexes
◆ Consolability, presence of tremors or jitteriness
◆ Gross and fine motor development

CHILDREN AND ADOLESCENTS

As during infancy, some adaptations in recorded history reflect the developmental progress of the child. Such modifications in recording the child's history are discussed next.

History

Past Medical History. Prenatal and neonatal history is less important as the child gets older. Birth weight and major neonatal problems are generally included in the history of an initial examination until the child reaches school age. If a health problem can be related to birth events, more detail is recorded, often summarized from old records, because the mother's recall may not be as accurate as time elapses.

Personal and Social History. Record how the child gets along with parents, siblings, and other children; his or her behavior in group situations; and any evidence of family problems. Include the principal caretaker, parents' relationship (e.g., married, divorced, separated, single parent, foster parent), education attainment of parents, dependence on relief or social agencies. Describe prevention strategies used by child and family.

For older children, record school performance: grade level, progress, adjustment to school, and parents' attitude toward education. Note any habits of the child, such as nail biting or thumb sucking; note hobbies, sports participation, clubs, and temperament.

For adolescents, add peer group activities, conflicts, sexual activity, alcohol or club/recreational drug use, concerns with identity and independence, self-esteem, favorite activities, type of job, and potential hazards. This may be summarized with the HEEADSSS tool. See Chapter 1.

Growth and Development. For toddlers and young children, list motor skills and language milestones attained, age toilet trained, and age weaned from bottle.

Physical Examination Findings. The physical findings are recorded in the same format used for adults and infants. Some additional notations related to development include the following:

Mental Status. Record mental status and cognitive development status.

Breasts. For females, record the Tanner stage of breast development.

Genitalia. Record the Tanner stage of pubic hair and genital development as appropriate. Record the sexual maturity rating.

Neurologic System. Findings should indicate developmental expectations of cerebellar function, cranial nerves, and deep tendon reflexes.

PREGNANT WOMEN

The organizational structure of the record does not vary from that of other adults; however, information about the pregnancy is added, and some aspects of the examination are modified.

History

History of Present Illness. List the gravidity and parity, last menstrual period, and expected delivery date. Describe details about specific problems such as bleeding or spotting, nausea, vomiting, fatigue, edema, illness, injury, surgery, or exposure to drugs, chemicals, radiation, or infections since conception.

Obstetric History. This additional history category should provide information on previous pregnancies, type of delivery, length of labor, complications in pregnancy, labor, postpartum; weight and gender of newborn; previous abortions.

Menstrual and Gynecologic History. Age at menarche, characteristics of cycle, unusual bleeding, use of contraceptives, sexual history, most recent Pap smear, infertility, exposure to diethylstilbestrol (DES).

Personal and Social History. In addition to the information usually obtained, include the adjustment to the pregnancy by the woman and her significant other, information about whether pregnancy was planned, acceptance by the father and family, any history of abuse, and father's role or other support available to the mother and child after delivery.

Physical Examination Findings

Abdomen
- Status of the pregnancy, fundal height in relation to dates
- Fetal heart rate, position, well-being, movement
- Contractions

Pelvic Region
- Pelvic measurements
- Uterine size
- During late pregnancy and labor: centimeters of dilation and effacement, station of the fetus, position of the fetal head or presenting part
- Leaking of fluid or rupture of membranes

OLDER ADULTS

The organizational structure, again, does not vary from that recorded for other adults. A few modifications in aspects of the history and physical examination are made as described in the following.

History

Personal and Social History. Describe the community and family support systems. Add the functional assessment of ability to prepare meals, manage personal affairs, and engage in social and other meaningful activities. Identify plans for advance directives and power of attorney for health care decisions.

Physical Examination Findings

General Assessment
- Extra time to assume positions for physical examination
- Position modifications needed for specific systems

Mental Status
- Functional assessment of cognitive function, memory, and reasoning and calculation

Skin

- Presence of common lesions of older age
- Turgor, resilience of skin
- Condition and thickness of nails, especially toenails
- Character and color of hair, baldness patterns

Chest and Lungs

- Change in chest shape and percussion tones
- Effect of chest shape on respiratory status

Heart and Blood Vessels

- Location of the apical pulse
- Characteristics of superficial vessels and distal pulses

Musculoskeletal System

- Posture and muscle mass changes
- Functional assessment of mobility and muscle strength

Neurologic System

- Functional assessment of fine motor movements
- Gait and balance, sensation

SAMPLE RECORDS

Information must be recorded as precisely as possible. Colorful language or expressive metaphors can be used, but select words for the patient's history carefully, because some words may have different implications. Health professionals have commonly used the term "denies" when a patient reports that no symptom has occurred. The term "denies" may imply a confrontational or unproductive relationship. It is better to write either "reports no" or "indicates no" symptoms, statements that more positively record the patient's cooperation in providing needed information.

AMBULATORY ADULT

See the sample record for the ambulatory adult.

Name: Martha Smith   **Date:** 11-30-05
Date of Birth: 5-22-1950
History Number: 54970B

PROBLEM LIST:

Problem #	Onset (date)	Problem	Inactive/resolved (date)
1	5/05	Pain and stiffness of hands, bilateral	
2	1995	Seasonal rhinitis	
3	1990	s/p Total abd. hysterectomy with oophorectomy	
4		Family history of diabetes	
5		Family history Alzheimer disease	
6		Family history glaucoma	

General Patient Information

Address: 841 Foxtrail Drive
          St. Louis, MO 63146

Home phone: (314) 555-6423
Social security number: 111-11-1111

Employer: Memorial Hospital

Position/title: Registered Nurse

Business address: 1050 Randolph Ctr.
          St. Louis, MO 63116

Business phone: (314) 747-0000

Age: 55
Gender: Female
Marital status: Married
Language: English, no special communication needs

Health insurance provider: Aetna
Member #: X45789

Continued

SOURCE AND RELIABILITY OF INFORMATION
Self—very reliable historian
Old record

CHIEF COMPLAINT
Time for annual examination. Has noticed pain in hands when doing needlework.

HISTORY OF PRESENT PROBLEM
Pain and stiffness in fingers and hands, began about 6 months ago but seems to be increasing in severity and with shorter time of activity. Dull, aching pain now occurs after 15 minutes of needlepoint or crocheting, right hand more than left hand. Pain ranges between 2 and 4 on a 10-point severity scale. Usually resolves with rest. Some stiffness in morning but does not currently interfere with ability to perform all job and household activities. Uses aspirin (650 mg every 4 hr) when pain does not resolve with rest; effective relief. Has not tried heat or ice. No other systemic symptoms such as fatigue, fever, or weight loss. No other joints affected. Has read about glucosamine and is considering trying it.

PAST MEDICAL HISTORY
Generally healthy
Hospitalizations, Illnesses, and Injuries. Hysterectomy for fibroids in 1990, usual childhood illnesses, no major adult illnesses, car crash 1995 without major injury.
Previous Health Care. Annual physical, hepatitis B vaccine series 2 years ago, Td booster 5 years ago, oral polio vaccine series in 1976, dental care every 4 months, vision exam every year. Pap smear and mammogram 6 months ago with no problems detected, 2 pregnancies (1972 and 1975), both vaginal delivery without complications.
Allergies. Hay fever in spring, no food or drug allergies known.
Family History. See pedigree below. No history of cancer, tuberculosis, blood dyscrasias, or respiratory, renal, thyroid, or psychiatric disorders.

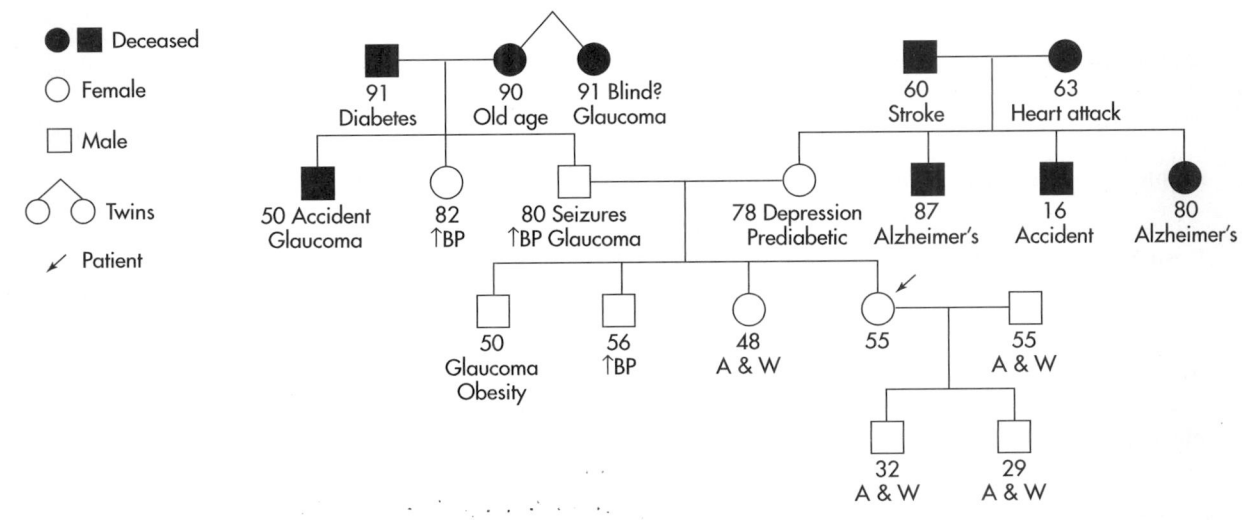

PERSONAL/SOCIAL HISTORY

Lives with husband, a psychologist in private practice, in 3-bedroom home in well-maintained neighborhood. Works as RN in hospital clinic 3 days a week. Has 2 sons, both married with 2 children each. Visits each at least once a month. Both parents still living, in retirement home in town, visits them 2 or 3 times a week. Active in church and local arts and crafts group. Needlepoint and quilting main hobbies.

Current Health Habits. Walks dog daily about ½ mile; 15 lb weight gain in last 2 years, tries dieting, loses a few pounds and then stops; no smoking or recreational drug use, 2 to 3 glasses of wine on weekends, 2 to 3 cups coffee and 1 glass iced tea daily.

Diet/Nutrition. Would like to lose 15 lb; currently 150 lb, 5'5"; diets sporadically; uses 1200 calorie diabetic exchange lists, usually has desired results when she persists, losing approximately 8 lb in 4 weeks; does own grocery shopping and cooking; rarely fries foods; binges on ice cream when traveling; eats in restaurants 2 to 3 times a week.

REVIEW OF SYSTEMS

General Constitutional Symptoms. No fever, chills, malaise; would like to lose 15 lb gained over past 2 years.

Skin, Hair, and Nails. Several flat nevi, no change in appearance noted; bathes daily without special skin preparations; washes hair once a week, permanent and colored; nails short, crack and split frequently.

Head and Neck. Periodic headaches, no more than once a month, related to tension, pain up neck and back of head, relieved by aspirin. No neck tenderness or stiffness currently, has had muscle spasm in past, some pain with car crash 10 years ago, no enlarged lymph nodes noted.

Eyes. Wears glasses for reading; no pain, swelling, tearing, or halos around lights. Sees optometrist yearly.

Ears. No change in hearing noted; no dizziness, sensitivity to noise, or pain; some pressure and popping in ears when hay fever symptoms occur; resolves with Allerest.

Nose and Sinuses. Hay fever in spring, postnasal drip, no problem with sense of smell. Uses Allerest for hay fever as needed.

Mouth and Throat. No sore throats, hoarseness, change in voice, no dental appliances, no difficulty eating or chewing food, brushes and flosses daily.

Breasts. No pain, tenderness, or nipple discharge; breast self-exam done when she remembers, about every 2 months; mammogram 6 months ago revealed no masses; no history of masses.

Cardiovascular. No difficulty performing regular activities, no shortness of breath or chest pain, last BP 126/82, no pain, tenderness, discoloration, temperature change, or swelling in extremities; wears support hose for work, some varicose veins.

Chest and Lungs. No history of asthma, bronchitis, or pneumonia; no breathing difficulties, cough, or pain. PPD at work 3 months ago, negative.

Endocrine. No history of changes in thyroid, skin, hair, or temperature preference; no polydipsia or polyuria; takes no estrogen replacement therapy; hot flashes about twice a day cause no distress.

Hematologic. No bleeding, excess bruising, anemia.

Lymphatic. No known lymph node enlargement.

Gastrointestinal. No diarrhea, constipation, blood in stool, or emesis; has bowel movement every other day, brown, formed, no pain; hemorrhoids during pregnancies only; indigestion occasionally after eating fried or rich foods, resolves with Gelusil. Uses no laxatives, tries to add bulk to daily food intake.

Genitourinary. Voids 5 or 6 times a day, light yellow, no change in odor or color, no complaint of nocturia or dysuria, good control of stream, no stress incontinence; no history of sexually transmitted infection; no known genital lesions, discharge, pain, itching, dyspareunia; satisfied with sexual activity, about twice a month.

painful sexual inter course

Continued

Musculoskeletal. No weakness, twitching, or pain other than in hands; no history of backache, fracture.

Neurologic. No problems with walking, balance, or sensations; no known changes in cognitive functioning; expresses concern with family history of Alzheimer disease and her possibility of developing the disorder.

Mental Status and Psychiatric. Coping well with stress of older parents requiring increasing care; no history of long-term depression; gets depressed and anxious occasionally about growing old, but feels this does not interfere with her ability to work or lead a productive life.

PHYSICAL EXAMINATION

General. 55-year-old white female, alert, cooperative, well groomed, communicates well, makes eye contact, and expresses appropriate concern throughout history.

      T 98.4° F, P 72, R 18

      BP 130/76 sitting L arm, 134/80 supine L arm, 132/78 sitting R arm

      Wt 66.2 kg (150 lb), Ht 165 cm (5 ft 5 in), about 50th percentile weight for height, medium frame,

      BMI = 25.0

Mental Status. Oriented to time, place, and person; reasoning and arithmetic calculations intact. Memory intact, Mini-mental score = 30; speech clear, smoothly enunciated; comprehends directions.

Skin, Hair, and Nails. Pink, soft, moist, turgor with instant recoil, no lesions, tenderness, or edema; nail beds pink without clubbing, uniform thickness; nails smooth, firmly adhered to nail bed, brisk capillary refill; hair with silky texture, thinning on crown, female distribution.

Head. Head erect and midline; scalp pink, freely movable without lesions or tenderness; well-spaced, symmetric facial features. Temporal arteries soft, nontender, no bruits.

Eyes. Brows, lids, and lashes evenly distributed; no tearing; conjunctivae pink without discharge; pupils react equally to light and accommodation; extraocular movements intact, no lid lag, no nystagmus; visual field equals examiner's, corneal light reflex equal bilaterally, red reflex present, discs cream colored with well-defined border bilaterally; arterial-venous ratio 2:5, no crossing changes noted; cornea, lens, and vitreous clear; retina pink, no hemorrhages or exudates; macula yellow; Snellen 20/20 each eye without glasses; near vision 20/40 each eye without glasses, 20/20 with glasses.

Ears. Auricles in proper alignment, without lesions, masses, or tenderness; canals with small amount dry cerumen; tympanic membranes gray, translucent, light reflex and bony landmarks present; no perforations. Rinne—air conduction > bone conduction bilaterally; Weber—no lateralization, repeats whispered words at 2 ft bilaterally.

Nose and Sinuses. No flaring of nares, septum slightly to left of midline, patent bilaterally, mucosa pink and moist, no polyps or discharge; correctly identified coffee, chocolate, and orange odors bilaterally; no frontal or maxillary sinus tenderness with palpation.

Throat and Mouth. Buccal mucosa pink and moist, no lesions, salivary glands nontender; 28 teeth in good repair, no movement; teeth 1, 16, 17, and 32 missing; gingivae slightly erythematous and spongy; tongue in midline without fibrillation, no lesions; uvula midline with elevation of soft palate; gag reflex intact; pharynx without erythema; no hoarseness; correctly identified sweet, salty, and sour tastes bilaterally.

Neck. Trachea midline, no tracheal tug, thyroid and cartilages move with swallowing, thyroid lateral borders palpable, no enlargement or nodules noted, lymph nodes nonpalpable, full range of motion and appropriate strength.

Chest and Lungs. AP diameter less than lateral with 1:2 ratio; muscle and respiratory effort symmetric without use of accessory muscles; inspiration-to-expiration ratio is 1:1; tactile fremitus symmetric; resonant percussion throughout; 4 cm excursion bilaterally; vesicular breath sounds throughout without adventitious sounds; even, quiet breathing.

Breasts. Moderate size, L slightly larger than R, nodular, granular consistency bilaterally, no masses palpated; nipples erect without discharge; areolas symmetric with Montgomery tubercles; no palpable axillary nodes; no dimpling, venous patterns symmetric.

Heart. Apical impulse barely palpable at 5th intercostal space, 4 cm from midsternal line, no heaves, lifts, or thrills, S_1 and S_2 heard without splitting, no murmurs, S_1 heard best at apex, S_2 heard best at base, apical impulse timed with radial pulse, no visible pulsations, no audible S_3, S_4, or murmur.

Blood Vessels. Pulse regular rhythm, smooth contour, no pulse deficit; jugular venous pulsation visible at sternal angle with 30-degree elevation; no carotid, renal, or abdominal bruits; no edema, swelling, or tenderness in lower extremities; Homans sign negative; lower extremities warm, pink with symmetric hair distribution; superficial varicosities in lower extremities, L leg more than R.

PULSE AMPLITUDE

	C	B	R	F	P	DP
L	2+	2+	2+	2+	2+	1+
R	2+	2+	2+	2+	2+	1+

Abdomen. Soft, rounded, faded 12-cm scar from umbilicus to symphysis pubis; aorta midline with no visible pulsation, no bruit; bowel sounds heard in all quadrants; tympanic percussion tones over epigastrium, remainder dull to percussion; liver span 6 cm at R midclavicular line by percussion; spleen percussed at L midaxillary line; liver, spleen, and kidney not palpable; no tenderness on palpation; no CVA tenderness; superficial abdominal reflexes intact.

Genital/Rectal. Deferred. Gyn exam 6 months ago.

Lymphatic. No palpable lymph nodes in neck, supraclavicular, axillary, epitrochlear, or inguinal areas.

Musculoskeletal. Heberden nodes at distal interphalangeal joints on both hands; good mobility of hands but tenderness when making a tight fist bilaterally; no swelling, heat, or erythema noted. Remainder of muscles appear symmetric, muscle strength appropriate and equal bilaterally, full range of active and passive motion, spine and extremities in good alignment, slight kyphosis.

Neurologic. Coordinated, smooth gait; negative Romberg sign; balance, rapid alternating movements, sensory functioning, and cranial nerves I-XII grossly intact; plantar flexion of toes bilaterally with plantar reflex, no clonus.

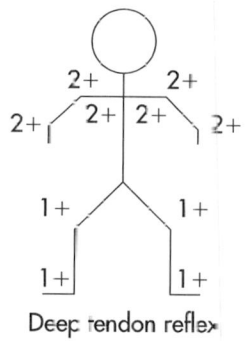

Deep tendon reflex
response

Continued

ASSESSMENT PLAN

Problem #1: Pain and stiffness in both hands

Assessment: Degenerative arthritis is the most likely diagnosis. This is supported by presence of Heberden nodes bilaterally and lack of systemic signs, which could suggest an inflammatory process. Pain is well controlled with aspirin. Since noninflammatory symptoms are evident, analgesia could be achieved with acetaminophen with less risk of gastrointestinal side effects. Plan to monitor liver enzymes at next visit. Glucosamine may help retard degeneration.

Dx Tests: None at present

Rx: Acetaminophen 325 mg, 2 tabs every 4 hr as needed, glucosamine, 500 mg 3 times a day for 3-month trial

Pt Ed: Discuss suspected pathophysiologic process of degenerative joint disease (DJD). Reassure that DJD pain can usually be successfully controlled with mild analgesics. Avoid use of alcohol with use of acetaminophen. If desired, use glucosamine for 3 months to see if effective. Recommend trials of heat and ice to augment analgesia. Return to clinic if increased signs/symptoms, any associated redness, swelling, or heat.

Problem #2: Seasonal rhinitis

Assessment: Mild nasal stuffiness every spring secondary to pollen exposure. Well controlled on nonprescription antihistamine/decongestant preparation.

Dx Tests: None at present

Rx: None at present

Pt Ed: Stay indoors as much as possible when pollen counts are elevated. If nonprescription agent does not control signs/symptoms, may try nonsedating antihistamine. Warned about sedating properties of many nonprescription preparations. Discussed increased risk of sinusitis when turbinates swell. To return to clinic if fever, facial pain, purulent nasal discharge develops.

Problem #3: s/p total abdominal hysterectomy (TAH)

Assessment: TAH with bilateral oophorectomy performed 1990 for fibroids per patient. Patient never supplemented with estrogen replacement therapy (ERT). Pt not symptomatic with hot flashes, but is at increased risk for osteoporosis and coronary heart disease (CHD). Will complete baseline evaluations and develop plan with patient.

Dx Tests: Baseline bone density test, fasting cholesterol and lipid profile

Rx: Ca supplement (nonprescription) as augment to diet to ensure 1500 mg Ca per day, Vit D 400 mg orally each day

Pt Ed: Discuss increased risk of CHD and osteoporosis secondary to early surgical menopause. Increase weight-bearing exercise. Will discuss individual plan after obtaining baseline studies.

Problem #4: Family history of diabetes

Assessment: No symptomatic evidence of hyperglycemia. Slightly obese.

Dx Tests: Fasting serum glucose, urinalysis

Rx: None at present

Pt Ed: Benefit of weight loss, goal to reach ideal body weight to avoid insulin insensitivity. Moderate exercise 3 or 4 times a week.

Problem #5: Family history of Alzheimer disease

Assessment: No evidence of cognitive deficit at present.

Dx Tests: None

Rx: None

Pt Ed: Return to clinic if memory problems or other cognitive difficulties develop.

Problem #6: Family history of glaucoma

Assessment: Sees optometrist on yearly basis. Will obtain latest tonometry screening values. No visual changes or objective signs of increased eye pressures.

Dx Tests: None

Rx: None

Pt Ed: Discuss importance of yearly glaucoma screening as glaucoma is a preventable cause of blindness. To report visual changes, eye pain immediately.

Progress Note Sample Write-Up. The patient in the previous POMR returns 2 months later (see the sample of a progress note).

SUBJECTIVE

cc: Pain in hands increasing

Since last seen in clinic, patient has noted more stiffness in hands each AM and pain with needlework after only 10 minutes. Pain relieved with acetaminophen but stiffness lasts several hours. Tried glucosamine for 3 months, but no improvement. Joint stiffness interfering with fine motor skills. No other joint involvement, fever, weight loss, swelling, redness, or heat of involved joints. No analgesic used today.

OBJECTIVE

T 98.2° F, P 88 reg, R 12 unlabored, BP 130/78, L arm supine

Extremities: Heberden nodes in distal interphalangeal joints bilaterally. Bouchard nodes in proximal interphalangeal joints right hand. No swelling or heat present. Mild tenderness to palpation of joints of 2nd digits bilat. Limitation of flexion in R hand, cannot make first without pain. No tenderness, heat, limited motion of other joints.

ASSESSMENT

Degenerative arthritis both hands, exacerbated by needlework and sewing. Will attempt to decrease symptoms with NSAID and rest of affected joints for 2 weeks. No contraindications to nonsteroidals evident. Consider extended-action NSAID.

PLAN

Dx Tests: None.

Rx: Ibuprofen 400 mg 4 times a day for 2-wk trial, then reduce dosage to ibuprofen 200 mg 4 times a day

Pt Ed: Medication schedule, warn of possibility of GI upset. May take meds with food. Discontinue glucosamine. To defer needlework and sewing until symptoms better controlled. Encouraged to try nonpharmacologic therapies (ice, heat) as degenerative joint disease is a chronic process. Return to clinic if no improvement or if symptoms worsen.

INFANT   See the sample record for an infant.

Name: Tom Mitchell   **Date:** 11-3-05
Date of Birth: 3-25-05
History Number: 49076M

PROBLEM LIST:

Problem #	Onset (date)	Problem	Inactive/resolved (date)

General Patient Information

Address: 749 Delta Circle, Apt. 5   **Home phone:** (410) 555-9307
         Baltimore, MD 21205   **Social security number:** 222-22-2222

Parent/Guardian's name: Anne Mitchell

Age: 7 months   **Health insurance provider:** Kaiser Permanente
Gender: Male   **Member #:** M57143

SOURCE AND RELIABILITY OF INFORMATION
Mother, reliable historian
Language: English, no special communication needs

CHIEF COMPLAINT
Needs immunizations.

PRESENT PROBLEM
No illnesses or concerns at present. Cold last month resolved without fever or sequelae. Overdue for third series of shots.

PAST MEDICAL HISTORY
Prenatal: Full-term infant, birth weight 7 lb 9 oz, 21 in, mother healthy throughout pregnancy, no x-ray examinations, prescription drugs, or health problems. Began care in third month, vaginal vertex delivery after 10 hours labor, spinal anesthesia, awake for delivery, baby breathed immediately, in regular nursery, home with mother on next day.
Health Care: Has attended well baby clinic since birth, goes to Dr. Green or hospital clinic for illness. DTaP-6-1-05, 8-8-05; IPV 6-1-05, 8-8-05; HIB 6-1-05, 8-8-05; HBV 4-10-05, 6-1-05, PCV 6-1-05, 8-8-05.

DIET/NUTRITION
Breast-fed since birth, feeds 3 times a day, uses supplemental feeding of Similac, 8 oz, 2 times a day in effort to begin weaning, seems content. Started cereal and fruit at 4 months of age, vegetables at 6 months of age, now introducing meat. Takes about 2 Tbsp each of cereal and fruit in AM and 2 Tbsp each of vegetable and meat in PM. Takes 3 oz juice and 3 oz water and teething cookies a day. Eats eagerly. Given ADC vitamins with iron.

PERSONAL/SOCIAL
Lives with parents and 4-year-old brother in 2-bedroom apartment, inner city neighborhood but parents concerned about increasing violence. Father employed as machinist, mother worked as secretary until Tom's birth, to return to work part time next week in temporary secretarial pool. Maternal GM to care for Tom during day while mother works. Lives close to grandparents, many family events, attends church fairly regularly. Money has been tight for last few months, but family has met major expenses. Tom was planned child, has been pleasure to family, some sibling rivalry with older son, father helps occasionally in care of infant, more in care of older son.

FAMILY HISTORY
Grandparents all living: maternal GF 55 years with hypertension, maternal GM 51 years A & W, paternal GF 60 years with myocardial infarction 2 years ago, paternal GM 58 with hypertension; mother 32 years and father 34 years, both healthy; aunts and uncles A & W, 1 brother 4 years of old with asthma. No known diabetes, cancer, tuberculosis, renal, seizure, psychiatric, or hereditary disorders.

GROWTH AND DEVELOPMENT
Sitting without support for 2 weeks, reaches for objects, passes object hand to hand, babbles and coos, has started scooting on floor, rolled over at 3 months.

REVIEW OF SYSTEMS
General. Happy infant, easy temperament, cries only when hungry or wet.
Skin, Hair, and Nails. Slight jaundice after birth, never enough to be treated; birthmark on back; fingernails fully formed.
Head and Neck. Holds head up well, turns head in all directions.
Eyes. Seems to follow mother around room with eyes; no crossed eyes noted; no tearing, redness, or discharge noted.
Ears. No infections, turns head toward loud noise or family member speaking.
Nose. One cold with clear to whitish discharge from nose, lasted 1 week, saw doctor, given nose drops and Triaminic Syrup.
Mouth and Throat. 2 front teeth, teething now, no difficulty sucking or swallowing.
Chest and Lungs. No problems breathing, noisy breathing with cold.
Cardiovascular. No known heart murmur, has never turned blue, does not tire easily with feeding, no excess perspiration.
Hematologic/Immunologic. No bleeding, bruises, no known anemia, has had only 1 cold, no swollen glands.
Gastrointestinal. No vomiting or diarrhea; spits up small amount of milk after feeding formula; bowel movement 2 times a day, light brown, mushy.
Genitourinary. Circumcised; strong urine stream, 10 wet or dirty diapers a day, no odor to urine; had hydrocele at birth, not noted 2 months ago.
Musculoskeletal. Moves all extremities, stands with support, left foot turned in at birth, seems straight now.
Neurologic. No seizures or tremors noted.

Continued

PHYSICAL EXAMINATION FINDINGS

General. 7-month-old black male, alert, happy, playful, responsive, and easily consoled by mother.

> T 37.1°C, P 100, R 26, BP 90/62 L arm by Doppler
>
> Wt 9.0 kg, 75%; length 70 cm, 50%; head circ. 45 cm, 75%

Skin. Soft, smooth, light brown, good turgor, mongolian spot over buttocks, café au lait spot 2 cm × 4 cm over R scapula, no lesions, nail beds pink.

Head. Normocephalic, anterior fontanel 1 cm × 2 cm, flat, posterior fontanel closed, scalp without lesions, sparse fine hair, facial features symmetric, well spaced.

Eyes. Conjunctivae pink without discharge, no excess tearing, PERRLA, follows object with eyes 180 degrees, no epicanthal folds, blinks to bright light, corneal light reflex symmetric, red reflex present bilaterally, discs visualized with clear margins, retina pink.

Ears. Auricles well formed, appropriate alignment with outer eye canthus; tympanic membranes pink, light reflex and bony landmarks present, mobile bilaterally; turns head to noise and mother's voice.

Nose. No discharge, nasal mucosa pink, nares patent bilaterally.

Mouth and Throat. Buccal mucosa pink and moist; 2 lower incisors present, 2 upper incisors erupting; palate intact, uvula midline and soft palate rises symmetrically with crying, pharynx without erythema; drooling saliva, sucks and swallows well.

Neck. Trachea midline; thyroid not palpable; supple, full passive range of motion; no palpable masses.

Chest and Lungs. Symmetric shape and expansion with respiration, no retractions, equal fremitus with crying, lungs clear to auscultation, even smooth respirations.

Heart and Blood Vessels. Apical impulse at 4th ICS, 3 cm from midsternal line; no heaves or thrills; S_1 heard loudest at apex, S_2 heard loudest at base, splitting of S_2 with inspiration, no murmurs; radial and femoral pulses strong and equal.

Abdomen. Soft, nontender, rounded, umbilical ring open 2 cm with hernia, bowel sounds heard all quadrants, liver palpable 1 cm below right costal margin at R midclavicular line, spleen and kidney not palpable, no other masses palpable, percussion note over epigastrium tympanic dullness over remainder of abdomen.

Genitalia. Circumcised, urethral opening on tip of glans, both testes descended, no hernia or hydrocele noted, voids with good stream, urine pale yellow.

Anus and Rectum. Adequate sphincter control, no fissures or cracks.

Lymphatic. Few shotty anterior cervical lymph nodes, 1 cm in diameter, no other lymph nodes palpable.

Musculoskeletal. Spine and extremities in alignment, full hip abduction bilaterally, muscle development symmetric, slight inward twisting of tibia bilaterally, weight bearing with support, 5 digits each hand and foot, all palmar creases present.

Neurologic. Strong grasp, suck, head control; patellar and biceps deep tendon reflexes 2+ and plantar reflex toes ↑↑ bilaterally, no clonus, cranial nerves II-XII intact; Denver II age-appropriate tasks passed.

ASSESSMENT

Healthy 7-month-old needing immunizations.

Mild internal tibial torsion, bilateral.

Umbilical hernia.

MANAGEMENT PLAN

DTaP #3, IPV #3, HIB #3, HBV #3, PCV #3, Influenza #1

Hematocrit and hemoglobin

Anticipatory guidance: nutrition, safety, fostering growth and development, shoes

Reevaluate tibial torsion and umbilical hernia at 12 months of age

EPISODIC NOTE SAMPLE WRITE-UP

In the following sample of an episodic note write-up, the patient is not known to you or the facility.

Name: Aretha Jones   **Date:** 12/07/05
ID: 6789
Patient identification: 21-year-old black female

SUBJECTIVE

cc. "Cold for 2 weeks"

HPI. Patient was well until 2 weeks ago when she developed intermittent nasal congestion and clear watery nasal discharge while at work during the day. Four days later, a dry cough developed, which became productive of small amounts of yellow sputum 1 week ago. Cough is more productive and copious on awakening in the AM. Nasal congestion clears within 1 hour of awakening. Has taken no nonprescription medications, no other therapeutic measures to relieve symptoms. No shortness of breath, dyspnea on exertion, hemoptysis, wheezing, facial pain, sore throat, ear pain, ear congestion, fever, chills, myalgias, or arthralgias.

Current Medications. Oral contraceptives for 4 years, daily multivitamin with iron

PMH. No history of asthma, heart disease, diabetes, seasonal allergies or frequent URIs, T & A age 3 for "frequent strep throats"

Social History. Full-time nursing student, doing well in college, lives in dorm with smoking roommate, patient has never smoked or used club/recreational drugs. Drinks 1 to 2 beers each weekend. CAGE negative.

OBJECTIVE

T 99.2° F, P 92 regular, R 12 unlabored, BP 118/68, L arm supine, no acute distress

Head. No sinus tenderness elicited with palpation

Eyes. Conjunctiva clear, no injection or exudate

Ears. Canals clear. TMs pearly gray, intact, with normal light reflex. Bony landmarks visible; there is no injection, exudate, or retraction evident.

Nose. Turbinates, red and moderately edematous. Discharge clear.

Throat. Pharynx mildly infected, tonsils surgically absent, no exudates or postnasal drip.

Neck. No palpable adenopathy in anterior, posterior triangles, submental, postauricular, or supraclavicular regions.

Chest. Chest symmetrical without deformities, percussion is resonant in all lung fields. Tactile fremitus equal bilaterally, diaphragm moves 4 cm with deep inspiration. Scattered rhonchi bilaterally that clear completely with cough leaving vesicular breath sounds all fields. No crackles or wheezes audible.

ASSESSMENT

Viral bronchitis: No evidence of respiratory compromise or systemic symptoms (fever, chills). Patient has no history of asthma and is a nonsmoker. She will therefore be treated symptomatically unless symptoms worsen or purulent sputum production lasts in excess of 3 weeks. Chest x-ray is not indicated at this time.

PLAN

Dx Tests: None

Rx: Increase hydration to a minimum of 10 glasses noncaffeinated liquids/day

Pt Ed: Discuss pathophysiology of assessed disease process. Promote respiratory hygiene: avoid smoke-filled environments. Call or return to clinic if symptoms do not improve in 1 week, if develops fever, chills, myalgias, ear pain, facial pain.

SUMMARY

As you begin to examine patients, it is often difficult to determine how to cluster information that will lead to a diagnosis. As a result, all collected information is initially part of the puzzle. With experience, you will be able to identify appropriate groupings of information, enabling you to better organize and synthesize the raw data. Your first attempts to write a complete history and physical examination will be lengthy and perhaps disorganized, but clinical experience will eventually lead to a more concise and organized record.

EMERGENCY OR LIFE-THREATENING SITUATIONS

An emergency situation, whether it be unresponsiveness, an acute medical condition, drug intoxication, or trauma, demands alterations in the usual sequence of history taking and examination. Life-threatening conditions must be rapidly identified and managed (Table 27-1). The steps to achieve this should take seconds, not minutes. Patients are assessed and treatment priorities established based on the physiologic condition and the stability of vital signs rather than on a specific diagnosis. A logical, sequential priority system must be implemented to provide an overall assessment of the patient. The Committee on Trauma of the American College of Surgeons and, in particular, its Subcommittee on Advanced Trauma Life Support have defined an approach for treating trauma patients that is applicable in other emergency situations. It is presented here in modified form.

The patient's vital functions must be determined quickly and efficiently through a rapid primary assessment with resuscitation of vital functions as necessary, followed by a more detailed secondary assessment. Only then is the initiation of definitive care begun. A primary survey involves a rapid assessment of the patient's physiologic status performed in a sequence known as the ABCs (*A*irway, *B*reathing, *C*irculation). It is worth noting that the terminology for the steps of the assessment process varies among professionals and with the continuing refinement of the specialty. O'Keefe et al (1998), for example, use initial assessment, focused history and physical examination, detailed physical examination, and ongoing assessment as guideposts in the process for emergency medical technicians.

THE ABCs OF PRIMARY ASSESSMENT

During the primary assessment, life-threatening conditions are identified, and simultaneous management is begun as soon as a problem is detected:

A   Airway assessment and management with cervical spine (C-spine) control is performed.
B   Breathing (ventilatory ability) is assessed and assisted ventilation is provided as needed.
C   Circulation is assessed and hemorrhage controlled or IV fluids are started as needed.
D   Disability (neurologic status) is assessed in terms of the patient's degree of responsiveness.
E   Exposure: Undress the patient as much as possible when trauma is apparent or suspected to identify all injuries. Do not hesitate to cut clothing away.

The immediate goal is to identify such life-threatening conditions as an airway obstruction, impaired ventilation and hypoxemia, hypovolemic shock, and hemorrhage. The primary assessment is interrupted to manage a life-threatening condition as soon as it is detected. Once the condition is stabilized, the primary assessment is continued. Repeat the primary assessment every 5 minutes during an emergency because physiologic status may change rapidly.

TABLE 27-1	Signs and Symptoms of Certain Life-Threatening Conditions		
	Definition	**Causes**	**Signs and Symptoms**
Upper airway obstruction	Compromise of airway space, resulting in impaired respiratory exchange	Foreign body Infection (e.g., epiglottitis) Tumor (e.g., goiter) Trauma Smoke inhalation Aspiration of chemicals (e.g., hydrocarbons)	Patient grasps neck Fatigue Severe dyspnea Tachypnea Stridor Hoarseness Dysphagia Sore throat Drooling Extreme anxiety Tripod positioning

Hypovolemic shock	Loss of fluid from intravascular space, resulting in inadequate tissue perfusion	Gastrointestinal bleeding
		Hemorrhage (trauma)
		Dehydration
		  Gastrointestinal fluid loss
		  Renal fluid loss
		  Cutaneous fluid loss (e.g., burns, perspiration)
		Internal fluid loss
		Ascites
			Anxiety
			Pallor
			Diaphoresis
			Oliguria
			Coma (alteration in mental status)
			Circulatory collapse
			Tachycardia
			Hypotension
			Delayed capillary refill

Hypoxemia	Severely reduced blood oxygen levels in major organs resulting from respiratory distress, poor tissue perfusion, ventilatory failure, or severe lung injury with increased permeability of alveoli	Aspiration
		Trauma (CNS)
		Increased intracranial pressure
		Drug overdose
		Disseminated intravascular coagulation
		Infection
		Toxins
		  Smoke
		  Volatile chemicals
		Shock
		Severe trauma
		Inadequate ventilation
		Upper airway obstruction
		Lower airway obstruction
		  Asthma
		  Chronic infection
		  Emphysema
		  Cystic fibrosis
			Severe dyspnea
			Cyanosis (pallor, mottling)
			Altered mental status (lethargy to coma; anxiety, combativeness may precede lethargy)
			Tachypnea
			Tachycardia

Status epilepticus	Seizures of any type that are protracted and recurrent without recovery of consciousness	Associated with a variety of epilepsies of uncertain cause: Convulsive types of every variety, generalized or partial Nonconvulsive types of every variety, petit mal or absence, psychomotor, or complex partial	Obvious convulsive movements with unresponsiveness when prolonged as much as 60 minutes Hypotension Cardiac dysrhythmias Fever
Status asthmaticus	A severe and prolonged asthma attack resisting usual therapeutic approaches; asthma itself characterized by dyspnea and wheezing, the result of widespread narrowing of the intrapulmonary airways; airways then defined as hyperreactive	A variety of physical, chemical, and pharmacologic stimuli	History of dyspnea and increasing use of medication over a period of many days Ability to get only a few words out between breaths Tachycardia (often more than 130 beats/min) Tachypnea (may be variable) Hypertension Dyspnea Hypoxemia Wheezing (unless airflow is so diminished that it obscures wheezing) Pulsus paradoxus greater than 20 mm Hg

Continued

TABLE 27-1	Signs and Symptoms of Certain Life-Threatening Conditions—cont'd			
	Definition	**Causes**		**Signs and Symptoms**
Increased intracranial pressure	The skull, a closed space, limits expansion of brain tissue or fluid (blood or CSF) volume, resulting in rising pressure with trauma or disease processes	Tumor or head trauma	Increased brain volume or mass	Headache (be especially wary with a child younger than 10 or 11 years); watch for Cushing triad, a drop in pulse rate, rising blood pressure, and irregular respirations, even Cheyne-Stokes
		Subdural or epidural hematoma Hypoxia Hypercapnia Vasodilators	Increased blood volume	Changes in mental status Lethargy Irritability Slowed responsiveness In severe circumstance, somnolence, stupor, coma
		Tumor Infection Seizures Anatomic defect	Increased CSF volume (hydrocephalus)	Seizures Syncope Meningismus Retinal hemorrhages Papilledema Cranial nerve palsy, particularly VI (abducens paralysis)
Ventilatory failure (i.e., hypercapnic respiratory failure)	Compromised exhalation of carbon dioxide because of alveolar hypoventilation	Upper airway obstruction Neurologic disorders Central nervous system compromise Drug overdose Increased intracranial pressure Upper cervical spinal cord involving third to fifth nerve roots serving diaphragm roots serving diaphragm Injury Phrenic nerve paralysis Neuromuscular disease Guillain-Barré disease (acute polyneuritis) Chest wall compromise Severe kyphoscoliosis Trauma with "flail chest" Pulmonary contusion		Apprehension, confusion Headache, occasionally; somnolence to coma (may be quite subtle if the process is chronic) Patient complaint of respiratory distress Slowed respiratory rate Paradoxic respiration

A secondary assessment is an in-depth, head-to-toe examination to identify anatomic problems, additional conditions that are potentially life-threatening, and the patient's previously diagnosed condition. This assessment begins only after all life-threatening conditions have been stabilized. The assessment is also interrupted for repeated primary assessment and if any life-threatening condition develops. In cases of trauma the secondary assessment is intended to identify the full range of injuries, with particular focus on body systems affected by the mechanism of injury.

Special procedures required for patient assessment, such as peritoneal lavage, radiologic evaluation, and laboratory studies, are also conducted during this secondary phase. Assessment of the eyes, ears, nose, mouth, rectum, and pelvis should not be neglected. This examination requires "tubes and fingers in every orifice."

PRIMARY ASSESSMENT

The primary assessment should be completed very rapidly and, with a stable patient, may take only 30 seconds. It may, however, take several minutes when the mechanism of injury leads you to suspect underlying critical conditions. The historical information obtained during the primary assessment is generally limited to the chief complaint.

Airway and Cervical Spine. The patency of the upper airway is assessed at the start by asking the patient a question. If the patient answers, this is a sign that the airway is open at this time (Box 27-1). It also gives some assurance at this point about the level of responsiveness. Keep the patient talking so that you know the airway is maintained.

If the patient does not respond, place your ear close to the patient's nose and mouth to detect any air movement (Fig. 27-1). Look for any blood, vomitus, teeth, or other foreign bodies that may be obstructing the airway. If the patient is supine, use a chin lift or jaw thrust to raise the tongue (the most common cause of airway obstruction) out of the oropharynx (Fig. 27-2). Remove blood, vomitus, or foreign bodies from the airway by suction. Endotracheal intubation is sometimes needed to control the airway.

In cases of actual or suspected trauma above the clavicle, it is necessary to control the cervical spine when performing any airway maneuvers or patient movement. Excessive movement of the cervical spine can convert a fracture or dislocation without neurologic damage to one with neurologic injury. The patient's head and neck, therefore, should never be hyperextended or hyperflexed to establish or maintain an airway. Control the cervical spine by manually maintaining the neck in a neutral position, in alignment with the body (Fig. 27-3). Neurologic examination alone does not eliminate the possibility of cervical spine injury. Ultimately, appropriate x-ray films of all seven cervical vertebrae must be obtained.

Breathing. Expose the patient's chest to assess ventilatory effort. Note the approximate rate and depth of respirations. Taking the time to count the respiratory rate is not generally appropriate during the primary survey. Bilateral chest movement should be synchronized with breathing. Use the stethoscope to assess the presence of breath sounds. Note any signs of res-

---

CLINICAL PEARL

A Reminder for Resuscitation

Airway management, assisted ventilation and chest compression, and other life-saving modalities for patient care should be initiated when the problem is identified, rather than after completion of the assessment.

BOX 27-1

ASSESSMENT OF AIRWAY PATENCY

Sources of Obstruction
- Foreign body
- Trauma: blunt or penetrating
- Infection: epiglottitis, croup, peritonsillar abscess, retropharyngeal abscess
- Inflammation: burn, smoke inhalation
- Tumor: thyroid, hemangioma, hematoma, squamous cell carcinoma, edema
- Neurologic lesion: vocal cord paralysis
- Congenital abnormalities: laryngeal web, tracheomalacia

Symptoms of Obstruction
- Respiratory distress: dyspnea, tachypnea
- Difficulty swallowing
- Pain, sometimes related directly to area of difficulty, sometimes diffuse
- Cough and associated strain or change in voice
- Restless behavior: inability to find a comfortable position
- Lethargy at times

Signs of Obstruction
- Hoarse voice and/or cough, sometimes characterized as a "bark"
- Anxiety: tense, deeply worried facies (may signal epiglottitis)
- Stridor: severity related to extent of obstruction and the patient's respiratory effort
  - Inspiratory: obstruction at the glottis, epiglottis
  - Expiratory: obstruction below the glottis (wheezing)
- Retraction
  - Suprasternal notch: obstruction at or above trachea
  - Intercostal and subcostal, below suprasternal notch: obstruction in bronchial tree or below
- Drooling (difficulty swallowing): obstruction at glottis or above
- Bleeding: hemoptysis, hematoma, particularly with trauma
- Subcutaneous emphysema, particularly with trauma
- Facial fracture, often palpable

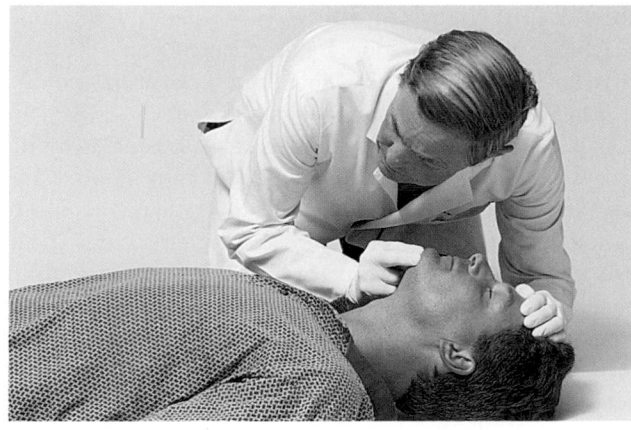

FIGURE 27-1
Look, listen, and feel for adequate breathing to assess patency of the upper airway.

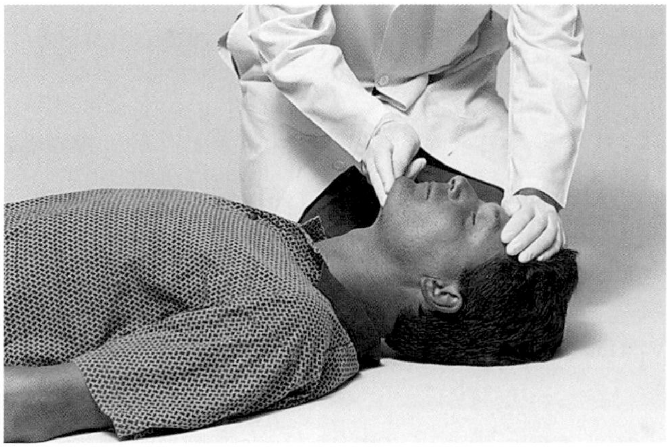

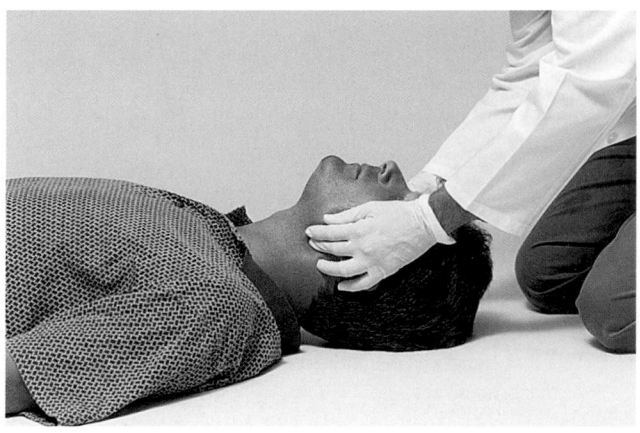

FIGURE 27-2
Use a chin lift to ensure an open airway.

FIGURE 27-3
Properly position both hands to maintain the head and neck in a neutral position, in alignment with the body.

piratory distress such as retractions, tachypnea, and cyanosis. Provide ventilatory assistance with 100% oxygen and ventilatory assistance with a bag-valve-mask as needed before continuing with the primary assessment.

In cases of trauma, look for bruising, paradoxic chest movement, and open chest wounds. Palpate the upper chest and neck for crepitation, a sign of air leakage into soft tissue. Bruising should alert you to the possibility of pulmonary contusion, which often results in a spontaneous pneumothorax. Open chest wounds should be covered to minimize the influx of atmospheric air until definitive treatment is available. Paradoxic chest movement may be associated with fractured ribs or a flail chest. This fracture should be stabilized immediately.

Circulation. Adequate circulation is needed to oxygenate the brain. Circulation can be impaired because of cardiac conditions, hemorrhage, dehydration, and other medical conditions. To assess peripheral perfusion and detect hypovolemic shock, note the skin color, presence and quality of pulses in and the temperature of the extremities, as well as the capil-

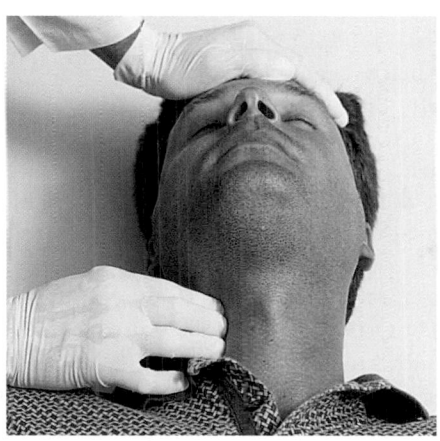

FIGURE 27-4
Check the carotid pulse to confirm circulation, one side at a time.

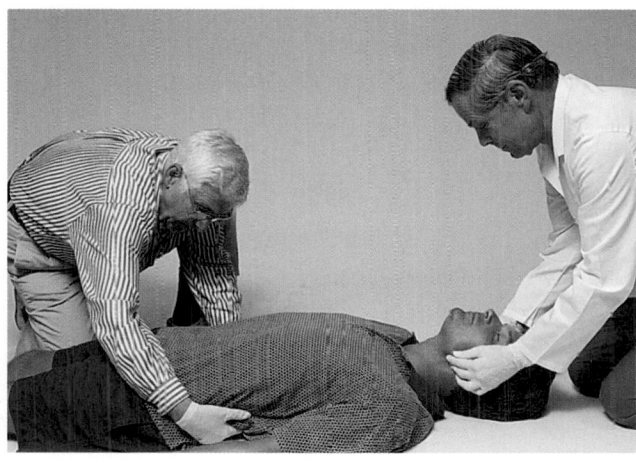

FIGURE 27-5
Quickly assess the entire body for bleeding sites.

lary refill time, because there may not be enough time for an adequate blood pressure determination.

Pulses should be detected in the distal extremities (i.e., radial, dorsalis pedis, or posterior tibial). If no pulses are detected at these sites, check the brachial and popliteal sites and then the femoral and carotid sites (Fig. 27-4). Diminished pulses in the distal sites indicate poor perfusion and hypovolemic shock. Generally, if the radial pulse is palpable, the systolic pressure will be greater than 80 mm Hg; if the femoral or carotid pulse is palpable, the systolic pressure will be greater than 70 mm Hg. To assess capillary refill, press firmly over a nail bed or bony prominence (e.g., chin, forehead, or sternum) until the skin blanches. Count the seconds it takes for color to return. A capillary refill time in excess of 2 seconds indicates poor perfusion.

Make a quick total body appraisal for bleeding sites, being especially careful to look and feel for dampness in dark clothing that may obscure hemorrhage (Fig. 27-5). Control bleeding before continuing the primary assessment, and estimate the amount of blood loss. Significant amounts of blood, enough to cause hypovolemic shock, can also be lost into the thoracic and abdominal cavities. Do not assume that there has not been hemorrhage simply because no blood is seen. Boluses of intravenous crystalloids are given if shock is identified.

Disability. A brief neurologic evaluation is performed, primarily to determine the patient's responsiveness or level of consciousness. (A more detailed neurologic evaluation is performed during the secondary assessment.) However, it is appropriate at this time to determine whether the patient is at one of these levels of responsiveness (the mnemonic AVPU: Alert; responsive to Verbal stimuli; responsive to Painful stimuli; or Unresponsive). A decrease in the level of consciousness may indicate hypoxemia or hypovolemic shock, necessitating a reevaluation of the patient's ABCs.

Exposure. In cases of trauma, the patient should be as completely undressed as possible to facilitate a brief body search for major injuries that may have been missed during the ABCs.

MNEMONICS

Patient's Level of Responsiveness: AVPU

A Alert
V Verbal stimuli: responsive to
P Painful stimuli: responsive to
U Unresponsive

SECONDARY ASSESSMENT

Mnemonics

Sections of the Health History: SAMPLE

S   Symptoms
A   Allergies
M   Medications or drugs of any type currently being taken by the patient
P   Past illnesses, such as diabetes, epilepsy, hypertension
L   Last meal
E   Events preceding the precipitating event

Check the vital signs before beginning the head-to-toe survey of the body in the search for additional injuries. Count the heart rate and respiratory rate, and determine the blood pressure. Initial observations of pulses and respirations to ensure their presence are obviously part of the primary assessment. (They may be counted at the end of the primary assessment.) Compare these values for the patient with those expected. It is important to recognize that vital sign values above or below those expected for the person's age are indicative of particular problems.

It is also appropriate at this time to quantify the patient's level of consciousness with the Glasgow Coma Scale (see Box 4-3). This score can be used for comparison with those computed during periodic reassessments to determine changes in the patient's level of consciousness.

History. Usually someone other than the examiner obtains an abbreviated history from the patient, family, emergency medical technicians, or scene bystanders. Pertinent information is then shared with the examiner during the assessment process. This abbreviated history should focus on information relevant to the emergency condition. A useful mnemonic is SAMPLE, reflecting the individual sections of the history.

Head and Neck. Inspect and palpate the head and scalp, looking for any depressions, bone instability, crepitus, lacerations, penetrating injuries, or drainage from the ears or nose. Clear or amber-colored drainage from the nose or ears may indicate a basilar skull fracture. Note any bruising around the eyes (raccoon eyes) or behind the ears (Battle sign), indicating a basilar skull fracture (Fig. 27-6).

Examine the eyes for pupillary size and responsiveness to light. Examine the retinas and conjunctivae for hemorrhage and the lens for dislocation. A quick visual examination of both eyes is performed by asking a conscious patient to read the words on the side of any container.

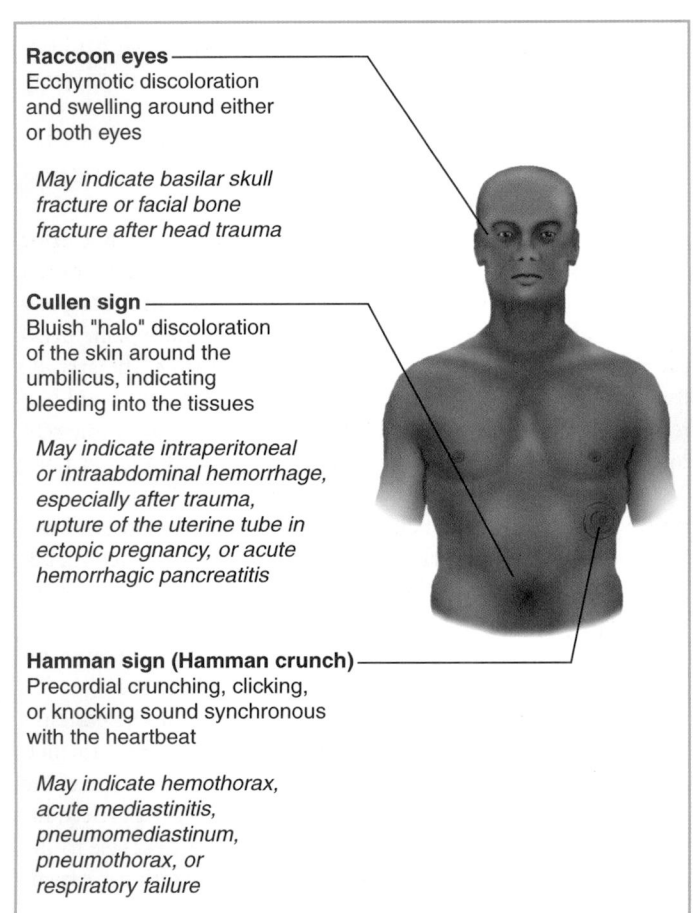

Raccoon eyes
Ecchymotic discoloration and swelling around either or both eyes

May indicate basilar skull fracture or facial bone fracture after head trauma

Cullen sign
Bluish "halo" discoloration of the skin around the umbilicus, indicating bleeding into the tissues

May indicate intraperitoneal or intraabdominal hemorrhage, especially after trauma, rupture of the uterine tube in ectopic pregnancy, or acute hemorrhagic pancreatitis

Hamman sign (Hamman crunch)
Precordial crunching, clicking, or knocking sound synchronous with the heartbeat

May indicate hemothorax, acute mediastinitis, pneumomediastinum, pneumothorax, or respiratory failure

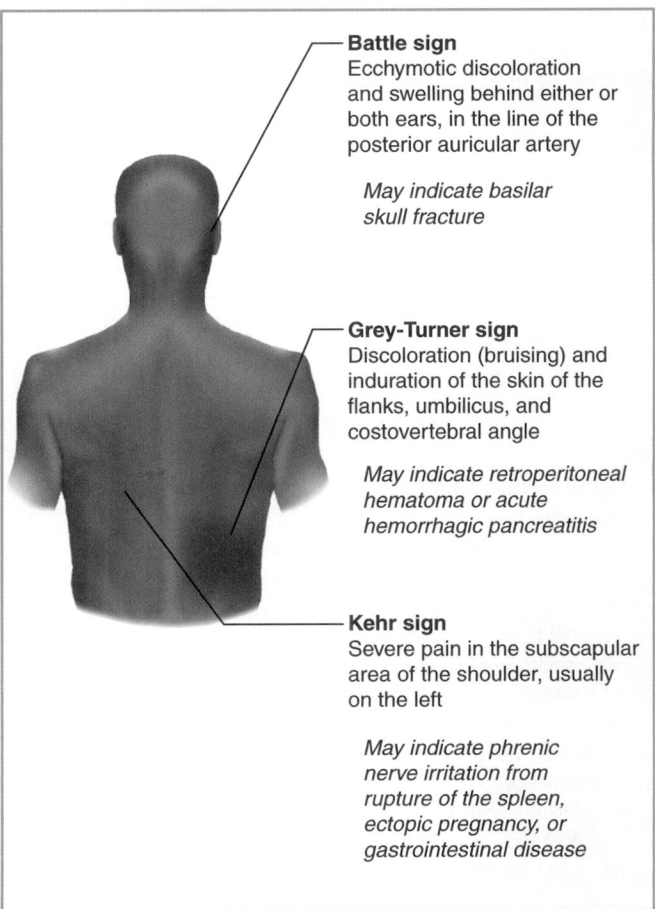

Battle sign
Ecchymotic discoloration and swelling behind either or both ears, in the line of the posterior auricular artery

May indicate basilar skull fracture

Grey-Turner sign
Discoloration (bruising) and induration of the skin of the flanks, umbilicus, and costovertebral angle

May indicate retroperitoneal hematoma or acute hemorrhagic pancreatitis

Kehr sign
Severe pain in the subscapular area of the shoulder, usually on the left

May indicate phrenic nerve irritation from rupture of the spleen, ectopic pregnancy, or gastrointestinal disease

FIGURE 27-6
Signs that indicate serious injury associated with trauma.

Inspect the neck for unexpected findings such as penetrating injury, bruising, and tracheal deviation from the midline, and palpate for deformity and crepitus. Be certain that the neck is manually maintained in neutral position until radiographic documentation confirming the absence of cervical injury has been obtained.

If the patient is wearing a helmet, it is difficult to determine when to obtain the film—before or after removing the helmet. Depending on the shape of the helmet, for example, a bike helmet, having the person supine for the film will put the neck out of alignment and potentially hyperflexed. In most instances, it is likely best to remove the helmet first, constantly assuring maintenance of the neutral position of the neck. During this two-person procedure, in-line manual stabilization of the neck is applied from below and the helmet is expanded laterally. In-line manual stabilization of the neck is then reestablished from above, and the patient is adequately immobilized. If the patient is wearing a motorcycle helmet, a lateral cervical spine film may be obtained before the helmet is removed if there is no evidence of respiratory distress. However, each situation must be carefully assessed because a helmet of any type is problematic.

Chest. Inspect the chest for bruising or obvious signs of deformity. Palpate the sternum, each rib, and clavicle. Blunt sternal pressure will be painful if any attached ribs are fractured. Patterns of bruising may indicate the mechanism of injury and may signal a possible pulmonary contusion.

Auscultate breath sounds at the apex, base, and midaxillary areas. Note any diminished or absent breath sounds, which may indicate a pneumothorax or hemothorax. Auscultate the heart for clarity of heart sounds. Distant, muffled heart sounds and distended neck veins may indicate cardiac tamponade, a life-threatening condition. In a noisy emergency department, heart sounds may be difficult to hear and hypovolemia may prevent distention of neck veins; therefore a narrow pulse pressure may be the only reliable indicator of cardiac tamponade.

Abdomen. Inspect the abdomen for bruising and distention. Gently palpate the abdomen, noting guarding and pain. Hollow organs in the abdomen are often ruptured with blunt trauma and result in occult hemorrhage; pain and distention may indicate an underlying hemorrhage.

Back. The back is briefly inspected for signs of injury. The patient must be log-rolled by three persons to maintain cervical spine stabilization as well as alignment of the thoracic and lumbar spine.

Extremities. Inspect and palpate all extremities for signs of fractures or deformities, crepitus, pain, and lack of spontaneous movement. Palpation of the bones with rotational or three-point pressure along the shaft helps identify fractures where alignment has been maintained. Note any wounds over the site of a suspected fracture, the possible indication of an open fracture. Palpate all peripheral pulses. It is particularly important to document skin temperature, capillary refill time, and the presence of a pulse in extremities with a suspected fracture.

Pelvic fractures are detected by placing downward pressure with the heels of the hands on both anterior superior iliac spines and on the symphysis pubis. Pain is readily evident. Pelvic fractures are associated with occult hemorrhage, which may become a life-threatening condition.

Rectum and Perineum. A rectal and perineal examination is essential to assess abdominal, pelvic, and neurologic injuries. The rectal examination is performed to detect blood within the bowel lumen, a high-riding prostate, pelvic fractures, the integrity of the abdominal wall, and the quality of sphincter tone.

Neurologic Examination. A more complete neurologic evaluation is performed once the patient's condition has been stabilized. Reassess the patient's Glasgow Coma Scale score. Then perform a more detailed motor and sensory evaluation. Note any paralysis or paresis, which suggests major injury to the spinal column or peripheral nervous system. Pain should be noted and the degree of its intensity recorded whenever possible.

Reevaluate the Patient. The patient must be reevaluated frequently so that any new signs and symptoms are not overlooked. A primary survey should be performed every 5 minutes and the results compared with those obtained in previous surveys. Vital signs must be monitored continuously. As life-threatening conditions are managed, other equally life-threatening problems may develop and less severe conditions may become evident. A high index of suspicion and constant alertness facilitate early recognition and management.

Physical Variations

Pediatric Priorities

Priorities for the infant and child are basically the same as for adults. Although blood volume, fluid requirements, and size may be smaller, and associated disease or the mechanism of injury may be different, the assessment sequence is the same. Remember, too, to keep the infant or child warm and to involve the parents as much as possible every step of the way.

Urgent or Emergent Threat. Sometimes there may be no obvious trauma, and the reason for a medical emergency may not be readily evident. On other occasions, the message is clear. Regardless, any situation (e.g., odor; Box 27-2), however subtle, that suggests a patient's increased vulnerability may indicate an urgent or emergent threat. Table 27-2 defines eight primary symptoms that may be associated with a life-threatening condition.

BOX 27-2

SMELL THE BREATH

Sometimes, when a situation is urgent, the patient's breath may have a distinctive odor that is a clue to the source of difficulty, a possible ingestion or poisoning.

Odor	Possible Source
Sweet, fruity	Chloroform, lacquer, salicylates
Fruity, alcohol	Ethyl alcohol, phenol
Pear-like, acrid	Chloral hydrate, paraldehyde
Halitosis	Amphetamine
Wintergreen	Methyl salicylate
Bitter almond	Cyanide, jetberry bush
Camphor	Mothballs (naphthalene)
Garlic	Phosphorus, arsenic, tellurium, parathion, malathion
Coal gas	Coal gas (associated with odorless but toxic carbon monoxide poisoning)
Metallic	Iodine
Rotten eggs	Hydrogen sulfide mercaptans
Shoe polish	Nitrobenzene
Stale tobacco	Nicotine
Burned rope	Marijuana
"Cloret's sign"	Lozenges (to cover up telltale odors!)

Modified from Wilson, 1997; and McMillan, Neiburg, Oski, 1977.

TABLE 27-2   **Symptoms and Risks of Serious and Life-Threatening Conditions**

Primary Symptoms	Possible Accompanying Symptoms	Possible Diagnosis	Risk
Sudden onset of unexplained shortness of breath	Persistent chest pain, sharp and stabbing, that worsens with breathing or coughing Faintness or actual fainting spell Cough with bloody sputum Swelling and pain in leg Cyanosis around the mouth Recently having been bed-bound for a long period Having sat in one position for a prolonged time, as in an overseas flight	Pulmonary embolism, usually from a site in the leg or pelvis	Two thirds of patients with a massive embolism die; intensive treatment of smaller embolism can limit the amount of damage to lung tissue.
Vomiting blood or black or dark brown material that resembles coffee grounds	Recurrent bouts of gnawing pain in the upper part of the abdomen Black or tarlike stool Loss of appetite Unexplained weight loss Weakness Paleness Progressive fatigue Increased awareness of the heartbeat (palpitations)	Bleeding ulcer of the stomach or duodenum, bleeding from esophageal varices	Possibly fatal hemorrhage.

TABLE 27-2	Symptoms and Risks of Serious and Life-Threatening Conditions—cont'd		
Primary Symptoms	**Possible Accompanying Symptoms**	**Possible Diagnosis**	**Risk**
Crushing pain in the center of the chest	Radiation of the pain to the arm(s), neck, or jaw Sweating Nausea and vomiting Shortness of breath Fainting Feeling of impending doom	Myocardial infarction	Mortality figures vary with the age of the patient and the location and extent of damage to the heart. Because most deaths occur within minutes or hours of the attack, the speed of treatment is crucial; rapid administration of anti-clotting drugs may limit some damage.
Severe throbbing pain in and around one blood-shot eye	Blurred vision in the affected eye Eyeball is both tender and firm to the touch Abnormal sensitivity to light Fixed and dilated pupil	Acute glaucoma	Delayed treatment can result in complete and permanent blindness in affected eye.
Flashes of light in the field of vision of one eye	Absence of pain in the affected eye Black cobweb-like floating spots Partial loss of vision spreading as a curtain-like shadow from the top or one side of the eye	Retinal detachment	Delayed treatment can result in further detachment extending to the area of most detailed vision (macula); permanent loss of central vision may result without treatment; detachment can cause blindness in the affected eye.
Sudden and progressively more severe abdominal pain	Nausea and vomiting Swollen or tender abdomen Severe constipation Temperature above 100° F (38° C)	Acute (surgical) abdomen (appendicitis, obstruction)	Delayed treatment can result in rupture or ischemic destruction of the involved organ and peritonitis.
Sudden feeling of weakness and unsteadiness that may result in momentary loss of consciousness	Loss of movement of arm(s) or leg(s) Numbness and/or tingling in any part of the body Excruciating headache Confusion Difficulty speaking Blurred or double vision, or loss of vision in one eye	Transient ischemic attack (TIA) or stroke (CVA)	TIA: although short-lived, it may signal an impending stroke; risk can be diminished with appropriate therapy. CVA: the outcome depends on the location and extent of the interruption of the blood supply. Overall, one third of strokes are fatal; one third leave some degree of permanent damage; one third have no long-lasting effect.
Difficult breathing that occurs suddenly (often in the middle of the night) and worsens rapidly	Restlessness, anxiety, and sense of doom Swollen ankles Cough producing frothy pink or brownish, blood-flecked sputum Audible bubbling sound when breathing Bluish lips and nail beds Profuse sweating	Pulmonary edema, related to a sudden left-sided heart failure	Delayed treatment can be fatal, although timely and appropriate therapy usually results in dramatic relief of acute symptoms.

Modified from The Johns Hopkins Medical Letter, 1990.

INJURY ASSESSMENT

If trauma is the root of the problem, a history of the injury or examination of the injury-producing mechanism may be helpful. Injuries can be divided into two basic types: blunt and penetrating. Each can be further classified according to the direction of energy force for blunt trauma and the degree of severity for penetrating trauma.

BLUNT TRAUMA

The severity of injury will vary according to the amount of energy transferred from an object to the human body. The direction of impact determines the pattern of injuries. The automobile accounts for the majority of severe blunt trauma cases and therefore is used as an example here. The emergency medical technicians or other first responders who were present at the scene should describe the appearance of the vehicle and the damage sustained to the passenger compartment.

On the basis of this information, the examiner can identify the portions of the body that absorbed the greatest transfer of energy. The following are some examples:

- A bent steering wheel and a bull's-eye fracture of the windshield should alert to the potential for C-spine injuries, brain injury, central flail chest, myocardial contusion, fractured spleen or liver, and posterior fracture or dislocation of the hip.

  In the event of brain injury, the delta V or change in force associated with deceleration of the brain's movement within the skull has a relationship with the severity of injury. The initial impact causes the *coup* injury closest to the point of impact. The impact of the brain on the opposite side of the skull *(contra-coup)* causes additional injury.
- A side impact may cause contralateral neck sprain, lateral flail chest, ruptured spleen or liver (depending on the side of impact), and fractured pelvis or acetabulum.
- Rear impact collision can result in neck injuries (i.e., cervical strain or whiplash).
- Persons ejected from a vehicle can sustain multiple injuries, including a cervical spine fracture and brain injury, depending on the part of the body that strikes first.
- An airbag injury commonly results in abrasions, sometimes severe, over arms, face, and neck; less commonly, particularly in small individuals, the force may cause life-threatening internal injuries. For this reason, infants and children should not ride in the front seat of a motor vehicle.

PENETRATING TRAUMA

The following two factors determine the type of injury and subsequent management:

- The region of the body sustaining the injury will anatomically determine the potential for specific organ injury.
- The transfer of energy is determined by the force of the penetrating object on impact. The amount of force is further measured by the velocity of the missile and the distance from the source (e.g., a 0.38 caliber handgun has a muzzle velocity of 850 feet per second). Energy transfer is also determined by the rate or change in speed once the missile is inside the patient's body and also by the frontal projection of the missile. In most penetrating injuries, the most important factor in determining energy is the speed of the missile.

BURNS

Burns should alert the examiner to the possibilities of smoke, heat, and toxic chemical inhalation and carbon monoxide poisoning. Airway inflammation may result with the potential of airway obstruction. Blunt trauma and fractures may also be associated with thermal injuries as a result of an explosion, falling debris, or the individual's attempts to escape the fire.

INFANTS AND CHILDREN

A smaller anatomy and differing physiologic responses to injury and acute illness by infants and children are important considerations when examining them during an emergency (Fig. 27-7; Box 27-3). For example, cardiac arrest is rarely a primary event in children as it is in adults. The child usually experiences respiratory and ventilatory failure that progresses to respiratory arrest first. Without rapid, appropriate intervention for the respiratory distress, a cardiac arrest occurs as a secondary event. Because cardiac arrest in children is complicated by prolonged hypoxemia and/or acidosis, resuscitation is seldom successful, even when expedi-

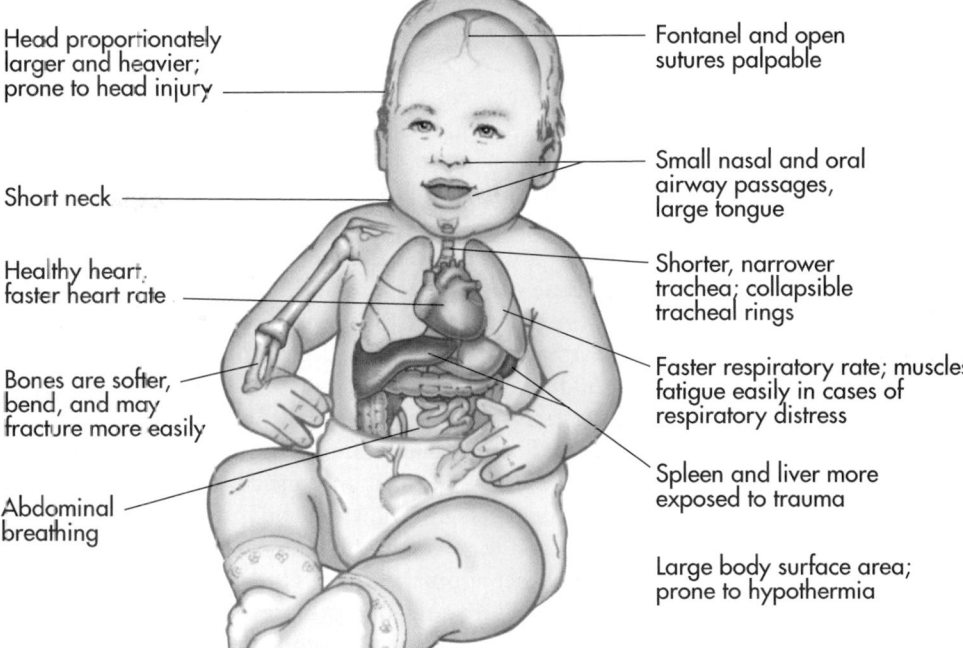

Head proportionately larger and heavier; prone to head injury

Short neck

Healthy heart, faster heart rate

Bones are softer, bend, and may fracture more easily

Abdominal breathing

Fontanel and open sutures palpable

Small nasal and oral airway passages, large tongue

Shorter, narrower trachea; collapsible tracheal rings

Faster respiratory rate; muscles fatigue easily in cases of respiratory distress

Spleen and liver more exposed to trauma

Large body surface area; prone to hypothermia

FIGURE 27-7
The unique anatomic and physiologic features of infants and young children.
Redrawn from Eichelberger et al, 1998.

BOX 27-3

FINDINGS THAT INDICATE A SENSE OF URGENCY IN INFANTS AND CHILDREN

Airway and Breathing
- Respiratory distress indicated by nasal flaring, retractions
- Respiratory rate >60, sustained, especially with oxygen administration
- Respiratory rate >20, especially in the presence of acute illness or with injury to the chest or abdomen
- Cyanosis: a late sign in respiratory failure, first seen in the mucous membranes of the mouth
- Stridor: upper airway obstruction
- Head bobbing: impending respiratory failure
- Prolonged expiration: reactive airway disease
- Grunting: alveolar collapse or loss of lung volume

Circulation
- Heart rate >160 or <80 (<5 years old)
- Heart rate >140 (>5 years old)
- Sinus tachycardia, sustained
- Bradycardia: sign of impending cardiac arrest
- Hypotension: late sign of hypovolemia that indicates decompensation (a decrease of 10 mm Hg is significant)
- Absence of peripheral pulses indicates poor tissue perfusion
- Absent central pulse is an ominous sign
- Capillary refill time: >2 seconds indicates poor tissue perfusion, hypothermia, constricted blood flow (perhaps the result of a tight cast)
- Mottling, pallor, and peripheral cyanosis are indicators of poor tissue perfusion, respiratory distress
- Diminished urinary output may indicate poor renal perfusion

Neurologic Disability
- Diminished level of consciousness (see Box 4-3)
- Agitation, anxiety
- Lethargy
- Irritability to passivity
- Unresponsiveness
- Failure to recognize parents
- Muscles: hypotonia and/or lost deep tendon reflexes may indicate hypoperfusion of the brain
- Generalized convulsions may indicate a seizure disorder, drug ingestion, hypoglycemia, hypertensive encephalopathy, severe renal dysfunction
- Pupil dilation may indicate increased intracranial pressure

tious. For this reason, repeated primary assessment of the child with respiratory distress is critical if deterioration is to be detected in time to allow adequate intervention.

During respiratory failure, carbon dioxide is not sufficiently blown off with hypoxia as the result. In the event of shock (poor tissue perfusion), blood is shunted to the vital organs, allowing the child a short period of physiologic compensation. Failure to reverse the hypoxia with 100% oxygen and assisted ventilation and to clear metabolites by improving circulation and tissue perfusion will result in hypoxemia, acidemia (low blood pH), and tissue acidosis. Early intervention usually prevents progression to cardiac arrest.

Cardiac monitoring may detect unexpected dysrhythmias, such as ventricular fibrillation, in children, who may well progress to cardiac arrest. Early detection is necessary if there is to be successful management (e.g., defibrillation) of such a condition.

Given the primary assessment, a secondary one may be more deliberate if the situation allows. Additional information is usually available:

- Parents usually know the child's weight in pounds. The conversion factor is 2.2 lb = 1 kg. If the weight is not known, estimate in kilograms: $8 + 1$ ($2 \times$ child's age in years). Another approach involves the now readily available "length-based resuscitation tapes." They afford a reasonably close estimate of weight as well as size of equipment, fluid volume, and drug doses appropriate for the child's length.
- The approximate expected systolic blood pressure for a child older than 1 year: $80 + (2 \times$ child's age in years). This calculated value can be used until the child is stabilized when comparison can be made with the actual expectation for age, gender, and height of the child.
- A crying child has, at that moment, a patent airway.
- Capillary refill is a marker for circulatory perfusion. A time greater than 2 seconds or greater than the time it takes to slowly say "capillary refill" suggests a problem.
- The mnemonic AVPU (p. 893) is helpful with children as well as with adults.
- Many aspects of physical examination in children discussed throughout the book are applicable in the emergency or life-threatening situation. Be mindful of the expected ways in which children differ physically from adults (Box 27-4).
- To the extent possible, try to keep an infant or child warm; use a radiant warmer if one is available.

Intervention, of course, must begin immediately in the event of a life-threatening situation but, given time and the opportunity, do the following:

- Attempt to establish rapport with the child consistent with the situation.
- Using the mnemonic SAMPLE (p. 894) as a base for history taking, and if an infant is still in the first few weeks of life, add questions about the mother's pregnancy and delivery, for example, due date, hypertension, vaginal bleeding.

STAYING WELL

PUT PREVENTION INTO PLAY

Health professionals have the responsibility to preserve their own health and sense of well-being. Malpractice suits challenge that effort. One way to avoid the irritability, inner tension, headache, fatigue, insomnia and gastrointestinal symptoms that often accompany a malpractice suit is to avoid them. Indeed, Stavroudis reminds us that the litigation stress syndrome is not uncommon. The five phases, she indicates, include denial ("I did my best, why me?), then anger (How dare they?), then bargaining (I promise, I'll do better from now on

if I get through this), followed by a period of depression (This will get worse!) and, finally, acceptance (I will get through this!).

The message is clear. Keeping precise and thorough records is one way to avoid such emotional trauma. That means accuracy, timeliness, and objectivity in records thoughtfully and logically prepared, never inappropriately altered, and always enhanced by excellent communication with your patients and your colleagues.

From Stavroudis, 2004; Charles, 1987.

♦ Consistent with age and condition, get as much information as possible from the child. For example, "Please show me with one finger where it hurts."

♦ Evaluate the meaning of signs and symptoms with deliberate speed (Box 27-5).

The Yale Observation Scales (Table 27-3) are a guide to the secondary assessment of a febrile child if you recognize the subjectivity and, hence, the possible variability in some of the observations, and if you recognize that the well-appearing infant or child may not be all that well. The higher the score, the more likely the child is ill, particularly when the sum approaches or is greater than 10. These observations are also helpful when a child is not febrile. As always, measures like this can aid but should not dictate final judgments.

BOX 27-4

WAYS IN WHICH CHILDREN DIFFER PHYSICALLY FROM ADULTS

Although children differ physically from adults, the closer they are in age to an adult, the more like an adult they become (Fig. 27-7).

Skin

- The skin is thinner, with less subcutaneous fat, and is less protective against burns and more likely to develop hypothermia.
- By age 10, the surface area relative to body mass is greater, more nearly approximating the adult relationship.

Head

- Until about age 4 years, the head is larger and heavier relative to the rest of the body.
- The bones of the skull are softer and are separated by fibrous tissue and cartilage until about age 5 years; this is somewhat protective against increased intracranial pressure, at least for a short time.
- The developing brain, particularly to age 5 years, is more vulnerable to injury, infection, and poisons.
- The dura, very firmly attached to the skull, has bridging veins to the brain which are apt to tear and bleed with inflicted injury. (child abuse).

Airway

- Nasal passages are relatively smaller and more easily obstructed with discharges or foreign bodies. Because newborns and young infants are obligate nose breathers, they are particularly vulnerable.
- The tongue is relatively larger and more easily able to obstruct the upper airway.
- The trachea is relatively much narrower and its cartilage more elastic and collapsible, and is therefore more vulnerable to edema, pressure, and inflammation; hyperextension or flexion can crimp and obstruct.
- The larynx is higher and more anterior, and is therefore more "available" for aspiration.

Chest and Lungs

- The rib cage is more elastic and flexible, less vulnerable to injury, and more apt to allow retraction during increased respiratory distress.

- Lung tissue is fragile and more easily contused.
- The mediastinum is more mobile and more vulnerable to tension pneumothorax.
- Chest muscles are not well developed. Their use, in addition to the expected diaphragmatic effort, suggests respiratory distress; they tire more easily with prolonged effort.
- The higher metabolic rate and greater oxygen requirement increase vulnerability to hypoxemia.

Heart and Circulation

- Infants and children have a relatively smaller total circulating blood volume, but will lose as much blood as will an adult from a similar laceration.
- When a significant blood or fluid volume is lost, children maintain their blood pressure longer than adults do; the pressure may be maintained even at the point of cardiac arrest.
- Bradycardia, usually the initial response to hypoxemia in neonates, may herald cardiac arrest.

Abdomen

- The liver and spleen are relatively larger and more vascular; thus they are less protected by the ribs and more susceptible to injury.

Extremities

- The not yet fully calcified bones of children are softer than those of adults until puberty and are perhaps more vulnerable to fracture.

Nervous System

- An infant is able to feel pain anywhere in the body, but cannot always localize or isolate it; older infants can push your hand away from a painful location.
- Children who appear passive in stressful situations and do not seek comforting reassurance from parents may have an altered, depressed level of consciousness; or, if alert, may be providing a clue to child abuse.

Modified from Eichelberger et al, 1998.

BOX 27-5

CLASSIC SIGNS OF PHYSIOLOGIC PROBLEMS IN CHILDREN

Pain
- Shallow breathing
- Irritable crying
- Splinting
- Facial expression change when touched or moved
- Resists movement
- Rigid posturing

Early Shock
- Tachycardia >130 beats/min
- Capillary refill >2 sec
- Pale, cool skin
- Altered level of consciousness
- Normal systolic blood pressure

Moderate Dehydration
- Sunken fontanel
- Pallor
- Doughy skin texture
- Dry mucous membranes

Respiratory Distress
- Nasal flaring
- Mottled, dusky skin color

- Tachypnea, shallow breathing
- Altered level of consciousness
- Sounds—stridor, hoarseness, muffled voice, wheezing
- Tripod positioning
- Retractions
- Asymmetric chest movement
- "See-saw" respirations

Late Shock
- Tachycardia >130 beats/min
- Capillary refill >5 sec
- Pallor, cold extremities
- Altered level of consciousness
- Systolic BP 80 mm Hg (except infants, whose systolic BP is often normally lower); sometimes, even in late shock, the pressure may be normal

Severe Dehydration
- Sunken fontanel
- Signs of shock
- Parched mucous membranes
- No tears (dry cry)
- Sunken eyeballs

Altered Level of Consciousness
- Combative
- Decreased responsiveness
- Lethargy
- Weak cry, moaning
- Personality change
- Does not recognize parents

Increased Intracranial Pressure
- Bulging fontanel (in infant)
- Altered level of consciousness
- High-pitched cry
- Change in vital signs (Note: Cushing's triad = hypertension with bradycardia and abnormal breathing)
- Irritable cry, impossible to distract or console child

From Eichelberger et al, 1998.

BOX 27-6

FORETHOUGHT AND PREPARATION

It is generally easier to limit the potentially dire consequences of an emergency situation if there is forethought and preparation. For example, as much as 20% of the combined adult and child population in the United States can be found in schools on any given day. The Emergency Cardiovascular Care Committee of the American Heart Association reminds us that life-threatening emergencies in schools, while relatively uncommon, do occur and, when they do, they need a planned, practiced, and efficient response with the provision of first aid, possible cardiopulmonary resuscitation (CPR), and even automated external defibrillation. Schools must have a well-developed, well-practiced emergency response plan including training in and equipment for CPR for the school nurse and other involved persons. One statistic underscores the point, the estimate that there are 0.5 to 1.0 possible episodes of sudden cardiac arrest per 876 million young person hours compared with 1 sudden cardiac arrest per 8.76 million adult person hours based on adult risk. That does not seem like a lot but it matters enormously to the affected student and to the people who may be in the position of caring for the crisis.

RECORDS AND LEGAL CONSIDERATIONS

RECORDS

Medical and legal problems commonly arise during emergency situations, and precise records are of aid to all concerned (Box 27-6). The patient record becomes a legal document and can be used in legal proceedings. It is a record of what you observed, evaluated, ordered, and performed; and conversely, what you did not: "If you didn't document it, you didn't do it." So be thorough, clear, and accurate, as well as concise. Pertinent negatives are as important as perti-

TABLE 27-3	Yale Observation Scales for Children		
Observation Item	**Reassuring (1 point)**	**Worrisome (3 points)**	**Ominous (5 points)**
Quality of cry	Strong, with expected tone OR Content and not crying	Whimpering OR Sobbing	Weak OR Moaning OR High pitched
Reaction to parental stimulation	Cries briefly then stops OR Content and not crying	Cries off and on	Continual cry OR Hardly responds
Awake or asleep	If awake, stays awake OR If asleep and stimulated, awakens quickly	Eyes close briefly, then awakens OR Awakens with prolonged stimulation	Falls asleep OR Will not rouse
Color	Pink	Pale extremities OR Acrocyanosis	Pale OR Cyanotic OR Mottled OR Ashen
Hydration	Appropriate skin turgor AND Eyes and mucous membranes moist	Appropriate skin turgor, eyes moist AND Mouth slightly dry	Skin doughy OR Tented AND Dry mucous membranes AND/OR Sunken eyes
Response (talk, smile) to social overtures	Smiles OR Consistently alert ($\leq$2 mo)	Brief smile OR Briefly alert ($\leq$2 mo)	No smile OR Face anxious, dull, expressionless OR Not alert ($\leq$2 mo)

Modified from McCarthy et al, 1985.
*The higher the score, the more likely the child is ill, particularly when the score approaches or is greater than 10.

nent positives. Chronologic reports using flow sheets help in the quick recording of assessment of changes in the patient's condition. Legibility is always essential. Write so that others can read; if that is not possible, print or type. Do not use any but the most conventional abbreviations. Do not erase a mistake; draw a line through the error so that it remains legible. Initial any corrections and date them.

CONSENT FOR TREATMENT

Consent is usually obtained before treatment. In life-threatening emergencies, the needed treatment should most often be given and formal consent obtained later. If forensic trauma is suspected, the personnel caring for the patient must preserve evidence. All items, such as bullets and clothing, must be saved for law enforcement personnel, with a documented chain of possession by health professionals.

ADVANCE DIRECTIVES, LIVING WILLS, AND DURABLE POWER OF ATTORNEY FOR HEALTH CARE

It is necessary to make a conscientious effort to learn whether a patient has left a formal statement of desired medical care in the event of an accident or illness that results in a cognitive impairment that preventing adequate participation in medical decision-making. A central concern involves the vigor with which life maintenance measures should be instituted. There is legal provision in most states for such statements (known as advance directives), usually in writing. There may also be a close relative or other trusted person to whom decision-making authority can be legally delegated in the form of a durable power of attorney for health care. Clearly, advance documentation of the patient's wishes in a so-called living will or even in a prior entry in a medical record can be helpful to those giving care, and to those persons with durable power of attorney.

> **BOX 27-7**
>
> **A PARTICULAR NEED FOR ADVANCE DIRECTIVES**
>
> The Patient Self-Determination Act has, since 1990, required that Medicaid and Medicare providers (hospitals, nursing homes, many health care agencies, prepaid health care organizations) inform patients of their rights under state law to make decisions to accept or refuse medical or surgical treatment, to establish advance directives, and to appoint a proxy, a health care agent, to act on their behalf in the event of an ultimate inability to communicate due to physical or cognitive compromise. Many nursing home patients, however, are among those who may not be able to understand these rights given the disturbing prevalence of mental disorders, particularly dementia, in this population. They then often need the assistance of family members. Health providers should, then, encourage the formulation of advance directives while patients are still competent to state their preferences and often before admission to a nursing home or other care facility.
>
> ———————
>
> Omnibus Budget Reconciliation Act [OBRA] of 1990 [Federal Patient Self-Determination Act]; Janovsky and Rovner, 1993.

Advance Directives. The purpose of an advance directive is to ensure that legally competent adult patients, generally those 18 years or older who are not mentally ill or under guardianship, may express their wishes regarding the extent of medical intervention in end-of-life circumstances (Box 27-7). It is now common practice to offer to all patients the possibility of preparing an advance directive and to ensure a reasonable effort to discover if such a directive exists in writing; these directives should be placed in the patient's medical record. Precise documentation is protective of the patient and provider and is essential. If there has not been a written advance directive, the patient's wishes as told to a health care provider, validated by a witness, and entered in the patient's record can be considered legally competent.

Living Wills. Such advance directives can be considered living wills. Living wills must have been completed voluntarily and, in general, must have been witnessed by two competent persons unrelated to the patient either directly or by marriage, without financial interest to be derived from the patient or the patient's estate, and without financial or other responsibilities for the patient's care either directly or indirectly.

The provisions of a living will may become applicable when the patient is in a terminal condition, which usually is validated by two physicians, both of whom have personally examined the patient. To be considered terminal, a condition must be incurable to a reasonable degree of certainty and, despite the application of life-sustaining procedures, give no evidence of a potential for recovery.

Although it is the patient's responsibility to bring attention to a living will, this is of course not always possible. Health care providers must make every effort to discover the patient's intentions and to abide by them. Certainly, if the provider cannot in conscience follow the patient's directive, it becomes a responsibility then to arrange for care with another provider.

The patient always has the right to revoke the declaration of a living will. This, too, is best done in writing and with witnesses.

Durable Power of Attorney for Health Care. The durable power of attorney gives a person selected by the patient the power to make health care decisions in the event that the patient's cognition is lost. That representative or agent then has the authority to decide with the provider what, if any, measures may be taken to sustain life or prolong dying artificially (e.g., tube feeding, antibiotics, and respirators). Again, it is generally required that two physicians validate that a condition is terminal or is likely to be terminal. It is important to note that the durable power of attorney for health care does not give authority for the patient's representative to handle other matters (e.g., financial or property). These can be left in the hands of yet another person. At times it is appropriate to suggest that a lawyer help the patient in the preparation of directives.

Clearly, advance documentation of a patient's wishes can be enormously helpful to those giving care and to those persons with durable power of attorney for health care. It imposes a grave responsibility complicated by the variety of possible ethical interpretations. Clearly stated wishes and candid, respectful involvement of everyone concerned smooths the way.

SUMMARY

Notably, diagnosis is not necessarily made before the initiation of treatment. Life-threatening physiologic indicators of disease or trauma are identified rapidly, leading to immediate management. The causes underlying these physiologic indicators—the diagnosis—can be determined after the condition of the patient is stabilized, and a thorough examination can then be performed.

Evaluation and care are divided into the following four phases:

1. Primary assessment: assessment of ABCs
   * *Airway* assessment and management: Perform C-spine control.
   * *Breathing* is assessed and ventilation is assisted as needed.
   * *Circulation* is assessed, with hemorrhage control or shock management.
   * *Disability:* Neurologic function is briefly evaluated.
   * *Exposure:* Completely undress the patient whenever possible but keep the patient warm, particularly an infant or child.
2. Resuscitation
   * The management of life-threatening problems identified in the primary survey is continued.
   * Mechanical monitoring is implemented.
3. Secondary assessment
   * Take the vital signs.
   * Develop the history, guided by the mnemonic SAMPLE. Total evaluation of the patient is performed in the following areas: head and skull, neck, chest, abdomen, rectum and perineum, and extremities (for fractures).
   * Complete neurologic examination is performed, along with appropriate x-ray examinations, laboratory tests, and special studies. "Tubes and fingers" are in every orifice.
4. Definitive care
   * After identifying and ascertaining the patient's injuries, managing life-threatening problems, and obtaining special studies, diagnosis and treatment specific to the condition can begin.
   * Heart rate, respiratory rate, level of consciousness, capillary refill time, and the assessment of central versus distal pulses all need a return to comfortable levels before you can relax; 100% oxygen, cervical immobilization, and the maintenance of core temperature are essential until the clinical situation stabilizes.

PHOTO AND ILLUSTRATION CREDITS

400 more self assessment picture tests in clinical medicine, Chicago, 1984, Year Book.

American Academy of Dermatology; available at http://www.aad.org; accessed January 2006.

American College of Rheumatology: *Clinical slide collection on the rheumatic diseases,* Atlanta, 1991, American College of Rheumatology.

Andrews JS: Making the most of the sports physical, *Contemp Pediatr* 14(3):196-197, 1997.

Ansell BM, Rudge S, Schaller JG: *Color atlas of pediatric rheumatology,* London, 1992, Mosby-Wolfe.

Ball JW, Bindler R: *Pediatric nursing; caring for children,* ed 3, Upper Saddle River NJ, 2003, Prentice Hall Health.

Ballard JL et al: New Ballard Score, expanded to include extremely premature infants, *J Pediatr* 119:413, 1991.

Baran R, Dawher RPR, Levene G: *Color atlas of the hair, scalp, and nails,* St Louis, 1991, Mosby.

Barkauskas VH et al: *Health and physical assessment,* ed 2, St Louis, 1998, Mosby.

Barkauskas VH et al: *Health and physical assessment,* ed 3, St Louis, 2002, Mosby.

Battaglia FC, Lubchenco LC: The practical classification of newborn infants by weight and gestational age, *J Pediatr* 71:159, 1967.

Battista EM: The assessment and management of chronic pain in the elderly: A guide for practice. *Adv Nurs Pract,* 10(11): 28-32, 2002.

Beeching NJ, Nye FJ: *Diagnostic picture tests in clinical infectious disease,* London, 1996, Mosby-Wolfe.

Belcher A: *Cancer nursing,* St Louis, 1993, Mosby.

Berne RM, Levy MN: *Principles of physiology,* ed 2, St Louis, 1996, Mosby.

Bingham BJG, Hawke M, Kwok P: *Atlas of clinical otolaryngology,* St Louis, 1992, Mosby.

Brooke P, Bullock R: Validation of a 6-item cognitive impairment test with a view to primary care, *Int J Geriatr Psychiatry* 14(11):936-940, 1999.

Bull TR: *A colour atlas of ENT diagnosis,* London, 1974, Wolfe Medical Publications.

Burke B: The dietary history as a tool in research, *J Am Diet Assoc* 23:1044-1046, 1947.

Canobbio MM: *Cardiovascular disorders,* St Louis, 1990, Mosby.

Centers for Disease Control and Prevention, National Center for Infectious Disease, Atlanta.

Chessell GSJ, Jamieson MJ, Morton RA, Petrie JC, Towler HMA: *Diagnostic picture tests in clinical medicine,* London, 1984, Wolfe Medical Publications.

Cohen BA: *Atlas of pediatric dermatology,* St Louis, 1993, Mosby.

Crouch JE: *Functional human anatomy and physiology,* ed 4, New York, 1985, Lea & Febiger.

Crouch JE, McClintic JR: *Human anatomy and physiology,* ed 2, New York, 1976, John Wiley & Sons.

D'Arcy CA, McGee S: Does this patient have carpal tunnel syndrome? *JAMA* 283(23):3110-3117, 2000.

DePalma AF: *Surgery of the shoulder,* ed 3, Philadelphia, 1983, JB Lippincott.

Dieppe P et al: *Arthritis and rheumatism in practice,* London, 1991, Gower.

Donaldson DD: *Atlas of the eye: the crystalline lens,* vol v, St Louis, 1976, Mosby.

Doughty DB, Jackson DB: *Gastrointestinal disorders,* St Louis, 1993, Mosby.

Dyken PR, Miller MD: *Facial features of neurologic syndromes,* St Louis, 1980, Mosby.

Dynski-Klein M: *Color atlas of pediatrics,* London, 1986, Wolfe Medical Publications.

Edge V, Miller M: *Women's health care,* St Louis, 1994, Mosby.

Eichelberger MR et al: *Pediatric emergencies: a manual for prehospital care providers,* Englewood Cliffs, NJ, 1998, Brady.

Ezrein D, Godden JO, Volpe R: *Systematic endocrinology,* ed 2, New York, 1979, Harper & Row.

Farrar WE et al: *Infectious diseases,* ed 2, London, 1992, Gower.

Folstein M et al: The meaning of cognitive impairment in the elderly, *J Am Geriatr Soc* 33:228, 1985.

Food and Nutrition Board, Institute of Medicine, 1992, Washington, DC.

Gallager HS et al: *The breast,* St Louis, 1978, Mosby.

Gardner HL: Cervical endometriosis, a lesion of increasing importance, *Am J Obstet Gynecol* 84:170, 1962.

Gardner HL, Kaufman RH: *Benign diseases of the vulva and vagina,* St Louis, 1969, Mosby.

Giddens JF: *Student workbook and laboratory manual to accompany Health Assessment for Nursing Practice,* St Louis, 1998, Mosby.

Goldman MP, Fitzpatrick RE: *Cutaneous laser surgery: the art and science of selective photothermolysis,* St Louis, 1994, Mosby.

Goodman RM, Gorlin RJ: *Atlas of the face in genetic disorders,* ed 2, St Louis, 1977, Mosby.

Grimes D: *Infectious diseases,* St Louis, 1991, Mosby.

Grossman SA et al: A comparison of the Hopkins Pain Rating Instrument with standard visual analogue and verbal descriptor scales in patients with cancer pain, *J Pain Symptom Manag* 7:196-203, 1992.

Guzzetta CD, Dossey BM: *Cardiovascular nursing: holistic practice,* St Louis, 1992, Mosby.

Habif TP: *Clinical dermatology,* ed 4, St Louis, 2004, Mosby.

Halstead CL et al: *Physical evaluation of the dental patient,* St Louis, 1982, Mosby.

Harris JA et al: *The measurement of man,* Minneapolis, 1930, University of Minnesota Press.

Hughes JG: *Synopsis of pediatrics,* ed 6, St Louis, 1984, Mosby.

Hylton C, Goldberg MF: Circumpapillary retinal ridge in the shaken-baby syndrome, *N Engl J Med* 351:170, 2004.

Johns Hopkins Hospital: *Harriet Lane handbook,* ed 15, Philadelphia, 2000, WB Saunders.

Jolly H: *Diseases of children,* ed 4, Oxford, 1981, Blackwell Scientific.

Kamal A, Brocklehurst JC: *Color atlas of geriatric medicine,* ed 2, St. Louis, 1992, Mosby.

Kaufman RH, Faro S: *Benign diseases of the vulva and vagina,* ed 4, St Louis, 1994, Mosby.

Korones SB: *High-risk newborn infants: the basis for intensive nursing care,* ed 4, St Louis, 1986, Mosby.

Lawrence CM, Cox NH: *Physical signs in dermatology: color atlas and text,* St Louis, 1993, Mosby.

Lemmi FO, Lemmi CAE: *Physical assessment findings CD-ROM,* Philadelphia, 2000, WB Saunders.

Lewis SM, Heitkemper MM, Dirksen SR: *Medical-surgical nursing: Assessment and management of clinical problems,* ed 6, St Louis, 2004, Mosby.

Lloyd-Davies RW et al: *Color atlas of urology,* ed 2, London, 1994, Mosby.

Lookingbill DP, Marks JG Jr: *Principles of dermatology,* ed 3, Philadelphia, 2000, WB Saunders.

Lowdermilk DL, Perry SE, Bobak IM: *Maternity and women's health care,* ed 6, St Louis, 1997, Mosby.

Lowdermilk DL, Perry SE: *Maternity and women's health care,* ed 8, St Louis, 2004, Mosby.

Lubchenco LC et al: Intrauterine growth in length and head circumference as estimated from live births at gestational ages from 26 to 42 weeks, *Pediatrics* 37:403, 1966.

Mansel R, Bundred N: *Color atlas of breast disease,* St Louis, 1995, Mosby.

Marks JG, DeLeo VA: *Contact and occupational dermatitis,* St Louis, 1992, Mosby.

Mazzaferri EL: *Endocrinology case studies,* ed 2, Flushing, NY, 1975, Medical Examination Publishing.

McCance KM, Huether SE: *Pathophysiology: the biologic basis for disease in adults and children,* ed 4, St Louis, 2002, Mosby.

McKusick VA: *Heritable disorders of connective tissues,* ed 4, St Louis, 1972, Mosby.

Medcom: *Selected topics in ophthalmology: Medcom clinical lecture guides,* Garden Grove, Calif, 1983, Medcom.

Meheus A, Ursi JP: *Sexually transmitted diseases,* Kalamazoo, Mich, 1982, The Upjohn Co.

Miyasaki-Ching CM: *Chasteen's essentials of clinical dental assisting,* ed 5, St Louis, 1997, Mosby.

Moore KL: *The developing human: clinically oriented embryology,* ed 2, Philadelphia, 1977, WB Saunders.

Morison M, Moffatt C: *A colour guide to the assessment and management of leg ulcers,* ed 2, St Louis, 1994, Mosby.

Morse SA, Moreland AA, Holmes KK: *Atlas of sexually transmitted diseases and AIDS,* ed 2, St Louis, 1996, Mosby.

Morse SA, Moreland AA, Holmes KK: *Atlas of sexually transmitted diseases and AIDS,* ed 3, St Louis, 2003, Mosby.

National Academy of Science, Institute of Medicine, Washington, DC. www.iom.edu.

Newell FW: *Ophthalmology: principles and concepts,* ed 6, St Louis, 1986, Mosby.

Newell FW: *Ophthalmology: principles and concepts,* ed 8, St Louis, 1996, Mosby.

Owen GM: Measurement, recording, and assessment of skin-fold thickness in childhood and adolescence: a report of a small meeting, *Am J Clin Nutr* 35:629, 1982.

Palay DA, Krachmer JH: *Ophthalmology for the primary care physician,* St Louis, 1997, Mosby.

Prior JA et al: *Physical diagnosis: the history and examination of the patient,* ed 6, St Louis, 1981, Mosby.

Ross Laboratories: *Nutrition screening initiative,* Washington, DC.

Rudy EB: *Advanced neurological and neurosurgical nursing,* St Louis, 1984, Mosby.

Saunders WH et al: *Nursing care in eye, ear, nose, and throat disorders,* ed 4, St Louis, 1979, Mosby.

Schneider HA et al: *Nutritional support of medical practice,* ed 2, New York, 1977, Harper & Row.

Sheikh JI, Yesavage JA: Geriatric depression scale: recent evidence and development of a shorter version, *Clin Gerontol* 5:165-172, 1986.

Sigler BA, Schuring LT: *Ear, nose, and throat disorders,* St Louis, 1993, Mosby.

Skarin AT: *Atlas of diagnostic oncology,* ed 2, London, 1996, Mosby-Wolfe.

Smith DW: *Growth and its disorders,* Philadelphia, 1977, WB Saunders.

Solodiuk J, Curley MA: Pain assessment in nonverbal children with severe cognitive impairments: The Individualized Numeric Rating Scale (INRS). *J Pediatr Nurs* 18(4): 295-299, 2003.

Stein HA, Slatt BJ, Stein RM: *The ophthalmic assistant: fundamentals and clinical practice,* ed 5, St Louis, 1988, Mosby.

Stein HA, Slatt BJ, Stein RM: *The ophthalmic assistant: fundamentals and clinical practice,* ed 6, St Louis, 1994, Mosby.

Stenchever M et al: *Comprehensive gynecology,* ed 4, St Louis, 2001, Mosby.

Stewart WD, Danto JL, Maddin S: *Dermatology: diagnosis and treatment of cutaneous disorders,* St Louis, 1978, Mosby.

Symonds EM, Macpherson MBA: *Color atlas of obstetrics and gynecology,* St Louis, 1994, Mosby.

Tanner JM, Davies PS: Clinical longitudinal standards for height and height velocity for North American Children, *J Pediatr* 107(3): 317-329, 1985.

Thibodeau GA, Patton KT: *Anatomy and physiology,* ed 5, St Louis, 2003, Mosby.

Thompson JM et al: *Mosby's clinical nursing,* ed 3, St Louis, 1993, Mosby.

Thompson JM et al: *Mosby's clinical nursing,* ed 4, St Louis, 1997, Mosby.

Thompson JM, Wilson SF: *Health assessment for nursing practice,* St Louis, 1996, Mosby.

Trevor-Roper PD, Curran PV: *The eye and its disorders,* ed 2, Oxford, 1984, Blackwell Scientific.

US Department of Agriculture, Center for Nutrition Policy and Promotion. Available at www.Mypyramid.gov. Accessed April 2005.

Van Wieringen JC et al: *Growth diagrams 1965 Netherlands. Second national survey on 0–24-year-olds,* Groningen, Netherlands, 1971, Wolters-Noordhoff.

Weston WL, Lane AT: *Color textbook of pediatric dermatology,* St Louis, 1991, Mosby.

Weston WL, Lane AT, Morelli JG: *Color textbook of pediatric dermatology,* ed 2, St Louis, 1996, Mosby.

White GM: *Color atlas of regional dermatology,* St Louis, 1994, Mosby.

Wilson JR, Carrington ER, Ledger WJ: *Obstetrics and gynecology,* ed 8, St Louis, 1987, Mosby.

Wilson JD, Walsh PC. In Harrison JH et al: *Campbell's urology,* ed 4, Philadelphia, 1979, WB Saunders.

Wilson SF, Giddens J: *Health assessment for nursing practice,* ed 3, St. Louis, 2005, Mosby.

Wilson SF, Thompson JM: *Respiratory disorders,* St Louis, 1990, Mosby.

Wong DL et al: *Whaley and Wong's nursing care of infants and children,* ed 6, St Louis, 1999, Mosby.

Wood NK, Goaz PW: *Differential diagnosis of oral lesions,* ed 4, St Louis, 1991, Mosby.

Yannuzzi LA, Guyer DR, Green WR: *The retina atlas,* St Louis, 1995, Mosby.

Zitelli BJ, Davis HW: *Atlas of pediatric physical diagnosis,* ed 3, St Louis, 1997, Mosby.

REFERENCES AND READINGS

Abbassi V: Growth and normal puberty, *Pediatrics* 102:507-511, 1998.

Abrams B, Pickett K: Maternal nutrition. In Creasey RK, Resnik R, editors: *Maternal-fetal medicine,* ed 4, Philadelphia, 1999, WB Saunders.

Acute Pain Management Guideline Panel: Acute pain management: operative or medical procedures and trauma. AHCPR Pub. No. 92-0032, Rockville, Md, 1992, Agency for Health Care Policy and Research, Public Health Service, US Department of Health and Human Services.

Adams JA: Evolution of a classification scale: medical evaluation of suspected child sexual abuse, *Child Maltreat* 6(1):31-36, 2001.

Adams MS, Niswander JD: Birth weight of North American Indians: a correlation and amplification, *Hum Biol* 45:351, 1973.

Adelman WP: Nicotine replacement therapy for teenagers, *Arch Pediatr Adolesc Med* 158:205-206, 2004.

Age-Related Eye Disease Study Research Group: A randomized, placebo-controlled clinical trial of high-dose supplementation with vitamins C and E, beta carotene, and zinc for age-related macular degeneration and vision loss, *Arch Ophthalmol* 119: 1417, 2000.

Agency for Healthcare Research and Quality: Criteria for determining disability in infants and children: failure to thrive, evidence report/technology assessment: No. 72, AHRQ Publication No. 03-E019, Rockville, Md, 2003, AHRQ. www.ahrq.gov/clinic/epcsums/fthrivesum. htm, accessed 6/10/04.

Ahuja V, Yencha MW, Lassen LF: Head and neck manifestations of gastroesophageal reflux disease, *Am Fam Physician* 60(3):873-880, 1999.

Alagaratnam TT, Wong J: Limitations of mammography in Chinese females, *Clin Radiol* 36(2):175-177, 1985.

American Academy of Audiology: Newborn hearing screening, 2002. www.audiology.org/professional/tech/eihbrochure.php, accessed 4/28/04.

American Academy of Ophthalmology: *Preferred practice pattern: Pediatric eye evaluations,* San Francisco, 2003, American Academy of Ophthalmology.

American Academy of Pediatrics and American Academy of Family Physicians: Clinical practice guideline: diagnosis and management of acute otitis media, 2004.www.aafp.org/x26481.xml, accessed 1/5/06.

American Academy of Pediatrics Committee on Child Abuse and Neglect: Guidelines for the evaluation of sexual abuse of children: subject review, *Pediatrics* 103(1):186-191, 1999.

American Academy of Pediatrics Committee on Infectious Disease: *Red book: report of the Committee on Infectious Disease,* ed 26, Elk Grove Village, Ill, 2003, American Academy of Pediatrics.

American Academy of Pediatrics Committee on Quality Improvement, Subcommittee on Developmental Dysplasia of the Hip: Clinical prac-

tice guideline: early detection of developmental dysplasia of the hip, *Pediatrics* 105(4):896-905, 2000.

American Academy of Pediatrics, Committee on Practice and Ambulatory Medicine and Section on Ophthalmology, American Association of Certified Orthoptists, American Association for Pediatric Ophthalmology and Strabismus, American Academy of Ophthalmology Policy Statement: Organizational principles to guide and define the child health care system and/or improve the health of all children, *Pediatrics* 111(4):902-907, 2003.

American Academy of Pediatrics, Committee on Sports Medicine and Fitness: Medical conditions affecting sports participation, *Pediatrics* 94(5):757, 2001.

American Academy of Pediatrics, Section on Sports Medicine and Fitness: Female athlete triad, *Sports Shorts* 8(July), 2002.

American Academy of Pediatrics: Sports preparticipation examination. In Dyment PG, editor: *Sports medicine: health care for young athletes,* ed 2, Elk Grove Village, Ill, 1991. American Academy of Pediatrics.

American Cancer Society: *Cancer facts and figures,* Atlanta, 2005, American Cancer Society. Available at www.cancer.org.

American Cancer Society: Early detection of cervical cancer, *CA Cancer J Clin* 52:375, 2002. Available at http://caonline.amercancersoc.org/cgi/content/full/52/6/375.

American College of Allergy, Asthma & Immunology (ACAAI): Latex allergies. Available at www.acaai.org/public/linkpages/latex.htm

American College of Gastroenterology: American College of Gastroenterology colon cancer resource kit for physicians and patients, 2004. www.acg.gi.org, accessed July 20, 2004.

American College of Obstetrics and Gynecology: Hypertension in pregnancy, *ACOG Tech Bull* 219(January), 1996.

American College of Pediatrics Policy Statement, 1999.

American Heart Association: Jones criteria (revised) for guidance in the diagnosis of rheumatic fever, *Circulation* 69:204A, 1984.

American Medical Association, Group on Science and Technology: Athletic preparticipation examinations for adolescents: report of the Board of Trustees, *Arch Pediatr Adolesc Med* 148:93, 1994.

American Medical Student Association, Standing Committee on Lesbian, Gay, and Bisexual People in Medicine: Taking a sensitive sexual history with the gay patient in mind, Report, 1991.

American Optometric Association: *Pediatric eye and vision examination reference guide for clinicians,* ed 2, St Louis, 2002, American Optometric Association.

American Psychiatric Association: *Diagnostic and statistical manual of mental disorders,* ed 4, Washington, DC, 1994, APA.

Amies AM, Miller L, Lee SK, Koutsky L: The effect of vaginal speculum lubrication on the rate of unsatisfactory cervical cytology diagnosis. *Obstet Gynecol* 100:889-892, 2002.

Anand SS et al: Does this patient have deep vein thrombosis? *JAMA* 279:1094, 1998.

Andrews JS: Making the most of the sports physical, *Contemp Pediatr* 14(3):182-205, 1997.

Angell M: Privilege and health: what is the connection? *N Engl J Med* 329(2):126-127, 1993.

Apantaku LM: Breast cancer diagnosis and screening, *Am Fam Physician* 62(3):596-602, 2000.

Arvidson CR: The adolescent gynecologic exam, *Pediatr Nurs* 25(1):71-74, 1999.

Athey J, Moody-Williams J: Serving disaster survivors: achieving cultural competence in crisis counseling, Washington, DC, 2000, Emergency Services and Disaster Relief Branch, Center for Mental Health Services, Substance Abuse and Mental Health Services Administration.

Attia MW et al: Performance of a predictive model for streptococcal pharyngitis in children, *Arch Pediatr Adolesc Med* 155:687-691, 2001.

Augustyn M et al: Silent victims: children who witness violence, *Contemp Pediatr* 12:35, 1995.

Auster S: Spirituality and medicine. Personal communication [from the Uniformed Services University of the Health Sciences], January 6, 2004.

Autotte PA: Folk medicine, *Arch Pediatr Adolesc Med* 149(9):949-950, 1995.

Axelsson G, Hedegard B: Torus mandibularis among Icelanders, *Am J Phys Anthropol* 54(3):383-389, 1981.

Babian R et al: Diagnostic testing for prostate cancer detection: less is best, *Urology* 41:5, 1993.

Badgett RG, Lucey CR, Mulrow CD: Can the clinical examination diagnose left-sided heart failure in adults? *JAMA* 277(21):1712-1719, 1997.

Ballock RT, Richards BS: Hip dysplasia: early diagnosis makes a difference, *Contemp Pediatr* 14:108, 1997.

Bamji M et al: Palpable lymph nodes in healthy newborns and infants, *Pediatrics* 78(4):573-575, 1986.

Barkauskas VH et al: *Health and physical assessment,* ed 3, St Louis, 2002, Mosby.

Barker LR: Division of General Internal Medicine, Hopkins Bayview Medical Center, Johns Hopkins University School of Medicine. Personal communication, 1996.

Barrone M, Wissow L, Varness T: Material prepared for pediatric communication seminars, 2003, at the Johns Hopkins School of Medicine, Baltimore, MD.

Berde CB, Sethna NF: Analgesics for the treatment of pain in children, *N Engl J Med* 347:1094-1103, 2002.

Berenson A et al: Inadequate weight gain among pregnant adolescents: risk factors and relationship to infant birth weight, *Am J Obstet Gynecol* 176:1220, 1997.

Berger JE and the Committee on Medical Liability: Consent by proxy for nonurgent pediatric care, *Pediatrics* 112:1186-1195, 2003.

Berger SE: *Horizontal woman,* New York, 1996, Houghton Mifflin.

Bergman AB: Pulse oximetry: good technology misapplied, *Arch Pediatr Adolesc Med* 158:594-595, 2004.

Binns HJ et al: Growth of Chicago-area infants 1985 through 1987: not what the curves predict, *Arch Pediatr Adolesc Med* 150:842, 1996.

Blackhall LJ et al: Ethnicity and attitudes toward patient autonomy, *JAMA* 274:820, 1996.

Blakeley JA, Ribeiro VES: Glucosamine and osteoarthritis, *Am J Nurs* 104(2), 54-59, 2004.

Blatt SD, Simms M: Foster care: special children, special needs, *Contemp Pediatr* 14:109-129, 1997.

Bliss M: *William Osler, a life in medicine,* p. 83, New York City, 1999, Oxford University Press.

Bluestone CD, Klein JO: *Otitis media in infants and children,* ed 2, Philadelphia, 2001, WB Saunders.

Boekeloo BO et al: Young adolescents' comfort with discussion about sexual problems with their physicians, *Arch Pediatr Adolesc Med* 150(11):1146-1152, 1996.

Borowsky IW, Ireland M: Parental screening for intimate partner violence by pediatricians and family physicians. *Pediatrics* 110:509-516, 2002.

Botash A: Pediatrics, child sexual abuse. January 9, 2004. www.emedicine.com, accessed 7/26/04, eMedicine.com, Inc.

Boustani M et al: Screening for dementia in primary care: a summary of the evidence for the U.S. Preventive Services Task Force, *Ann Intern Med* 138, 927-937, 2003.

Bowers AC, Thompson JM: *Clinical manual of health assessment,* ed 4, St Louis, 1992, Mosby.

Brace RA, Resnik R: Maternal dynamics and disorders of amniotic fluid. In Creasey RK, Resnik R, editors: *Maternal-Fetal Medicine,* ed 4, Philadelphia, WB Saunders, 1999.

Bradford BJ: Don't let our youth go down tobacco road, *Contemp Pediatr* 9:96, 1992.

Brandt MM, Wahl WL: Liberal use of CT scanning helps to diagnose appendicitis in adults, *Am Surg* 69(9):727-731, 2003.

Branski SH: Delirium in hospitalized geriatric patients, *Am J Nurs* 98(4):16D-16L, 1998.

Brooke P, Bullock R: Validation of a 6-item cognitive impairment test with a view to primary care, *Int J Geriatr Psychiatry* 14(11):936-940, 1999.

Brothwell DR, Carbonell VM, Goose DH: Congenital absence of teeth in human populations. In Brothwell DR, editor: *Dental anthropology,* Tarrytown, NY, 1963, Pergamon Press.

Brown JE, Carlson M: Nutrition and multi-fetal pregnancy, *J Am Diet Assoc* 100(3):343-348, 2000.

Brown MS, Hurlock JT: Preparation of the breast for breast feeding, *Nurs Res* 24:448, 1975.

Brown-Jones LC, Orr OP: Enlisting parents as allies against depression, *Contemp Pediatr* 13:6, 1996.

Burchard KW, Rowland-Morin PA: A new method of assessing the interpersonal skills of surgeons, *Acad Med* 65(4):274-276, 1990.

Burrow GN, Duffy TP: *Medical complications during pregnancy,* ed 6, Philadelphia, 2004, WB Saunders.

Butz AM et al: Infant health care utilization predicted by pattern of prenatal care, *Pediatrics* 92:50, 1993.

Bynum DT: Clinical snapshot: gout, *Am J Nurs* 97(7):36-37, 1997.

Cadarette SM et al: Development and validation of the Osteoporosis Risk Assessment Instrument to facilitate selection of women for bone densitometry, *Can Med Assoc J* 162(9):1289-1294, 2000.

Callahan CM: The benefit of the doubt, *JAMA* 264:341, 1990.

Caputo GM et al: Assessment and management of foot disease in patients with diabetes, *N Engl J Med* 331(13):854-860, 1994.

Carbajal R, Lenclen R, Gajdos V, Jugie M, Paupe A: Crossover trial of analgesic efficacy of glucose and pacifier in very preterm infants during subcutaneous injections, *Pediatrics* 110:389-393, 2002.

Carli P, De Giorgi V, B Giannotti B: Dermoscopy as a second step in the diagnosis of doubtful pigmented skin lesions: how great is the risk of missing a melanoma? *J Eur Acad Dermatol Venereol* 15(1):24, 2001.

Carrese JA, Rhodes LA: Western bioethics on the Navajo reservation: benefit or harm? *JAMA* 274:826, 1995.

Casselman CW, Crutcher RA, Jadusingh IH. Use of water-soluble gel in obtaining the cervical cytologic smear. Letter, *Acta Cytol* 41(6):1861-1862, 1997.

Castiglia PT: Depression in children, *J Pediatr Health Care* 14(2):73-75, 2000.

Caufield C: A developmental approach to hearing screening in children, *Pediatr Nurs* 4:39, 1978.

Centers for Disease Control and Prevention: Food borne illness. www.cdc.gov/ncidod/dbmd/diseaseinfo/foodborneinfections_g.htm, accessed 7/22/04.

Centers for Disease Control and Prevention: Hepatitis. www.cdc.gov/ncidod/diseases/hepatitis/index.htm, revised 12/1/05.

Centers for Disease Control and Prevention, National Immunization Program: Pneumococcal polysaccharide vaccine: what you need to know, 1997. www.cdc.gov/nip/publications/VIS/vis-ppv.pdf, accessed 1/14/05.

Centers for Disease Control and Prevention: Prostate cancer. www.cdc.gov/cancer/prostate/index.htm, accessed 8/31/04.

Centers for Disease Control and Prevention: Standard Precautions. www.cdc.gov/ncidod/dhqp/guidelines.html, updated September 2005.

Centers for Disease Control and Prevention: Travelers' diarrhea. www.cdc.gov/travel/diarrhea.htm, accessed 7/22/04.

Centers for Disease Control and Prevention: Public health emergency preparedness and response. www.bt.cdc.gov/Agent/Agentlist.asp, 2004.

Centers for Disease Control and Prevention: Transmission-based precautions. www.cdc.gov/ncidod/dhqp/gl_isolation.html, updated April 2005.

Chang S, Tzeng S, Cheng J, Chie W: Height and weight change across menarche of schoolgirls with early menarche, *Arch Pediatr Adolesc Med* 154(9):880-884, 2000.

Charles SC: Malpractice suits: their effects on doctors, patients, and families, *J Med Assoc Ga*, 1987.

Chernick V, editor: *Kendig's disorders of the respiratory tract in children,* ed 5, Philadelphia, 1990, WB Saunders.

Christensen FC, Rayburn WF: Fetal movement counts, *Obstet Gynecol Clin North Am* 26(4):607-621, 1999.

Christianson RE et al: Incidence of congenital anomalies among white and black live births with long-term follow-up, *Am J Public Health* 71:1333, 1981.

Chrzastek-Spruch H, Wolanski N, Wrebiakowski H: Socioeconomic and endogenous factors in growth of 11 year old children from Lublin, *Collegium Anthropologium* 8:57, 1984.

Chumlea W et al: Age at menarche and racial comparisons in US girls, *Pediatrics* 111:110-113, 2003. www.pediatrics.org/cgi/content/full/111/1/110.

Churgay CA: Diagnosis and treatment of pediatric foot deformities, *Am Fam Physician* 47(4):883-889, 1993.

Coles R: *The call of stories: teaching and the moral imagination,* Boston, 1989, Houghton Mifflin.

Collins JW Jr, David RJ: Differential survival rates among low birth weight black and white infants in a tertiary care hospital, *Epidemiology* 1:16, 1990.

Connelly JE: Emotions and clinical decisions, *SGIM News* 13:1, 1990.

Cooper-Patrick L, Crum RM, Ford DE: Identifying suicidal ideation in general medical patients, *JAMA* 272:1757, 1994.

Criddle LM, Bonnono C, Fisher SK: Standardizing stroke assessment using the National Institutes of Health Stroke Scale, *J Emerg Nursing* 26(6):541-546, 2003.

Crigger N, Forbes W: Assessing neurologic function in older adults, *Am J Nurs* 97:37, 1997.

Crowell DH et al: Race, ethnicity and birth-weight Hawaii 1983 to 1986, *Hawaii Med J* 51:242, 1992.

Crowley W et al: Receptor gene plays key role in regulating puberty, *N Engl J Med* 349:1589-1592, 1614-1627, 2003.

Crum R et al: Population-based norms for the Mini-Mental State Examination by age and education level, *JAMA* 269(18):2386-2391, 1993.

Cugell DW: Lung sound nomenclature, *Am Rev Respir Dis* 136:1016, 1987.

Cullum CM, Rosenberg RN: Memory loss—when is it Alzheimer disease? *JAMA* 279(21):1689-1690, 1996.

Culture and chronic illness: raising children with disabling conditions in a culturally diverse world: proceedings of a conference, *Pediatrics* 91(5 Pt 2):1025-1081, 1993.

Cunningham G et al: *Williams obstetrics,* ed 22, Columbus, Ohio, 2005, McGraw-Hill.

Curative Health Services: *The curative footsense 5.07 monofilament,* East Setauket, NJ, 1996, Curative Health Services.

Dahlberg AO: Analyses of the American Indian dentition. In Brothwell DR, editor: *Dental anthropology,* Tarrytown, NY, 1963, Pergamon Press.

Dains JE, Bauman LC, Scheibel P: Common problems of the musculoskeletal system. In Dains JE, Baumann LC, Scheibel P: *Advanced health assessment and clinical diagnosis in primary care,* St Louis, 1998, Mosby.

Dains JE, Baumann LC, Scheibel P: *Advanced health assessment and clinical diagnosis in primary care,* ed 2, St Louis, 2003, Mosby.

Daniels SR, Khoury PR, Morrison JA: The utility of body mass index as a measure of body fatness in children and adolescents: differences by race and gender, *Pediatrics* 99(6):804-807, 1997.

D'Arcy CA, McGee S: Does this patient have carpal tunnel syndrome? *JAMA* 283(23):3110-3117, 2000.

Dasgupta A: Review of abnormal laboratory test results and toxic effects due to use of herbal medicines, *Am J Clin Pathol* 120:127-137, 2003.

Davies R: *World of wonders,* New York, 1977, Penguin.

Davies T, Mills C: Personal communication, 15 September 1997.

Deering CG: To speak or not to speak: self-disclosure with patients, *Am J Nurs* 99:34-38, 1999.

Defer TM: An evidence-based approach to low back pain in primary care, *Adv Stud Med* 4(3):135-148, 2004.

Delves PJ, Roitt IM: The immune system, *N Engl J Med* 343:108-116, 2000.

Des Jardin T, Burton GG: *Clinical manifestations and assessment of respiratory disease,* ed 3, St Louis, 1995, Mosby.

DeSwiet MD: The respiratory system. In Hytten F, Chamberlain G, editors: *Clinical physiology in obstetrics,* ed 2, Boston, 1991, Blackwell Scientific.

Dewey KG et al: Height and weight of Southeast Asian preschool children in northern California, *Am J Public Health* 76:806, 1986.

DiClemente C, Prochaska J: Toward a comprehensive transtheoretical model of change. In Miller WR, Healther N, editors: *Treating addictive behaviors,* New York, 1998, Plenum Press.

Dietary Guidelines for Americans 2005. www.health.gov/dietaryguidelines/dga2005/document/.

DiFrancesco E: Getting teens to talk to you, *Pediatric News,* Aug 19, 1992.

Dillon MJ: Investigation and management of hypertension in children: a personal perspective, *Pediatr Nephrol* 1(1):59-68, 1987.

Dodd V: Gestational age assessment, *Neonatal Network* 15(1):27-36, 1996.

Donnelly WJ: Medical language as symptoms: doctor talk in teaching hospitals, *Perspect Biology Med* 30:81, 1986.

Dowd R, Cavalieri RJ: Help your patient live with osteoporosis, *Am J Nurs* 99(4):55, 57-60, 1999.

Drolett B et al: The hair collar sign: marker for cranial dysraphism, *Pediatrics* 96(2 Pt 1):309-313, 1995.

Druzin ML, Gabbe SG, Reed KL: Antepartum fetal evaluation. In Gabbe SG, Niebyl JR, Simpson JL, editors: *Obstetrics: normal and problem pregnancies,* ed 4, London, 2002, Churchill Livingstone.

Eddy DM: The anatomy of a decision, *JAMA* 263:441, 1990.

Edge V, Miller M: *Women's health care,* St Louis, 1994, Mosby.

Edwards L et al: Pregnancy complications and birth outcomes in obese and normal weight women: effects of gestational weight changes, *Obstet Gynecol* 87(3):389-394, 1996.

Eichelberger MR et al: *Pediatric emergencies: a manual for prehospital care providers,* Englewood Cliffs, NJ, 1998, Brady.

Ellen J: Adolescent care: what are the challenges? *Adv Studies Med* 4(2B):S122-S127, 2004.

Elmore JG et al: Ten-year risk of false positive screening mammograms and clinical breast examinations, *N Engl J Med* 338(16):1089-1096, 1998.

Elster A et al: Racial and ethnic disparities in health care for adolescents, *Arch Pediatr Adolesc Med* 157:867-874, 2003.

Emanuel EJ, Emanuel LL: Four models of the physician-patient relationship, *JAMA* 267:2221, 1992.

Emergency Cardiovascular Care Committee, American Heart Association: Policy statement: response to cardiac arrest and selected life-threatening medical emergencies: the medical emergency response plan for schools, *Pediatrics* 113:155-168, 2004.

Erickson MJ, Hill TD, Siegel RM: Barriers to domestic violence screening in the pediatric setting, *Pediatrics* 108:98-102, 2001.

Esteban-Santillan C et al: Clock drawing test in very mild Alzheimer's disease, *J Am Geriatr Soc* 46(10):1266-1269, 1998.

Ewing JA: Detecting alcoholism, the CAGE questionnaire, *JAMA* 252:1905, 1984.

Fai FV et al: Assessment of fetal health should be based on maternal perception of clusters rather than episodes of fetal movements, *J Obstet Gynecol Res* 22:299, 1996.

Falkner G, Tanner J: *Human growth I: principles and prenatal growth,* New York, 1978, Plenum Press.

FDA approves technetium (99m Tc) Fanolesomab, NeutroSpec (murine monoclonal antibody to CD15) for the scintigraphic imaging of patients with equivocal signs and symptoms of appendicitis who are five years of age or older. www.fda.gov/cder/previous_news.htm, July 7, 2004.

Fedullo PF, Tapson VF: The evaluation of suspected pulmonary embolism, *N Engl J Med* 349:1247-1256, 2003.

Feldhaus KM et al: Accuracy of 3 brief screening questions for detecting partner violence in the emergency department, *JAMA* 277(17):1400-1401, 1997.

Feldmann J, Middleman A: Adolescent sexuality and sexual behavior, *Curr Opin Obstet Gynecol* 14(5):489-493, 2002.

Ferreyra S, Hughes K: *Table manners: a guide to the pelvic examination for disabled women and health care providers,* Alameda/San Francisco, 1982, Planned Parenthood.

Ferrini R, Woolf S: Screening for prostate cancer in American Men, American College of Preventive Medicine Practice Policy Statement, *Am J Prevent Med* 15:18-84, 1998.

Ferro RT et al: A nonoperative approach to shoulder impingement syndrome, *Adv Studies Med* 3(9):518-528, 2003.

Fetters MD: The family in medical decision making: Japanese perspectives, *J Clin Ethics* 9:132-146, 1998.

Fisher B et al: Tamoxifen for prevention of breast cancer: report of the National Surgical Adjuvant Breast and Bowel Project P-1 Study, *J Natl Cancer Inst* 16;90(18):1371-1388, 1998.

Folstein M et al: The meaning of cognitive impairment in the elderly, *J Am Geriatr Soc* 33:228, 1985.

Folstein MF, Folstein SE, McHugh PR: "Mini-Mental State": a practical method for grading the cognitive state of patients for the clinician, *J Psychiatric Res* 12:189, 1975.

Ford CA, Millstein SG: Delivery of confidentiality assurances to adolescents by primary care physicians, *Arch Pediatr Adolesc Med* 151(5):505-509, 1997.

Fosarelli P: Children and the development of faith: implications for pediatric practice. *Contemp Pediatr* 20:85-98, 2003.

Foster TA et al: Anthropometric and maturation measurements of children, ages 5 to 14 years, in a biracial community: the Bogalusa Heart Study, *Am J Clin Nutr* 30:582, 1977.

Fox GN: Teaching first trimester uterine sizing, *J Fam Pract* 21(5):400-401, 1985.

Franklin SS et al: Is pulse pressure useful in predicting risk for coronary heart disease? *Circulation* 100:354, 1999.

Freeman JM: The three-cent neurologic exam and other tools for an era of managed care, *Contemp Pediatr* 14:153, 1997.

Fried LP et al: Untangling the concepts of disability, frailty, and comorbidity: implications for improved targeting and care, *J Gerontol* 59:255-263, 2004.

Fried LP et al: Frailty in older adults: evidence for a phenotype, *J Gerontol* 56A:M146-M156, 2001.

Fried LP: *Functional assessment: the role of the clinician:* presented as part of Annual Geriatrics Symposium at The Johns Hopkins Medical Institutions, February 3-8, 1992.

Frisancho A: New norms of upper limb fat and muscle areas for assessment of nutritional status, *Am J Clin Nutr* 34:2540, 1981.

Frisancho AR: New standards of weight and body composition by frame size and height for assessment of nutritional status of adults and the elderly, *Am J Clin Nutr* 40:808, 1984.

Froehling DA et al: Does this dizzy patient have a serious form of vertigo? *JAMA* 271(5):385-388, 1994.

Gabbe S, Niebyl J, Simpson J: *Obstetrics: Normal and problem pregnancies,* ed 4, Philadelphia, 2002, Churchill Livingstone.

Gallagher RP et al: Melanocytic nevus density in Asian, Indo-Pakistani, and white children: the Vancouver Mole Study, *J Am Acad Dermatol* 25(3):507, 1991.

Gallagher-Allred CR: *Implementing nutrition screening and intervention strategies,* Washington, DC, 1993, Nutrition Screening Initiative.

Gallo AM: Osteoporosis and children at risk with genetic hypercalciuria, *Image J Nurs Sch* 28:368, 1996.

Gambert S: Screening for prostate cancer, *Int Urol Nephrol* 33:249-257, 2001.

Gans B: Breast and nipple pain in early stages of lactation, *Br Med J* 5100:830, 1958.

Gardosi J, Francis A: Controlled trial of fundal height measurement plotted on customised antenatal growth charts, *Br J Obstet Gynaecol* 104(4):309-317, 1999.

Garn SM, Clark DC, Guire KE: Level of fatness and size attainment, *Am J Phys Anthropol* 40:447, 1974.

Garner JS: Hospital Infection Control Practices Advisory Committee: Guideline for isolation precautions in hospitals, *Infect Control Hosp Epidemiol* 17:53, 1996a.

Garner JS: Hospital Infection Control Practices Advisory Committee: Guideline for isolation precautions in hospitals, *Am J Infect Control* 24:24-52, 1996b.

Garrick JG: Sports medicine, *Pediatr Clin North Am* 24:737, 1977.

Glascoe FP, Macias MM: How you can implement the AAP's new policy on developmental and behavioral screening. *Contemp Pediatr* 20:85-102, 2003.

Goldberg B et al: Preparticipation sports assessment: an objective evaluation, *Pediatrics* 66(5):736, 1980.

Goldenring JM, Rosen DS: Getting into adolescent heads, an essential update, *Contemp Pediatr* 21:64-90, 2004.

Goodenough-Harris Drawing Test, Psychological Corporation, 757 Third Ave, New York, NY 10017.

Gordon MC: Maternal physiology in pregnancy. In Gabbe SG, Niebyl JR, Simpson JL, editors: *Obstetrics: normal and problem pregnancies,* ed 4, London, 2002, Churchill Livingstone.

Gotzsche PC, Olsen O: Is screening for breast cancer with mammography justifiable? *Lancet* 355(9198):129-134, 2000.

Gradin M et al: Pain reduction at venipuncture in newborns: oral glucose compared with local anesthetic cream, *Pediatrics* 110:1053-1057, 2002.

Grant A: *Nutritional assessment guidelines,* ed 2, Seattle, 1979, Author.

Green M, Stuy MZ: Persistent symptoms: how to end the frustration, *Contemp Pediatr* 9:104, 1992.

Green M: The 10-minute visit: anything but routine, *Contemp Pediatr* 9:53, 1992.

Griffith LSC, Seidel HM: *Clinical history and physical examination,* Baltimore, 1986, Johns Hopkins School of Medicine.

Gross RH: The pediatric orthopaedic examination. In Morrissy RT, Weinstein SL, editors: *Lovell & Winter's pediatric orthopaedics,* ed 4, Philadelphia, 1996, Lippincott-Raven.

Grundy S et al: Implications of recent clinical trials for the National Cholesterol Education Program Adult Treatment Panel III Guidelines, *Circulation* 110:227-239, 2004. Available at http://www.circulationaha.org.

Guilbert TW, Taussig LM: Doctor, he's been coughing for a month: is it serious? *Contemp Pediatr* 15:155-172, 1998.

Guo SS et al: Weight-for-length reference data for preterm, low-birth-weight infants. *Arch Pediatr Adolesc Med* 150:964-970, 1996.

Guttmacher AE, Collins FS, Carmona RA: The family history—more important than ever. *N Engl J Med* 351:2333-2336, 2004.

Guzzetta CD, Dossey BM: *Cardiovascular nursing: holistic practice,* St Louis, 1992, Mosby.

Hagman J: Diagnosis and treatment of depression in adolescence, *Adolesc Health Update* 13:1-8, 2001.

Hahn BA: Children's health: racial and ethnic differences in the use of prescription medications, *Pediatrics* 95(5):727-732, 1995.

Haka-Ikse K, Mian M: Sexuality in children, *Pediatr Rev* 14:10, 1993.

Halffman CM, Scott CR, Pedersen PO: Palatine torus in the Greenlandic Norse, *Am J Phys Anthropol* 88(2):145-161, 1992.

Hall ET: *The hidden dimension,* Garden City, NY, 1969, Anchor Books, Doubleday.

Haller CA, Benowitz NL: Adverse cardiovascular and central nervous system events associated with dietary supplements containing ephedra alkaloids, *N Engl J Med* 343:1833-1842, 2000.

Hamill PV, Johnston FE, Lemeshow S: Body weight, stature, and sitting height: white and Negro youths 12-17 years, *Vital Health Stat* 11:1, 1973.

Hardie GE et al: Ethnic differences: word descriptors used by African-American and white asthma patients during induced bronchoconstriction, *Chest* 117(4):935-943, 2000.

Harer WB, Valenzuela G Jr, Lebo D: Lubrication of the vaginal introitus and speculum does not affect Papanicolaou smears, *Obstet Gynecol* 100(5 Pt 1):887-888, 2002.

Harris RP et al: Screening for prostate cancer. Systematic Evidence Review No. 16 (Prepared by the Research Triangle Institute—University of North Carolina Evidence-based Practice Center under Contract No. 290-97-0011). Rockville, Md: Agency for Healthcare Research and Quality. December 2001. Available at www.ncbi.nlm.nih.gov/books/bv.fcgi?rid=hstat3.Chapter3159.

Harris RP, Lohr KN: Screening for prostate cancer: an update of the evidence for the U.S. Preventive Services Task Force, *Ann Intern Med* 137:917-929, 2002.

Hartmann LC et al: Efficacy of bilateral prophylactic mastectomy in BRCA1 and BRCA2 gene mutation carriers, *J Natl Cancer Inst* 93(21):1633-1637, 2001.

Harvey AM et al: *The principles and practice of medicine,* ed 22, Norwalk, Conn, 1988, Appleton & Lange.

Harvey WP: *Cardiac pearls,* pp. 62-64, Newton, NJ, Laennec Publishing, 1943.

Hawkins JL, Chestnut DH, Gibbs CP: Obstetric anesthesia. In Gabbe SG, Niebyl JR, Simpson JL: *Obstetrics: normal and problem pregnancies,* ed 4, London, 2002, Churchill Livingstone.

Hedley AA et al: Prevalence of overweight and obesity among US children, adolescents, and adults, 1999-2002, *JAMA* 291(23):2847-2850, 2004.

Hellmann DB: Eurekapenia: a disease of medical residency training programs, *Pharos* Spring, 24-26, 2003.

Henderson et al: Smallpox as a biological weapon: medical and public health management. Working Group on Civilian Biodefense, *JAMA* 281(22):2127-2137, 1999.

Hennigan L, Kollar LM, Rosenthal SL: Methods for managing pelvic examination anxiety: individual differences and relaxation techniques, *J Pediatr Health Care* 14(1):9-12, 2000.

Herman-Giddens ME et al: Secondary sexual characteristics and menses in young girls seen in office practice: a study from the pediatric research in office setting network, *Pediatrics* 99:505, 1997.

Herr KA: Pain assessment in cognitively impaired older adults. *Am J Nurs* 102:65-68, 2002.

Hershko DD et al: The role of selective computed tomography in the diagnosis and management of suspected acute appendicitis. *Am Surg* 68(11):1003-1007, 2002.

Herzog LW: Prevalence of lymphadenitis of the head and neck in infants and children, *Clin Pediatr* 22:485, 1983.

Hilliard AA et al: Occam's razor versus saint's triad, *N Engl J Med* 350:599-603, 2004.

Hirsch ED Jr: *Cultural literacy: what every American needs to know,* Boston 1987, Houghton Mifflin.

Hirschfield RMA, Russell JM: Assessment and treatment of suicidal patients, *N Engl J Med* 337:910-915, 1997.

Hitchcock JM, Wilson HS: Personal risking: lesbian self-disclosure of sexual orientation to professional health care providers, *Nurs Res* 41:178 1992.

Hoberman A, Paradise JL: Acute otitis media: diagnosis and management in the year 2000, *Pediatric Ann* 29(10):609-620, 2000.

Hockenberry MJ et al: *Nursing care of infants and children,* ed 7, St Louis, 2003, Mosby.

Hockenberry MJ: *Wong's essentials of pediatric nursing,* ed 7, St Louis, 2005, Mosby.

Hodgson SF, Johnston CC: *AACE clinical practice guidelines for the prevention of postmenopausal osteoporosis,* Brandamore, Penn, 1998, Herrin Communications.

Hoekelman RA et al: *Primary pediatric care,* ed 3, St Louis, 1997, Mosby.

Horner G: Sexual behavior in children. Normal or not? *J Pediatr Health Care,* 18(2):57-64, 2004.

Hubert PM: Revealing patient concerns, *Am J Nurs* 98:16H-16L, 1998.

Huether SE, Leo J: Pain, temperature regulation, sleep, and sensory function. In McCance KL, Huether SE: *Pathophysiology: the biologic basis for disease in adults and children,* ed 4, St Louis, 2002, Mosby.

Hulsey TC, Levkoff AH, Alexander GR: Birth weights of infants of black and white mothers without pregnancy complications, *Am J Obstet Gynecol* 164(part 1):1299, 1991.

Humphrey LL et al: Breast cancer screening: a summary of the evidence for the U.S. Preventive Services Task Force, *Ann Intern Med* 137(5):347-360, 2002.

Iams JD: Preterm birth. In Gabbe SG, Niebyl JR., Simpson JL: *Obstetrics: normal and problem pregnancies,* ed 4, London, 2002, Churchill Livingstone.

Ibraimov IA: Brief communication: cerumen phenotypes in certain populations of Eurasia and Africa, *Am J Phys Anthropol* 84:209, 1991.

Ikegami N: Functional assessment and its place in health care, *N Engl J Med* 332(9):598-599, 1995.

Ilic D et al: Screening for prostatic cancer (Protocol for a Cochrane Review). Updated 18 February 2004, *The Cochrane Library* 3, 2004.

Inglesby TV et al: Anthrax as a biological weapon: medical and public health management. Working Group on Civilian Biodefense, *JAMA* 281(18):1735-1745, 1999.

Institute of Medicine: Dietary reference intakes tables, 2004, the National Academy of Sciences. Available at www.iom.edu/file.asp?id=21372.

Isaacson G: Sinusitis in childhood, *Pediatr Clin North Am* 43:1297, 1996.

Jacobson A: Research for practice: saving limbs with Semmes-Weinstein monofilament, *Am J Nurs* 99(2):76, 1999.

Jacobson RD: Approach to the child with weakness or clumsiness, *Pediatr Clin North Am* 45(1):145-168, 1998.

James HE: Neurologic evaluation and support of the child with acute brain insult, *Pediatr Ann* 15(1):17, 1986.

James WD, Carter JM, Rodman OG: Pigmentary demarcation lines: a population survey: *J Am Acad Dermatol* 16(3, part 1):584, 1987.

Janofsky JS, McCarthy RJ, Folstein MF: The Hopkins Competency Assessment Test: a brief method for evaluating patients' capacity to give informed consent, *Hospital Community Psychiatry* 43:132-136, 1992.

Janofsky JS, Rovner BW: Prevalence of advance directives and guardianship in nursing home patients, *J Geriatr Psychiatr Neurol* 6:214-216, 1993.

Jantz JW, Blosser CD, Fruechting LA: A motor milestone change noted with a change in sleep position, *Arch Pediatr Adolesc Med* 151:565, 1997.

Jarvis A, Gorlin RJ: Minor orofacial abnormalities in an Eskimo population, *Oral Surg* 33:417, 1972.

Jecker NS, Carrese JA, Pearlman RA: Caring for patients in cross-cultural settings, *Hastings Center Report* 25:6, 1995.

Jellinck MS et al: Psychosocial aspects of ambulatory pediatrics, *Curr Probl Pediatr* 20:623, 1990.

Jellinck MS et al: The difficult parent—and the difficult physician, *Contemp Pediatr* 8:118, 1991.

Jerant AF et al: Early detection and treatment of skin cancer, *Am Fam Physician* 62(2):357-368, 375-376, 2000.

Johns Hopkins Medical Letter, p. 3, May 1990.

Johns Hopkins University Center for Civilian Biodefense Studies, 2001. Available at www.hopkins-biodefense.org/index.html.

Johns RJ, Fortuin NJ, Wheeler PS: The collection and evaluation of clinical information. In Harvey AM et al, editors: *Principles and practice of medicine,* ed 22, Norwalk, Conn, 1988, Appleton & Lange.

Johnson TS et al: Reliability of three length measurement techniques in term infants, *Pediatr Nurs* 25(1):13-17, 1999.

Johnson T, Niebyl JR: Preconception and prenatal care. In Gabbe SG, Niebyl JR, Simpson JL, editors: *Obstetrics: normal and problem pregnancies,* ed 4, London, 2002, Churchill Livingstone.

Jones AK: Primary care management of acute low back pain, *Nurse Pract* 22:50, 1997.

Judge R, Zuidema G, Fitzgerald F: *Clinical diagnosis,* ed 5, Boston, 1988, Little, Brown.

Kahn JA, Emans SJ: Gynecologic examination of the prepubertal girl, *Contemp Pediatr* 16(3):148-159, 1999.

Kain CD, Reilly N, Schultz ED: The older adult: a comparative assessment, *Nurs Clin North Am* 25:833, 1990.

Kakarla N, Bradshaw KD: Disorders of pubertal development: precocious puberty, *Semin Reprod Med* 21(4):339-351, 2003.

Kaplowitz PB, Oberfield SE, and the Drug and Therapeutics and Executive Committees of the Lawson Wilkins Pediatric Endocrine Society: Reexamination of the age limits for defining when puberty is precocious in girls in the United States: implications for evaluation and treatment, *Pediatrics* 104(4):936-941, 1999.

Kass-Wolff J, Wilson E: Pediatric gynecology: assessment strategies and common problems, *Semin Reprod Med* 21(4):329-338, 2003.

Katzman R et al: Validation of a short orientation-memory-concentration test of cognitive impairment, *Am J Psychiatry* 140(6):734-739, 1983.

Keith NM, Wagner HP, Barker NW: Some different types of essential hypertension: their course and prognosis, *Am J Med Sci* 197:337, 1939.

Keller C, Stevens KR: Childhood obesity: measurement and risk assessment, *Pediatr Nurs* 22:494, 1996.

Kemper KJ, Rivara FP: Parents in jail, *Pediatrics* 92(2):261-264, 1993.

Kennedy CT, Kyle P: Skin diseases. In James DK et al, editors: *High risk pregnancy: management options,* ed 2, Philadelphia, 1999, WB Saunders.

Kerker BD et al: Identification of violence in the home, *Arch Ped Adolesc Med* 154:457-462, 2000.

Kernan WN et al: Phenylpropanolamine and the risk of hemorrhagic stroke, *N Engl J Med* 343:1826-1832, 2000.

Khandker RK et al: A decision model and cost-effectiveness analysis of colorectal cancer screening and surveillance guidelines for average-risk adults, *Int J Technol Assess Health Care* 16(3):799-810, 2000.

Kipper SL et al: Neutrophil-specific 99mTc-labeled anti-CD15 monoclonal antibody imaging for diagnosis of equivocal appendicitis, *J Nucl Med* 41:447-455, 2000.

Klebanoff MA et al: Pre-term and small for gestational-age birth across generations, *Am J Obstet Gynecol* 176:521, 1997.

Klein JD et al: Adolescents' risky behavior and mass media use, *Pediatrics* 92:24, 1993.

Kleinman A, Eisenberg L, Good B: Clinical lessons from anthropological and cross-cultural research, *Ann Intern Med* 88:251, 1978.

Kluckhohn C: *Culture and behavior,* New York, 1962, The Free Press.

Kluckhohn F: Dominant and variant value orientation. In Brink P, editor: *Transcultural nursing: a book of readings,* Englewood Cliffs, NJ, 1976, Prentice-Hall.

Knight JR et al: A new brief screen for adolescent substance abuse, *Arch Pediatr Adolesc Med* 153:591-596, 1999.

Knight JR et al: Reliabilities of short substance abuse screening tests among adolescent medical patients, *Pediatrics* 105(4 Pt 2):948-953, 2000.

Kolata G: Is frailty inevitable? Some experts say no, *The New York Times* November 19, 2002, D5.

Koop CE: *The Surgeon General's letter on child sexual abuse,* Rockville, Md, 1988, U.S. Department of Health and Human Services, Public Health Service.

Kopp VJ: Letter to the editor: Diagnoses, *N Engl J Med* 337:941-942, 1997.

Koutures CG, Landry GL: The acutely injured knee, *Pediatr Ann* 26:50, 1997.

Krajicek MJ, Tomlinson AT: *Detection of developmental problems in children,* ed 2, Baltimore, 1983, University Park Press.

Kuczmarski MF, Kuczmarski RJ, Najjar M: Descriptive anthropometric reference data for older Americans, *J Am Diet Assoc* 100:59-66, 2000.

Lancaster T, Stead LF: Individual behavioural counseling for smoking cessation, *The Cochrane Library* 3, 2004.

Lanham DM et al: Accuracy of tympanic temperature readings in children under 6 years of age, *Pediatr Nurs* 25(1):39-42, 1999.

Lapinsky S: Cardiopulmonary changes in pregnancy: what you need to know, *Women's Health in Primary Care* 2:353, 1999.

Lawrence J et al: Development of a tool to assess neonatal pain, *Neonatal Network* 12:59-66, 1993.

Leitzmann MF et al: Subsequent risk of prostate cancer, *JAMA* 291:1578, 2004.

Lembo NJ et al: Bedside diagnosis of systolic murmurs, *N Engl J Med* 318:1572, 1988.

Leung AKC, Kellner JD: Acute sinusitis in children: diagnosis and management, *J Pediatr Health Care* 18(2):72-76, 2004.

Levin J: When doctors question kids (letter to editor), *N Engl J Med* 323:1569, 1990.

Lin WS: Physical growth of Chinese school children 7-18 years, in 1985, *Ann Hum Biol* 19:41, 1992.

Lipman TH et al: Assessment of growth by primary health care providers, *J Pediatr Health Care* 14(4):166-171, 2000.

Lively MW: Making sure young athletes are fit to compete in Special Olympics, *Contemp Pediatr* 20:101-107, 2003.

Lowdermilk DL, Perry SE: *Maternity and women's health care,* ed 8, St Louis, 2004, Mosby.

Lowrey GH: *Growth and development of children,* ed 8, Chicago, 1986, Mosby.

Lurie N et al: Preventive care for women: does the sex of the physician matter? *N Engl J Med* 329(7):478-482, 1993.

Lyketsos CG: Dementia and Alzheimer's disease: Part 1: Evaluation and diagnosis, *Adv Studies Med* 4(6):297-306, 2004.

Lynch SH: Elder abuse: what to look for and how to intervene, *Am J Nurs* 97:27-32, 1997.

Lyon RM, Street CC: Pediatric sports injury: when to refer or x-ray, *Pediatr Clin North Am* 45(1):221-244, 1998.

Mace JW et al: The child with an unusual odor; a clinical resume, *Clin Pediatr* 15(1):57-62, 1976.

Mackie RM et al: The use of the dermatoscope to identify early melanoma using the three-colour test, *Br J Dermatol* 146(3):481, 2002.

Malina RM, Hamill PV, Lemeshow S: Body dimensions and proportions, white and Negro children 6-11 years, *Vital Health Stat* 11:1, 1974.

Malina RM, Zavaleta AN, Little BB: Body size, fatness, and leanness of Mexican American children in Brownsville, Texas: changes between 1972 and 1983, *Am J Public Health* 77:573, 1987.

Mallory MD et al: Bronchiolitis management preferences and the influence of pulse oximetry and respiratory rate on the decision to admit, *Pediatrics* [serial on line] 111:e45-e51, 2003.

Mankin KP, Zimbler S: Gait and leg alignment: what's normal and what's not, *Contemp Pediatr* 14(11):41-70, 1997.

Mann JM: Medicine and public health, ethics and human rights, *Hastings Center Report* May-June:6-13, 1997.

Mann DR, Plant TM: Leptin and pubertal development, *Semin Reprod Med* 20(2):93-102, 2002.

Manning ML: Health assessment of the early adolescent, *Nurs Clin North Am* 25:923, 1990.

Marcus CL: Does your child snore? *Contemp Pediatr* 15(2):101-115, 1998.

Marder MZ: The standard of care for oral diagnosis as it relates to oral cancer, *In Compendium* 19:569-582, 1998.

Margileth AM, Hadfield TL: A new look at old cat-scratch, *Contemp Pediatr* 7:25, 1990.

Martin JL, Crump EP: Leukoedema of the buccal mucosa in Negro children and youth, *Oral Surg* 34:49, 1972.

Matsunaga E: The dimorphism in human normal cerumen, *Ann Hum Genet* 25:273, 1962.

Mattson JE: The language of pain, *Reflections on Nursing Leadership,* 4th quarter, 11-14, 2000.

Mayer BW, Coulter M: Partner abuse of adult women, *Am J Nurs* 102:May (Critical Care Extra), 2002.

Maynard CK: Differentiate depression from dementia, *Nurse Pract* 28(3),18-27, 2003.

Mays RM, Gillon JE: Autism in young children: an update, *J Pediatr Health Care* 7:17, 1993.

McCaffery M, Pasero C: Teaching patients to use a numerical pain-rating scale, *Am J Nurs* 99:22, 1999.

McCance KL, Huether SE: *Pathophysiology: the biologic basis for disease in adults and children,* ed 5, St Louis, 2006, Mosby.

McCarthy PL et al: History and observation variables in assessing febrile children, *Pediatrics* 65:1090, 1985.

McCarty DJ: *Arthritis and allied conditions: a textbook of rheumatology,* ed 2, Philadelphia, 1993, Lea & Febiger.

McClain N et al: Evaluation of sexual abuse in the pediatric patient, *J Pediatr Health Care* 14(3):93-102, 2000.

McGee S: *Evidence-based physical diagnosis,* Philadelphia, 2001, WB Saunders.

McMillan JA, Neiburg PL, Oski FA: *The whole pediatrician catalogue,* vol 1, Philadelphia, 1977, WB Saunders.

McMillan JA, Stockman JA, Oski FA: *The whole pediatric catalogue,* vol 3, Philadelphia, 1982, WB Saunders.

Melzack R et al: Labour is still painful after prepared childbirth training, *Can Assoc Med J* 125:357, 1981.

Mendelson M, Lang R: Pregnancy and cardiovascular disease. In Barron WM, Lindheimere MD, Davison JM, editors: *Medical disorders during pregnancy,* St Louis, 2000, Mosby.

Merz ML et al: Tooth diameters and arch perimeters in a black and white population, *Am J Orthod Dentofacial Orthop* 100(1):53-58, 1991.

Meskin LH, Gorlin RJ, Isaacson RJ: Abnormal morphology of the soft palate: the prevalence of cleft uvula, *Cleft Palate J* 1:342, 1965.

Meuller DH, Burke F: Vitamin and mineral therapy. In Morrison G, Hark L, editors: *Medical nutrition and disease,* Cambridge, 1996, Blackwell Science.

Migliori ME, Gladstone GJ: Determination of the normal range of exophthalmometric values for black and white adults, *Am J Ophthalmol* 98:438, 1984.

Mills MV et al: The use of osteopathic manipulative treatment as adjuvant therapy in children with recurrent acute otitis media, *Arch Pediatr Adolesc Med* 157:861-866, 2003.

Modigliani RM: Gastrointestinal and pancreatic disorders. In Barron WM, Lindheimer MD, editors: *Medical disorders during pregnancy,* ed 3, St Louis, 2000, Mosby.

Molitch M: Pituitary, thyroid, adrenal, and parathyroid disorders. In Barron WM, Lindheimer MD, editors: *Medical disorders during pregnancy,* ed 3, St Louis, 2000, Mosby.

Monga M: Maternal cardiovascular and renal adaptation to pregnancy. In Creasey RK, Resnik R, editors: *Maternal-fetal medicine,* ed 4, Philadelphia, 1999, WB Saunders.

Moody CW: Male child sexual abuse, *J Pediatr Health Care* 13(3 Pt 1):112-119, 1999.

Morrow M: The evaluation of common breast problems, *Am Fam Physician* 61(8):2371-2378, 2000.

Moyer LA, Mast EE, Alter MJ: Hepatitis C: Part II. Prevention counseling and medical evaluation, *Am Fam Physician* 59(2):349-354, 357, 1999.

MyPyramid USDA Food Guide Pyramid. Available at www.mypyramid. gov. Accessed January 2006.

National Cancer Institute (NCI) and the National Surgical Adjuvant Breast and Bowel Project (NSABP) Biostatistics Center: Breast Cancer Risk Assessment Tool. Available at bcra.nci.nih.gov/brc.

National Cancer Institute Task Force Announces New Cervical Cancer Screening Guidelines, Jan 22, 2003. Available at www.cancer.gov/ newscenter/pressreleases/cervicalscreen, accessed August 1, 2004.

National Cancer Institute, Prostate Cancer Screening, modified 12/15/2003. Available at www.nci.nih.gov/cancertopics/screening/ prostate, accessed December 2005.

National Cancer Institute: NCAB issues mammography screening recommendations (3/97), rex.nci.nih.gov/INTRFCE_GIFS/MASSMED_ INTR_DOC.htm, June 22, 1998.

National Cancer Institute: Questions and answers about mammography screening (3/97), www.icic.nci/nih.gov/clinpdq/detec; answers_about_mammography_screening.hml#1, Sept 16, 1997.

National Center for Health Statistics (1996), National Health and Nutrition Examination Survey III (1988-1994).Available at www.cdc.gov/nchs/about/major/nhanes/datalink.htm, accessed Jan 20, 2002.

National Center for Health Statistics: Advance report of final natality statistics, 1979, *Monthly Vital Stat Rep* 30:1, 1981.

National Center for Infectious Diseases: Epidemiology and prevention of viral hepatitis a to e, on-line slide set. Available at www.cdc.gov/ ncidod/diseases/hepatitis/slideset/httoc.htm, accessed Aug 22, 1997.

National Center for Infectious Diseases: hepatitis fact sheets. Available at www.cdc. gov/ncidod/diseases/hepatitis/hepatitis.htm, August 22, 1997.

National Cholesterol Education Program (NCEP) Expert Panel on Detection, Evaluation, and Treatment of High Blood Cholesterol in Adults (Adult Treatment Panel III): Executive summary of the third report, *JAMA* 285(19):2486-2497, 2001.

National High Blood Pressure Education Program Working Group on High Blood Pressure in Children and Adolescents: The fourth report on the diagnosis, evaluation, and treatment of high blood pressure in children and adolescents, *Pediatrics* 114(2): 555-576, 2004.

National Institute for Occupational Safety and Health (NIOSH): Alert: Preventing allergic reaction to natural rubber latex in the workplace, Pub. No. 97-135, June 1997a, DHHS (NIOSH), Washington, DC.

National Institute for Occupational Safety and Health (NIOSH): Latex allergy facts. June 1997b, Doc. No. 705006. Available at www.cdc.gov/niosh/latexfs.html.

National Institutes of Health: Practical guide to the identification, evaluation, and treatment of overweight and obesity in adults, 2000, developed by the North American Association for the Study of Obesity and the National Heart, Lung, and Blood Institute, Bethesda, MD.

National Institutes of Health: The seventh report of the Joint National Committee on Prevention, Detection, Evaluation, and Treatment of High Blood Pressure (JNC7), National Heart, Lung, and Blood Institute, NIH Pub. No. 04-5230, 2004, NIH.

Nawaz H et al: Concordance of clinical findings and clinical judgment in the diagnosis of streptococcal pharyngitis, *Acad Emerg Med* 7(10):1104-1109, 2000.

Nuss R, Manco-Johnson MJ: Venous thrombosis: issues for the pediatrician, *Contemp Pediatr* 17:75, 2000.

Obel J: Losing the touch: as technology and medical education change, doctors may lose the ability to perform physical exams, *The Washington Post,* June 17, 2003.

O'Hanlon-Nichols T: Basic assessment series: A review of the adult musculoskeletal system, *Am J Nurs* 98(6):48-52, 1998.

O'Keefe MF et al: *Emergency care,* ed 8, Upper Saddle River, NJ, 1998, Brady/Prentice Hall.

Omnibus Budget Reconciliation Act [OBRA] of 1990 [Federal Patient Self-Determination Act], Pub. L No. 101-508, Sections 4206 and 4751 [Medicare and Medicaid].

Pachter LM et al: Home-based therapies for the common cold among European American and ethnic minority families: the interface between alternative/complementary and folk medicine, *Arch Pediatr Adolesc Med* 152(11):1083-1088, 1998.

Pachter LM, Dworkin PH: Maternal expectations about normal child development in 4 cultural groups, *Arch Ped Adolesc Med* 151:1144-1150, 1997.

Pachter LM: Practicing culturally sensitive pediatrics, *Contemp Pediatr* 14:139-154, 1997.

Papiernik E et al: Ethnic differences in duration of pregnancy, *Ann Hum Biol* 13:259, 1986.

Park MK, Menard SW, Yuan C: Comparison of auscultatory and oscillometric blood pressures, *Arch Pediatr Adolesc Med* 155:50-54, 2001.

Patrick D et al: Increased CT scan utilization does not improve the diagnostic accuracy of appendicitis in children, *J Pediatr Surg* 38(5):659-662, 2003.

Pawson EG, Petrakis NL: Comparisons of breast pigmentation among women of different racial groups, *Hum Biol* 47:441, 1975.

Pearce KF et al: Cytopathological findings on vaginal Papanicolaou smears after hysterectomy for benign gynecologic disease, *N Engl J Med* 335(21):1559-1562, 1996.

Peck EB, Ullrich HD: *Children and weight: a changing perspective,* Berkeley, CA, 1985, Nutrition Communications Associates.

Pedigree Standardization Task Force of the National Society of Genetic Counselors and Bennett RL et al: Recommendations for standardized human pedigree nomenclature, *Am J Hum Genet* 56:745-752, 1995.

Penninger J: Urinary incontinence: new approaches to age-old problems, *Greater Houston Nursing* 1:2, 1993.

Perez J et al: Liberal use of computed tomography scanning does not improve diagnostic accuracy in appendicitis, *Am J Surg* 185(3):194-197, 2003.

Perkins HS, Supik JD, Hazuda HP: Cultural differences among health professionals, *J Clin Ethics* 9:108-117, 1998.

Peters R, Flack M: Hypertensive disorders of pregnancy, *J Obstet Gynecol Neonat Nurs* 33:209, 2004.

Petit J, Barkhaus PE: Evaluation and management of polyneuropathy: a practical approach, *Nurse Pract* 22:131, 1997.

Petrakis NL: Cerumen genetics and human breast cancer, *Science* 173:347, 1971.

Pickering TG et al: Recommendations for blood pressure measurement in humans: an AHA scientific statement from the Council on High Blood Pressure Research Professional and Public Education Subcommittee, *J Clin Hypertension* 7:102, 2005.

Plant SM: Boundary violations in professional-client relationships: overview and guidelines for prevention, *Sexual and Marital Therapy* 12:79, 1997.

Pletcher SD, Goldberg AN: The diagnosis and treatment of sinusitis, *Adv Studies Med* 3(9):495-506, 2003.

Prazor GE, Friedman SB: An office-based approach to adolescent psychosocial issues, *Contemp Pediatr* 14:59, 1997.

Puchalski CM, Romer AL: Taking a spiritual history allows clinicians to understand patients more fully, *J Palliat Med* 3:129-137, 2000.

Quality Standards Subcommittee of the American Academy of Neurology: The management of concussion in sports (practice parameter), *Neurology* 48:581-585, 1997.

Quill TE: Recognizing and adjusting to barriers in doctor-patient communication, *Ann Intern Med* 112:51, 1989.

Rabins PV: Research update: mild cognitive impairment (MCI)—definition, diagnosis, and treatment possibilities, *Adv Studies Med* 4(6):290-296, 2004.

RADAR: A domestic violence intervention, 1992, Massachusetts Medical Society, Waltham, MA.

Raj GV, Wiener JS: Varicoceles in adolescents: when to observe, when to intervene, *Contemp Pediatr* 21:39, 2004.

Rampen FHJ, de Wit PEJ: Racial differences in mole proneness, *Acta Derm Venereol* 69:234, 1989.

Rampen FHJ: Nevocytic nevi and skin complexion, *Dermatologia* 176:111, 1988.

Ramsburg KL: Rheumatoid arthritis, *Am J Nurs* 100(11):40-43, 2000.

Rapini D: The skin and pregnancy. In Creasey RK, Resnik R, editors: *Maternal-fetal medicine*, ed 4, Philadelphia, 1999, WB Saunders.

Rathore SS, Wang Y, Krumholz HM: Sex based differences in the effect of digoxin for the treatment of heart failure, *N Engl J Med* 347:1403-1410, 2002.

Ravussin E, Tataranni PA: Dietary fat and human obesity, *J Am Diet Assoc* 97:S42, 1997.

Ravussin E, Tataranni PA: Dietary fat and human obesity. In Williams CL, Williams GM, editors: *Reducing dietary fat: putting theory into practice*, Chicago, 1997, American Dietetic Association.

Reifsnider E, Gill S: Nutrition for the childbearing years, *J Obstet Gynecol Neonat Nurs* 29(1):43-55, 2000.

Rennard SI: Looking at the patient—approaching the problem of COPD, *N Engl J Med* 350:965-966, 2004.

Resnick MB et al: Effect of birth weight, race, and sex on survival of low birth weight infants in neonatal intensive care, *Am J Obstet Gynecol* 161:184, 1989.

Revere C, Hasty R: Diagnostic and characteristic signs of illness and injury, *J Emerg Nurs* 19(2):137-139, 1993.

Rex DK et al: Colorectal cancer prevention 2000: screening recommendations of the American College of Gastroenterology, *Am J Gastroenterol* 95(4):868-877, 2000.

Rhodes LA: Norms of culture in a "culture" of norms, *Arch Pediatr Adolesc Med* 157:1155-1156, 2003.

Rice VH, Stead LF: Nursing interventions for smoking cessation. *The Cochrane Library* 3, 2004.

Rich EC, Burke W, Heaton CJ: Reconsidering the family history in primary care, *J Gen Intern Med* 19:273-280, 2004.

Richardson JL et al: Relationship between after school care of adolescents and substance abuse, risk taking, depressed mood, and academic achievement, *Pediatrics* 92:22, 1993.

Riggs SR, Alario A: *RAFFT questions: project ADEPT manual*, Providence RI, 1987, Brown University.

Risser AL, Mazur LJ: Use of folk remedies in a Hispanic population, *Arch Pediatr Adolesc Med* 149(9):978-981, 1995.

Rivara FP, Wasserman AL: Teaching psychosocial issues to pediatric house officers, *J Med Educ* 59:45, 1984.

Roberts JM: Pregnancy-related hypertension. In Creasey RK, Resnik R, editors: *Maternal-fetal medicine*, ed 4, Philadelphia, 1999, WB Saunders.

Robinson CH, Weigley ES, Mueller DH, editors: *Basic nutrition and diet therapy*, ed 7, Upper Saddle River, NJ, 1993, Prentice Hall.

Roche AF et al: Reference data for weight/stature in Mexican Americans from the Hispanic Health and Nutrition Survey (HHANES 1982-1984), *Am J Clin Nutr* 51:917S, 1990.

Rose LC: Recognizing neoplastic skin lesions: a photo guide, *Am Fam Physician* 58(4):873-884, 887-888, 1998.

Rose VL: CDC issues new recommendations for the prevention and control of hepatitis C virus infection, *Am Fam Physician* 59(5):1321-1323, 1999.

Rudy EB: *Advanced neurological and neurosurgical nursing*, St Louis, 1984, Mosby.

Ryan AS et al: Median skinfold thickness distributions and fat-wave patterns in Mexican-American children from the Hispanic Health and Nutrition Survey (HHANES 1982-1984), *Am J Clin Nutr* 51:925S, 1990.

Ryan C, Futterman D: Caring for gay and lesbian teens, *Contemp Pediatr* 15:107-130, 1998.

Sackett DL et al: Evidence-based medicine: what it is and what it isn't, *Br Med J* 312:71, 1996.

Samiy AH, Douglas RG Jr, Barondess JA: *Textbook of diagnostic medicine*, Philadelphia, 1987, Lea & Febiger.

Sapar JR: *Headache disorders: current concepts and treatment strategies*, Boston, 1983, PSG Publishing.

Saphis J: Human genetics: constructing a family pedigree, *Am J Nurs* 102(7):44-49, 2002.

Saslow D et al: American Cancer Society guideline for the early detection of cervical neoplasia and cancer, *CA Cancer J Clin* 52:342-362, 2002.

Schairer C et al: Menopausal estrogen and estrogen-progestin replacement therapy and breast cancer risk, *JAMA* 283(4):485-491, 2000.

Schaumann BF, Peagler FD, Gorlin RJ: Minor craniofacial anomalies among a Negro population, *Oral Surg Oral Med Oral Pathol* 29(4):566-575, 1970.

Schroeder AR et al: Impact of pulse oximetry and oxygen therapy on length of stay in bronchiolitis hospitalizations, *Arch Pediatr Adolesc Med* 158:527-530, 2004.

Schulman KA et al: The effects of race and sex on physician recommendations for cardiac catheterization, *N Engl J Med* 340(8):618-626, 1999.

Schutte JE: Growth differences between lower and middle income black male adolescents, *Hum Biol* 52:193, 1980.

Scott M, Gelhot AR: Gastroesophageal reflux disease: diagnosis and management, *Am Fam Physician* 59(5):1161-1169, 1199, 1999.

Seidel HM: On paternalism, *Pediatr Ann* 21:295, 1992.

Selfridge J, Sanning SS: The accuracy of the tympanic membrane thermometer in detecting fever in infants aged 3 months and younger in the emergency department setting, *J Emerg Nurs* 19:2, 1993.

Serlin M et al: What sexually transmitted disease screening method does the adolescent prefer? *Arch Pediatr Adolesc Med* 156:588-591, 2002.

Shah S et al: Risk of bacteremia in young children with pneumonia treated as outpatients, *Arch Pediatr Adolesc Med* 157:389-393, 2003.

Shaper A: Obesity and cardiovascular disease. In Chadwick D, Cardew G, editors: *The origins and consequences of obesity*, Chichester, 1996, CIBA Foundation Symposium 201.

Shapiro J, Roper J, Schulzinger J: Managing delirious patients, *Nursing* 93:78, 1993.

Shapiro W: Hemolytic uremic syndrome. Available at www.emedicine.com June 18, 2004, accessed July 22, 2004.

Shaw BA, Gerardi JA, Hennrikus WL: Avoiding the pitfalls of orthopedic disorders, *Contemp Pediatr* 15(6):122-135, 1998.

Shay DK et al: Bronchiolitis-associated mortality and estimates of respiratory syncytial virus–associated deaths among US children, *J Infect Dis* 183:16-22, 2001.

Sherin KM et al: HITS: A short domestic violence screening tool for use in a family practice setting, *Fam Med* 30(7):508-512, 1998.

Sherry B et al: Evaluation of and recommendations for growth references for very low birth weight (1500 grams) infants in the United States, *Pediatrics* 111(4):750-758, 2003.

Shinitzky HE, Kub J: The art of motivating behavioral change: the use of motivational interviewing to promote health, *Public Health Nurs* 18(3):178-185, 2001.

Shipman JJ: *Mnemonics and tactics in surgery and medicine,* ed 2, Chicago, 1984, Mosby.

Shoaf SC: What your patient's mouth may be telling you, *Clin Rev* 13(8):41-48, 2003.

Siegler R: *Children's thinking,* Englewood Cliffs, NJ, 1991, Prentice-Hall.

Silagy C, Stead LF: Physician advice for smoking cessation. *The Cochrane Library* 3, 2004.

Simel DL: The clinical examination: an agenda to make it more rational, *JAMA* 277:572, 1997.

Siminoski K: Does this patient have a goiter? *JAMA* 273:813, 1995.

Sin DD et al: The relationship between birthweight and childhood asthma, *Arch Pediatr Adolesc Med* 158:60-64, 2004.

Singer P: *A darwinian left: politics, evolution and cooperation,* Yale University Press, New Haven, Conn, 1999, Yale University Press.

Skinner J et al: Racial, ethnic and geographic disparities in rates of knee arthroplasty among Medicare patients, *N Engl J Med* 349:1350-1359, 2003.

Sloan RP et al: Should physicians prescribe religious activities? *N Engl J Med* 342:1913-1916, 2000.

Smith AC III, Kleinman S: Managing emotions in medical school: students' contacts with the living and the dead, *Soc Psychol Q* 52:56, 1989.

Smith-Alnimer M, Watford MF: Alcohol withdrawal and delirium tremens, *Am J Nurs* 104(5):72a-72g, 2004.

Smith DM et al: *Preparticipation physical evaluation,* ed 2, Minneapolis, 1997, McGraw-Hill.

Smith R et al: American Cancer Society guidelines for the early detection of cancer, *CA Cancer J Clin* 53:27-43, 2003.

Smith W: Fibromyalgia syndrome, *Nurs Clin North Am* 33(4):653-668, 1998.

Sokol RJ, Martier SS, Ager JW: The TACE questions: practical prenatal detection of risk drinking, *Am J Obstet Gynecol* 160:863, 1989.

Sprague J: Vision screening. In Krajicek M, Tomlinson AIT, editors: *Detection of developmental problems in children,* ed 2, Baltimore, 1983, University Park Press.

Stang J: Adolescent physical growth and development: implications for pregnancy. In Story M, Stang J, editors: *Nutrition and the pregnant adolescent,* Minneapolis, 2000, University of Minnesota.

Starr NB, Poland C, Dean JA: Malocclusion: how important is that bite? *J Pediatr Health Care* 13:245-247, 1999.

Stashwick C: When you suspect an eating disorder, *Contemp Pediatr* 13:124, 1996.

Stavroudis L: Medical malpractice grand rounds presentation, The Johns Hopkins Children's Center, May 31, 2004.

Stellwagen LM et al: Look for the "stuck baby" to identify congenital torticollis, *Contemp Pediatr* 21:55, 2004.

Stevens B et al: Premature infant pain profile: development and initial validation, *Clin J Pain* 12:13-22, 1996.

Stiell IG et al: Decision rules for the use of radiography in acute ankle injuries: refinement and prospective validation, *JAMA* 269(9):1127-1132, 1993.

Stiell IG et al: Prospective validation of a decision rule for the use of radiography in acute knee injuries, *JAMA* 275(8):641-642, 1996.

Strauss KF: American Indian school children height and weight survey, *The Provider* 18:1, 1993.

Stulc DM: The family as a bearer of culture. In Cookfair JM, editor: *Nursing process and practice in the community,* St Louis, 1991, Mosby.

Subcommittee on Military Weight Management, Committee on Military Nutrition Research, and Food and Nutrition Board of the Institute of Medicine: Factors that influence body weight (pp. 43-60) In *Weight management: state of science and opportunities for military programs.* Washington, DC, 2003, National Academies Press.

Subcommittee on the Tenth Edition of the RDAs, Food and Nutrition Board: *Recommended dietary allowances,* ed 10, Washington, DC, 1989, National Academy Press.

Suchman AL et al: A model of empathic communication in the medical interview, *JAMA* 277:678-682, 1997.

Sugarman RA: Structure and function of the neurologic system. In McCance KL, Huether SE, editors: *Pathophysiology: the biologic basis for disease in adults and children,* ed 4, St Louis, 2002, Mosby.

Sutter K et al: Reliability of head circumference measurements in preterm infants, *Pediatr Nurs* 23(5):485-490, 1997.

Tachdjian MO: Clinical pediatric orthopedics: the art of diagnosis and principles of management, Stamford, Conn, 1997, Appleton & Lange.

Taddio A et al: Effect of neonatal circumcision on pain response during subsequent routine vaccination, *Lancet* 349:599-603, 1997.

Tanner JM, Davies PS: Clinical longitudinal standards for height and height velocity for North American children, *J Pediatr* 107(3):317-329, 1985.

Tanner JM: *Foetus into man: physical growth from conception to maturity,* ed 2, Cambridge, Mass, 1990, Harvard University Press.

Taylor GA: *Neuroimaging techniques in pediatrics,* a lecture, Baltimore, 1989, The Johns Hopkins Medical Institutions.

Taylor L, Willies-Jacobo LJ: The culturally competent pediatrician: respecting ethnicity in your practice, *Contemp Pediatr* 20:83-105, 2003.

Teasdale G, Jennett B: Assessment of coma and impaired consciousness: a practical scale, *Lancet* 2:81-84, 1974.

Teoh TG, Fisk NM: Hydramnios, oligohydramnios. In James DK et al, editors: *High risk pregnancy: management options,* ed 2, Philadelphia, 1999, WB Saunders.

Theophilopoulos EP, Barrett DJ: Getting a grip on the pediatric hip, *Contemp Pediatr* 15(11):43-65, 1998.

Thibodeau GA, Patton KT: *Anatomy and physiology,* ed 5, St Louis, 2003, Mosby.

Thomas SP: Anger: the mismanaged emotion, *Dermatol Nurs* 15:351-357, 2003.

Thomas DB et al: Randomized Trial of Breast Self-Examination in Shanghai: final results, *J Natl Cancer Inst* 94(19):1445-1457, 2002.

Thompson JK, Cohen ME: Studies on the normal circulation in normal pregnancy: II—Vital capacity observations in normal pregnant women, *Surg Gynecol Obstet* 66:591, 1938.

Thompson JM et al: *Mosby's clinical nursing,* ed 4, St Louis, 1997, Mosby.

Thomson M: Heavy birthweight in Native Indians of British Columbia, *Can J Public Health* 81:443, 1990.

Tinetti ME: Performance-oriented assessment of mobility problems in elderly patients, *J Am Geriatr Soc* 34(2):119-126, 1986.

Trauner DA: *Childhood neurological problems: a textbook for health professionals,* Chicago, 1979, Mosby.

Tunnesen WW Jr: *Signs and symptoms in pediatrics,* Philadelphia, 1999, Lippincott Williams and Wilkins.

US Department of Health and Human Services, Washington, DC.

US Preventive Health Services Task Force: Screening for depression: recommendations and rationale, *Am J Nurs* 102(7):77-80, 2002.

US Preventive Health Services Task Force: Screening for dementia: recommendations and rationale, *Am J Nurs* 103(9), 87-95, 2003.

US Preventive Health Services Task Force: Screening for colorectal cancer: recommendations and rationale, *Ann Intern Med* 137(2):129-131, 2002.

US Preventive Services Task Force: Screening for osteoporosis in postmenopausal women: recommendations and rationale, *Am J Nurs* 103(1):73-80, 2003.

US Preventive Services Task Force: Screening for cervical cancer, January 2003. Available at www.ahrq.gov/clinic/uspstf/uspscerv.htm, accessed August 1, 2004.

Varcarolis EM: *Psychiatric nursing clinical guide: assessment tools and diagnosis,* Philadelphia, 1999, WB Saunders.

Veille JC, Kitzman DW, Bacevice AF: Effects of pregnancy on the electrocardiogram in healthy subjects during exercise, *Am J Obstet Gynecol* 175:1360, 1996.

Videlefsky A: Routine vaginal cuff smear testing in post-hysterectomy patients with benign uterine conditions: when is it indicated? *J Am Board Fam Pract* 13(4):233-238, 2000.

Wagley PF: Counselling the patient contemplating suicide, *Hum Med* 8:317, 1992.

Wagner JM, McKinney WP, Carpenter JL: Does this patient have appendicitis? *JAMA* 276(19):1589-1594, 1996.

Walsh S: Cardiovascular disease in pregnancy: a nursing approach, *J Cardiovasc Nurs* 2(4):53-64, 1988.

Wardlaw GM, Insel PM, Seyler MF: *Contemporary nutrition,* ed 2, St Louis, 1994, Mosby.

Waring WW, Jeansonne LO: *Practical manual of pediatrics,* ed 2, St Louis, 1982, Mosby.

Warner PH, Rowe T, Whipple B: Shedding light on the sexual history, *Am J Nurs* 99:34-40, 1999.

Wasserman HP: *Ethnic pigmentation: historical, physiological and chemical aspects,* New York, 1974, American Elsevier.

Weinberger S, Weiss S: Pulmonary diseases. In Burrow G, Duffy T, editors: *Medical complications of pregnancy,* ed 5, Philadelphia, 1999, WB Saunders.

Weiner CP, Baschat AA: Fetal growth restriction: evaluation and management. In James DK et al, editors: *High risk pregnancy: management options,* ed 2, Philadelphia, 1999, WB Saunders.

Weiss BD, Coyne C: Communicating with patients who cannot read, *N Engl J Med* 337:272-273, 1997.

Werk LN, Bauchner H, Chessare JB: Medicine for the millennium: demystifying EBM, *Contemp Pediatr* 16:87-107, 1999.

Wharton P, Mowrer DE: Prevalence of cleft uvula among school children in kindergarten through grade five, *Cleft Palate J* 29:10, 1992.

Whooley MA, Simon GE: Managing depression in medical outpatients, *N Engl J Med* 343:1942-1950, 2000.

Wiens L et al: Chest pain in otherwise healthy children and adolescents is frequently caused by exercise-induced asthma, *Pediatrics* 90(3):350-353, 1992.

Williams JW Jr et al: Clinical evaluation for sinusitis. Making the diagnosis by history and physical examination, *Ann Intern Med* 117(9): 705-710, 1992.

Williams JW, Simel DL: Does this patient have sinusitis? Diagnosing sinusitis by history and physical examination, *JAMA* 270(10):1242-1246, 1993.

Wilson HS, Kneisl CR: *Psychiatric nursing,* ed 3, Menlo Park, Calif, 1988, Addison-Wesley Publishing.

Wilson MEH: Keeping quiet, *Arch Pediatr Adolesc Med* 152:1054-1055, 1999.

Wilson MEH: Odor (unusual body and urine). In Hoekelman RA et al, editors: *Primary pediatric care,* ed 3, St Louis, 1997, Mosby.

Wilson SF, Giddens JF: *Health assessment for nursing practice,* ed 3, St Louis, 2005, Mosby.

Winawer S: Colorectal cancer screening and surveillance: clinical guidelines and rationale—update based on new evidence, *Gastroenterology* 124(2):544-560, 2003.

Winkleby MA et al: Effects of an advocacy intervention to reduce smoking among teenagers, *Arch Pediatr Adolesc Med* 158:269-275, 2004.

Wisner KL, Parry BL, Piontek CM: Postpartum depression, *N Engl J Med* 347:194-199, 2002.

Wong DL et al: *Whaley and Wong's nursing care of infants and children,* ed 6, St Louis, 1999, Mosby.

World Health Organization: Energy and protein requirements: report of a Joint FAO/WHO/UNU expert consultation, *Technical Report Series* 724, Geneva, 1985, WHO.

World Health Organization: Foodborne and waterborne health risks. Available at www.who.int/ith/chapter03_02.html, accessed July 22, 2004.

Wright RJ: Identification of violence in the community pediatric setting, *Arch Ped Adolesc Med* 154:431-433, 2000.

Yip R, Li Z, Chong WH: Race and birth weight: the Chinese example, *Pediatrics* 87:688, 1991.

Zardawi IM et al: Effects of lubricant gel on conventional and liquid-based cervical smears, Letter, *Acta Cytol* 47(4):704-705, 2003.

Zhang J, Savitz DA: Preterm birth subtypes among blacks and whites, *Epidemiology* 3:428, 1992.

Zitelli BJ, Davis HW: *Atlas of pediatric physical diagnosis,* ed 4, St. Louis, 2002, Mosby.

Zlatnik F et al: Vaginal ultrasound as an adjunct to cervical digital examination in women at risk for early delivery, *Gynecol Obstet Invest* 51(1):12-16, 2001.

Zoorob R et al: Cancer screening guidelines, *Am Fam Physician* 63(6):1101-1112. Available at www.aafp.org/afp, accessed Aug 31, 2004.

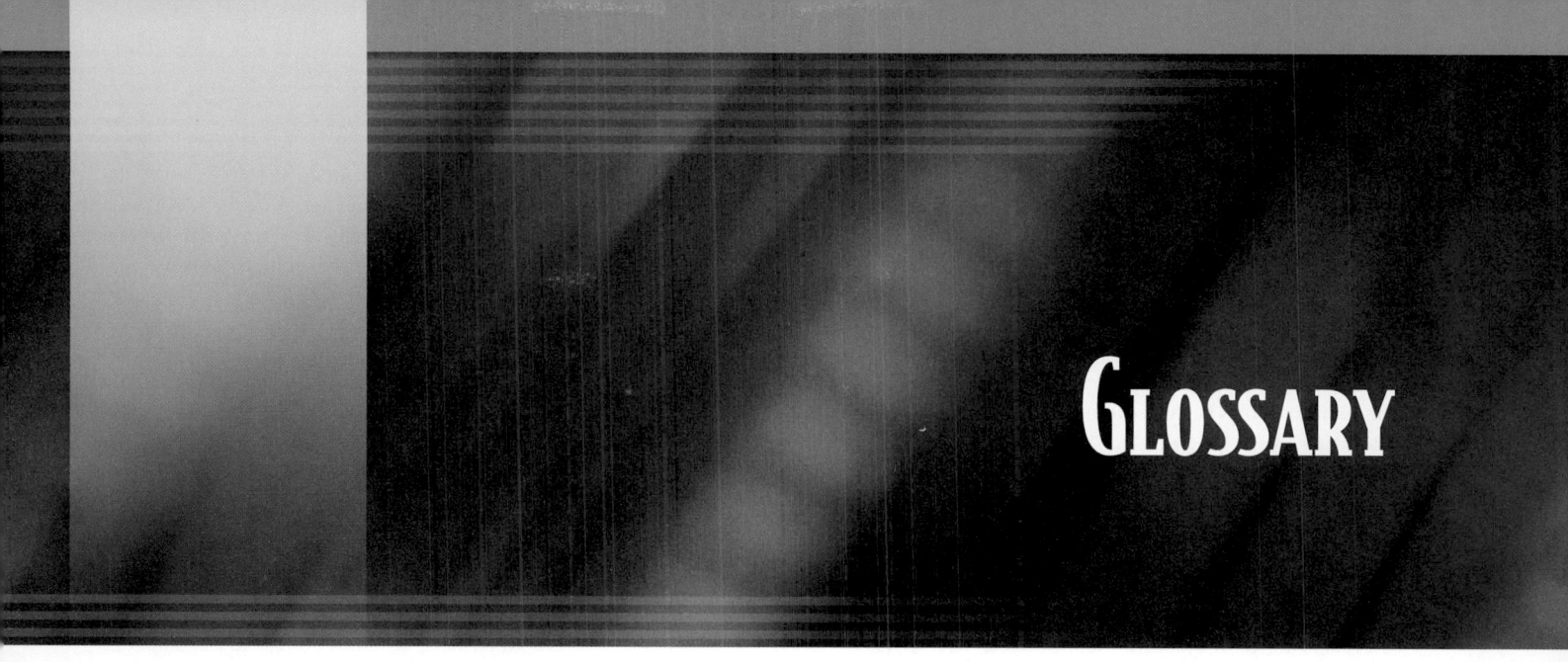

GLOSSARY

abduction: Movement of the limbs toward the lateral plane or away from the axial line of a limb.

abruptio placenta: Premature separation of the placenta during pregnancy or labor before delivery of the fetus.

accommodation: Adjustment of the eye for various distances through modification of the lens curvature; negative accommodation is adjustment for far vision by relaxation of ciliary muscle; positive accommodation is adjustment for near vision by contraction of ciliary muscle.

acini cells: Milk-producing alveoli located in the glandular tissue of the breast.

adduction: Movement of the limbs toward the medial plane of the body or toward the axial line of a limb.

adenitis: Inflammation of a lymph node or a group of lymph nodes.

adnexa: Appendages (e.g., adnexa uteri are the structures adjacent to the uterus, including the ovaries, fallopian tubes, and uterine ligaments).

adventitious: Accidental or acquired, not natural or hereditary; located away from the usual place.

agoraphobia: Fear of being in an open, crowded or public place.

alveolar ridge: Bony prominence of the maxilla and mandible that supports the teeth or dentures.

amblyopia: Reduced vision in an eye that appears structurally normal and without detectable cause when examined, including inspection with an ophthalmoscope.

amenorrhea: Absence of menses.

anacrotic: The upstroke of the pulse, which also implies a "notch" or "shoulder" on the upstroke.

anesthesia: Partial or complete loss of sensation.

aneurysm: A balloon-like swelling of the wall of an artery, vein, or heart; generally the result of a congenital defect in the wall or degenerative disease or infection (e.g., atherosclerosis or syphilis); dissecting aneurysm is longitudinal splitting of the arterial wall from hemorrhage.

angle of Louis: (Sternal angle) the angle between the manubrium and the body of the sternum.

anhedonia: The state in which a person appears to be involved in pleasurable activities, but feels no pleasure associated with those activities.

annulus: A ring or circular structure; e.g., tympanic annulus is a fibrous ring around the tympanic membrane that looks whiter and denser than the membrane itself.

anosmia: Absence of the sense of smell.

antalgic: Painful limp in which the patient shortens the time on the affected extremity.

anthropometry: Measurement of the size, weight, and proportions of the human body.

apex beat: The visible or palpable pulsation made by the apex of the left ventricle as it strikes the chest wall in systole; usually located in the fifth left intercostal space, several centimeters to the left of the median line (midsternal line).

aphakia: A condition in which part or all of the crystalline lens of the eye is absent, usually because of surgical removal for the treatment of cataracts.

aphasia: Impairment of language function in which speech or writing is not understood (receptive or sensory), words cannot be formed (expressive), or a combination of both.

apical: Pertaining to the apex or the area of the apex (top or tip) of a body, organ, or part.

apnea: A temporary halt to breathing.

appropriate for gestational age: A weight classification of newborns associated with better health outcomes, the weight falling between the 10th and 90th percentiles on the intrauterine growth curve for the newborn's calculated gestational age.

apraxia: Inability to execute a skilled or learned motor act, not related to paralysis or lack of comprehension; caused by a lesion in the cerebral cortex.

arrhythmia (see dysrhythmia): A deviation from the expected rhythm of the heart.

arteriovenous fistula: A pathologic direct communication between an artery and a vein without an intervening capillary bed.

arteriovenous shunt: The passage of blood directly from an artery to a vein, without an intervening capillary network.

articulation: The ability to pronounce speech sounds, words, and thoughts clearly and fluently; the junction of two or more bones; contact of the occlusal surfaces of the teeth.

ascites: Abnormal intraperitoneal accumulation of serous fluid.

asterixis: Postural tremor characterized by nonrhythmic, flapping movements of wide amplitude; extended wrist or fingers suddenly and briefly flex and then return to their original position.

astigmatism: An abnormal condition in which the light rays cannot be focused clearly in a point on the retina because of an irregular curvature of the cornea or lens.

ataxia: Impaired ability to coordinate muscular movement, usually associated with staggering gait and postural imbalance.

atelectasis: Incomplete expansion of the lung, either congenital or acquired.

athetosis: Slow, twisting, writhing movements, with larger amplitude than chorea, that commonly involve the hands.

atrioventricular valve: Refers to the tricuspid or mitral valves.

Austin Flint murmur: A presystolic murmur, not unlike that of mitral stenosis, best heard at the apex of the heart; caused by aortic insufficiency.

autonomic nervous system: The portion of the nervous system that regulates involuntary functions supporting life; divided into the sympathetic and parasympathetic nervous systems.

baroreceptor: Sensory nerves within the walls of the atria, vena cava, aortic arch, and carotid sinus that monitor blood pressure change.

barrel chest: Increased anteroposterior diameter of the chest, often with some degree of kyphosis; commonly seen with COPD.

Bartholin glands: (Vestibular glands) mucus-secreting glands located posterolaterally to the vaginal opening.

bifurcated: Having two branches, tines, or prongs.

bigeminal pulse: A pulse in which two beats occur in rapid succession so that they seem coupled and distinct from the succeeding set of two. Each set is separated by a longer interval.

bisferiens pulse: The double-peaked systolic pulse. An arterial pulse with two palpable peaks, the second stronger than the first, but not markedly so; detected in instances of decreased arterial tension.

borborygmi: Rumbling, gurgling, tinkling noises heard on auscultation of the abdomen as a result of hyperactive intestinal peristalsis.

bossing: Bulging of the frontal areas of the skull; associated with prematurity and rickets.

boutonnière deformity: Fixed flexion of the proximal interphalangeal joint associated with hyperextension of the distal interphalangeal joint.

bradycardia: A heart rate less than 60 beats per minute.

bradykinesia: Slowing of voluntary and involuntary movements.

bradypnea: Slower than expected respiratory rate.

bronchial breathing: Harsh breathing characterized by prolonged high-pitched expiration with a tubular quality; often heard when lung tissue is consolidated.

bronchial fremitus: Adventitious pulmonary or voice sounds palpable over the chest or audible to the ear.

bronchiectasis: Persistent dilation of bronchi or bronchioles as a consequence of inflammatory disease, obstruction, or congenital abnormality.

bronchiolitis: (Bronchopneumonia) inflammation of the bronchioles, caused by bacteria or viruses.

bronchogenic: Originating from the bronchi.

bronchophony: An exaggeration of vocal resonance emanating from a bronchus surrounded by consolidated lung tissue.

bronchopulmonary dysplasia: A form of chronic lung disease of uncertain cause sometimes seen in children who have had intensive respiratory support during the neonatal period.

bronchovesicular: Pertaining to bronchial tubes and alveoli.

bruit: An unexpected audible swishing sound or murmur over an artery or vascular organ.

bruxism: Compulsive unconscious grinding of the teeth.

bubo: Inflammation and swelling of one or a group of lymph nodes, particularly in the groin or axilla, often accompanied by suppuration.

buccal mucosa: Mucous membrane inside the mouth.

bundle of His: A small band of modified heart muscle fibers that originates at the atrioventricular node and passes through the right atrioventricular junction to the interventricular septum, where the fibers divide into right and left branches and enter the respective ventricles; this bundle carries the atrial contractual rhythm to the ventricles; an interruption results in some degree of heart block.

bunion: Unexpected prominence of the medial aspect of the first metatarsal head, with bursa formation, resulting in lateral or valgus deviation of the great toe.

bursa: Disk-shaped, fluid-filled synovial sacs that develop at points of friction around joints, between tendons, cartilage, and bone; they decrease friction and promote ease of motion.

canthus: The angle at the medial or lateral margin of the eyelid; the medial canthus opens into a small space containing openings to the lacrimal duct.

caput succedaneum: An edematous swelling of the scalp of the newborn resulting from labor.

cardiac cycle: The complete sequence of cardiac action occurring from one heartbeat to the next, including both systole and diastole.

cardiac impulse: The thrust of the ventricles against the chest wall as a result of cardiac contraction.

cardiac output: The amount of blood ejected by the heart, usually stated in liters per minute, calculated by stroke volume × number of heartbeats per unit of time.

cardiac reserve: The heart's ability to respond to demands that exceed ordinary circumstances.

carrying angle: The angle at which the humerus and radius articulate.

cellulitis: Inflammation of soft or connective tissue that causes a watery exudate to spread through the tissue spaces.

cephalhematoma: A subperiosteal hemorrhage, usually benign, along one of the cranial bones; it generally results from birth trauma.

cheilitis: Inflammation and cracking of the lips.

chemoreceptor: Any cell that is activated by a change in its chemical milieu and thereby originates a flow of nervous impulses; nerve cells sensitive to changes in the composition of the blood or cerebrospinal fluid.

choanae: A pair of posterior openings between the nasal cavity and the nasopharynx.

chordee: Ventral curvature of the penis caused by a fibrous band of tissue, often associated with hypospadias or gonorrhea.

chorea: Purposeless, involuntary rapid movements associated with muscle weakness and behavioral change; these are not tics, athetosis, or hyperkinesis. Chorea is often a delayed manifestation of rheumatic fever and may be confused with manifestations of Huntington chorea, systemic lupus erythematosus, Wilson disease, and drug reactions.

choreiform movements: Brief, rapid, jerky, irregular, and involuntary movements that occur at rest or interrupt normal coordinated movements; most often involve the face, head, lower arms, and hands.

choroid: The thin, highly vascular membrane covering the posterior five sixths of the eye between the retina and sclera.

cicatricial: Composed of scar tissue that is avascular, pale, and contracted.

ciliary body: The thickened part of the vascular tunic of the eye that joins the iris with the anterior portion of the choroid.

circumcorneal: Around the cornea.

circumduction: Circular movement of a limb (e.g., the shoulder) or the eye.

circumlocution: The use of pantomime, nonverbal expressions, or word substitutions to avoid revealing that a word has been forgotten.

clang association: Word choice based on sound so that words rhyme in a nonsensical way.

claudication: The condition resulting from muscle ischemia due to decreased arterial blood flow to an area and characterized by intermittent pain and limping.

clonus: Rapidly alternating involuntary contraction and relaxation of skeletal muscles.

coarctation: Constriction, stricture, stenosis, or narrowing, as of the aorta.

cochlea: A coiled bony structure within the inner ear; it contains the organ of Corti and perforations for the passage of the cochlear division of the auditory nerve.

cognition: The mental process of knowing, thinking, learning, and judging.

colic: Gradual onset of pain that increases in crescendo fashion until it reaches a peak of severity, then slowly subsides.

colostrum: Yellow, milky secretion from the breast that precedes the onset of true lactation; composed primarily of serum and white blood cells.

concha: A structure that is shell-shaped; the deep cavity in the auricle of the external ear containing the auditory canal meatus.

conductive hearing loss: Reduction in hearing acuity relating to interference of sound being transmitted through the outer and middle ear.

confabulation: Fabrication of detailed, plausible experiences and events to cover gaps in memory.

conjunctivitis: Inflammation of the conjunctiva caused by infectious agents or by allergies.

consolidation: Solidification of part of the lung into a firm, dense mass, particularly when the alveoli fill with fluid as a result of inflammation.

contracture: Permanent fixed flexion of a joint resulting from atrophy and shortening of muscles or from loss of skin elasticity.

coryza: Rhinitis; inflammation of the nasal mucous membranes, accompanied by swelling of the mucosa and nasal discharge.

crackle: A general term for an unexpected sound heard on auscultation of the chest; sometimes used to describe crepitus heard on auscultation (see Box 13-7).

craniotabes: An unusual softness of the skull in infants with hydrocephalus and rickets; the skull feels brittle and has a Ping-Pong ball—snapping sensation when firmly pressed.

crepitus: A crinkly, crackling, grating feeling or sound in the joints, skin, or lungs; the quality of sound is simulated by Rice Krispies in milk; the quality of touch is somewhat simulated by rubbing hair between the fingers.

croup: An inflammation of the larynx, causing swelling of the vocal chords and sometimes severe obstruction; characterized by harsh, difficult breathing, stridor, and a hoarse cough; usually occurs in young children.

cryptorchidism: Failure of one or both testicles to descend into the scrotum.

cyanosis: A bluish or purplish color (may range from slight to intense) of the skin and mucous membranes because of insufficient oxygen levels in the blood.

deafness: Partial or complete loss of hearing.

decerebrate posturing: Rigid extension of all four extremities with hyperpronation of the forearms and plantar flexion of the feet.

dermatome: The area of skin innervated by a single posterior spinal nerve.

development: The process of growth and differentiation; the acquisition of function associated with cell differentiation and maturation of individual organ systems.

dextrocardia: Location of the heart in the right hemithorax, either by displacement from disease or congenital mirror-image reversal.

diastole: That time between two contractions of the heart when the muscles relax, allowing the chambers to fill with blood; diastole of the atria precedes that of the ventricles; diastole alternates, usually in a regular rhythm, with systole.

dicrotic notch: The notch in a pulse tracing between two elevations for each pulse beat.

dicrotic pulse: The double-peaked pulse; the second peak is usually weaker than the first and diastolic in timing.

diplopia: Double vision caused by defective function of the extraocular muscles or a disorder of the nerves that innervate the muscles.

dizziness: (Vertigo) sensation of an inability to maintain normal balance in a standing or sitting position.

dorsiflexion: Backward bending or flexion of a joint.

dysarthria: Defective articulation secondary to a motor deficit involving the lips, tongue, palate, or pharynx.

dysfunctional uterine bleeding (DUB): Abnormal uterine bleeding not associated with tumor, inflammation, pregnancy, trauma, or hormonal imbalance; a diagnosis is given only after these causes are ruled out.

dyspareunia: Difficult or painful sexual intercourse.

dysphagia: Difficulty in swallowing.

dysphonia: A disorder in voice volume, such as hoarseness.

dyspnea: Difficult and labored breathing, shortness of breath.

dysrhythmia: Unexpected variation in the regular rhythm of the heart.

ecchymosis: (Bruise) discoloration of the skin or mucous membrane as the result of hemorrhage into subcutaneous tissue.

echolalia: Automatic and meaningless repetition of another's words or phrases.

edema: Excessive accumulation of fluid in the cells, tissues, or serous cavities of the body.

edentulous: Without teeth.

effacement: The shortening of the vaginal portion of the cervix and thinning of its walls as it is stretched and dilated during labor.

effusion: Loss of fluid from the blood vessels or lymphatics into the tissues or a body cavity.

ejection murmur: A diamond-shaped systolic murmur occupying most but not necessarily all of systole; produced by the ejection of blood into the aorta or pulmonary artery.

electrocardiogram (ECG): A graphic record of the heart's electrical currents obtained with an electrocardiograph.

embolism: Obstruction of an artery by a blood clot or foreign matter.

emphysema: Pathologic accumulation of air in tissue or organs, especially the lungs.

encephalocele: A congenital gap in the skull, usually with herniation of the brain or meninges.

endocardium: The innermost membrane lining the heart cavities that is continuous with the lining of the blood vessels; its slippery surface eases the flow of blood.

epicardium: The inner visceral layer of the serous pericardium lying directly on the heart, forming the outermost layer of the heart wall.

epigastrium: The upper central region of the abdomen between the costal margins and a line drawn horizontally across the lowest costal margin.

epispadias: A congenital defect resulting in the urethra opening on the dorsum of the penis.

epulis: A tumor on the gingiva.

erythema marginatum: A distinctive evanescent pink rash, a rare manifestation of rheumatic fever. The erythematous areas have pale centers and round or serpiginous margins; they vary in size and appear mainly on the trunk and extremities, never on the face. The erythema is transient and migratory and may be induced by application of heat.

esotropia: (Cross-eye) the inward or nasal deviation of an eye.

eustachian tube: The cartilaginous and bony passage between the nasopharynx and the middle ear that allows equalization of air pressure between the inner ear and external pressure.

exotropia: (Walleye) the outward or temporal deviation of an eye.

extension: Movement that increases the angle between two adjoining bones to 180 degrees, bringing a limb toward a straight line.

external rotation: Lateral turning of a limb.

exudate: Fluid that has escaped from tissue or capillaries, usually after injury or inflammation, typically containing protein and white blood cells.

facies: Expression or appearance of the face; often used to describe characteristic expressions of disease states or congenital anomalies.

fasciculation: A localized, uncoordinated twitching of a single muscle group innervated by a single motor nerve filament; it is visible or palpable.

fibrosis: The formation of excessive connective tissue as an attempt to repair damage or as a reaction to foreign material, resulting in scarring and thickening.

flaccid: Muscles that are weak, soft, and flabby, lacking expected muscle tone.

flail chest: A flapping, unfixed chest wall caused by loss of stability of the thoracic cage after fractures of the sternum and/or ribs.

flank: The posterior part of the body below the ribs and above the ilium.

flatulence: The presence of excessive air or gases in the stomach or intestines, causing abdominal distention and resulting in rectal passage.

flexion: Movement that decreases the angle between two articulating bones, bending the limb.

floater: One or more spots that appear to drift in front of the eye; caused by a shadow cast on the retina by vitreous debris or separation of the vitreous humor from the retina.

fluctuant: A wavelike motion that is felt when a structure containing liquid is palpated.

fluency: Articulate speech that flows easily.

flutter: A rapid vibration or pulsation that impedes appropriate function.

fontanels: Membranous spaces at the juncture of an infant's cranial bones that later ossify.

foramen ovale: The communication between the two atria of the fetal heart; if it remains patent, blood shunts between the atria after birth, usually from left to right.

Fordyce spots: Ectopic sebaceous glands of the buccal mucosa appearing as small yellow-white raised lesions.

fornix: Arched structure (e.g., the vaginal fornix is the recess between the cervix and the vaginal wall); although one continuous structure, the vaginal fornix is anatomically divided into the anterior, posterior, and lateral fornices.

fourchette: Ridges of tissue formed by the fusion of the labia minora at the posterior aspect of the vulva.

fovea centralis: A tiny pit in the center of the macula lutea that is the area of clearest vision, permitting light to fall on the cones; it appears as an oval yellow spot on the retina and is free of blood vessels.

fremitus: A tremor vibration in any part of the body, detectable on palpation.

frenulum, lingual: Band of tissue that attaches the ventral surface of the tongue to the floor of the mouth.

friction rub: A sound audible through the stethoscope, resulting from the rubbing of opposed, inflamed serous surfaces.

functional assessment: Measurement of the abilities and activities used to perform the activities of daily living necessary for survival, vocational and social pursuits, and leisure activities.

galea aponeurotica: The fibrous sheet or tendonous material connecting the frontalis and occipitalis muscles over the skull.

gaussian distribution: A frequency distribution of observations and/or events that results in a plotted curve having the shape of a bell, reasonable symmetry, and the potential for infinite extent in either direction.

gestational age: Fetal age of a newborn, calculated from the number of completed weeks since the first day of the mother's last menstrual period to the date of birth.

gingivae: Gums of the mouth.

glaucoma: An abnormal condition of elevated pressure within an eye resulting from obstruction of the outflow of aqueous humor.

glottis: Pertaining to the vocal apparatus of the larynx, the true vocal cords, and the opening between them.

goiter: Cystic or fibrous enlargement of the thyroid gland, often related to thyroid dysfunction.

Graham Steell murmur: An early diastolic murmur of pulmonic insufficiency secondary to pulmonary hypertension.

graphesthesia: The ability to recognize symbols, shapes, numbers, and letters traced on the skin.

hallucination: A sensation (hearing, sight, smell, taste, or touch) perceived by a person while awake that is not caused by external stimuli.

helix: The prominent outer rim of the auricle of the ear.

hemangioma: A benign tumor of newly formed blood vessels that may occur anywhere in the body, most readily noticed in the skin and subcutaneous tissues.

hemianesthesia: Loss of sensation on one side of the body.

hemiplegia: Loss of motor function and sensation (paralysis) on one side of the body.

hemodynamic: Pertaining to the movement of blood and other aspects of the circulation.

hemoptysis: Coughing up blood or bloodstained sputum from the respiratory tree.

hernia: Protrusion of an organ or tissue through an opening in the muscle wall.

hilus of the lung: A hollow depression on the mediastinal surface of each lung, which is the point of entry of the bronchus, blood vessels, nerves, and lymphatics.

hirsutism: Excessive hair growth, especially an adult male pattern of hair distribution in women; usually related to heredity, hormonal dysfunction, porphyria, or medications.

holodiastolic: Occupying all of diastole.

holosystolic: Occupying all of systole.

Homans sign: Pain or discomfort behind the knee or in the calf when the ankle is gently dorsiflexed while the knee is flexed; it suggests thrombosis of the leg veins.

homonymous hemianopia: Defective vision in half of the visual field, occurring on the same side in each eye.

hydramnios: A condition of pregnancy characterized by an excess of amniotic fluid.

hydrocephaly: Enlargement of the head by an excessive accumulation of fluid dilating the cerebral ventricles, thinning the cerebral cortex, and causing separation of the cranial bones.

hyperesthesia: Unusual increased sensitivity to sensory stimuli, such as touch or pain.

hyperextension: A position of maximum extension.

hyperkeratosis: Overgrowth of the cornified layer of the skin or the cornea.

hyperkinesia: Excessive muscular activity; hyperactivity.

hypermenorrhea: Excessive bleeding during a menstrual period of usual duration.

hyperopia: (Farsightedness) a refractive error in which light rays entering the eye are focused behind the retina.

hyperpnea: Respiration that is deeper and more rapid than expected.

hyperresonance: Greater than expected resonance that is lower pitched in response to percussion of the chest wall or abdomen.

hyperthyroidism: Excessive activity of the thyroid gland with an increase in thyroid secretion.

hyperventilation: A state in which an increased amount of air enters the lungs, usually a result of deep and rapid breathing; if severe, it leads to alkalosis with the excessive loss of carbon dioxide.

hypesthesia: Decreased sensitivity to sensory stimuli such as touch and pain.

hypokinesia: Unusually diminished muscular activity.

hypomenorrhea: Decreased amount of menstrual flow.

hypospadias: A congenital defect in which the urethra opens on the ventral surface of the penis rather than on the glans.

hypotension: A condition in which arterial blood pressure is lower than expected.

hypothyroidism: Diminished activity of the thyroid gland with consequent reduction of thyroid hormone.

incus: One of the three ossicles of the middle ear, lying between the malleus and stapes.

induration: Excessive hardening or firmness of any body site.

infarction: An acute interruption to the blood supply of a part of the body by thrombi, emboli, extrinsic pressure, or twisting of blood vessels resulting in tissue death at the involved site.

infrapatellar fat pad: The soft tissue palpable in front of the joint space on either side of the patellar tendon.

intermittent claudication: Cramping pain and limping commonly in the calf brought on by walking; caused by ischemia of the muscles, usually from atheroma that narrows the leg's arteries.

internal rotation: Medial turning of a limb.

intertriginous: An area where opposing skin surfaces touch and may rub, such as skin folds in the axillae, groin, inner thighs, and beneath large breasts.

introitus: The vaginal opening.

isthmus: A narrow band of tissue connecting the two lateral lobes of the thyroid.

Janeway lesions (spots): Tiny hemorrhagic spots, a bit raised or nodular, occurring principally on the palms and soles, suggesting subacute bacterial endocarditis.

joint instability: An unusual increase in joint mobility.

jugular pulse: A pulsation in the jugular vein resulting from waves transmitted from the right side of the heart via circulating blood.

keratin: A scleroprotein that is the primary constituent of epidermis, hair, and nails.

Kiesselbach plexus: A convergence of small, fragile arteries and veins located superficially on the anterosuperior portion of the nasal septum.

Koplik spots: Small red spots with bluish-white centers on the buccal mucosa opposite the molar teeth, appearing in the prodromal stage of measles.

kyphosis: An increased convex curvature of the thoracic spine.

lactation: The production and secretion of milk from the breasts.

large for gestational age (LGA): A weight classification of newborns associated with poorer health outcomes, the weight falling above the 90th percentile on the intrauterine growth curve for the infant's calculated gestational age.

leukoplakia: Circumscribed, firmly attached, thick white patches on the tongue and other mucous membranes, often occurring as a precancerous growth.

lobule: A small lobe; the soft, lower, pendulous portion of the auricle of the ear.

locking: Inability to fully extend the joint, or stiffness after being in one position for an extended time.

log-rolling: Keeping the body of the patient rigid, that is, similar to a log, while being turned.

lordosis: Accentuation of the lumbar curvature of the spine.

lymphangioma: A tumor composed of lymphatic vessels that vary in size and are often dilated

lymphangitis: Inflammation of lymph vessels from bacterial infection of an extremity, characterized by fine red streaks running from the area of infection toward the groin or axilla.

lymphedema: Swelling, particularly of subcutaneous tissues, caused by obstruction of the lymphatic system and accumulation of interstitial fluid.

macroglossia: Excessively large tongue.

malleus: One of the three ossicles of the middle ear, connected to the tympanic membrane.

malocclusion: Inappropriate contact between the teeth of the upper and lower jaws.

McBurney point: In acute appendicitis, extreme sensitivity over the appendix, approximately 2 inches above the right anterosuperior iliac spine, on a line between that spine and the umbilicus.

meconium: First stools of the newborn; viscous, sticky, dark green, usually sterile and odorless.

mediastinum: The space in the thoracic cavity behind the sternum and between the two pleural sacs; contains the remaining thoracic organs and structures.

medulla oblongata: The lowest subdivision of the brainstem, immediately adjacent to the spinal cord.

menarche: The first menstruation and initiation of cyclic menstrual function.

meninges: One of three membrane layers (dura mater, pia mater, and arachnoid) that enclose the brain and spinal cord.

meningomyelocele: A protrusion of the meninges and spinal cord through a defect in the vertebral column.

menorrhagia: Excessive bleeding during a menstrual period that is longer in duration than usual

metrorrhagia: Menstrual bleeding at irregular intervals, sometimes prolonged, but of expected amount.

microcephaly: An unusually small head of a newborn.

midaxillary line: A vertical line drawn midway between the anterior and posterior axillary folds.

midclavicular line: A vertical line drawn through the midpoint of the clavicle.

midsternal line: A vertical line drawn through the middle of the sternum.

miosis: Contraction of the pupil to less than 2 mm in diameter.

mitral valve: The heart valve between the left atrium and left ventricle consisting of two cusps; it allows blood to flow into the ventricle and prevents backflow.

Montgomery tubercles: Enlarged sebaceous glands located on the areola of the breast.

mucopurulent: An exudate that contains both pus and mucus.

murmur: A heart sound audible with the stethoscope, generated by disruptions in the passage of blood within the heart or blood vessels.

Murphy sign: Pain on inspiration during palpation of the liver and gallbladder that causes the patient to stop inspiration; usually a sign of gallbladder disease.

muscle tone: Level of tension or consistency of muscle mass.

myalgia: Tenderness or pain in muscle.

myocardium: The middle and thickest of the three layers of the wall of the heart, consisting of cardiac muscle.

myopia: (Nearsightedness) a condition resulting from a refractive error in which light rays entering the eye are brought into focus in front of the retina.

myxedema: A condition caused by hypothyroidism characterized by dry, waxy skin, coarse hair, intolerance to cold, cognitive impairment, and slowing of the relaxation phase of deep tendon reflexes.

nasal polyp: Boggy, dependent mucosa that is rounded and elongated, and projects into the nasal cavity.

nasopharynx: The portion of the pharynx extending from the posterior nares to the level of the soft palate.

neologism: A word used by a person with a mental disorder that is understood only by that person.

neurogenic: Arising from or caused by the nervous system.

nevus: A circumscribed skin lesion that is presumed to be genetic; the excess or deficient tissue may involve epidermal or connective tissue, nerve elements, or vascular elements; the nevus may be pigmented or nonpigmented.

nocturia: Urination at night; the individual is awakened from sleep by the need to void.

nuchal rigidity: Resistance to flexion of the neck, seen in individuals with meningitis.

nystagmus: Involuntary rhythmic movements of the eyes; the oscillations may be horizontal, vertical, rotary, or mixed.

oligomenorrhea: Infrequent menstruation.

oncotic pressure: The pressure difference between the osmotic pressure of blood and that of tissue fluid or lymph; an important force in maintaining balance between blood and surrounding tissues.

onycholysis: The loosening of the nails starting at the border.

oropharynx: Division of the pharynx extending from behind the soft palate dorsally to the upper edge of the epiglottis.

orthostatic: Referring to an upright body position; orthostatic edema develops after standing; orthostatic hypotension occurs when the patient stands erect.

Osler nodes: Small, tender, swollen areas, varying in color from pink or red to bluish, generally in the fleshy pads of fingers or toes, or in the thenar or hypothenar prominences; findings indicating subacute bacterial endocarditis.

ossification: The formation of bone.

otorrhea: Discharge, especially a purulent one, from the ear.

pack-years of smoking: An index risk for cardiac and pulmonary problems; calculated by multiplying number of years of smoking by number of packs smoked each day.

palpebral fissures: The elliptical opening between the upper and lower eyelids.

palpitation: Beating of the heart so vigorous that the patient is aware of it; causes include exertion, emotional stress, hyperthyroidism, and various heart diseases.

papillae: Small nipple-shaped projections; papillae on the dorsal portion of the tongue contain the taste buds.

papilledema: Edema of the optic disc resulting in loss of definition of the disc margin; the cause often is increased intracranial pressure.

paradoxic pulse: Variation in systolic pressure with respiration, diminishing with inspiration and increasing with expiration; also known as pulsus paradoxus.

paraphrasia: Speech that is incoherent or incomprehensible, but that could be meaningful when carefully interpreted by a psychotherapist.

parasternal: Situated close to or beside the sternum.

parasympathetic nervous system: The division of the autonomic nervous system responsible for the protection, conservation, and restoration of body resources.

parenchyma: The functional cells of an organ, as distinguished from the supporting connective tissue framework.

paresthesia: Unusual sensation such as numbness, tingling, or burning.

parietal: Referring to inner walls of any body cavity.

paroxysm: A sudden sharp spasm, convulsion, or attack; a sudden relapse of disease.

peak height velocity: The time during pubescence at which the tempo of growth is greatest.

peau d'orange: Dimpling of the skin that gives it the appearance of the skin of an orange.

pectoriloquy: A striking transmission of voice sounds through the pulmonary structures, so that they are clearly audible through the stethoscope; commonly occurs from lung consolidation.

pectus carinatum: (Pigeon chest) forward protrusion of the sternum.

pectus excavatum: (Funnel chest) depression of the sternum.

pedunculated: Having a stalk or stem that acts as a means of connection.

pericardium: The fibroserous membrane covering the heart and roots of the great vessels.

perineum: The region between the thighs, in the female between the vulva and the anus and in the male between the scrotum and the anus.

peristalsis: The wavelike motion by which the alimentary tract propels its contents.

petechiae: Purple or red pinpoint spots on the skin, the result of minute hemorrhages into the dermal or submucosal layers.

Peyer patches: Collections of closely packed lymphoid follicles, forming elevations on the mucous membrane of the small intestine.

philtrum: The vertical groove in the midline above the upper lip.

photophobia: Increased sensitivity to light; the condition is prevalent in albinism and disorders of the conjunctiva and cornea.

pica: A craving to eat nonfood substances such as dirt, clay, or starch; may occur with some nutritional deficiency states, pregnancy, or mental disorders.

pilonidal: Pertaining to the sacrococcygeal area.

pitch: A quality of sound that typifies its highness or lowness of tone, as determined by the frequency of vibrations.

plantar flexion: Extension of the foot so that the forepart is lower than the ankle.

pleura: The serous membranes covering the lungs (visceral pleura) and lining the inner aspect of the pleural cavity (parietal pleura).

pleural cavity: The potential space between the usually closely opposed parietal and visceral layers of the pleura.

pleurisy: Inflammation of the pleura, often associated with pneumonia.

plumbism: Lead poisoning.

pneumothorax: Accumulation of air or gas in the pleural space.

polydactyly: Extra digits on the hands or feet.

polymenorrhea: Increased frequency of menstruation not consistently associated with ovulation.

postauricular: Behind the auricle of the ear.

posterior axillary line: A vertical line drawn inferiorly from the posterior axillary fold.

postmenopausal bleeding: Menstrual bleeding occurring 1 year or more after menopause.

postterm infant: An infant born after 41 completed weeks of gestation.

postural hypotension: (Orthostatic hypotension) the presence of low blood pressure when the patient stands erect.

preauricular: In front of the auricle of the ear.

precordium: That area of the thorax situated over the heart.

prepuce: The foreskin of the penis.

presbyopia: Hyperopia and impaired near vision from loss of lens elasticity, generally developing during middle age.

preterm infant: An infant born before 37 weeks' gestation.

prodromal event: An early sign or warning of a developing disorder.

prognathism: Protrusion of the jaws, causing malocclusion of the teeth.

pronate: The act of assuming a prone position; applied to the hand, the act of turning the palm backward or downward by medially rotating the forearm; applied to the foot, turning the medial edge of the foot lower and outward by eversion and abduction of the tarsal and metatarsal joints.

proprioception: The sensation of position and muscular activity originating from within the body, which provides awareness of posture, movement, and changes in equilibrium.

proptosis, proptotic: Bulging or protrusion of an organ, such as the eyes.

pruritus: An itching sensation producing the urge to scratch.

ptosis: Prolapse of an organ or part; drooping of the upper eyelid.

pubarche: Beginning growth of pubic hair, breasts, and genitals.

pulmonary pressure: The blood pressure in the pulmonary artery.

pulmonary valve: The valve at the junction of the pulmonary artery and right ventricle consisting of three half-moon–shaped cusps; it prevents blood from regurgitating into the ventricle.

pulse: The palpable, rhythmic expansion and contraction of an artery, the result of an increased thrust of blood into the circulation each time the heart contracts; it is readily felt in the arterial component of the systemic circulation and also occurs in veins (e.g., jugular vein) and highly vascular organs (e.g., liver).

punctum: The tiny aperture in the margin of each eyelid that opens into a lacrimal duct.

purpura: Brownish-red or purple discolorations on the skin as the result of hemorrhage into the tissue; also a group of disorders characterized by purpura.

pyrosis: Epigastric burning sensation; heartburn.

QRS complex: The central deflections of the electrocardiogram representing the activity of the ventricles.

radiculopathy: Nerve root pain.

rale: (See crackle) a general term for an unexpected sound heard on auscultation of the chest; sometimes used to denote crepitus heard on auscultation.

regurgitation: A backward flowing (e.g., the blood between the chambers of the heart or between the great vessels and the heart).

retrognathia: Position of the jaws behind the frontal plane of the forehead.

rhonchus: A dry, coarse sound in the bronchial tubes heard on auscultation of the chest, the result of partial obstruction; a sonorous rhonchus is low pitched; a sibilant rhonchus is high pitched and squeaky.

rigidity: A condition of hardness and inflexibility.

saccular: Pouched; shaped like a sac.

scapular line: A vertical line drawn through the inferior angle of the scapula.

sclerosis: Hardening or induration of body tissues, which can be the result of inflammation, particularly when it is prolonged.

scoliosis: Lateral curvature of the spine.

scotoma: A loss of vision in a defined area in one or both eyes; shimmering film appearing as an island in the visual field, often occurring as a prodromal symptom.

scrotal raphe: The line of union of the two halves of the scrotum; often more highly pigmented than the surrounding tissue.

sebum: A thick substance secreted by the sebaceous glands that consists of fat and epithelial debris.

semilunar valve: Refers to the pulmonic or aortic valves.

sensorineural hearing loss: Reduction in hearing acuity related to a defect in the inner ear or damage to the eighth cranial nerve.

sessile: Attached by a base rather than a stalk; a sessile lesion adheres closely to the surface of the skin or mucosa (see pedunculated).

shunt, left to right: Referring to a diversion of blood from the left side of the heart to the right (e.g., from a septal defect) or from the systemic circulation to the pulmonary circulation (e.g., from a patent ductus arteriosus).

sibilant: Having the character of a hiss or whistle.

sign: An objective finding perceived by the examiner.

simian crease: A single palmar crease associated with Down syndrome.

sinus dysrhythmia: An increase in heart rate with inspiration. It is a physiologic response to decreased left ventricular volume during inspiration producing a cyclic irregularity with each inspiration.

sinus rhythm: The expected regular cardiac rhythm stimulated by the sinoatrial node.

situs inversus: The inversion or transposition of the body viscera so that the heart is on the right and the liver on the left; the chest and abdominal contents become mirror images of the usual.

Skene glands: (Paraurethral glands) mucus-secreting glands that open onto the vestibule on each side of the urethra.

small for gestational age (SGA): A weight classification of newborns associated with poorer health outcomes, the weight falling below the 10th percentile on the intrauterine growth curve for the infant's calculated gestational age.

smegma: Sebaceous material secreted by the glans penis and epithelial cells desquamated from the prepuce; it appears as a cheesy white material.

spasm: Involuntary contraction of a muscle or group of muscles, interfering with usual function of that particular muscle group.

spastic: Increased muscle tone, spasms, or uncontrolled contractions of skeletal muscles causing stiff, awkward movements.

spotting: Small amounts of intermenstrual bloody vaginal discharge ranging from pink to dark brown.

sprain: Traumatic injury to the tendons, muscles, or ligaments around a joint.

stapes: One of the three ossicles of the middle ear, connected to the inner ear.

steatorrhea: Frothy, foul-smelling fecal matter that floats because of its high fat content; associated with malabsorption syndromes.

stellate: Shaped like a star; arranged in a rosette.

stereognosis: The ability to recognize objects by the sense of touch.

striae: Streaks or lines; skin striae result from weakening of the elastic tissue associated with pregnancy, weight gain, rapid growth periods, and high levels of corticosteroids.

stridor: A harsh, high-pitched sound during respiration caused by laryngeal or tracheal obstruction.

stroke volume: The amount of blood pumped out of one ventricle of the heart as the result of a single contraction.

stroke Common term indicating a sudden neurologic impairment of varying degree usually related to a more or less sudden interruption of blood flow to the brain as from hemorrhage, thrombosis, or embolism.

GLOSSARY

stroma: The supportive connective tissue framework of an organ as distinguished from the functional tissue (parenchyma).

sty: A purulent infection of a meibomian gland of the eyelid, often caused by a staphylococcal organism.

subaortic stenosis: Congenital narrowing of the outflow tract of the left ventricle caused by a ring of fibrous tissue or hypertrophy of the muscular septum just below the aortic valve.

subcutaneous emphysema: The presence of air or gas beneath the skin.

subcutaneous nodules: Firm and painless nodules discovered in the presence of acute rheumatic fever. These nodules occur only rarely and, when they do, usually in the presence of carditis. They appear over the extensor surfaces of certain joints, particularly the elbows, knees, and wrists; over the spinous processes of the thoracic and lumbar vertebrae; and in the suboccipital area. The skin over these nodules moves freely and is not inflamed.

subgaleal: The area underlying the galea aponeurotica.

subjective data: That information collected during the interview with the patient or a significant other.

subluxation: Partial or incomplete dislocation.

sulcus: A shallow groove or depression on the surface of an organ (e.g., the median sulcus of the prostate gland separating the two lateral lobes).

supernumerary nipples: Extra nipples usually not associated with underlying glandular tissue located along the embryonic mammary ridge.

supinate: To assume a supine position; applied to the arm, the act of turning the palm forward or upward by laterally rotating the forearm; applied to the foot, the act of raising the medial margin of the foot.

sutures: A fibrous joint in which the bones are closely approximated, as between the infant's cranial bones, permitting expansion of the skull for brain growth.

swan neck deformity: Hyperextension of the proximal interphalangeal joint with fixed flexion of the distal interphalangeal joint.

sympathetic nervous system: The division of the autonomic nervous system that activates responses to physiologic or psychologic stress.

symptom: The subjective indication of disease perceived by the patient.

syndactyly: Webbing between the digits of the hands or feet.

systole: The part of the cardiac cycle during which the heart contracts, particularly the ventricles, resulting in a forceful flow of blood into both the systemic and pulmonary circulations.

tachycardia: Rapid heart rate greater than 100 beats per minute.

tachypnea: Rapid, usually shallow, breathing.

tactile fremitus: A tremor or vibration in any part of the body detected on palpation.

tail of Spence: Upper outer tail of the breast that extends into the axilla.

term infant: An infant born between 37 and 41 weeks' gestation.

terminal hair: The pigmented coarse hair that grows on the scalp, axilla, pubis, and in males, the face.

thelarche: The beginning of female pubertal breast development.

thrill: A palpable vibration or tremor resulting from a cardiac murmur or a disruption in vascular blood flow.

thrombophlebitis: Inflammation of the wall of a vein associated with thrombus formation.

thrombosis: The formation or presence of a blood clot within a blood vessel or within one of the cavities of the heart.

thyrotoxicosis: A disease caused by excessive quantities of thyroid hormones.

tic: An involuntary movement or spasm of a small group of muscles that may be aggravated by stress or anxiety; sometimes momentarily controllable.

tinnitus: An auditory sensation in the absence of sound heard in one or both ears, such as ringing, buzzing, hissing, or clicking.

tocolysis: Suppression of premature labor with drugs.

tonus: Expected state of muscle tone, maintained by partial contraction or alternate contraction and relaxation of neighboring muscle fibers in a group of muscles.

tophus: A chalky deposit of uric acid crystals around joints or on the external ear; associated with gout.

tragus: The cartilaginous projection of the ear anterior to the auditory canal meatus.

transient ischemic attack (TIA): A transient episode of cerebral dysfunction, rapid (within minutes) in onset; usually due to vasospasm, hypotension, or a variety of events producing an ischemia which resolves usually in less than 24 hours; most often referable to the areas served by carotid and/or vertebrobasilar arteries.

transient tachypnea of the newborn: A self-limited neonatal respiratory problem characterized by a rapid respiratory rate and associated with maternal treatment with narcotics or analgesics during labor, premature labor and, at times, cesarean delivery.

tremor: Rhythmic, purposeless, quivering movements resulting from involuntary alternate contraction and relaxation of opposing muscle groups.

tricuspid valve: A heart valve between the right atrium and right ventricle, consisting of three cusps, that allows blood to flow to the ventricle and prevents backflow.

turbinates: Extensions of the ethmoid bone located along the lateral wall of the nose, covered by erectile mucous membrane.

tympanic membrane: (Eardrum) a membranous structure separating the external ear from the middle ear.

umbo: Landmark on the tympanic membrane created by the attachment of the tympanic membrane to the malleus.

valgus: A position in which part of a limb is twisted outward away from the midline.

Valsalva maneuver: Forced expiratory effort against a closed airway (i.e., closed mouth and nose or glottis).

varicosity: An unnaturally swollen, often tortuous, blood or lymph vessel.

varus: A position in which part of a limb is twisted inward toward the midline.

vascular: Referring to blood vessels.

vasoconstriction: A narrowing in the caliber of a blood vessel.

vasomotor: Referring to control over the dilation and constriction of blood vessels.

vasopressor: Stimulating contraction of the muscular tissues of the capillaries and arteries, causing a rise in blood pressure.

vellus hair: The soft, nonpigmented hair that covers the body.

velocity of growth: The rate of growth or change in growth measurements over a period of time.

venous hum: A continuous musical murmur heard on auscultation over the major veins at the base of the neck, particularly when a patient is anemic, upright, and looking to the contralateral side; also heard in the healthy individual, particularly the young.

venous thrombosis: Formation or presence of a blood clot within a vein.

ventilation: The movement of air into and out of the lungs, resulting in the exchange of gases between the lungs and the air.

vertigo: Sensation of dizziness, either of spinning oneself or of external objects whirling around oneself.

vesicular breath sounds: Expected breathing sounds when the patient is healthy and free of respiratory embarrassment.

vestibular function: Balance.

vestibule: The almond-shaped area enclosed by the labia minora laterally, extending from the clitoris to the fourchette anteroposteriorly.

Virchow node: (Signal or sentinel node) a firm supra-clavicular lymph node, particularly on the left, so enlarged that it is palpable.

virilization: The process by which a female acquires male secondary sexual characteristics, usually as a result of adrenal dysfunction.

vulva: (Pudendum) the visible external female genitalia consisting of the mons pubis, labia, clitoris, vaginal orifice, vestibule, and vestibular glands.

water-hammer pulse: Full, forcible impulse and immediate collapse, providing a jerking sensation; characteristic of aortic regurgitation.

webbing: Skin folds in the neck from the acromion to the mastoid; associated with chromosomal anomalies.

whispered pectoriloquy: The transmission of a whisper in the same way as that of more readily audible speech, commonly detected when the lung is consolidated by pneumonia (see pectoriloquy).

whoop: The noisy spasm of inspiration that terminates the paroxysms of coughing characteristic of pertussis (whooping cough); caused by a sudden, sharp increase in tension of the vocal chords.

winged scapula: An outward prominence of the scapula caused by disruption of its nerves or muscles.

word salad: Meaningless, disconnected word choices often used by a person with schizophrenia or some other problem of disorientation.

xanthelasma: Xanthoma located on the eyelids.

xanthoma: Small, flat, yellowish skin plaques, the result of lipid deposition in histiocytes (cells of the reticuloendothelial system).

xiphodynia: Pain in the cartilage of the xiphoid process.

APPENDIX A

CONVERSION TABLES

Length

Inches	Centimeters	Centimeters	Inches
1	2.54	1	0.4
2	5.08	2	0.8
4	10.16	3	1.2
6	15.24	4	1.6
8	20.32	5	2.0
10	25.40	6	2.4
20	50.80	8	3.1
30	76.20	10	3.9
40	101.60	20	7.9
50	127.00	30	11.8
60	152.40	40	15.7
70	177.80	50	19.7
80	203.20	60	23.6
90	228.60	70	27.6
100	254.00	80	31.5
150	381.00	90	35.4
200	508.00	100	39.4

1 inch = 2.54 cm
1 cm = 0.3937 inch

Weight

Pounds	Kilograms	Kilograms	Pounds
1	0.5	1	2.2
2	0.9	2	4.4
4	1.8	3	6.6
6	2.7	4	8.8
8	3.6	5	11.0
10	4.5	6	13.2
20	9.1	8	17.6
30	13.6	10	22
40	18.2	20	44
50	22.7	30	66
60	27.3	40	88
70	31.8	50	110
80	36.4	60	132
90	40.9	70	154
100	45.4	80	176
150	66.2	90	198
200	90.8	100	220

1 lb = 0.454 kg
1 kg = 2.204 lb

APPENDIX

B

TEMPERATURE EQUIVALENTS

Celsius*	Fahrenheit	Celsius*	Fahrenheit
34.0	93.2	38.6	101.4
34.2	93.6	38.8	101.8
34.4	93.9	39.0	102.2
34.6	94.3	39.2	102.5
34.8	94.6	39.4	102.9
35.0	95.0	39.6	103.2
35.2	95.4	39.8	103.6
35.4	95.7	40.0	104.0
35.6	96.1	40.2	104.3
35.8	96.4	40.4	104.7
36.0	96.8	40.6	105.1
36.2	97.1	40.8	105.4
36.4	97.5	41.0	105.8
36.6	97.8	41.2	106.1
36.8	98.2	41.4	106.5
37.0	98.6	41.6	106.8
37.2	98.9	41.8	107.2
37.4	99.3	42.0	107.6
37.6	99.6	42.2	108.0
37.8	100.0	42.4	108.3
38.0	100.4	42.6	108.7
38.2	100.7	42.8	109.0
38.4	101.1	43.0	109.4

From Hoekelman, 1997.
*To convert Celsius to Fahrenheit: $(9/5 \times \text{Temperature}) + 32$.
To convert Fahrenheit to Celsius: $5/9 \times (\text{Temperature} - 32)$.

HEIGHT/WEIGHT TABLES AND CHARTS

Growth curves are needed to determine the appropriateness of an infant's or a child's height, weight, and head circumference for age. Clues to significant health problems are sometimes revealed because the child is not growing as expected. These growth curves can be used for a one-time assessment, but they become more valuable if used over time to plot the child's growth pattern.

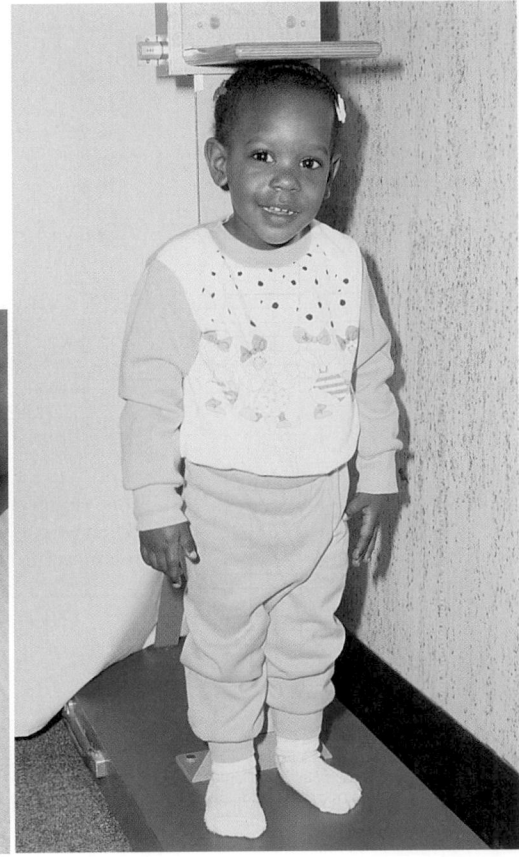

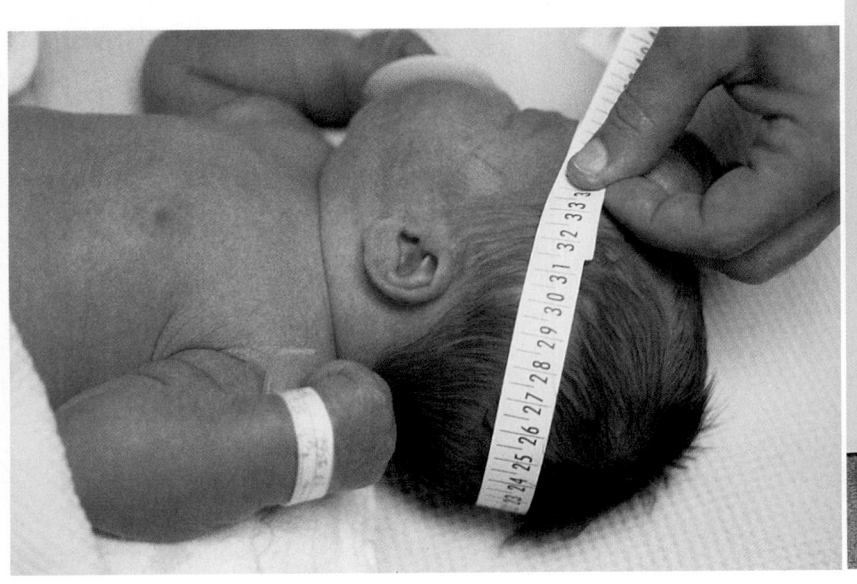

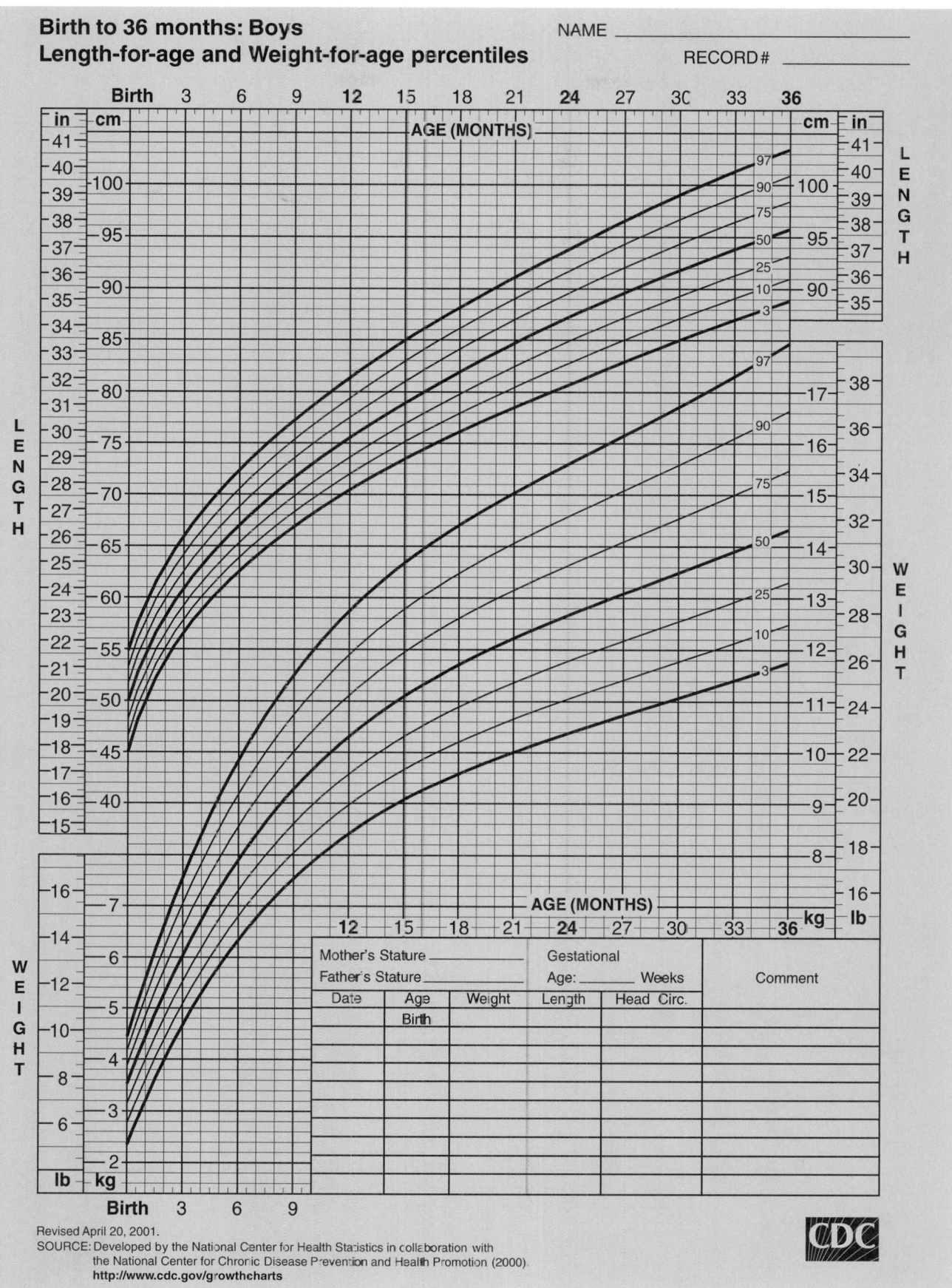

FIGURE C-1
Physical growth curves for children ages birth to 36 months: Boys.

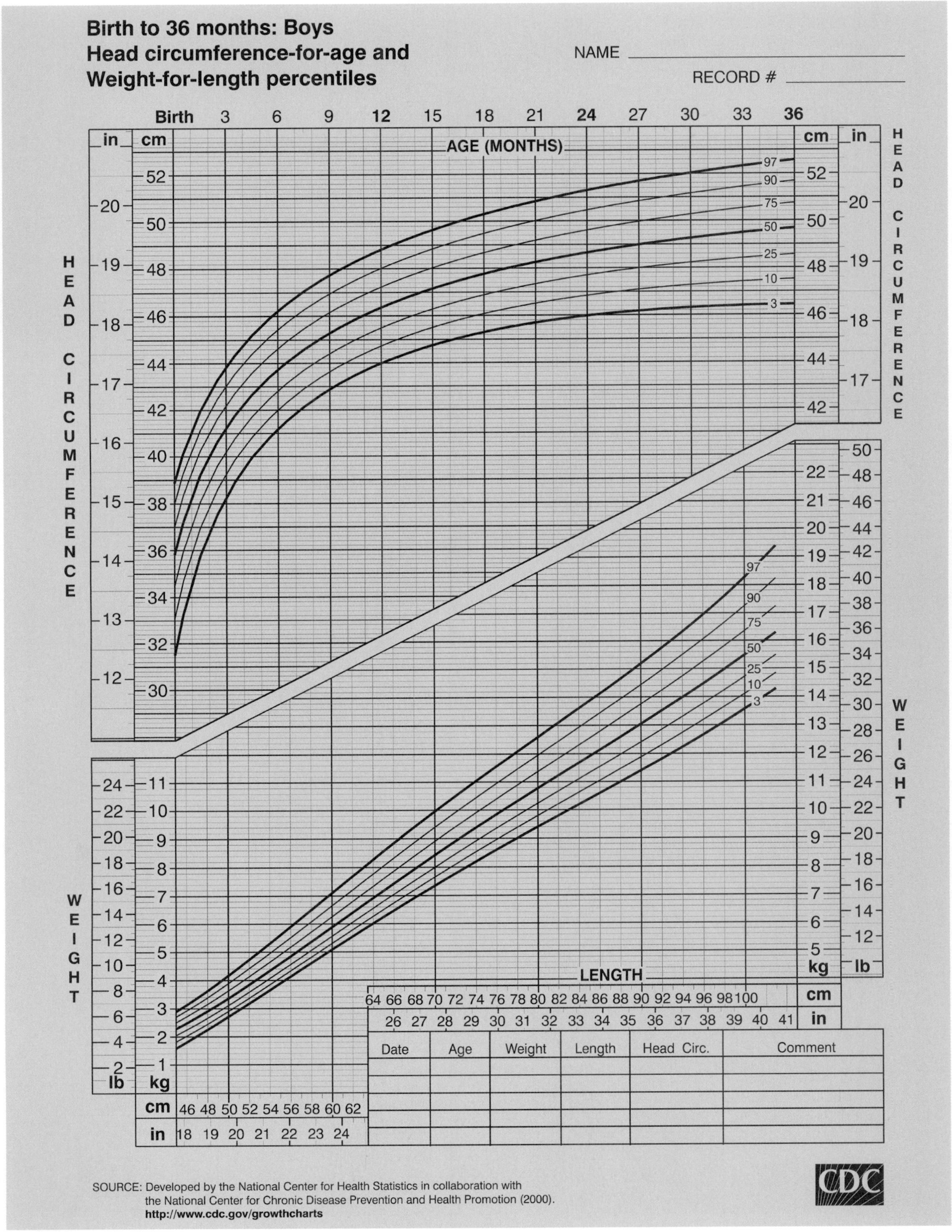

Birth to 36 months: Boys
Head circumference-for-age and
Weight-for-length percentiles

NAME _____

RECORD # _____

AGE (MONTHS)

Birth   3   6   9   12   15   18   21   24   27   30   33   36

HEAD CIRCUMFERENCE

in	cm		cm	in
20	52	97	52	20
19	50	90	50	19
18	48	75	48	18
17	46	50	46	17
16	44	25	44	
15	42	10	42	
14	40	3		
13	38			
12	36			
	34			
	32			
	30			

LENGTH

97
90
75
50
25
10
3

WEIGHT

in	cm		cm	in
		50	22	48
			21	46
			20	44
			19	42
			18	40
			17	38
			16	36
			15	34
			14	32
			13	30
			12	28

WEIGHT

lb	kg
24	11
22	10
20	9
18	8
16	7
14	6
12	5
10	4
8	3
6	2
4	
2	1
lb	kg

LENGTH

cm 64 66 68 70 72 74 76 78 80 82 84 86 88 90 92 94 96 98 100

in   26 27 28 29 30 31 32 33 34 35 36 37 38 39 40 41

kg	lb
11	24
10	22
9	20
8	18
7	16
6	14
5	12
kg	lb

Date	Age	Weight	Length	Head Circ.	Comment

cm 46 48 50 52 54 56 58 60 62

in   18 19 20 21 22 23 24

SOURCE: Developed by the National Center for Health Statistics in collaboration with
the National Center for Chronic Disease Prevention and Health Promotion (2000).
http://www.cdc.gov/growthcharts

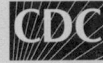

FIGURE C-1—cont'd

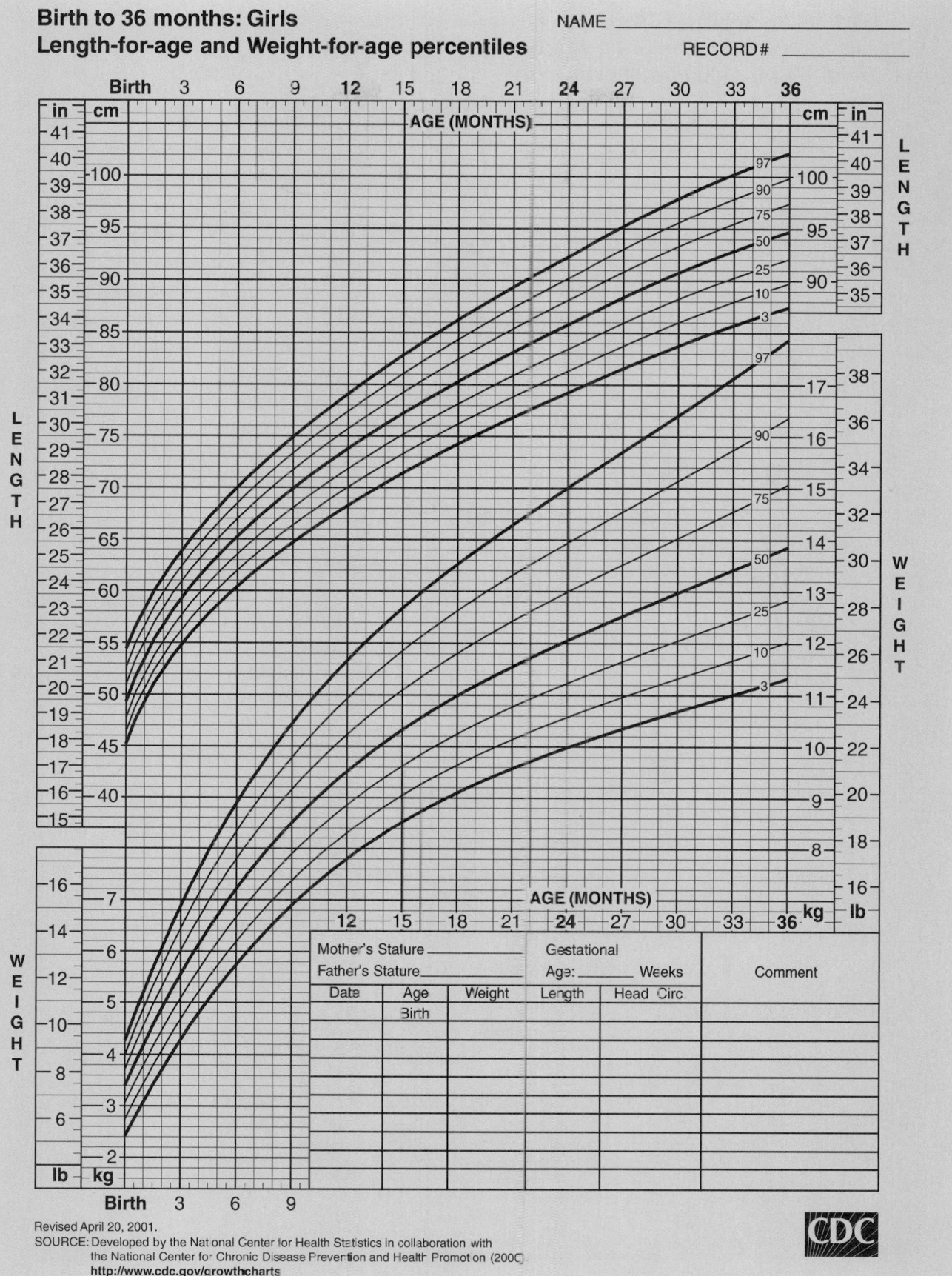

Birth to 36 months: Girls
Length-for-age and Weight-for-age percentiles

NAME _____

RECORD # _____

Revised April 20, 2001.
SOURCE: Developed by the National Center for Health Statistics in collaboration with
the National Center for Chronic Disease Prevention and Health Promotion (2000)
http://www.cdc.gov/growthcharts

FIGURE C-2
Physical growth curves for children ages birth to 36 months: Girls.

APPENDIX

Birth to 36 months: Girls
Head circumference-for-age and
Weight-for-length percentiles

NAME _____

RECORD # _____

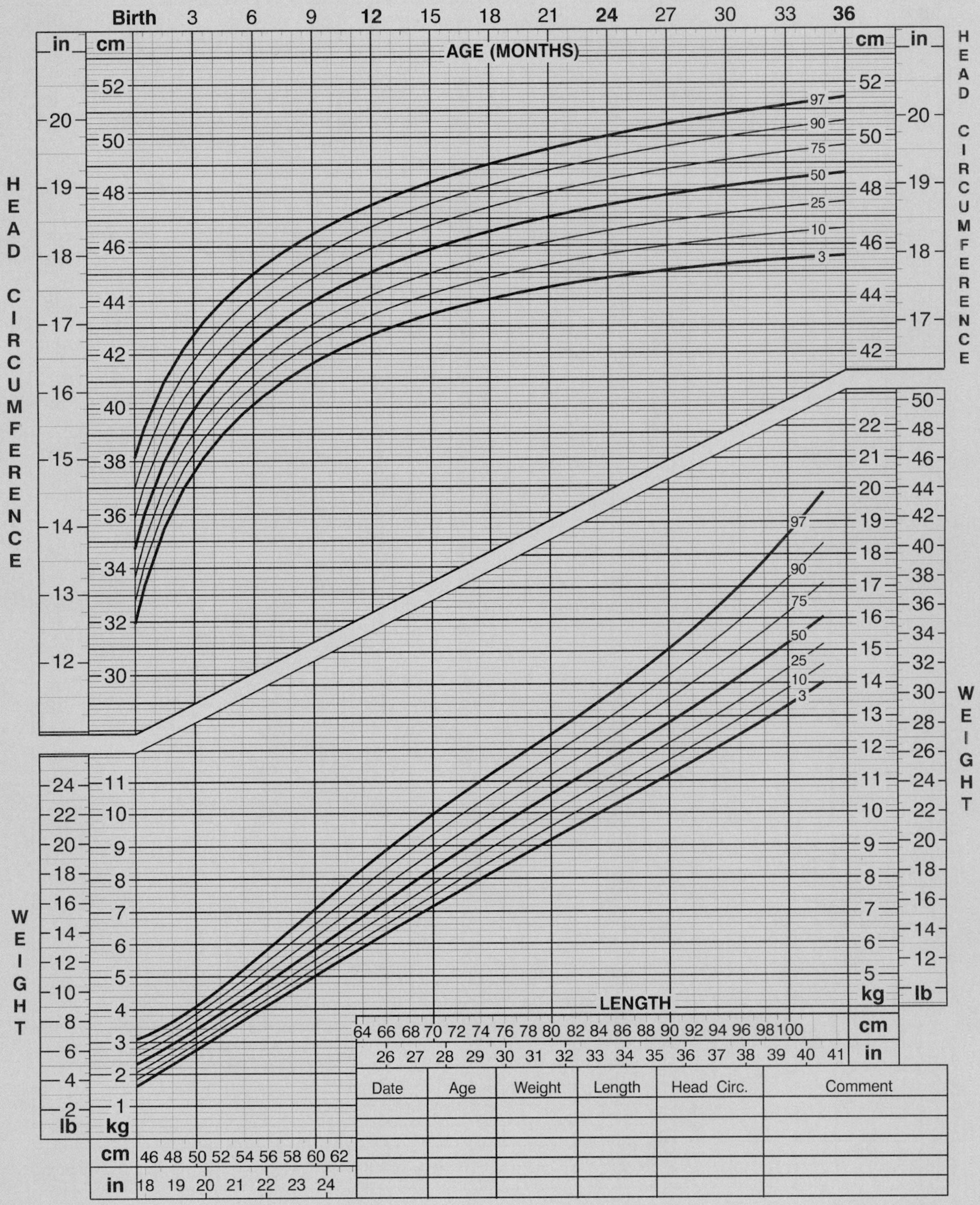

AGE (MONTHS)

Birth 3 6 9 12 15 18 21 24 27 30 33 36

HEAD CIRCUMFERENCE

| | | | | |
|97|
|90|
|75|
|50|
|25|
|10|
|3|

WEIGHT

LENGTH

Date	Age	Weight	Length	Head Circ.	Comment

SOURCE: Developed by the National Center for Health Statistics in collaboration with
the National Center for Chronic Disease Prevention and Health Promotion (2000).
http://www.cdc.gov/growthcharts

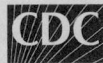

FIGURE C-2—cont'd

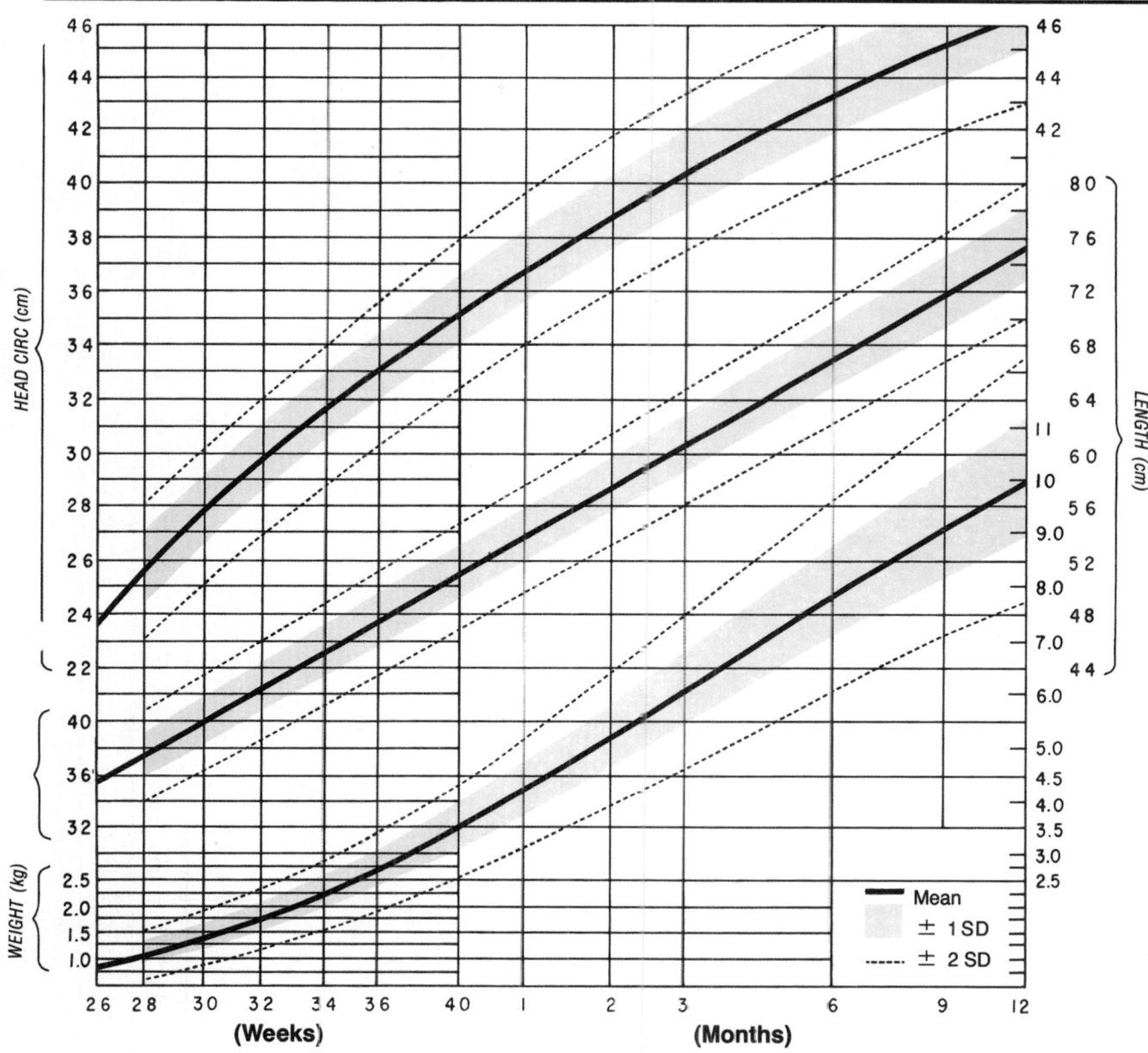

GROWTH RECORD FOR INFANTS*
BIRTH TO 1 YEAR,
SEXES COMBINED

NAME: _____

DATE OF BIRTH: _____

I.D. NO.: _____

DATE	AGE	LENGTH	WEIGHT	HEAD CIRC	DATE	AGE	LENGTH	WEIGHT	HEAD CIRC

*Adapted with permission: Babson SG, Benda GI: Growth graphs for the clinical assessment of infants of varying gestational age. *J Pediatr* 1976;89:814-820.

Provided as a service of

The Ross Hospital Formula System™

ROSS   **ROSS PRODUCTS DIVISION**
ABBOTT LABORATORIES
COLUMBUS, OHIO 43215-1724

G413(0.05)/FEBRUARY 1996   LITHO IN USA

FIGURE C-3
Physical growth curves for premature infants ages birth to 1 year: Boys and girls combined.

APPENDIX

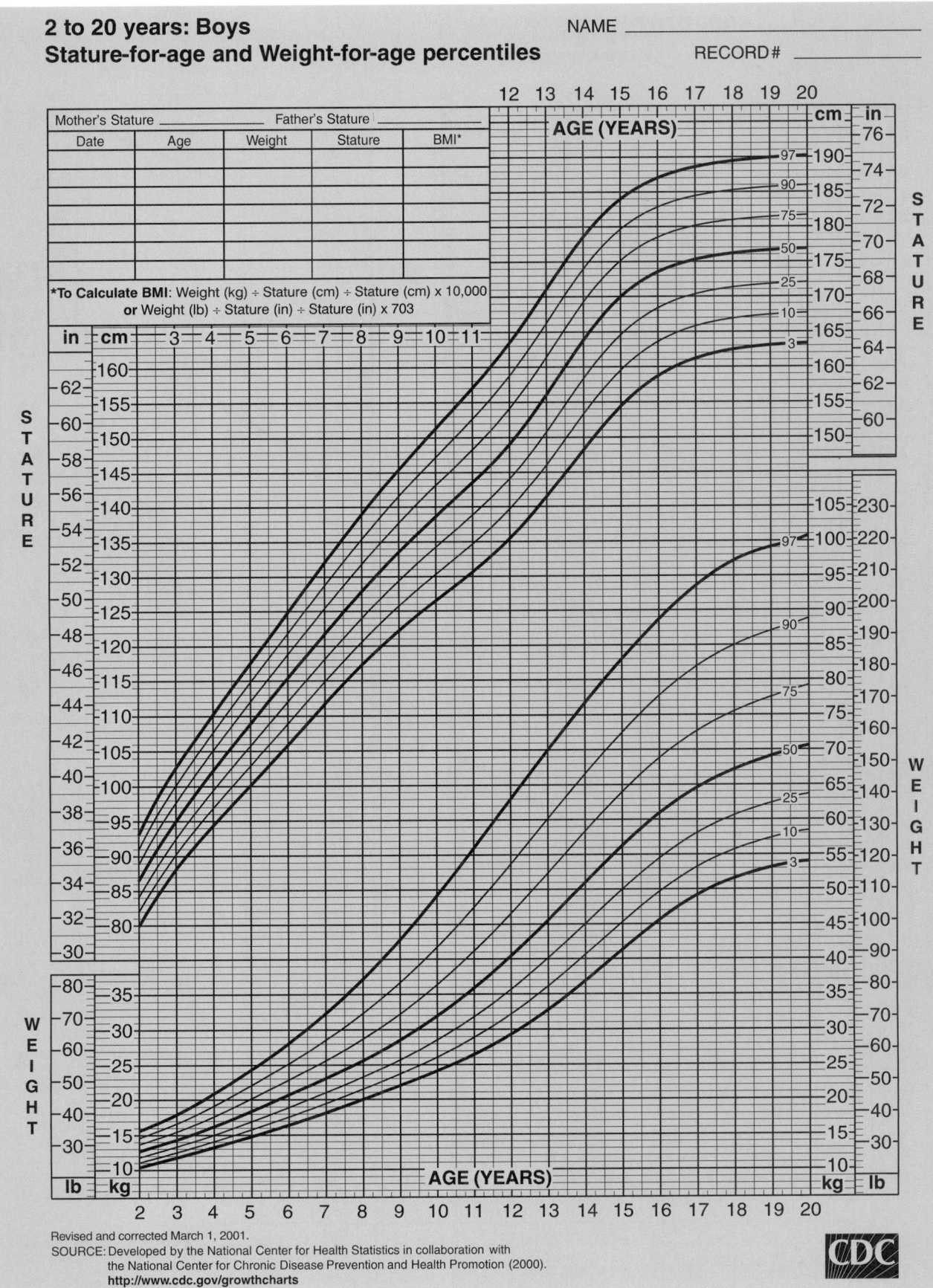

2 to 20 years: Boys
Stature-for-age and Weight-for-age percentiles

NAME _____

RECORD # _____

Revised and corrected March 1, 2001.
SOURCE: Developed by the National Center for Health Statistics in collaboration with the National Center for Chronic Disease Prevention and Health Promotion (2000).
http://www.cdc.gov/growthcharts

FIGURE C-4
Physical growth curves for ages 2 to 20 years: Boys.

2 to 20 years: Boys
Body mass index-for-age percentiles

NAME _____

FECORD# _____

Date	Age	Weight	Stature	BMI*	Comments

*To Calculate BMI: Weight (kg) ÷ Stature (cm) ÷ Stature (cm) x 10,000
or Weight (lb) ÷ Stature (in) ÷ Stature (in) x 703

BMI

35
34
33
32
31
30
29
28
27
26
25
24
23
22
21
20
19
18
17
16
15
14
13
12

97
95
90
85
75
50
25
10
3

BMI

27
26
25
24
23
22
21
20
19
18
17
16
15
14
13
12

kg/m²   **AGE (YEARS)**   kg/m²

2 3 4 5 6 7 8 9 10 11 12 13 14 15 16 17 18 19 20

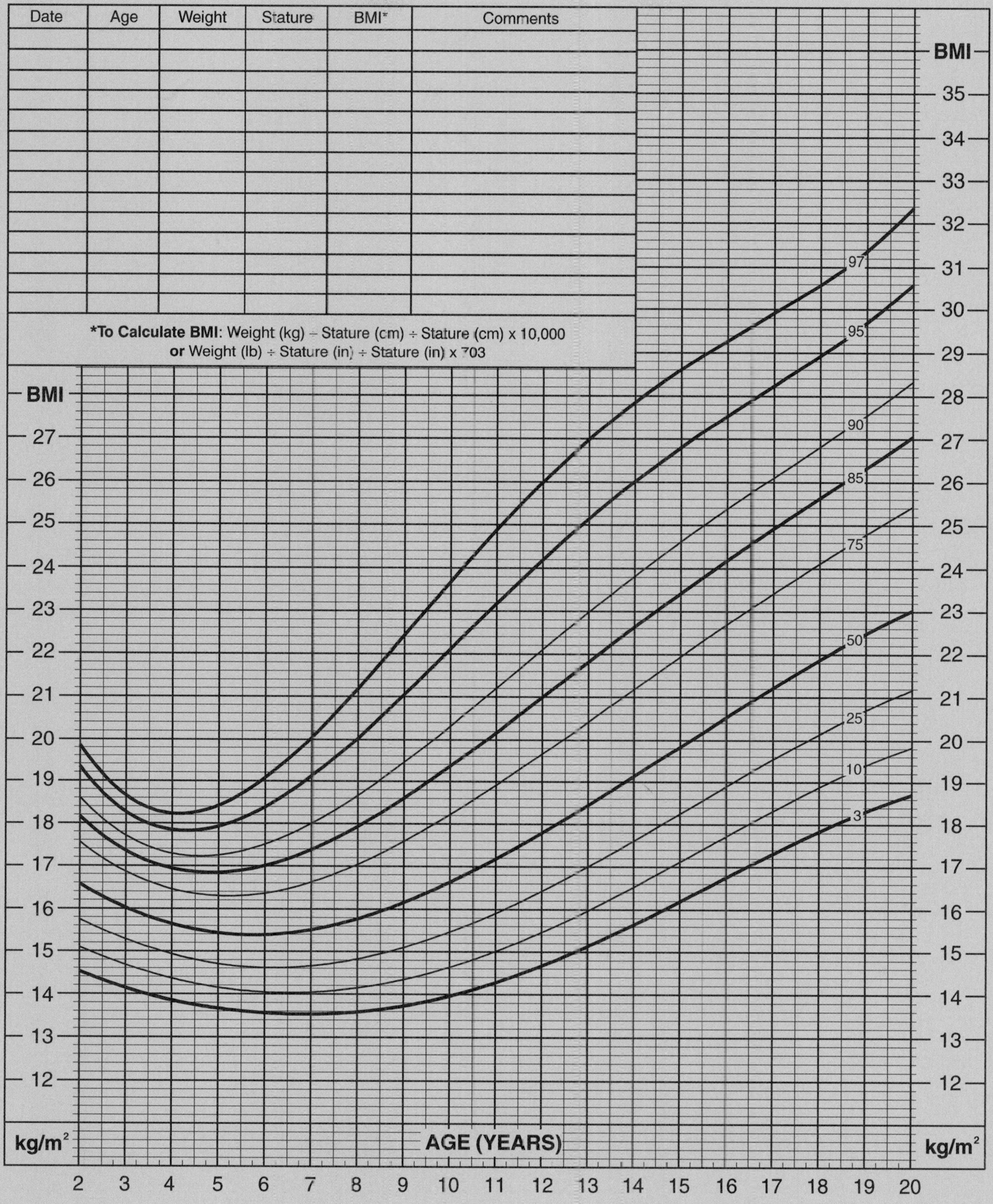

SOURCE: Developed by the National Center for Health Statistics in collaboration with
the National Center for Chronic Disease Prevention and Health Promotion (2000).
http://www.cdc.gov/growthcharts

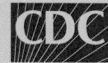

FIGURE C-4—cont'd

APPENDIX

Weight-for-stature percentiles: Boys

NAME _____

RECORD # _____

Date	Age	Weight	Stature	Comments

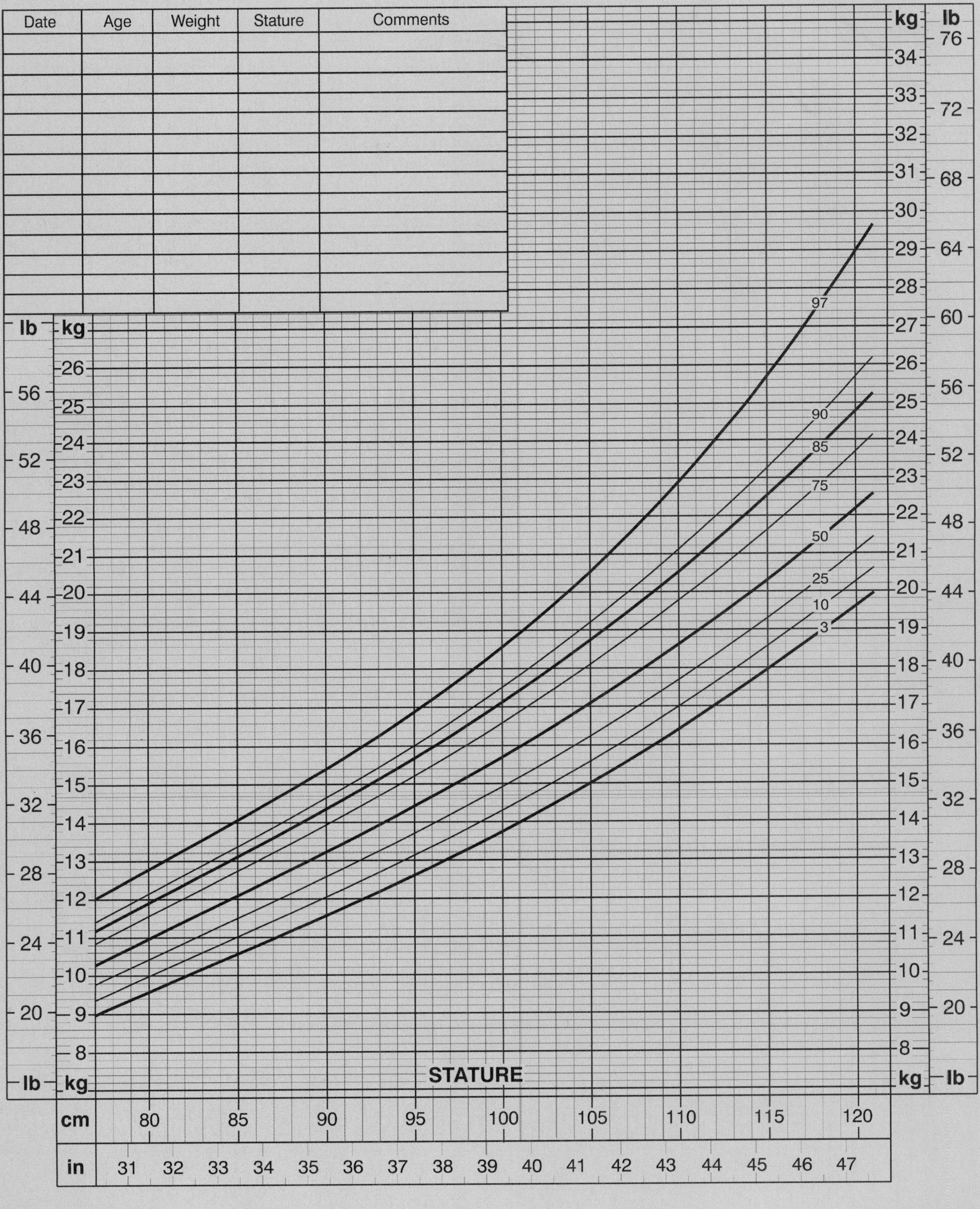

STATURE

SOURCE: Developed by the National Center for Health Statistics in collaboration with
the National Center for Chronic Disease Prevention and Health Promotion (2000).
http://www.cdc.gov/growthcharts

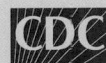

FIGURE C-4—cont'd

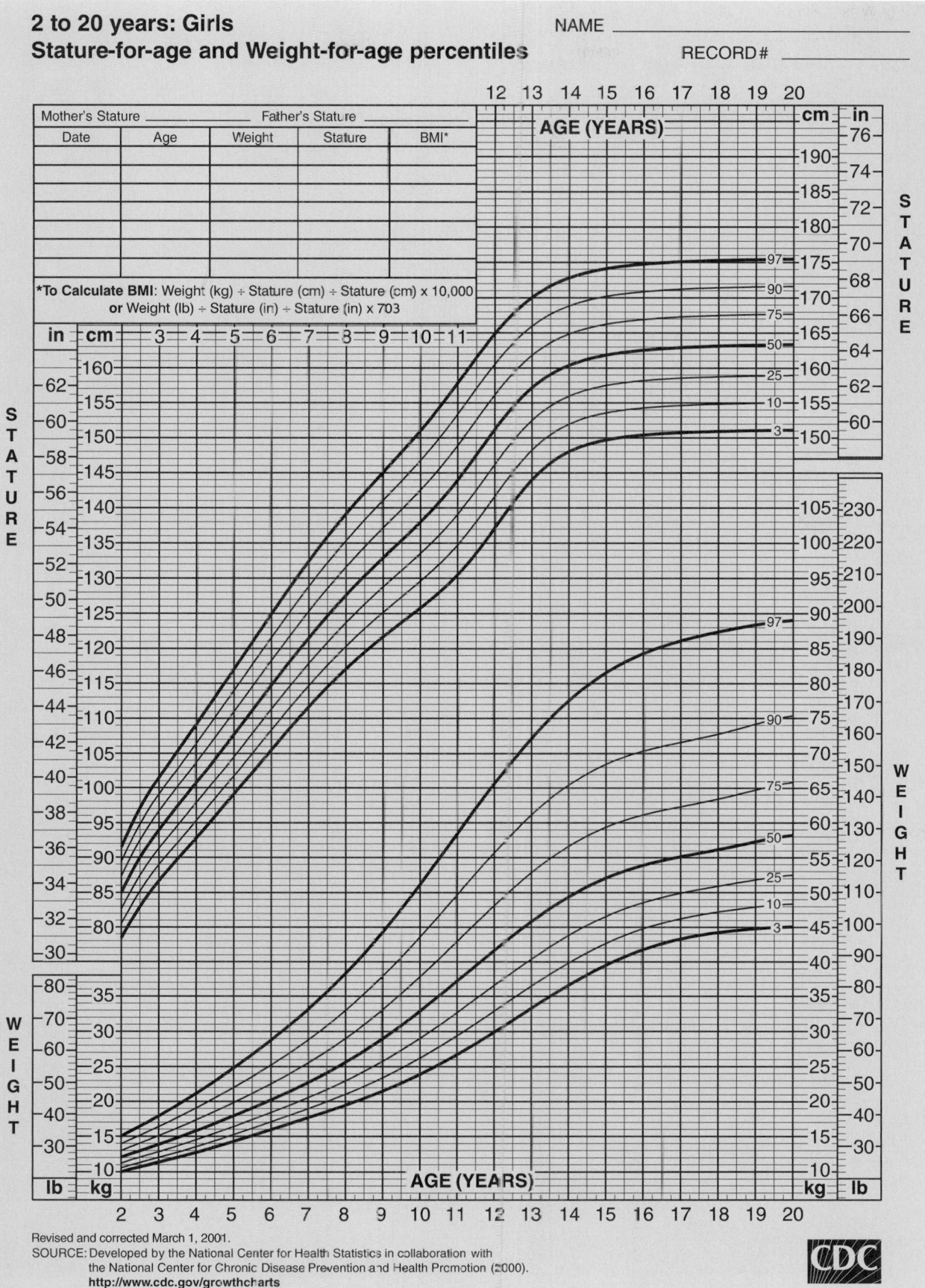

2 to 20 years: Girls
Stature-for-age and Weight-for-age percentiles

NAME _____

RECORD # _____

Revised and corrected March 1, 2001.
SOURCE: Developed by the National Center for Health Statistics in collaboration with
the National Center for Chronic Disease Prevention and Health Promotion (2000).
http://www.cdc.gov/growthcharts

FIGURE C-5
Physical growth curves for ages 2 to 20 years: Girls

2 to 20 years: Girls
Body mass index-for-age percentiles

NAME _____

RECORD # _____

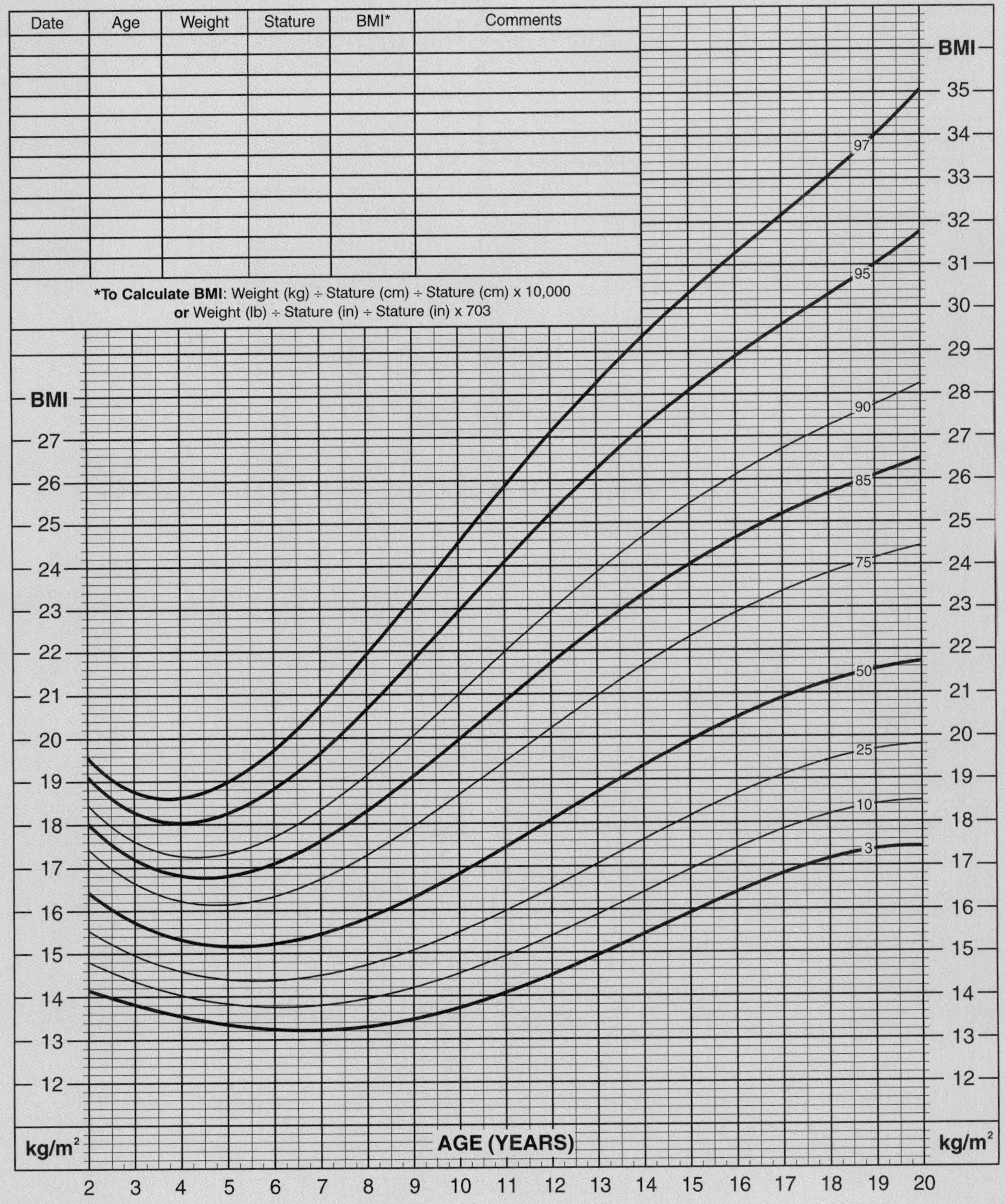

Date	Age	Weight	Stature	BMI*	Comments

*To Calculate BMI: Weight (kg) ÷ Stature (cm) ÷ Stature (cm) x 10,000
or Weight (lb) ÷ Stature (in) ÷ Stature (in) x 703

BMI

kg/m²

AGE (YEARS)

BMI

kg/m²

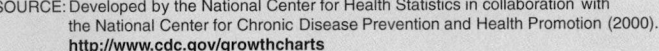

SOURCE: Developed by the National Center for Health Statistics in collaboration with
the National Center for Chronic Disease Prevention and Health Promotion (2000).
http://www.cdc.gov/growthcharts

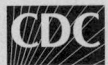

FIGURE C-5—cont'd

NAME ____________________

Weight-for-stature percentiles: Girls

RECORD # ____________

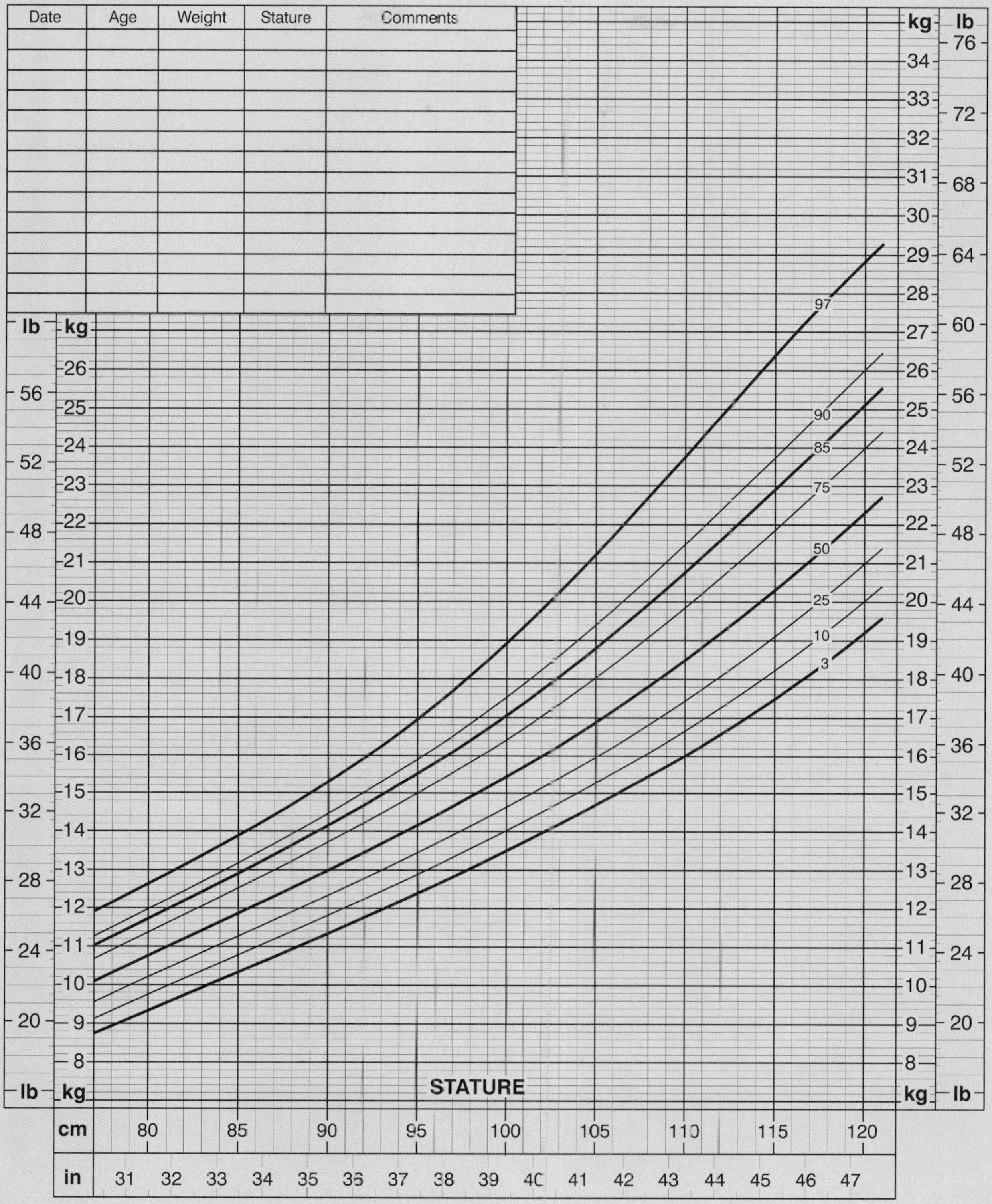
Date
Age
Weight
Stature
Comments
lb
kg
97
90
85
75
50
25
10
3
STATURE
cm
80 85 90 95 100 105 110 115 120
in
31 32 33 34 35 36 37 38 39 40 41 42 43 44 45 46 47
kg: 8 9 10 11 12 13 14 15 16 17 18 19 20 21 22 23 24 25 26 27 28 29 30 31 32 33 34
lb: 20 24 28 32 36 40 44 48 52 56 60 64 68 72 76

SOURCE: Developed by the National Center for Health Statistics in collaboration with the National Center for Chronic Disease Prevention and Health Promotion (2000)
http://www.cdc.gov/growthcharts

CDC

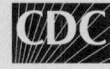

FIGURE C-5—cont'd

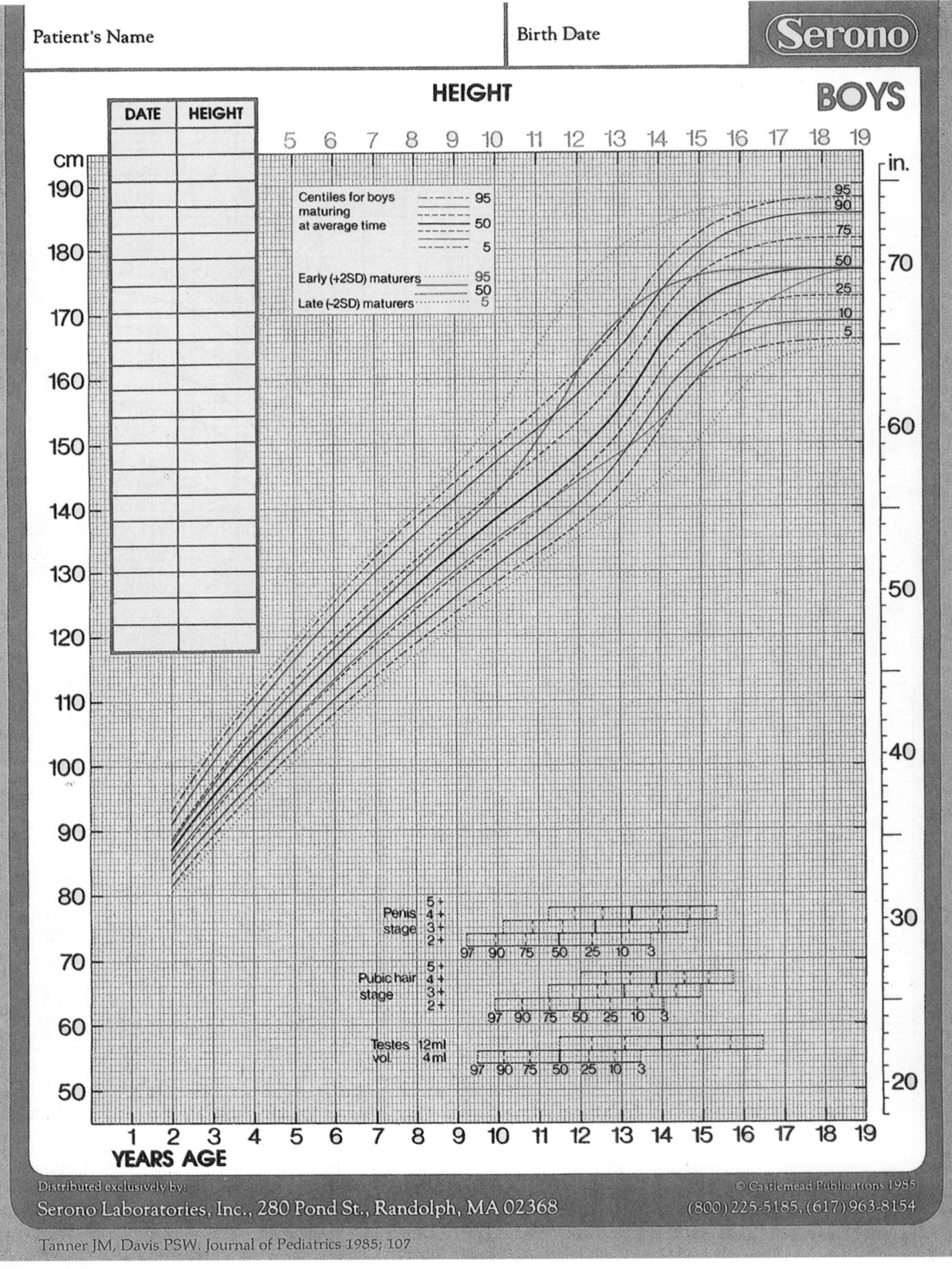

FIGURE C-6
Physical growth curves for children and adolescents ages 2 to 19 years, for height and sexual development: Boys.
From Tanner, Davies, 1985.

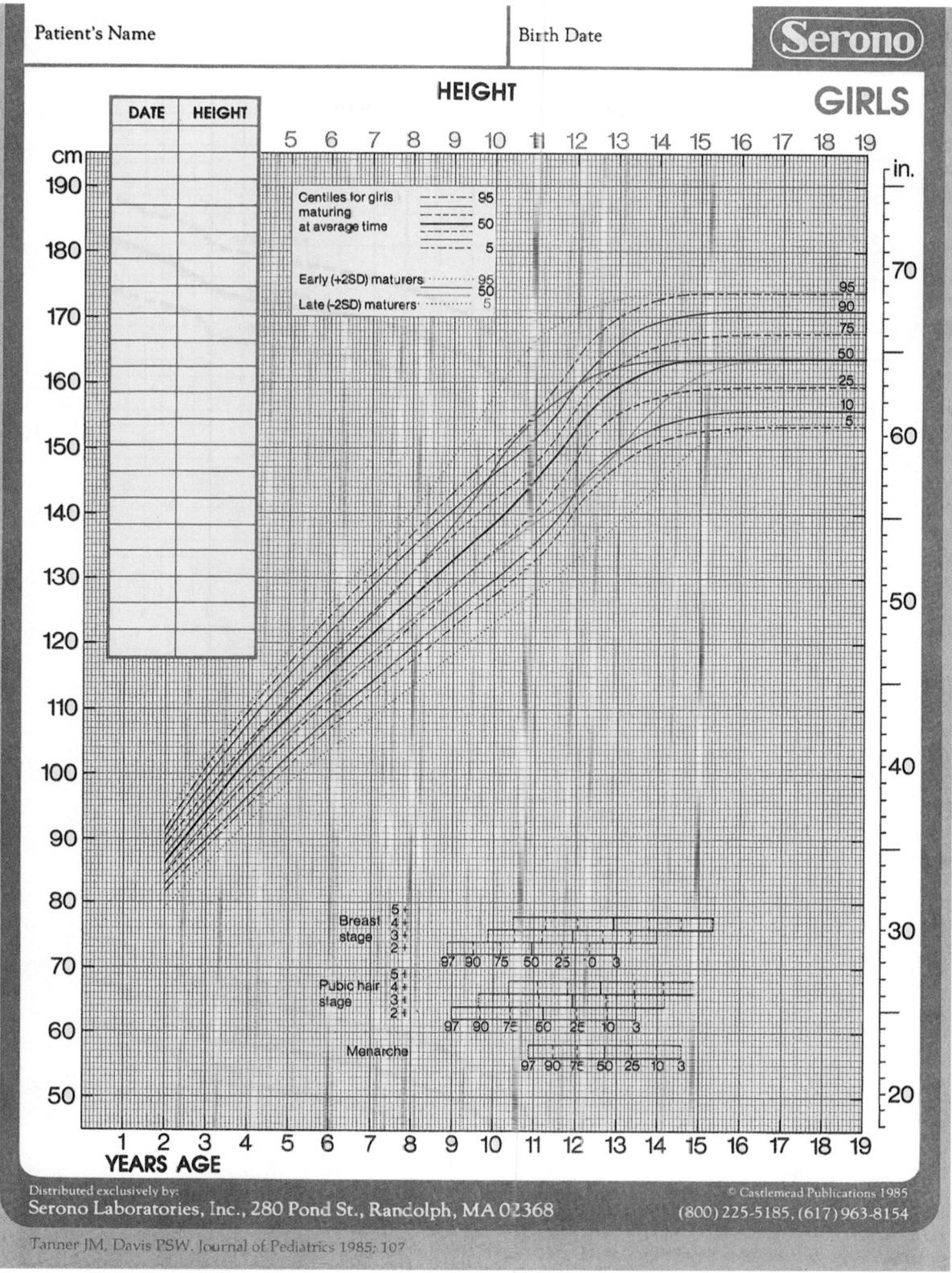

FIGURE C-6—cont'd
Physical growth curves for children and adolescents ages 2 to 19 years, for height and sexual development: Girls.
From Tanner, Davies, 1985.

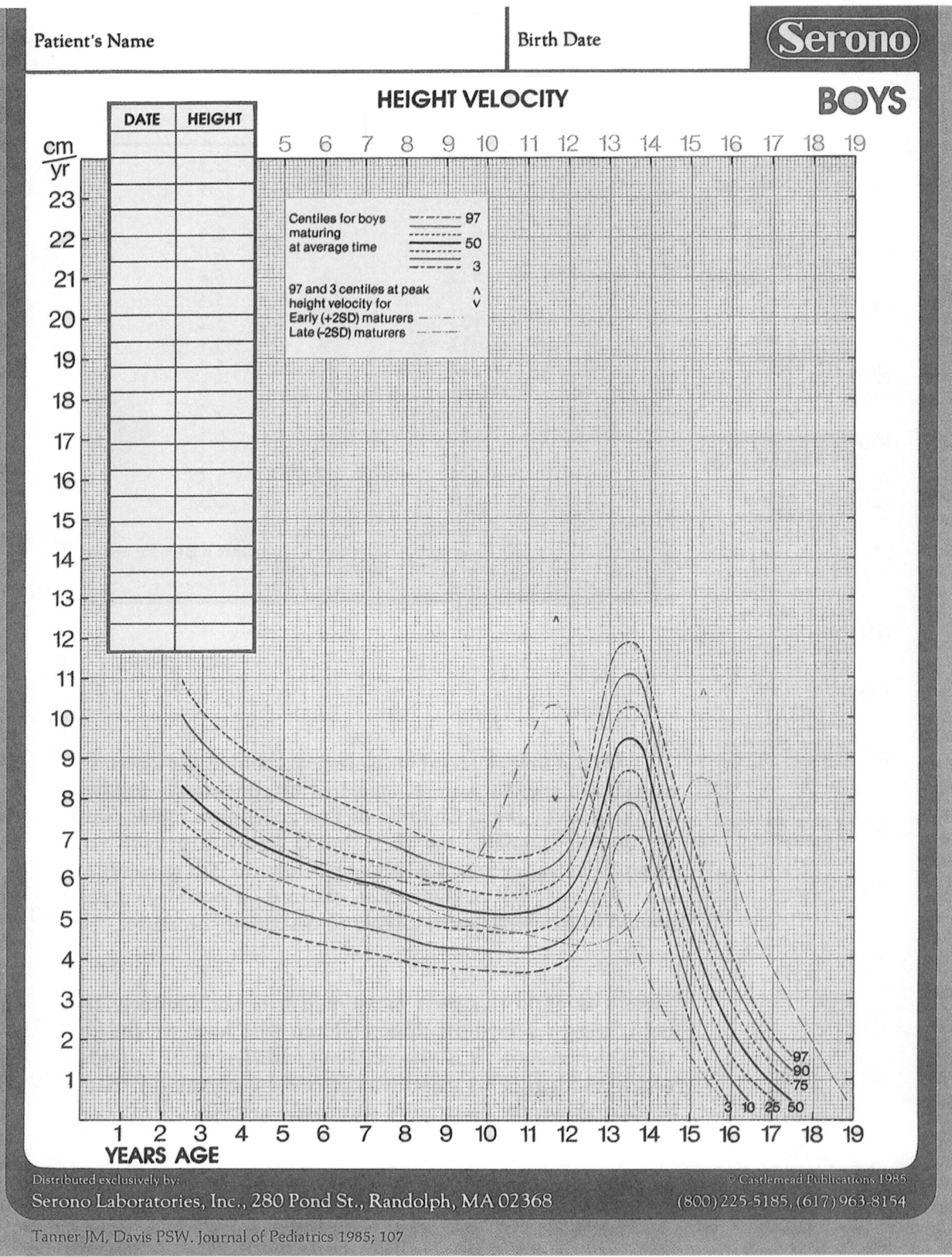

FIGURE C-7
Height velocity growth curves: Boys.
From Tanner, Davies, 1985.

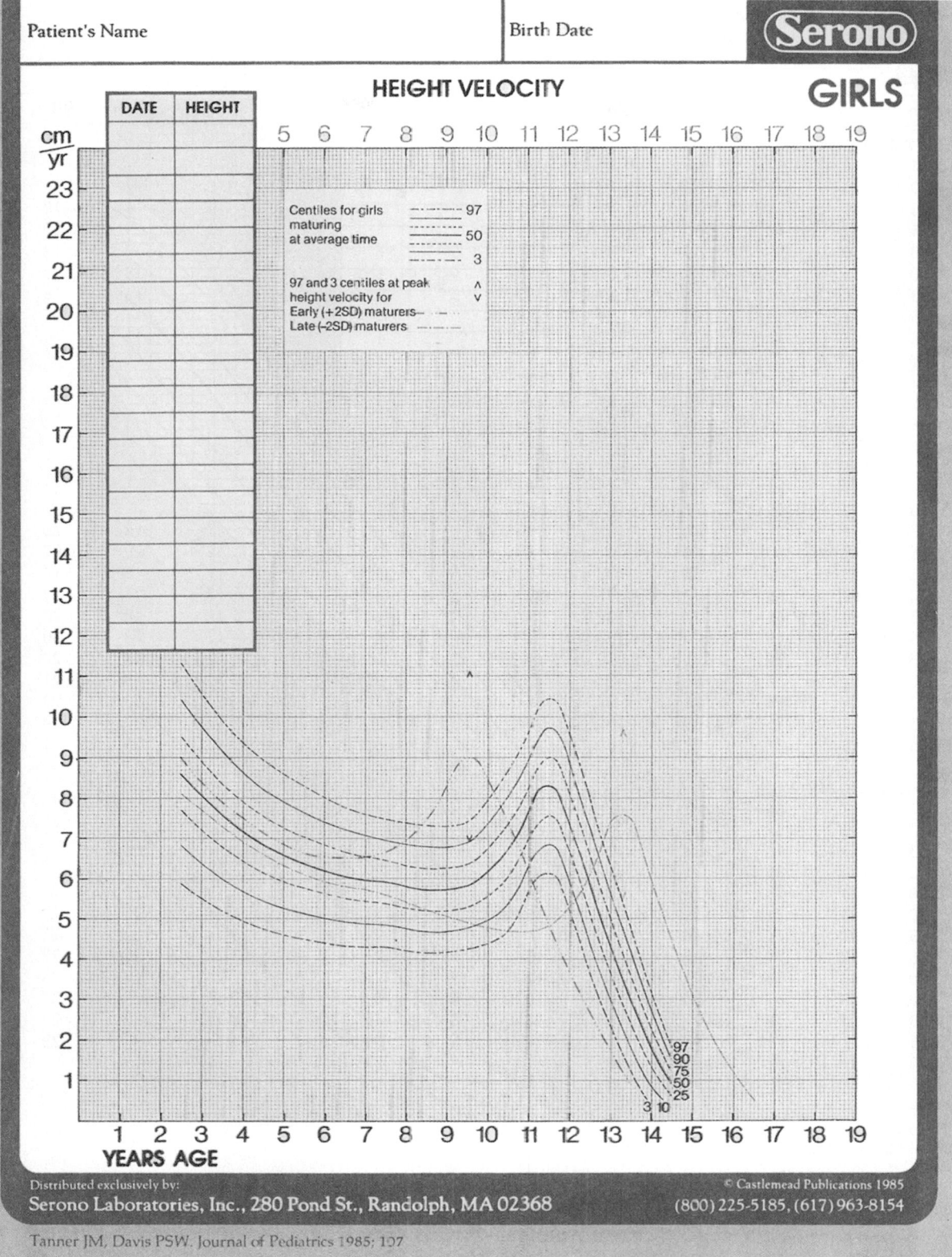

FIGURE C-7—cont'd
Height velocity growth curves: Girls.
From Tanner, Davies, 1985.

TABLE C-1 — Selected Percentiles of Weight and Triceps Skinfold Thickness for U.S. Men Ages 25 to 54 Years*

Height			Weight (kg)				Triceps (mm)						
In	Cm	5th	15th	50th	85th	95th	5th	10th	15th	50th	85th	90th	95th
SMALL FRAMES, MEN													
62	157	46	52	64	71	77				11			
63	160	48	53	61	70	79			6	10	17		
64	163	49	55	66	76	80		5	5	10	16	18	
65	165	52	58	66	77	84	4	5	6	11	17	19	21
66	168	56	59	67	78	84	5	6	6	11	18	18	20
67	170	56	62	71	82	88	5	6	6	11	18	20	22
68	173	56	62	71	79	85	5	6	6	10	15	16	20
69	175	57	65	74	84	88		6	6	11	17	20	
70	178	59	67	75	87	90			7	10	17		
71	180	60	70	76	79	91			7	10	16		
72	183	62	67	74	87	93				10			
73	185	63	69	79	89	94							
74	188	65	71	80	90	96							
MEDIUM FRAMES, MEN													
62	157	51	58	68	81	87				15			
63	160	52	59	71	82	89				11			
64	163	54	61	71	83	90		6	6	12	18	20	
65	165	59	65	74	87	94	5	7	8	12	20	22	25
66	168	58	65	75	85	93	5	6	7	11	16	18	22
67	170	62	68	77	89	100	5	7	7	13	21	23	28
68	173	60	66	78	89	97	4	5	7	11	18	20	24
69	175	63	68	78	90	97	5	6	7	12	18	20	24
70	178	64	70	81	90	97	5	6	7	12	18	20	23
71	180	62	70	81	92	100	4	5	7	12	19	21	25
72	183	68	74	84	97	104	5	7	7	12	20	22	26
73	185	70	75	85	100	104	6	7	8	12	20	24	27
74	188	68	77	88	100	104		6	9	13	21	23	
LARGE FRAMES, MEN													
62	157	57	66	82	99	108							
63	160	58	67	83	100	109							
64	163	59	68	84	101	110							
65	165	60	69	79	102	111				14			
66	168	60	75	84	103	112		9		14	30		
67	170	62	71	84	102	113		7	10	11	23	27	
68	173	63	76	86	101	114		9	10	14	22	23	
69	175	68	74	89	103	114	6	7	8	15	25	29	32
70	178	68	74	87	106	114	7	7	7	14	23	25	30
71	180	73	82	91	113	123	6	8	10	15	25	27	31
72	183	73	78	91	109	121	5	6	7	12	20	22	25
73	185	72	79	93	106	116	5	6	7	13	19	22	31
74	188	69	82	92	105	120			8	12	19		

Modified from Frisancho, 1984.

*Data from National Center for Health Statistics, 1981.

| TABLE C-2 | Selected Percentiles of Weight and Triceps Skinfold Thickness for U.S. Women Ages 25 to 54 Years* |

Height			Weight (kg)					Triceps (mm)						
In	Cm	5th	15th	50th	85th	95th	5th	10th	15th	50th	85th	90th	95th
SMALL FRAMES, WOMEN													
58	147	37	43	52	58	66		12	13	24	30	33	
59	150	42	44	53	63	72	8	11	14	21	29	36	37
60	152	42	45	53	63	70	8	11	12	21	28	29	33
61	155	44	47	54	64	72	11	12	14	21	28	31	34
62	157	44	48	55	63	70	10	12	14	20	28	31	34
63	160	46	49	55	65	79	10	11	13	20	27	30	36
64	163	49	51	57	67	74	10	13	13	20	28	30	34
65	165	50	53	60	70	80	12	13	14	22	29	31	34
66	168	46	54	58	65	74			12	19	30		
67	170	47	52	59	70	76				18			
68	173	48	53	62	71	77				20			
69	175	49	54	63	72	78							
70	178	50	55	64	73	79							
MEDIUM FRAMES, WOMEN													
58	147	41	50	63	77	79			20	25	40		
59	150	47	52	66	76	85	15	19	21	30	37	40	40
60	152	47	52	60	77	85	14	15	17	26	35	37	41
61	155	47	51	61	73	86	11	14	15	25	34	36	42
62	157	49	52	61	73	83	12	14	16	24	34	36	40
63	160	49	53	62	77	88	12	13	15	24	33	35	38
64	163	50	54	62	76	87	11	14	15	23	33	36	40
65	165	52	55	63	75	89	12	14	15	22	31	34	38
66	168	52	55	63	75	83	11	13	14	22	31	33	37
67	170	54	57	65	79	88	12	13	15	21	29	30	35
68	173	58	60	67	77	87	10	14	15	22	31	32	36
69	175	49	60	68	79	87		11	12	19	29	31	
70	178	50	57	70	80	37				19			
LARGE FRAMES, WOMEN													
58	147	56	67	86	105	117							
59	150	56	67	78	105	116			36				
60	152	55	66	87	104	116			38				
61	155	54	66	81	105	115		25	26	36	48	50	
62	157	59	65	81	103	113	16	19	22	34	48	48	50
63	160	58	67	83	105	119	18	20	22	34	46	48	51
64	163	59	63	79	102	112	16	20	21	32	43	45	49
65	165	59	63	81	103	114	17	20	21	31	43	46	48
66	168	55	62	75	95	107	13	17	18	27	40	43	45
67	170	58	65	80	100	114	13	16	17	30	41	43	49
68	173	51	66	76	104	111		16	20	29	37	40	
69	175	50	68	79	105	111			21	30	42		
70	178	50	61	76	99	110				20			

Modified from Frisancho, 1984.
*Data from National Center for Health Statistics, 1981.

TABLE C-3	Weight by Height for All Men Ages 50 Years and Older*		
Height (in) by Age Group	**Percentile**		
	15th	**50th**	**85th**
50-59 YEARS			
<65	140.8	159.5	177.5
65	123.6	170.1	215.0
66	146.3	173.4	198.5
67	156.4	177.6	207.0
68	166.2	191.7	225.5
69	164.1	184.1	223.0
70	166.4	196.3	229.1
71	168.0	190.0	224.5
72 and over	175.5	205.8	251.6
60-69 YEARS			
<65	133.8	155.9	177.9
65	139.1	157.8	185.0
66	146.4	170.6	197.1
67	139.5	172.7	197.7
68	151.7	183.4	212.7
69	159.6	192.2	222.0
70	167.4	195.0	229.0
71	167.5	205.3	232.7
72 and over	178.0	203.0	240.1
70-79 YEARS			
<65	129.4	153.3	181.7
65	133.5	162.3	189.1
66	136.1	159.3	193.2
67	150.2	172.1	194.7
68	146.7	170.9	211.2
69	151.5	181.9	211.2
70 and over	160.8	186.8	220.3
80-89 YEARS			
<65	119.2	140.8	159.2
65	126.5	151.8	170.7
66	139.7	161.0	189.1
67	133.1	160.2	183.7
68	145.8	167.7	189.9
69	146.5	172.4	200.2
70 and over	141.6	171.5	203.5

From Kuczmarski, Kuczmarski, Najjar, 2000.
*Data from the National Center for Health Statistics, 2002.

TABLE C-4	Percentiles for Triceps Skinfold Thickness for Men Over 50 Years of Age*						
	Triceps Skinfold Thickness (mm)						
Age	**10th**	**15th**	**25th**	**50th**	**75th**	**85th**	**90th**
50-59 years	7.5	8.0	9.4	12.6	16.0	18.7	21.8
60-69 years	7.7	8.5	10.1	12.7	17.1	20.2	23.1
70-79 years	7.3	7.9	9.0	12.4	16.0	18.8	20.6
80-89 years	6.6	7.6	8.7	11.2	13.8	16.2	18.0

From Kuczmarski, Kuczmarski, Najjar, 2000.
*Data from the National Center for Health Statistics, 2002.

TABLE C-5	Weight for Height for All Women Ages 50 Years and Older*		
Height (in) by Age Group	Percentile		
	15th	**50th**	**85th**
50-59 YEARS			
<60	112.2	147.2	181.1
60	112.5	143.5	187.0
61	123.2	153.6	194.0
62	120.0	145.7	191.3
63	130.2	155.1	211.0
64	134.1	165.0	203.2
65	126.1	158.1	182.5
66	142.0	182.0	200.4
67 and over	137.9	171.1	226.5
60-69 YEARS			
<60	115.4	135.0	165.9
60	114.3	140.7	178.2
61	117.2	142.0	179.2
62	119.9	147.4	193.6
63	116.0	153.9	189.5
64	129.9	158.4	193.9
65	134.6	159.2	209.7
66	129.7	160.9	202.1
67 and over	142.7	171.3	207.8
70-79 YEARS			
<60	97.4	125.8	163.2
60	107.4	133.4	164.1
61	116.3	140.4	179.5
62	117.5	141.2	180.4
63	125.8	152.9	183.1
64	131.3	159.2	192.4
65 and over	130.8	154.4	189.5
80-89 YEARS			
<60	96.1	119.0	147.1
60	106.5	132.9	155.0
61	112.3	138.8	159.7
62	110.3	132.0	155.9
63	120.0	140.8	170.7
64	121.3	139.7	170.4
65 and over	112.6	155.7	201.8

From Kuczmarski, Kuczmarski, Najjar, 2000.
*Data from the National Center for Health Statistics, 2002.

TABLE C-6	Percentiles for Triceps Skinfold Thickness for Women Over 50 Years of Age*						
Age	Triceps Skinfold Thickness (mm)						
	10th	**15th**	**25th**	**50th**	**75th**	**85th**	**90th**
50-59 years	16.4	18.3	20.6	26.7	32.1	35.2	37.0
60-69 years	14.5	15.9	18.2	24.1	29.7	32.9	34.9
70-79 years	12.5	14.0	16.4	21.8	27.7	30.6	32.1
80-89 years	9.3	11.1	13.1	18.1	23.3	26.4	28.9

From Kuczmarski, Kuczmarski, Najjar, 2000.
*Data from National Center for Health Statistics, 2002.

DENVER II DEVELOPMENTAL SCREENING TOOL

The Denver II Developmental Screening Tool is a standardized screening tool widely used to assess an infant's or a child's development between birth and 6 years of age. Fine and gross motor skills, language, and personal-social skills are all assessed. Recording the screening results can be done repeatedly on the same Denver II form for a child, enabling the examiner to mark the child's developmental progress over time.

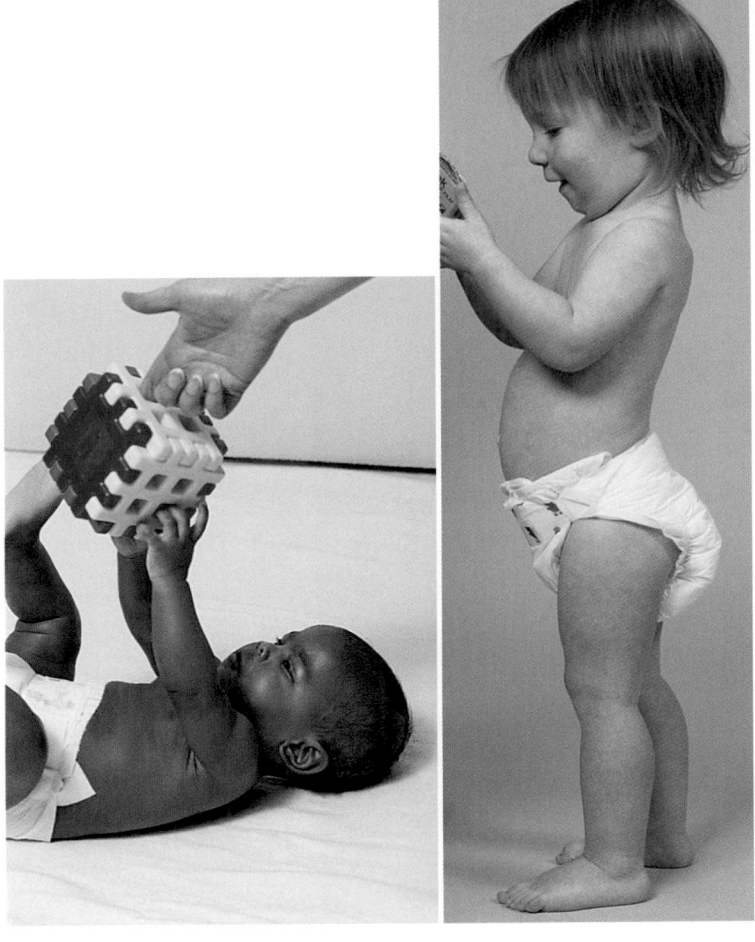

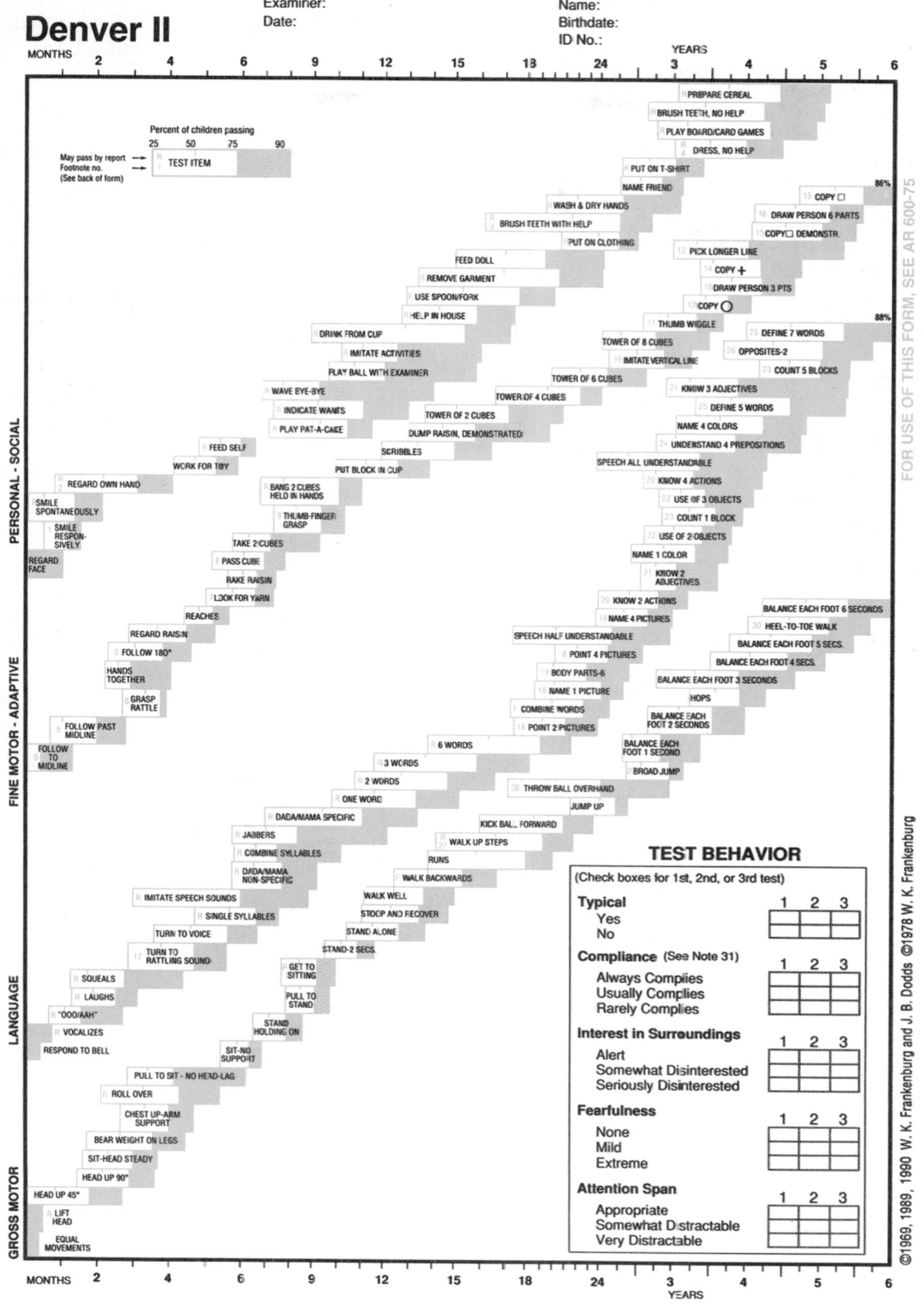

DIRECTIONS FOR ADMINISTRATION

1. Try to get child to smile by smiling, talking or waving. Do not touch him/her.
2. Child must stare at hand several seconds.
3. Parent may help guide toothbrush and put toothpaste on brush.
4. Child does not have to be able to tie shoes or button/zip in the back.
5. Move yarn slowly in an arc from one side to the other, about 8" above child's face.
6. Pass if child grasps rattle when it is touched to the backs or tips of fingers.
7. Pass if child tries to see where yarn went. Yarn should be dropped quickly from sight from tester's hand without arm movement.
8. Child must transfer cube from hand to hand without help of body, mouth, or table.
9. Pass if child picks up raisin with any part of thumb and finger.
10. Line can vary only 30 degrees or less from tester's line.
11. Make a fist with thumb pointing upward and wiggle only the thumb. Pass if child imitates and does not move any fingers other than the thumb.

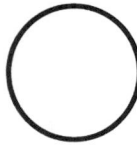 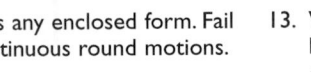 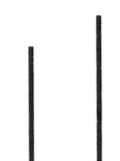 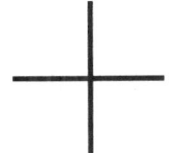 

| 12. Pass any enclosed form. Fail continuous round motions. | 13. Which line is longer? (Not bigger.) Turn paper upside down and repeat. (pass 3 of 3 or 5 of 6) | 14. Pass any lines crossing near midpoint. | 15. Have child copy first. If failed, demonstrate. |

When giving items 12, 14, and 15, do not name the forms. Do not demonstrate 12 and 14.

16. When scoring, each pair (2 arms, 2 legs, etc.) counts as one part.
17. Place one cube in cup and shake gently near child's ear, but out of sight. Repeat for other ear.
18. Point to picture and have child name it. (No credit is given for sounds only.) If fewer than 4 pictures are named correctly, have child point to picture as each is named by tester.

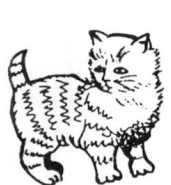 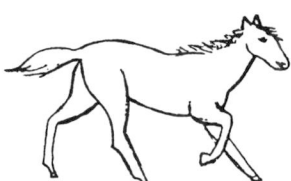 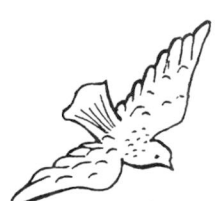 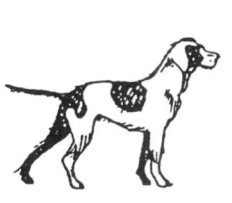 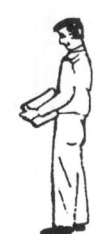

19. Using doll, tell child: Show me the nose, eyes, ears, mouth, hands, feet, tummy, hair. Pass 6 of 8.
20. Using pictures, ask child: Which one flies?... says meow?... talks?... barks?... gallops? Pass 2 of 5, 4 of 5.
21. Ask child: What do you do when you are cold?... tired?... hungry? Pass 2 of 3, 3 of 3.
22. Ask child: What do you do with a cup? What is a chair used for? What is a pencil used for? Action words must be included in answers.
23. Pass if child correctly places and says how many blocks are on paper. (1, 5).
24. Tell child: Put block **on** table; **under** table; **in front** of me, **behind** me. Pass 4 of 4. (Do not help child by pointing, moving head or eyes.)
25. Ask child: What is a ball? ... lake? ... desk? ... house? ... banana? ... curtain? ... fence? ... ceiling? Pass if defined in terms of use, shape, what it is made of, or general category (such as banana is fruit, not just yellow). Pass 5 of 8, 7 of 8.
26. Ask child: If a horse is big, a mouse is ___? If fire is hot, ice is ___? If the sun shines during the day, the moon shines during the ___? Pass 2 of 3.
27. Child may use wall or rail only, not person. May not crawl.
28. Child must throw ball overhand 3 feet to within arm's reach of tester.
29. Child must perform standing broad jump over width of test sheet (8 1/2 inches).
30. Tell child to walk forward, ⚬⚬⚬⚬⚬⚬→ heel within 1 inch of toe. Tester may demonstrate. Child must walk 4 consecutive steps.
31. In the second year, half of normal children are non-compliant.

OBSERVATIONS:

APPENDIX E

DIETARY REFERENCE INTAKES

The following dietary reference intake charts are included in this appendix on the following pages:

* Dietary Reference Intakes: Macronutrients (includes Energy, Carbohydrate, Fiber, Fat, Fatty Acids, Cholesterol, Protein and Amino Acids)
* Dietary Reference Intakes: Vitamins
* Dietary Reference Intakes: Elements

Dietary Reference Intakes (DRIs): Recommended Intakes for Individuals, Macronutrients
Food and Nutrition Board, Institute of Medicine, National Academies

Life Stage Group	Total Water[a] (L/d)	Carbohydrate (g/d)	Total Fiber (g/d)	Fat (g/d)	Linoleic Acid (g/d)	α-Linolenic Acid (g/d)	Protein[b] (g/d)
Infants							
0–6 mo	0.7*	60*	ND	31*	4.4*	0.5*	9.1*
7–12 mo	0.8*	95*	ND	30*	4.6*	0.5*	**13.5**
Children							
1–3 y	1.3*	**130**	19*	ND	7*	0.7*	**13**
4–8 y	1.7*	**130**	25*	ND	10*	0.9*	**19**
Males							
9–13 y	2.4*	**130**	31*	ND	12*	1.2*	**34**
14–18 y	3.3*	**130**	38*	ND	16*	1.6*	**52**
19–30 y	3.7*	**130**	38*	ND	17*	1.6*	**56**
31–50 y	3.7*	**130**	38*	ND	17*	1.6*	**56**
51–70 y	3.7*	**130**	30*	ND	14*	1.6*	**56**
> 70 y	3.7*	**130**	30*	ND	14*	1.6*	**56**
Females							
9–13 y	2.1*	**130**	26*	ND	10*	1.0*	**34**
14–18 y	2.3*	**130**	26*	ND	11*	1.1*	**46**
19–30 y	2.7*	**130**	25*	ND	12*	1.1*	**46**
31–50 y	2.7*	**130**	25*	ND	12*	1.1*	**46**
51–70 y	2.7*	**130**	21*	ND	11*	1.1*	**46**
> 70 y	2.7*	**130**	21*	ND	11*	1.1*	**46**
Pregnancy							
14–18 y	3.0*	**175**	28*	ND	13*	1.4*	**71**
19–30 y	3.0*	**175**	28*	ND	13*	1.4*	**71**
31–50 y	3.0*	**175**	28*	ND	13*	1.4*	**71**
Lactation							
14–18 y	3.8*	**210**	29*	ND	13*	1.3*	**71**
19–30 y	3.8*	**210**	29*	ND	13*	1.3*	**71**
31–50 y	3.8*	**210**	29*	ND	13*	1.3*	**71**

NOTE: This table presents Recommended Dietary Allowances (RDAs) in **bold** type and Adequate Intakes (AIs) in ordinary type followed by an asterisk (*). RDAs and AIs may both be used as goals for individual intake. RDAs are set to meet the needs of almost all (97 to 98 percent) individuals in a group. For healthy infants fed human milk, the AI is the mean intake. The AI for other life stage and gender groups is believed to cover the needs of all individuals in the group, but lack of data or uncertainty in the data prevent being able to specify with confidence the percentage of individuals covered by this intake.
[a] Total water includes all water contained in food, beverages, and drinking water.
[b] Based on 0.8 g/kg body weight for the reference body weight.

Dietary Reference Intakes (DRIs): Additional Macronutrient Recommendations
Food and Nutrition Board, Institute of Medicine, National Academies

Macronutrient	Recommendation
Dietary cholesterol	As low as possible while consuming a nutritionally adequate diet
Trans fatty acids	As low as possible while consuming a nutritionally adequate diet
Saturated fatty acids	As low as possible while consuming a nutritionally adequate diet
Added sugars	Limit to no more than 25% of total energy

SOURCE: *Dietary Reference Intakes for Energy, Carbohydrate, Fiber, Fat, Fatty Acids, Cholesterol, Protein, and Amino Acids* (2002).

Dietary Reference Intakes (DRIs): Recommended Intakes for Individuals, Vitamins
Food and Nutrition Board, Institute of Medicine, National Academies

Life Stage Group	Vit A (µg/d)[a]	Vit C (mg/d)	Vit D (µg/d)[b,c]	Vit E (mg/d)[d]	Vit K (µg/d)	Thiamin (mg/d)	Riboflavin (mg/d)	Niacin (mg/d)[e]	Vit B_6 (mg/d)	Folate (µg/d)[f]	Vit B_{12} (µg/d)	Pantothenic Acid (mg/d)	Biotin (µg/d)	Choline[g] (mg/d)
Infants														
0–6 mo	400*	40*	5*	4*	2.0*	0.2*	0.3*	2*	0.1*	65*	0.4*	1.7*	5*	125*
7–12 mo	500*	50*	5*	5*	2.5*	0.3*	0.4*	4*	0.3*	80*	0.5*	1.8*	6*	150*
Children														
1–3 y	**300**	**15**	5*	**6**	30*	**0.5**	**0.5**	**6**	**0.5**	**150**	**0.9**	2*	8*	200*
4–8 y	**400**	**25**	5*	**7**	55*	**0.6**	**0.6**	**8**	**0.6**	**200**	**1.2**	3*	12*	250*
Males														
9–13 y	**600**	**45**	5*	**11**	60*	**0.9**	**0.9**	**12**	**1.0**	**300**	**1.8**	4*	20*	375*
14–18 y	**900**	**75**	5*	**15**	75*	**1.2**	**1.3**	**16**	**1.3**	**400**	**2.4**	5*	25*	550*
19–30 y	**900**	**90**	5*	**15**	120*	**1.2**	**1.3**	**16**	**1.3**	**400**	**2.4**	5*	30*	550*
31–50 y	**900**	**90**	5*	**15**	120*	**1.2**	**1.3**	**16**	**1.3**	**400**	**2.4**	5*	30*	550*
51–70 y	**900**	**90**	10*	**15**	120*	**1.2**	**1.3**	**16**	**1.7**	**400**	**2.4**[h]	5*	30*	550*
> 70 y	**900**	**90**	15*	**15**	120*	**1.2**	**1.3**	**16**	**1.7**	**400**	**2.4**[h]	5*	30*	550*
Females														
9–13 y	**600**	**45**	5*	**11**	60*	**0.9**	**0.9**	**12**	**1.0**	**300**	**1.8**	4*	20*	375*
14–18 y	**700**	**65**	5*	**15**	75*	**1.0**	**1.0**	**14**	**1.2**	**400**[i]	**2.4**	5*	25*	400*
19–30 y	**700**	**75**	5*	**15**	90*	**1.1**	**1.1**	**14**	**1.3**	**400**[i]	**2.4**	5*	30*	425*
31–50 y	**700**	**75**	5*	**15**	90*	**1.1**	**1.1**	**14**	**1.3**	**400**[i]	**2.4**	5*	30*	425*
51–70 y	**700**	**75**	10*	**15**	90*	**1.1**	**1.1**	**14**	**1.5**	**400**	**2.4**[h]	5*	30*	425*
> 70 y	**700**	**75**	15*	**15**	90*	**1.1**	**1.1**	**14**	**1.5**	**400**	**2.4**[h]	5*	30*	425*
Pregnancy														
14–18 y	**750**	**80**	5*	**15**	75*	**1.4**	**1.4**	**18**	**1.9**	**600**[j]	**2.6**	6*	30*	450*
19–30 y	**770**	**85**	5*	**15**	90*	**1.4**	**1.4**	**18**	**1.9**	**600**[j]	**2.6**	6*	30*	450*
31–50 y	**770**	**85**	5*	**15**	90*	**1.4**	**1.4**	**18**	**1.9**	**600**[j]	**2.6**	6*	30*	450*
Lactation														
14–18 y	**1,200**	**115**	5*	**19**	75*	**1.4**	**1.6**	**17**	**2.0**	**500**	**2.8**	7*	35*	550*
19–30 y	**1,300**	**120**	5*	**19**	90*	**1.4**	**1.6**	**17**	**2.0**	**500**	**2.8**	7*	35*	550*
31–50 y	**1,300**	**120**	5*	**19**	90*	**1.4**	**1.6**	**17**	**2.0**	**500**	**2.8**	7*	35*	550*

NOTE: This table (taken from the DRI reports, see www.nap.edu) presents Recommended Dietary Allowances (RDAs) in **bold type** and Adequate Intakes (AIs) in ordinary type followed by an asterisk (*). RDAs and AIs may both be used as goals for individual intake. RDAs are set to meet the needs of almost all (97 to 98 percent) individuals in a group. For healthy breastfed infants, the AI is the mean intake. The AI for other life stage and gender groups is believed to cover needs of all individuals in the group, but lack of data or uncertainty in the data prevent being able to specify with confidence the percentage of individuals covered by this intake.

[a] As retinol activity equivalents (RAEs). 1 RAE = 1 µg retinol, 12 µg β-carotene, 24 µg α-carotene, or 24 µg β-cryptoxanthin. The RAE for dietary provitamin A carotenoids is twofold greater than retinol equivalents (RE), whereas the RAE for preformed vitamin A is the same as RE.

[b] As cholecalciferol. 1 µg cholecalciferol = 40 IU vitamin D.

[c] In the absence of adequate exposure to sunlight.

[d] As α-Tocopherol. α-Tocopherol includes *RRR*-α-tocopherol, the only form of α-tocopherol that occurs naturally in foods, and the *2R*-stereoisomeric forms of α-tocopherol (*RRR*-, *RSR*-, *RRS*-, and *RSS*-α-tocopherol) that occur in fortified foods and supplements. It does not include the *2S*-stereoisomeric forms of α-tocopherol (*SRR*-, *SSR*-, *SRS*-, and *SSS*-α-tocopherol), also found in fortified foods and supplements.

[e] As niacin equivalents (NE). 1 mg of niacin = 60 mg of tryptophan; 0–6 months = preformed niacin (not NE).

[f] As dietary folate equivalents (DFE). 1 DFE = 1 µg food folate = 0.6 µg of folic acid from fortified food or as a supplement consumed with food = 0.5 µg of a supplement taken on an empty stomach.

[g] Although AIs have been set for choline, there are few data to assess whether a dietary supply of choline is needed at all stages of the life cycle, and it may be that the choline requirement can be met by endogenous synthesis at some of these stages.

[h] Because 10 to 30 percent of older people may malabsorb food-bound B_{12}, it is advisable for those older than 50 years to meet their RDA mainly by consuming foods fortified with B_{12} or a supplement containing B_{12}.

[i] In view of evidence linking folate intake with neural tube defects in the fetus, it is recommended that all women capable of becoming pregnant consume 400 µg from supplements or fortified foods in addition to intake of food folate from a varied diet.

[jk] It is assumed that women will continue consuming 400 µg from supplements or fortified food until their pregnancy is confirmed and they enter prenatal care, which ordinarily occurs after the end of the periconceptional period—the critical time for formation of the neural tube.

Dietary Reference Intakes (DRIs): Recommended Intakes for Individuals, Elements
Food and Nutrition Board, Institute of Medicine, National Academies

Life Stage Group	Calcium (mg/d)	Chromium (μg/d)	Copper (μg/d)	Fluoride (mg/d)	Iodine (μg/d)	Iron (mg/d)	Magnesium (mg/d)	Manganese (mg/d)	Molybdenum (μg/d)	Phosphorus (mg/d)	Selenium (μg/d)	Zinc (mg/d)	Potassium (g/d)	Sodium (g/d)	Chloride (g/d)
Infants															
0–6 mo	210*	0.2*	200*	0.01*	110*	0.27*	30*	0.003*	2*	100*	15*	2*	0.4*	0.12*	0.18*
7–12 mo	270*	5.5*	220*	0.5*	130*	11	75*	0.6*	3*	275*	20*	3	0.7*	0.37*	0.57*
Children															
1–3 y	500*	11*	340	0.7*	90	7	80	1.2*	17	460	20	3	3.0*	1.0*	1.5*
4–8 y	800*	15*	440	1*	90	10	130	1.5*	22	500	30	5	3.8*	1.2*	1.9*
Males															
9–13 y	1,300*	25*	700	2*	120	8	240	1.9*	34	1,250	40	8	4.5*	1.5*	2.3*
14–18 y	1,300*	35*	890	3*	150	11	410	2.2*	43	1,250	55	11	4.7*	1.5*	2.3*
19–30 y	1,000*	35*	900	4*	150	8	400	2.3*	45	700	55	11	4.7*	1.5*	2.3*
31–50 y	1,000*	35*	900	4*	150	8	420	2.3*	45	700	55	11	4.7*	1.5*	2.3*
51–70 y	1,200*	30*	900	4*	150	8	420	2.3*	45	700	55	11	4.7*	1.3*	2.0*
>70 y	1,200*	30*	900	4*	150	8	420	2.3*	45	700	55	11	4.7*	1.2*	1.8*
Females															
9–13 y	1,300*	21*	700	2*	120	8	240	1.6*	34	1,250	40	8	4.5*	1.5*	2.3*
14–18 y	1,300*	24*	890	3*	150	15	360	1.6*	43	1,250	55	9	4.7*	1.5*	2.3*
19–30 y	1,000*	25*	900	3*	150	18	310	1.8*	45	700	55	8	4.7*	1.5*	2.3*
31–50 y	1,000*	25*	900	3*	150	18	320	1.8*	45	700	55	8	4.7*	1.5*	2.3*
51–70 y	1,200*	20*	900	3*	150	8	320	1.8*	45	700	55	8	4.7*	1.3*	2.0*
>70 y	1,200*	20*	900	3*	150	8	320	1.8*	45	700	55	8	4.7*	1.2*	1.8*
Pregnancy															
14–18 y	1,300*	29*	1,000	3*	220	27	400	2.0*	50	1,250	60	13	4.7*	1.5*	2.3*
19–30 y	1,000*	30*	1,000	3*	220	27	350	2.0*	50	700	60	11	4.7*	1.5*	2.3*
31–50 y	1,000*	30*	1,000	3*	220	27	360	2.0*	50	700	60	11	4.7*	1.5*	2.3*
Lactation															
14–18 y	1,300*	44*	1,300	3*	290	10	360	2.6*	50	1,250	70	14	5.1*	1.5*	2.3*
19–30 y	1,000*	45*	1,300	3*	290	9	310	2.6*	50	700	70	12	5.1*	1.5*	2.3*
31–50 y	1,000*	45*	1,300	3*	290	9	320	2.6*	50	700	70	12	5.1*	1.5*	2.3*

NOTE: This table presents Recommended Dietary Allowances (RDAs) in **bold type** and Adequate Intakes (AIs) in ordinary type followed by an asterisk (*). RDAs and AIs may both be used as goals for individual intake. RDAs are set to meet the needs of almost all (97 to 98 percent) individuals in a group. For healthy breastfed infants, the AI is the mean intake. The AI for other life stage and gender groups is believed to cover needs of all individuals in the group, but lack of data or uncertainty in the data prevent being able to specify with confidence the percentage of individuals covered by this intake.

SOURCES: *Dietary Reference Intakes for Calcium, Phosphorous, Magnesium, Vitamin D, and Fluoride* (1997); *Dietary Reference Intakes for Thiamin, Riboflavin, Niacin, Vitamin B_6, Folate, Vitamin B_{12}, Pantothenic Acid, Biotin, and Choline* (1998); *Dietary Reference Intakes for Vitamin C, Vitamin E, Selenium, and Carotenoids* (2000); *Dietary Reference Intakes for Vitamin A, Vitamin K, Arsenic, Boron, Chromium, Copper, Iodine, Iron, Manganese, Molybdenum, Nickel, Silicon, Vanadium, and Zinc* (2001); and *Dietary Reference Intakes for Water, Potassium, Sodium, Chloride, and Sulfate* (2004). These reports may be accessed via http://www.nap.edu.

NUTRITION SCREENING FORMS

The following forms are included in this appendix:

* *Level I Screen,* a nutritional screen, which can be used for adults or healthy older adults. It includes a *BMI nomogram* for determining body mass index.
* *Level II Screen,* a more detailed nutritional screen that can be used with older adults or those at nutritional risk.
* *Determine Your Nutritional Health,* a quick and easy screening form to determine whether an individual is at nutritional risk. It discusses the warning signs of nutritional risk and can be used for patient education.
* *A One-Day (24-Hour) Record of Food Intake* and a *Food Diary,* both of which can be used to obtain an individual's food intake to allow estimation of the adequacy of the diet.

Level I Screen

Body Weight

Measure height to the nearest inch and weight to the nearest pound. Record the values below and mark them on the Body Mass Index (BMI) scale to the right. Then use a straight edge (ruler) to connect the two points and circle the spot where this straight line crosses the center line (body mass index). Record the number below.

Healthy adults should have a BMI between 18.5 and 24.9.

Height (in):_____
Weight (lbs):_____
Body Mass Index:_____
(number from center column)

Check any boxes that are true for the individual:

☐ Has lost or gained 10 pounds (or more) in the past 6 months.

☐ Body mass index <18.5

☐ Body mass index >24.9

For the remaining sections, please ask the individual which of the statements (if any) is true for him or her and place a check by each that applies.

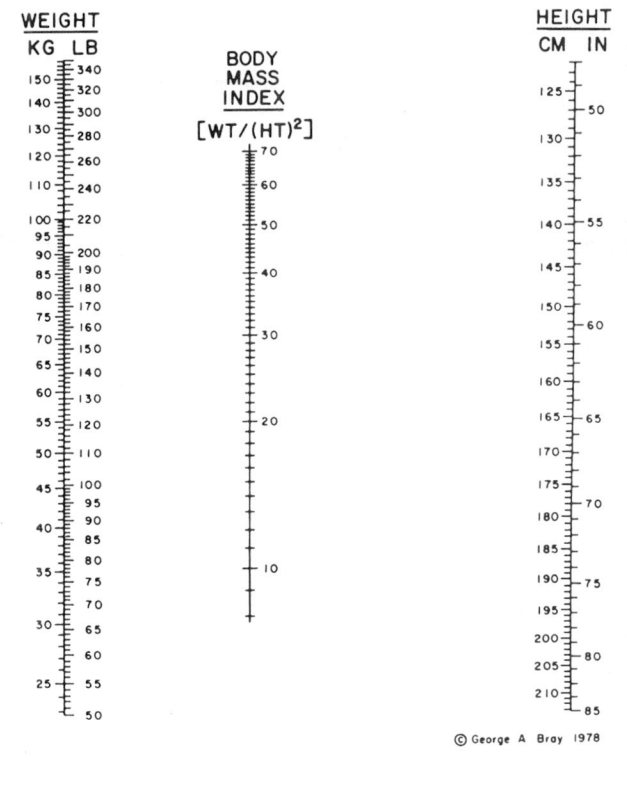

NOMOGRAM FOR BODY MASS INDEX

© George A Bray 1978

Eating Habits

☐ Does not have enough food to eat each day

☐ Usually eats alone

☐ Does not eat anything on one or more days each month

☐ Has poor appetite

☐ Is on a special diet

☐ Eats vegetables two or fewer times daily

☐ Eats milk or milk products once or not at all daily

☐ Eats fruit or drinks fruit juice once or not at all daily

☐ Eats breads, cereals, pasta, rice, or other grains five or fewer times daily

☐ Has difficulty chewing or swallowing

☐ Has more than one alcoholic drink per day (if woman); more than two drinks per day (if man)

☐ Has pain in mouth, teeth, or gums

LEVEL I SCREEN   Name: Date:

APPENDIX

A health care provider should be contacted if the individual has gained or lost 10 pounds unexpectedly or without intending to during the past 6 months. A health care provider should also be notified if the individual's body mass index is above 27 or below 22.

Living Environment

☐ Lives on an income of less than $6000 per year (per individual in the household)

☐ Lives alone

☐ Is housebound

☐ Is concerned about home security

☐ Lives in a home with inadequate heating or cooling

☐ Does not have a stove and/or refrigerator

☐ Is unable or prefers not to spend money on food (<$25-30 per person spent on food each week)

Functional Status

Usually or always needs assistance with (check each that apply):

☐ Bathing

☐ Dressing

☐ Grooming

☐ Toileting

☐ Eating

☐ Walking or moving about

☐ Traveling (outside the home)

☐ Preparing food

☐ Shopping for food or other necessities

If you have checked one or more statements on this screen, the individual you have interviewed may be at risk for poor nutritional status. Please refer this individual to the appropriate health care or social service professional in your area. For example, a dietitian should be contacted for problems with selecting, preparing, or eating a healthy diet, or a dentist if the individual experiences pain or difficulty when chewing or swallowing. Those individuals whose income, lifestyle, or functional status may endanger their nutritional and overall health should be referred to available community services: home-delivered meals, congregate meal programs, transportation services, counseling services (alcohol abuse, depression, bereavement, etc.), home health care agencies, day care programs, etc.

Please repeat this screen at least once each year--sooner if the individual has a major change in his or her health, income, immediate family (e.g., spouse dies), or functional status.

Level II Screen

Complete the following screen by interviewing the patient directly and/or by referring to the patient chart. If you do not routinely perform all of the described tests or ask all of the listed questions, please consider including them but do not be concerned if the entire screen is not completed. Please try to conduct a minimal screen on as many older patients as possible, and please try to collect serial measurements, which are extremely valuable in monitoring nutritional status. Please refer to the manual for additional information.

Anthropometrics

Measure height to the nearest inch and weight to the nearest pound. Record the values below and mark them on the Body Mass Index (BMI) scale to the right. Then use a straight edge (paper, ruler) to connect the two points and circle the spot where this straight line crosses the center line (body mass index). Record the number below; healthy older adults should have a BMI between 18.5 and 24.9; check the appropriate box to flag an abnormally high or low value.

Height (in):_____
Weight (lbs):_____
Body Mass Index
(weight/height^2):_____

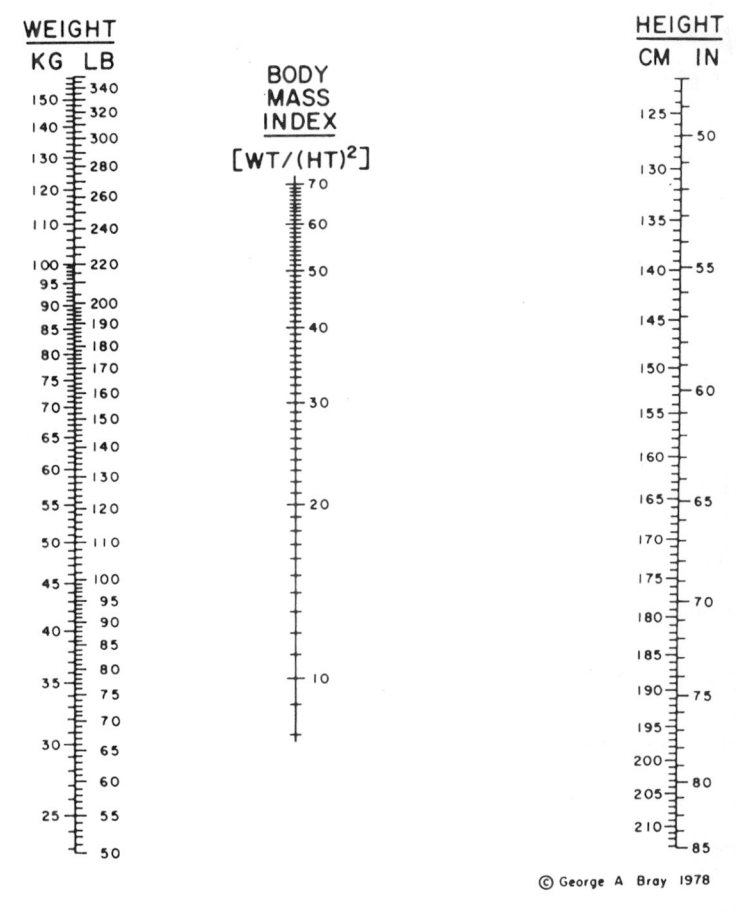

NOMOGRAM FOR BODY MASS INDEX

© George A Bray 1978

Please place a check by any statement regarding BMI and recent weight loss that is true for the patient.

❑ Body mass index <18.5

❑ Body mass index >24.9

❑ Has lost or gained 10 pounds (or more) of body weight in the past 6 months

Record the measurement of mid-arm circumference to the nearest 0.1 centimeter and of triceps skinfold to the nearest 2 millimeters.

Mid-Arm Circumference (cm):_____
Triceps Skinfold (mm):_____
Mid-Arm Muscle Circumference (cm):_____

Refer to the table and check any abnormal values:

❑ Mid-arm muscle circumference <10th percentile

❑ Triceps skinfold <10th percentile

❑ Triceps skinfold >95th percentile

Note: Mid-arm circumference (cm) − (0.314 × triceps skinfold [mm])= Mid-arm *muscle* circumference (cm)

For the remaining sections, please place a check by any statements that are true for the patient.

Laboratory Data

❑ Serum albumin below 3.5 g/dL

❑ Serum cholesterol below 120 mg/dL

❑ Serum cholesterol above 200 mg/dL

Drug Use

❑ Three or more prescription drugs, OTC medications, and/or vitamin/mineral supplements daily

Clinical Features

Presence of (check each that apply):

❏ Problems with mouth, teeth, or gums

❏ Difficulty chewing

❏ Difficulty swallowing

❏ Angular stomatitis

❏ Glossitis

❏ History of bone pain

❏ History of bone fractures

❏ Skin changes (dry, loose, nonspecific lesions, edema)

		Men		*Women*	
Percentile		55-65 y	65-75 y	55-65 y	65-75 y
Arm circumference (cm)					
10th		27.3	26.3	25.7	25.2
50th		31.7	30.7	30.3	29.9
95th		36.9	35.5	38.5	37.3
Arm muscle circumference (cm)					
10th		24.5	23.5	19.6	19.5
50th		27.8	26.8	22.5	22.5
95th		32.0	30.6	28.0	27.9
Triceps skinfold (mm)					
10th		6	6	16	14
50th		11	11	25	24
95th		22	22	38	36

From: Frisancho AR. *New norms of upper limb fat and muscle areas for assessment of nutritional status.* Am J Clin Nutr 1981; 34:2540-2545. © 1981 American Society for Clinical Nutrition.

Eating Habits

❏ Does not have enough food to eat each day

❏ Usually eats alone

❏ Does not eat anything on one or more days each month

❏ Has poor appetite

❏ Is on a special diet

❏ Eats vegetables two or fewer times daily

❏ Eats milk or milk products once or not at all daily

❏ Eats fruit or drinks fruit juice once or not at all daily

❏ Eats breads, cereals, pasta, rice, or other grains five or fewer times daily

❏ Has more than one alcoholic drink per day (if woman); more than two drinks per day (if man)

Living Environment

❏ Lives on an income of less than $6000 per year (per individual in the household)

❏ Lives alone

❏ Is housebound

❏ Is concerned about home security

❏ Lives in a home with inadequate heating or cooling

❏ Does not have a stove and/or refrigerator

❏ Is unable or prefers not to spend money on food (<$25-30 per person spent on food each week)

Functional Status

Usually or always needs assistance with (check each that apply):

❏ Bathing

❏ Dressing

❏ Grooming

❏ Toileting

❏ Eating

❏ Walking or moving about

❏ Traveling (outside the home)

❏ Preparing food

❏ Shopping for food or other necessities

Mental/Cognitive Status

❏ Clinical evidence of impairment, e.g. MMSE <26

❏ Clinical evidence of depressive illness, e.g., Geriatric Depression Scale >5

Patients in whom you have identified one or more major indicator of poor nutritional status require immediate medical attention; if minor indicators are found, ensure that they are known to a health professional or to the patient's own physician. Patients who display risk factors of poor nutritional status should be referred to the appropriate health care or social service professional (dietitian, nurse, dentist, case manager, etc.).

DETERMINE YOUR NUTRITIONAL HEALTH

The Warning Signs of poor nutritional health are often overlooked. Use this checklist to find out if you or someone you know is at nutritional risk.

Read the statements in the Nutrition Checklist below. Circle the number in the YES column for those that apply to you or to someone you know. For each yes answer, score the number in the box. Total your nutritional score.

	Yes
I have an illness or condition that made me change the kind and/or amount of food I eat.	2
I eat fewer than 2 meals per day.	3
I eat few fruits or vegetables, or milk products.	2
I have 3 or more drinks of beer, liquor, or wine almost every day.	2
I have tooth or mouth problems that make it hard for me to eat.	2
I don't always have enough money to buy the food I need.	4
I eat alone most of the time.	1
I take 3 or more different prescribed or over-the-counter drugs a day.	1
Without wanting to, I have lost or gained 10 pounds in the last 6 months.	2
I am not always physically able to shop, cook, and/or feed myself.	2
TOTAL	

TOTAL YOUR NUTRITIONAL SCORE. IF IT'S:

0-2   **Good!** Recheck your nutritional score in 6 months.

3-5   **You are at moderate nutritional risk.** See what can be done to improve your eating habits and lifestyle. Your office on aging, senior nutrition program, senior citizens center, or health department can help. Recheck your nutritional core in 3 months.

6 or more   **You are at high nutritional risk.** Bring this checklist the next time you see your doctor, dietitian, or other qualified health or social service professional. Talk with them about any problems you may have. Ask for help to improve your nutritional health.

Remember that warning signs suggest risk but do not represent diagnosis of any condition. See the next page to learn more about the Warning Signs of poor nutritional health.

The Nutrition Checklist is based on the Warning Signs described below. Use the word <u>DETERMINE</u> to remind you of the Warning Signs:

Disease: Any disease, illness or chronic condition that causes you to change the way you eat, or makes it hard for you to eat, puts your nutritional health at risk. Four out of five adults have chronic diseases that are affected by diet. Confusion or memory loss that keeps getting worse is estimated to affect one out of five or more older adults. This can make it hard to remember what, when, or even if you've eaten. Feeling sad or depressed, which happens to about one in eight older adults, can cause big changes in appetite, digestion, energy level, weight, and well-being.

Eating poorly: Eating too little and eating too much both lead to poor health. Eating the same foods day after day or not eating fruit, vegetables, and milk products daily will also cause poor nutritional health. One in five adults skips meals daily. Only 13% of adults eat the minimum amount of fruit and vegetables needed. One in four older adults drinks too much alcohol. Many health problems become worse if you drink more than one or two alcoholic beverages per day.

Tooth loss/mouth pain: A healthy mouth, teeth, and gums are needed to eat. Missing, loose, or rotten teeth or dentures that don't fit well or cause mouth sores make it hard to eat.

Economic hardship: As many as 40% of older Americans have incomes of less than $6,000 per year. Having less—or choosing to spend less—than $25 to $30 per week for food makes it very hard to get the foods you need to stay healthy.

Reduced social contact: One third of all older people live alone. Being with people daily has a positive effect on morale, well-being, and eating.

Multiple medicines: Many older Americans must take medicines for health problems. Almost half of older Americans take multiple medicines daily. Growing old may change the way we respond to drugs. The more medicines you take, the greater the chance of side effects such as increased or decreased appetite, change in taste, constipation, weakness, drowsiness, diarrhea, nausea, and others. Vitamins or minerals when taken in large doses act like drugs and can cause harm. Alert your doctor to everything you take.

Involuntary weight loss/gain: Losing or gaining a lot of weight when you are not trying to do so is an important warning sign that must not be ignored. Being overweight or underweight also increases your chance of poor health.

Needs assistance in self-care: Although most older people are able to eat, one of every five has trouble walking, shopping, buying, and cooking food, especially as they get older.

Elder years above age 80: Most older people lead full and productive lives. But as age increases, risk of frailty and health problems increase. Checking your nutritional health regularly makes good sense.

Modified from materials developed and distributed by the Nutrition Screening Initiative, a project of The American Academy of Family Physicians, The American Dietetic Association, and The National Council on the Aging, Inc.

The Nutrition Screening Initiative
1010 Wisconsin Avenue, NW Suite 800
Washington, DC 20007

The Nutrition Screening Initiative is funded in part by a grant from Ross Laboratories, a division of Abbott Laboratories.

A ONE-DAY (24-HOUR) RECORD OF FOOD INTAKE

NAME _____ DATE OF RECORD _____

BREAKFAST   Time Eaten _____

Food/Beverage	Type and/or Method of Preparation (List Ingredients)	Amount
MILK		
FRUIT Fresh, canned, sweetened, etc.		
CEREAL _____ with milk _____ with sugar _____ other	Brand_____	
BREAD _____ margarine/butter _____ mayonnaise _____ other	White _____ Whole wheat _____	
EGGS		
MEAT or OTHER PROTEIN		
BEVERAGE _____ with milk _____ with sugar _____ other		
OTHER FOODS		

Did you eat a mid-morning snack?   Yes _____ No _____   If yes, time? _____
(list foods and beverages eaten)

_____

_____

NOON MEAL   Time Eaten _____

Food/Beverage	Type and/or Method of Preparation (List Ingredients)	Amount
SOUP		
BREAD _____ margarine/butter _____ mayonnaise _____ other	White_____ Whole wheat_____	
_____ MEAT _____ EGG _____ FISH _____ CHEESE		
VEGETABLES _____ cooked _____ raw _____ topping/seasoning (butter, white sauce, cheese sauce, etc.)		
SALAD _____ dressing (brand, etc.)		
FRUIT Fresh, canned, sweetened, etc.		
MILK		
BEVERAGE _____ with milk _____ with sugar _____ other		
DESSERT		
OTHER FOODS		

Did you eat an afternoon snack?   Yes _____ No _____   If yes, time? _____
(list foods and beverages eaten)

_____

_____

EVENING MEAL   Time Eaten _____

Food/Beverage	Type and/or Method of Preparation (List Ingredients)	Amount
MAIN DISH _____ meat _____ cheese _____ poultry _____ other protein _____ pasta _____ rice		
VEGETABLES _____ cooked _____ raw _____ topping/seasoning (butter, white sauce, cheese sauce, etc.)		
SALAD _____ dressing (brand, etc.)		
BREAD _____ margarine/butter _____ mayonnaise _____ other	White_____ Whole wheat_____	
FRUIT Fresh, canned, sweetened, etc.		
MILK		
BEVERAGE _____ with milk _____ with sugar _____ other		
DESSERT		
OTHER FOODS		

Did you eat an evening snack?   Yes _____   No _____   If yes, time? _____
(list foods and beverages eaten)

_____

_____

FOOD DIARY

Name_____Date_____

Time	Food type and amount	Where eaten and with whom	Other activity while eating	How you feel before eating (e.g., anxious, bored, tired, angry, depressed)

ANTHROPOMETRIC MEASUREMENTS

TABLE G-1	Body Weight in Pounds According to Height and Body Mass Index												
	Body Mass Index (kg per m²)												
	19.0	20.0	21.0	22.0	23.0	24.0	25.0	26.0	27.0	28.0	29.0	30.0	35.0	40.0
Height (inches)	**Body Weight (pounds)**													
58.0	90.7	95.5	100.3	105.0	109.8	114.6	119.4	124.1	128.9	133.7	138.5	143.2	167.1	191.0
59.0	93.9	98.8	103.8	108.7	113.6	118.6	123.5	128.5	133.4	138.3	143.3	148.2	172.9	197.6
60.0	97.1	102.2	107.3	112.4	117.5	122.6	127.7	132.9	138.0	143.1	148.2	153.3	178.8	204.4
61.0	100.3	105.6	110.9	116.2	121.5	126.8	132.0	137.3	142.6	147.9	153.2	158.4	184.8	211.3
62.0	103.7	109.1	114.6	120.0	125.5	130.9	136.4	141.9	147.3	152.8	158.2	163.7	191.0	218.2
63.0	107.0	112.7	118.3	123.9	129.6	135.2	140.8	146.5	152.1	157.7	163.4	169.0	197.2	225.3
64.0	110.5	116.3	122.1	127.9	133.7	139.5	145.3	151.2	157.0	162.8	168.6	174.4	203.5	232.5
65.0	113.9	119.9	125.9	131.9	137.9	143.9	149.9	155.9	161.9	167.9	173.9	179.9	209.9	239.9
66.0	117.5	123.7	129.8	136.0	142.2	148.4	154.6	160.8	166.9	173.1	179.3	185.5	216.4	247.3
67.0	121.1	127.4	133.8	140.2	146.5	152.9	159.3	165.7	172.0	178.4	184.8	191.1	223.0	254.9
68.0	124.7	131.3	137.8	144.4	151.0	157.5	164.1	170.6	177.2	183.8	190.3	196.9	229.7	262.5
69.0	128.4	135.2	141.9	148.7	155.4	162.2	168.9	175.7	182.5	189.2	196.0	202.7	236.5	270.3
70.0	132.1	139.1	146.1	153.0	160.0	166.9	173.9	180.8	187.8	194.7	201.7	208.6	243.4	278.2
71.0	135.9	143.1	150.3	157.4	164.6	171.7	178.9	186.0	193.2	200.3	207.5	214.6	250.4	286.2
72.0	139.8	147.2	154.5	161.9	169.2	176.6	183.9	191.3	198.7	206.0	213.4	220.7	257.5	294.3
73.0	143.7	151.3	158.8	166.4	174.0	181.5	189.1	196.7	204.2	211.8	219.3	226.9	264.7	302.5
74.0	147.7	155.4	163.2	171.0	178.8	186.5	194.3	202.1	209.9	217.6	225.4	233.2	272.0	310.9
75.0	151.7	159.7	167.7	175.6	183.6	191.6	199.6	207.6	215.6	223.5	231.5	239.5	279.4	319.4
76.0	155.8	164.0	172.2	180.4	188.6	196.8	205.0	213.2	221.4	229.5	237.7	245.9	286.9	327.9

From U.S. Department of Health and Human Services, 1992.
NOTE: A body mass index (BMI) of 25 is classified as overweight, and 30 is classified as obesity in the National Health and Nutrition Examination Survey (NHANES II).

TABLE G-2	Midarm Muscle Circumference Percentiles (mm) for Males						
Age Group	5th	10th	25th	50th	75th	90th	95th
1-2	110	113	119	127	135	144	147
2-3	111	114	122	130	140	146	150
3-4	117	123	131	137	143	148	153
4-5	123	126	133	141	148	156	159
5-6	128	133	140	147	154	162	169
6-7	131	135	142	151	161	170	177
7-8	137	139	151	160	168	177	190
8-9	140	145	154	162	170	182	187
9-10	151	154	161	170	183	196	202
10-11	156	160	166	180	191	209	221
11-12	159	165	173	183	195	205	230
12-13	167	171	182	195	210	223	241
13-14	172	179	196	211	226	238	245
14-15	189	199	212	223	240	260	264
15-16	199	204	218	237	254	266	272
16-17	213	225	234	249	269	287	296
17-18	224	231	245	258	273	294	312
18-19	226	237	252	264	283	298	324
19-25	238	245	257	273	289	309	321
25-35	243	250	264	279	298	314	326
35-45	247	255	269	286	302	318	327
45-55	239	249	265	281	300	315	326
55-65	236	245	260	278	295	310	320
65-75	223	235	251	263	284	298	306

Data from Frisancho, 1981.

TABLE G-3	Midarm Muscle Circumference Percentiles (mm) for Females						
Age Group	5th	10th	25th	50th	75th	90th	95th
1-2	105	111	117	124	132	139	143
2-3	111	114	119	126	133	142	147
3-4	113	119	124	132	140	146	152
4-5	115	121	128	136	144	152	157
5-6	125	128	134	142	151	159	165
6-7	130	133	138	145	154	166	171
7-8	129	135	142	151	160	171	176
8-9	138	140	151	160	171	183	194
9-10	147	150	158	167	180	194	198
10-11	148	150	159	170	180	190	197
11-12	150	158	171	181	196	217	223
12-13	162	166	180	191	201	214	220
13-14	169	175	183	198	211	226	240
14-15	174	179	190	201	216	232	247
15-16	175	178	189	202	215	228	244
16-17	170	180	190	202	216	234	249
17-18	175	183	194	205	221	239	257
18-19	174	179	191	202	215	237	245
19-25	179	185	195	207	221	236	249
25-35	183	188	199	212	228	246	264
35-45	186	192	205	218	236	257	272
45-55	187	193	206	220	238	260	274
55-65	187	196	209	225	244	266	280
65-75	185	195	208	225	244	264	279

Data from Frisancho, 1981.

TABLE G-4	Midarm Muscle Area Percentiles (mm²) for Males						
Age Group	5th	10th	25th	50th	75th	90th	95th
1-2	956	1014	1133	1278	1447	1644	1720
2-3	973	1040	1190	1345	1557	1690	1787
3-4	1095	1201	1357	1484	1618	1750	1853
4-5	1207	1264	1408	1579	1747	1926	2008
5-6	1298	1411	1550	1720	1884	2089	2285
6-7	1360	1447	1605	1815	2056	2297	2493
7-8	1497	1548	1808	2027	2246	2494	2886
8-9	1550	1664	1895	2089	2296	2628	2788
9-10	1811	1884	2067	2288	2657	3053	3257
10-11	1930	2027	2182	2575	2903	3486	3882
11-12	2016	2156	2382	2670	3022	3359	4226
12-13	2216	2339	2649	3022	3496	3968	4640
13-14	2363	2546	3044	3553	4061	4502	4794
14-15	2830	3147	3586	3963	4575	5368	5530
15-16	3138	3317	3788	4481	5134	5631	5900
16-17	3625	4044	4352	4951	5753	6576	6980
17-18	3998	4252	4777	5286	5950	6886	7726
18-19	4070	4481	5066	5552	6374	7067	8355
19-25	4508	4777	5274	5913	6660	7606	8200
25-35	4694	4963	5541	6214	7067	7847	8436
35-45	4844	5181	5740	6490	7265	8034	8488
45-55	4546	4946	5589	6297	7142	7918	8458
55-65	4422	4783	5381	6144	6919	7670	8149
65-75	3973	4411	5031	5716	6432	7074	7453

Data from Frisancho, 1981.

TABLE G-5	Midarm Muscle Area Percentiles (mm²) for Females						
Age Group	5th	10th	25th	50th	75th	90th	95th
1-2	885	973	1084	1221	1378	1535	1621
2-3	973	1029	1119	1269	1405	1595	1727
3-4	1014	1133	1227	1396	1563	1690	1846
4-5	1058	1171	1313	1475	1644	1832	1958
5-6	1238	1301	1423	1596	1825	2012	2159
6-7	1354	1414	1513	1683	1877	2182	2323
7-8	1330	1441	1602	1815	2045	2332	2469
8-9	1513	1566	1808	2034	2327	2657	2996
9-10	1723	1788	1976	2227	2571	2987	3112
10-11	1740	1784	2019	2296	2583	2873	3093
11-12	1784	1987	2316	2612	3071	3739	3953
12-13	2092	2182	2579	2904	3225	3655	3847
13-14	2269	2426	2657	3130	3529	4061	4568
14-15	2418	2562	2874	3220	3704	4294	4850
15-16	2426	2518	2847	3248	3689	4123	4756
16-17	2306	2567	2865	3248	3718	4353	4946
17-18	2442	2674	2996	3336	3883	4552	5251
18-19	2396	2538	2917	3243	3694	4461	4767
19-25	2538	2728	3026	3406	3877	4439	4940
25-35	2661	2826	3198	3573	4138	4806	5541
35-45	2750	2948	3359	3783	4428	5240	5877
45-55	2784	2956	3378	3858	4520	5375	5964
55-65	2784	3063	3477	4045	4750	5632	6247
65-75	2737	3018	3444	4019	4739	5566	6214

Data from Frisancho, 1981.

A & P	Anterior and posterior; auscultation and percussion
A & W	Alive and well
abd	Abdomen; abdominal
a̅c̅	Before meals
ADL	Activities of daily living
AJ	Ankle jerk
AK	Above knee
ANS	Autonomic nervous system
AP	Anteroposterior
bid	Twice a day
BK	Below knee
BP	Blood pressure
BPH	Benign prostatic hypertrophy
BS	Bowel sounds; breath sounds
c̅	With
CAD	Coronary artery disease
CC	Chief complaint
CHD	Childhood disease; congenital heart disease; coronary heart disease
CHF	Congestive heart failure
CNS	Central nervous system
c/o	Complains of
COPD	Chronic obstructive pulmonary disease
CV	Cardiovascular
CVA	Costovertebral angle; cerebrovascular accident
CVP	Central venous pressure
Cx	Cervix
D & C	Dilation and curettage
D/C	Discontinued
DM	Diabetes mellitus
DOB	Date of birth
DOE	Dyspnea on exertion
DTRs	Deep tendon reflexes
DUB	Dysfunctional uterine bleeding
Dx	Diagnosis
ECG, EKG	Electrocardiogram; electrocardiograph
EENT	Eye, ear, nose, and throat
ENT	Ear, nose, and throat
EOM	Extraocular movement
FB	Foreign body
FH	Family history
FROM	Full range of motion
FTT	Failure to thrive
Fx	Fracture
GB	Gallbladder
GE	Gastroesophageal
GI	Gastrointestinal
GU	Genitourinary
GYN	Gynecologic
HA	Headache
HCG	Human chorionic gonadotropin
HEENT	Head, eyes, ears, nose, and throat
HPI	History of present illness
Hx	History
ICS	Intercostal space
IOP	Intraocular pressure
IUD	Intrauterine device
IV	Intravenous
JVP	Jugular venous pressure
KJ	Knee jerk
KUB	Kidneys, ureters, and bladder
lat	Lateral
LCM	left costal margin
LE	Lower extremities
LLL	Left lower lobe (lung)
LLQ	Left lower quadrant (abdomen)
LMD	Local medical doctor
LMP	Last menstrual period
LOC	Loss of consciousness; level of consciousness

LS	Lumbosacral; lumbar spine	PMH	Past medical history
LSB	Left sternal border	PMI	Point of maximum impulse; point of maximum intensity
LUL	Left upper lobe (lung)		
LUQ	Left upper quadrant (abdomen)	PMS	Premenstrual syndrome
M	Murmur	prn	As necessary
MAL	Midaxillary line	Pt	Patient
MCL	Midclavicular line	PVC	Premature ventricular contraction
MGF	Maternal grandfather	q	Every
MGM	Maternal grandmother	qd	Every day
MSL	Midsternal line	qh	Every hour
MVA	Motor vehicle accident	qod	Every other day
NA	No answer; not applicable	RCM	Right costal margin
N & T	Nose and throat	REM	Rapid eye movement
N & V	Nausea and vomiting	RLL	Right lower lobe (lung)
NKA	No known allergies	RLQ	Right lower quadrant (abdomen)
NPO	Nothing by mouth	RML	Right middle lobe (lung)
NSR	Normal sinus rhythm	ROM	Range of motion
OD	Oculus dexter; right eye	ROS	Review of systems
OM	Otitis media	RSB	Right sternal border
OS	Oculus sinister; left eye	RUL	Right upper lobe (lung)
OTC	Over the counter	RUQ	Right upper quadrant (abdomen)
OU	Oculus uterque; both eyes	$\bar{s}$	Without
$\bar{p}$	After	SCM	Sternocleidomastoid
P & A	Percussion and auscultation	SQ	Subcutaneous
$\overline{pc}$	After meals	Sx	Symptoms
PE	Physical examination	T & A	Tonsillectomy and adenoidectomy
PERRLA	Pupils equal, round, react to light and accommodation	TM	Tympanic membrane
		TPR	Temperature, pulse, and respiration
PGF	Paternal grandfather	UE	Upper extremities
PGM	Paternal grandmother	URI	Upper respiratory infection
PI	Present illness	UTI	Urinary tract infection
PID	Pelvic inflammatory disease	WD	Well developed
PMD	Private medical doctor	WN	Well nourished

WORD PARTS

Word Parts Commonly Used as Prefixes

Word Part	Meaning	Word Part	Meaning
a-	Without, not	inter-	Between
af-	Toward	intra-	Within
an-	Without, not	iso-	Same, equal
ante-	Before	macro-	Large
anti-	Against; resisting	mega-	Large; million(th)
auto-	Self	mes-	Middle
bi-	Two; double	meta-	Beyond, after
circum-	Around	micro-	Small; million(th)
co-, con-	With; together	milli-	Thousandth
contra-	Against	mono-	One (single)
de-	Down from, undoing	neo-	New
dia-	Across, through	non-	Not
dipl-	Twofold, double	oligo-	Few, scanty
dys-	Bad; disordered; difficult	ortho-	Straight; correct, normal
ectop-	Displaced	para-	By the side of; near
ef-	Away from	per-	Through
em-, en-	In, into	peri-	Around; surrounding
endo-	Within	poly-	Many
epi-	Upon	post-	After
eu-	Good	pre-	Before
ex-, exo-	Out of, out from	pro-	First; promoting
extra-	Outside of	quadr-	Four
hapl-	Single	re-	Back again
hem-, hemat-	Blood	retro-	Behind
hemi-	Half	semi-	Half
hom(e)o-	Same; equal	sub-	Under
hyper-	Over; above	super-, supra-	Over, above, excessive
hypo-	Under; below	trans-	Across; through
infra-	Below, beneath	tri-	Three; triple

From Thibodeau, Patton, 2003.

Word Parts Commonly Used as Suffixes

Word Part	Meaning	Word Part	Meaning
-al, -ac	Pertaining to	-malacia	Softening
-algia	Pain	-megaly	Enlargement
-aps, -apt	Fit; fasten	-metric, -metry	Measurement, length
-arche	Beginning; origin	-oid	Like; in the shape of
-ase	Signifies an enzyme	-oma	Tumor
-blast	Sprout; make	-opia	Vision, vision condition
-centesis	A piercing	-oscopy	Viewing
-cide	To kill	-ose	Signifies a carbohydrate (especially a sugar)
-clast	Break; destroy		
-crine	Release; secrete	-osis	Condition, process
-ectomy	A cutting out	-ostomy	Formation of an opening
-emesis	Vomiting	-otomy	Cut
-emia	Refers to blood condition	-penia	Lack
-flux	Flow	-philic	Loving
-gen	Creates; forms	-phobic	Fearing
-genesis	Creation; production	-phragm	Partition
-gram	Something written	-plasia	Growth, formation
-graph(y)	To write, draw	-plasm	Substance, matter
-hydrate	Containing H_2O (water)	-plasty	Shape; make
-ia, -sia	Condition; process	-plegia	Paralysis
-iasis	Abnormal condition	-pnea	Breath, breathing
-ic, -ac	Pertaining to	-(r)rhage, -(r)hagia	Breaking out, discharge
-in	Signifies a protein	-(r)rhaphy	Sew, suture
-ism	Signifies "condition of"	-(r)rhea	Flow
-itis	Signifies "inflammation of"	-some	Body
-lemma	Rind; peel	-tensin, -tension	Pressure
-lepsy	Seizure	-tonic	Pressure, tension
-lith	Stone; rock	-tripsy	Crushing
-logy	Study of	-ule	Small, little
-luna	Moon; moonlike	-uria	Refers to urine condition

From Thibodeau, Patton, 2003.

Word Parts Commonly Used as Roots

Word Part	Meaning	Word Part	Meaning
acro-	Extremity	lys-	Break apart
aden-	Gland	mal-	Bad
alveol-	Small hollow cavity	melan-	Black
angi-	Vessel	men-, mens-, (menstru-)	Month (monthly)
arthr-	Joint	muta-	Change
asthen-	Weakness	my-, myo-	Muscle
bar-	Pressure	myc-	Fungus
bili-	Bile	myel-	Marrow
brachi-	Arm	nat-	Birth
brady-	Slow	natr-	Sodium
bronch-	Air passage	nephr-	Nephron, kidney
capn-	Smoke	neur-	Nerve
carcin-	Cancer	noct-, nyct-	Night
card-	Heart	ocul-	Eye
cephal-	Head, brain	odont-	Tooth
cerv-	Neck	onco-	Cancer
chem-	Chemical	ophthalm-	Eye
chol-	Bile	orchid-	Testis
chondr-	Cartilage	osteo-	Bone
corp-	Body	oto-	Ear
cortico-	Pertaining to cortex	ov-, oo-	Egg
crani-	Skull	oxy-	Oyxgen
crypt-	Hidden	path-	Disease
cusp-	Point	ped-	Children
cut(an)-	Skin	phag-	Eat
cyan-	Blue	pharm-	Drug
cyst-	Bladder	phleb-	Vein
cyt-	Cell	photo-	Light
dactyl-	Fingers, toes (digits)	physio-	Nature (function) of
dendr-	Tree; branched	plex-	Twisted; woven
dent-	Tooth	pneumo-	Air, breath
derm-	Skin	pneumon-	Lung
diastol-	Relax; stand apart	pod-	Foot
dips-	Thirst	poie-	Make; produce
ejacul-	To throw out	presby-	Old
electr-	Electrical	proct-	Rectum
enter-	Intestine	pseud-	False
eryth(r)-	Red	psych-	Mind
esthe-	Sensation	pyel-	Pelvis
febr-	Fever	ren-	Kidney
gastr-	Stomach	rhino-	Nose
gingiv-	Gums	rigor-	Stiffness
glomer-	Wound into a ball	sarco-	Flesh; muscle
gloss-	Tongue	scler-	Hard
gluc-	Glucose, sugar	semen-, semin-	Seed; sperm
glutin-	Glue	sept-	Contamination
glyc-	Sugar (carbohydrate): glucose	sin-	Cavity; recess
hepat-	Liver	som-	Sound
hist-	Tissue	spiro-, spire-	Breathe
hydro-	Water	stat-, stas-	A standing, stopping
hyster-	Uterus	syn-	Together
iatr-	Treatment	systol-	Contract; stand together
kal-	Potassium	tachy-	Fast
kary-	Nucleus	therm-	Heat
kerat-	Cornea	thromb-	Clot
lact-	Milk; milk production	tox-	Poison
lapar-	Abdomen	troph-	Grow; nourish
leuk-	White	tympan-	Drum
lig-	To tie, bind	varic-	Enlarged vessel
lip-	Lipid (fat)	vas-	Vessel, duct

From Thibodeau, Patton, 2003.

APPENDIX J

ENGLISH-TO-SPANISH TRANSLATION GUIDE: KEY MEDICAL QUESTIONS

The following is a guide to help you complete the history and examination of Spanish-speaking patients. Initial questions presented are general ones used at the beginning of the examination. Questions for pain assessment follow. The remainder of the translations are arranged in order of the body systems. Each system's section contains basic vocabulary, questions used for history taking, and instructions that would facilitate examination. The intent of this guide is to offer an array of questions and phrases from which the examiner can choose as appropriate for assessment.

HINTS FOR PRONUNCIATION OF SPANISH WORDS

1. *h* is silent.
2. *j* is pronounced as *h*.
3. *ll* is pronounced as a *y* sound.
4. *r* is pronounced with a trilled sound, and *rr* is trilled even more.
5. *v* is pronounced with a *b* sound.
6. A *y* by itself is pronounced with a long *e* sound.
7. Accent marks over the vowel indicate the syllable that is to be stressed.

INTRODUCTORY

I am _____.	Soy _____.
What is your name?	¿Cómo se llama usted?
I would like to examine you now.	Quisiera examinarlo(a) ahora. (Note (a) when speaking to female)

GENERAL

How do you feel?	¿Cómo se siente?
Good	Bien
Bad	Mal
Do you feel better today?	¿Se siente mejor hoy?
Where do you work?	¿Dónde trabaja? (Cuál es su profesión o trabajo?) (¿Qué hace usted?)
Are you allergic to anything?	¿Tiene usted algerias?
Medications, foods, insect bites?	¿Medicinas, alimentos, picaduras de insectos?
Do you take any medications?	¿Toma usted algunas medicinas?
Do you have any drug allergies?	¿Es usted alérgico(a) a algún médicamento?
Do you have a history of . . .	¿Padece usted enfermedad . . .
Heart disease?	del corazón?
Diabetes?	del diabetes?
Epilepsy?	la epilepsia?
Bronchitis?	de bronquitis?
Emphysema?	de enfsema?
Asthma?	de asma?

PAIN

Have you any pain?	¿Tiene dolor?
Where is the pain?	¿Dónde está el dolor?
Do you have any pain here?	¿Tiene usted dolor aquí?
How severe is the pain?	¿Qué tan fuerte es el dolor?
Mild, moderate, sharp, or severe?	¿Ligero, moderado, agudo, o severo?
What were you doing when the pain started?	¿Qué hacía usted cuando le comenzó el dolor?
Have you ever had this pain before?	¿Ha tenido este dolor antes?
	(¿Ha sido siempre así?)
Do you have a pain in your side?	¿Tiene usted dolor en el costado?
Is it worse now?	¿Está peor ahora?
Does it still hurt?	¿Le duele todavía?
Did you feel much pain at the time?	¿Sintió mucho dolor entonces?
Show me where.	Muéstreme dónde.
Does it hurt when I press here?	¿Le duele cuando aprieto aquí?

HEAD

Vocabulary

Head	La cabeza
Face	La cara

History

How does your head feel?	¿Cómo siente la cabeza?
Have you any pain in the head?	¿Le duele la cabeza?
Do you have headaches?	¿Tiene usted dolores de cabeza?
Do you have migraines?	¿Tiene usted migrañas?
What causes the headaches?	¿Qué le causa los dolores de cabeza?

Examination

Lift up your head.	Levante la cabeza.

EYES

Vocabulary

Eye	El ojo

History

Have you had pain in your eyes?	¿Ha tenido dolor en los ojos?
Do you wear glasses?	¿Usa usted anteojos/gafas/lentes/espejuelos?
Do you wear contact lenses?	¿Usa usted lentes de contacto?
Can you see clearly?	¿Puede ver claramente?
Better at a distance?	¿Mejor a cierta distancia?
Do you sometimes see things double?	¿Ve las cosas doble algunas veces?
Do you see things through a mist?	¿Ve las cosas nubladas?
Were you exposed to anything that could	¿Fue expuesto a cualquier cosa que pudiera
have injured your eye?	haberle dañado el ojo?
Do your eyes water much?	¿Le lagrimean mucho los ojos?

Examination

Look up.	Mire para arriba.
Look down.	Mire para abajo.
Look toward your nose.	Mírese la nariz.
Look at me.	Míreme.
Tell me what number it is.	Dígame qué número es éste.
Tell me what letter it is.	Dígame qué letra es ésta.

EARS/NOSE/THROAT

Vocabulary

Ears	Los oídos
Eardrum	El tímpano
Laryngitis	La laringitis
Lip	El labio
Mouth	La boca
Nose	La naríz
Tongue	La lengua

History

Do you have any hearing problems?	¿Tiene usted problemas de oir?
Do you use a hearing aid?	¿Usa usted un audífono?
Do you have ringing in the ears?	¿Le zumban los oídos?
Do you have allergies?	¿Tiene alergias?
Do you use dentures?	¿Usa usted dentadura postiza?
Do you have any loose teeth, removable bridges, or any prosthesis?	¿Tiene dientes flojos, dientes postizos, o cualquier prostesis?
Do you have a cold?	¿Tiene usted un resfriado/resfrío?
Do you have sore throats frequently?	¿Le duele la garganta con frecuencia?
Have you ever had a strep throat?	¿Ha tenido alguna vez infección de la garganta?

Examination

Open your mouth.	Abra la boca.
I want to take a throat culture. This will not hurt.	Quiero hacer un cultivo de la garganta. Esto no le va a doler.

CARDIOVASCULAR

Vocabulary

Heart	El corazón
Heart attack	El ataque al corazón
Heart disease	La enfermedad del corazón
Heart murmur	El soplo del corazón
High blood pressure	Alta presión

History

Have you ever had any chest pain? Where?	¿Ha tenido alguna vez dolor de pecho? ¿Dónde?
Do you notice any irregularity of heartbeat or any palpitations?	¿Nota cualquier latido o palpitación irregular?
Do you get short of breath? When?	¿Tiene usted problemas con la respiración? ¿Cuándo?
Do you take medicine for your heart? How often?	¿Toma medicina para el corazón? ¿Con qué frecuencia?
Do you know if you have high blood pressure?	¿Sabe usted si tiene la presión alta?
Is there a history of hypertension in your family?	¿En su familia, se encuentran varias personas con alta presión?
Do you take medicine for high blood pressure? How often?	¿Toma medicina para la presión alta? ¿Con qué frecuencia?
Are any of your limbs swollen? Hands, feet, legs?	¿Están hinchados algunos de sus miembros? ¿Manos, pies, piernas?
How long have they been swollen like this?	¿Desde cuándo están hinchados así? (¿Qué tanto tiempo tiene usted con esta hinchazón?)

Examination

| Let me feel your pulse. | Déjeme tomarle el pulso. |
| I am going to take your blood pressure now. | Le voy a tomar la presión ahora. |

RESPIRATORY

Vocabulary

| Chest | El pecho |
| Lungs | Los pulmones |

History

Do you smoke?	¿Fuma usted?
How many packs a day?	¿Cuántos paquetes al día?
Have you any difficulty in breathing?	¿Tiene dificultad al respirar?
How long have you been coughing?	¿Desde cuándo tiene tos?
Do you cough up phlegm?	¿Al toser, escupe usted flema(s)?
What is the color of your expectorations?	¿Cuándo usted escupe, qué color es?
White/Green	Blanco/Verde
Do you cough up blood?	¿Al toser, arroja usted sangre?
Do you wheeze?	¿Le silba a usted el pecho?

Examination

Take a deep breath.	Respire profundo.
Breathe normally.	Respire normalmente.
Cough.	Tosa.
Cough again.	Tosa otra vez.

GASTROINTESTINAL

Vocabulary

Abdomen	El abdomen
Intestines/bowels	Los intestinos/las entrañas
Liver	El hígado
Nausea	Náusea
Gastric ulcer	La úlcera gástrica
Stomach	El estómago, la panza, la barriga
Stomachache	El dolor de estómago

History

What foods disagree with you?	¿Qué alimentos le caen mal?
Do you get heartburn?	¿Suele tener ardor en el pecho?
Do you have indigestion often?	¿Tiene indigestión con frecuencia?
Are you going to vomit?	¿Va a vomitar (arrojar)?
Do you have blood in your vomit?	¿Tiene usted vómitos con sangre?
Do you have abdominal pain?	¿Tiene dolor en el abdomen?
How are your stools?	¿Cómo son sus defecaciones?
Are they regular?	¿Son regulares?
Have you noticed their color?	¿Se ha fijado en el color?
Are you constipated?	¿Está estreñido?
Do you have diarrhea?	¿Tiene diarrea?

GENITOURINARY

Vocabulary

Genitals	Los genitales
Penis	El pene, el miembro
Kidney	El riñón
Urine	La orina

History

| Have you any difficulty passing water? | ¿Tiene dificultad en orinar? |
| Do you pass water involuntarily? | ¿Orina sin querer? |

Do you have a urethral discharge?	¿Tiene secreción de la uretra?
Do you have burning with urination?	¿Tiene ardor al orinar?

ANUS, RECTUM, AND PROSTATE

Vocabulary

Abdomen	El abdomen
Intestines/bowels	Los intestinos/las entrañas
Nausea	Náusea
Stomach	El estómago, la panza, la barriga
Stomachache	El dolor de estómago
Urine	La orina

History

Are you going to vomit?	¿Va a vomitar (arrojar)?
Do you have abdominal pain?	¿Tiene dolor en el abdomen?
How are your stools?	¿Cómo son sus defecaciones?
Are they regular?	¿Son regulares?
Have you noticed their color?	¿Se ha fijado en el color?
Are you constipated?	¿Está estreñido?
Do you have diarrhea?	¿Tiene diarrea?
Have you any difficulty passing water?	¿Tiene dificultad en orinar?
Do you have a urethral discharge?	¿Tiene secreción de la uretra?
Do you have burning with urination?	¿Tiene ardor al orinar?

MUSCULOSKELETAL

Vocabulary

Ankle	El tobillo
Arm	El brazo
Back	La espalda
Bones	Los huesos
Elbow	El codo
Finger	El dedo
Foot	El pie
Fracture	La fractura
Hand	La mano
Hip	La cadera
Knee	La rodilla
Leg	La pierna
Muscles	Los músculos
Rib	La costilla
Shoulder	El hombro
Thigh	El muslo

History

Did you fall, and how did you fall?	¿Se cayó, y cómo se cayó?
How did this happen?	¿Cómo sucedio esto?
How long ago?	¿Cúanto tiempo hace?

Examination

Raise your arm.	Levante el brazo.
Raise it more.	Más alto.
Now the other.	Ahora el otro.
Stand up and walk.	Párese y camine.
Straighten your leg.	Enderece la pierna.
Bend your knee.	Doble la rodilla.
Push	Empuje
Pull	Jale
Up	Arriba
Down	Abajo

In/out	Adentro/afuera
Rest	Descanse
Kneel	Arrodíllese

NEUROLOGIC

Vocabulary

Brain	El cerebro
Dizziness	El vértigo, el mareo
Epilepsy	La epilepsia
Fainting spell	El desmayo
Unconsciousness	La insensibilidad (inconsciente)

History

Have you ever had a head injury?	¿Ha tenido alguna vez daño a la cabeza?
Do you have convulsions?	¿Tiene convulsiones?
Do you have tingling sensations?	¿Tiene hormigueos?
Do you have numbness in your hands, arms, or feet?	¿Siente entumecidos las manos, los brazos, o los pies?
Have you ever lost consciousness?	¿Perdió alguna vez el sentido? (inconsciente)
For how long?	¿Por cuánto tiempo?
How often does this happen?	¿Con qué frecuencia ocurre esto?

Examination

Squeeze my hand.	Apriete mi mano.
Can you not do it better than that?	¿No puede hacerlo más fuerte?
Turn on your left/right side.	Voltéese al lado izquierdo/al lado derecho.
Roll over and sit up over the edge of the bed.	Voltéese y siéntese sobre el borde de la cama.
Stand up slowly. Put your weight only on your right/left foot.	Párese despacio. Ponga peso sólo en la pierna derecha/izquierda.
Take a step to the side.	Dé un paso al lado.
Turn to your left/right.	Doble a la izquierda/derecha.
Is this hot or cold?	¿Está frío o caliente esto?
Am I sticking you with the point or the head of the pin?	¿Le estoy pinchando con el punto o la cabeza del alfiler?

ENDOCRINE/ REPRODUCTIVE

Vocabulary

Genitals	Los genitales
Uterus	El útero, la matríz
Vagina	La vagina

History

Have you had any problems with your thyroid?	¿Ha tenido alguna vez problemas con el tiroides?
Have you noticed any significant weight gain or loss?	¿Ha notado pérdida o aumento de peso?

Women:

How old were you when your periods started?	¿Cuántos años tenía cuando tuvo la primera regla?
How many days between periods?	¿Cuántos dias entre las reglas?
When was your last menstrual period?	¿Cuándo fue su última regla?
Have you ever been pregnant?	¿Ha estado embarazada?
How many children do you have?	¿Cuántos hijos tiene?
When was your last Pap smear?	¿Cuándo fue su última prueba de Papanicolau?
Would you like information on birth control methods?	¿Quiere usted información sobre los métodos del control de la natalidad?
Do you have a vaginal discharge?	¿Tiene secreción vaginal?

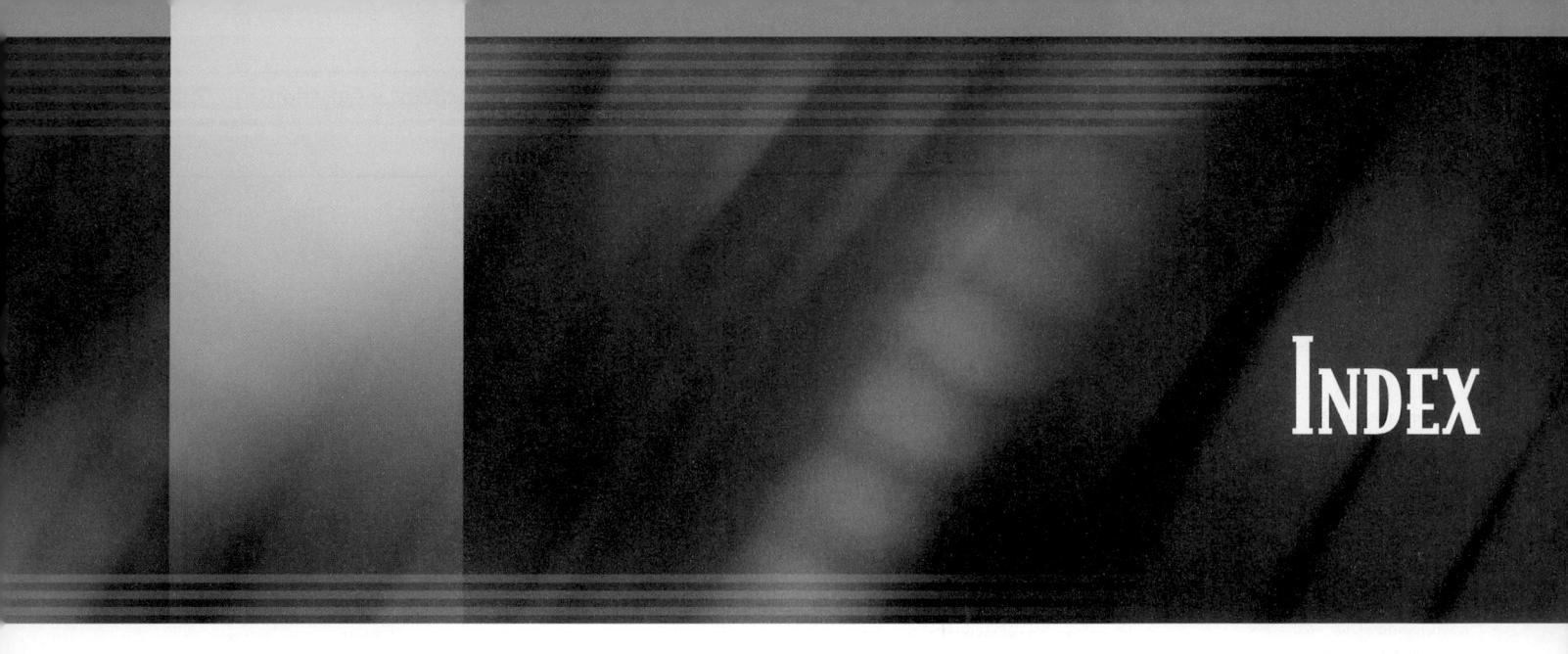

INDEX

b indicates boxed material, *f* indicates illustrations, and
t indicates tables.

SPECIAL FEATURES

Continued

DIFFERENTIAL DIAGNOSIS

EVIDENCE-BASED PRACTICE IN PHYSICAL EXAMINATION

STAYING WELL

Please see preceding page.